Edited by
Pavel Anzenbacher and
Ulrich M. Zanger

Metabolism of Drugs and Other Xenobiotics

Related Titles

Smith, D. A., Allerton, C., Kalgutkar, A. S., van de Waterbeemd, H., Walker, D. K.

Pharmacokinetics and Metabolism in Drug Design

2012

ISBN: 978-3-527-32954-0

Bernhard, D. (ed.)

Cigarette Smoke Toxicity

Linking Individual Chemicals to Human Diseases

2011

ISBN: 978-3-527-32681-5

Testa, B., Krämer, S. D.

The Biochemistry of Drug Metabolism

Two Volume Set

2010

ISBN: 978-3-906390-55-0

Mumtaz, M. (ed.)

Principles and Practice of Mixtures Toxicology

2010

ISBN: 978-3-527-31992-3

van de Waterbeemd, H., Testa, B. (eds.)

Drug Bioavailability

Estimation of Solubility, Permeability, Absorption and Bioavailability

2009

ISBN: 978-3-527-32051-6

Edited by Pavel Anzenbacher and Ulrich M. Zanger

Metabolism of Drugs and Other Xenobiotics

WILEY-VCH

WILEY-VCH Verlag GmbH & Co. KGaA

The Editors

Prof. Pavel Anzenbacher
Palacky University at Olomouc
Dept. Pharmacology
Hnevotinska str. 3
779 00 Olomouc
Czech Republic

Prof. Dr. Ulrich M. Zanger
University of Stuttgart (IKP)
Inst. of Clinical Pharmacology
Auerbachstr. 112
70376 Stuttgart
Germany

Cover
Nabumetone bound in the active site of cytochrome P450 1A2 (Anzenbacherova, Berka et al., 17th Intl. Conference Cytochromes P450, Manchester 2011).

The structure has been supplied by Dr. Karel Berka.

Library of Congress Card No.: applied for

British Library Cataloguing-in-Publication Data
A catalogue record for this book is available from the British Library.

Bibliographic information published by the Deutsche Nationalbibliothek
The Deutsche Nationalbibliothek lists this publication in the Deutsche Nationalbibliografie; detailed bibliographic data are available on the Internet at <http://dnb.d-nb.de>.

Print ISBN: 978-3-527-32903-8
ePDF ISBN: 978-3-527-63091-2
ePub ISBN: 978-3-527-64632-6
mobi ISBN: 978-3-527-64633-3
oBook ISBN: 978-3-527-63090-5

Cover Design Adam-Design, Weinheim
Typesetting Toppan Best-set Premedia Limited, Hong Kong
Printing and Binding Markono Print Media Pte Ltd, Singapore

Contents

Preface

Lecturis salutem!

The editors of this new book, *Metabolism of Drugs and Other Xenobiotics*, are happy to greet all actual and prospective readers.

Why is drug metabolism of interest to so many researchers and medical professionals? Rudolf Buchheim, the founder of modern pharmacology, anticipated one of the major reasons as early as 1859:

> *In order to understand the actions of drugs it is an absolute necessity to have knowledge of the transformations they undergo in the body. It is obvious that we must not judge drugs according to the form and amount administered, but rather according to the form and amount which actually is eliciting the action.* (R. Buchheim, Lehrbuch der Arzneimittellehre, Voss, Leipzig, 1859, p. 19).

However, there are already quite a few books on drug metabolism – so why should there be another one?

One reason is, of course, that new drugs and other xenobiotic chemicals are constantly being produced by our industry; another is the pace of today's science, which even in a more than a hundred-year-old discipline discovers new fascinating and important facts at exponential speed. However, the most compelling reason, at least to us, was the idea that came up during discussions with Frank Weinreich from Wiley VCH in 2009, to present this wildly complex topic of xenobiotic metabolism in a new and more practical way, that is, by drug class. The intention was to give readers the opportunity to get complete information on a given substance in one place (and not distributed among different chapters on enzymes and reactions), as well as to compare different substances in the same therapeutic group with respect to their metabolic pathways. Both can be of advantage, for example, to estimate pharmacokinetic variability based on the genetic and non-genetic factors that influence the involved enzyme(s), or to compare alternative drugs with respect to their biotransformation pathways. A further important aspect was not only to cover therapeutic drugs, but also to present a rather comprehensive overview of the xenobiotic chemical world, including recreational and abused drugs, natural plant and food constituents, as well as industrial chemicals and pollutants.

We divided the book's 25 chapters into four parts: part I contains nine chapters that describe the major drug metabolizing enzyme and transporting protein systems, along with chapters that deal with general aspects of xenobiotic metabolism, regulation, and pharmacogenomics. Part II contains, after a general introduction, five chapters that describe the metabolism of over 300 clinically used drugs in five major therapeutic groups, as well as unique chapters on the two major socially accepted drugs, nicotine and alcohol, and an overview on illegal drugs of abuse. Part III presents the metabolism of natural compounds, such as plant terpenoids and flavonoids, in addition to food components and supplements, an often neglected area of growing importance. The final section then describes the metabolism of a wide variety of industrial products, environmental pollutants, and agrochemicals such as insecticides.

Nevertheless, the book is by no means exhaustive, and it does not cover the scope extensively, as this would not be possible in a single book. Thus, several important therapeutic areas are not included, and many other xenobiotics from different areas are unmentioned as well. Nevertheless, we hope that the selection we chose provides an interesting read and a useful desktop reference for a diverse spectrum of specialists and researchers, including clinical and experimental pharmacologists, pharmacists or toxicologists, as well as a helpful guide for those who try to find their way into this fascinating field. Although we did our best to avoid mistakes, omissions (particularly of important references), and inconsistencies, we apologize if you may find any.

We would like to express sincere thanks to our contributors. It was not an easy task to cover this broad field but we are confident that they are among the best experts in their fields, and we are very proud to have them as authors. We would also like to thank our co-workers and our families for their patience when we were deeply immersed in the preparation of our chapters and proofs, having even less time for them than usual. Last but not least, this book would not have been possible without the work of numerous people at Wiley VCH, and we would like to thank them all for their cooperation, patience, and tremendously good job.

Olomouc and Stuttgart, January 2012 *Pavel Anzenbacher and Uli Zanger*

List of Contributors

Pavel Anzenbacher
Palacky University at Olomouc
Faculty of Medicine and Dentistry
Department of Pharmacology and
Inst. Mol. and Translational Medicine
Hnevotinska st. 3, Olomouc, 775 15
Czech Republic

Eva Anzenbacherová
Palacky University at Olomouc
Faculty of Medicine and Dentistry
Department of Medical Chemistry and
Biochemistry
Hnevotinska st. 3, Olomouc, 775 15
Czech Republic

Pierre Baumann
Université de Lausanne
Centre Hospitalier Universitaire
Vaudois
Department of Psychiatry
Site de Cery
1008 Prilly-Lausanne
Switzerland

Hiltrud Brauch
Dr. Margarete Fischer-Bosch Institute
of Clinical Pharmacology
Auerbachstrasse 112
70376 Stuttgart
Germany

Janet K. Coller
University of Adelaide
School of Medical Sciences
Discipline of Pharmacology
Adelaide, 5005
Australia

Michael W.H. Coughtrie
University of Dundee
Ninewells Hospital & Medical School
Medical Research Institute
Dundee, DD1 9SY, Scotland
UK

Alice L. Crane
State University of New York at
Buffalo
Department of Pharmacology and
Toxicology
Buffalo, NY 14214
USA

Chantal Csajka
University of Lausanne
University Hospital Center
Division of Clinical Pharmacology and
Toxicology
1011 Lausanne
Switzerland

Laurent Decosterd
University of Lausanne
University Hospital Center
Division of Clinical Pharmacology and Toxicology
1011 Lausanne
Switzerland

Miroslav Dostalek
University of Rhode Island
College of Pharmacy
Department of Biomedical and Pharmaceutical Sciences
Clinical Pharmacokinetic Research Laboratory
41 Lower College Road
Kingston, RI 02881
USA
Simcyp Limited
Blades Enterprise Centre
John Street
S2 4SU Sheffield
UK

Zdenek Dvorak
Palacky University
Faculty of Science
Department of Cell Biology and Genetics
Slechtitelu 11
783 71 Olomouc
Czech Republic

Corie A. Ellison
State University of New York at Buffalo
Department of Pharmacology and Toxicology
Buffalo, NY 14214
USA

F. Peter Guengerich
Vanderbilt University School of Medicine
Department of Biochemistry and Center in Molecular Toxicology
638 Robinson Research Building
2200 Pierce Avenue
Nashville, TN 37232-0146
USA

Christoph Hiemke
Klinik für Psychiatrie und PsychotherapieUniversitätsmedizin Mainz
Untere Zahlbacher Str. 8
55131 Mainz
Germany

Petr Hodek
Charles University Prague
Department of Biochemistry
Albertov 2030
Prague, 128 40 Praha 2
Czech Republic

Sandra Kalthoff
Professor of Gastroenterology and Hepatology
Hannover Medical School
Department of Gastroenterology, Hepatology and Endocrinology
Carl-Neuberg-Str. 1
30625 Hannover
Germany

Kathrin Klein
Dr. Margarete Fischer-Bosch Institute of Clinical Pharmacology
Auerbachstrasse 112
70376 Stuttgart
Germany

Miroslav Machala
Veterinary Research Institute
Department of Toxicology,
Pharmacology and Immunotherapy
Hudcova 70
621 00 Brno
Czech Republic

Oriol Manuel
University Hospital Center
Service of Infectious Diseases and
Transplantation Center
1011 Lausanne
Switzerland

Oscar Marchetti
University of Lausanne
University Hospital Center
Service of Infectious Diseases
1011 Lausanne
Switzerland

Hans H. Maurer
Saarland University
Institute of Experimental and Clinical
Pharmacology and Toxicology
Department of Experimental and
Clinical Toxicology
66421 Homburg (Saar)
Germany

Markus R. Meyer
Saarland University
Institute of Experimental and Clinical
Pharmacology and Toxicology
Department of Experimental and
Clinical Toxicology
66421 Homburg (Saar)
Germany

Sebastian Mueller
University of Heidelberg
Centre of Alcohol Research and
Salem Medical Centre
Department of Medicine
Zeppelinstraße 11-33
69121 Heidelberg
Germany

Michael Murray
University of Sydney
Faculty of Pharmacy
Pharmacogenomics and Drug
Development Group
Sydney, NSW 2006
Australia

Tadashi Namisaki
Dr. Margarete Fischer-Bosch Institute
of Clinical Pharmacology
Auerbachstrasse 112
70376 Stuttgart
Germany

Anne T. Nies
Dr. Margarete Fischer-Bosch Institute
of Clinical Pharmacology
Auerbachstrasse 112
70376 Stuttgart
Germany

James R. Olson
State University of New York at
Buffalo
Department of Pharmacology and
Toxicology/Department of Social and
Preventive Medicine
Buffalo, NY 14214
USA

Alexandr Parlesak
Technical University of Denmark
Department of Systems Biology
Søltofts Plads
Bldg. 224
2800 Lyngby
Denmark

Claudia Resch
Dr. Margarete Fischer-Bosch Institute of Clinical Pharmacology
Auerbachstrasse 112
70376 Stuttgart
Germany

Stephan Riedmaier
Dr. Margarete Fischer-Bosch Institute of Clinical Pharmacology
Auerbachstrasse 112
70376 Stuttgart
Germany

Jessica Rieger
Dr. Margarete Fischer-Bosch Institute of Clinical Pharmacology
Auerbachstrasse 112
70376 Stuttgart
Germany

Elke Schaeffeler
Dr. Margarete Fischer-Bosch Institute of Clinical Pharmacology
Auerbachstrasse 112
70376 Stuttgart
Germany

Matthias Schwab
Dr. Margarete Fischer-Bosch Institute of Clinical Pharmacology
Auerbachstrasse 112
70376 Stuttgart
Germany
and
Institute of Experimental and Clinical Pharmacology and Toxicology
Department of Clinical Pharmacology
University Hospital
Otfried-Müller-Str. 45
72076 Tübingen
Germany

Helmut K. Seitz
University of Heidelberg
Centre of Alcohol Research and Salem Medical Centre
Departement of Medicine
Zeppelinstraße 11-33
69121 Heidelberg
Germany

Andrew A. Somogyi
University of Adelaide
School of Medical Sciences
Discipline of Pharmacology
Adelaide, 5005
Australia

Anna-Katarina Stark
Karolinska Institutet
National Institute of Environmental Medicine
171 11 Stockholm
Sweden

Marie Stiborova
Charles University Prague
Department of Biochemistry
Albertov 2030
Prague, 128 40 Praha 2
Czech Republic

Christian P. Strassburg
Hannover Medical School
Department of Gastroenterology,
Hepatology and Endocrinology
Carl-Neuberg-Str. 1
30625 Hannover
Germany

Amalio Telenti
University of Lausanne
University Hospital Center
Institute of Microbiology
1011 Lausanne
Switzerland

Rachel F. Tyndale
University of Toronto
Departments of Psychiatry,
Pharmacology and Toxicology
Centre for Addiction and Mental
Health
1 King's College Circle
Toronto, Ontario M5S 1A8
Canada

Jan Vondráček
Veterinary Research Institute
Department of Toxicology
Hudcova 70
621 00 Brno
Czech Republic

Bingfang Yan
University of Rhode Island
Department of Biomedical and
Pharmaceutical Sciences
Kingston, RI 02881
USA

Ulrich M. Zanger
Dr. Margarete Fischer-Bosch Institute
of Clinical Pharmacology
Auerbachstrasse 112
70376 Stuttgart
Germany

Andy Z.X. Zhu
University of Toronto
Departments of Psychiatry,
Pharmacology and Toxicology
Centre for Addiction and Mental
Health
1 King's College Circle
Toronto, Ontario M5S 1A8
Canada

Part One
Biochemistry and Molecular Genetics of Drug Metabolism

1
Drug-Metabolizing Enzymes – An Overview

Pavel Anzenbacher and Eva Anzenbacherová

1.1
Introduction: Fate of a Drug in the Human Body

Drugs and, more generally, all substances foreign to the human body enter the organism in many ways. Intentional administration of a drug implies that the route of administration is selected depending on the clinical status of the patient, on the target tissue or organ, and on the chemical nature of the drug. For example, highly ionized compounds cannot easily penetrate barriers such as that of the gastrointestinal tract and therefore should be administered parenterally. Peptides or proteins are degraded to a great extent in the gastrointestinal tract by the action of hydrolytic enzymes and hence are often given to patients in ways other than the most common oral route (e.g., by intranasal application). Intravenous application implies an immediate interaction of a drug with plasma enzymes (e.g., carboxyesterases).

In many cases, the enzymes performing the biotransformation of a drug are needed to convert a parent drug (a prodrug) to the active molecule. Lovastatin – a hypolipidemic drug – is a good example of this process as it requires metabolic activation by carboxyesterases. Carboxyesterases in the plasma, liver microsomes, and liver cytosol convert 18, 15, and 67%, respectively, of the orally given drug to the active hydroxyacid molecule [1].

In general, after its administration a drug should be absorbed; subsequently, it is distributed in the body, often it is also metabolized, and finally excreted. These processes determine the pharmacokinetics of a drug; in other words, the time course of the drug level in the tissue or organ of interest.

The majority of drugs are administered orally and, hence, the uptake of a drug from the gastrointestinal tract is the most frequent way of drug absorption; consequently, the action of liver (and intestinal) drug-metabolizing enzymes starts already in the process of absorption, even before the drug reaches the systemic circulation. The enzymes of drug biotransformation often lower the amount of drug available in the systemic circulation by converting it into metabolites (active, inactive, or with an altered activity) – this process is known as the "first-pass effect." The enzymes of drug biotransformation often decide the biological availability of

Metabolism of Drugs and Other Xenobiotics, First Edition. Edited by Pavel Anzenbacher, Ulrich M. Zanger.

a drug (i.e., the level of a drug available at the site of its action). This book focuses on drug metabolism and on the respective enzymes responsible for this process.

However, this is not the only role of drug-metabolizing enzymes. Changes in drug metabolism may be responsible for the incidence of adverse reactions to drugs, such as when a drug's metabolism is blocked by another compound (e.g., due to competition with another drug – then the level of the "victim" drug may increase and even exceed the toxic levels) or, on the contrary, by induction of drug-metabolizing enzymes. Then, the metabolism of another drug ("victim"), metabolized by the same enzyme, is quicker and it may fail to reach its therapeutic range. This type of drug–drug interaction has been intensively studied as it is a potential reason for failure of pharmacotherapy [2]. The situation may be further heavily influenced by genetic predisposition of a patient to metabolize the respective drug, such as in many examples of drugs metabolized by cytochromes P450 (CYPs). This is, for example, the case for antidepressants metabolized by CYP form 2D6, where the genetically determined ability of a patient to metabolize the drug may lead to effective dose variations approaching an order of magnitude [3]. For example, when a slowly metabolizing patient on a somewhat lower dose of the "victim" drug takes another drug metabolized by the same CYP2D6 enzyme, both the effects of drug interaction caused by the competition for the enzyme active site and the pharmacogenetic predisposition come into play, and the patient could easily be overdosed. This is why this book deals not only with the respective enzymes and drugs, but also with the pharmacogenetic implications of patients' predispositions to variations in drug metabolism.

1.2 Classification Systems of Drug-Metabolizing Enzymes According to Different Criteria

Drug-metabolizing enzymes have been traditionally grouped into two main classes, reflecting the fact that a drug is often primarily transformed to a more polar metabolite either by insertion of a polar group into the molecule (e.g., by hydroxylation) or by liberation of an already present functional group (e.g., by demethylation of a hydroxymethyl derivative yielding a free hydroxyl). These "first-phase" reactions are in most cases followed by conjugation reactions ("second phase") during which the molecule is typically attached to a more polar molecule to facilitate its excretion. Since 1959 when Williams [4] introduced this terminology, it has been shown (with progress in elucidation of the drug metabolic pathways of many drugs) that there are possibly more exceptions to this general rule than expected; for example, some "phase II" reactions may not be preceded by "phase I" biotransformation – morphine that is glucuronidated directly or paracetamol (acetaminophen) that is also predominantly glucuronidated or conjugated with sulfate (Figure 1.1) [5].

The original concept of the drug or its metabolite being converted to an even more polar molecule in the "phase II" process is also not generally valid. As has

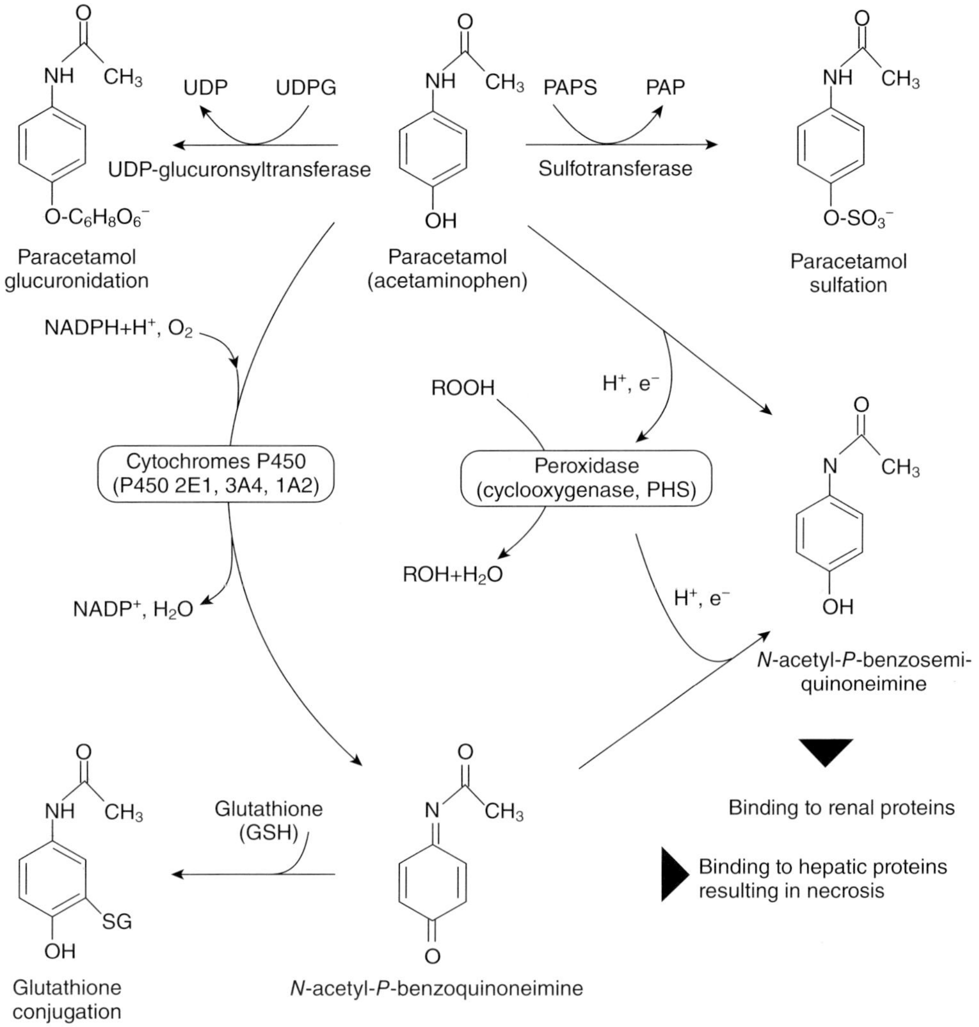

Figure 1.1 Pathways of paracetamol (acetaminophen) metabolism. Paracetamol is primarily converted to a sulfate or glucuronide by SULT (with a PAPS coenzyme) and UGT, UDPG is the UDP-glucuronide; oxidation reactions catalyzed by CYPs or peroxidase lead to the formation of reactive toxic products; for detoxication, conjugation with glutathione (GSH) by GST is available under physiological conditions [5].

been recently pointed out, for example, the *N*-acetylation of aromatic amines or the methylation of catechols usually decreases the water solubility of the resulting compounds [6].

The apparent complexity of this problem is also reflected in a classification of biotransformation reactions suggested in [6] based on the chemical nature of the process:

i) Oxidations, including reactions mediated by CYPs and peroxidases, but also by alcohol hydrogenases and others.

ii) Reductions, performed by, for example, ketoreductases and azoreductases.

iii) Conjugations, limited, however, to reactions in which the electrophilic nucleoside-containing cofactors (such as adenosine triphosphate, activated sulfate 3′-phosphoadenosine-5′-phosphosulfate (PAPS), acetyl-CoA, UDP-glucuronic acid, *S*-adenosylmethionine, etc.) play a crucial role in interactions with nucleophilic sites in a xenobiotic molecule (e.g., the amino or hydroxy group).

iv) Nucleophilic trapping processes, when electrophilic xenobiotics react with cellular nucleophiles – often represented by water or by glutathione (including formation of protein and DNA adducts).

Clearly, the future will show whether the new classification is more viable than the original one.

Figure 1.1 gives an introduction to drug metabolism processes by showing the pathways of paracetamol metabolism. Reactions of the "first phase" involve oxidation of the parent molecule to quinone structures catalyzed by CYPs and peroxidase (cyclooxygenase (COX, also called prostaglandin H synthase); the conjugation processes are both sulfation and glucuronidation (the majority of paracetamol is metabolized by these two reactions) as well as a detoxication reaction by conjugation of glutathione to the toxic and reactive *N*-acetyl-*p*-benzoquinone imine (NAPQI).

In the first part of this book, the focus is on the main classes of biotransformation enzymes without attempting to divide or group them into categories. As in most textbooks, the description will start with CYPs as they represent the most important family of drug-metabolizing enzymes. Formation of adducts of activated xenobiotics with biological macromolecules (proteins, DNA, but also polysaccharides) as well as with other structures is not covered here since the aim of this book is to give the interested professional information on the interaction of drugs with enzymes of metabolism and on the related consequences.

1.3 Overview of the Most Important Drug-Metabolizing Enzymes

1.3.1 CYPs

CYPs are the best known drug-metabolizing enzymes [7]. They deserve this attention – more than three-quarters of all known drug oxidations are catalyzed by CYPs and this is certainly not the final count. The oxidation reactions are started by one-electron reduction of the heme iron central atom, which is followed by binding of molecular oxygen. In other words: (i) CYPs are proteins that possess heme in their active site (just as with hemoglobin or other cytochromes), (ii) their function needs electrons to be supplied from a suitable source – another protein having the ability to transfer electrons from NADPH to CYPs (for drug-metabolizing microsomal CYPs, in most cases a flavoprotein), and, finally, (iii) the heme iron should be able to bind molecular oxygen (no wonder – as in hemoglobin), but in this particular case it should be endowed with "magical" force to split the dioxygen and activate it. This "extra" force is provided by donation of electron density coming from a sulfur atom serving as the sixth ligand of the heme iron. To refresh the chemistry of hemes, an iron atom can be bound to six partner atoms or ligands; here, in the resting state, four bonds are occupied by nitrogen atoms of the heme, the fifth bond joins the heme iron to a negatively charged sulfur atom ("thiolate" sulfur) of a Cys amino acid residue from the protein chain and the sixth bond is with an oxygen from a water molecule present in the active center (during the catalytic process, a dioxygen is bound here). The result can be described by a relatively simple equation summarizing the reaction in which the molecular oxygen (dioxygen) is activated and split, yielding a water molecule and a monooxygenated (mostly hydroxylated) substrate. Very recently, the crucial intermediate of this process, the Fe(IV) oxo porphyrin radical species (so-called Compound I of the heme enzymes) has been prepared in high yield from microbial CYP119 [8]. A detailed description of the catalytic mechanism is given in Chapter 2. The reaction summarizing most of the processes in which the CYP enzymes take part can be written as:

$$\mathrm{NADPH} + \mathrm{H}^+ + \mathrm{R{-}H} + \mathrm{O}_2 \rightarrow \mathrm{NADP}^+ + \mathrm{H_2O} + \mathrm{R{-}OH}$$

The reaction involves the source of electrons (reduced NADPH cofactor with a proton H^+), a substrate (R–H), dioxygen, and oxidized $NADP^+$, water, and a monooxygenated or hydroxylated molecule of substrate (R–OH).

CYP enzymes metabolizing xenobiotics are localized in many tissues, typically in the liver, intestines, lung, and kidney, but also in the brain, heart, and nasal mucosa. Subcellular localization of these enzymes is mainly in microsomes (formed after cell disruption from the endoplasmic reticulum); however, drug-metabolizing CYPs are present also in cellular membranes and mitochondria [9].

In most cases, the products (i.e., metabolites) are welcome as the drugs should be easier to conjugate after hydroxylation (e.g., with a polar residue of glucuronic acid) or excreted as hydroxy derivatives. However, in many cases the metabolites formed by monooxygenation are harmful to the body or, more precisely, the products of the CYPs-mediated reaction are further converted to species that lead to toxic responses of organism or are involved in mechanisms underlying serious diseases (e.g., initiation of chemical carcinogenesis) [5]. Typical cases of such processes are the formation of reactive NAPQI (which binds covalently to proteins of liver and kidney, Figure 1.1) from paracetamol or generation of reactive dihydrodiol epoxide of benzo[*a*]pyrene as well as activation of *N*-nitrosamines leading to the formation of reactive carbenium ions that bind to bases of nucleic acids.

The aim of this introduction is to provide basic information on this highly important class of drug-metabolizing enzymes; a more fundamental discussion on CYPs is the subject of Chapter 2. Clinical implications will be given, as a rule, in the respective chapters with individual classes of drugs and active substances.

1.3.2
Peroxidases

With the exception of glutathione peroxidases (selenium-containing enzymes), the majority of peroxidases are hemoproteins (like CYPs) that can couple the reduction of hydrogen peroxide (more generally, peroxides) to oxidation of another substrates, such as drugs and other xenobiotics [10]. This cooxidation reaction is typical for prostaglandin H synthase (Figure 1.2), better known by the name COX [11].

The CYP and peroxidase enzyme systems are generally considered to be the most important groups of enzymes involved in the bioactivation of potentially toxic compounds, producing either electrophilic or radical metabolites known to be related to chemical carcinogenesis and toxicity [10].

For example, aflatoxin B_1 is converted by CYP as well as by peroxidases to its 8,9-epoxide, which causes liver tumors or renal papilla neoplasia [5]. Another example of the participation of peroxidase (here, prostaglandin H synthase) as well as of CYP in drug toxicity is the well-known formation of NAPQI (Figure 1.1) from paracetamol, leading to the hepatotoxicity (and to the nephrotoxicity) of this drug [5, 12]. Prostaglandin H synthase itself is an enzyme exhibiting two types of catalytic activities: COX as well as peroxidase activity. This is why this enzyme (or, more precisely, these enzymes as there are at least two known forms – the first constitutively expressed in many tissues and the second inducible, for example, by cytokines such as interleukin-1β or by bacterial endotoxins) is known as COX (COX1, 2, or 3 for the respective forms). Both activities require the activation of the oxygen moiety (Figure 1.2). In the first step, two molecules of oxygen are inserted into the substrate molecule (arachidonic acid) – one forming a cyclic endoperoxide bridge and the second inserted into the molecule of arachidonic acid to create a hydroperoxide group. In the peroxidase reaction, the

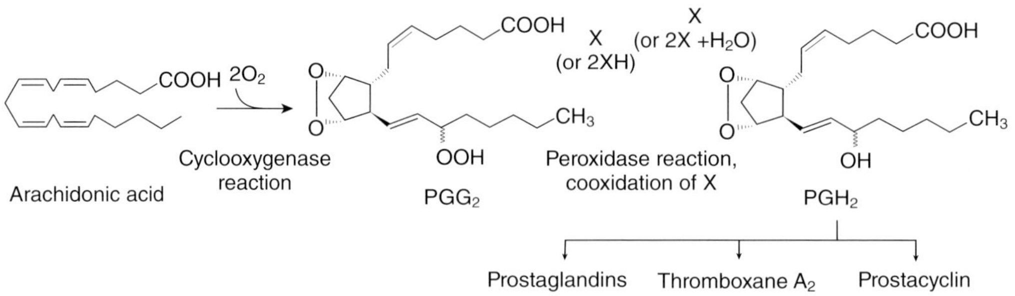

Figure 1.2 Schematic description of reactions catalyzed by prostaglandin H synthase (COX). Prostaglandins PGG_2 and PGH_2 are formed; the reactions involve activation of molecular oxygen and cooxidation of cosubstrate X.

OOH hydroperoxide group is reduced to an OH group; simultaneously, a substrate is cooxidized either by insertion of an oxygen atom or into a radical that may then undergo further reaction (for reviews on peroxidases and COXs, see [13–15]). Cyclophosphamide – an antineoplastic drug – is a typical example of a drug causing lung damage due to its oxidative biotransformation [16]. Activation of cyclophosphamide is known to proceed via CYPs; however, in this study the lung toxicity has been shown to be caused by cooxidation through the action of the COX enzyme because typical inhibitors of the CYP enzymes have not interfered with biomarkers of drug toxicity.

Prostaglandin H synthase or COX is in fact unique among peroxidases due to its mechanism of action. Metabolism of drugs and other xenobiotics is often realized by the action of ubiquitous peroxidases, such as myeloperoxidase of polymorphonuclear leukocytes (neutrophils), eosinophil peroxidase, or lactoperoxidase. Hydroperoxide substrates of these peroxidases are typically formed from hydrogen peroxide, which is a product of cellular respiration; its level is controlled by scavenging mechanisms (e.g., by glutathione peroxidase or catalase). Myeloperoxidase has been implicated in reactions leading to inactivation of the anticancer anthracyclines doxorubicin and daunorubicin [17]. However, another anthracycline-derived drug – mitoxantrone has been shown to exhibit particular effectiveness against tumors expressing high levels of heme peroxidases (myeloid leukemia, and breast and ovarian carcinoma); a recent systematic *in vitro* study has demonstrated the formation of oxidized derivatives of mitoxantrone from covalent complexes with DNA leading to DNA strand breakage and inhibition of topoisomerase II [18]. These studies open the possibility that certain types of solid tumors (lymphoma, and prostate and breast carcinoma) secreting peroxidases may activate mitoxantrone by this mechanism; in other words, that the mechanism of mitoxantrone action may be understood in terms of peroxidase/hydrogen peroxide-mediated reactions.

Airway peroxidases such as myeloperoxidase and lactoperoxidase, which are naturally present in these tissues, can apparently contribute to peroxidative metabolism of phenolic β_2-adrenoreceptor agonists such as salbutamol, fenoterol, and terbutaline [19]. Under inflammatory conditions associated with asthma, these drugs function as substrates for airway peroxidases and the resulting products (of a radical nature) may result in diminishing therapeutic efficacy of the drug [20]. Myeloperoxidase-catalyzed reactions (i.e., oxidations by the myeloperoxidase/hydrogen peroxide/Cl^- system generating HOCl) were also found to be the most probable reason of leukopenia (agranulocytosis) observed as an adverse effect after treatment with many drugs such as ticlopidine, clozapine, aminopyrine, dapsone, sulfonamides, or procainamide (e.g., see [21, 22]). In many countries, patients who are prescribed clozapine must be nationally registered in order to monitor white blood cell counts and absolute neutrophil counts. Idiosyncratic drug reactions including agranulocytosis seem to be generally caused by several factors and have more mechanisms underlying the process; however, formation of reactive metabolites typically by peroxidases and CYPs, which subsequently act as antigens, seems to be one of the most frequent ones [23].

1.3.3
Flavin Monooxygenases

Non-CYP (and nonheme)-mediated oxidative biotransformation plays an important role in the metabolism of xenobiotics. Among enzymes possessing the flavin moiety, the microsomal flavin monooxygenases (FMOs), molybdenum-containing hydroxylases (xanthine oxidase (XO) and aldehyde oxidase (AO) (Section 1.3.4)), and FAD-dependent amine oxidases (Section 1.3.5) should be discussed. As a rule, however, these enzymes have many endogenous substrates, which means that the possibility of interactions of drugs metabolized by these enzymes with natural substrates should be considered. A review of FAD-dependent enzymes participating in the metabolic oxidation of xenobiotics has been published recently [24].

FMOs were considered as "sister enzymes" of CYPs as they also catalyze microsomal NADPH-dependent *N*- or *S*-monooxygenation by activated oxygen. The reactive oxygen species (ROS) originates from a dioxygen molecule bound to reduced flavin, yielding a hydroperoxide moiety (Figure 1.3). Contrary to CYPs, which can insert the oxygen atom into a non-nucleophilic substrate, FMOs catalyze monooxygenation of compounds that have in their structures a highly polarizable nucleophilic N or S heteroatom. Tertiary amines are then converted to *N*-oxides, secondary amines to hydroxylamines or *N*-oxides, and primary amines also to derivatives of hydroxylamine or to oximes. Thiols (possessing a free SH group) are oxidized to disulfides by joining two sulfur atoms by an -S–S- bridge; sulfur atoms in compounds of the R–S–R′ structure are converted by FMOs to

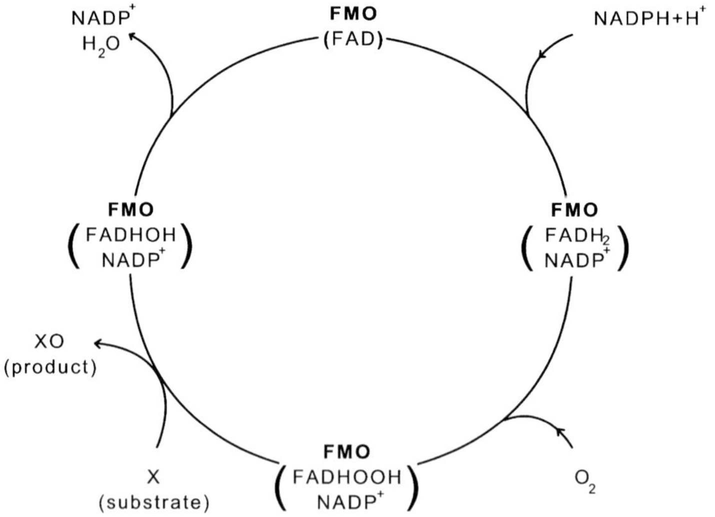

Figure 1.3 Scheme of FMO catalytic cycle; the enzyme possesses the FAD cofactor that undergoes reduction, then binds the molecular oxygen forming a hydroperoxide; subsequently, it is converted to a hydroxy form and finally is regenerated in its resting state.

S-oxides. An analogous reaction takes place at the phosphorus atom; a *P*-oxide is the product [5].

FMO enzymes are in principle inducible [25], at least in rats, by ligands of aryl hydrocarbon receptor (AhR) [26] and are also regulated by different factors such as nitric oxide [27]. Their pharmacogenetics is rather complex. There are five known forms in humans (FMO1–5); their genes are clustered on chromosome 1 [28]. Most humans are homozygous for a nonsense mutation that inactivates FMO2. However, a substantial proportion of sub-Saharan Africans expresses a functional FMO2, and thus are is predicted to respond differently to drugs and other foreign chemicals. FMO3 is a well-known liver enzyme, catalyzing the oxygenation of drug substrates such as clozapine, amphetamine, metamphetamine, sulindac, tamoxifen, and nicotine [28, 29]. Loss-of-function mutations of *FMO3* cause a disorder called trimethylaminuria – also known as fish odor syndrome, because these individuals are not able to metabolize this compound to the odorless *N*-oxide. More common variants that decrease enzyme activity are associated with increased drug efficacy [5, 30].

1.3.4
Other Oxidases: Amine Oxidases, and Molybdenum-Containing XO and AO

Amine oxidases – monoamine oxidase (MAO, typically mitochondrial), diamine oxidase (DAO), and polyamine oxidase (PAO, mostly cytosolic) – mediate oxidative deamination of primary, secondary, and tertiary amines, and their substrates hence are both of natural origin (endobiotics), such as 5-hydroxytryptamine (serotonin, substrate of MAO), putrescine (substrate of DAO), or spermine (substrate of PAO), as well as of foreign origin (xenobiotics, e.g., drugs) [24, 31]. Amine oxidases MAO and PAO typically possess flavin cofactor (FAD); products of these reactions are dehydrogenated and further oxidized. For example, propranolol – a β-blocking agent – forms two metabolites by two different forms of CYPs (CYP2D6 and CYP2C19): a hydroxylated product and a dealkylated primary amine, which is further oxidized by MAO to an aldehyde (in parallel, ammonia is formed with hydrogen peroxide) [32]. Activity of MAO is primarily associated with inactivation of neurotransmitters; its dysfunction (either increased or diminished activity) is associated with neurological disorders (such as depression, schizophrenia, and migraine). Interestingly, its activity seems to be suppressed in the adipose tissue of obese patients [33].

DAO is often employed as a clinical indicator of the integrity of intestinal mucosa. It is not a flavoenzyme; instead, it has a copper atom and trihydroxyphenylalanine quinone as cofactors. Among its natural substrates, histamine is probably the most important [34]. Drug substrates are rare.

Molybdenum-containing flavoenzymes or molybdenum hydroxylases (i.e., XO (more precisely, xanthine oxidase/dehydrogenase) and AO (aldehyde oxidase)), are cytosolic metalloflavoproteins catalyzing among their endogenous functions also oxidation and reduction of many drugs and xenobiotics. The molybdoenzymes possess not only the Mo(VI) ion bound to oxygen and sulfur atoms and the FAD coenzyme, but also two Fe_2S_2 iron–sulfur centers. Detailed mechanisms of their redox reactions are hence not simple and not fully understood yet; what is known is that the substrate is bound directly to the molybdenum atom by a Mo–C bond and that the oxygen atom for hydroxylations or, in general, for insertion to substrate molecule, is taken from a water molecule present in the active site [5, 35]. Electrons flow either to the NAD^+ (dehydrogenase reaction) or to the oxygen atom with ROS formed (XO reaction). Among reactions catalyzed by the XO enzyme, conversion of purines ultimately to uric acid, and its participation in the metabolism of the immunomodulating drugs azathioprine and 6-mercaptopurine are often listed (see also methyltransferases below and Figure 1.4). In this respect, it should be recalled here that the deposition of uric acid in joints and other places is the cause of inflammatory arthritis known as gout. Allopurinol is the leading antigout drug, which is *de facto* a prodrug metabolized in the first step by XO and AO to oxypurinol that then subsequently inhibits the XO enzyme directly, thus reducing the formation of uric acid [36]. Febuxostat – a novel nonpurine selective inhibitor of XO – has been introduced recently [37]. There are not many drugs known to be metabolized by XO or AO; the acyclovir prodrug 6-deoxyacyclovir is an example of a prodrug activated by XO into its active compound [38]. The AO enzyme has been recently found to metabolize a drug called FK3453 in humans and in experimental animals [39]. Both molybdoenzymes – XO and AO – are able to interact with flavonoids, acting as inhibitors of these enzymes [40]. Interestingly, in a medium with low partial pressure of oxygen and in the presence of easily oxidized substrates (in fact "cosubstrates"), the AO may catalyze the reduction of, for example, azo or nitro groups [5].

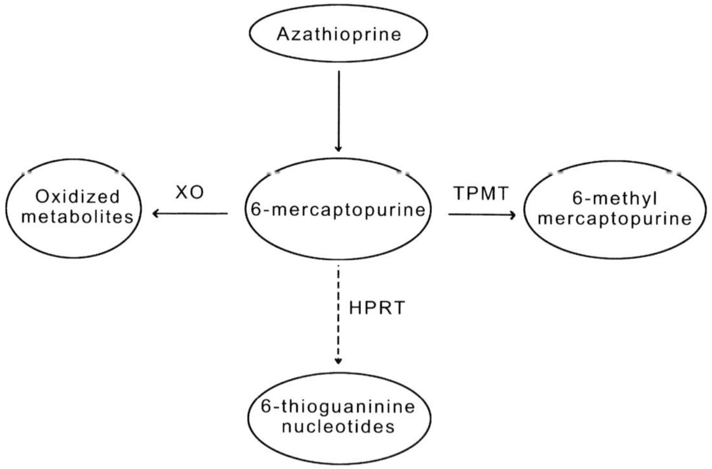

Figure 1.4 Metabolic conversion of azathioprine and 6-mercaptopurine. Levels of 6-thioguanine nucleotides are controlled by xanthine oxidase (XO) and/or thiopurine S-methyl transferase (TPMT). Hypoxanthine-guanine phosphoribosyl transferase (HPRT) participates in the formation of 6-thioguanine nucleotides.

1.3.5
NADPH Oxidase, NAD(P)H Oxidoreductase, and Dihydropyridine Dehydrogenase

Two oxidoreductases should be mentioned here as they represent a bridge to reductive processes in xenobiotic metabolism. First, the NADPH oxidase is a cell membrane-bound enzyme catalyzing the production of superoxide from oxygen and NADPH. It is a family of enzymes comprised of membrane proteins with both a heme and flavin moiety of which five isoenzymes were described, and of other cytosolic subunits [41]. This complex enzyme exhibits only one known function–generation of superoxide and ROS in general. Rather than searching for drugs metabolized by this enzyme, the pharmacologic interest is in finding an inhibitor or class of inhibitors of this enzyme as the generation of ROS is connected with many pathologies (hypertension, diabetes, atherosclerosis, and inflammation, just to name the most important) [42].

The second enzyme is the NAD(P)H oxidoreductase, also named DT-diaphorase since it can use both NADH (abbreviated DPNH in earlier literature) and NADPH (abbreviated TPNH earlier) as sources of electrons for reduction of its typical substrates, quinones [43]. The soluble cytosolic enzyme is a dimer of two identical subunits, each containing the FAD moiety, and in humans is coded by four genes in four forms; the most active (and important) is the form labeled NQO1 (NADPH: quinone oxidoreductase-1). Interestingly, it is itself polymorphic, which has important consequences for the metabolism of drugs by this enzyme (i.e., quinone anticancer agents). As the NQO enzyme is more active in cancer cells, activation of anticancer drugs by NQO leading to formation of cytotoxic products is a way that may lead to the development of a novel class of anticancer agents [44]. This is the mechanism of activation of mitomycin C, which is, however, not the best substrate of NQO; the most promising drug of this class seems to be RH1 (possessing a quinone moiety), which has been recently shown to exhibit promising pharmacodynamic and pharmacokinetic properties [45]. In the same study, a patient homozygous for an inactive allele has been shown not to respond as expected. The enzyme is inducible by two mechanisms, one of which involves the AhR (see Chapter 8) which means that its expression is controlled by the same mechanisms as that of, for example, CYP1A1 or glutathione *S*-transferases (GSTs) and UDP-glucuronosyltransferases (UGTs) [46].

Dihydropyridine dehydrogenase (DPD) is the last enzyme to be discussed here. It is a cytosolic enzyme that is highly conserved among mammals, being a homodimer with each subunit having one FAD, one FMN, and four 4Fe–4S clusters [47]. The DPD gene exhibits many mutations and polymorphisms, which may lead to defective activities of this enzyme and hence to increased levels of drugs such as 5-fluorouracil (reduced by DPD to fluorodihydrouracil). Unfortunately, high levels of this drug, known for its narrow therapeutic window, result in hematotoxicity and gastrointestinal toxicity [48].

5-Fluorouracil is the standard treatment for stage II–IV colon cancer. As already been mentioned, DPD metabolizes 5-fluorouracil to inactive 5-fluorodihydrouracil, which means a lowering of the level of the parent drug and simultaneously also a lowering of the formation of fluorouracil derivatives (nucleotide analogs) that enter RNA and DNA of cancer cells causing the desired anticancer effect. As the cancer cells grow rapidly, the cytotoxic effect of fluorouracil derivatives should be primarily observed in them. DPD was also the reason for lethal drug interactions caused by concomitant administration of two drugs – 5-fluorouracil and sorivudine (an antiviral drug used to treat herpes zoster) – in Japan almost 20 years ago. Sorivudine – a uracil derivative – was converted by gut flora to an intermediate that was further reduced by DPD to a compound covalently bound to this enzyme. Sorivudine thus inhibited DPD, which in turn resulted in elevated and lethal levels of 5-fluorouracil [49].

1.3.6
Reductases

Reductive processes are common in cells, and are not limited just to tissues and compartments with a lower partial pressure of oxygen (as in the intestines with gut microflora reducing and splitting azo groups to amines [5]). As has been mentioned earlier, many oxidoreductases are able to catalyze the reduction of substrates such as azo or nitro derivatives (aldehyde oxidase), quinones (NAD(P)H oxidoreductase, DT-diaphorase), uracil derivatives (DPD) or unsaturated aldehydes (CYPs) and halogenated hydrocarbons (e.g., reductive dehalogenation of halothane by CYPs). However, the main task of (mostly cytosolic) NAD(P)H-dependent reductases is to reduce carbonyl groups of ketones and aldehydes. These enzymes belong to two protein superfamilies – aldo-keto reductases (AKRs) and short-chain dehydrogenase/reductases (SDRs) [50, 51].

AKRs are soluble enzymes, acting as NAD(P)H oxidoreductases; 10 enzymes were found in man. AKRs are involved in the reduction of aldehydes and ketones to primary and secondary alcohols, and their substrates are either detoxified or activated. For example, they contribute to tobacco-induced carcinogenesis by activating *trans*-dihydrodiols of polycyclic aromatic compounds to reactive quinones; they also participate in the detoxication of aflatoxin-derived aldehydes and lipid peroxides [50].

To date, the SDRs constitute a superfamily of nearly 50 000 mostly soluble cytosolic enzymes in all domains of life [51, 52]. Three SDRs, NADPH-dependent carbonyl reductases, are known in humans, namely carbonyl reductases 1, 3, and 4 (abbreviated as CBR1, CBR3, and CBR4; according to the nomenclature of SDRs, the systematic names of these enzymes are SDR21C1, SDR21C2, and SDR45C). The CBR2 enzyme was found only in rodents and pigs. CBR1 is known to reduce a variety of aldehydes, ketones, and quinones such as the anthracycline-based anticancer drugs doxorubicin and daunorubicin. It has been shown recently that resistance to these drugs correlates with increased activity of CBR1 [53]. This enzyme is also known for its participation in the reduction of haloperidol and related structures (haloperidol metabolism is rather complicated and includes glucuronidation, reduction, as well as oxidation by CYP enzymes [54]). Interestingly, the expression and activity of CBR1 has been found to be increased in tumor tissues [52]. CBR3 shares high structural similarity to CBR1; however, its activity towards most of the CBR1 substrates is lower, as is the number of its known substrates. Contrary to most of the CBRs, CBR4 is localized in the mitochondrial matrix and its substrates are predominantly quinones; however, daunorubicin is a poor substrate of this enzyme.

1.3.7 Conjugating Enzymes

Enzymes helping to join two molecules, one being a xenobiotic and the other a helping particle such as glutathione or a UDP-glucuronic acid, with the aim of facilitating the excretion of the xenobiotic part of the conjugate, are usually named phase II enzymes and will be treated here as one group of drug-metabolizing enzymes, regardless of the fact of whether the xenobiotic binds by a nucleophilic (e.g., an amino or hydroxyl group) or by an electrophilic site of its molecule (e.g., as in conjugation to glutathione) (see also Figure 1.1). Only several, more or less classical examples of these reactions will be listed here, as detailed discussions of individual enzymes and their importance for drug metabolism are given in the following chapters.

UDP glycosyltransferases, including UGTs, are a superfamily of enzymes transferring (at the expense of energy supplied by the UDP) a sugar moiety to another particle forming a glycosidic bond [55]. When the sugar moiety is represented by glucuronic acid, then as a result of the glucuronidation reaction, the drug is bound to glucuronic acid by a glycosidic bond (i.e., at the C1 carbon atom of the carbohydrate),whereas the acid, carboxylic group at the C6 position, thanks to which the glucuronic acid exhibits polar properties, is free and thus enables better excretion. There are four families of genes coding the UGTs found in the human genome (UGT1, 2, 3, and 8).

Mammals utilize six sugar nucleotide donors for UGTs: UDP-glucuronic acid, UDP-glucose, UDP-galactose, UDP-*N*-acetylglucosamine, UDP-*N*-acetylgalactosamine, and UDP-xylose. For conjugation reactions with drugs, UDP-glucuronic acid is utilized as a donor; the UGTs of family 1 and 2 that need this donor molecule are the well-known "UGTs." Put another way, the abbreviation "UGT" has a broader meaning than solely "glucuronyltransferase," as it encompasses also the two other UGT families that, however, catalyze mostly reactions involving UDP-*N*-acetylglucosamine (UGT3) or UDP-galactose (UGT8) [56, 57]. The focus in this book is hence on the UGTs of families 1 and 2.

Drugs are glucuronidated by enzymes of both the UGT1A and UGT2B subfamily (the UGT2A enzymes are rare and their role in drug metabolism is marginal). In both these families of microsomal proteins, pharmacogenetic variants of the respective enzymes have been described in detail (see Chapter 3 and the web site http://www.pharmacogenomics.pha.ulaval.ca/sgc/ugt_alleles). Paracetamol (Figure 1.1), oxazepam, or morphine are typical examples of substrates for UGT1A6 and UGT2B7 [57]. As glucuronidation is the most common type of drug conjugation [57, 58], its clinical importance, including the pathways of drug elimination and evaluation of the possible drug interactions, is relatively high.

Methods of studying drug interactions that are able to provide data on the specificity of drug–enzyme interactions involve, for example, *in vitro* studies with purified or, more often, recombinant enzymes, making it possible to identify the respective form of a particular enzyme (e.g., CYP or UGT) responsible for the drug metabolism, or studies with microsomal preparations examining possible inhibition of a prototypic activity of a particular drug-metabolizing enzyme by another drug acting as an inhibitor. For UGTs, more or less specific substrates and inhibitors for the most important UGTs have been identified [57, 59]. As an example, an analysis of quantitative prediction of *in vivo* drug interaction based on *in vitro* data was presented with fluconazole (a selective UGT2B7 inhibitor) and zidovudine [60]. Complexity and difficulty in interpretation of drug interaction studies with UGTs and CYPs has been recently demonstrated in a study describing the inhibition of CYP enzyme (CYP2C8) by glucuronide of the interacting drug (gemfibrozil, formed by UGT2B7 and 1A3) leading to increased levels of another concomitantly administered drug, repaglinide; leading to an order of magnitude increase of the repaglinide bioavailability due to inhibited CYP2C8 [61].

It is not only the pharmacogenetics that may significantly influence the ability of a human subject to glucuronidate the respective substrates. Recent studies have found another factor affecting the efficacy with which the drugs are glucuronidated and, hence, excreted from the human body. Namely, induction of UGT enzymes via the AhR (see also Chapter 8). For example, a very recent paper has documented that drinking coffee induces expression of glucuronosyltransferases including the already mentioned form UGT1A3 in the liver and stomach via the AhR and nuclear factor erythroid 2-related factor 2 (Nrf2) pathways [62].

Sulfotransferases (SULTs) are members of a superfamily of enzymes catalyzing transfer of a sulfonyl moiety (SO_3H or, more generally, SO_3^- anion) from the universal donor PAPS to an acceptor group possessing an O, N, or S nucleophilic atom. Hence, the name is *de facto* not correct because the transferred group is a sulfonate, not a sulfate (SO_4H); however, it remains in use for practical reasons. SULTs were formerly classified by their subcellular localization as either cytosolic or membrane-bound. Sulfonate conjugation is important also from the ontogenetic point of view: the human fetus does not possess a functional UGT transcript until week 20 of gestation [63]; on the contrary, cytosolic fetal liver fractions exhibit SULT activities towards drug substrates such as paracetamol [64].

SULTs are known to participate in conjugation reactions involving endogenous (hormones, neurotransmitters) and exogenous compounds (xenobiotics, including drugs). They are present in the main organs involved in interaction with xenobiotics [5, 65]. Human SULT1A1, which represents over a half of liver SULTs and is the major form present in the kidney [65], catalyzes sulfate conjugation primarily of phenolic xenobiotics such as paracetamol (Figure 1.1). Thanks to this property, and also thanks to its remarkable thermostability, it was formerly called phenol SULT or thermostable phenol SULT [66]. Human monoamine-preferring SULT (SULT1A3, present in the kidney, small intestine, and lungs [65]) catalyzes sulfate conjugation of phenolic monoamines, including neurotransmitters such as dopamine, noradrenaline (norepinephrine), and serotonin, as well as conjugation of phenolic drugs [67]. Human SULT1E1 – the major form in the lungs – plays a major role in sulfation of estrogens [68] and human hydroxysteroid SULT (SULT2A1, present in the liver, but also in the lungs, small intestine, and to a lesser extent in the kidneys) is important for regulation of dehydroepiandrosterone and other hydroxysteroid hormones [65, 69].

Inhibition of SULTs may interfere with their ability to detoxify xenobiotics, as well as with other processes in which sulfated (more precisely, sulfonated) compounds play a role. For example, an inhibitory effect of nonsteroidal anti-inflammatory agents such as nimesulide or piroxicam on SULT1A1 was described recently; other drugs of this class (sulindac, ibuprofen) act as inhibitors of the SULT1E1 enzyme [70]. Studies with flavonoids and related polyphenols present in food including beverages have shown that many compounds of this and similar structure such as curcumin or quercetin are inhibitors of SULT enzymes [71]; SULT1A1 and SULT1A3 have been recently shown to be inhibited by grapefruit juice, green tea, black tea, and oolong tea [72]. Interestingly, inhibition of SULT may be beneficial: Some compounds (e.g., safrole) may be bioactivated by sulfation and the subsequent reactions may lead to electrophilic nitrenium or carbenium ions that bind to DNA, hence initiating the process of chemical carcinogenesis; inhibition of the respective SULT by flavonoids from the diet in such cases helps to protect the organism [73].

Induction, regulation of biosynthesis, and effects of gene polymorphism are usual factors complicating the study of drug metabolism efficacy and toxicity. These aspects that should be taken into account also with SULTs are largely covered in Chapter 4.

N-acetyltransferases (NATs) are cytosolic enzymes found typically in the liver, but also in other tissues, catalyzing in two steps the transfer of an acetyl group from acetyl-CoA at first to a Cys residue of the enzyme and, in the next step, the transfer of the acetyl group from the enzyme to the amino group of a substrate. Typical substrates are aromatic amines and hydrazides; aliphatic primary amines are rarely substrates of these enzymes. Interestingly, the products – acetylated amines – are often less hydrophilic than the substrates, which is seemingly in contrast with the general concept of making the xenobiotic more polar to be excreted. However, the elimination process is more complex and the properties of the protein transporters following the conjugation should also be taken into account – these proteins may prefer acetylated substrates.

NATs became well known for their genetic polymorphism already more than 50 years ago (for a review, see, e.g., [74]). The concept of the slow and rapid or fast acetylator phenotype was known in the pharmacology of the antituberculotic isoniazide, and was in fact the beginning of the era of clinical pharmacogenetics. In humans, there are two known genes coding for NATs – for NAT1 and NAT2 – with 85% homology of nucleotide sequences; the respective proteins exhibit a certain overlap, but they have distinctly different substrate specificity. Typical substrates of NAT1 are *p*-aminosalicylic acid, *p*-aminobenzoic acid, and sulfamethoxazole;

ATP, formation of acyl-AMP conjugate); (ii) formation of acyl-CoA (by acyl-CoA synthetase (more correctly, ATP-dependent acid : CoA ligase, which catalyzes both the first steps)), and (iii) ligation of the amino acid (Gly, but also Gln or taurine) with the CoA-activated acyl to get the conjugate by formation of the acyl carbonyl-NH (α-amino group from the amino acid as glycine) peptide-like bond. The third step is catalyzed by acyl-CoA : amino acid *N*-acyltransferase; CoA is liberated. Reactions with xenobiotics including drugs occur in mitochondria where the corresponding enzymes as well as the ATP are available. Conjugated drugs (e.g., hippuric acid, product with benzoic acid conjugated to glycine) are excreted in urine, which is the last step of this detoxication process – there are no known pathways leading to reactive nucleophiles as it is the case with glucuronidation, glutathione conjugation, *N*-acetylation by NAT, or sulfation.

This introduction does not claim to be an exhaustive list of all reactions – only those enzyme systems that are most important have been discussed here, and only the basic characteristics and the principles covered. The following chapters will give more detailed information focusing on selected enzymes of drug metabolism.

Acknowledgments

The authors wish to thank the Grant Agency of the Czech Republic (grants **305/09/0535**, **P303/12/G163**) and **CZ.1.05/2.1.00/01.00300** for financial support. The authors also wish to thank Dr J. Strojil for critical reading of this manuscript.

References

1 Tang, B.K. and Kalow, W. (1995) Variable action of lovastatin by hydrolytic enzymes in human plasma and liver. *Eur. J. Clin. Pharmacol.*, **47**, 449–451.

2 Bachmann, K.A., Lewis, J.D., Fuller, M.A., and Bonfiglio, M.F. (eds) (2004) *Drug Interaction Handbook*, 2nd edn, Lexi-Comp, Hudson, OH.

3 Kirchheiner, J. and Seeringer, A. (2007) Clinical implications of pharmacogenetics of cytochrome P450 drug metabolizing enzymes. *Biochem. Biophys. Acta*, **1170**, 489–494.

4 Williams, R.T. (1959) *Detoxication Mechanisms: The Mechanism and Detoxication of Drugs, Toxic Substances, and Other Organic Compounds*, 2nd edn, Chapman & Hall, London.

5 Parkinson, A. (2001) Biotransformation of xenobiotics, in *Casarett and Doull's Toxicology: The Basic Science of Poisons*, 6th edn (ed. C.D. Klaasen), McGraw-Hill, New York, pp. 133–224.

6 Josephy, P.D., Guengerich, F.P., and Miners, J.O. (2005) "Phase I" and "Phase II" drug metabolism: terminology that we should phase out? *Drug Metab. Rev.*, **37**, 575–580.

7 Guengerich, F.P. (2005) Human cytochromes P450, in *Cytochrome P450. Structure, Mechanism and Biochemistry*, 3rd edn (ed. P.R. Ortiz de Montellano), Kluwer/Plenum, New York, pp. 473–535.

8 Rittle, J. and Green, M.T. (2010) Cytochrome P450 compound I: capture, characterization, and C–H bond

activation kinetics. *Science*, **330**, 933–937.

9 Neve, E.P. and Ingelman-Sundberg, M. (2010) Cytochrome P450 protein: retention and distribution from the endoplasmic reticulum. *Curr. Opin. Drug Discov. Dev.*, **13**, 78–85.

10 Walsh, J.S. and Miwa, G.T. (2011) Bioactivation of drugs: risk and drug design. *Annu. Rev. Pharmacol. Toxicol.*, **51**, 145–167.

11 Marnett, L.J., Wlodawer, P., and Samuelsson, B. (1975) Co-oxygenation of organic substrates by the prostaglandin synthetase of sheep vesicular gland. *J. Biol. Chem.*, **250**, 8510–8517.

12 Harvison, P.J., Egan, R.W., Gale, P.H., Christian, G.D., Hill, B.S., and Nelson, S.D. (1988) Acetaminophen and analogs as cosubstrates and inhibitors of prostaglandin H synthase. *Chem. Biol. Interact.*, **64**, 251–266.

13 O'Brien, P.J. (2000) Peroxidases. *Chem. Biol. Interact.*, **129**, 113–139.

14 Furtmüller, P.G., Zederbauer, M., Jantschko, W., Helm, J., Bogner, M., Jakopitsch, C., and Obinger, C. (2006) Active site structure and catalytic mechanisms of human peroxidases. *Arch. Biochem. Biophys.*, **445**, 199–213.

15 Wang, P., Bai, H.-W., and Zhu, B.T. (2010) Structural basis for certain naturally occurring bioflavonoids to function as reducing co-substrates of cyclooxygenase I and II. *PLoS One*, **5**, 1–11.

16 Smith, R.D. and Kehrer, J.P. (1991) Cooxidation of cyclophosphamide as an alternative pathway for its bioactivation and lung toxicity. *Cancer Res.*, **51**, 542–548.

17 Reszka, K.J., Wagner, B.A., Teesch, L.M., Britigan, B.E., Spitz, D.R., and Burns, C.P. (2005) Inactivation of anthracyclines by cellular peroxidase. *Cancer Res.*, **65**, 6346–6353.

18 Brück, T.B. and Brück, D.W. (2011) Oxidative metabolism of the anti-cancer agent mitoxantrone by horseradish, lacto- and lignin peroxidase. *Biochimie*, **93**, 217–226.

19 Reszka, K.J., Sallans, L., Macha, S., Brown, K., McGraw, D.W., Kovacic, M.B., and Britigan, B.E. (2011) Airway peroxidases catalyze nitration of the β_2-agonist salbutamol and decrease its pharmacological activity. *J. Pharmacol. Exp. Ther.*, **336**, 440–449.

20 Reszka, K.J., McGraw, D.W., and Britigan, B.E. (2009) Peroxidative metabolism of β_2-agonists salbutamol and fenoterol and their analogs. *Chem. Res. Toxicol.*, **22**, 1137–1150.

21 Liu, Y.C. and Uetrecht, J.P. (2000) Metabolism of ticlopidine by activated neutrophils: implications for ticlopidine/ induced agranulocytosis. *Drug Metab. Dispos.*, **28**, 726–730.

22 Liu, Y.C. and Uetrecht, J.P. (1995) Clozapine is oxidized by activated human neutrophils to a reactive nitrenium ion that irreversibly binds in the cells. *J Pharmacol. Exp.Ther.*, **275**, 1476–1483.

23 Uetrecht, J. (2008) Idiosyncratic drug reactions: past, present, and future. *Chem. Res. Toxicol.*, **21**, 84–92.

24 Strolin Benedetti, M. (2011) FAD-dependent enzymes involved in the metabolic oxidation of xenobiotics. *Ann. Pharm. Fr.*, **69**, 45–52.

25 Phillips, I.R. and Shephard, E.A. (2008) Flavin-containing monooxygenases: mutations, disease and drug response. *Trends Pharmacol. Sci.*, **29**, 294–230.

26 Celsius, T., Pansoy, A., Matthews, J., Okey, A.B., Henderson, M.C., Krueger, S.K., and Williams, D.E. (2010) Flavin-containing monooxygenase-3: induction by 3-methylcholanthrene and complex regulation by xenobiotic chemicals in hepatoma cells and mouse liver. *Toxicol. Appl. Pharmacol.*, **247**, 60–69.

27 Park, C.S., Baek, H.M., Chung, W.G., Lee, K.H., Ryu, S.D., and Cha, Y.N. (1999) Suppression of flavin-containing monooxygenase 1 by overproduced nitric oxide in rat. *Mol. Pharmacol.*, **56**, 507–514.

28 Crettol, S., Petrovic, N., and Murray, M. (2010) Pharmacogenetics of phase I and phase II drug metabolism. *Curr. Pharm. Des.*, **16**, 204–219.

29 Cashman, J.R. (2008) Role of flavin-containing monooxygenase in drug

development. *Expert Opin. Drug Metab. Toxicol.*, **4**, 1507–1521.

30 Motika, M.S., Zhang, J., Zheng, X., Riedler, K., and Cashman, J.R. (2009) Novel variants of the human flavin-containing monooxygenase 3 (FMO3) gene associated with trimethylaminuria. *Mol. Genet. Metab.*, **97**, 128–135.

31 Benedetti, M.S. and Dostert, P. (1994) Contribution of amine oxidases to the metabolism of xenobiotics. *Drug Metab. Rev.*, **26**, 507–535.

32 Wu, X., Noda, A., Noda, H., and Imamura, Y. (2001) Side chain metabolism of propranolol: involvement of monoamine oxidase and aldehyde reductase in the metabolism of *N*-desisopropylpropranolol to propranolol glycol in rat liver. *Comp. Biochem. Physiol. C*, **129**, 361–368.

33 Visentin, V., Prévot, D., De Saint Front, V.D., Morin-Cussac, N., Thalamas, C., Galitzky, J., Valet, P., Zorzano, A., and Carpéné, C. (2004) Alteration of amine oxidase activity in adipose tissue of obese subjects. *Obes. Res.*, **12**, 547–555.

34 McGrath, A.P., Caradoc-Davies, T., Collyer, C.A., and Guss, J.M. (2010) Correlation of active site metal content in human diamine oxidase with trihydroxyphenylalanine quinone cofactor biogenesis. *Biochemistry*, **49**, 8316–8324.

35 Rettie, A.R. and Fisher, M.B. (1999) Transformation enzymes: oxidative; non-P450, in *Handbook of Drug Metabolism* (ed. T.R. Woolf), Dekker, New York, pp. 131–151.

36 Roberts, R.L., Gearry, R.B., and Barclay, M.L. (2010) Allopurinol-thiopurine combination therapy in inflammatory bowel disease. are there genetic clues to this puzzle? *Pharmacogenomics*, **11**, 1505–1508.

37 Takano, Y., Hase-Aoki, K., Horiuchi, H., Zhao, L., Kasahara, Y., Kondo, S., and Becker, M.A. (2005) Selectivity of febuxostat, a novel non-purine inhibitor of xanthine oxidase/xanthine dehydrogenase. *Life Sci.*, **76**, 1835–1847.

38 Krenitsky, T.A., Hall, W.W., de Miranda, P., Beauchamp, L.M., Schaeffer, H.J., and Whiteman, P.D. (1984) 6-Deoxyacyclovir: a xanthine-oxidase-activated prodrug of acyclovir. *Proc. Natl. Acad. Sci. USA*, **81**, 3209–3213.

39 Akabane, T., Tanaka, K., Irie, M., Terashita, S., and Teramura, T. (2011) Case report of extensive metabolism by aldehyde oxidase in humans: pharmacokinetics and metabolite profile of FK3453 in rats, dogs, and humans. *Xenobiotica*, **41**, 372–384.

40 Rashidi, M.R. and Nazemiyeh, H. (2010) Inhibitory effects of flavonoids on molybdenum hydroxylases activity. *Expert Opin. Drug Metab. Toxicol.*, **6**, 133–152.

41 Bedard, K. and Krause, K.-H. (2007) The NOX family of ROS-generating NADPH oxidases: physiology and pathophysiology. *Physiol. Rev.*, **87**, 245–312.

42 Wind, S., Beuerlein, K., Eucker, T., Müller, H., Scheurer, P., Armitage, M.E., Ho, H., Schmidt, H.H.H.W., and Wingler, K. (2010) Comparative pharmacology of chemically distinct NADPH oxidase inhibitors. *Br. J. Pharmacol.*, **161**, 885–898.

43 Riley, R.J. and Workman, P. (1992) DT-diaphorase and cancer chemotherapy. *Biochem. Pharmacol.*, **43**, 1657–1669.

44 Danson, S., Ward, T.H., Butler, J., and Ranson, M. (2004) DT-diaphorase: a target for new anticancer drugs. *Cancer Treat. Rev.*, **30**, 437–449.

45 Danson, S.J., Johnson, P., Ward, T.H., Dawson, M., Denneny, O., Dickinson, G., Aarons, L., Watson, A., Jowle, D., Cummings, J., Robson, C., Halbert, G., Dive, C., and Ranson, M. (2011) Phase I pharmacokinetic and pharmacodynamic study of the bioreductive drug RH1. *Ann. Oncol.*, **22**, 1653–1660.

46 Ma, Q., Kinneer, K., Bi, Y., Chan, J.Y., and Kan, Y.W. (2004) Induction of murine NAD(P)H : quinone oxidoreductase by 2,3,7,8-tetrachlorodibenzo-*p*-dioxin requires the CNC (cap "n" collar) basic leucine zipper transcription factor Nrf2 (nuclear factor erythroid 2-related factor 2): cross-interaction between AhR (aryl hydrocarbon receptor) and Nrf2 signal transduction. *Biochem. J.*, **377**, 205–213.

47 Dobritzsch, D., Schneider, G., Schnackerz, K.D., and Lindquist, Y. (2001) Crystal structure of dihydropyrimidine dehydrogenase, a

major determinant of the pharmacokinetics of the anti-cancer drug 5-fluorouracil. *EMBO J.*, **20**, 650–660.

48 van Kuilenburg, A.B.P. (2004) Dihydropyrimidine dehydrogenase and the efficacy and toxicity of 5-fluorouracil. *Eur. J. Cancer*, **40**, 939–950.

49 Kanamitsu, S.-I., Ito, K., Okuda, H., Ogura, K., Watabe, T., Muro, K., and Sugiyama, Y. (2000) Prediction of *in vivo* drug–drug interactions based on mechanism-based inhibition from *in vitro* data: inhibition of 5-fluorouracil metabolism by (*E*)-5-(2-bromovinyl)uracil. *Drug Metab. Dispos.*, **28**, 467–474.

50 Jin, Y. and Penning, T.M. (2007) Aldo-keto reductases and bioactivation/detoxication. *Annu. Rev. Pharmacol. Toxicol.*, **47**, 263–292.

51 Hoffmann, F. and Maser, E. (2007) Carbonyl reductases and pluripotent hydroxysteroid dehydrogenases of the short-chain dehydrogenase/reductase superfamily. *Drug Metab. Rev.*, **39**, 87–144.

52 Malátková, P., Maser, E., and Wsól, V. (2010) Human carbonyl reductases. *Curr. Drug Metab.*, **11**, 639–658.

53 Ax, W., Soldan, M., Koch, L., and Maser, E. (2000) Development of daunorubicin resistance in tumour cells by induction of carbonyl reduction. *Biochem. Pharmacol.*, **59**, 293–300.

54 Kalgutkar, A.S., Taylor, T.J., Venkatakrishnan, K., and Isin, E.M. (2003) Assessment of the contributions of CYP3A4 and CYP3A5 in the metabolism of antipsychotic agent haloperidol to its potentially neurotoxic pyridinium metabolite and effect of antidepressants on the bioactivation pathway. *Drug Metab. Dispos.*, **31**, 243–249.

55 Mackenzie, P.I., Bode, K.W., Burchell, B., Guillemette, C., Ikushiro, S., Iyanagi, T., Miners, J.O., Owens, I.S., and Nebert, D.W. (2005) Nomenclature update for the mammalian UDP glycosyltransferase (UGT) gene superfamily. *Pharmacogenet. Genomics*, **15**, 677–685.

56 Mackenzie, P.I., Rogers, A., Elliot, D.J., Chan, N., Hulin, J.A., Miners, J.O., and Meech, R. (2011) The novel UDP glycosyltransferase 3A2: cloning, catalytic properties, and tissue distribution. *Mol. Pharmacol.*, **79**, 482–488.

57 Kiang, T.K.L., Ensom, M.H.H., and Chang, T.K.H. (2005) UDP-glucuronosyltransferases and clinical drug–drug interactions. *Pharmacol. Ther.*, **106**, 97–132.

58 Jančová, P., Anzenbacherova, E., and Anzenbacher, P. (2010) Phase II drug metabolizing enzymes. *Biomed. Pap. Med. Fac. Univ. Palacky Olomouc Czech. Repub.*, **154**, 103–116.

59 Uchaipichat, V., Mackenzie, P.I., Elliot, D.J., and Miners, J.O. (2006) Selectivity of substrate (trifluoperazine) and inhibitor (amitriptyline, androsterone, canrenoic acid, hecogenin, phenylbutazone, quinidine, quinine, and sulfinpyrazone) "probes" for human UDP-glucuronosyltransferases. *Drug Metab. Dispos.*, **34**, 449–456.

60 Uchaipichat, V., Winner, L.K., Mackenzie, P.I., Elliot, D.J., Williams, J.A., and Miners, J.O. (2006) Quantitative prediction of *in vivo* inhibitory interactions involving glucuronidated drugs from *in vitro* data: the effect of fluconazole on zidovudine glucuronidation. *Br. J. Clin. Pharmacol.*, **61**, 427–439.

61 Honkalammi, J., Niemi, M., Neuvonen, P.J., and Backman, J.T. (2011) Mechanism-based inactivation of CYP2C8 by gemfibrozil occurs rapidly in humans. *Clin. Pharmacol. Ther.*, **89**, 579–586.

62 Kalthoff, S., Ehmer, U., Freiberg, N., Manns, M.P., and Strassburg, C.P. (2010) Coffee induces expression of glucuronosyltransferases via the aryl hydrocarbon receptor and Nrf2 in liver and stomach. *Gastroenterology*, **139**, 1699–1710.

63 Strassburg, C.P., Strassburg, A., Kneip, S., Barut, A., Tukey, R.H., Rodeck, B., and Manns, M.P. (2002) Developmental aspects of human hepatic drug glucuronidation in young children and adults. *Gut*, **50**, 259–265.

64 Ring, J.A., Ghabrial, H., Ching, M.S., Smallwood, R.A., and Morgan, D.J. (1999) Fetal hepatic drug elimination. *Pharmacol. Ther.*, **84**, 429–445.

65 Riches, Z., Stanley, E.L., Bloomer, J.C., and Coughtrie, M.W. (2009) Quantitative

evaluation of the expression and activity of five major sulfotransferases (SULTs) in human tissues: the SULT pie. *Drug Metab. Dispos.*, **37**, 2255–2261.

66 Falany, C.N., Zhuang, W., and Falany, J.L. (1994) Characterization of expressed human phenol-sulfating phenolsulfotransferase: effect of mutating cys70 on activity and thermostability. *Chem. Biol. Interact.*, **92**, 57–66.

67 Lu, J.H., Li, H.T., Liu, M.C., Zhang, J.P., Li, M., An, X.M., and Chang, W.R. (2005) Crystal structure of human sulfotransferase SULT1A3 in complex with dopamine and 3′-phosphoadenosine 5′-phosphate. *Biochem. Biophys. Res. Commun.*, **335**, 417–423.

68 Her, C., Aksoy, I.A., Kimura, S., Brandriff, B.F., Wasmuth, J.J., and Weinshilboum, R.M. (1995) Human estrogen sulfotransferase gene (STE): cloning, structure, and chromosomal localization. *Genomics*, **29**, 16–23.

69 Otterness, D.M., Wieben, E.D., Wood, T.C., Watson, W.G., Madden, B.J., McCormick, D.J., and Weinshilboum, R.M. (1992) Human liver dehydroepiandrosterone sulfotransferase: molecular cloning and expression of cDNA. *Mol. Pharmacol.*, **41**, 865–872.

70 King, R.S., Ghosh, A.A., and Wu, J. (2006) Inhibition of human phenol and estrogen sulfotransferase by certain non-steroidal anti-inflammatory agents. *Curr. Drug Metab.*, **7**, 745–753.

71 Pacifici, G.M. (2004) Inhibition of human liver and duodenum sulfotransferases by drugs and dietary chemicals: a review of the literature. *Int. J. Clin. Pharmacol. Ther.*, **42**, 488–495.

72 Nishimuta, H., Ohtani, H., Tsujimoto, M., Ogura, K., Hiratsuka, A., and Sawada, Y. (2007) Inhibitory effects of various beverages on human recombinant sulfotransferase isoforms SULT1A1 and SULT1A3. *Biopharm. Drug Dispos.*, **28**, 491–500.

73 Huang, C., Chen, Y., Zhou, T., and Chen, G. (2009) Sulfation of dietary flavonoids by human sulfotransferases. *Xenobiotica*, **39**, 312–322.

74 Wormhoudt, L.W., Commandeur, J.N.M., and Vermeulen, N.P.E. (1999) Genetic polymorphisms of human *N*-acetyltransferase, cytochrome P450, glutathione-*S*-transferase and epoxide hydrolase enzymes: relevance to xenobiotic metabolism and toxicity. *CRC Crit. Rev. Toxicol.*, **29**, 59–124.

75 Kawamura, A., Graham, J., Mushtaq, A., Tsiftsoglou, S.A., Vath, G.M., Hanna, P.E., Wagner, C.R., and Sim, E. (2005) Eukaryotic arylamine *N*-acetyltransferase. Investigation of substrate specificity by high-throughput screening. *Biochem. Pharmacol.*, **69**, 347–359.

76 Grant, D.M., Blum, M., Beer, M., and Meyer, U.A. (1991) Monomorphic and polymorphic human arylamine *N*-acetyltransferases: a comparison of liver isoenzymes and expressed products of two cloned genes. *Mol. Pharmacol.*, **39**, 184–191.

77 Sim, E., Payton, M., Noble, M., and Minchin, R. (2000) An update on genetic, structural and functional studies of arylamine *N*-acetyltransferases in eucaryotes and procaryotes. *Hum. Mol. Genet.*, **9**, 2435–2441.

78 Oakley, A. (2011) Glutathione transferases: a structural perspective. *Drug Metab. Rev.*, **43**, 138–151.

79 Wheeler, J.B., Stourman, N.V., Thier, R., Dommermuth, A., Vuilleumier, S., Rose, J.A., Armstrong, R.N., and Guengerich, F.P. (2001) Conjugation of haloalkanes by bacterial and mammalian glutathione transferases: mono- and dihalomethanes. *Chem. Res. Toxicol.*, **14**, 1118–1127.

80 Josephy, P.D. (2010) Genetic variations in human glutathione transferase enzymes: significance for pharmacology and toxicology. *Hum. Genomics Proteomics*, **2010**, 876940.

81 Hukkanen, J., Jacob, P., III, and Benowitz, N.L. (2005) Metabolism and disposition kinetics of nicotine. *Pharmacol. Rev.*, **57**, 79–115.

82 Saletu, M., Anderer, P., Hogl, B., Saletu-Zyhlarz, G., Kunz, A., Poewe, A., and Saletu, B. (2003) Acute double-blind, placebo-controlled sleep laboratory and clinical follow-up studies with a combination treatment of rr-L-dopa and sr-L-dopa in restless legs syndrome. *J. Neural Transm.*, **110**, 611–626.

83 Zhu, B.T. (2002) Catechol-*O*-methyltransferase (COMT)-mediated methylation metabolism of endogenous bioactive catechols and modulation by endobiotics and xenobiotics: importance in pathophysiology and pathogenesis. *Curr. Drug Metab.*, **3**, 321–349.

84 Weinshilboum, R.M. (2006) Pharmacogenomics: catechol *O*-methyltransferase to thiopurine *S*-methyltransferase. *Cell. Mol. Neurobiol.*, **26**, 539–561.

85 Valente, N.L., Vallada, H., Cordeiro, Q., Bressan, R.A., Andreoli, S.B., Mari, J.J., and Mello, M.F. (2011) Catechol-*O*-methyltransferase (COMT) val158met polymorphism as a risk factor for PTSD after urban violence. *Mol. Neurosci.*, **43**, 516–523.

86 Reuter, M., Frenzel, C., Walter, N.T., Market, S., and Montag, C. (2011) Investigating the genetic basis of altruism: the role of the COMT Val158Met polymorphism. *Soc. Cogn. Affect. Neurosci.*, **6**, 662–668.

87 Wang, L. and Weinshilboum, R. (2006) Thiopurine *S*-methyltransferase pharmacogenetics: insights, challenges and future directions. *Oncogene*, **25**, 1629–1638.

88 Knights, K.M., Sykes, M.J., and Miners, J.O. (2007) Amino acid conjugation: contribution to the metabolism and toxicity of of xenobiotic carboxylic acids. *Expert Opin. Drug Metab. Toxicol.*, **3**, 159–168.

2
Cytochromes P450

F. Peter Guengerich

2.1
Introduction and Historical Perspective

The cytochrome P450 field developed out of the study of the metabolism of drugs, steroids, and carcinogens. For instance, reactions with carcinogens were known in the 1940s [1]. The concept and stoichiometry of mixed function oxidation (Eq. 2.1):

$$NAD(P)H + H^+ + O_2 + R \rightarrow NADP^+ + H_2O + RO \quad (2.1)$$

were developed for other enzyme systems by Mason and Hayaishi [2, 3]. In 1956, Williams noted an unusual peak with a wavelength maximum near 450 nm, and this observation was first reported by Klingenberg and Garfinkel [4, 5]. Sato and Omura further characterized this pigment in 1962 and termed it "P450," indicating a "pigment" with a Soret absorption based at 450 nm [6], and the name has been retained (Figure 2.1). The relationship between this pigment and mixed-function oxidation was established in 1965 by Cooper *et al.* [8] with studies on the 21-hydroxylation of a steroid in adrenal cortex microsomes. The inhibition of the reaction by CO was reversed most effectively using light with a wavelength of 450 nm, consistent with the view that this protein is responsible for the hydroxylation reaction. During the 1960s several other lines of investigation showed the roles of P450 enzymes in drug oxidation reactions and evidence began to accumulate that more than one form of P450 might be present in a tissue, especially the liver–known to be the major organ in which P450 was found. Another development was the inducibility of P450s in rat liver, which had been recognized at the level of certain catalytic activities [9], and which explained some experimental [10] and clinical [11] observations regarding chemical carcinogenesis and drug metabolism.

In the 1960s, the basic understanding of the P450 systems was meager, in the context of the current state of the art. One advance was the discovery of P450 in bacteria and the characterization of the $P450_{cam}$ system (P450 101A1) from *Pseudomonas putida* [12]. The P450 and its two accessory proteins were readily purified, and have been used as a model for other P450s. For instance, the electron transfer

Metabolism of Drugs and Other Xenobiotics, First Edition. Edited by Pavel Anzenbacher, Ulrich M. Zanger.

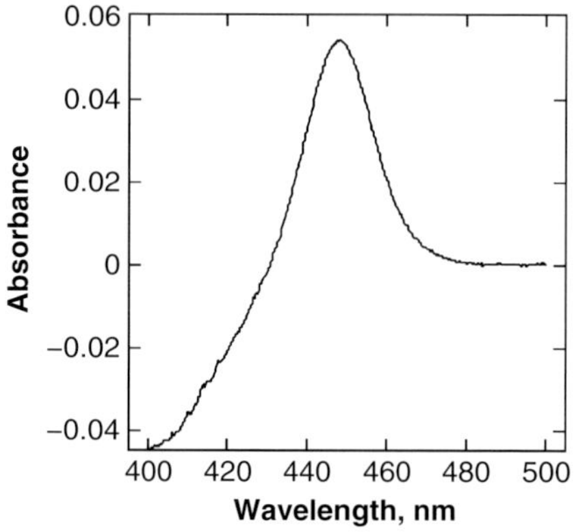

Figure 2.1 Difference spectrum of P450 [7]. A sample of rat liver P450 1A1 was divided into two cuvettes and one was saturated with CO gas. The two cuvettes were balanced in an Amino DW2a/OLIS spectrophotometer using the automatic baseline correction mode. The corrected baseline was recorded. After addition of $Na_2S_2O_4$ as indicated in the text the final difference spectrum was obtained. The calculations yield 0.59 nmol P450/ml and 0.03 nmol cytochrome P420/ml.

system was characterized in detail [13] and P450 101A1 was the first P450 for which a crystal structure was obtained [14]. In 1968, Coon and Lu succeeded in solubilizing rabbit liver microsomes with detergent, separating the P450 and the NADPH-P450 reductase and phospholipids by chromatography, and then reconstituting catalytic activity by combining the components [15]. Subsequent work in the laboratories of Coon and Sato led to purification of rabbit liver P450s to electrophoretic homogeneity [16, 17].

Subsequently, numerous P450 enzymes were purified from rabbit and rat liver [18–20]. Later, several of what are now considered the major human P450s were purified from liver microsomes [21–23]. The introduction of recombinant DNA methods led to the first sequence analysis of a P450 [24]. Subsequently, mammalian P450s were heterologously expressed in mammalian [25] and bacterial [26, 27] systems. Early work showed that some chemicals, including carcinogens [9] and drugs [11], could induce P450. The development of sequencing methods for DNA, other recombinant DNA technology, and useful cell culture methods have facilitated advances in the field of P450 regulation.

Exactly how P450s oxidize chemicals was difficult to understand, particularly when the protein components had not yet been purified. In the late 1970s, the concept developed that a high-valent iron–oxygen complex is involved, not mobile species of reactive oxygen. Seminal studies with P450 and substrates that could report mechanistic events led to the development of a mechanism involving abstraction of a hydrogen atom (or electron) by a perferryl-oxo intermediate (formally FeO^{3+}) and “oxygen rebound” to yield the product [28, 29]. The (bacterial) P450 101A1 crystal structure was solved in 1987 [30] and led to considerable insight into the catalytic specificity of a P450. Subsequently, several other bacterial P450 structures were solved and, in 1999, Johnson's group published the structure of a rabbit P450 [31]. Today crystal structures of all of the major human P450s involved in drug metabolism are available (*vide infra*).

(For a collection of classic P450 papers published in *The Journal of Biological Chemistry*, see the web site: http://www.jbc.org/site/collections/p450/classics/60s70s.xhtml.)

2.2 Nomenclature and Gene Organization

As soon as evidence for the existence of multiple forms of P450 began to appear, names of individual forms developed in multiple laboratories, including the terms "P450" and "P448" (based on small, but reproducible wavelength differences in the Soret CO complexes when only two P450s were considered to be present [32]). With the separation of many individual hepatic P450s [33] and the known number of steroid-oxidizing P450s with trivial names related to function (e.g., $P450_{scc}$, aromatase), the nomenclature soon became rather unwieldy.

When it became feasible to determine nucleotide sequences of cDNAs and genes, a nomenclature system was proposed based on sequence identity. (It is appropriate to refer to (%) sequence identity or similarity, depending on methods and algorithms, but not (%) sequence homology. Two sequences are either homologous or not [34].) Sequences that are 40% or more identical are in the same family (i.e., P450 Family 2; Figure 2.2) [35]. When two sequences are more than 55% identical, they are placed in the same subfamily (e.g., P450 2C; Figure 2.2). The final number indicates the individual P450 (e.g., P450 2C8; Figure 2.2).

This system has served the field well, in general, but there are some nuances to consider. Cytochromes P450 are abbreviated "P450" or "CYP, " but the latter is somewhat problematic in that cyclophilins also use the same abbreviation– a search for "CYP" will also include cyclophilins. If the abbreviation CYP is used, the convention is to use italics to indicate the gene. Small letters are used

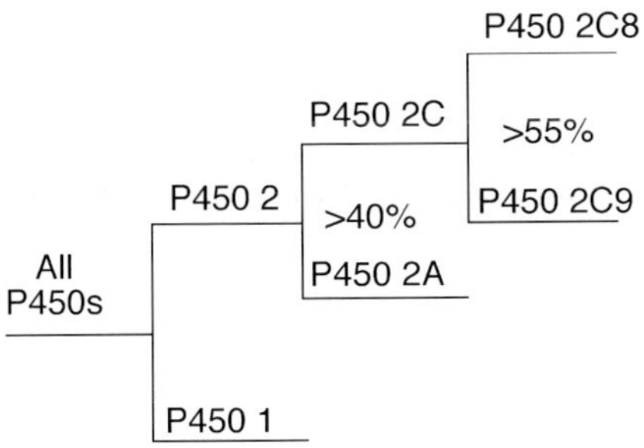

Figure 2.2 Nomenclature basis for P450s and classification into families (e.g., Family 2) and subfamilies (Family 2C) on the basis of sequence identity [35].

to designate mouse genes (*Cyp*). Another point that should be made is that it is no longer appropriate to refer to individual P450s as "isozymes" or "isoforms," any more than grouping all flavoprotein oxidases with such a term. The term isozymes refers to enzymes that have the same substrate and product, and therefore is only be appropriate for restricted comparisons. (Regarding jargon and conventions, the use of the terms "phase I, II, III, etc." is discouraged regarding different aspects of drug metabolism, for reasons discussed elsewhere [36].)

In some subfamilies, the individual P450s have numbers denoting individual enzymes for each species; for example, humans have P450s 3A4, 3A5, 3A7, and 3A43, but rats have P450s 3A2, 3A9, 3A18, 3A23, 3A62, and 3A73. In principle, all species are given the identical name (e.g., 1A2) when the function is conserved across species (e.g., 1A2, 2E1), although the conservation of function is definitely not exact in many of these cases (e.g., see [37]).

With regard to gene organization, the P450s vary in terms of number of introns. Usually, the P450s within a particular subfamily share similar intron/exon organizational patterns. The conserved exons seem to correspond to important structural domains within P450s. Some of the P450s are proposed to result from gene duplications (i.e., nonreciprocal exchange of nucleotide sequences between similar genes). For further discussion of genomic organization, see Nelson *et al.* [38].

To some extent the P450s can be classified in terms of function. One approach to the 57 human P450s is presented in Table 2.1. About a quarter of the P450s are involved in the metabolism of sterols. These P450s are highly conserved and regu-

Table 2.1 Classification of human P450s based on major substrate class[a].

Sterols	Xenobiotics	Fatty acids	Eicosanoids	Vitamins	Unknown
1B1	1A1	2J2	4F2	2R1	2A7
7A1	1A2	4A11	4F3	24A1	2S1
7B1	2A6	4B1	4F8	26A1	2U1
8B1	2A13	4F12	5A1	26B1	2W1
11A1	2B6		8A1	26C1	3A43
11B1	2C8			27B1	4A22
11B2	2C9				4F11
17A1	2C18				4F22
19A1	2C19				4V2
21A2	2D6				4X1
27A1	2E1				4Z1
39A1	2F1				20A1
46A1	3A4				27C1
51A1	3A5				
	3A7				

a) This classification is somewhat arbitrary in some cases (e.g., P450s 1B1 and 27A1 could be grouped in either of two different categories).

lated, and the levels do not vary much among individuals. Studies with transgenic mice and human clinical experience show the importance of these P450s in normal physiology and reproduction [39].

In contrast, the roughly one-quarter of the P450s involved in the metabolism of xenobiotics do not appear to have critical physiological functions. Levels of these P450s can vary considerably among individuals and the complete absence of some of these P450s does not seem to be a serious problem (e.g., P450 2D6, *vide infra*). Some of the P450s in this group may catalyze the oxidation of endogenous compounds, but it is not clear that this is physiologically relevant (e.g., P450 3A4 testosterone 6β-hydroxylation), in that the enzyme levels can vary widely without obvious physiological effects.

Some P450s oxidize fatty acids efficiently, especially in the 4F subfamily. Such oxidation may contribute to overall clearance, although the overall fractional contribution is not known. Some of the oxidation products of fatty acids do have biological activities, and may be important in hypertension and other conditions, (e.g., some epoxides and compounds derived from them) [40]. However, nonselective oxidation products such as ω-1, ω-2, and ω-3 hydroxylated fatty acids have no clear functions of their own.

Five P450s function in the metabolism of eicosanoids. Three of these oxidize leukotrienes [41]. The other two P450s do not catalyze mixed-function oxidation reactions *per se*, but rather the rearrangement of prostaglandin H_2 to prostacyclin I_2 (P450 5A1) or thromboxane A_2 (P450 8A1). These P450s appear to be important, particularly the latter two.

At least six P450s have roles in the oxidation of fat-soluble vitamins (A and D). Several of these P450s have been shown to be important (e.g., deficiency of P450 27B1 is associated with vitamin D-dependent rickets type I) [39].

The remainder of the P450s (roughly a quarter) are termed "orphans," in the sense that these do not have homes. At least three of these (2A7, 3A43, and 4A22) show very little expression and may not be relevant, even it they are not true pseudogenes. mRNA localization studies have been done with most of the orphan P450s, although with conflicting results in some cases (little immunochemical localization has been done, i.e., protein expression level). Some reactions of these orphan P450s have been identified [42], but the relevance of any is not clear yet. For more information about the orphans P450s and approaches to discerning their functions, see [43].

The classification in Table 2.1 is imperfect in the sense that some P450s can be placed in more than one category. For instance, P450 1B1 catalyzes estrogen hydroxylation and its absence is associated with glaucoma (although these phenomena are not necessarily related), but the enzyme also activates a wide variety of procarcinogens [44]. Another point is that many P450s will catalyze low rates of oxidations of fatty acids, often rather nondescript reactions [45, 46], but the significance is not clear. The overlap of these activities among the P450s precludes definitive transgenic mouse studies in some cases (also, the correspondence of mouse and human P450s is not clear in some of the complex P450 subfamilies).

The above discussion of the P450s is focused on the human enzymes, but studies with experimental animals are important in drug development (and domestic animals in veterinary research). Mice have 103 P450 genes (obviously making many direct comparisons with the 57 human P450s problematic) and the number of P450 genes in other mammals is probably in the range of 40–120. Information on the P450 genes of many organisms is available at http://drnelson.uthsc.edu/cytochromeP450.html.

2.3 Regulation

Most of the mammalian P450 enzymes are regulated in one way or another. The focus here will be on the P450s involved in the metabolism of xenobiotics (Table 2.1), in that many of the drugs of interest are not only potential P450 substrates, but also inducers.

2.3.1 Transcriptional Regulation

Much of the regulation of P450s occurs at the transcriptional level (i.e., the rate of synthesis of mRNA). A general model is presented (Figure 2.3) where binding of a ligand activates a receptor. In most cases this activated receptor then binds

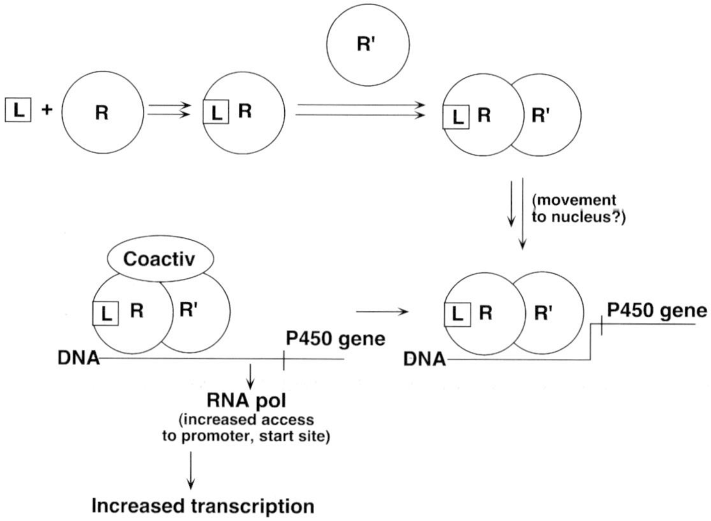

Figure 2.3 Generalized mechanism of P450 induction by enhanced transcription. L, ligand; R, receptor; R′, heterodimer component for binding the receptor R; Coactiv, coactivator protein; pol, RNA polymerase [47].

another protein to form a heterodimer, which then occupies a specific position in the 5′ upstream region of the P450 gene. In some cases coactivators are recruited to the complex. The process opens the promoter segment of the gene to RNA polymerase, which then copies the DNA to form RNA. This general model (Figure 2.3) is applicable in several cases.

i) In the aryl hydrocarbon receptor (AhR) system the receptor is the AhR protein, the ligand is 2,3,7,8-tetrachlorodibenzo-*p*-dioxin (TCDD), a polycyclic hydrocarbon such as benzo[*a*]pyrene, or another structurally related entity, and the heterodimeric protein is the AhR nuclear translocator (ARNT) protein. Heat shock protein (hsp) 90 is displaced when the ligand binds. The AhR–ARNT complex binds to one or more xenobiotic-responsive element (XRE) sites in the 5′ region of the genes coding for P450s 1A1, 1A2, or 1B1 (or any of a number of other non-P450 genes). The system is more complex than this, in that there is a second AhR protein that binds ligand but does not activate the AhR repressor [48], several coactivators have been identified or proposed, and there is some "cross-talk" with estrogen receptors. TCDD is extremely toxic in some animal species and the current consensus is that the AhR system is necessary for toxicity, but not sufficient.

ii) The peroxisome proliferator-activated receptor (PPAR)-α system is involved in inducing P450 4A enzymes in several species, as well as a number of peroxisomal enzymes involved in fatty acid metabolism and peroxisomal proliferation. The ligands are fatty acids or a variety of xenobiotic chemicals (e.g., fibrates, phthalates) and the heterodimer is a retinoid X receptor (RXR), charged with a (retinoid) ligand of its own.

iii) The pregnane X receptor (PXR) regulates the important human P450 3A4 and some of the animal orthologs. The ligands include certain endogenous or artificial steroids, certain macrolide antibiotics, and many other drugs. The heterodimer is an RXR protein (with a ligand). There is also cross-talk with the P450 2C subfamily genes.

Much of the regulation of the P450 2C subfamily proteins is driven by the constitutive androgen receptor (CAR) protein, which is rather unusual. Some strong inducers are ligands (e.g., TCPOBOPOP [49]), but most inducers of this system apparently do not act by binding as ligands; they somehow induce phosphorylation of CAR at a specific site to facilitate its movement into the nucleus, followed by interaction with a liganded RXR protein to induce transcription of P450 subfamily 2B and 2C proteins. Again, there is some cross-talk with the PXR system for these P450s (and 3A subfamily enzymes).

The roles of coactivator proteins have already been alluded to. These are important in considering tissue-specific gene expression and also which cell lines can be used for induction assays. Hepatocyte nuclear factor (HNF)-4α is a coactivator of P450 3A4 [50] and the human P450 1A2 gene contains a (half) HNF-1 consensus site, contributing to the liver-selective expression of these P450s. Thus, cell lines known to express these coactivators should be used for induction assays.

In addition to P450 induction, downregulation can also occur. Early studies with rats showed that some P450s can be downregulated an order of magnitude by some of the chemicals commonly used to induce other P450s [33]. This phenomenon has been shown to have a basis at the level of reduced mRNA synthesis [51], although the mechanism is not yet understood at a more fundamental level.

Another complex type of regulation is gender specificity. This phenomenon can be quite dramatic in rodents and can be modulated by castration/hormone supplementation regimes [52]. The basis of this effect appears to be the gender specificity of patterns of growth hormone release and certain factors (e.g., cytostatic proteins) [53]. Gender-specific P450 differences are much less dramatic in humans than rodents [54]. The gender differences in rodent P450s (e.g., rat P450 2C11 and 2C12) can be important in evaluating metabolism and toxicity in animal models and extrapolation to humans.

2.3.2
Post-Translational and Epigenetic Regulation

Although transcriptional regulation may seem complex, it is still more straightforward than several alternate mechanisms. mRNA stability has been proposed as one mechanism of the induction of P450 2E1 by ethanol and other chemicals [55, 56].

MicroRNAs have been explored in many facets of gene regulation, including P450s. Yokoi's group has shown that (i) miR-27b attenuates expression of P450 1B1 [57] and (ii) that miR-378 attenuates expression of P450 2E1 [58]. The latter finding is significant in the context of the difficulties in understanding the regulation of P450 2E1 (*vide supra*). Also of note are reports on the regulation of human PXR and HNF-4α, which regulate P450 3A4 and other P450s, by microRNAs [59, 60].

Methylation of cytosine in CpG islands has been considered as a mechanism of gene regulation for several P450s and there is some evidence for a role in several cases, including P450s 1A1, 1A2, 1B1, 2E1, and 2W1 [61, 62]. CpG islands are also found in potentially relevant regions of the *CYP2A6*, *CYP2C19*, *CYP2D6*, *CYP2J2*, *CYP2R1*, and *CYP2S1* genes [61], but these have not been investigated as much.

Histone modification has also been considered as a possible epigenetic regulatory mechanism. Some evidence for a role in regulation has been presented in the cases of the human *CYP1A1* and *CYP1B1* genes [61, 62].

2.3.3
Post-Translational Regulation

Presently, there is limited evidence for major roles for post-translational regulation of P450s, at least in comparison to some other enzyme systems.

The insertion of the prosthetic group heme is an obligatory post-translational modification of all P450s. Based on the available crystal structures of P450, the heme is sequestered deep within the protein and only degraded by heme oxygenase (to biliverdin and CO) after release, presumably due to protein degradation [63]. Abnormalities in heme synthesis could block the production of heme to the extent that P450 function would be impaired and there is evidence that this can be achieved in animal models (e.g., with Co^{2+} [64]), but how common this is in humans is unknown except in the case of porphyria [65].

Phosphorylation has been studied with some of the P450s. The presence of substrates or inducers has been reported to block phosphorylation of Ser129 of P450 2E1 and lead to protein stabilization [55]. However, site-directed mutagenesis (S129A) did not change the half-life of P450 2E1 in cell culture [66]. Phosphorylation of P450 2E1 has also been reported to be involved in targeting this P450 to mitochondria [67]. Phosphorylation of P450 2D6 has also been implicated in targeting of that protein to mitochondria and some polymorphic variants lack the ability to undergo phosphorylation [68]. The phosphorylation of rat P450 2B1 has been reported to attenuate its catalytic activity [69] and also its targeting to mitochondria [70].

Apparently the only report of P450 glycosylation is with P450 19A1 – the steroid aromatase [71]. However, an active enzyme can be expressed in bacteria [72, 73], presumably in the absence of glycosylation. Specific searches for glycosylation of several major rat P450s were negative [33, 74].

Ubiquination has been implicated in the degradation of P450s, particularly P450 3A4 [75, 76]. Phosphorylation has also been implicated in the ubiquitin-dependent proteasomal degradation of P450 3A4 [77]. However, the role of ubiquination in P450 processing appears to vary. Ubiquination of (rat) P450s 2D1 and 2C11 is important, but this is not the case for P450 2E1 [75].

There are many kinds of post-translational modification of proteins (more than 100). Today it is possible to use mass spectrometry to systematically search for modification of peptides, but to the author's knowledge this has not been done.

Finally, evidence exists that some microsomal P450s undergo proteolytic processing to expose mitochondrial targeting signals (in the N-terminal sequence). For instance, this process occurs with rat P450 1A1 with a cytosolic endoprotease [70, 78, 79]. As mentioned earlier, phosphorylation also plays a role in mitochondrial targeting of these microsomal P450s [68, 70]. As pointed out earlier, this mitochondrial trafficking is relevant as evidenced by the finding of 1–47% of P450 2D6 in the mitochondria of human livers, depending upon single nucleotide polymorphisms (SNPs) [68, 80].

2.4 Polymorphisms

In a very general sense, polymorphism refers to interindividual variations. In the most commonly used definition, it refers to genetic polymorphisms (i.e., not due to induction and other environmental effects). The most common genetic polymorphisms are SNPs (single base changes), although gene deletions and other complex variations are known.

Genetic polymorphisms are significant in experimental animals as well as humans. Particularly in outbred animals, polymorphisms may exist and give rise to strain variations (e.g., rat P450 2B1 [81]). These differences may be important in the selection of a species as a model in drug development, and lead to issues regarding the metabolism and toxicity of drugs and other chemicals. Mouse SNPs can be used in quantitative trait loci (QTLs) linkage studies to define genes relevant to certain diseases [82, 83].

Most of the work on polymorphisms has been done with human systems because of the recent interest in the human genome, personalized medicine, and so on. What is the significance of a SNP in a gene? The answer is that variation can yield a result. However, before proceeding further, it is important to note that *most* SNPs do not result in phenotyptic changes. The (positive) fraction has been estimated at around 10% [84].

How can a SNP alter the expression at catalytic function of a P450 (or other protein)? At least four mechanisms are relevant:

i) Nonsynonymous changes in the protein-coding region may lead to amino acid substitutions that alter the catalytic activity of a P450 (or do so indirectly by destabilizing the protein). An example is the *3 variant of human P450 2C9, where the I359L variation affects activity towards some substrates [85].

ii) A change in the coding region could affect the regulation of the gene, in terms of the DNA not being translated as efficiently (aside from introduction of a nonsense codon in the coding region). Although this possibility seems straightforward, there are few if any good examples reported yet.

iii) SNPs at splice sites can lead to poor intron processing of the initial RNA transcript and no mRNA. This is the major defect recognized for the "poor metabolizer" phenotypes for P450s 2D6 and 2C19 [86, 87].

iv) SNPs can also be responsible for gene duplication. The most prominent example is the *CYP2D6* gene, which has been found to have up to 13 copies of the gene [88]. In this case the levels of production of the mRNA and P450 2D6 protein are accordingly around 13-fold higher, leading to the "ultra-rapid metabolizer" phenotype. These individuals, as the name indicates, clear all P450 2D6 substrates much more rapidly than normal.

Research on human P450 polymorphisms really began in the 1970s with the studies of Smith *et al.* on debrisoquine metabolism [89], with concurrent work by Eichelbaum's group on sparteine [90] and the group of Lennard and Tucker on debrisoquine [91] leading to the same phenomenon. Today, more than 100 *CYP2D6* polymorphisms are known. P450 polymorphisms are compiled on the web site www.cypalleles.ki.se.

The ready access to published (and other) information on the web site greatly facilitates access to compilations of information about P450 polymorphisms. However, several points should be made:

i) The phenotypic effects of many of the changes have not been reported.

ii) When amino acid substitutions are the result of SNPs in the coding region, the phenotypic effect may be dependent upon the substrate and reaction. For instance, the *CYP2C9*3* genotype has been reported to attenuate the P450 2C9 oxidations of warfarin and tolbutamide, but not diclofenac [92–94].

iii) With P450s that are often regarded to be "not highly polymorphic" there are still polymorphisms and some may have important phenotypes. For instance, the *CYP3A4*20* is a frameshift that accordingly eliminates activity [95] and the *CYP3A4*17* allele (F189S) has variable phenotypes depending on the substrate [96]. Regarding P450 3A4, some human liver samples devoid of the enzyme are known in the literature [54, 97], although the genotypes have not been reported.

2.5 Protein Structure

Some crystals of bacterial P450 101A1 (P450$_{cam}$) had already been obtained in 1972 in Gunsalus' laboratory, but did not diffract, and the structure was reported in 1985 [14, 30]. The next reported P450 crystal structure was bacterial P450 102A1 in 1993 [98]. For many years after, the structural literature consisted of efforts to fit the primary sequences of mammalian P450s into the bacterial structures and predict substrate binding [99]. In 1999, Johnson's laboratory reported the crystallization and determination of a structure of a rabbit P450 2C5 derivative [31]. Since then, numerous human P450 structures have been solved (Table 2.2) – as well as many other mammalian and bacterial ones – most with ligands in place.

P450s are defined by the characteristic FXXGXXXCXG element, with the Cys acting as the axial ligand to the heme iron (thus the nitric oxide synthases are not considered P450s, even though they have an axial Cys ligand and show similar spectral properties). Most P450s, but not all (e.g., *Streptomyces coelicolor* P450 157C1 [125]) contain an EXXR sequence – the function of which is unknown. Among the characterized P450s (including the bacterial ones) there are 12 common helices (A–L) plus four β-sheet regions (Figure 2.4). Some P450s contain additional helices. The I- and L-helices make contact with the heme, and are relatively well conserved. In some cases the I-helix is bent (e.g., *Mycobacterium tuberculosis* P450 51A1) [126].

The N-terminal hydrophobic tail present in most of the eukaryotic P450s helps anchor these into the membrane. Evidence also exists for signal recognition particle and "halt/transfer" elements in the N-terminus to facilitate membrane insertion. In several cases it has been possible to delete much of the N-terminus in bacterial expression of mammalian P450s and retain functional activity. The general dogma is that interaction of P450s and NADPH-P450 reductase is enhanced in membranes because both proteins are inserted, but at higher protein concentrations the protein–protein interactions of these proteins are facilitated through a

Table 2.2 Structures of human P450s.

P450	References
1A2	[100]
1B1	[101]
2A6	[102, 103]
2A13	[104]
2B6	[105]
2C8	[106, 107]
2C9	[108, 109]
2C19	[110]
2D6	[101, 111]
2E1	[112, 113]
2R1	[114]
3A4	[115–117]
8A1	[118, 119]
19A1	[120]
24A1	[121]
46A1	[122, 123]
51A1	[124]

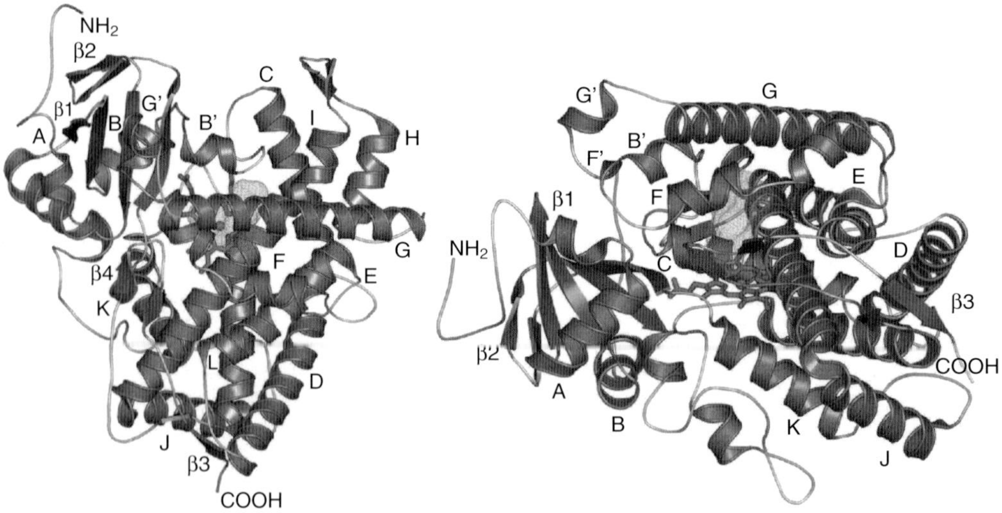

Figure 2.4 Crystal structure of human P450 1A2 (α-NF complex), showing two views [100].

mass action effect. Care is needed in comparing protein interactions in bacterial and mammalian enzymes, but there is evidence that some elements other than the N-terminal tail have roles in binding of P450s to membranes [127, 128].

In 1992, Gotoh defined six "substrate recognition sequences" (SRS regions) in P450s, based upon the crystal structure of bacterial P450 101A1 and alignments of mammalian family 2 P450 sequences [129]. This analysis has proven to be useful and is generally supported in the mammalian P450 crystal structures now available. However, the point has been made by Johnson that the "length" of each SRS region (and its predictability) varies among the P450s. In the P450s with large and more flexible active sites (e.g., P450 3A4) the SRS regions are less defined and predictable.

Most P450s contain a Thr residue in the I-helix (corresponding to Thr252 in bacterial P450 101A1). Originally, site-directed mutagenesis studies with P450 101A1 showed that this Thr is critical for proton donation to the $Fe^{2+} \cdot O_2^-$ complex (and for ultimate formation of FeO^{3+} and productive coupling) [130, 131]. The high pK_a of Thr is a problem with this explanation, however. Further, site-directed mutagenesis with the unnatural amino acid Thr-*O*-methyl ether yields a functional protein [132]. Also, several P450s do not contain this Thr [127]. A more current view is that the Thr residue is one of several ways of facilitating the protonation of the $Fe^{2+} \cdot O_2^-$ complex in P450s. The conserved Thr has also been postulated to play a more structural role (e.g., forming a "bubble" for O_2 binding in the I-helix).

The size of active sites varies considerably, from around 190 Å^3 in P450 2E1 [112] to 1385 Å^3 in P450 3A4 [116] and 1438 Å^3 in P450 2C8 [106] – at least a 7-fold range (Figure 2.5). Another issue is the shape of the active site. In P450s with small active sites this is less an issue, although our own group has shown that doing two conservative mutations with P450 2A6 (N297Q and I300V), without changing the M_r of the protein, can greatly expand the size of the active site, and allow new substrates and reactions [134]. P450s 2C8 and 3A4 have similar active site volumes (*vide supra*), but the shape of the former is more elongated and defined, limiting its access to many substrates that can be oxidized by P450 3A4.

Several P450 crystal structures have been reported with two ligands present, including human P450s 2C8 [107] and 3A4 [117], and bacterial P450s 107A1 [135]

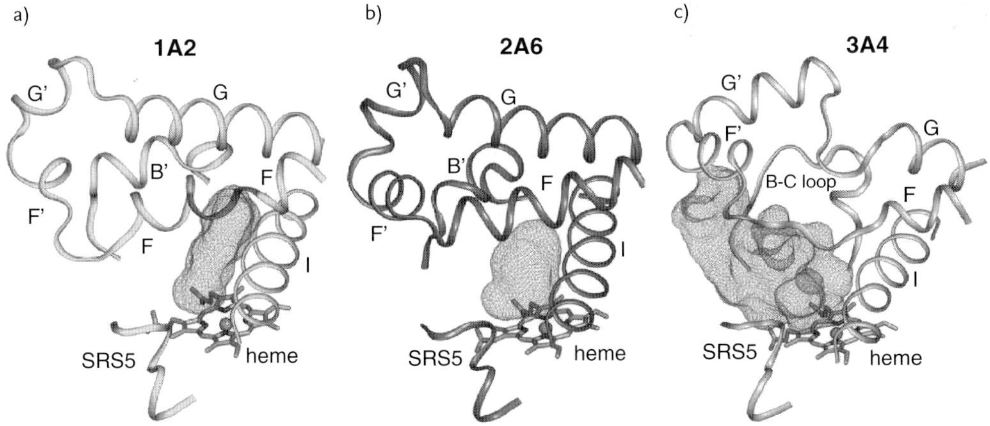

Figure 2.5 Crystal structures of some human P450s, showing the binding sites [128]. The calculated volumes of the active sites are listed for each. (a) P450 1A2 (375 Å^3) [100], (b) P450 2A6 (260 Å^3) [102, 133], and (c) P450 3A4 (1385 Å^3) [116].

and 158A2 [136]. In the case of P450 3A4, this behavior may be relevant to the cooperative behavior seen in some of the reactions.

Another issue regarding the P450 structures is the "malleability" or "plasticity" of the proteins [137]. The crystal structures of several of the P450s obtained to date have demonstrated structural changes upon binding of substrates, particularly the mammalian "xenobiotic-metabolizing" P450s (Table 2.1). Moreover, the protein backbones are varied in structures with different ligands (e.g., [117]). Thus, predicting the binding of another substrate for a P450 *de novo* is still not trivial, particularly with those with larger sites (e.g., P450 3A4). The flexibility of the active site has been linked with the I-helix; that is, in the more rigid P450s (e.g., P450 1A2, 2A6, and 2C8) the I-helix forms one side of the active site, but this is not the case with P450 3A4. However, even P450 2E1, with its small active site, is capable of new conformations to accommodate fatty acids [113].

In some cases the crystal structures of P450–substrate complexes are consistent with catalytic activity. However, this is not necessarily always the case – adding another level of complexity to the prediction of function. One example is the α-naphthoflavone–human P450 1A2 structure [100]. The only oxidation product of α-naphthoflavone is the 5,6-epoxide [138] and in the crystal structure this part of the molecule is furthest away from the heme iron. Thus, the structure does not represent a productive complex with this substrate. As discussed earlier, the catalytic efficiency of a P450 (or other enzyme) is the product of the on-rate times the probability of the encounter leading to a reaction yielding the product. The low catalytic efficiency of many P450 reactions may be attributed to the existence of multiple binding modes, with some unproductive ones being energetically favorable and competing for productive binding.

Some unusual aspects of P450 structures have been noted and are still under investigation. One is the "reverse" orientation of the heme in *S. coelicolor* P450 154A1 [139]. Another is an *S. coelicolor* P450 without the general EXXR sequence mode (*vide supra*) [125].

2.6
Catalytic Mechanisms

The oxidation of substrates involves two parts: (i) the activation of oxygen and (ii) the subsequent oxidation of the substrate. Most of the events shown in Figure 2.6 are involved in the former aspect.

Substrate binding (step **1**) is fast in many cases (i.e., nearly diffusion-limited). However, recent studies with several P450s indicate that the process is at least two-step and the latter stage, yielding a change in the iron d_5 orbital distribution from low-spin to high-spin, is relatively slow. This spin change is associated with the removal of the distal ligand to the iron, H_2O, and related to conformational changes in the protein known to be related to substrate binding (as discerned by crystallography). Not all P450 substrates yield the spin-state change, however [46, 140]. In some cases the binding of a substrate can lower the oxidation/reduction

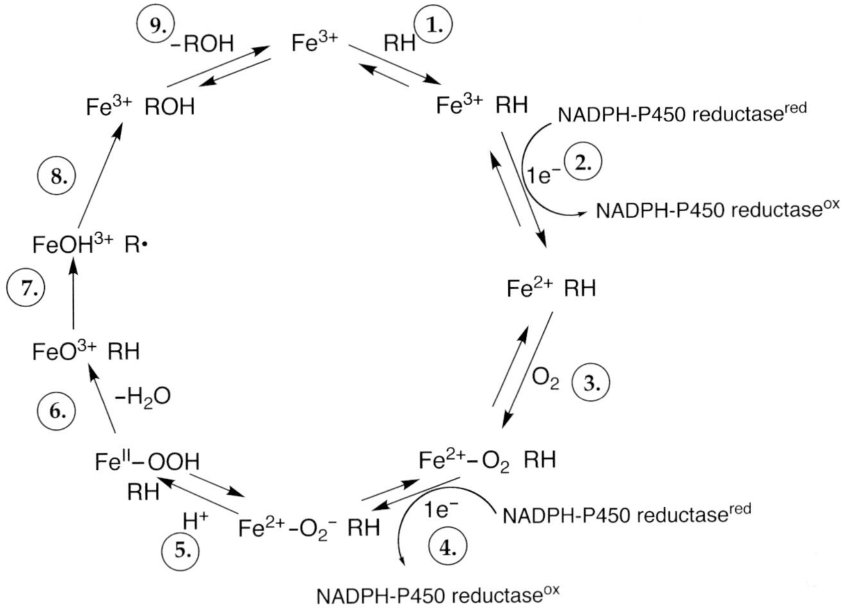

Figure 2.6 General mechanism of P450 catalysis.

potential ($E_{m,7}$) of a P450 [141, 142], making reduction more thermodynamically favorable, although this phenomenon is not universal [140, 143].

The next step is reduction by NADPH-P450 reductase (step **2**). The electronic possibilities of the diflavin reductase are complex [144]. Hydride ions from NADPH reduce the FAD component of the reductase and electrons pass on to the FMN. The consensus is that during catalytic turnover it is the three-electron reduced form of the reductase ($FMNH_2/FADH^{\cdot}$) that donates the electron to P450. With some P450s electron transfer to the P450 is slow in the absence of substrate and facilitated by substrate; some P450s are reduced rapidly with or without substrate [73, 145]. The concentration of NADPH-P450 reductase in rat liver is less than 10% of the total P450 and in some cases the rate of reduction is probably rate-limiting, at least in microsomal systems [146].

Ferrous P450 binds oxygen in step **3**, in a process that is probably limited only by the rate of diffusion of oxygen in the protein. This electronic state is formally identical to oxyhemoglobin, but is unstable at this state. The rates of decomposition (to $O_2^{-\cdot}$?) vary considerably and can also be influenced by the presence of substrate [147].

Step **4** (of Figure 2.6) involves the input of the "second" electron (from NADPH-P450 reductase) in the P450 FeO_2^{2+} complex, in a reaction competitive with decomposition. In some cases there is evidence that another microsomal protein, cytochrome b_5 (which is also reduced by NADPH-P450 reductase as well as NADH-b_5 reductase) can provide this electron [148, 149]. However, in other cases where

b_5 is stimulatory, the b_5 effects are probably more complex and may not involve electron transfer [149]. Rates of this step have not been measured in many cases [150].

The succeeding steps have not been analyzed in great detail because of their difficulty, and much of our insight has been gained from work with biomimetic models [151] and, to some extent, theoretical calculations [152]. The two-electron reduced P450–oxygen complex (FeO_2^-) is protonated, utilizing a proton network including a generally conserved Thr residue (*vide supra*). This network also facilitates the heterolytic scission of the peroxide bond.

The resulting entity is formally FeO^{3+}, with most evidence favoring an electronic distribution with Fe(IV) and the other positive charge distributed in the porphyrin ring. Almost all P450 oxidations can be rationalized in the context of reactions with this entity (Figure 2.7). For instance, in carbon hydroxylation the generally accepted mechanism involves abstraction of a hydrogen atom, creating an excipient $FeOH^{3+}$–carbon radical pair. "Oxygen rebound" involves homolytic scission of the Fe–O bond, with the hydroxyl radical added to the carbon radical to form the product. Reactions with low-potential heteroatoms are similar although there is strong evidence the initial reaction is one-electron abstraction followed by rearrangement and the oxygen transfer [155–158]. The oxidation of π-bonded systems has several possibilities. The general consensus is that a σ-complex (with a C–O bond) is formed and rearranges, and the possibility of initial electron transfer should still be considered. The σ-complex shown in Figure 2.7 can yield an epoxide, explain several heme adducts derived from olefins, and explain 1,2-migrations seen with unsaturated systems [159], including acetylenes [160].

Some alternatives have been presented to the above system. One is the existence of two spin-states of FeO^{3+}, with a high-spin form involved in some of the reactions, but a low-spin form explaining others [152]. According to the theory, the spin-state course of a P450 reaction will be dictated by a unique combination of interactions between each P450 and each substrate [152]. However, all considerations of these proposals are theoretical and definitive experiments to test these have not been developed.

Other alternative proposals involve the entities on the route to FeO^{3+} in Figure 2.6 (i.e., FeO_2^+ and FeO_2H^{2+}). These intermediates are termed peroxy ferric species. Arguments in favor of [161] and against [162] their involvement in carbon hydroxylations have been made. The most common applications of these peroxyferryl species have been made in cases involving oxidations of aldehydes, beginning with P450 19A1 (aromatase) [163, 164]. The mechanism can explain the conversion of an aldehyde to formic acid [163, 165], although FeO^{3+}-based mechanisms can be considered as alternatives [166]. A key tenet of the FeO_2^-/aldehyde mechanism (which is a modified Bayer–Villiger reaction) is the report of Akhtar *et al.* [163] that ^{18}O from O_2 is incorporated into formic acid, which was done with placental microsomes [163], but to the best of the author's knowledge has not been attempted with purified P450 19A1. Some other mechanisms have also been proposed, but have only limited support [167, 168].

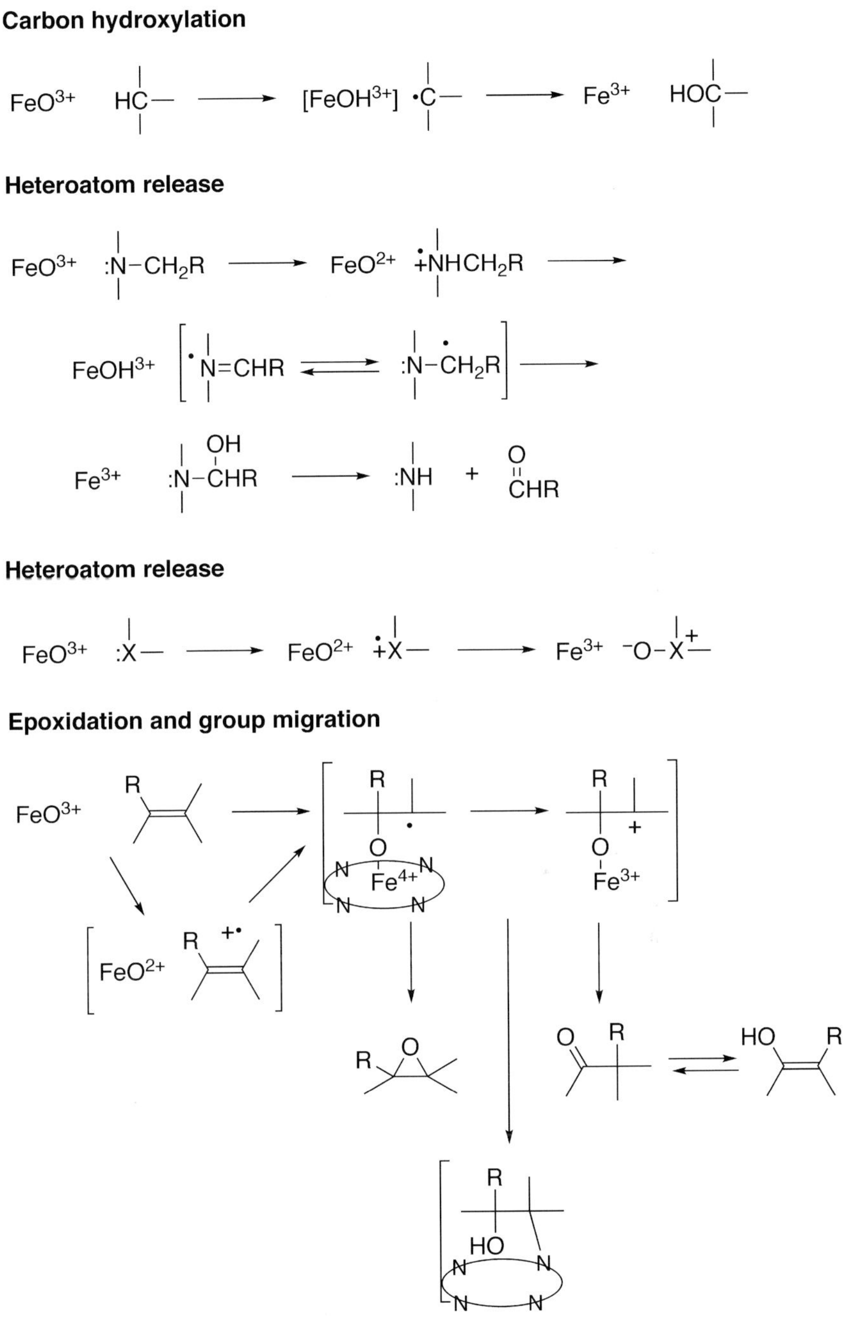

Figure 2.7 Various P450 oxidation reactions described with a unified chemical mechanism [153, 154].

The final step in the overall catalytic cycle (step **7** of Figure 2.6) is product release. Historically, this has been considered to be fast and experimental evidence has been obtained [169]. Given the similarity of P450 substrates and products, it is presumed that the path through the enzyme (and the residues that interact) is similar to the substrate entrance route. Although one can propose separate entrance (substrate) and egress/exit (product) routes, there is no experimental evidence that there are separate routes. In several cases in which rates have been measured, the rates of substrate and product leaving and rebinding to P450s are much faster than substrate oxidation [169].

However, there are some cases in which slow steps follow product formation. One is ethanol oxidation by P450 2E1, in which burst kinetics are observed [148, 170]. The first oxidation (ethanol to acetaldehyde) is part of a two-step sequence (followed by oxidation of acetaldehyde to acetic acid). In that case [170], and in the oxidation of dimethyl and diethyl nitrosamines to aldehydes and then carboxylic acids, pulse-chase experiments showed a lack of equilibration of the intermediate aldehyde with the medium (with P450 2A6 [171]). Thus, for some reason these aldehydes do not rapidly dissociate from these two P450s, although it appears not to be an issue of apparent affinity *per se* [170, 171]. Interestingly, pulse-chase studies with the human steroid aromatase (P450 19A1) showed equilibration of the intermediates (including the aldehyde) with the medium [73].

Finally, some mention should be made of kinetic deuterium isotope effects, particularly in light of the recent interest in using deuterated drugs to slow metabolism *in vivo* [172]. Kinetic isotope effects are complex and an extensive discussion of the subject is beyond the scope of this chapter [173]. A kinetic deuterium isotope effect is simply the ratio of the rate of a reaction with a substrate containing (for our purposes) a C–H bond compared to the rate with the same substrate containing a C–D bond. The intrinsic isotope effect is the isotope effect of the isolated rate constant for the bond-breaking step (i.e., step **6** in Figure 2.6). If this is the rate-limiting step in the cycle (the slowest one) then an isotope effect will be seen for the overall conversion of substrate to product. However, if C–H bond breaking is a fast step (not rate-limiting), then substituting deuterium (C–D) will have little effect on the rate of the overall conversion of substrate to product. This is the gist of the system, although analysis becomes more complex when also considering the contributions of rate constants of back reactions and rates of nonproductive breakdown of oxygenated complexes (e.g., FeO_2^{2+} to $O_2^{-\cdot}$ and H_2O_2) and the reduction of FeO^{3+} to yield H_2O [174]. The design of kinetic isotope effect experiments can produce various comparisons [145], but the most relevant here are studies that will estimate the intrinsic isotope effect (e.g., competition of two hydrogens at an archival site, with consideration of secondary isotope effects), and comparison of k_{cat} and K_m in separate reactions with substrates containing C–H and C–D bonds (noncompetitive intermolecular experiment). If the latter value (usually termed $^D[V/K]$) approximates the intrinsic isotope effect then the isotope effect is said to be fully expressed [175]. Observed isotope effects in P450 reactions vary from near unity to more than 15 [145, 176, 177]. In some cases high intrinsic isotope effects have been found, but they are attenuated in noncompetitive intermolecular experiments (e.g., testosterone 6β-hydroxylation by P450 3A4). The theoretical maximum deuterium isotope effect is about 7 [178], but higher values can be observed. Some are the result of nonclassical quantum mechanical tunneling, but clear evidence for a role of tunneling has been presented in P450 reactions.

2.7
What Determines P450 Catalytic Selectivity?

The question of catalytic selectivity is one that applies to all enzymes and there are some special considerations with P450s. It is clear that the classic Fischer view of a "lock-and-key" model of enzymes [179], still often promoted in introductory biochemistry courses due to its simplicity, is inadequate for explaining many enzymes today and certainly for predicting all P450 reactions. Thus, we must consider not only the "fit" of a substrate in an enzyme (i.e., as a ligand), but also additional events. The real question is how to determine the number of reactions possible with a given substrate and the rates of each (i.e., the rates of oxidation at each possible atom of the substrate). As with all enzymes, the catalytic efficiency k_{cat}/K_m (for each possible reaction) is the diffusion-limited on-rate (k_{on}) multiplied by the probability of that reaction occurring (which can be related to the transition state barrier) [178, 180].

In light of the growing availability of P450 crystal structures, some general points can be made about structure (*vide supra*) and substrate complementarity. The P450s are globular structures and the heme is clearly inside the protein in all structures. As the active oxidant is an Fe–O complex, a particular atom of the substrate must be within a few angstroms of the (Fe)O atom to be oxidized. In most cases seen to date, moving the substrate into a position for oxidation requires movement of the protein. Some of the "xenobiotic-metabolizing" P450s such as P450s 2A6 and 2E1 have relatively small active sites, which are rather rigid. Getting a substrate within the active site of P450 2A6 appears to require opening and closing, and the off-rate (k_{off}) has been estimated at $6\,s^{-1}$ for coumarin [169]. Thus, we have a picture of the P450 opening and closing 6 times/s. With other P450s such as 2C8 and 3A4, the active site is much larger (around 7-fold for P450s 2C8 and 3A4) [107, 116]. These P450s vary in their behavior, but with both it is difficult to predict binding modes because of the large space. With both of the latter two P450s there is some crystal evidence that at least two substrates can fit concurrently [107, 117]. Further, at least in the case of P450 3A4 there is evidence that at least some element of induced fit occurs. Crystal structures of P450 3A4 with different ligands show adaptation of amino acids to include different ligands [117]. Such behavior has even been reported for P450 2E1 [112, 113].

With several of the P450s (but not all [169]), there is evidence that multiple events occur to move the substrate from the periphery of the protein into the active site (i.e., near the Fe–O complex) [73, 146, 181–183]. This phenomenon may be related to some P450 3A4 structures with progesterone bound on the periphery [115]. In summary, we have a difficult time predicting where, on a substrate, a reaction will occur. An example is seen in the α-naphthoflavone–P450 1A2 crystal structure [100] where the only known site of oxidation is farthest away from the iron atom [183].

One of the issues, which needs to be considered with each reaction that has the potential to occur (within the confines of how close each atom of a potential substrate can get to the Fe–O complex), is what will limit the rate of the (putative) reaction. With P450s, there are three major possibilities for rate-limiting steps: (i) O_2 activation, (ii) Fe–O reaction, and (iii) competing rates of back reactions and nonproductive side-reactions, particularly the production of reduced oxygen species ($O_2^{\cdot-}$, H_2O_2, H_2O).

Although the literature discussion of rate-limiting steps in P450 reaction is over 40 years old, the work has often not been very systematic nor have all possibilities been fully considered. Structure–activity relationships can be useful (e.g., Hammett relationships [184]), but must be considered in the context that steric (or any) changes may change the juxtaposition of the substrates in the active site and influence the results. The experience in this laboratory is that kinetic deuterium isotope effects, when considered appropriately, can provide important information. With a number of human (and animal) P450s the observed kinetic deuterium isotope effects seen in noncompetitive intermolecular experiments [145, 175] are large, often greater than 10 [145, 169, 171, 185, 186]. When compared with estimates of the intrinsic kinetic deuterium isotope effects (${}^{D}k$), there is generally high expression of the isotope effects. Thus, the most straightforward conclusion is that the rate of C–H bond breaking is limiting. The result could be due to either poor geometry for C–H bond cleavage (hydrogen atom abstraction) or inherently weak abstraction potential due to some other reason.

One of the faster reactions of P450 3A4–testosterone hydroxylation (several sites)–showed an intrinsic kinetic isotope effect (greater than 15 for 6β-hydroxylation), but attenuated kinetic deuterium isotope effects [177], suggesting that another step of the reaction is rate-limiting. The fastest known reaction of a mammalian P450 is P450 7A1-mediated cholesterol 7α-hydroxylation [187]. Recent work in this laboratory has shown a k_{cat} of 180 min^{-1} and k_{cat}/K_m of 2.4×10^6 M^{-1} s^{-1} [146], with no observed kinetic isotope effect. Kinetic models indicate that even though the rate of first electron reduction is rapid (around 10 s^{-1} for fast phase), this is the most rate-limiting step. Thus, in comparing the fast and slow P450 reactions, a driving feature is the ease of substrate oxidation (with steric and chemical issues), but when the ease of this reaction is optimal then oxygen activation can become rate-limiting.

One point often neglected in the enzyme kinetics literature is consideration of the rates of back-reactions and abortive side-reactions, so that there is not a single rate-limiting step [188]. These considerations have previously been considered in the context of "commitment to catalysis" [175]. The P450 system has been known to waste NADPH in the partial reduction of O_2 since at least 1957 [189]. Coon's laboratory also demonstrated, by balance analysis, that H_2O was also produced [174, 190]. Thus, the overall rates of product formation can be considered in the context of competition with abortive O_2 reduction. The experience in this laboratory has been that the rates of abortive oxygen reduction are relatively similar among different (mammalian) P450s, at least when measured *in vitro*. (It is not clear that this is a dominant process *in vivo*, as judged by isoprostane measurements [191, 192].)

Thus, P450 reactions can be viewed as a competition between abortive oxygen reaction and oxidation of organic substrates by the activated oxygen complex. A better fit will improve complementarity and if the complementarity is great enough (e.g., P450 7A1) then the oxygen activation process will become rate-limiting.

Many P450 reactions are sequential–an initial product is oxidized again to yield a final product. One question has been how processive these reactions are–does the first product leave the enzyme and then rebind before being further oxidized (distributive) or does it remain on the enzyme throughout the sequence (processive)? In the cases of ethanol oxidation (to acetic acid) (P450 2E1), and dimethyl and diethyl nitrosamines (P450 2A6), there is evidence that a considerable fraction of the intermediate aldehyde does not leave the enzyme [170, 171]. Modeling studies also suggest the distributive nature of pyrene oxidation (to dihydroxypyrenes) by P450 1A2. The three-step conversion of androgens to estrogens by P450 19A1 was almost completely distributive [73], which might seem surprising compared with the more processive nature of the oxidation of ethanol and nitrosamines (*vide supra*). Exactly why the aldehydes do not leave the P450s (2A6, 2E1) is unclear, in that they were not found to have any inherently high intrinsic affinity [170, 171]. Exactly how processive several other P450 oxidations of steroids are is still unclear [193].

A final question in this section is whether it will be possible to predict P450 reactions, in light of recent information about P450 structures. The concerns about protein flexibility have already been mentioned. Nevertheless, a number of knowledge-based systems have been advanced, some commercially. For more discussions of the usefulness of these systems, see [194]. Systems based on either P450 structures or ease of oxidation at different atoms have value, as do algorithms based only on previous experience with similar compounds. The results indicate the difficulty of predicting the major site of oxidation, although the predictions rise considerably in picking only the top three sites. An experienced drug metabolism scientist could achieve a similar (or slightly better) record in the referenced analysis. As more information becomes available, the prospects for picking sites of oxidation may improve. However, predicting absolute rates *de novo* will continue to be difficult.

2.8 Oxidative Stress and P450s

As discussed above, the abortive breakdown of P450 intermediates generates $O_2^{-\cdot}$ and H_2O_2, which together can generate $HO^{\cdot}$ in the presence of transition metals. *In vitro* reactions are not well coupled and even under the best experimental conditions the coupling efficiency (ratio of product/NADPH consumed) is usually below

50% (i.e., most of the electrons are used to reduce O_2 to H_2O_2 and H_2O) [73, 169, 174]. This is not only the case with the "drug-metabolizing" P450s, but also those that use endogenous substrates, such as P450s 7A1 and 19A1 [73, 146]. The large degree of uncoupling is also seen in liver microsomes [195].

A plethora of literature is available about oxidative stress and much has been written about the contribution of the P450s to the overall burden. However, the overwhelming majority of this literature is with *in vitro* systems (subcellular preparations and cultured cells) and many of the *in vivo* (whole animal) studies have used unvalidated biomarkers of oxidative stress. Isoprostane formation is considered the most reliable marker of oxidative stress [196] and has been applied in studies designed to evaluate the effect of P450 induction on oxidative stress. In work with rats treated with classical P450 inducers, only phenobarbital elevated the level of liver or urinary isoprostanes [191]. The phenobarbital effect is considered to involve P450 induction because treatment of the rats with 1-aminobenztriazole blocked the increase [191]. Studies with transgenic mice yielded similar results, with the selective phenobarbital effect attributable in part to concurrent effects on pyridine nucleotide-dependent systems for protecting against reduced oxygen species [192].

These studies argue that P450s are not involved in large-scale production of reactive oxygen species *in vivo*, at least not in the absence of highly uncoupling substrates. Although P450 2E1 has been purported to be the most uncoupled P450, neither induction of P450 2E1 with isoniazid [191, 192] nor comparisons with transgenic P450 2e1$^{-/-}$ mice showed any changes in liver or urinary isoprostanes [192]. Collectively these studies argue against a role of P450s in inducing oxidative stress, in general, although the work cannot rule out localized action in specialized cells or organelles [197].

2.9
Relevance in Drug Metabolism and Clinical Medicine

Analyses with sets of drugs and drug candidates of two pharmaceutical companies both suggest that P450s are involved in around 75% of the enzymatic reactions in drug metabolism (Figure 2.8). Of these P450 reactions, most are oxidations and roughly 90% could be attributed to a set of five P450s (1A2, 2C9, 2C19, 2D6, and 3A4). Assignments of catalytic activities to individual P405s can be done with a battery of approaches [200], including (*in vitro*) inhibitors (Table 2.3) and diagnostic marker activities for correlation analyzes (Table 2.4).

The major clinical issues with P450s involve two aspects: (i) deficiencies in the P450s involved in the metabolism of endogenous compounds, especially steroids and fat-soluble vitamins (Table 2.1), and (ii) issues with the metabolism of drugs, including drug–drug interactions.

Issues involving metabolism of endogenous compounds have been discussed at more length elsewhere [39]. For instance, endocrine disorders have been associated with the absence of function of several P450s involved in steroid metabolism

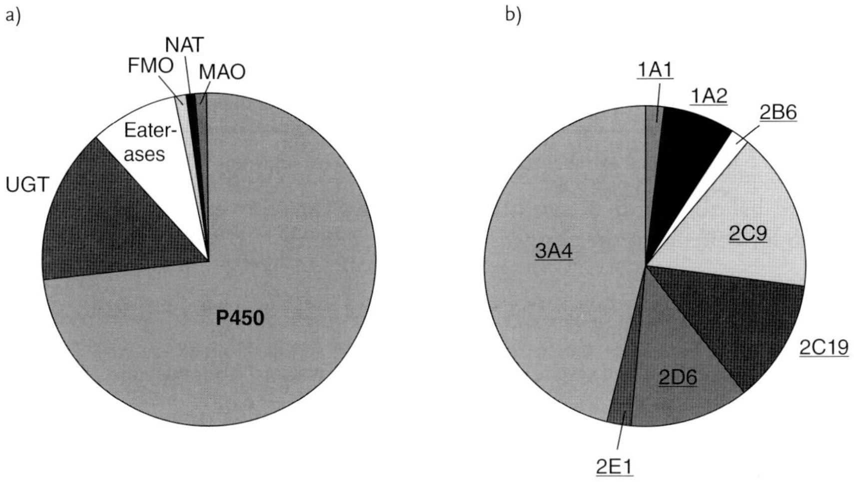

Figure 2.8 (a) Fractions of (metabolized) drugs that undergo biotransformation by individual enzyme systems. UGT, UDP-glucuronosyltransferase; FMO, flavin-containing monooxygenase; NAT, *N*-acetyltransferase; MAO, monoamine oxidase. (b) Contribution of individual P450s to biotransformation of drugs. The five major P450s involved in the metabolism of drugs in these two studies are underlined [198, 199].

Table 2.3 Useful selective inhibitors of human P450 enzymes (see also [201]).

P450 1A1	7,8-benzoflavone (but see [202] regarding P450 1A2)
	ellipticine
	1-(1-propynyl)pyrene
	2-(1-propynyl)phenanthrene
P450 1A2	7,8-benzoflavone
	furafylline
	fluvoxamine
P450 1B1	7,8-benzoflavone
	2-ethynylpyrene
P450 2A6	diethyldithiocarbamate (see [203])
P450 2C9	sulfaphenazole
	tienilic acid
P450 2D6	quinidine
P450 2E1	aminoacetonitrile
	4-methylpyrazole
	diethyldithiocarbamate (see [203])
P450 3A4	troleandomycin
	ketoconazole
	gestodene

the author's knowledge no defining clinical evidence has been presented yet with humans. *In vitro* studies suggest that this phenomenon is highly unpredictable [92] and, if it does occur *in vivo* with humans, could be rather problematic.

During the past 25 years there has been an explosion of knowledge regarding human P450s, and this has been used extensively in drug development and medical practice. In the period 1964–1985 the leading cause of attrition of drug candidates was poor human pharmacokinetic properties [221]. More recent estimates have reduced the issue to below 10% [222]. Some of the ways in which this knowledge is utilized include:

i) The knowledge base is utilized in early phases of both drug discovery and development. *In vitro* human P450 systems (microsomes, hepatocytes, and recombinant P450s) are used in conjunction with diagnostic inhibitors and marker assays (Tables 2.3 and 2.4). Compounds with very rapid rates of disappearance (low "metabolic stability") and strong inhibitors are generally removed from development early, as are those for which the metabolism is dependent primarily upon a single major (highly) polymorphic P450. Regarding inhibitors, it is also common to carefully analyze for mechanism-based inactivation ("time-dependent inhibition") before advancing compounds.

ii) Warning labels and contraindication statements can be developed on the basis of knowledge about P450s involved in the metabolism of a particular P450. For instance, the possibility exists that any P450 3A4 substrate will show an interaction with grapefruit juice.

iii) Doses to patients can be adjusted based on knowledge of P450s, plus information on response to other drugs, other concurrent medications, and even race.

iv) Side-effect problems with drugs can be treated in a more logical manner. For instance, if a patient has a problem with one drug cleared primarily due to P450 2D6 metabolism, prescribing another P450 2D6 substrate-drug might be discerned from knowledge about the drug history of a patient. The dose of a P450 3A4-metabolized drug can be adjusted lower if the prescribing physician is aware that a strong (P450 3A4) inducer is being used concurrently.

v) "Personalized medicine" is a concept that has been discussed for more than a decade. In principle, all of the knowledge presented above could be applied to individual patients if enough genetic information (or phenotypic results) were available. The broad application of such approaches has not occurred yet, although such knowledge now guides drug development programs. Further direct applications of genotyping and drug adjustment are most likely to occur in cases of cancer and life-threatening diseases, in which cost is less of an issue.

References

1 Mueller, G.C. and Miller, J.A. (1948) The metabolism of 4-dimethylaminoazobenzene by rat liver homogenates. *J. Biol. Chem.*, **176**, 535–544.

2 Mason, H.S. (1957) Mechanisms of oxygen metabolism. *Science*, **125**, 1185–1190.

3 Hayaishi, O. (ed.) (1974) *Molecular Mechanisms of Oxygen Activation*, Academic Press, New York.

4 Klingenberg, M. (1958) Pigments of rat liver microsomes. *Arch. Biochem. Biophys.*, **75**, 376–386.

5 Garfinkel, D. (1958) Studies on pig liver microsomes. I. Enzymic and pigment composition of different microsomal fractions. *Arch. Biochem. Biophys.*, **77**, 493–509.

6 Omura, T. and Sato, R. (1962) A new cytochrome in liver microsomes. *J. Biol. Chem.*, **237**, 1375–1376.

7 Guengerich, F.P. and Bartleson, C.J. (2007) Analysis and characterization of enzymes and nucleic acids, in *Principles and Methods of Toxicology*, 5th edn (ed. A.W. Hayes), CRC Press, Boca Raton, FL, pp. 1981–2048.

8 Cooper, D.Y., Levine, S., Narasimhulu, S., Rosenthal, O., and Estabrook, R.W. (1965) Photochemical action spectrum of the terminal oxidase of mixed function oxidase systems. *Science*, **147**, 400–402.

9 Conney, A.H., Miller, E.C., and Miller, J.A. (1956) The metabolism of methylated aminoazo dyes. V. Evidence for induction of enzyme synthesis in the rat by 3-methylcholanthrene. *Cancer Res.*, **16**, 450–459.

10 Richardson, H.L., Stier, A.R., and Borsos-Nachtnebel, E. (1952) Liver tumor inhibition and adrenal histologic responses in rats to which 3′-methyl-4-dimethylaminoazobenzene and 20-methylcholanthrene were simultaneously administered. *Cancer Res.*, **12**, 356–361.

11 Remmer, H. (1959) The acceleration of evipan oxidation and the demethylation of methylaminopyrine by barbiturates. *Naunyn Schmiedebergs Arch. Exp. Pathol. Pharmakol.*, **237**, 296–307.

12 Katagiri, M., Ganguli, B.N., and Gunsalus, I.C. (1968) A soluble cytochrome P-450 functional in methylene hydroxylation. *J. Biol. Chem.*, **243**, 3543–3546.

13 Tyson, C.A., Lipscomb, J.D., and Gunsalus, I.C. (1972) The roles of putidaredoxin and P-450_{cam} in methylene hydroxylation. *J. Biol. Chem.*, **247**, 5777–5784.

14 Poulos, T.L., Finzel, B.C., Gunsalus, I.C., Wagner, G.C., and Kraut, J. (1985) The 2.6-Å crystal structure of *Pseudomonas putida* cytochrome P-450. *J. Biol. Chem.*, **260**, 16122–16130.

15 Lu, A.Y.H. and Coon, M.J. (1968) Role of hemoprotein P-450 in fatty acid ω-hydroxylation in a soluble enzyme system from liver microsomes. *J. Biol. Chem.*, **243**, 1331–1332.

16 van der Hoeven, T.A., Haugen, D.A., and Coon, M.J. (1974) Cytochrome P-450 purified to apparent homogeneity from phenobarbital-induced rabbit liver microsomes: catalytic activity and other properties. *Biochem. Biophys. Res. Commun.*, **60**, 569–575.

17 Imai, Y. and Sato, R. (1974) A gel-electrophoretically homogeneous preparation of cytochrome P-450 from liver microsomes of phenobarbital-pretreated rabbits. *Biochem. Biophys. Res. Commun.*, **60**, 8–14.

18 Haugen, D.A., van der Hoeven, T.A., and Coon, M.J. (1975) Purified liver microsomal cytochrome P-450: separation and characterization of multiple forms. *J. Biol. Chem.*, **250**, 3567–3570.

19 Ryan, D., Lu, A.Y.H., West, S., and Levin, W. (1975) Multiple forms of cytochrome P-450 in phenobarbital- and 3-methylcholanthrene-treated rats. *J. Biol. Chem.*, **250**, 2157–2163.

20 Guengerich, F.P. (1978) Separation and purification of multiple forms of microsomal cytochrome P-450. Partial characterization of three apparently homogeneous cytochromes P-450

prepared from livers of phenobarbital- and 3-methylcholanthrene-treated rats. *J. Biol. Chem.*, **253**, 7931–7939.

21 Distlerath, L.M., Reilly, P.E.B., Martin, M.V., Davis, G.G., Wilkinson, G.R., and Guengerich, F.P. (1985) Purification and characterization of the human liver cytochromes P-450 involved in debrisoquine 4-hydroxylation and phenacetin *O*-deethylation, two prototypes for genetic polymorphism in oxidative drug metabolism. *J. Biol. Chem.*, **260**, 9057–9067.

22 Shimada, T., Misono, K.S., and Guengerich, F.P. (1986) Human liver microsomal cytochrome P-450 mephenytoin 4-hydroxylase, a prototype of genetic polymorphism in oxidative drug metabolism. Purification and characterization of two similar forms involved in the reaction. *J. Biol. Chem.*, **261**, 909–921.

23 Guengerich, F.P., Martin, M.V., Beaune, P.H., Kremers, P., Wolff, T., and Waxman, D.J. (1986) Characterization of rat and human liver microsomal cytochrome P-450 forms involved in nifedipine oxidation, a prototype for genetic polymorphism in oxidative drug metabolism. *J. Biol. Chem.*, **261**, 5051–5060.

24 Fujii-Kuriyama, Y., Mizukami, Y., Kawajiri, K., Sogawa, K., and Muramatsu, M. (1982) Primary structure of a cytochrome P-450: coding nucleotide sequence of phenobarbital-inducible cytochrome P-450 cDNA from rat liver. *Proc. Natl. Acad. Sci. USA*, **79**, 2793–2797.

25 Zuber, M.X., Simpson, E.R., and Waterman, M.R. (1986) Expression of bovine 17α-hydroxylase cytochrome P-450 cDNA in nonsteroidogenic (COS 1) cells. *Science*, **234**, 1258–1261.

26 Larson, J.R., Coon, M.J., and Porter, T.D. (1991) Alcohol-inducible cytochrome P-450IIE1 lacking the hydrophobic NH_2-terminal segment retains catalytic activity and is membrane-bound when expressed in *Escherichia coli*. *J. Biol. Chem.*, **266**, 7321–7324.

27 Barnes, H.J., Arlotto, M.P., and Waterman, M.R. (1991) Expression and enzymatic activity of recombinant cytochrome P450 17α-hydroxylase in *Escherichia coli*. *Proc. Natl. Acad. Sci. USA*, **88**, 5597–5601.

28 Groves, J.T., McClusky, G.A., White, R.E., and Coon, M.J. (1978) Aliphatic hydroxylation by highly purified liver microsomal cytochrome P-450: evidence for a carbon radical intermediate. *Biochem. Biophys. Res. Commun.*, **81**, 154–160.

29 Rittle, J. and Green, M.T. (2010) Cytochrome P450 compound I: capture, characterization, and C–H bond activation kinetics. *Science*, **330**, 933–937.

30 Poulos, T.L., Finzel, B.C., and Howard, A.J. (1987) High-resolution crystal structure of cytochrome $P450_{cam}$. *J. Mol. Biol.*, **195**, 687–700.

31 Williams, P.A., Cosme, J., Sridhar, V., Johnson, E.F., and MeRee, D.E. (2000) Mammalian microsomal cytochrome P450 monooxygenase: structural adaptations for membrane binding and functional diversity. *Mol. Cell*, **5**, 121–131.

32 Alveres, A.P., Schilling, G., Levin, W., and Kuntzman, R. (1967) Studies on the induction of CO-binding pigments in liver microsomes by phenobarbital and 3-methylcholanthrene. *Biochem. Biophys. Res. Commun.*, **29**, 521–526.

33 Guengerich, F.P., Dannan, G.A., Wright, S.T., Martin, M.V., and Kaminsky, L.S. (1982) Purification and characterization of liver microsomal cytochromes P-450: electrophoretic, spectral, catalytic, and immunochemical properties and inducibility of eight isozymes isolated from rats treated with phenobarbital or β-naphthoflavone. *Biochemistry*, **21**, 6019–6030.

34 Reeck, G.R., de Haën, C., Teller, D.C., Doolittle, R.F., Fitch, W.M., Dickerson, R.E., Chambon, P., McLachlan, A.D., Margoliash, E., Jukes, T.H., and Zuckerkandl, E. (1987) "Homology" in proteins and nucleic acids: a terminology muddle and a way out of it. *Cell*, **50**, 667.

35 Nebert, D.W., Adesnik, M., Coon, M.J., Estabrook, R.W., Gonzalez, F.J., Guengerich, F.P., Gunsalus, I.C.,

Johnson, E.F., Kemper, B., Levin, W., Phillips, I.R., Sato, R., and Waterman, M.R. (1987) The P450 gene superfamily: recommended nomenclature. *DNA*, **6**, 1–11.

36 Josephy, P.D., Guengerich, F.P., and Miners, J.O. (2005) Phase 1 and phase 2 drug metabolism: terminology that we should phase out. *Drug Metab. Rev.*, **37**, 579–584.

37 Turesky, R.J., Constable, A., Richoz, J., Vargu, N., Markovic, J., Martin, M.V., and Guengerich, F.P. (1998) Differences in activation of heterocyclic aromatic amines by rat and human liver microsomes and by rat and human cytochromes P450 1A2. *Chem. Res. Toxicol.*, **11**, 925–936.

38 Nelson, D.R., Zeldin, D.C., Hoffman, S.M., Maltais, L.J., Wain, H.M., and Nebert, D.W. (2004) Comparison of cytochrome P450 (CYP) genes from the mouse and human genomes, including nomenclature recommendations for genes, pseudogenes and alternative-splice variants. *Pharmacogenetics*, **14**, 1–18.

39 Nebert, D.W. and Russell, D.W. (2002) Clinical importance of the cytochromes P450. *Lancet*, **360**, 1155–1162.

40 Capdevila, J., Holla, V.R., and Falck, J.R. (2005) Cytochrome P450 and the metabolism and bioactivation of arachidonic acid and eicosanoids, in *Cytochrome P450: Structure, Mechanism, and Biochemistry*, 3rd edn (ed. P.R. Ortiz de Montellano), Kluwer/Plenum, New York, pp. 531–551.

41 Kikuta, Y., Kusunose, E., and Kusunose, M. (2002) Prostaglandin and leukotriene omega-hydroxylases. *Prostaglandins Other Lipid Mediat.*, **68–69**, 345–362.

42 Guengerich, F.P., Tang, Z., Cheng, Q., and Salamanca- Pinzón, S.G. (2011) Approaches to deorphanization of human and microbial cytochrome P450 enzymes. *Biochem. Biophys. Acta*, **1814**, 139–145.

43 Guengerich, F.P., Tang, Z., Salamanca- Pinzón, S.G., and Cheng, Q. (2010) Characterizing proteins of unknown function: orphan cytochrome P450s as a paradigm. *Mol. Interv.*, **10**, 153–163.

44 Shimada, T., Hayes, C.L., Yamazaki, H., Amin, S., Hecht, S.S., Guengerich, F.P., and Sutter, T.R. (1996) Activation of chemically diverse procarcinogens by human cytochrome P450 1B1. *Cancer Res.*, **56**, 2979–2984.

45 Niwa, T., Murayama, N., and Yamazaki, H. (2009) Oxidation of endobiotics mediated by xenobiotic-metabolizing forms of human cytochrome P450. *Curr. Drug Metab.*, **10**, 700–712.

46 Tang, Z., Martin, M.V., and Guengerich, F.P. (2009) Elucidation of functions of human cytochrome P450 enzymes: identification of endogenous substrates in tissue extracts by LC-MS metabolomics and isotopic labeling approaches. *Anal. Chem.*, **81**, 3071–3078.

47 Guengerich, F.P. (2010) Cytochrome P450 enzymes, in *Biotransformation*, 2nd edn (ed. F.P. Guengerich), Elsevier, Oxford, pp. 41–76.

48 Mimura, J., Ema, M., Sogawa, K., and Fujii-Kuriyama, Y. (1999) Identification of a novel mechanism of regulation of Ah (dioxin) receptor function. *Genes Dev.*, **13**, 20–25.

49 Swales, K., Kakizaki, S., Yamamoto, Y., Inoue, K., Kobayashi, K., and Negishi, M. (2005) Novel CAR-mediated mechanism for synergistic activation of two distinct elements within the human cytochrome P450 2B6 gene in HepG2 cells. *J. Biol. Chem.*, **280**, 3458–3466.

50 Tirona, R.G., Lee, W., Leake, B.F., Lan, L.B., Cline, C.B., Lamba, V., Parviz, F., Duncan, S.A., Inoue, Y., Gonzalez, F.J., Schuetz, E.G., and Kim, R.B. (2003) The orphan nuclear receptor HNF4α determines PXR- and CAR-mediated xenobiotic induction of CYP3A4. *Nat. Med.*, **9**, 220–224.

51 Lee, C. and Riddick, D.S. (2000) Transcriptional suppression of cytochrome P450 2C11 gene expression by 3-methycholanthrene. *Biochem. Pharmacol.*, **59**, 1417–1423.

52 Waxman, D.J., Dannan, G.A., and Guengerich, F.P. (1985) Regulation of rat hepatic cytochrome P-450: age-dependent expression, hormonal imprinting, and xenobiotic inducibility of sex-specific isoenzymes. *Biochemistry*, **24**, 4409–4417.

53 Waxman, D.J. and Holloway, M.G. (2009) Sex differences in the expression of hepatic drug metabolizing enzymes. *Mol. Pharmacol.*, **76**, 215–228.

54 Yang, X., Zhang, B., Molony, C., Chudin, E., Hao, K., Zhu, J., Gaedigk, A., Suver, C., Zhong, H., Leeder, J.S., Guengerich, F.P., Strom, S.C., Schuetz, E., Rushmore, T.H., Ulrich, R.G., Slatter, J.G., Schadt, E.E., Kasarskis, A., and Lum, P.Y. (2010) Genetic and genomic analysis of cytochrome P450 enzyme activities in human liver. *Genome Res.*, **20**, 1020–1036.

55 Eliasson, E., Johansson, I., and Ingelman-Sundberg, M. (1990) Substrate-, hormone-, and cAMP-regulated cytochrome P450 degradation. *Proc. Natl. Acad. Sci. USA*, **87**, 3225–3229.

56 Kim, H., Putt, D.A., Zanger, R.C., Wolf, C.R., Guengerich, F.P., Hollenberg, P.F., and Novak, R.F. (2001) Differential induction of rat hepatic cytochromes P450 3A1, 3A2, 2B1, 2B2, and 2E1 in response to pyridine treatment. *Drug Metab. Dispos.*, **29**, 353–360.

57 Tsuchiya, Y., Nakajima, M., Takagi, S., Taniya, T., and Yokoi, T. (2006) MicroRNA regulates the expression of human cytochrome P450 1B1. *Cancer Res.*, **66**, 9090–9098.

58 Mohri, T., Nakajima, M., Fukami, T., Takamiya, M., Aoki, Y., and Yokoi, T. (2010) Human CYP2E1 is regulated by miR-378. *Biochem. Pharmacol.*, **79**, 1045–1052.

59 Takagi, S., Nakajima, M., Mohri, T., and Yokoi, T. (2008) Post-transcriptional regulation of human pregnane X receptor by micro-RNA affects the expression of cytochrome P450 3A4. *J. Biol. Chem.*, **283**, 9674–9680.

60 Takagi, S., Nakajima, M., Kida, K., Yamaura, Y., Fukami, T., and Yokoi, T. (2010) MicroRNAs regulate human hepatocyte nuclear factor 4α, modulating the expression of metabolic enzymes and cell cycle. *J. Biol. Chem.*, **285**, 4415–4422.

61 Gomez, A. and Ingleman-Sundberg, M. (2009) Epigenetic and microRNA-dependent control of cytochrome P450 expression: a gap between DNA and protein. *Pharmacogenomics*, **10**, 1067–1076.

62 Beedanagari, S.R., Taylor, R.T., Bui, P., Wang, F., Nickerson, D.W., and Hankinson, O. (2010) Role of epigenetic mechanisms in differential regulation of the dioxin-inducible human CYP1A1 and CYP1B1 genes. *Mol. Pharmacol.*, **78**, 608–616.

63 Yamazaki, H., Shimada, T., Martin, M.V., and Guengerich, F.P. (2001) Stimulation of cytochrome P450 reactions by apo-cytochrome b_5. Evidence against transfer of heme from cytochrome P450 3A4 to apo-cytochrome b_5 or heme oxygenase. *J. Biol. Chem.*, **276**, 30885–30891.

64 Drummond, G.S. and Kappas, A. (1982) The cytochrome P-450-depleted animal: an experimental model for *in vivo* studies in chemical biology. *Proc. Natl. Acad. Sci. USA*, **79**, 2384–2388.

65 Ortiz de Montellano, P.R. and Correia, M.A. (1983) Suicidal destruction of cytochrome P-450 during oxidative drug metabolism. *Annu. Rev. Pharmacol. Toxicol.*, **23**, 481–503.

66 Freeman, J.E. and Wolf, C.R. (1994) Evidence against a role for serine 129 in determining murine cytochrome p450 Cyp2e-1 protein levels. *Biochemistry*, **33**, 13963–13966.

67 Robin, M.A., Anandatheerthavarada, H.K., Biswas, G., Sepuri, N.B., Gordon, D.M., Pain, D., and Avadhani, N.G. (2002) Bimodal targeting of microsomal CYP2E1 to mitochondria through activation of an N-terminal chimeric signal by cAMP-mediated phosphorylation. *J. Biol. Chem.*, **277**, 40583–40593.

68 Sangar, M.C., Anandatheerthavarada, H.K., Prabu, S.K., Martin, M.V., Guengerich, F.P., and Aradhani, N.G. (2009) Identification of genetic variants of human cytochrome P450 2D6 with impaired mitochondrial targeting. *Mol. Genet. Metab.*, **99**, 90–97.

69 Oesch-Bartlomowicz, B., Richter, B., Becker, R., Vogel, S., Padma, P.R., Hengstler, J.G., and Oesch, F. (2001) cAMP-dependent phosphorylation of CYP2B1 as a functional switch for cyclophosphamide activation and its

hormonal control *in vitro* and *in vivo*. *Int. J. Cancer*, **94**, 733–742.

70 Anandatheerthavarada, H.K., Vijayasarathy, C., Bhagwat, S.V., Miswas, G., Mullick, J., and Avadhani, N.G. (1999) Physiological role of the N-terminal processed P4501A1 targeted to mitochondria in erythromycin metabolism and reversal of erythromycin-mediated inhibition of mitochondrial protein synthesis. *J. Biol. Chem.*, **274**, 6617–6625.

71 Shimozawa, O., Sakaguchi, M., Ogawa, H., Harada, N., Mihara, K., and Omura, T. (1993) Core glycosylation of cytochrome P-450$_{arom}$: evidence for localization of N terminus of microsomal cytochrome P-450 in the lumen. *J. Biol. Chem.*, **268**, 21399–21402.

72 Kagawa, N., Cao, Q., and Kusano, K. (2003) Expression of human aromatase (CYP19) in *Escherichia coli* by N-terminal replacement and induction of cold stress response. *Steroids*, **68**, 205–209.

73 Sohl, C.D. and Guengerich, F.P. (2010) Kinetic analysis of the three-step steroid aromatse reaction of human cytochrome P450 19A1. *J. Biol. Chem.*, **285**, 17734–17743.

74 Armstrong, R.N., Pinto-Coelho, C., Ryan, D.E., Thomas, P.E., and Levin, W. (1983) On the glycosylation state of five rat hepatic microsomal cytochrome P-450 isozymes. *J. Biol. Chem.*, **258**, 2106–2108.

75 Correia, M.A., Sadeghi, S., and Mundo-Paredes, E. (2005) Cytochrome P450 ubiquitination: branding for the proteolytic slaughter? *Annu. Rev. Pharmacol. Toxicol.*, **45**, 439–464.

76 Kim, S.M., Acharya, P., Engel, J.C., and Correia, M.A. (2010) Liver cytochrome P450 3A ubiquitination *in vivo* by GP78/autocrine motility factor receptor (AMFR) and C-terminus of HSP70-interacting protein (CHIP) E3 ubiquitin ligases: physiological and pharmacological relevance. *J. Biol. Chem.*, **285**, 35866–35877.

77 Wang, Y., Liao, M., Hoe, N., Acharya, P., Deng, C., Krutchinsky, A.N., and Correia, M.A. (2009) A role for protein phosphorylation in cytochrome P450 3A4 ubiquitin-dependent proteasomal degradation. *J. Biol. Chem.*, **284**, 5671–5684.

78 Addya, S., Anandatheerthavarada, H.K., Biswas, G., Bhagwat, S.V., Mullick, J., and Avadhani, N.G. (1997) Targeting of NH_2-terminal-processed microsomal protein to mitochondria: a novel pathway for the biogensis of hepatic mitochondrial P450$_{MT2}$. *J. Cell Biol.*, **139**, 589–599.

79 Bhagwat, S.V., Biswas, G., Anandatheerthavarada, H.K., Addya, S., Pandak, W., and Avadhani, N.G. (1999) Dual targeting property of the N-terminal signal sequence of P4501A1. Targeting of heterologous proteins to endoplasmic reticulum and mitochondria. *J. Biol. Chem.*, **274**, 24014–24022.

80 Sangar, M.C., Anandatheerthavarada, H.K., Tang, W., Prabu, S.K., Martin, M.V., Dostalek, M., Guengerich, F.P., and Avadhani, N.G. (2009) Targeting of human cytochrome P450 2D6 to the mitochondrial compartment: identification of genetic variants with impaired mitochondrial targeting. *FEBS J.*, **276**, 3440–3453.

81 Kedzie, K.M., Balfour, C.A., Escobar, G.Y., Grimm, S.W., He, Y., Pepperl, D.J., Regan, J.W., Stevens, J.C., and Halpert, J.R. (1991) Molecular basis for a functionally unique cytochrome P450IIB1 variant. *J. Biol. Chem.*, **266**, 22515–22521.

82 Chesler, E.J., Rodriguez-Zas, S.L., and Mogil, J.S. (2001) *In silico* mapping of mouse quantitative trait loci. *Science*, **294**, 2423.

83 Churchill, G.A., Airey, D.C., Allayee, H., Angel, J.M., Attie, A.D., Beatty, J., Beavis, W.D., Belknap, J.K., Bennett, B., Berrettini, W., Bleich, A., Bogue, M., Broman, K.W., Buck, K.J., Buckler, E., Burmeister, M., Chesler, E.J., Cheverud, J.M., Clapcote, S., Cook, M.N., Cox, R.D., Crabbe, J.C., Crusio, W.E., Darvasi, A., Deschepper, C.F., Doerge, R.W., Farber, C.R., Forejt, J., Gaile, D., Garlow, S.J., Geiger, H., Gershenfeld, H., Gordon, T., Gu, J., Gu, W., de Haan, G., Hayes, N.L., Heller, C., Himmelbauer, H., Hitzemann, R., Hunter, K., Hsu, H.C., Iraqi, F.A.,

Ivandic, B., Jacob, H.J., Jansen, R.C., Jepsen, K.J., Johnson, D.K., Johnson, T.E., Kempermann, G., Kendziorski, C., Kotb, M., Kooy, R.F., Llamas, B., Lammert, F., Lassalle, J.M., Lowenstein, P.R., Lu, L., Lusis, A., Manly, K.F., Marcucio, R., Matthews, D., Medrano, J.F., Miller, D.R., Mittleman, G., Mock, B.A., Mogil, J.S., Montagutelli, X., Morahan, G., Morris, D.G., Mott, R., Nadeau, J.H., Nagase, H., Nowakowski, R.S., O'Hara, B.F., Osadchuk, A.V., Page, G.P., Paigen, B., Paigen, K., Palmer, A.A., Pan, H.J., Peltonen-Palotie, L., Peirce, J., Pomp, D., Pravenec, M., Prows, D.R., Qi, Z., Reeves, R.H., Roder, J., Rosen, G.D., Schadt, E.E., Schalkwyk, L.C., Seltzer, Z., Shimomura, K., Shou, S., Sillanpaa, M.J., Siracusa, L.D., Snoeck, H.W., Spearow, J.L., Svenson, K., Tarantino, L.M., Threadgill, D., Toth, L.A., Valdar, W., de Villena, F.P., Warden, C., Whatley, S., Williams, R.W., Wiltshire, T., Yi, N., Zhang, D., Zhang, M., and Zou, F. (2004) The Collaborative Cross, a community resource for the genetic analysis of complex traits. *Nat. Genet.*, **36**, 1133–1137.

84 Shen, M.R., Jones, I.M., and Mohrenweiser, H. (1998) Nonconservative amino acid substitution variants exist at polymorphic frequency in DNA repair genes in healthy humans. *Cancer Res.*, **58**, 604–608.

85 Lee, C.R., Goldstein, J.A., and Pieper, J.A. (2002) Cytochrome P450 2C9 polymorphisms: a comprehensive review of the in-vitro and human data. *Pharmacogenetics*, **12**, 251–263.

86 Gonzalez, F.J., Skoda, R.C., Kimura, S., Umeno, M., Zanger, U.M., Nebert, D.W., Gelboin, H.V., Hardwick, J.P., and Meyer, U.A. (1988) Characterization of the common genetic defect in humans deficient in debrisoquine metabolism. *Nature*, **331**, 442–446.

87 de Morais, S.M.F., Wilkinson, G.R., Blaisdell, J., Nakamura, K., Meyer, U.A., and Goldstein, J.A. (1994) The major genetic defect responsible for the polymorphism of *S*-mephenytoin metabolism in humans. *J. Biol. Chem.*, **269**, 15419–15422.

88 Johansson, I., Lundqvist, E., Bertilsson, L., Dahl, M.L., Sjoqvist, F., and Ingelman-Sundberg, M. (1993) Inherited amplification of an active gene in the cytochrome P450 *CYP2D* locus as a cause of ultrarapid metabolism of debrisoquine. *Proc. Natl. Acad. Sci. USA*, **90**, 11825–11829.

89 Mahgoub, A., Idle, J.R., Dring, L.G., Lancaster, R., and Smith, R.L. (1977) Polymorphic hydroxylation of debrisoquine in man. *Lancet*, **ii**, 584–586.

90 Eichelbaum, M., Spannbrucker, N., and Dengler, H.J. (1979) Influence of the defective metabolism of sparteine on its pharmacokinetics. *Eur. J. Clin. Pharmacol.*, **16**, 189–194.

91 Tucker, G.T., Silas, J.H., Iyun, A.O., Lennard, M.S., and Smith, A.J. (1977) Polymorphic hydroxylation of debrisoquine. *Lancet*, **ii**, 718.

92 Guengerich, F.P. (2005) Human cytochrome P450 enzymes, in *Cytochrome P450: Structure, Mechanism, and Biochemistry*, 3rd edn (ed. P.R. Ortiz de Montellano), Kluwer /Plenum, New York, pp. 377–530.

93 Takanashi, K., Tainaka, H., Kobayashi, K., Yasumori, T., Hosakawa, M., and Chiba, K. (2000) CYP2C9 Ile^{359} and Leu^{359} variants: enzyme kinetic study with seven substrates. *Pharmacogenetics*, **10**, 95–104.

94 Yasar, U., Eliasson, E., Forslund-Bergengren, C., Tybring, G., Gadd, M., Sjoqvist, F., and Dahl, M.L. (2001) The role of CYP2C9 genotype in the metabolism of diclofenac *in vivo* and *in vitro*. *Eur. J. Clin. Pharmacol.*, **57**, 729–735.

95 Westlind-Johnsson, A., Hermann, R., Huennemeyer, A., Hauns, B., Lahu, G., Nassr, N., Zech, K., Ingelman-Sundberg, M., and von Richter, O. (2006) Identification and characterization of CYP3A4*20, a novel rare CYP3A4 allele without functional activity. *Clin. Pharmacol. Ther.*, **79**, 339–349.

96 Dai, D., Tang, J., Rose, R., Hodgson, E., Bienstock, R.J., Mohrenweiser, H.W., and Goldstein, J.A. (2001) Identification of variants of CYP3A4 and characterization of their abilities to

metabolize testosterone and chlorpyrifos. *J. Pharmacol. Exp. Ther.*, **299**, 825–831.

97 Guengerich, F.P. and Turvy, C.G. (1991) Comparison of levels of several human microsomal cytochrome P-450 enzymes and epoxide hydrolase in normal and disease states using immunochemical analysis of surgical liver samples. *J. Pharmacol. Exp. Ther.*, **256**, 1189–1194.

98 Ravichandran, K.G., Boddupalli, S.S., Hasemann, C.A., Peterson, J.A., and Deisenhofer, J. (1993) Crystal structure of hemoprotein domain of P450 BM-3, a prototype for microsomal P450's. *Science*, **261**, 731–736.

99 Lewis, D.F.V., Lake, B.G., George, S.G., Dickins, M., Eddershaw, P.J., Tarbit, M.H., Beresford, A.P., Goldfarb, P.S., and Guengerich, F.P. (1999) Molecular modeling of CYP family enzymes CYP1A1, CYP1A2, CYP1A6, and CYP1B1 based on sequence homology with CYP102. *Toxicology*, **139**, 53–79.

100 Sansen, S., Yano, J.K., Reynald, R.L., Schoch, G.A., Griffin, K.J., Stout, C.D., and Johnson, E.F. (2007) Adaptations for the oxidation of polycyclic aromatic hydrocarbons exhibited by the structure of human P450 1A2. *J. Biol. Chem.*, **282**, 14348–14355.

101 Johnson, E.F., Wang, A., Savas, U., and Stout, C.D. (2010) Analysis of P450 structure–function relations in drug metabolism using x-ray crystallography. *Ninth Meeting of the International Society for the Study Xenobiotics, Istanbul*, abstract S10.

102 Yano, J.K., Hsu, M.H., Griffin, K.J., Stout, C.D., and Johnson, E.F. (2005) Structures of human microsomal cytochrome P450 2A6 complexed with coumarin and methoxsalen. *Nat. Struct. Mol. Biol.*, **12**, 822–823.

103 Yano, J.K., Denton, T.T., Cerny, M.A., Zhang, X., Johnson, E.F., and Cashman, J.R. (2006) Synthetic inhibitors of cytochrome P-450 2A6: inhibitory activity, difference spectra, mechanism of inhibition, and protein cocrystallization. *J. Med. Chem.*, **49**, 6987–7001.

104 Smith, B.D., Sanders, J.L., Porubsky, P.R., Lushington, G.H., Stout, C.D., and Scott, E.E. (2007) Structure of the human lung cytochrome P450 2A13. *J. Biol. Chem.*, **282**, 17306–17313.

105 Gay, S.C., Shah, M.B., Talakad, J.C., Maekawa, K., Roberts, A.G., Wilderman, P.R., Sun, L., Yang, J.Y., Huelga, S.C., Hong, W.X., Zhang, Q., Stout, C.D., and Halpert, J.R. (2010) Crystal structure of a cytochrome P450 2B6 genetic variant in complex with the inhibitor 4-(4-chlorophenyl)imidazole at 2.0-A resolution. *Mol. Pharmacol.*, **77**, 529–538.

106 Schoch, G.A., Yano, J.K., Wester, M.R., Griffin, K.J., Stout, C.D., and Johnson, E.F. (2004) Structure of human microsomal cytochrome P450 2C8: evidence for a peripheral fatty acid binding site. *J. Biol. Chem.*, **279**, 9497–9503.

107 Schoch, G.A., Yano, J.K., Sansen, S., Dansette, P.M., Stout, C.D., and Johnson, E.F. (2008) Determinants of cytochrome P450 2C8 substrate binding: structures of complexes with montelukast, troglitazone, felodipine, and 9-*cis*-retinoic acid. *J. Biol. Chem.*, **283**, 17227–17237.

108 Wester, M.R., Yano, J.K., Schoch, G.A., Yang, C., Griffin, K.J., Stout, C.D., and Johnson, E.F. (2004) The structure of human cytochrome P450 2C9 complexed with flurbiprofen at 2.0-Å resolution. *J. Biol. Chem.*, **279**, 35630–35637.

109 Williams, P.A., Cosme, J., Ward, A., Angove, H.C., Matak Vinkovic, D., and Jhoti, H. (2003) Crystal structure of human cytochrome P450 2C9 with bound warfarin. *Nature*, **424**, 464–468.

110 Johnson, E.F., Sansen, S., Reynald, R.L., and Stout, C.D. (2008) X-ray crystallography as a tool for understanding P40 2C structure-function relationships. *17th International Symposium on Microsomes and Drug Oxidations, Saratoga Springs, NY.*

111 Rowland, P., Blaney, F.E., Smyth, M.G., Jones, J.J., Leydon, V.R., Oxbrow, A.K., Lewis, C.J., Tennant, M.G., Modi, S., Eggleston, D.S., Chenery, R.J., and Bridges, A.M. (2006) Crystal structure of

human cytochrome P450 2D6. *J. Biol. Chem.*, **281**, 7614–7622.

112 Porubsky, P.R., Meneely, K.M., and Scott, E.E. (2008) Structures of human cytochrome P-450 2E1. Insights into the binding of inhibitors and both small molecular weight and fatty acid substrates. *J. Biol. Chem.*, **283**, 33698–33707.

113 Porubsky, P.R., Battaile, K.P., and Scott, E.E. (2010) Human cytochrome P450 2E1 structures with fatty acid analogs reveal a previously unobserved binding mode. *J. Biol. Chem.*, **285**, 22282–22290.

114 Strushkevich, N.V., Min, J., Jones, G., Plotnikov, A., Usanov, S., and Park, H.-W. (2007) Structure of CYP2R1 in complex with vitamin D_3. *15th International Conference on Cytochromes P450: Biochemistry, Biophysics, Functional Genomics, Bled.*

115 Williams, P.A., Cosme, J., Vinkovic, D.M., Ward, A., Angove, H.C., Day, P.J., Vonrhein, C., Tickle, I.J., and Jhoti, H. (2004) Crystal structures of human cytochrome P450 3A4 bound to metyrapone and progesterone. *Science*, **305**, 683–686.

116 Yano, J.K., Wester, M.R., Schoch, G.A., Griffin, K.J., Stout, C.D., and Johnson, E.F. (2004) The structure of human microsomal cytochrome P450 3A4 determined by X-ray crystallography to 2.05 Å resolution. *J. Biol. Chem.*, **279**, 38091–38094.

117 Ekroos, M. and Sjogren, T. (2006) Structural basis for ligand promiscuity in cytochrome P450 3A4. *Proc. Natl. Acad. Sci. USA*, **103**, 13682–13687.

118 Chiang, C.W., Yeh, H.C., Wang, L.H., and Chan, N.L. (2006) Crystal structure of the human prostacyclin synthase. *J. Mol. Biol.*, **364**, 266–274.

119 Li, Y.C., Chiang, C.W., Yeh, H.C., Hsu, P.Y., Whitby, F.G., Wang, L.H., and Chan, N.L. (2008) Structures of prostacyclin synthase and its complexes with substrate analog and inhibitor reveal a ligand-specific heme conformation change. *J. Biol. Chem.*, **283**, 2917–2926.

120 Ghosh, D., Griswold, J., Erman, M., and Pangborn, W. (2009) Structural basis for androgen specificity and oestrogen synthesis in human aromatase. *Nature*, **457**, 219–223.

121 Annalora, A.J., Goodin, D.B., Hong, W.X., Zhang, Q., Johnson, E.F., and Stout, C.D. (2010) Crystal structure of CYP24A1, a mitochondrial cytochrome P450 involved in vitamin D metabolism. *J. Mol. Biol.*, **396**, 441–451.

122 Mast, N., White, M.A., Bjorkhem, I., Johnson, E.F., Stout, C.D., and Pikuleva, I.A. (2008) Crystal structures of substrate-bound and substrate-free cytochrome P450 46A1, the principal cholesterol hydroxylase in the brain. *Proc. Natl. Acad. Sci. USA*, **105**, 9546–9551.

123 Mast, N., Charvet, C., Pikuleva, I.A., and Stout, C.D. (2010) Structural basis of drug binding to CYP46A1, an enzyme that controls cholesterol turnover in the brain. *J. Biol. Chem.*, **285**, 31783–31795.

124 Strushkevich, N., Usanov, S., and Park, H.-W. (2009) Crystal structure of human lanosteroal 14α-demethylase (CYP51) in complex with ketoconazole. *16th International Conference on Cytochrome P450: Biochemistry, Biophysics, Biotechnology, Nago*, abstract P-33.

125 Rupasinghe, S., Schuler, M.A., Kagawa, N., Yuan, H., Lei, L., Zhao, B., Kelly, S.L., Waterman, M.R., and Lamb, D.C. (2006) The cytochrome P450 gene family CYP157 does not contain EXXR in the K-helix reducing the absolute conserved P450 residues to a single cysteine. *FEBS Lett.*, **580**, 6338–6342.

126 Podust, L.M., Poulos, T.L., and Waterman, M.R. (2001) Crystal structure of cytochrome P450 14α-sterol demethylase (CYP51) from *Mycobacterium tuberculosis* in complex with azole inhibitors. *Proc. Natl. Acad. Sci. USA*, **98**, 3068–3073.

127 Hasemann, C.A., Kurumbail, R.G., Boddupalli, S.S., Peterson, J.A., and Deisenhofer, J. (1995) Structure and function of cytochromes P450: a comparative analysis of three crystal structures. *Structure*, **2**, 41–62.

128 Poulos, T.L., and Johnson, E.F. (2005) Structures of cytochrome P450 enzymes, in *Cytochrome P450: Structure, Mechanism, and Biochemistry*, 3rd edn

(ed. P.R. Ortiz de Montellano), Kluwer / Plenum, New York, pp. 87–114.

129 Gotoh, O. (1992) Substrate recognition sites in cytochrome P450 family 2 (CYP2) proteins inferred from comparative analysis of amino acid and coding nucleotide sequences. *J. Biol. Chem.*, **267**, 83–90.

130 Imai, M., Shimada, H., Watanabe, Y., Matsushima-Hibiya, Y., Makino, R., Koga, H., Horiuchi, T., and Ishimura, Y. (1989) Uncoupling of the cytochrome P-450_{cam} monooxygenase reaction by a single mutation, threonine-252 to alanine or valine: a possible role of the hydroxy amino acid in oxygen activation. *Proc. Natl. Acad. Sci. USA*, **86**, 7823–7827.

131 Martinis, S.A., Atkins, W.M., Stayton, P.S., and Sligar, S.G. (1989) A conserved residue of cytochrome P-450 is involved in heme-oxygen stability and activation. *J. Am. Chem. Soc.*, **111**, 9252–9253.

132 Kimata, Y., Shimada, H., Hirose, T., and Ishimura, Y. (1995) Role of Thr-252 in cytochrome $P450_{CAM}$: a study with unnatural amino acid mutagenesis. *Biochem. Biophys. Res. Commun.*, **208**, 96–102.

133 Sansen, S., Hsu, M.H., Stout, C.D., and Johnson, E.F. (2007) Structural insight into the altered substrate specificity of human cytochrome P450 2A6 mutants. *Arch. Biochem. Biophys.*, **464**, 197–206.

134 Wu, Z., Podust, L.M., and Guengerich, F.P. (2005) Expansion of substrate specificity of cytochrome P450 2A6 by mutagenesis. *J. Biol. Chem.*, **280**, 41090–41100.

135 Cupp-Vickery, J., Anderson, R., and Hatziris, Z. (2000) Crystal structures of ligand complexes of $P450_{eryF}$ exhibiting homotropic cooperativity. *Proc. Natl. Acad. Sci. USA*, **97**, 3050–3055.

136 Zhao, B., Guengerich, F.P., Bellamine, A., Lamb, D.C., Izumikawa, M., Funa, N., Lei, L., Podust, L.M., Sundamoorthy, M., Reddy, L.M., Kelly, S.L., Stec, D., Voehler, M., Falck, J.R., Moore, B.S., Shimada, T., and Waterman, M.R. (2005) Binding of two flaviolin substrate molecules, oxidative coupling, and crystal structure of *Streptomyces coelicolor* A3(2) cytochrome P450 158A2. *J. Biol. Chem.*, **280**, 11599–11607.

137 Guengerich, F.P. (2006) A malleable catalyst dominates the metabolism of drugs. *Proc. Natl. Acad. Sci. USA*, **103**, 13565–13566.

138 Bauer, E., Guo, Z., Ueng, Y.-F., Bell, L.C., and Guengerich, F.P. (1995) Oxidation of benzo[*a*]pyrene by recombinant human cytochrome P450 enzymes. *Chem. Res. Toxicol.*, **8**, 136–142.

139 Podust, L.M., Bach, H., Kim, Y., Lamb, D.C., Arase, M., Sherman, D.H., Kelly, S.L., and Waterman, M.R. (2004) Comparison of the 1.85 Å structure of CYP154A1 from *Streptomyces coelicolor* A3(2) with the closely related CYP154C1 and CYPs from antibiotic biosynthetic pathways. *Protein Sci.*, **13**, 255–268.

140 Guengerich, F.P. (1983) Oxidation-reduction properties of rat liver cytochrome P-450 and NADPH-cytochrome P-450 reductase related to catalysis in reconstituted systems. *Biochemistry*, **22**, 2811–2820.

141 Sligar, S.G., Cinti, D.L., Gibson, G.G., and Schenkman, J.B. (1979) Spin state control of the hepatic cytochrome P450 redox potential. *Biochem. Biophys. Res. Commun.*, **90**, 925–932.

142 Das, A., Grinkova, Y.V., and Sligar, S.G. (2007) Redox potential control by drug binding to cytochrome P 450 3A4. *J. Am. Chem. Soc.*, **129**, 13778–13779.

143 Huang, Y.Y., Hara, T., Sligar, S., Coon, M.J., and Kimura, T. (1986) Thermodynamic properties of oxidation-reduction reactions of bacterial, microsomal, and mitochondrial cytochromes P-450: an entropy–enthalpy compensation effect. *Biochemistry*, **25**, 1390–1394.

144 Bhattacharyya, A.K., Lipka, J.J., Waskell, L., and Tollin, G. (1991) Laser flash photolysis studies of the reduction kinetics of NADPH : cytochrome P-450 reductase. *Biochemistry*, **30**, 759–765.

145 Guengerich, F.P., Krauser, J.A., and Johnson, W.W. (2004) Rate-limiting steps in oxidations catalyzed by rabbit cytochrome P450 1A2. *Biochemistry*, **43**, 10775–10788.

146 Shinkyo, R. and Guengerich, F.P. (2011) Cytochrome P450 7A1 cholesterol 7α-hydroxylation. Individual reaction steps in the catalytic cycle and rate-limiting ferric iron reduction. *J. Biol. Chem.*, **286**, 4632–4643.

147 Denisov, I.G., Grinkova, Y.V., McLean, M.A., and Sligar, S.G. (2007) The one-electron autoxidation of human cytochrome P450 3A4. *J. Biol. Chem.*, **282**, 26865–26873.

148 Bell, L.C. and Guengerich, F.P. (1997) Oxidation kinetics of ethanol by human cytochrome P450 2E1. Rate-limiting product release accounts for effects of isotopic hydrogen substitution and cytochrome b_5 on steady-state kinetics. *J. Biol. Chem.*, **272**, 29643–29651.

149 Yamazaki, H., Komatsu, T., Ohyama, K., Nakamura, M., Asahi, S., Shimada, N., Guengerich, F.P., Nakajima, A., and Yokoi, T. (2002) Roles of NADPH-P450 reductase and apo- and holo-cytochrome b_5 on xenobiotic oxidations catalyzed by 12 recombinant human cytochrome P450s expressed in membranes of *Escherichia coli*. *Protein Expr. Purif.*, **24**, 329–337.

150 Zhang, H., Hamdane, D., Im, S.C., and Waskell, L. (2008) Cytochrome b_5 inhibits electron transfer from NADPH-cytochrome P450 reductase to ferric cytochrome P450 2B4. *J. Biol. Chem.*, **283**, 5217–5225.

151 Groves, J.T. (2006) High-valent iron in chemical and biological oxidations. *J. Inorg. Biochem.*, **100**, 434–447.

152 Shaik, S., Kumar, D., de Visser, S.P., Altun, A., and Thiel, W. (2005) Theoretical perspective on the structure and mechanism of cytochrome P450 enzymes. *Chem. Rev.*, **105**, 2279–2328.

153 Guengerich, F.P. and Macdonald, T.L. (1984) Chemical mechanisms of catalysis by cytochromes P-450: a unified view. *Acc. Chem. Res.*, **17**, 9–16.

154 Guengerich, F.P. and Macdonald, T.L. (1993) Sequential electron transfer reactions catalyzed by cytochrome P-450 enzymes, in *Advances in Electron Transfer Chemistry*, vol. 3 (ed. P.S. Mariano), JAI Press, Greenwich, CT, pp. 191–241.

155 Augusto, O., Beilan, H.S., and Ortiz de Montellano, P.R. (1982) The catalytic mechanism of cytochrome P-450: spin-trapping evidence for one-electron substrate oxidation. *J. Biol. Chem.*, **257**, 11288–11295.

156 Bondon, A., Macdonald, T.L., Harris, T.M., and Guengerich, F.P. (1989) Oxidation of cycloalkylamines by cytochrome P-450. Mechanism-based inactivation, adduct formation, ring expansion, and nitrone formation. *J. Biol. Chem.*, **264**, 1988–1997.

157 Guengerich, F.P., Yun, C.-H., and Macdonald, T.L. (1996) Evidence for a one-electron oxidation mechanism in *N*-dealkylation of *N,N*-dialkylanilines by cytochrome P450 2B1. Kinetic hydrogen isotope effects, linear free energy relationships, comparisons with horseradish peroxidase, and studies with oxygen surrogates. *J. Biol. Chem.*, **271**, 27321–27329.

158 Sato, H. and Guengerich, F.P. (2000) Oxidation of 1,2,4,5-tetramethoxybenzene to a cation radical by cytochrome P450. *J. Am. Chem. Soc.*, **122**, 8099–8100.

159 Liebler, D.C. and Guengerich, F.P. (1983) Olefin oxidation by cytochrome P-450: evidence for group migration in catalytic intermediates formed with vinylidene chloride and *trans*-1-phenyl-1-butene. *Biochemistry*, **22**, 5482–5489.

160 Komives, E.A. and Ortiz de Montellano, P.R. (1987) Mechanism of oxidation of π bonds by cytochrome P-450: electronic requirements of the transition state in the turnover of phenylacetylenes. *J. Biol. Chem.*, **262**, 9793–9802.

161 Chandrasena, R.E., Vatsis, K.P., Coon, M.J., Hollenberg, P.F., and Newcomb, M. (2004) Hydroxylation by the hydroperoxy-iron species in cytochrome P450 enzymes. *J. Am. Chem. Soc.*, **126**, 115–126.

162 Derat, E., Kumar, D., Hirao, H., and Shaik, S. (2006) Gauging the relative oxidative powers of compound I, ferric-hydroperoxide, and the ferric-hydrogen peroxide species of cytochrome P450 toward C–H hydroxylation of a radical clock substrate. *J. Am. Chem. Soc.*, **128**, 473–484.

163 Akhtar, M., Calder, M.R., Corina, D.L., and Wright, J.N. (1982) Mechanistic studies on C-19 demethylation in oestrogen biocynthesis. *Biochem. J.*, **201**, 569–580.
164 Cole, P.A. and Robinson, C.H. (1988) A peroxide model reaction for placental aromatase. *J. Am. Chem. Soc.*, **110**, 1284–1285.
165 Vaz, A.D.N., Roberts, E.S., and Coon, M.J. (1991) Olefin formation in the oxidative deformylation of aldehydes by cytochrome P-450. Mechanistic implications for catalysis by oxygen-derived peroxide. *J. Am. Chem. Soc.*, **113**, 5886–5887.
166 Hackett, J.C., Brueggemeier, R.W., and Hadad, C.M. (2005) The final catalytic step of cytochrome P450 aromatase: a density functional theory study. *J. Am. Chem. Soc.*, **127**, 5224–5237.
167 Collman, J.P., Chien, A.S., Eberspacher, T.A., and Brauman, J.I. (1998) An agostic alternative to the P-450 rebound mechanism. *J. Am. Chem. Soc.*, **120**, 425–426.
168 Newcomb, M., Shen, R., Choi, S., Toy, P.H., Hollenberg, P.F., Vaz, A.D.N., and Coon, M.J. (2000) Cytochrome P450-catalyzed hydroxylation of mechanistic probes that distinguish between radicals and cations. Evidence for cationic but not for radical intermediates. *J. Am. Chem. Soc.*, **122**, 2677–2686.
169 Yun, C.-H., Kim, K.-H., Calcutt, M.W., and Guengerich, F.P. (2005) Kinetic analysis of oxidation of coumarins by human cytochrome P450 2A6. *J. Biol. Chem.*, **280**, 12279–12291.
170 Bell-Parikh, L.C. and Guengerich, F.P. (1999) Kinetics of cytochrome P450 2E1-catalyzed oxidation of ethanol to acetic acid via acetaldehyde. *J. Biol. Chem.*, **274**, 23833–23840.
171 Chowdhury, G., Calcutt, M.W., and Guengerich, F.P. (2010) Oxidation of *N*-nitrosodimethylamine and *N*-nitrosodiethylamine by human cytochrome P450 2A6: sequential oxidation to carboxylic acids and analysis of reaction steps. *J. Biol. Chem.*, **285**, 8031–8044.
172 Yarnell, A.T. (2009) Heavy-hydrogen drugs turn heads, again. *Chem. Eng. News*, **87**, 36–39.
173 Cook, P.F. and Cleland, W.W. (2007) *Enzyme Kinetics and Mechanism*, Garland, New York, pp. 225–364.
174 Gorsky, L.D., Koop, D.R., and Coon, M.J. (1984) On the stoichiometry of the oxidase and monooxygenase reactions catalyzed by liver microsomal cytochrome P-450: products of oxygen reduction. *J. Biol. Chem.*, **259**, 6812–6817.
175 Northrop, D.B. (1982) Deuterium and tritium kinetic isotope effects on initial rates. *Methods Enzymol.*, **87**, 607–625.
176 Yun, C.-H., Miller, G.P., and Guengerich, F.P. (2000) Rate-determining steps in phenacetin oxidations by human cytochrome P450 1A2 and selected mutants. *Biochemistry*, **39**, 11319–11329.
177 Krauser, J.A. and Guengerich, F.P. (2005) Cytochrome P450 3A4-catalyzed testosterone 6β-hydroxylation: stereochemistry, kinetic deuterium isotope effects, and rate-limiting steps. *J. Biol. Chem.*, **280**, 19496–19506.
178 Fersht, A. (1999) *Structure and Mechanism in Protein Science*, Freeman, New York, pp. 116–118.
179 Fischer, E. (1894) Einfluss der Configuration auf die Wirkung der Enzyme. *Ber. Dtsch. Chem. Ges.*, **27**, 2985–2993.
180 Frey, P.A. and Hegeman, A.D. (2007) *Enzymatic Reaction Mechanisms*, Oxford University Press, New York.
181 Isin, E.M. and Guengerich, F.P. (2006) Kinetics and thermodynamics of ligand binding by cytochrome P450 3A4. *J. Biol. Chem.*, **281**, 9127–9136.
182 Isin, E.M. and Guengerich, F.P. (2007) Multiple sequential steps involved in the binding of inhibitors to cytochrome P450 3A4. *J. Biol. Chem.*, **282**, 6863–6874.
183 Sohl, C.D., Isin, E.M., Eoff, R.L., Marsch, G.A., Stec, D.F., and Guengerich, F.P. (2008) Cooperativity in oxidation reactions catalyzed by cytochrome P450 1A2. Highly cooperative pyrene hydroxylation and

multiphasic kinetics of ligand binding. *J. Biol. Chem.*, **283**, 7293–7308.

184 Burka, L.T., Guengerich, F.P., Willard, R.J., and Macdonald, T.L. (1985) Mechanism of cytochrome P-450 catalysis. Mechanism of *N*-dealkylation and amine oxide deoxygenation. *J. Am. Chem. Soc.*, **107**, 2549–2551.

185 Yun, C.-H., Miller, G.P., and Guengerich, F.P. (2001) Oxidations of *p*-alkoxyacylanilides by human cytochrome P450 1A2: structure-activity relationships and simulation of rate constants of individual steps in catalysis. *Biochemistry*, **40**, 4521–4530.

186 Guengerich, F.P., Miller, G.P., Hanna, I.H., Sato, H., and Martin, M.V. (2002) Oxidation of methoxyphenethylamines by cytochrome P450 2D6. Analysis of rate-limiting steps. *J. Biol. Chem.*, **277**, 33711–33719.

187 Nakayama, K., Puchkaev, A., and Pikuleva, I.A. (2001) Membrane binding and substrate access merge in cytochrome P450 7A1, a key enzyme in degradation of cholesterol. *J. Biol. Chem.*, **276**, 31459–31465.

188 Johnson, K.A. (2008) Role of induced-fit in enzyme specificity: a molecular forward/reverse switch. *J. Biol. Chem.*, **283**, 26297–26301.

189 Gillette, J.R., Brodie, B.B., and La Du, B.N. (1957) The oxidation of drugs by liver microsomes: on the role of TPNH and oxygen. *J. Pharmacol. Exp. Ther.*, **119**, 532–540.

190 Nordblom, G.D. and Coon, M.J. (1977) Hydrogen peroxide formation and stoichiometry of hydroxylation reactions catalyzed by highly purified liver microsomal cytochrome P-450. *Arch. Biochem. Biophys.*, **180**, 343–347.

191 Dostalek, M., Brooks, J.D., Hardy, K.D., Milne, G.L., Moore, M.M., Sharma, S., Morrow, J.D., and Guengerich, F.P. (2007) *In vivo* oxidative damage in rats is associated with barbiturate response but not other cytochrome P450 inducers. *Mol. Pharmacol.*, **72**, 1419–1424.

192 Dostalek, M., Hardy, K.D., Milne, G.L., Morrow, J.D., Chen, C., Gonzalez, F.J., Gu, J., Ding, X., Johnson, D.A., Johnson, J.A., Martin, M.V., and Guengerich, F.P. (2008) Development of oxidative stress by cytochrome P450 induction in rodents is selective for barbiturates and related to loss of pyridine nucleotide-dependent protective systems. *J. Biol. Chem.*, **283**, 17147–17157.

193 Guengerich, F.P., Sohl, C.D., and Chowdhury, G. (2011) Multi-step oxidations catalyzed by cytochrome P450 enzymes: processive vs. distributive kinetics and the issue of carbonyl oxidation. *Arch. Biochem. Biophys.*, **507**, 126–134.

194 Afzelius, L., Arnby, C.H., Broo, A., Carlsson, L., Isaksson, C., Jurva, U., Kjellander, B., Kolmodin, K., Nilsson, K., Raubacher, F., and Weidolf, L. (2007) State-of-the-art tools for computational site of metabolism predictions: comparative analysis, mechanistical insights, and future applications. *Drug Metab. Rev.*, **39**, 61–86.

195 Kuthan, H. and Ullrich, V. (1982) Oxidase and oxygenase function of the microsomal cytochrome P450 monooxygenase system. *Eur. J. Biochem.*, **126**, 583–588.

196 Kadiiska, M.B., Gladen, B.C., Baird, D.D., Graham, L.B., Parker, C.E., Ames, B.N., Basu, S., Fitzgerald, G.A., Lawson, J.A., Marnett, L.J., Morrow, J.D., Murray, D.M., Plastaras, J., Roberts, L.J., 2nd, Rokach, J., Shigenaga, M.K., Sun, J., Walter, P.B., Tomer, K.B., Barrett, J.C., and Mason, R.P. (2005) Biomarkers of oxidative stress study III. Effects of the nonsteroidal anti-inflammatory agents indomethacin and meclofenamic acid on measurements of oxidative products of lipids in CCl_4 poisoning. *Free Radic. Biol. Med.*, **38**, 711–718.

197 Bansal, S., Liu, C.-P., Sepuri, N.B.V., Anandatheerthavarada, H.K., Guengerich, F.P., and Avadhani, N.G. (2010) Mitochondria-targeted cytochrome P450 2E1 preferentially induces oxidative damage and augments alcohol mediated mitochodrial dysfunction in cultured cells. *J. Biol. Chem.*, **285**, 24609–24619.

198 Williams, J.A., Hyland, R., Jones, B.C., Smith, D.A., Hurst, S., Goosen, T.C., Peterkin, V., Koup, J.R., and Ball, S.E. (2004) Drug–drug interactions for

UDP-glucuronosyltransferase substrates: a pharmacokinetic explanation for typically observed low exposure (AUC_i/AUC) ratios. *Drug Metab. Dispos.*, **32**, 1201–1208.

199 Wienkers, L.C. and Heath, T.G. (2005) Predicting *in vivo* drug interactions from *in vitro* drug discovery data. *Nat. Rev. Drug Discov.*, **4**, 825–833.

200 Guengerich, F.P. and Shimada, T. (1991) Oxidation of toxic and carcinogenic chemicals by human cytochrome P-450 enzymes. *Chem. Res. Toxicol.*, **4**, 391–407.

201 Correia, M.A. (2005) Inhibition of cytochrome P450 enzymes, in *Cytochrome P450: Structure, Mechanism, and Biochemistry*, 3rd edn (ed. P.R. Ortiz de Montellano), Kluwer/Plenum, New York, pp. 247–322.

202 Shimada, T., Yamazaki, H., Foroozesh, M., Hopkins, N.E., Alworth, W.L., and Guengerich, F.P. (1998) Selectivity of polycyclic inhibitors for human cytochromes P450 1A1, 1A2, and 1B1. *Chem. Res. Toxicol.*, **11**, 1048–1056.

203 Yamazaki, H., Inui, Y., Yun, C.-H., Guengerich, F.P., and Shimada, T. (1992) Cytochrome P450 2E1 and 2A6 enzymes as major catalysts for metabolic activation of *N*-nitrosodialkylamines and tobacco-related nitrosamines in human liver microsomes. *Carcinogenesis*, **13**, 1789–1794.

204 Chovan, J.P., Ring, S.C., Yu, E., and Baldino, J.P. (2007) Cytochrome P450 probe substrate metabolism kinetics in Sprague Dawley rats. *Xenobiotica*, **37**, 459–473.

205 Sahakitrungruang, T., Huang, N., Tee, M.K., Agrawal, V., Russell, W.E., Crock, P., Murphy, N., Migeon, C.J., and Miller, W.L. (2009) Clinical, genetic, and enzymatic characterization of P450 oxidoreductase deficiency in four patients. *J. Clin. Endocrinol. Metab.*, **94**, 4992–5000.

206 Brodie, A.M.H. (1985) Aromatase inhibition and its pharmacologic implications. *Biochem. Pharmacol.*, **34**, 3213–3219.

207 Ingelman-Sundberg, M. (2008) Pharmacogenomic biomarkers for prediction of severe adverse drug reactions. *N. Engl. J. Med.*, **358**, 637–639.

208 Bolt, H.M., Bolt, M., and Kappus, H. (1977) Interaction of rifampicin treatment with pharmacokinetics and metabolism of ethinyloestradiol in man. *Acta Endocrinol.*, **85**, 189–197.

209 Schwarz, U.I., Buschel, B., and Kirch, W. (2003) Unwanted pregnancy on self-medication with St. John's wort despite hormonal contraception. *Br. J. Clin. Pharmacol.*, **55**, 112–113.

210 Guengerich, F.P. (1988) Oxidation of 17α-ethynylestradiol by human liver cytochrome P-450. *Mol. Pharmacol.*, **33**, 500–508.

211 Yun, C.-H., Okerholm, R.A., and Guengerich, F.P. (1993) Oxidation of the antihistaminic drug terfenadine in human liver microsomes: role of cytochrome P450 3A(4) in *N*-dealkylation and *C*-hydroxylation. *Drug Metab. Dispos.*, **21**, 403–409.

212 Woosley, R.L., Chen, Y., Freiman, J.P., and Gillis, R.A. (1993) Mechanism of the cardiotoxic actions of terfenadine. *JAMA*, **269**, 1532–1536.

213 Sevior, D.K., Hokkanen, J., Tolonen, A., Abass, K., Tursas, L., Pelkonen, O., and Ahokas, J.T. (2010) Rapid screening of commercially available herbal products for the inhibition of major human hepatic cytochrome P450 enzymes using the N-in-one cocktail. *Xenobiotica*, **40**, 245–254.

214 Bailey, D.G., Spence, J.D., Munoz, C., and Arnold, J.M.O. (1991) Interaction of citrus juices with felodipine and nifedipine. *Lancet*, **337**, 268–269.

215 Wiebel, F.J., Leutz, J.C., Diamond, L., and Gelboin, H.V. (1971) Aryl hydrocarbon (benzo[*a*]pyrene) hydroxylase in microsomes from rat tissues: differential inhibition and stimulation by benzoflavones and organic solvents. *Arch. Biochem. Biophys.*, **144**, 78–86.

216 Anders, M. (1968) Acetone enhancement of microsomal aniline *para*-hydroxylase activity. *Arch. Biochem. Biophys.*, **126**, 269–275.

217 Guengerich, F.P., Kim, B.-R., Gillam, E.M.J., and Shimada, T. (1994) Mechanisms of enhancement and

inhibition of cytochrome P450 catalytic activity, in *Proceedings of the 8th International Conference on Cytochrome P450: Biochemistry, Biophysics, and Molecular Biology* (ed. M. C. Lechner), John Libbey Eurotext, Paris, pp. 97–101.

218 Shou, M., Grogan, J., Mancewicz, J.A., Krausz, K.W., Gonzalez, F.J., Gelboin, H.V., and Korzekwa, K.R. (1994) Activation of CYP3A4: evidence for the simultaneous binding of two substrates in a cytochrome P450 active site. *Biochemistry*, **33**, 6450–6455.

219 Lasker, J.M., Huang, M.-T., and Conney, A.H. (1982) *In vivo* activation of zoxazolamine metabolism by flavone. *Science*, **216**, 1419–1421.

220 Tang, W. and Stearns, R.A. (2001) Heterotropic cooperativity of cytochrome P450 3A4 and potential drug–drug interactions. *Curr. Drug Metab.*, **2**, 185–198.

221 Prentis, R.A., Lis, Y., and Walker, S.R. (1988) Pharmaceutical innovation by the seven UK-owned pharmaceutical companies (1964–1985). *Br. J. Clin. Pharmacol.*, **25**, 387–396.

222 Kola, I. and Landis, J. (2004) Can the pharmaceutical industry reduce attrition rates? *Nat. Rev. Drug Discov.*, **3**, 711–715.

3
UDP-Glucuronosyltransferases

Christian P. Strassburg and Sandra Kalthoff

3.1
Introduction

The discovery and subsequent characterization of UDP-glucuronosyltransferases (UGTs) was initiated by biochemical experiments studying the formation of glucuronides. In this metabolic process termed glucuronidation, UDP-glucuronic acid is utilized as a cosubstrate to generate hydrophilic glucuronides from non-membrane-associated substrates. In higher organisms it serves as an important process of metabolism and detoxification that is evolutionarily well conserved. Thus, the majority of vertebrate species are capable of generating glucuronides from a broad array of substrates [1]. Dutton isolated and described UDP-glucuronic acid in 1953 [2], which led the way to the characterization and purification of transferase proteins capable of glucuronide formation, first in rodents and later in man [3–5]. UGTs (EC 2.4.1.17) utilize UDP-glucuronic acid as a sugar donator and transfer glucuronic acid to the respective substrate compound, which generates β-glucuronidase-sensitive β-D-glucopyranosiduronic acids (glucuronides).

3.2
A Simple Phenotype: Unconjugated Nonhemolytic Hyperbilirubinemia and Glucuronidation

Fifty years before Dutton's key experiments, Gilbert and Lereboulet had described an abnormality characterized by fluctuating, low-level unconjugated nonhemolytic hyperbilirubinemia [6]. This anomaly is found with high prevalence among the white population. The syndrome was also reported by Meulengracht in 1946 and by Arias in 1962 [7], leading to the designation Gilbert–Meulengracht syndrome (GMS) in parts of the literature. Jaundice represents a clinical symptom of potentially serious liver dysfunction, which has prompted intense studies of

Metabolism of Drugs and Other Xenobiotics, First Edition. Edited by Pavel Anzenbacher, Ulrich M. Zanger.

GMS and to its inclusion into standard hepatological textbooks [8]. GMS is generally described as a benign variant of the norm leading to transient unconjugated hyperbilirubinemia [9]. This view is founded on the observation that GMS is not associated with chronic liver inflammation, histological changes, or progressive fibrosis. In 1991, the "bilirubin transferase" was identified [10] and linked to a life-threatening variant (defect) of bilirubin conjugation, Crigler–Najjar syndrome [11], which is fatal when left untreated and when bilirubin glucuronidation activity is absent (Crigler–Najjar syndrome type 1). As a consequence of the data provided by genotyping analyses and the genome project, GMS, which affects about 10% of white individuals, has received a genetic link to a frequent genetic polymorphism–a TA insertion into the promoter of the human *UGT1A1* gene designated UGT1A1*28 [12]. However, the concept of an uncomplicated abnormality should be viewed with caution [13] based on the pharmacogenetics associated with this seemingly benign clinical phenotype [8]. To appreciate this, the structure, organization, function, regulation, and pharmacogenetics of the responsible genes and their gene products require detailed consideration, and this chapter will focus primarily on the human *UGT1A* gene locus, where *UGT1A1* is encoded.

3.3
Organization of UGTs and the *UGT1A* Gene Locus

The driving force of the discovery of the *UGT1A* supergene family encoded on chromosome 2q37 [14] has been unconjugated intermittent hyperbilirubinemia (GMS) and Crigler–Najjar syndrome. The metabolic importance of UGTs is a simple reaction leading to the conjugation of target substrates with glucuronic acid, which facilitates their subsequent biliary or renal elimination as water-soluble glucuronides [15]. With few exceptions, compounds conjugated with glucuronic acid are biologically inactive. Over 50 UGTs have meanwhile been identified in different vertebrate species. Hundreds of chemically diverse compounds, including dietary constituents, pharmaceutical drugs, endogenous hormones, bile acids, and the heme catalytic byproduct bilirubin, as well as aromatic hydrocarbons, flavonoids, and environmental mutagens, have been observed to be substrates for glucuronidation. This promiscuous substrate choice is a result of the UGTs' ability to catalyze glucuronide formation using hydroxy, carbonyl, sulfuryl, carboxyl, and amine groups [15] (Figure 3.1).

In humans, 15 UGT transcripts have been identified and divided into two families based upon sequence homology [16]. *UGT2* genes are located on chromosome 4q13 and 4q28, consist of six exons, and preferentially glucuronidate endobiotic substrates including steroids and bile acids. In contrast, the *UGT1A* gene locus has been mapped to chromosome 2q37, and enables the transcription of individual gene products sharing a common C-terminal portion of 280 amino acids and an exon 1 encoded divergent N-terminal portion of approximately 250 amino acids [17] (Figure 3.2). Utilizing a strategy of exon sharing, potentially nine functional

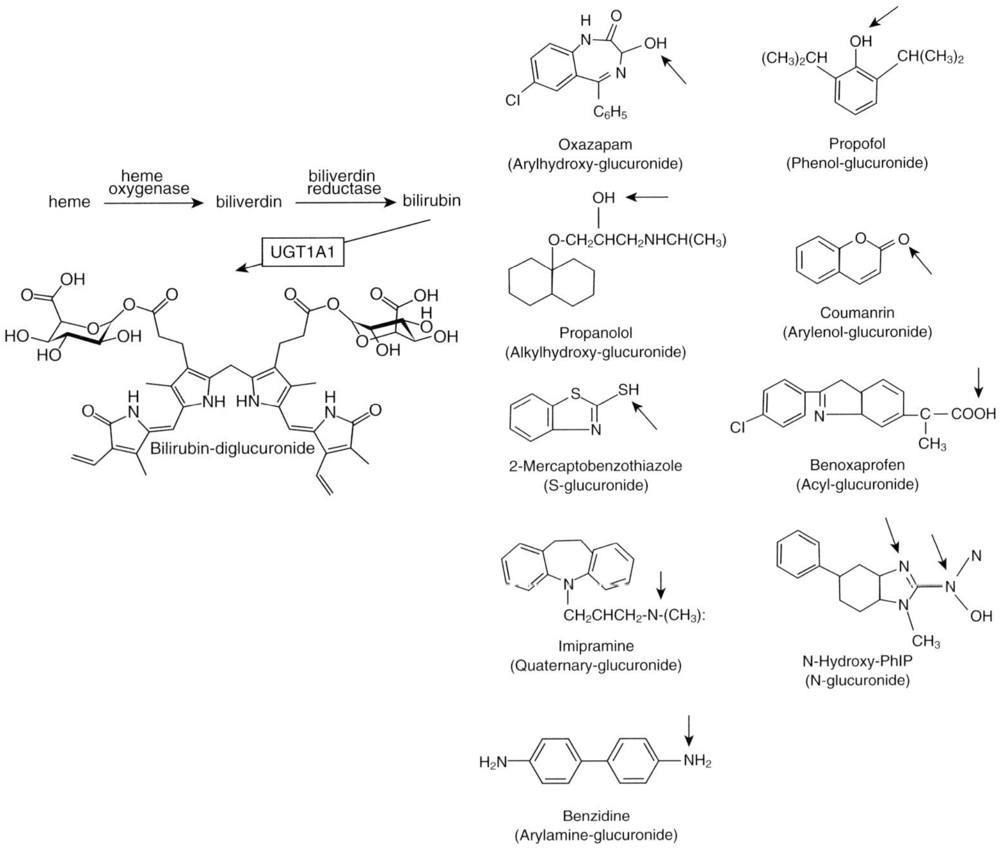

Figure 3.1 Glucuronidation of bilirubin and catalysis from heme. The production of bilirubin glucuronides is reduced in the absence of adequate activity of UGT1A1, leading to unconjugated hyperbilirubinemia. In addition, the different biochemical groups for glucuronide formation are shown.

exon 1 sequences can be combined with the constant exons 2–5, leading to individual UGT1A transcripts [14]. The tissue-specific and individual regulation of the *UGT1A* first exons has been extensively characterized in the human hepatogastrointestinal tract. In human liver, transcripts of UGT1A1, UGT1A3, UGT1A4, UGT1A6, and UGT1A9 have been detected and cloned, whereas UGT1A7 (esophagus, stomach), UGT1A8 (esophagus, colon), and UGT1A10 (esophagus, bile ducts, stomach, colon) transcripts have been identified exclusively in extrahepatic epithelial tissues [18–23]. A later study additionally described UGT1A5 transcripts [24]. The genetic organization of the *UGT1A* gene locus therefore enables tissue specificity and most likely accounts for the broad spectrum of substrates for glucuronidation in man [21, 25]. This is also characterized by a considerable overlap of substrate specificities, which has been demonstrated by studies with recombinant

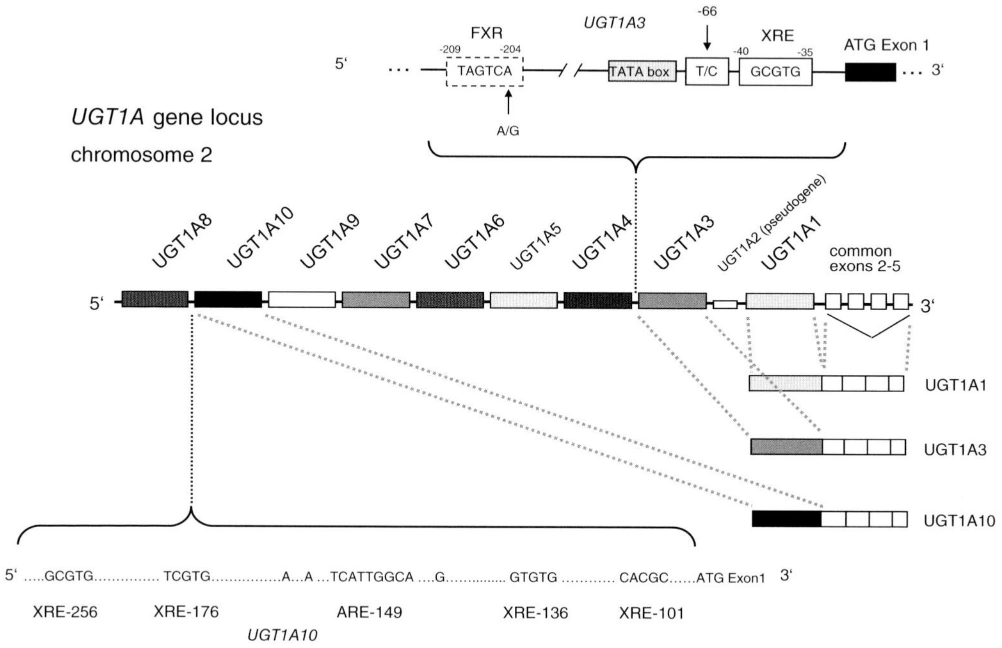

Figure 3.2 Graphic representation of the human *UGT1A* gene locus encoding the UGT1A enzymes (not to scale). Individual first exons are positioned at the 5′ end of the chromosome and common exons 2–5 at the 3′ end. Individual exon 1 sequences are combined with the exon 2–5 sequence, which is present in every UGT1A transcript; the intervening sequence of the primary transcript is eliminated by splicing. Examples of UGT1A1, UGT1A3, and UGT1A10 transcription are shown. For *UGT1A3* and *UGT1A10*, identified binding motifs for transcriptional regulation are shown. These include XREs, AREs, and the FXR. For the *UGT1A3* gene (top), SNPs are indicated by arrows.

UGT proteins and experimentally can confound functional studies of individual UGT proteins [26].

3.4
UGT1A Gene Nomenclature

The nomenclature of the *UGT1A* genes and proteins utilizes the comparison of sequences and evolutionary divergence [27]. A human *UGT* gene is named using the root abbreviation *UGT* (*Ugt* in mice and *Drosophila*), which is followed by an Arabic number representing the family, a letter designating the subfamily, and an Arabic number indicating the individual gene within the family or subfamily (i.e., "human *UGT1A1*" and "mouse *Ugt1a1*"). An international nomenclature committee compiles and updates the current nomenclature of the *UGT* supergene family, and is accessible on the world-wide web at http://www.

pharmacogenomics.pha.ulaval.ca/sgc/ugt_alleles. In recent years increasing numbers of allelic UGT variants have been identified, characterized, and reported. These variants are designated by separation of gene and allele by an asterisk followed by an Arabic number and upper-case Roman letters with less than four characters to name the allele (e.g., UGT1A1*2, UGT1A7*2B). The sequence of a gene comprises the sequence from 5 kb upstream relative to the transcription start site to 500 bp downstream of the last exon. In cases in which a regulatory element positioned further away has been characterized, this area is also considered part of the gene (Figure 3.2). A unique allele is expected to contain nucleotide changes that result in at least one amino acid change in the resulting protein. For sequence designations in flanking regions of the exons the base A in the initiation codon ATG is designated +1 and the base before A is numbered −1. A "wild-type" allele of a specific *UGT* gene is defined as the sequence of the first allele sequenced and should be designated as *1 (or *1a, and *1b in case of slightly variant sequences). A summary of variant alleles of the *UGT1A1*, *UGT1A3*, and *UGT1A7* genes are given in Tables 3.1–3.3.

3.5
Human *UGT1A* Gene Locus and Sequence Variability

The *UGT1A* locus (Figure 3.2) spans approximately 200 kbp, likely having evolved by a series of gene duplication events. This is suggested by the high homology of clustered UGTs such as *UGT1A3*, *UGT1A4*, and *UGT1A5*, as well as *UGT1A7*, *UGT1A8*, *UGT1A9*, and *UGT1A10* [16]. *Cis*-acting promoter elements of individual *UGT1As* and their corresponding first exons are in close proximity to each other. Genetic variability within the *UGT1A* gene locus is surprisingly common and has obviously been conserved during the process of evolutionary development. *UGT1A* genotyping has reported over 100 single nucleotide polymorphisms (SNPs) within the promoter regions and the *UGT1A* coding sequence, many of which are found to be in linkage disequilibrium with each other, and are found at individual allelic frequencies of up to 40–50% of the general population [46, 48, 57]. Studies have shown that haplotypes of numerous of these *UGT1A* variants occur simultaneously [46, 55, 58–60], influencing glucuronidation by expressing proteins with altered function [46, 50, 51], or by modulating transcriptional regulation [12, 55, 61–64], or both (Tables 3.1–3.3). Owing to of this potential to influence drug metabolism and the disposition to unwanted drug side-effects, *UGT* genes have attracted considerable attention for pharmacogenetic studies. Therefore, in an individual with GMS presenting with an easily distinguishable phenotype of hyperbilirubinemia, the actual complete genotype is likely to be far more complex than the clinically visible modulation of bilirubin glucuronidation alone would suggest (Table 3.4 and Figure 3.3) [13]. In view of the available genotyping and functional analyses, variants of the *UGT1A1* gene but also of the *UGT1A3* and *UGT1A7* genes exhibit high frequencies and functional as well as transcriptional alterations. Therefore, *UGT1A1*, *UGT1A3*, and *UGT1A7* will be discussed in more detail in the following sections.

Table 3.1 Selected genetic variants of the *UGT1A1* gene.

Allele	Nucleotides	Amino acids	UGT1A exon	Activity *in vivo*	Activity *in vitro*	Reference	Syndrome
UGT1A1*1	NA	NA	NA	wild-type	wild-type	[10]	–
UGT1A1*2	877(T>A)/878–890del	frameshift/deletion	2	absent	absent	[11]	Crigler–Najjar 1
UGT1A1*3	1124(C>T)	S375F	4	inactive	inactive	[28]	Crigler–Najjar 1
UGT1A1*4	1069(C>T)	Q357X	3	inactive	inactive	[29]	Crigler–Najjar 1
UGT1A1*5	991(C>T)	Q331X	2	absent	inactive	[28]	Crigler–Najjar 1
UGT1A1*6	211(G>A)	G71R	1	reduced	reduced	[30]	–
UGT1A1*7	1456(T>G)	Y486D	5	reduced	reduced	[30]	Crigler–Najjar 2
UGT1A1*8	625(C>T)	R209W	1	4.4%	reduced	[31]	Crigler–Najjar 2
UGT1A1*9	992(A>G)	Q331R	2	reduced	reduced	[32]	Crigler–Najjar 2
UGT1A1*10	1021(C>T)	R341X	3	absent	absent	[33]	Crigler–Najjar 1
UGT1A1*11	923(G>A)	G308E	2	inactive	absent	[34, 35]	Crigler–Najjar 1
UGT1A1*12	524(T>A)	L175Q	1	38.4%	reduced	[36]	Crigler–Najjar 2
UGT1A1*13	508–510del	F170del	1	inactive	inactive	[37]	Crigler–Najjar 1
UGT1A1*14	826(G>C)	G276R	1	inactive	inactive	[36]	Crigler–Najjar 1
UGT1A1*15	529(T>C)	C177R	1	inactive	inactive	[36]	Crigler–Najjar 1
UGT1A1*16	1070(A>G)	Q357R	3	absent	absent	[35]	Crigler–Najjar 1
UGT1A1*17	1143(C>G)	S381R	4	absent	absent	[35]	Crigler–Najjar 1
UGT1A1*18	1201(G>C)	A401P	4	absent	absent	[35]	Crigler–Najjar 1
UGT1A1*19	1005(G>A)	W335X	3	absent	absent	[35]	Crigler–Najjar 1
UGT1A1*20	1102(G>A)	A368T	4	absent	absent	[35]	Crigler–Najjar 1
UGT1A1*21	1223insG	frameshift	4	absent	absent	[35]	Crigler–Najjar 1
UGT1A1*22	872(C>T)	A291V	2	absent	absent	[35]	Crigler–Najjar 1

UGT1A1*23	1282(A>G)	K426E	**4**	absent	absent	[35]	Crigler–Najjar 1
UGT1A1*24	1309(A>T)	K437X	**5**	absent	absent	[35]	Crigler–Najjar 1
UGT1A1*25	840(C>A)	C280X	1	absent	absent	[38]	Crigler–Najjar 1
UGT1A1*26	973delG	frameshift	**2**	absent	absent	[36]	Crigler–Najjar 2
UGT1A1*27	686(C>A)	P229Q	1	reduced	reduced	[39]	Gilbert's
UGT1A1*28	A(TA)6TAA to A(TA)7TAA	NA	*promoter*	reduced	reduced	[12]	Gilbert's
UGT1A1*36	A(TA)6TAA to A(TA)5TAA	NA	*promoter*	increased	increased	[40]	–
UGT1A1*37	A(TA)6TAA to A(TA)8TAA	NA	*promoter*	reduced	reduced	[40]	Crigler–Najjar 2
UGT1A1*29	1099(C>G)	R367G	**4**	reduced	reduced	[39]	Gilbert's
UGT1A1*60	–3279(T>G)	NA	*promoter*	–	–	[41]	Gilbert's
UGT1A1*62	247(T>C)	F83L	1	–	–	[42]	Gilbert's
UGT1A1*64	488–491dupACCT	frameshift	1	reduced	–	[43]	Gilbert's
UGT1A1*65	–1126(C>T)	NA	*promoter*	reduced	–	[43]	Gilbert's
UGT1A1*66	997-82(T>C)	NA	intron 2	–	–	[43]	Gilbert's
UGT1A1*67	–85 to –83 ins CAT	NA	*promoter*	–	–	[44]	Gilbert's
UGT1A1*68	–63(G>C)		*promoter*	reduced	reduced	[44]	Gilbert's
UGT1A1*69	476(T>C)	I159T	1	normal	–	[44]	Gilbert's
UGT1A1*70	962(C>G)	A321G	**2**	normal	–	[44]	Gilbert's
UGT1A1*72	1075(G>A)	D359N	**3**	normal	–	[44]	Gilbert's
UGT1A1*73	1091(C>T)	P364L	**4**	normal	–	[44]	Gilbert's

Bold entries indicate variants in the common exons (see Figure 3.1) with an impact on all UGT1A gene transcripts, italic entries indicate promoter variants.

Table 3.2 Genetic variants of the *UGT1A3* gene.

Allele	Promoter nucleotide change	Coding nucleotide change	Amino acid change	Transcription level	Activity *in vivo*	Activity *in vitro*	Reference
UGT1A3*1a	reference sequence	reference sequence	reference sequence	normal	normal	normal	
UGT1A3*1b	reference sequence	537(T>C)	D179D	normal	–	–	[45]
UGT1A3*1c	reference sequence	477(A>G)	A159A	normal	–	–	[45]
UGT1A3*1d	reference sequence	81(G>A)	E27E	normal	–	–	[45]
UGT1A3*1e	–581(C>T)	reference sequence	reference sequence	low	–	–	[45]
UGT1A3*1f	–581(C>T)	81(G>A)	E27E	low	–	–	[45]
UGT1A3*2a	–758(A>G)/–751(T>C)/–581(C>T)/–204(A>G)/–66(T>C)	31(T>C)/81(G>A)/140(T>C)/477(A>G)	W11R/E27E/V47A/A159A	low	–	normal	[45, 46]
UGT1A3*2b	–758(A>G)/–751(T>C)/–581(C>T)/–204(A>G)/–148(T>C)/–66(T>C)	31(T>C)/81(G>A)/140(T>C)/477(A>G)	W11R/E27E/V47A/A159A	low	–	high	[45, 47]
UGT1A3*2c	–758(A>G)/–751(T>C)/–581(C>T)/–553(G>A)/–204(A>G)/–66(T>C)	31(T>C)/81(G>A)/140(T>C)/234(A>G)/477(A>G)	W11R/E27E/V47A/T78T/A159A	low	–	–	[45]
UGT1A3*2d	–758(A>G)/–751(T>C)/–581(C>T)/–553(G>A)/–204(A>G)/–66(T>C)	31(T>C)/81(G>A)/140(T>C)/477(A>G)	W11R/E27E/V47A/A159A	low	–	–	[45]
UGT1A3*2e	reference sequence	31(T>C)/81(G>A)/140(T>C)	W11R/E27E/V47A	low	–	–	[45]

UGT1A3*3a	−758(A>G)/−581(C>T)/−204(A>G)/−66(T>C)	31(T>C)/81(G>A)/477(A>G)	W11R/E27E/A159A	low	–	normal	[45, 46]
UGT1A3*3b	NA	31(T>C)/81(G>A)/477(A>G)	W11R/E27E/A159A	NA	–	–	[47]
UGT1A3*4a	NA	133(C>T)	R45W	NA	–	low	[47]
UGT1A3*5a	NA	17(A>G)/31(T>C)/81(G>A)/477(A>G)	Q6R/W11R/E27E/A159A	NA	–	inter mediate	[47]
UGT1A3*6a	−758(A>G)/−751(T>C)/−581(C>T)/−204(A>G)/−66(T>C)	31(T>C)/81(G>A)/140(T>C)/477(A>G)/808(A>G)	W11R/E27E/V47A/A159A/M270V	low	–	low	[45]
UGT1A3*7a	−758(A>G)/−751(T>C)/−581(C>T)/−204(A>G)/−66(T>C)	328(T>A)	F110I	low	–	inter mediate	[45]
UGT1A3*8a	reference sequence	473(C>T)	A158V	normal	–	low	[45]
UGT1A3*9a	−758(A>G)/−751(T>C)/−581(C>T)/−204(A>G)/−66(T>C)	31(T>C)/81(G>A)/477(A>G)/622(A>C)	W11R/E27E/A159A/M208L	low	–	inter mediate	[45]
UGT1A3*10a	reference sequence	140(T>C)	V47A	normal	–	inter mediate	[45]
UGT1A3*10b	−581(C>T)	140(T>C)	V47A	low	–	–	[45]
UGT1A3*11a	NA	31(T>C)/81(G>A)/140(T>C)/342(G>A)/477(A>G)	W11R/E27E/V47A/M114I/A159A	NA	–	inter mediate	[48]

UGT1A3*7a and UGT1A3*9a are found in only 1/500 individuals.

Table 3.3 Genetic variants of the *UGT1A7* gene.

Allele	Promoter nucleotide change	Coding nucleotide change	Amino acid change	Function	Activity *in vivo*	Activity *in vitro*	Reference
UGT1A7*1a				wild-type		high	[22]
UGT1A7*1b	–70(G>A)						[49]
UGT1A7*2		387(T>G)/391(C>A)/392(G>A)	N129K/R131K			high	[50, 51]
UGT1A7*3		387(T>G)/391(C>A)/392(G>A)/622(T>C)	N129K/R131K/W208R			low	[50, 51]
UGT1A7*4		622(T>C)	W208R			low	[50, 51]
UGT1A7*5		343(G>A)	G115S			low	[52]
UGT1A7*6		417(G>C)	E139D			high	[52]
UGT1A7*7		387(T>G)/391(C>A)/392(G>A)/417(G>C)	N129K/R131K/E139D			high	[52]
UGT1A7*8		387(T>G)/391(C>A)/392(G>A)/417(G>C)/622(T>C)	N129K/R131K/E139D/W208R			low	[52]
UGT1A7*9		343(G>A)/387(T>G)/391(C>A)/392(G>A)	G115S/N129K/R131K			low	[52]
UGT1A7*10		386(A>G)/387(T>G)/391(C>A)/392(G>A)/622(T>C)	N129R/R131K/W208R				[53]
UGT1A7*11		392(G>A)	R131Q				[54]
UGT1A7*12	–57(T>G)	622(T>C)/760(C>T)	W208R/R254X			70% reduction of luciferase activity	[55]
UGT1A7*13		828(C>A)	N276K				[48]
UGT1A7*14		422(G>C)	C141S				[56]

Table 3.4 Likely non-UGT-associated abnormalities affecting drug metabolism in GMS.

Abnormality	Potential mechanism	Reference
Reduced indocyanine green clearance	altered transport	[65, 66]
Reduced bromosulphthalein clearance	altered transport	[67]
Impaired hepatic bilirubin uptake	altered transport, SCLO1B1?	[68]
Impaired tolbutamide clearance	altered hepatic uptake?	[69]
	genome-wide association of hyperbilirubinemia with *UGT1A1* and *SCLO1B1*	[70]

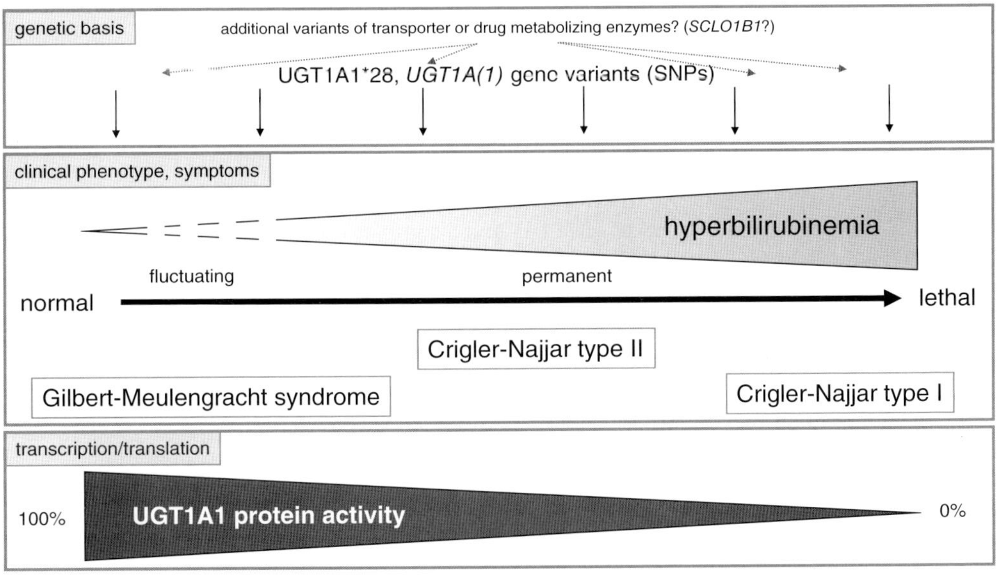

Figure 3.3 Summary of the continuous syndrome of hereditary unconjugated hyperbilirubinemia, which has three clinically distinguished degrees of severity: GMS, and Crigler–Najjar type 2 and type 1 disease. This distinction is not evidence of differing pathophysiological mechanisms. Variability at the *UGT1A1* gene locus leads to a continuous spectrum of altered bilirubin conjugation without clear diagnostic thresholds. In addition, there is evidence not only for associated variability regarding other *UGT1A* genes, but also for changes in hepatic transport (see Table 3.4).

3.6
Glucuronidation of Bilirubin

The hydrophobic tetrapyrrole bilirubin represents the endpoint of heme catabolism (Figure 3.1). Only 5% exists as the excretable bilirubin (di)glucuronide. In 1991, the bilirubin conjugating transferase, UGT1A1, was identified and cloned [10]. Although the UGT1A4 cDNA, which was cloned at the same time, encoded a protein that had a low bilirubin UGT activity *in vitro*, it has become evident that UGT1A1 is the major bilirubin UGT in humans. This is surprising in light of the aforementioned number of different human UGTs and their considerable overlap of substrate specificities. The initial studies of unconjugated hyperbilirubinemia in patients with Crigler–Najjar type 1 disease, which are characterized by a complete loss of bilirubin glucuronidation, provided evidence for coding region mutations within exons 2, 3, and 4 of the *UGT1A* gene locus (Figure 3.3 and Table 3.1) [17, 28, 29]. Mutant alleles of the common *UGT1A* exons 2–5 affect all transcripts generated by the *UGT1A* locus, both hepatic and extrahepatic, and this was viewed as the reason for the complete absence of bilirubin glucuronide formation in Crigler–Najjar disease type 1. In addition, the Gunn rat represented a model with the analogous features [71]. The detection of exon 1 mutations in Crigler–Najjar type 2 disease, characterized by a decrease of bilirubin conjugation activity to below 30%, but not its complete absence, appeared to confirm this hypothesis [31]. However, the discovery of mutations in the first exon of *UGT1A1* in patients with Crigler–Najjar type 1 disease [37] has demonstrated that this can result in the selective inactivation of UGT1A1 and a complete absence of bilirubin conjugation in humans despite the considerable redundancy of catalytic activity and tissue-specific expression of human UGT gene products. This finding is significant for two reasons: (i) it confirms that UGT1A1 is the only biologically relevant bilirubin UGT and that none of the unaffected *UGT1A* or *UGT2B* genes can substitute for this activity, and (ii) no alternative pathway exists for the effective detoxification and elimination of bilirubin in humans, with perhaps the exception of the much less-effective generation of hydrophilic lumirubin by photoisomeration. Consequently, the *UGT1A1* gene has moved to the center of attention in unconjugated hyperbilirubinemia. To date, 113 variant allelic genotypes have been identified (UGT1A1*1–UGT1A1*113). When functions of the *UGT1A1* gene are considered, it is important to keep in mind that in Crigler–Najjar type 1 as well as in type 2 disease variant alleles can affect all five exons. For the hyperbilirubinemic phenotype, homozygous or compound heterozygous mutant alleles are required. The alteration of an individual exon 1 would affect only this specific isoform, whereas an alteration of any of the exons 2–5 would affect the entire group of UGT1A enzymes because this portion is present in all UGT1A gene transcripts as delineated above. More than 45 of the UGT1A1 variants have been identified in the exon 2–5 region, which also implicates their potential effect on glucuronidation by all other proteins encoded by the *UGT1A* gene locus and therefore for glucuronidation throughout the body in general. Based on the complexity of this organization and its variants it is important to realize that Gilbert's syndrome represents one end of a spectrum that continuously extends to the most severe phenotype of Crigler–Najjar disease type 1, which is fatal and completely lacks bilirubin glucuronidation and UGT1A1 activity [9] (Figure 3.3).

3.7
UGT1A1 Gene

UGT1A1 is the only physiological enzyme capable of forming water-soluble bilirubin glucuronides [72], which then undergo biliary or renal elimination from the body. Bilirubin itself is not water-soluble and cannot be excreted. Apart from bilirubin glucuronidation, UGT1A1 has several other endogenous and exogenous substrates [15]. These include 2-hydroxy-estrone and estradiol, and a number of therapeutic drugs such as ethinylestradiol, gemfibrozil, metabolites of irinotecan, simvastatin, and buprenorphine. Furthermore, mutagenic xenobiotics such as *N*-OH-PhIP (PhIP = 2-amino-1-methyl-6-phenylimidazo[4,5-*b*]pyridine) and benzo[*a*]pyrenes undergo conjugation and detoxification by UGT1A1 [73]. Based on these functional considerations, alterations in UGT1A1 activity are capable of modulating drug metabolism and the disposition towards environmental mutagens. The significance of this is evident when the number of genetic UGT1A1 variants is considered: to date 113 variants have been reported, which lead to differing degrees of functional variation (Table 3.1). The best studied is UGT1A1*28 which leads to a $A(TA)_7TAA$ promoter sequence differing from the more prevalent $A(TA)_6TAA$. This reduces *UGT1A1* transcription by 70% [12]. UGT1A1*$28^{+/+}$ is found in 12% of Scottish [74], 16% of European [12], 12% of Indian [75], 8% of Egyptian [58], and 23% of African-American subjects [40]. In China and Japan, the frequencies are lower [75, 76]. A promoter variant comprising seven TA repeats is not the only permutation detected. The UGT1A1*36 variant exhibits $A(TA)_5TAA$, leading to an increase in UGT1A1 transcription; the UGT1A1*37 exhibits $A(TA)_8TAA$, leading to reduced transcription and has been associated with Crigler–Najjar disease type 2 [40]. These findings suggest an inverse association of the number of TA repeats with the transcriptional activity of the *UGT1A1* promoter. The differing UGT1A1*28 frequencies in geographically and evolutionary distinct populations suggests that there is ethnic diversity. This is further substantiated by the finding of variants such as UGT1A1*6 (leading to G71R in exon 1) [30], UGT1A1*7 (Y486D in exon 1) [30], UGT1A1*27 (P229Q in exon 1) [39], and UGT1A1*62 (F83L in exon 1) in Asians – although occurring only at frequencies of 1–3% – and not in Caucasoids or Africans [77]. These data show that the Gilbert's phenotype is not only associated with the frequent Caucasoid genotype UGT1A1*28, but is also reported to occur with evolutionary conserved and distinct variants, including UGT1A1*27 [39], UGT1A1*29 [39], UGT1A1*60 [41], UGT1A1*64–70 [43, 44], and UGT1A1*72–73 [44, 78], which affect exons 1, 2, 3, 4, the *UGT1A1* promoter, and intron 2 (Table 3.1). In most carriers of these variants *in vivo* enzymatic UGT1A1 activity is reduced, in UGT1A1*36 it is increased, and in UGT1A1*68–73 no differences were detectable [40, 44, 78]. *UGT1A1* regulation and function (variant protein sequence and activity level) are therefore fine tuned by a considerable variety of possible variants in humans (Table 3.4). However, these data only show one side of the coin. The real challenge is the presence of haplotypes including more than one of these genetic variations. Haplotypes including the common UGT1A1*28 (promoter) allele as well as UGT1A1*27 (exon 1), variation at −3279(T>G), and UGT1A1*91–93 (promoter) have been identified showing that promoter SNPs and coding variants can coexist in the same patient [79]. This explains in part why the clinical phenotype of hyperbilirubinemia is generally observed in about 5–9% of the general Caucasoid population, while 10–16% are homozygous for UGT1A1*28. This also has implications for the prediction of drug toxicity based on only one pharmacogenetic marker such as UGT1A1*28. Among this group of individuals the association with other genetic *UGT1A1* variants will modulate the phenotype of observable GMS and under drug treatment with compounds targeted for glucuronidation will affect the severity of a potential disposition to toxic side-effects. To render the issue even more complex, these associations will include haplotypes including *UGT1A* genes other than *UGT1A1*, which has been shown for the association of SNPs of *UGT1A1*, *UGT1A3*, *UGT1A6*, and *UGT1A7* [48, 57–60]. Recent studies furthermore suggest that individual SNPs in a specific *UGT1A* gene influence the activities of other genes. This has been reported for the UGT1A1*7 variant (exon 5 effect) as well as for the combination of promoter as well as coding region SNPs of *UGT1A1*, *UGT1A3*, and *UGT1A7* [60, 77, 80, 81].

3.8 Is There an Advantage or Risk Associated with *UGT1A1* Variability?

In view of the high allelic frequency of homozygous or compound heterozygous genetic variants of the *UGT1A1* gene worldwide it is an interesting evolutionary question whether their inheritance confers an advantage for the carriers (Table 3.5). The vast majority of reports describe risk constellations associated with the

Table 3.5 *UGT1A1* genetic variants and potential for disease disposition.

UGT1A1 variant	Disease association	Comment	Reference
Risk factor for disease disposition			
UGT1A1*6	CRC	increased risk of CRC with additional UGT1A7*3 variant (OR 2.34)	[82]
UGT1A1*6	development of metastases in CRC	increased risk of metastases with additional UGT1A7*3 variant (OR 6.83)	[82]
UGT1A1*28	gall stones	UGT1A1*28 in patients with cystic fibrosis increases risk	[83]

Table 3.5 (*Continued*)

UGT1A1 variant	Disease association	Comment	Reference
UGT1A1*28	gall stones	homozygous UGT1A1*28 and spherocytosis increases risk (no control group in study)	[84]
UGT1A1*28	gall stones	each TA repeat increases bilirubin by 21% and cholelithiasis by 87% in patients with sickle cell disease; no effect of hemoxigenase 1; risk of pigment gall stones increased	[85, 86]
Potential risk factor for disease disposition			
UGT1A1*28	breast cancer (especially estrogen receptor-negative) in premenopausal women	no association in whites	[87, 88]
UGT1A1*28	breast cancer in women <40 years	no association with estrogen receptor status	[89]
UGT1A1*28 UGT1A1 haplotypes	endometrial cancer	no overall association but trend towards an inverse association of UGT1A1*28 and endometrial cancer	[90]
Protective factor in disease disposition			
UGT1A1*28	endometrial cancer	decreased risk of cancer, strongest association in premenopausal women (OR 0.39)	[91]
UGT1A1*28	Hodgkin's lymphoma	presence of the UGT1A1*28 allele increases overall survival (RR 2.54), freedom from progression (RR 2.7), and time to treatment failure (RR 2.37)	[92]
UGT1A1*28 (bilirubin levels)	intermittent claudication	association of variant with hyperbilirubinemia and low bilirubin with increased intermittent claudication, no association with variant directly	[93]
UGT1A1*28	cardiovascular disease	conditional linkage analysis based on cardiovascular disease, bilirubin levels, and TA repeats in UGT1A1: TA repeats appear as likely key position for risk	[94]
UGT1A1*28	coronary heart disease	Framingham study data: hyperbilirubinemia and homozygous UGT1A1*28 has two-thirds lower risk of coronary heart disease (and cardiovascular disease)	[95]

RR, risk ratio.

presence of GMS, but unconjugated hyperbilirubinemia has also been studied and proposed to represent a protective factor.

3.9
UGT1A1 Gene and Pharmacogenetic Protection

3.9.1
Cardiovascular Disease

Hemoxigenase-1 and bilirubin have been suggested to exert vasodilator and antioxidant actions, respectively, which are believed to reduce the effects and development of atherosclerosis [96]. Higher bilirubin levels have been found to be associated with a lower atherosclerosis and cancer risk, but also with a higher risk of neurological abnormalities [93, 97]. In the Framingham Heart Study higher bilirubin levels and the presence of the UGT1A1*28 allele were associated with a lower risk of cardiovascular disease [95], which may be an effect of the mentioned antioxidant properties. In an animal model it was recently shown that the inhibition of bilirubin metabolism by indinavir attenuated angiotensin II-mediated hypertension in mice, thereby linking hyperbilirubinemia to hypertension as one of the major risk factors for cardiovascular disease [98]. From these data a genetic advantage regarding one of the major causes of death in man may be associated with mild hyperbilirubinemia present in individuals with GMS. The modulation of bilirubin levels may therefore represent an attractive potential therapeutic target for future drug intervention strategies for cardiovascular diseases [94, 99]. Herbal preparations can exert inhibitory effects on UGT1A1 activity [100]. However, a recent study also showed that citrus fruit reduced bilirubin levels in women with UGT1A1*28 [101]. These effects and potential drug interventions still require more studies [102, 103].

3.9.2
Cancer

Antioxidant mechanisms are attractive candidates for the modulation of neoplastic initiation. It is therefore plausible to speculate whether the presence of higher levels of bilirubin and lower activities of the bilirubin transferase may protect from malignancy (Table 3.5). In a case control study in 2004, lower UGT1A1 activity represented by UGT1A1*28 was associated with a lower risk of endometrial cancer [91]. The same authors recently showed that *UGT1A1* variants did not lead to an increased risk of endometrial cancer with a trend towards protection [90]. In Hodgkin's lymphoma, which is usually a well treatable malignancy, a study analyzing 313 patients for glutathione *S*-transferase (GST), cytochrome P450 (CYP), and *UGT1A1* variants found an association of the UGT1A1*28 allele with a superior prognosis indicating that UGT1A1*28 may influence the prognosis in Hodgkin's lymphoma [92]. The exact mechanisms of these association studies need to be elucidated and the associations replicated, but they provide intriguing examples of potentially protective properties of Gilbert's syndrome that may explain the evolutionary conservation of these genetic variants and their prevalent frequency.

3.10 *UGT1A1* Gene and Pharmacogenetic Risks

3.10.1 Disposition to Drug Toxicity

A more immediate impact of GMS has emerged in recent years regarding pharmacotherapy with drugs that exhibit a narrow therapeutic spectrum as well as commonly prescribed and used drugs, which thus have a high potential for unwanted side-effects (Table 3.6). This significance of GMS and its associated variants carries a considerable potential for patient morbidity, utilization of medical resources, drug development, and economic impact.

UGT1A1 is involved in the glucuronidation of commonly used pharmaceuticals, which include gemfibrocil, ezetimibe, simvastatin, atorvastatin, cerivastatin, ethinylestradiol, buprenorphine, ibuprofen, and ketoprofen [111–114, 116, 117, 119]. GMS may also play a role in drug treatment with drugs such as ribavirin that lead to hemolysis, because of the inherently reduced glucuronidation capacity of ensuing bilirubin [118]. A prominent example is the anticancer drug irinotecan [55, 104, 120].

Regarding the pharmacogenetics of Gilbert's disease and drug side-effects, there are two examples with a potential to influence the future administration of drugs and potentially the drug licensing process: irinotecan, the 7-ethyl-10-hydroxycamptothecin (SN-38) metabolite of which is a UGT substrate, and atazanavir, which is not a substrate for glucuronidation, but nevertheless conveys a significant risk of unwanted jaundice by means of UGT inhibition. They are examples of a direct and an indirect pharmacogenetic influence of *UGT1A1* variants on drug safety.

3.10.1.1 Irinotecan Toxicity

Irinotecan (camptothecin) represents a standard treatment option for metastatic colorectal cancer (CRC) and other solid tumors. The prodrug irinotecan is converted to SN-38 by ubiquitously expressed carboxylesterases. SN-38 has a 100-fold higher antitumor activity [121]. SN-38 is mainly inactivated by UGT1A proteins, which generate nontoxic SN-38 glucuronides that are eliminated via bile and urine [122]. Irinotecan has a narrow therapeutic range, and leads to side-effects such as myelosuppression (mainly leukopenia and thrombocytopenia) and diarrhea [123] observed in 29–44% of patients [124], and often resulting in the necessity to discontinue or lower the dose of the drug.

Based on irinotecan detoxification by UGT1A1 these side-effects have been linked to genetic variations of UGT activity present in GMS (UGT1A1*28) [104–

Table 3.6 GMS and unwanted drug reactions.

		References
GMS	UGT1A1*28 (main variant in white population)	[12, 74]
	hyperbilirubinemia (genome-wide association study)	[70, 94]
Established toxicity reactions	irinotecan risk alleles:	[80, 104–106]
	UGT1A1*28 (A(TA)$_7$TAA), UGT1A7*3 (N129K/R131K/W208R), UGT1A7*12 (–57T>G) main risk allele in Japanese: UGT1A1*6 (211 G>A)	[107]
	atazanavir risk alleles: UGT1A1*28 (A(TA)$_7$TAA), UGT1A3*2a (–66T>C), UGT1A7*3 (N129K/R131K/W208R), UGT1A7*12 (–57T>G)	[60, 108]
	indinavir risk alleles: UGT1A1*28 (A(TA)$_7$TAA), UGT1A3*2a (–66T>C), UGT1A7*3 (N129K/R131K/W208R), UGT1A7*12 (–57T>G)	[108–110]
UGT1A1 substrates (potential risk?)	gemfibrozil[a)]	[111]
	ezetimibe	[112]
	simvastatin, atorvastatin, cerivastatin[a)]	[113]
	ethinylestradiol	[114]
	buprenorphine	[115]
	fulvestrant	[116]
	ibuprofen, ketoprofen	[117]
	interferon + ribavirin	[118]
Nutritional impact on UGT1A1	increase of UGT1A1 activity in women with UGT1A1*28 by citrus fruit and Rutaceae	[101]
	kampo and Japanese medicinal herbs inhibit SN-38 and β-estradiol-3 glucuronidation	[100]

a) A severe drug reaction due to the inhibition of glucuronidation (UGT1A1) and CYP2C8 and CYP2C9 when both drugs were combined led to the withdrawal of cerivastatin [111].

106, 125]. However, regarding the predisposition for irinotecan toxicity by UGT1A1*28, conflicting results have been reported. In one study with 66 patients, UGT1A1*28 variants were not found to predict all cases of irinotecan-associated neutropenia [105]. Rouits *et al.* demonstrated in a cohort of 75 patients that UGT1A1*28 had an impact on irinotecan-induced neutropenia, but not on gastrointestinal toxicity, whereas Marcuello *et al.* observed in 95 irinotecan-treated patients a significant association between UGT1A1*28 and diarrhea, but not neutropenia [126, 127]. Moreover, Carlini *et al.* failed to observe an association between irinotecan-induced side-effects and UGT1A1*28, and conversely reported an opposing trend based on six patients with GMS without any observed adverse event [128]. These studies suggested that additional factors may contribute to the estimation of irinotecan toxicity, possibly owing to additional UGT1A proteins with SN-38 activity. In addition, it has become obvious that the dose of irinotecan is relevant [129]. There is also racial diversity and in Japanese patients UGT1A1*6 appears to be a major risk factor in particular for neutropenia [107].

The UGT1A7 protein exhibits an about 5-fold higher specific activity with SN-38 than UGT1A1 [55, 130]. SNPs at the *UGT1A7* gene locus alter enzyme activity and/or transcription [50, 51, 55]. It has also been shown in Gunn rats that intestinal UGTs and not only hepatic UGTs such as UGT1A1 appear to be critical for irinotecan-induced toxicity [131]. Reported analyses of the *UGT1A7* gene sequence have identified three SNPs in the coding region at base pair positions 129, 131 (UGT1A7 N129K R131K) and 208 (W208R), which result in functionally altered UGT1A7*3 protein variants with a reduced glucuronidation activity [50, 51]. In addition, UGT1A7*12 (UGT1A7-57T/G, TATA-box variant) leads to a 70% reduction of transcriptional activity [55] and UGT1A7*12 was found to occur in linkage disequilibrium with UGT1A7*3 (W208R). SNP association studies further showed an association of homozygous UGT1A7*12 in 75% with homozygous UGT1A1*28 [55]. Against this background a recent study demonstrated that the combination of variants of *UGT1A1* and *UGT1A7* can be used to predict irinotecan toxicity [80]. In a low-dose irinotecan treatment study with 105 genotyped CRC patients, an association of toxicity with UGT1A1*28 alone was not detected, whereas *UGT1A7* variants alone were associated with diarrhea, thrombocytopenia, and dose reductions. When the markers were combined the haplotype was superior for the prediction of thrombocytopenia, leukocytopenia, and drug dose reductions in this study. In a different study, *UGT1A7* was also identified as a marker for toxicity in irinotecan patients [81]. These data may help to explain the controversial results obtained with the analysis of UGT1A1*28 alone and demonstrate that a combination of markers may improve toxicity prediction. However, now that genotyping for UGT1A1*28 and other variants is widely available [132] prospective studies with different dose regimens are required to conclusively answer the question of the role of genotyping before irinotecan therapy. In clinical practice, genotyping can be performed by sequencing or more conveniently by TaqMan® allelic discrimination [132]; the commercially available INVADER® assay has been approved by the US Food and Drug Administration. From an interventional point of view it will be interesting to develop strategies to induce glucuronidation activity, which has been recently shown to occur by coffee exposure even in the presence of the GMS polymorphisms [133].

3.10.1.2 Jaundice in Protease Inhibitor Therapy (Atazanavir and Indinavir)

Hyperbilirubinemia is frequently observed in patients during treatment with antiretroviral protease inhibitors (i.e., atazanavir or indinavir) [108, 109]. In many instances drug reactions occur when a single enzyme/pathway is the primary route of elimination of a drug such as in irinotecan toxicity. In the case of atazanavir the drug is not a significant substrate for glucuronidation, but is capable of inhibiting UGT proteins, which include UGT1A1, UGT1A3, and UGT1A4 [134].

In the presence of the UGT1A1*28 variant atazanavir-treated patients were shown to develop variable degrees of hyperbilirubinemia, linking this toxic reaction to GMS [108]. In a study of 106 HIV-positive patients treated with atazanvir all subjects were genotyped and jaundice associated with the presence of UGT1A1*28, UGT1A3*2 as well as with UGT1A7*12 and UGT1A7*3 [60]. UGT1A1*28 alone was found to be a poor predictor of atazanvir-associated jaundice. However, when all five individual SNPs were combined, the probability of jaundice was well predicted. This example identifies a haplotype of variants of the *UGT1A1*, *UGT1A3*, and *UGT1A7* genes, which includes the UGT1A1*28 GMS variant. When these five variants were present as a homozygous trait, hyperbilirubinemia exceeded 85 μmol/l (World Health Organization grade 4) in atazanavir-treated patients. Homozygous carriers of all five variants amount to 9.6% of the white population, which is just below the prevalence of GMS (16%) and represents a significant proportion of the population who carry this risk haplotype. These data demonstrate that the side-effects of atazanavir treatment are associated with the presence of a haplotype of five functional UGT variants spanning three *UGT1A* genes, which are found among the group of GMS patients. It also shows that inhibition of UGT enzymes (e.g., by immunosuppressants and protease inhibitors) is an important mechanism of unwanted side-effects, which is aggravated in the presence of activity-reducing genetic variants [60]. A similar association was recently observed in a second study that analyzed patients who developed jaundice during indinavir therapy, which confirms the potentially predictive role of this haplotype [110]. In view of the ongoing licensing process of new-generation anti-hepatitis C virus drugs, the protease inhibitor-associated hyperbilirubinemia is likely to be of continued significance. In addition, complex associations of UGT1A1*28 with numerous other genes are a possibility that requires further analyses [13, 135].

3.11 *UGT1A1* Variability and Cancer Risk

UGT1A1 is capable of glucuronidating estrogens as well as benzo[*a*]pyrene metabolites [136, 137]. Reduced glucuronidation of estrogens and mutagens in tissues carrying UGT1A1*28 promoter variants is therefore hypothesized to influence the development of hormone- as well as carcinogen-associated diseases such as neoplastic transformation.

3.11.1
CRC

In a case control study the risk for developing CRC was associated with UGT1A1*6 (G71R in exon 1). The analysis of 268 Chinese patients with CRC compared to 441 control subjects identified an odd's ratio (OR) of 2.03 in individuals carrying the UGT1A1*6 variant [82]. A combination of UGT1A1*6 with UGT1A7 variants increased the OR to 2.34 in that study [82].

3.11.2
Breast Cancer

In a case control study with 200 patients, a 1.8-fold increase of invasive breast cancer risk was reported for postmenopausal women with UGT1A1*28 [87], which was not confirmed in a later larger study involving 455 patients [88]. Interestingly, a later study reported a reduced breast cancer risk associated with UGT1A1*28 [138]. Geographically determined variability becomes evident in a large Chinese study of 1047 patients that associated UGT1A1*28 with an elevated breast cancer risk in women under 40 years of age, irrespective of estrogen receptor status [89]. However, this study looked only at UGT1A1*28, but not at the other low-frequency alleles present in Asians.

These examples of case control studies analyzing the risk of neoplastic disease related to genetic variation of UGT1A1*28 show that a single variable is not likely to conclusively predict the true risk, and that *UGT1A1* variants – although conferring a low individual risk disposition – require future haplotype and multigene analyses. These should take additional factors into account that are independent of genetic background, such as age and, in cases of breast cancer, hormone receptor status.

3.12
UGT1A3 Gene

The activity of the UGT1A3 gene product has been determined by cloning and recombinant expression in cell culture [139]. It is expressed in the intestine and to a lower degree in the liver [18]. Expression levels in the stomach and the large intestine are also lower [21, 22]. Catalytic activity studies demonstrate a substrate spectrum, which includes xenobiotics such as polyaromatic hydrocarbons including hydroxylated benzo[*a*]pyrenes [139], amines [140], nonsteroidal anti-inflammatory drugs such as ibuprofen, flurbiprofen, and ketoprofen [117], statins [113], flavonoids [140], bile acids [141], estrogens [47], vitamin D derivatives [142], ezetimibe [112], and the platelet-derived growth factor receptor tyrosine kinase inhibitor 6,7-(dimethoxy-2,4-dihydroindeno[1,2-*c*]pyrazol-3-yl)-(3-fluoro-phenyl)-amine [143].

Genetic polymorphisms located within the *UGT1A3* gene exon 1 sequence (UGT1A3*2, UGT1A3*3) have been identified [45–47] and found to lead to functional alterations of the expressed UGT1A3 protein [47] (Table 3.2). The identified SNP variants W11R and V47A were found to occur in Caucasians with a frequency between 35 and 44%. Based on the activity profile and the high frequency of variants in the general Caucasoid population, a role for drug metabolism and possibly for cancer disposition would appear plausible. So far, a study with 258 hepatocellular carcinomas (HCCs) and 470 healthy control subjects failed to find an association [46]. However, *UGT1A3* promoter and coding exon variants are part of the *UGT1A* haplotype predisposing to jaundice in atazanavir- and indinavir-treated individuals [60, 110] (Tables 3.2 and 3.6). The UGT1A3*2 variant has recently been linked to increased atorvastatin lactonization *in vivo* [144].

3.13 *UGT1A7* Gene

The UGT1A7 cDNA was cloned in 1997 [22] following the analysis of UGT1A expression in liver and the gastrointestinal tract [19–21, 23, 145]. UGT1A7 is not expressed in human liver, but transcripts are detected in orolaryngeal tissue, esophagus, stomach, and pancreas. The hypothesis of these analyzes was the assumption that glucuronidation would represent an important metabolic feature not only of the liver, but also of the mucosal barrier of the gastrointestinal tract, and would therefore be specifically regulated to perform organ-specific glucuronidation requirements at the point of entry of xenobiotic material. In line with the exclusively extrahepatic UGT1A7 expression profile in epithelial tissues of the gastrointestinal tract with direct contact to extrinsic food-borne materials and compounds, UGT1A7 exhibits an activity spectrum encompassing numerous xenobiotics. UGT1A7 catalyzes the glucuronidation of phenols, anthraquinones, flavones, naphthol structures, and coumarin structures [19, 137, 146]. Importantly, UGT1A7 forms glucuronides and leads to the detoxification of mutagens including polyaromatic hydrocarbons such as hydroxylated benzo[*a*]pyrenes and heterocyclic amines such as PhIP [19, 137, 146], which have epidemiologically been identified as human carcinogens for a variety of cancers [147–151]. UGT1A7 is also a major transferase for the glucuronidation of the irinotecan metabolite SN-38 [55, 130]. *UGT1A7* variants and the risk in drug therapy is discussed above (*UGT1A1* gene) in the context of *UGT1A* risk haplotypes [55, 60, 80, 110]. A role for chemical carcinogenesis based on the detoxification of mutagens and procarcinogens by glucuronidation has been suggested by a number of studies [152–157], and has recently been further pursued in a genome-wide association analysis (bladder carcinoma) [158] as an interesting hypothesis (Table 3.7). In HCC the downregulation of UGT1A mRNA and protein expression was reported leading to the reduction of benzo[*a*]pyrene metabolite glucuronidation [178]. However, these

Table 3.7 UGT1A variants and disease association studies.

UGT isoform	UGT variant	Base change (amino acid change)	Tumor association	OR	Population	Study scale (patients/ controls)	Comment	Reference
UGT1A1	*6	211 G>A (G71R)	CRC	2.03	Taiwanese	n = 268/441	increased risk of CRC with additional UGT1A7*3 variant (OR 2.34)	[82]
			development of metastases in CRC	4.90	Taiwanese	n = 268/441	increased risk of metastases with additional UGT1A7*3 variant (OR 6.83)	[82]
	*28	$-52(TA)_7$	breast cancer (especially estrogen receptor-negative) in premenopausal women	1.80	African-Americans	n = 200/200	no association in Caucasians (n = 455/609)	[87, 88]
			breast cancer in women <40 years	1.70	Chinese	n = 1047/1083	no association with estrogen receptor status	[89]
			decreased risk of endometrial cancer	0.72	US-American	n = 222/666	strongest association in premenopausal women (OR 0.39)	[91]
UGT1A3			no association with cancer reported to date				no association with HCC in German Caucasoid population (n = 80/82)	[46]
UGT1A4			no association with cancer reported to date				no association with HCC in German Caucasoid population (n = 71/83), no significant association with cancer in Japanese population (n = 88/60)	[46, 159]

(Continued)

Table 3.7 (*Continued*)

UGT isoform	UGT variant	Base change (amino acid change)	Tumor association	OR	Population	Study scale (patients/controls)	Comment	Reference
UGT1A6	*2/*3		no association with cancer reported to date				no association with CRC in Caucasian population ($n = 371/415$)	[53]
		541 A>G/552 A>C (T181A/R184S)	decreased risk of colon adenoma in aspirin users	0.66	US-American	$n = 474/563$, $n = 1062$	no association in non-aspirin users; no significant association in UK group ($n = 500$) for aspirin/nonsteroidal anti-inflammatory drug users	[160–162]
			reduced risk of recurrence of colorectal neoplasia	RR 0.68	Caucasian	$n = 546$	no effect of aspirin intake	[163]
UGT1A7	*2 and/or *3	387 T>G/391 C>A (/622 T>C)	CRC	2.0	Caucasian	$n = 371/415$	association found for age- and gender-matched control and cancer groups	[53]
			liver cirrhosis	5.23	Taiwanese	$n = 263/159$	higher OR (7.50) for advanced liver cirrhosis (Child–Pugh B/C)	[164]
			HCC	1.50		$n = 217/291$	highest OR (3.06) for low-activity genotypes	[165]
		(−57 T>G/) 387 T>G/391 C>A (/622 T>C)	HCC in hepatitis B carriers	4.95 (*2) 1.45 (*3)	Korean	$n = 244/314$ (+223 HBV-positive patients)	association between UGT1A7*2 and HCC only in the absence of additional polymorphisms at bp −341 and bp 756; increased HCC risk for haplotype other than wild-type (OR 1.67 for heterozygous, OR 1.85 for homozygous)	[166]

*3	387 T>G/391 C>A/622 T>C	proximal gastrointestinal tract cancer	2.02	German Caucasian	$n = 76/210$		[167]
		CRC	2.75	German Caucasian	$n = 78/210$	genotyping data deviates from Hardy–Weinberg equilibrium	[51]
		development of metastases in CRC	4.90	Taiwanese	$n = 268/441$	increased risk of metastases with additional UGT1A1*6 variant (OR 6.83), in combination also increased risk of CRC (OR 2.34)	[82]
		HCC	1.52	German Caucasian	$n = 107/270$	association with HCC in male cohort without viral hepatitis; OR lower than in earlier study with smaller HCC/control group ($n = 59/70$); no association in HCC patients with viral hepatitis	[168], and unpublished data [169])
		HCC	3.4	French Caucasian	$n = 165/142$	association between UGT1A7*3/*3 genotype and HCC only in patients with viral hepatitis	[170]
		pancreatic cancer	1.98	Caucasian	$n = 52/235$	initial pancreas study: genotyping deviates from Hardy–Weinberg equilibrium; no association found in larger study ($n = 236/1409$) or Italian cohort ($n = 61/105$)	[54, 145, 169, 171]
		lung cancer	4.02	Japanese	$n = 113/178$	association applies to homozygous UGT1A7*3 carriers only	[172]

(Continued)

Table 3.7 (*Continued*)

UGT isoform	UGT variant	Base change (amino acid change)	Tumor association	OR	Population	Study scale (patients/controls)	Comment	Reference
	*2 and/or *3 and/or *4	(387 T>G/391 C>A) (/622 T>C)	CRC	1.59	Chinese	$n = 140/280$	highest association with alcohol drinking (OR 3.14) and cigarette smoking (OR 3.39)	[173]
	*3/*3, *3/*4, *4/*4	(387 T>G/391 C>A/) 622 T>C genotypes correspond to low-activity variants	orolaryngeal cancer	6.2 2.8	African-American and Caucasian	$n = 194/388$	highest risk for heavy smokers with low activity genotype, no effect of alcohol intake	[174]
			CRC (only with additional high intake of heterocyclic amines)	2.40	African-American and white	$n = 197/202$ $n = 203/210$	association with regard to heterocyclic amine intake	[175]
			HCC	2.33	Japanese	$n = 122/158$	all subjects were positive for hepatitis C	[176]
UGT1A8			no association with cancer reported to date				no association with CRC in Caucasoid population ($n = 371/415$)	[53]
UGT1A9			no association with cancer reported to date				no association with pancreatic cancer in Italian cohort ($n = 61/105$)	[171]
UGT1A10	*2	415 G>A (E139K)	decreased risk of orolaryngeal cancer	0.29	African-American	$n = 115/115$	no association of 730C>A (L244I) variant (1A10*4) with orolaryngeal cancer to be found in same study population (OR 0.94)	[177]

findings did not answer the question whether glucuronidation may be an initial permissive feature predisposing to the development of neoplastic transformation in a tissue exposed to mutagens. This hypothesis was more intensively studied, when low-carcinogen-metabolizing activity genetic variants of the *UGT1A7* gene were identified and characterized, namely UGT1A7*3 combining three amino acid substitutions in exon 1 (N129K/R131K and W208R) [50, 51]. A series of case control studies were reported that examined UGT1A7*3 in luminal gastrointestinal and HCC, known to develop in association with carcinogen exposure such as tobacco smoke-borne mutagens.

3.13.1 CRC

In 2002, in an initial study of 78 Caucasoid CRC patients without Amsterdam criteria and 210 healthy controls, an association with UGT1A7*3 detected by polymerase chain reaction (PCR) and direct resequencing was reported with an OR of 2.75 [51]. In this study the genotyping data obtained by PCR amplification and subsequent resequencing deviated from Hardy–Weinberg equilibrium possibly because of primer colocalization with an at-the-time unknown additional SNP [55, 169]. However, in a subsequent larger study with 474 CRC patients and 563 healthy controls, which also included variants of UGT1A1, UGT1A6, UGT1A8 as well as GST, genotyping with a different method (by PCR and restriction fragment length polymorphism (RFLP)) identified an age- and gender-adjusted risk associated with UGT1A7 variants (OR 2.4), as well as an influence of UGT1A6 variants [53]. Tang *et al.* described an OR of 4.9 in 268 Taiwanese CRC patients genotyped by RFLP for the development of metastases and also a CRC association with UGT1A1*6 as well as with combinations of UGT1A7 variants (including the −57T>G promoter variant) and UGT1A1*6 [82]. In African-Americans ($n = 197$) and American white ($n = 203$) cohorts the association with UGT1A7*3 determined by TaqMan PCR and RFLP was detectable when the group was stratified for heterocyclic amine intake [175]. In a Chinese study of 140 CRC patients the overall UGT1A7 variant association detected by RFLP and allele-specific PCR exhibited an OR of 1.59, but when alcohol consumption and cigarette smoking was taken into account the OR increased to 3.14 and 3.39, respectively [173]. These last two observations are particularly interesting regarding the initial hypothesis of a carcinogen metabolism-dependent carcinogenesis risk. Overall, UGT1A7*3 appears to represent a low risk factor allele for CRC in combination with environmental factors and also in combination with other polymorphic variants of the *UGT1A* genes.

3.13.2 HCC

A significant association of HCC of viral and nonviral etiology with UGT1A7*3 in 59 Caucasoid patients analyzed by PCR and resequencing was initially reported in

2001 [168]. In 2004, using the same methodology, 122 HCC patients with hepatitis C were analyzed leading to a similar association with an OR of 2.33 [176]. The methods used in both studies lead to genotyping results that deviate from Hardy–Weinberg equilibrium, which may be the result of SNP and amplication primer colocalization in the noncoding UGT1A7 region [55, 169]. In a later study with 217 Chinese patients genotyped by different methodology (PCR and RFLP), logistic regression identified male gender, hepatitis B virus infection, and low-activity *UGT1A7* genotypes (OR 3.06) as HCC risk factors [165]. In this study, UGT1A7*3 was associated with an earlier age of HCC manifestation in males. Regarding the different etiologies of HCC encompassing viral and nonviral underlying diseases, association studies have reported differential findings. In a French study of 165 HCC patients genotyped by 5′ nuclease allelic discrimination an association of UGT1A7*3 was identified only in patients with HCC related to chronic viral infection (OR 3.4) [170]. A similar association was found in a Korean study with 244 HCC patients with chronic hepatitis B infection, who were genotyped by PCR and resequencing to determine *UGT1A7* gene variant haplotypes and compared to 223 hepatitis B patients without HCC and 314 normal healthy controls [166]. In this cohort an OR of 1.45 for HCC development was reported in individuals with *UGT1A7* variant haplotypes. These data suggest that *UGT1A7* gene variants with low-carcinogen-metabolizing activity are a risk marker for HCC development in Caucasoid as well as Asian individuals, but that etiology and the selection of patient cohorts is essential. Further studies are required to elucidate the association of carcinogen-associated factors and their dimension in the overall risk for HCC – a tumor that in recent years has developed into a rapidly increasing health problem worldwide and remains difficult to predict in risk groups with chronic liver diseases.

3.13.3
Pancreatic Cancer

An association of UGT1A7*3 with pancreatic cancer was reported in 52 Caucasian patients in 2003 [145], but these findings were not reproduced in a larger multinational study with 236 patients with pancreatic cancer [54] and an Italian study with 61 patients [171]. Other *UGT1A* variants were also studied and failed to show significant associations. These data indicate that variants of the *UGT1A7* gene and other *UGT1A* polymorphisms do not appear to play a significant role as risk factor for pancreatic cancer.

In this context the issue of genotyping methodology has been discussed [169, 179]. The high frequency of variants at the *UGT1A* gene locus has the potential to influence primer-based genotyping strategies, when variants colocalize with primer binding areas potentially affecting the fidelity of the PCR amplification reactions and leading to an amplification bias. Some of the studies reported nearly a decade ago show that the genotyping results deviate from Hardy–Weinberg equilibrium apart from being studies on small cohorts [51, 145, 168, 176]. Later studies employing different methodology identified significant associations with

HCC with lower OR values. Genotyping in cancer patients has been reported utilizing a variety of approaches, which include PCR and resequencing, TaqMan PCR allelic discrimination, RFLP, and others. In view of the multitude of differing experimental approaches applied in the above-mentioned allelic association studies in cancer, the hypothesis of carcinogen metabolism and its genetically determined variability as a risk factor for neoplastic transformation is strongly suggested, although not relevant for all tumor types. The fact that studies report differing OR values, degrees of significance, and negative studies is also likely to be significantly influenced by evolutionary geographical factors and by the selection of patient cohorts with different risk factors, such as exposure to dietary, environmental, and tobacco smoke mutagens. In addition, it is being increasingly recognized that haplotypes of different markers detected simultaneously play an important role. A good example of variable risk factors is HCC, the etiology of which encompasses metabolic, toxic, genetic, and viral etiologies in addition to the presence of cirrhosis, indicating a diverse spectrum of potential factors contributing to carcinogenesis, and their relevance in the presence of alterations in xenobiotic metabolism by glucuronidation.

3.14 Transcriptional Regulation of *UGT1A* Genes

For future studies of UGT regulation and function, and to assess the impact of glucuronidation on metabolism in different physiological situations and during drug therapy, detailed knowledge of the signal transduction pathways and transcriptional regulation is required. This is of increased importance in view of the multitude of non-coding-region SNPs identified in the *UGT1A* gene locus, which may alter physiological control of glucuronidation (Figure 3.4) and may be significant for the discovery of drugable modulators of *UGT1A* transcription and activity.

3.15 Aryl Hydrocarbon Receptor/Aryl Hydrocarbon Receptor Nuclear Translocator Regulation of *UGT1A* Genes

Aryl hydrocarbon receptor (AhR)/AhR nuclear translocator (ARNT) regulation of drug-metabolizing enzymes has been intensively studied for the *CYP* genes. Evidence suggests that *UGT1A* genes are also transcriptionally activated by this pathway via xenobiotic-responsive elements (XREs) within *cis*-acting promoter elements of the individual *UGT1A* genes. AhR regulation of *UGT1A* expression was demonstrated in rats, in which a GCGTG core sequence was identified 134 bp upstream of the *UGT1A1* first exon [180]. The human *UGT1A4* (and other *UGT1As*) promoter exhibits identical motifs in proximity to the ATG codon. This suggests that this pathway of regulation has been conserved during evolution not

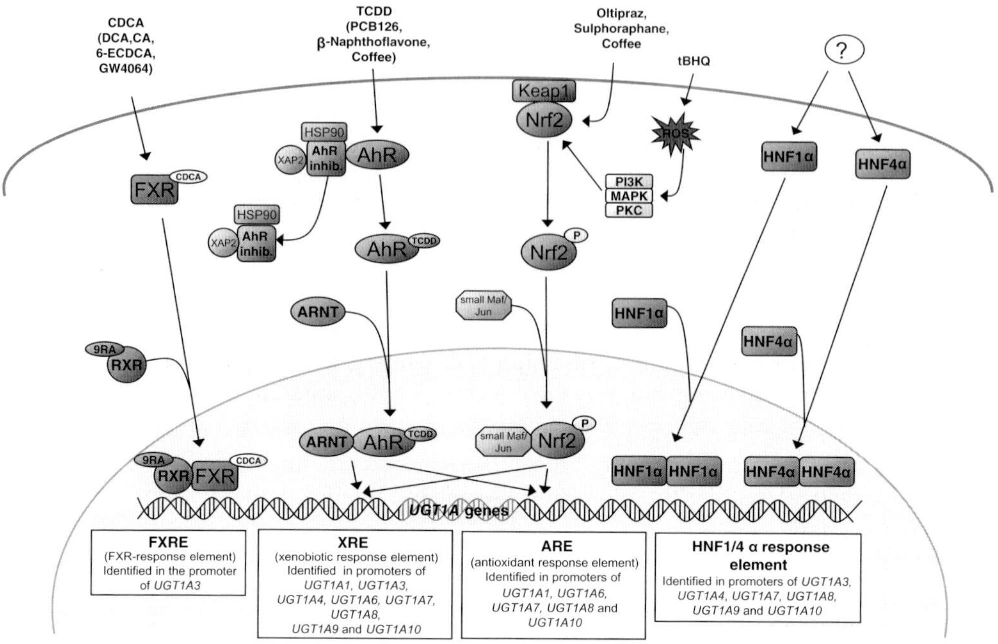

Figure 3.4 Graphic summary of transcriptional regulation of the *UGT1A* genes by FXR, AhR, Nrf2, and HNFs using their respective DNA-binding elements within *UGT1A* promoter sequence. Note that AhR and Nrf2 have been shown to each utilize both XREs as well as AREs.

only across different *UGT1A* genes, but also across species. In humans, AhR regulation has been demonstrated for *UGT1A6* [181, 182] and *UGT1A1* [183, 184]. Similar findings have also been reported for the rat *Ugt1a6* gene [185]. Xenobiotic inducibility of UGTs was first demonstrated in rodents [186] and had been debated in human glucuronidation because the induction experiment results were not reproducible in all laboratories. It was hypothesized to contrast the significant induction levels demonstrated for CYP regulation [187, 188]. A study on *UGT1A4* gene promoter function showed two SNPs located at –219(C>T) and –163(G>A) upstream of the ATG codon, and that activation by 2,3,7,8-tetrachlorodibenzo-*p*-dioxin (TCDD) was significantly reduced in individuals carrying a variant –163A/–219T genotype compared to those with the –163G/–219C genotype (wild-type) [61]. An analysis of the *UGT1A3* gene also demonstrated XRE-mediated regulation of transcription by AhR, indicating environmental stimuli-dependent responses of glucuronidation in man [189]. *UGT1A* genes are clearly activated by signal transduction involving AhR, and for some *UGT1A* genes an interaction between AhR and nuclear factor erythroid 2-related factor 2 (Nrf2) was described (see below).

3.16 Regulation by Hepatic Nuclear Factors

Hepatocyte nuclear factors (HNFs) play an important role in the activation of several *UGT1A* isoforms [190, 191]. By interacting with other transcription factors they appear to contribute to tissue-specific expression profiles. HNFs were first described in the liver, but are actually expressed in a variety of extrahepatic tissues [192, 193]. Depending on the cellular background, HNF-1α and HNF-4α are capable of binding to promoter elements of different genes [194]. Together with other transcription factors (such as HNF-6, small heterodimeric partner (SHP), or liver X receptor (LXR)) they are believed to participate in a complex regulatory network that controls tissue-specific expression of different genes [194]. HNF-1α and caudal-related homeodomain protein-2 (Cdx2) are involved in intestinal expression of *UGT1A8* and *UGT1A10* [195]. HNF-1α also plays a role for the regulation of *UGT1A3* [189]. HNF-1α and HNF-4α are also involved in the expression of liver-expressed *UGT1A9* [195–197], and a recent report indicates that *UGT1A7* is also regulated by shared HNF-1α and HNF-4α signal transduction [198]. In contrast to liver-expressed *UGT1A9*, transcriptional activation of *UGT1A7* by HNF-4α was found to be lower and dependent on higher HNF-4α concentrations, which may contribute to the observed tissue-specific expression patterns. In rats, activation of *Ugt1a7* by HNF-1 has also been described [199]. However, in contrast to the human homolog, rat *Ugt1a7* is expressed in the liver, suggesting an involvement of regulatory elements potentially different from those in humans.

3.17 Regulation by the Farnesoid X Receptor

A key mechanism of transcriptional regulation of bile acid homeostasis (and cholestasis) involves nuclear receptor proteins, which function as ligand-inducible transcription factors affecting CYP7A1, conjugating transferases, and ABC transporter protein expression. Activated nuclear receptors include the pregnane X receptor (PXR) [200], the vitamin D receptor (VDR) [201], the constitutive androstane receptor (CAR) [202, 203], and the farnesoid X receptor (FXR) [200], but bile acid also leads to an activation of the c-Jun N-terminal kinase (JNK) cascade [204, 205], the G-protein-coupled receptor TGR5 [206], and the regulation of the mitogen-activated protein kinase (MAPK) pathway [207]. Bile acids are substrates of UGT proteins leading to more hydrophilic and therefore less toxic bile acid glucuronides [141, 208–210]. UGT1A3 catalyzes the C24-glucuronidation of chenodeoxycholic acid (CDCA), lithocholic acid (LCA), and hyodeoxycholic acid (HDCA) by forming acyl glucuronides [141, 211]. Therefore, CDCA is a substrate for glucuronidation by UGT1A3 [141], which is expressed in the liver, intestine, and large bowel [18, 19, 22], representing a similar expression profile as FXR, which is present in the liver, intestine, kidney, and adrenal glands [212–214]. Regulation of *UGT1A3* and not the highly similar *UGT1A4* gene by *cis*-acting FXR elements was observed and found to be dependent on the presence of a SNP at −204 bp leading to an A>G change within the identified FXR responsive element half-site (BARE) [63]. Interestingly, this bile acid- and FXR-dependent regulation of *UGT1A3* provides a functional biochemical link of endogenous (bile acid) substrate metabolism with xenobiotic metabolism because *UGT1A3* is also a target gene for AhR-mediated regulation, which is associated with an XRE located at −35 to −40 bp [189]. It can be speculated that an additional activation of *UGT1A3* by xenobiotics and AhR would influence CDCA glucuronidation, impacting the feedback mechanisms of transcriptional control of CDCA glucuronidation by its substrate.

3.18
Regulation by Nuclear Factor Erythroid 2-Related Factor 2

The identification of *UGT1A* regulation by Nrf2 indicates an important role in oxidative and antioxidative defense mechanisms [215]. In the absence of antioxidants, the cytoplasmic transcription factor Nrf2 is bound to its inhibitor Keap1. Upon oxidative stress or by stimulation with antioxidants (e.g., sulforaphane or oltipraz) Nrf2 dissociates from Keap1, translocates into the nucleus, and binds as a heterodimer with small Maf proteins to DNA antioxidant response elements (ARE: TGACNNNGC) in the promoter of potential target genes [216–218]. Nrf2 mainly activates (upregulates) phase II enzymes, leading an increased elimination of reactive molecules. In mice, *Ugt1a1*, *Ugt1a5*, and *Ugt1a6* are regulated by Nrf2 [219]. In the human *UGT1A1* promoter, a functional ARE was identified adjacent to a phenobarbital response enhancer module at position −3431 [220]. Studies of the *UGT1A6* gene have showed that induction by AhR was dependent on a neighboring ARE site, which indicates that an involvement of Nrf2 is also relevant for AhR-mediated gene regulation [182]. Cross-talk between AhR and Nrf2 was confirmed by studies in Nrf2 knockout mice showing that the activation of different phase II enzymes including Ugt1a5 and Ugt1a9 by TCDD was abolished in $Nrf2^{-/-}$ mice [221]. Recently, the coordinated regulation between Nrf2 and AhR was shown for the human *UGT1A8* and *UGT1A10* genes. Transcriptional regulation of these two genes was directly dependent on the simultaneous presence of AhR and Nrf2, whereas AhR-mediated activation of the liver-expressed *UGT1A9* gene was independent of Nrf2 [133, 215].

3.19
Regulation by Splice Variants

As outlined above, the nine first exons can be combined with four common exons (exons 2–5) during the splicing process to produce UGT1A transcripts. Recently, a novel exon (exon 5b) was identified in the common shared region [222]. Exons 5a and 5b are alternatively spliced to generate two variant UGT1A proteins – the classical isoform 1 or UGT1A_i1 and the new isoform 2 or UGT1A_i2. This process potentially leads to the generation of 18 different proteins encoded at the *UGT1A* gene locus. With little exception the novel and classical transcripts are almost always coexpressed, but expression levels of the novel transcripts are usually lower. An isoform 2 protein lacks the characteristic hydrophobic transmembrane domain (residues 445–530) encoded by exon 5a. The 10-amino-acid sequence encoded by the newly discovered exon 5b contains a di-Lys motif, which may be responsible for retention in the endoplasmic reticulum, as well as four positively charged residues that may promote the interaction of the protein with negatively charged ER membranes. Despite a colocalization of the novel isoforms and as well as classical isoforms, *in vitro* experiments show that the i2 proteins are enzymatically inactive [222]. In addition, the i2 proteins reduce the activity of the classical UGT1A proteins by 15–79% [223]. This repressive effect is achieved by direct binding of i2 to i1 proteins, thereby generating inactive i1–i2 complexes that appear to act as dominant inhibitors with a negative effect only the velocity of the glucuronidation reaction [223]. Since the mRNA and proteins of the alternative UGT1A splice variants are differentially expressed in different human tissues, these splice mechanism variants may represent an additional possibility to modulate cellular responses to exo- and endogenous stimuli. In tumor tissue, there is a heterogeneous expression of i1 and i2 proteins, with decreased levels of i1 and i2 in colon cancer specimens and increased expression of i2 proteins in liver tumors. The differences in the expression pattern of i1 and i2 proteins may be relevant to human liver and colon cancer tumorigenesis [224].

3.20 Animal Models to Study *UGT1A* Genes

The Gunn rat – a mutant strain of the Wistar rat – was first described in 1938. Its liver lacks UGT1A1 activity because of the deletion of a single guanosine base in the *Ugt1a1* gene that results in a frameshift and premature stop codon [71, 225]. The unconjugated bilirubin concentration in serum of the Gunn rat is significantly higher than that of normal rats. In 1952, the Gunn rat was established as an animal model for human Crigler–Najjar type I disease [226]. Apart from lacking bilirubin glucuronidation, Gunn rats show a deficit of multiple hepatic glucuronidation activities, which include the glucuronidation of 3-methylcholanthrene-inducible phenolic substrates and digitoxigenin monodigitoxiside. In contrast, glucuronidation activity toward steroids, chloramphenicol, and morphine is relatively normal [227]. The Gunn rat contributed to the biochemical characterization of the unconjugated hyperbilirubinemia caused by mutations in the *Ugt1a* gene locus. Furthermore, the Gunn rat model is also useful for the development of therapeutic strategies for the treatment of congenital hyperbilirubinemia in patients with Crigler–Najjar type I disease. However, it is not evident if the results from experiments with the Gunn rat model can be transferred to man. Therefore, an animal model carrying a human *UGT1A* gene locus was required and, in 2005, a humanized transgenic *UGT1* mouse model (Tg-*UGT1*-mouse) exhibiting the entire human *UGT1* locus was developed by Chen *et al.* [183]. The expression of the nine *UGT1A* genes closely resembles the expression patterns of human tissues. The regulation of human *UGT1A*s by PXR, AhR, LXR, and peroxisome proliferator-activated receptor (PPAR)-α in Tg-UGT1-mice was shown by gene expression analyses [183, 228, 229]. Expanding on this model a $Ugt1^{-/-}$ mouse model was developed by interrupting mouse exon 4 sequence (*Ugt1a* gene locus). Newborn $Ugt1^{-/-}$ mice developed 40–60 times higher levels of unconjugated bilirubin than $Ugt1^{+/-}$ or wild-type mice. The extremely high bilirubin levels in $Ugt1^{-/-}$ mice are comparable to the levels observed in patients with Crigler–Najjar type 1 disease and are fatal in neonatal $Ugt1^{-/-}$ mice within the first 2 weeks of life. No Ugt1a mRNA expression is detectable in those mice, resulting in a complete absence of Ugt1a enzymes in liver microsomes. The loss of Ugt1a function in $Ugt1^{-/-}$ mice leads to a syndrome that can serve as a model to further investigate toxicity associated with unconjugated bilirubin and the impact of this disease in humans [230]. Finally, in 2010, humanized mice were developed that express the human *UGT1A* gene locus in an Ugt1-null background to improve predictions of human UGT1A-dependent drug clearance by excluding potential mouse-related Ugt1a interactions. Concurrently, humanized *UGT1A* mice were developed that express the Gilbert's UGT1A1*28 allele (Tg(UGT1A1*28)$Ugt1^{-/-}$ mice). The glucuronidation activity (V_{max}) for SN-38 was 5-fold decreased in Tg(UGT1A1*28) $Ugt1^{-/-}$ mice compared to wild-type TgUGT1A mice [231]. Thus, Tg(UGT1A1*28) $Ugt1^{-/-}$ mice can serve as a pharmacokinetic model to further investigate the effects of decreased UGT1A1 expression on drug metabolism. In the future it will be necessary to develop transgenic mice carrying complex haplotypes of *UGT1A* variants, and to study the effects on *UGT1A* signaling and transcriptional regulation.

3.21 Outlook

The human *UGT1A* gene locus has a unique organization, and a remarkable number and frequency of variant genotypes. Metabolism by glucuronidation is influenced by complex genotypes and signal transduction pathways, which are linked to the simple clinical phenotype of GMS. This together with Crigler–Najjar disease has been one of the driving forces of the investigation of *UGT1A* genes and gene products, their genetic variants, and their regulation. The evaluation of *UGT1A* alleles as markers of cancer risk prediction is ongoing. The improvement of drug safety and the future establishment of individualized pharmacotherapy depend on the identification and characterization of such risk constellations. So far, most research efforts have been undertaken to identify risk factors and their functional consequences by studying variant proteins with coding sequence alterations and variants of the sequence portions responsible for transcriptional regulation. It has been shown in a number of studies that the *UGT1A1* gene (and other

UGTs) is inducible, which includes nuclear receptor-mediated signaling [180, 191, 220, 232, 233]. Inducibility can be dependent on the presence of SNPs [61]. Induction in humans is clinically possible [133, 234, 235]. The further analysis of transcriptional regulation of the *UGT1A* genes will offer the potential for therapeutic intervention by identifying drugable inducers that could be administered in individuals at risk or coadministered with potentially side-effect-prone drugs. Suggestions to incorporate pharmacogenomic data such as the above-mentioned examples and tests into the drug-approval process are a first step, which will in future contribute to individualized therapy and risk assessment.

Acknowledgments

C.P.S. is supported by the Deutsche Forschungsgemeinschaft grants **TRR77 project A4** and **SFB621 project C3**.

References

1 Dutton, G.J. (1956) Uridine diphosphate glucuronic acid as glucuronyl donor in the synthesis of ester, aliphatic and steroid glucuronides. *Biochem. J.*, **64**, 693–701.

2 Dutton, G.J. and Storey, I.D. (1953) The isolation of a compound of uridine diphosphate and glucuronic acid from liver. *Biochem. J.*, **53**, xxxvii–xxxviii.

3 Dutton, G.J. (1961) The mechanism of glucuronide formation. *Biochem. Pharmacol.*, **6**, 65–71.

4 Burchell, B., Leakey, J., and Dutton, G.J. (1975) Relationship between activation of "detoxicating" enzymes in stored broken-cell preparations and in autolysing liver. *Enzyme*, **20**, 156–164.

5 Dutton, G.J., Leakey, J.E., and Pollard, M.R. (1981) Assays for UDPglucuronyltransferase activities. *Methods Enzymol.*, **77**, 383–391.

6 Gilbert, A. and Lereboullet, P. (1901) La cholamae simple familiale. *Sem. Med.*, **21**, 241–248.

7 Arias, I.M. (1962) Chronic unconjugated hyperbilirubinemia without signs of overt hemolysis in adolescents and adults. *J. Clin. Invest.*, **41**, 2233–2245.

8 Strassburg, C.P. (2010) Hyperbilirubinemia syndromes (Gilbert–Meulengracht, Crigler–Najjar, Dubin–Johnson, and Rotor syndrome). *Best Pract. Res. Clin. Gastroenterol.*, **24**, 555–571.

9 Strassburg, C.P. and Manns, M.P. (2000) Jaundice, genes and promoters. *J. Hepatol.*, **33**, 476–479.

10 Ritter, J.K., Crawford, J.M., and Owens, I.S. (1991) Cloning of two human liver bilirubin UDP-glucuronosyltransferase cDNAs with expression in COS-1 cells. *J. Biol. Chem.*, **266**, 1043–1047.

11 Ritter, J.K., Yeatman, M.T., Ferreira, P., and Owens, I.S. (1992) Identification of a genetic alteration in the code for bilirubin UDP-glucuronosyltransferase in the UGT1 gene complex of a Crigler–Najjar type I patient. *J. Clin. Invest.*, **90**, 150–155.

12 Bosma, P.J., Chowdhury, J.R., Bakker, C., Gantla, S., de Boer, A., Oostra, B.A., Lindhout, D., Tytgat, G.N., Jansen, P.L., Oude Elferink, R.P., *et al.* (1995) The genetic basis of the reduced expression of bilirubin UDP-glucuronosyltransferase 1 in Gilbert's syndrome. *N. Engl. J. Med.*, **333**, 1171–1175.

13 Strassburg, C.P. (2010) Gilbert–Meulengracht's syndrome and pharmacogenetics: is jaundice just the

tip of the iceberg? *Drug Metab. Rev.*, **42**, 162–175.

14 Gong, Q.H., Cho, J.W., Huang, T., Potter, C., Gholami, N., Basu, N.K., Kubota, S., Carvalho, S., Pennington, M.W., Owens, I.S., *et al.* (2001) Thirteen UDPglucuronosyltransferase genes are encoded at the human UGT1 gene complex locus. *Pharmacogenetics*, **11**, 357–368.

15 Tukey, R.H. and Strassburg, C.P. (2000) Human UDP-glucuronosyltransferases: metabolism, expression, and disease. *Annu. Rev. Pharmacol. Toxicol.*, **40**, 581–616.

16 Tukey, R.H. and Strassburg, C.P. (2001) Genetic multiplicity of the human UDP-glucuronosyltransferases and regulation in the gastrointestinal tract. *Mol. Pharmacol.*, **59**, 405–414.

17 Ritter, J.K., Chen, F., Sheen, Y.Y., Tran, H.M., Kimura, S., Yeatman, M.T., and Owens, I.S. (1992) A novel complex locus UGT1 encodes human bilirubin, phenol, and other UDP-glucuronosyltransferase isozymes with identical carboxyl termini. *J. Biol. Chem.*, **267**, 3257–3261.

18 Strassburg, C.P., Kneip, S., Topp, J., Obermayer-Straub, P., Barut, A., Tukey, R.H., and Manns, M.P. (2000) Polymorphic gene expression and interindividual variation of UDP-glucuronosyltransferase activity in human small intestine. *J. Biol. Chem.*, **275**, 36164–36171.

19 Strassburg, C.P., Manns, M.P., and Tukey, R.H. (1998) Expression of the UDP-glucuronosyltransferase 1A locus in human colon. Identification and characterization of the novel extrahepatic UGT1A8. *J. Biol. Chem.*, **273**, 8719–8726.

20 Strassburg, C.P., Nguyen, N., Manns, M.P., and Tukey, R.H. (1998) Polymorphic expression of the UDP-glucuronosyltransferase UGT1A gene locus in human gastric epithelium. *Mol. Pharmacol.*, **54**, 647–654.

21 Strassburg, C.P., Nguyen, N., Manns, M.P., and Tukey, R.H. (1999) UDP-glucuronosyltransferase activity in human liver and colon. *Gastroenterology*, **116**, 149–160.

22 Strassburg, C.P., Oldhafer, K., Manns, M.P., and Tukey, R.H. (1997) Differential expression of the UGT1A locus in human liver, biliary, and gastric tissue: identification of UGT1A7 and UGT1A10 transcripts in extrahepatic tissue. *Mol. Pharmacol.*, **52**, 212–220.

23 Strassburg, C.P., Strassburg, A., Nguyen, N., Li, Q., Manns, M.P., and Tukey, R.H. (1999) Regulation and function of family 1 and family 2 UDP-glucuronosyltransferase genes (UGT1A, UGT2B) in human oesophagus. *Biochem. J.*, **338**, 489–498.

24 Finel, M., Li, X., Gardner-Stephen, D., Bratton, S., Mackenzie, P.I., and Radominska-Pandya, A. (2005) Human UDP-glucuronosyltransferase 1A5: identification, expression, and activity. *J. Pharmacol. Exp. Ther.*, **315**, 1143–1149.

25 Strassburg, C.P., Strassburg, A., Kneip, S., Barut, A., Tukey, R.H., Rodeck, B., and Manns, M.P. (2002) Developmental aspects of human hepatic drug glucuronidation in young children and adults. *Gut*, **50**, 259–265.

26 Strassburg, C.P., Kalthoff, S., and Ehmer, U. (2008) Variability and function of family 1 uridine-5′-diphosphate glucuronosyltransferases (UGT1A). *Crit. Rev. Clin. Lab. Sci.*, **45**, 485–530.

27 Mackenzie, P.I., Owens, I.S., Burchell, B., Bock, K.W., Bairoch, A., Belanger, A., Fournel-Gigleux, S., Green, M., Hum, D.W., Iyanagi, T., *et al.* (1997) The UDP glycosyltransferase gene superfamily: recommended nomenclature update based on evolutionary divergence. *Pharmacogenetics*, **7**, 255–269.

28 Bosma, P.J., Chowdhury, J.R., Huang, T.J., Lahiri, P., Elferink, R.P., Van Es, H.H., Lederstein, M., Whitington, P.F., Jansen, P.L., and Chowdhury, N.R. (1992) Mechanisms of inherited deficiencies of multiple UDP-glucuronosyltransferase isoforms in two patients with Crigler–Najjar syndrome, type I. *FASEB J.*, **6**, 2859–2863.

29 Bosma, P.J., Chowdhury, N.R., Goldhoorn, B.G., Hofker, M.H., Oude Elferink, R.P., Jansen, P.L., and

Chowdhury, J.R. (1992) Sequence of exons and the flanking regions of human bilirubin–UDP-glucuronosyltransferase gene complex and identification of a genetic mutation in a patient with Crigler–Najjar syndrome, type I. *Hepatology*, **15**, 941–947.

30 Aono, S., Yamada, Y., Keino, H., Hanada, N., Nakagawa, T., Sasaoka, Y., Yazawa, T., Sato, H., and Koiwai, O. (1993) Identification of defect in the genes for bilirubin UDP-glucuronosyltransferase in a patient with Crigler–Najjar syndrome type II. *Biochem. Biophys. Res. Commun.*, **197**, 1239–1244.

31 Bosma, P.J., Goldhoorn, B., Oude Elferink, R.P., Sinaasappel, M., Oostra, B.A., and Jansen, P.L. (1993) A mutation in bilirubin uridine 5′-diphosphate-glucuronosyltransferase isoform 1 causing Crigler–Najjar syndrome type II. *Gastroenterology*, **105**, 216–220.

32 Moghrabi, N., Clarke, D.J., Boxer, M., and Burchell, B. (1993) Identification of an A-to-G missense mutation in exon 2 of the UGT1 gene complex that causes Crigler–Najjar syndrome type 2. *Genomics*, **18**, 171–173.

33 Moghrabi, N., Clarke, D.J., Burchell, B., and Boxer, M. (1993) Cosegregation of intragenic markers with a novel mutation that causes Crigler–Najjar syndrome type I: implication in carrier detection and prenatal diagnosis. *Am. J. Hum. Genet.*, **53**, 722–729.

34 Erps, L.T., Ritter, J.K., Hersh, J.H., Blossom, D., Martin, N.C., and Owens, I.S. (1994) Identification of two single base substitutions in the UGT1 gene locus which abolish bilirubin uridine diphosphate glucuronosyltransferase activity *in vitro*. *J. Clin. Invest.*, **93**, 564–570.

35 Labrune, P., Myara, A., Hadchouel, M., Ronchi, F., Bernard, O., Trivin, F., Chowdhury, N.R., Chowdhury, J.R., Munnich, A., and Odievre, M. (1994) Genetic heterogeneity of Crigler–Najjar syndrome type I: a study of 14 cases. *Hum. Genet.*, **94**, 693–697.

36 Seppen, J., Bosma, P.J., Goldhoorn, B.G., Bakker, C.T., Chowdhury, J.R., Chowdhury, N.R., Jansen, P.L., and Oude Elferink, R.P. (1994) Discrimination between Crigler–Najjar type I and II by expression of mutant bilirubin uridine diphosphate-glucuronosyltransferase. *J. Clin. Invest.*, **94**, 2385–2391.

37 Ritter, J.K., Yeatman, M.T., Kaiser, C., Gridelli, B., and Owens, I.S. (1993) A phenylalanine codon deletion at the UGT1 gene complex locus of a Crigler–Najjar type I patient generates a pH-sensitive bilirubin UDP-glucuronosyltransferase. *J. Biol. Chem.*, **268**, 23573–23579.

38 Aono, S., Yamada, Y., Keino, H., Sasaoka, Y., Nakagawa, T., Onishi, S., Mimura, S., Koiwai, O., and Sato, H. (1994) A new type of defect in the gene for bilirubin uridine 5′-diphosphate-glucuronosyltransferase in a patient with Crigler–Najjar syndrome type I. *Pediatr. Res.*, **35**, 629–632.

39 Aono, S., Adachi, Y., Uyama, E., Yamada, Y., Keino, H., Nanno, T., Koiwai, O., and Sato, H. (1995) Analysis of genes for bilirubin UDP-glucuronosyltransferase in Gilbert's syndrome. *Lancet*, **345**, 958–959.

40 Beutler, E., Gelbart, T., and Demina, A. (1998) Racial variability in the UDP-glucuronosyltransferase 1 (UGT1A1) promoter: a balanced polymorphism for regulation of bilirubin metabolism? *Proc. Natl. Acad. Sci. USA*, **95**, 8170–8174.

41 Sugatani, J., Yamakawa, K., Yoshinari, K., Machida, T., Takagi, H., Mori, M., Kakizaki, S., Sueyoshi, T., Negishi, M., and Miwa, M. (2002) Identification of a defect in the UGT1A1 gene promoter and its association with hyperbilirubinemia. *Biochem. Biophys. Res. Commun.*, **292**, 492–497.

42 Sutomo, R., Laosombat, V., Sadewa, A.H., Yokoyama, N., Nakamura, H., Matsuo, M., and Nishio, H. (2002) Novel missense mutation of the UGT1A1 gene in Thai siblings with Gilbert's syndrome. *Pediatr. Int.*, **44**, 427–432.

43 Costa, E., Vieira, E., Martins, M., Saraiva, J., Cancela, E., Costa, M., Bauerle, R., Freitas, T., Carvalho, J.R., Santos-Silva, E., *et al.* (2006) Analysis of the UDP-glucuronosyltransferase gene

in Portuguese patients with a clinical diagnosis of Gilbert and Crigler–Najjar syndromes. *Blood Cells Mol. Dis.*, **36**, 91–97.

44 Farheen, S., Sengupta, S., Santra, A., Pal, S., Dhali, G.K., Chakravorty, M., Majumder, P.P., and Chowdhury, A. (2006) Gilbert's syndrome: high frequency of the $(TA)_7$ TAA allele in India and its interaction with a novel CAT insertion in promoter of the gene for bilirubin UDP-glucuronosyltransferase 1 gene. *World J. Gastroenterol.*, **12**, 2269–2275.

45 Caillier, B., Lepine, J., Tojcic, J., Menard, V., Perusse, L., Belanger, A., Barbier, O., and Guillemette, C. (2007) A pharmacogenomics study of the human estrogen glucuronosyltransferase UGT1A3. *Pharmacogenet. Genomics*, **17**, 481–495.

46 Ehmer, U., Vogel, A., Schutte, J.K., Krone, B., Manns, M.P., and Strassburg, C.P. (2004) Variation of hepatic glucuronidation: novel functional polymorphisms of the UDP-glucuronosyltransferase UGT1A4. *Hepatology*, **39**, 970–977.

47 Iwai, M., Maruo, Y., Ito, M., Yamamoto, K., Sato, H., and Takeuchi, Y. (2004) Six novel UDP-glucuronosyltransferase (UGT1A3) polymorphisms with varying activity. *J. Hum. Genet.*, **49**, 123–128.

48 Thomas, S.S., Li, S.S., Lampe, J.W., Potter, J.D., and Bigler, J. (2006) Genetic variability, haplotypes, and htSNPs for exons 1 at the human UGT1A locus. *Hum. Mutat.*, **27**, 717.

49 Saeki, M., Saito, Y., Jinno, H., Sai, K., Ozawa, S., Kurose, K., Kaniwa, N., Komamura, K., Kotake, T., Morishita, H., *et al.* (2006) Haplotype structures of the UGT1A gene complex in a Japanese population. *Pharmacogenomics J.*, **6**, 63–75.

50 Guillemette, C., Ritter, J.K., Auyeung, D.J., Kessler, F.K., and Housman, D.E. (2000) Structural heterogeneity at the UDP-glucuronosyltransferase 1 locus: functional consequences of three novel missense mutations in the human UGT1A7 gene. *Pharmacogenetics*, **10**, 629–644.

51 Strassburg, C.P., Vogel, A., Kneip, S., Tukey, R.H., and Manns, M.P. (2002) Polymorphisms of the UDP-glucuronosyltransferase (UGT) 1A7 gene in colorectal cancer. *Gut*, **50**, 851–856.

52 Villeneuve, L., Girard, H., Fortier, L.C., Gagne, J.F., and Guillemette, C. (2003) Novel functional polymorphisms in the UGT1A7 and UGT1A9 glucuronidating enzymes in Caucasian and African-American subjects and their impact on the metabolism of 7-ethyl-10-hydroxycamptothecin and flavopiridol anticancer drugs. *J. Pharmacol. Exp. Ther.*, **307**, 117–128. Epub 2003 Aug 2027.

53 Van Der Logt, E.M., Bergevoet, S.M., Roelofs, H.M., Van Hooijdonk, Z., Te Morsche, R.H., Wobbes, T., De Kok, J.B., Nagengast, F.M., and Peters, W.H. (2004) Genetic polymorphisms in UDP-glucuronosyltransferases and glutathione *S*-transferases and colorectal cancer risk. *Carcinogenesis*, **19**, 19.

54 Verlaan, M., Drenth, J.P., Truninger, K., Koudova, M., Schulz, H.U., Bargetzi, M., Kunzli, B., Friess, H., Cerny, M., Kage, A., *et al.* (2005) Polymorphisms of UDP-glucuronosyltransferase 1A7 are not involved in pancreatic diseases. *J. Med. Genet.*, **42**, e62.

55 Lankisch, T.O., Vogel, A., Eilermann, S., Fiebeler, A., Krone, B., Barut, A., Manns, M.P., and Strassburg, C.P. (2005) Identification and characterization of a functional TATA box polymorphism of the UDP glucuronosyltransferase 1A7 gene. *Mol. Pharmacol.*, **67**, 1732–1739.

56 Fujita, K., Ando, Y., Nagashima, F., Yamamoto, W., Endo, H., Kodama, K., Araki, K., Miya, T., Narabayashi, M., and Sasaki, Y. (2006) Novel single nucleotide polymorphism of UGT1A7 gene in Japanese. *Drug Metab. Pharmacokinet.*, **21**, 75–78.

57 Maitland, M.L., Grimsley, C., Kuttab-Boulos, H., Witonsky, D., Kasza, K.E., Yang, L., Roe, B.A., and Di Rienzo, A. (2006) Comparative genomics analysis of human sequence variation in the UGT1A gene cluster. *Pharmacogenomics J.*, **6**, 52–62.

58 Kohle, C., Mohrle, B., Munzel, P.A., Schwab, M., Wernet, D., Badary, O.A., and Bock, K.W. (2003) Frequent co-occurrence of the TATA box mutation associated with Gilbert's syndrome (UGT1A1*28) with other polymorphisms of the UDP-glucuronosyltransferase-1 locus (UGT1A6*2 and UGT1A7*3) in Caucasians and Egyptians. *Biochem. Pharmacol.*, **65**, 1521–1527.

59 Lampe, J.W., Bigler, J., Horner, N.K., and Potter, J.D. (1999) UDP-glucuronosyltransferase (UGT1A1*28 and UGT1A6*2) polymorphisms in Caucasians and Asians: relationships to serum bilirubin concentrations. *Pharmacogenetics*, **9**, 341–349.

60 Lankisch, T.O., Moebius, U., Wehmeier, M., Behrens, G., Manns, M.P., Schmidt, R.E., and Strassburg, C.P. (2006) Gilbert's disease and atazanavir: from phenotype to UDP-glucuronosyltransferase haplotype. *Hepatology*, **44**, 1324–1332.

61 Erichsen, T.J., Ehmer, U., Kalthoff, S., Lankisch, T.O., Müller, T.M., Munzel, P.A., Manns, M.P., and Strassburg, C.P. (2008) Genetic variability of aryl hydrocarbon receptor (AhR)-mediated regulation of the human UDP glucuronosyltransferase (UGT) 1A4 gene. *Toxicol. Appl. Pharmacol.*, **230**, 252–260.

62 Gardner-Stephen, D.A. and Mackenzie, P.I. (2007) Isolation of the UDP glucuronosyltransferase 1A3 and 1A4 proximal promoters and characterization of their dependence on the transcription factor hepatocyte nuclear factor 1 alpha. *Drug Metab. Dispos.*, **35**, 116–120.

63 Erichsen, T.J., Aehlen, A., Ehmer, U., Kalthoff, S., Manns, M.P., and Strassburg, C.P. (2010) Regulation of the human bile acid UDP-glucuronosyltransferase 1A3 by the farnesoid X receptor and bile acids. *J. Hepatol.*, **52**, 570–578.

64 Matsui, K., Maruo, Y., Sato, H., and Takeuchi, Y. (2010) Combined effect of regulatory polymorphisms on transcription of UGT1A1 as a cause of Gilbert syndrome. *BMC Gastroenterol.*, **10**, 57.

65 Martin, J.F., Vierling, J.M., Wolkoff, A.W., Scharschmidt, B.F., Vergalla, J., Waggoner, J.G., and Berk, P.D. (1976) Abnormal hepatic transport of indocyanine green in Gilbert's syndrome. *Gastroenterology*, **70**, 385–391.

66 Testa, R., Bardellini, E., Borzone, S., Montani, P., Risso, D., Bindi, P., Caglieris, S., Campo, N., Alvarez, S., Pireddu, M., *et al.* (1995) Caffeine clearance in subjects with constitutional unconjugated hyperbilirubinemia. *Ital. J. Gastroenterol.*, **27**, 129–132.

67 Berk, P.D., Blaschke, T.F., and Waggoner, J.G. (1972) Defective bromosulfophthalein clearance in patients with constitutional hepatic dysfunction (Gilbert's syndrome). *Gastroenterology*, **63**, 472–481.

68 Macklon, A.F., Savage, R.L., and Rawlins, M.D. (1979) Gilbert's syndrome and drug metabolism. *Clin. Pharmacokinet.*, **4**, 223–232.

69 Carulli, N., Ponz de Leon, M., Mauro, E., Manenti, F., and Ferrari, A. (1976) Alteration of drug metabolism in Gilbert's syndrome. *Gut*, **17**, 581–587.

70 Johnson, A.D., Kavousi, M., Smith, A.V., Chen, M.H., Dehghan, A., Aspelund, T., Lin, J.P., van Duijn, C.M., Harris, T.B., Cupples, L.A., *et al.* (2009) Genome-wide association meta-analysis for total serum bilirubin levels. *Hum. Mol. Genet.*, **18**, 2700–2710.

71 Iyanagi, T. (1991) Molecular basis of multiple UDP-glucuronosyltransferase isoenzyme deficiencies in the hyperbilirubinemic rat (Gunn rat). *J. Biol. Chem.*, **266**, 24048–24052.

72 Bosma, P.J., Seppen, J., Goldhoorn, B., Bakker, C., Oude Elferink, R.P., Chowdhury, J.R., Chowdhury, N.R., and Jansen, P.L. (1994) Bilirubin UDP-glucuronosyltransferase 1 is the only relevant bilirubin glucuronidating isoform in man [published erratum appears in *J. Biol. Chem.* 1994 269, 2542]. *J. Biol. Chem.*, **269**, 17960–17964.

73 Fang, J.L. and Lazarus, P. (2004) Correlation between the UDP-glucuronosyltransferase (UGT1A1) TATAA box polymorphism and carcinogen detoxification phenotype: significantly decreased glucuronidating

activity against benzo(*a*)pyrene-7,8-dihydrodiol(–) in liver microsomes from subjects with the UGT1A1*28 variant. *Cancer Epidemiol. Biomarkers Prev.*, **13**, 102–109.

74 Monaghan, G., Ryan, M., Seddon, R., Hume, R., and Burchell, B. (1996) Genetic variation in bilirubin UDP-glucuronosyltransferase gene promoter and Gilbert's syndrome. *Lancet*, **347**, 578–581.

75 Balram, C., Sabapathy, K., Fei, G., Khoo, K.S., and Lee, E.J. (2002) Genetic polymorphisms of UDP-glucuronosyltransferase in Asians: UGT1A1*28 is a common allele in Indians. *Pharmacogenetics*, **12**, 81–83.

76 Ando, Y., Chida, M., Nakayama, K., Saka, H., and Kamataki, T. (1998) The UGT1A1*28 allele is relatively rare in a Japanese population. *Pharmacogenetics*, **8**, 357–360.

77 Udomuksorn, W., Elliot, D.J., Lewis, B.C., Mackenzie, P.I., Yoovathaworn, K., and Miners, J.O. (2007) Influence of mutations associated with Gilbert and Crigler–Najjar type II syndromes on the glucuronidation kinetics of bilirubin and other UDP-glucuronosyltransferase 1A substrates. *Pharmacogenet. Genomics*, **17**, 1017–1029.

78 Sai, K., Saeki, M., Saito, Y., Ozawa, S., Katori, N., Jinno, H., Hasegawa, R., Kaniwa, N., Sawada, J., Komamura, K., *et al.* (2004) UGT1A1 haplotypes associated with reduced glucuronidation and increased serum bilirubin in irinotecan-administered Japanese patients with cancer. *Clin. Pharmacol. Ther.*, **75**, 501–515.

79 Innocenti, F., Grimsley, C., Das, S., Ramirez, J., Cheng, C., Kuttab-Boulos, H., Ratain, M.J., and Di Rienzo, A. (2002) Haplotype structure of the UDP-glucuronosyltransferase 1A1 promoter in different ethnic groups. *Pharmacogenetics*, **12**, 725–733.

80 Lankisch, T.O., Schulz, C., Zwingers, T., Erichsen, T.J., Manns, M.P., Heinemann, V., and Strassburg, C.P. (2008) Gilbert's syndrome and irinotecan toxicity: combination with UDP-glucuronosyltransferase 1A7 variants increases risk. *Cancer Epidemiol. Biomarkers Prev.*, **17**, 695–701.

81 Cecchin, E., Innocenti, F., D'Andrea, M., Corona, G., De Mattia, E., Biason, P., Buonadonna, A., and Toffoli, G. (2009) Predictive role of the UGT1A1, UGT1A7, and UGT1A9 genetic variants and their haplotypes on the outcome of metastatic colorectal cancer patients treated with fluorouracil, leucovorin, and irinotecan. *J. Clin. Oncol.*, **27**, 2457–2465.

82 Tang, K.S., Chiu, H.F., Chen, H.H., Eng, H.L., Tsai, C.J., Teng, H.C., and Huang, C.S. (2005) Link between colorectal cancer and polymorphisms in the uridine-diphosphoglucuronosyltransferase 1A7 and 1A1 genes. *World J. Gastroenterol.*, **11**, 3250–3254.

83 Wasmuth, H.E., Keppeler, H., Herrmann, U., Schirin-Sokhan, R., Barker, M., and Lammert, F. (2006) Coinheritance of Gilbert syndrome-associated UGT1A1 mutation increases gallstone risk in cystic fibrosis. *Hepatology*, **43**, 738–741.

84 del Giudice, E.M., Perrotta, S., Nobili, B., Specchia, C., d'Urzo, G., and Iolascon, A. (1999) Coinheritance of Gilbert syndrome increases the risk for developing gallstones in patients with hereditary spherocytosis. *Blood*, **94**, 2259–2262.

85 Vasavda, N., Menzel, S., Kondaveeti, S., Maytham, E., Awogbade, M., Bannister, S., Cunningham, J., Eichholz, A., Daniel, Y., Okpala, I., *et al.* (2007) The linear effects of alpha-thalassaemia, the UGT1A1 and HMOX1 polymorphisms on cholelithiasis in sickle cell disease. *Br. J. Haematol.*, **138**, 263–270.

86 Haverfield, E.V., McKenzie, C.A., Forrester, T., Bouzekri, N., Harding, R., Serjeant, G., Walker, T., Peto, T.E., Ward, R., and Weatherall, D.J. (2005) UGT1A1 variation and gallstone formation in sickle cell disease. *Blood*, **105**, 968–972.

87 Guillemette, C., Millikan, R.C., Newman, B., and Housman, D.E. (2000) Genetic polymorphisms in uridine diphospho-glucuronosyltransferase 1A1 and association with breast cancer

among African Americans. *Cancer Res.*, **60**, 950–956.

88 Guillemette, C., De Vivo, I., Hankinson, S.E., Haiman, C.A., Spiegelman, D., Housman, D.E., and Hunter, D.J. (2001) Association of genetic polymorphisms in UGT1A1 with breast cancer and plasma hormone levels. *Cancer Epidemiol. Biomarkers Prev.*, **10**, 711–714.

89 Adegoke, O.J., Shu, X.O., Gao, Y.T., Cai, Q., Breyer, J., Smith, J., and Zheng, W. (2004) Genetic polymorphisms in uridine diphospho-glucuronosyltransferase 1A1 (UGT1A1) and risk of breast cancer. *Breast Cancer Res. Treat.*, **85**, 239–245.

90 McGrath, M., Lepine, J., Lee, I.M., Villeneuve, L., Buring, J., Guillemette, C., and De Vivo, I. (2009) Genetic variations in UGT1A1 and UGT2B7 and endometrial cancer risk. *Pharmacogenet. Genomics*, **19**, 239–243.

91 Duguay, Y., McGrath, M., Lepine, J., Gagne, J.F., Hankinson, S.E., Colditz, G.A., Hunter, D.J., Plante, M., Tetu, B., Belanger, A., *et al.* (2004) The functional UGT1A1 promoter polymorphism decreases endometrial cancer risk. *Cancer Res.*, **64**, 1202–1207.

92 Ribrag, V., Koscielny, S., Casasnovas, O., Cazeneuve, C., Brice, P., Morschhauser, F., Gabarre, J., Stamatoullas, A., Lenoir, G., and Salles, G. (2009) Pharmacogenetic study in Hodgkin lymphomas reveals the impact of UGT1A1 polymorphisms on patient prognosis. *Blood*, **113**, 3307–3313.

93 Rantner, B., Kollerits, B., Anderwald-Stadler, M., Klein-Weigel, P., Gruber, I., Gehringer, A., Haak, M., Schnapka-Kopf, M., Fraedrich, G., and Kronenberg, F. (2008) Association between the UGT1A1 TA-repeat polymorphism and bilirubin concentration in patients with intermittent claudication: results from the CAVASIC study. *Clin. Chem.*, **54**, 851–857.

94 Lin, J.P., Schwaiger, J.P., Cupples, L.A., O'Donnell, C.J., Zheng, G., Schoenborn, V., Hunt, S.C., Joo, J., and Kronenberg, F. (2009) Conditional linkage and genome-wide association studies identify UGT1A1 as a major gene for anti-atherogenic serum bilirubin levels–The Framingham Heart Study. *Atherosclerosis*, **206**, 228–233.

95 Lin, J.P., O'Donnell, C.J., Schwaiger, J.P., Cupples, L.A., Lingenhel, A., Hunt, S.C., Yang, S., and Kronenberg, F. (2006) Association between the UGT1A1*28 allele, bilirubin levels, and coronary heart disease in the Framingham Heart Study. *Circulation*, **114**, 1476–1481.

96 Siow, R.C., Sato, H., and Mann, G.E. (1999) Heme oxygenase–carbon monoxide signalling pathway in atherosclerosis: anti-atherogenic actions of bilirubin and carbon monoxide? *Cardiovasc. Res.*, **41**, 385–394.

97 Rigato, I., Ostrow, J.D., and Tiribelli, C. (2005) Bilirubin and the risk of common non-hepatic diseases. *Trends Mol. Med.*, **11**, 277–283.

98 Vera, T., Granger, J.P., and Stec, D.E. (2009) Inhibition of bilirubin metabolism induces moderate hyperbilirubinemia and attenuates ANG II dependent hypertension in mice. *Am. J. Physiol. Regul. Integr. Comp. Physiol.*, **297**, R738–R743.

99 Schwertner, H.A. and Vitek, L. (2008) Gilbert syndrome, UGT1A1*28 allele, and cardiovascular disease risk: possible protective effects and therapeutic applications of bilirubin. *Atherosclerosis*, **198**, 1–11.

100 Katoh, M., Yoshioka, Y., Nakagawa, N., and Yokoi, T. (2009) Effects of Japanese herbal medicine, Kampo, on human UGT1A1 activity. *Drug Metab. Pharmacokinet.*, **24**, 226–234.

101 Saracino, M.R., Bigler, J., Schwarz, Y., Chang, J.L., Li, S., Li, L., White, E., Potter, J.D., and Lampe, J.W. (2009) Citrus fruit intake is associated with lower serum bilirubin concentration among women with the UGT1A1*28 polymorphism. *J. Nutr.*, **139**, 555–560.

102 Kapitulnik, J. (2004) Bilirubin: an endogenous product of heme degradation with both cytotoxic and cytoprotective properties. *Mol. Pharmacol.*, **66**, 773–779.

103 Gajdos, V., Petit, F.M., Perret, C., Mollet-Boudjemline, A., Colin, P., Capel, L., Nicaud, V., Evans, A., Arveiler, D.,

Parisot, F., *et al.* (2006) Further evidence that the UGT1A1*28 allele is not associated with coronary heart disease: the ECTIM Study. *Clin. Chem.*, **52**, 2313–2314.

104 Ando, Y., Saka, H., Asai, G., Sugiura, S., Shimokata, K., and Kamataki, T. (1998) UGT1A1 genotypes and glucuronidation of SN-38, the active metabolite of irinotecan. *Ann. Oncol.*, **9**, 845–847.

105 Innocenti, F., Undevia, S.D., Iyer, L., Chen, P.X., Das, S., Kocherginsky, M., Karrison, T., Janisch, L., Ramirez, J., Rudin, C.M., *et al.* (2004) Genetic variants in the UDP-glucuronosyltransferase 1A1 gene predict the risk of severe neutropenia of irinotecan. *J. Clin. Oncol.*, **22**, 1382–1388.

106 Iyer, L., King, C.D., Whitington, P.F., Green, M.D., Roy, S.K., Tephly, T.R., Coffman, B.L., and Ratain, M.J. (1998) Genetic predisposition to the metabolism of irinotecan (CPT-11). Role of uridine diphosphate glucuronosyltransferase isoform 1A1 in the glucuronidation of its active metabolite (SN-38) in human liver microsomes. *J. Clin. Invest.*, **101**, 847–854.

107 Onoue, M., Terada, T., Kobayashi, M., Katsura, T., Matsumoto, S., Yanagihara, K., Nishimura, T., Kanai, M., Teramukai, S., Shimizu, A., *et al.* (2009) UGT1A1*6 polymorphism is most predictive of severe neutropenia induced by irinotecan in Japanese cancer patients. *Int. J. Clin. Oncol.*, **14**, 136–142.

108 Rotger, M., Taffe, P., Bleiber, G., Gunthard, H.F., Furrer, H., Vernazza, P., Drechsler, H., Bernasconi, E., Rickenbach, M., and Telenti, A. (2005) Gilbert syndrome and the development of antiretroviral therapy-associated hyperbilirubinemia. *J. Infect. Dis.*, **192**, 1381–1386.

109 Zucker, S.D., Qin, X., Rouster, S.D., Yu, F., Green, R.M., Keshavan, P., Feinberg, J., and Sherman, K.E. (2001) Mechanism of indinavir-induced hyperbilirubinemia. *Proc. Natl. Acad. Sci. USA*, **98**, 12671–12676.

110 Lankisch, T.O., Behrens, G., Ehmer, U., Mobius, U., Rockstroh, J., Wehmeier, M., Kalthoff, S., Freiberg, N., Manns, M.P., Schmidt, R.E., *et al.* (2009) Gilbert's syndrome and hyperbilirubinemia in protease inhibitor therapy – an extended haplotype of genetic variants increases risk in indinavir treatment. *J. Hepatol.*, **50**, 1010–1018.

111 Ogilvie, B.W., Zhang, D., Li, W., Rodrigues, A.D., Gipson, A.E., Holsapple, J., Toren, P., and Parkinson, A. (2006) Glucuronidation converts gemfibrozil to a potent, metabolism-dependent inhibitor of CYP2C8: implications for drug–drug interactions. *Drug Metab. Dispos.*, **34**, 191–197.

112 Ghosal, A., Hapangama, N., Yuan, Y., Achanfuo-Yeboah, J., Iannucci, R., Chowdhury, S., Alton, K., Patrick, J.E., and Zbaida, S. (2004) Identification of human UDP-glucuronosyltransferase enzyme(s) responsible for the glucuronidation of ezetimibe (Zetia). *Drug Metab. Dispos.*, **32**, 314–320.

113 Prueksaritanont, T., Subramanian, R., Fang, X., Ma, B., Qiu, Y., Lin, J.H., Pearson, P.G., and Baillie, T.A. (2002) Glucuronidation of statins in animals and humans: a novel mechanism of statin lactonization. *Drug Metab. Dispos.*, **30**, 505–512.

114 Ebner, T., Remmel, R.P., and Burchell, B. (1993) Human bilirubin UDP-glucuronosyltransferase catalyzes the glucuronidation of ethinylestradiol. *Mol. Pharmacol.*, **43**, 649–654.

115 King, C.D., Green, M.D., Rios, G.R., Coffman, B.L., Owens, I.S., Bishop, W.P., and Tephly, T.R. (1996) The glucuronidation of exogenous and endogenous compounds by stably expressed rat and human UDP-glucuronosyltransferase 1.1. *Arch. Biochem. Biophys.*, **332**, 92–100.

116 Chouinard, S., Tessier, M., Vernouillet, G., Gauthier, S., Labrie, F., Barbier, O., and Belanger, A. (2005) Inactivation of the pure antiestrogen fulvestrant and other synthetic estrogen molecules by UGT1A enzymes expressed in the breast tissue. *Mol. Pharmacol.*, **69**, 908–920.

117 Kuehl, G.E., Lampe, J.W., Potter, J.D., and Bigler, J. (2005) Glucuronidation of nonsteroidal anti-inflammatory drugs:

identifying the enzymes responsible in human liver microsomes. *Drug Metab. Dispos.*, **33**, 1027–1035.

118 Deterding, K., Grungreiff, K., Lankisch, T.O., Potthoff, A., Bahr, M.J., Manns, M.P., Wedemeyer, H., and Strassburg, C.P. (2009) Gilbert's syndrome and antiviral therapy of hepatitis C. *Ann. Hepatol.*, **8**, 246–250.

119 King, C.D., Rios, G.R., Green, M.D., MacKenzie, P.I., and Tephly, T.R. (1997) Comparison of stably expressed rat UGT1.1 and UGT2B1 in the glucuronidation of opioid compounds. *Drug Metab. Dispos.*, **25**, 251–255.

120 Innocenti, F., Vokes, E.E., and Ratain, M.J. (2006) Irinogenetics: what is the right star? *J. Clin. Oncol.*, **24**, 2221–2224.

121 Kawato, Y., Aonuma, M., Hirota, Y., Kuga, H., and Sato, K. (1991) Intracellular roles of SN-38, a metabolite of the camptothecin derivative CPT-11, in the antitumor effect of CPT-11. *Cancer Res.*, **51**, 4187–4191.

122 Tukey, R.H., Strassburg, C.P., and Mackenzie, P.I. (2002) Pharmacogenomics of human UDP-glucuronosyltransferases and irinotecan toxicity. *Mol. Pharmacol.*, **62**, 446–450.

123 Innocenti, F. and Ratain, M.J. (2003) Irinotecan treatment in cancer patients with UGT1A1 polymorphisms. *Oncology*, **17**, 52–55.

124 Douillard, J.Y., Cunningham, D., Roth, A.D., Navarro, M., James, R.D., Karasek, P., Jandik, P., Iveson, T., Carmichael, J., Alakl, M., *et al.* (2000) Irinotecan combined with fluorouracil compared with fluorouracil alone as first-line treatment for metastatic colorectal cancer: a multicentre randomised trial. *Lancet*, **355**, 1041–1047.

125 Gagne, J.F., Montminy, V., Belanger, P., Journault, K., Gaucher, G., and Guillemette, C. (2002) Common human UGT1A polymorphisms and the altered metabolism of irinotecan active metabolite 7-ethyl-10-hydroxycamptothecin (SN-38). *Mol. Pharmacol.*, **62**, 608–617.

126 Marcuello, E., Altes, A., Menoyo, A., Del Rio, E., Gomez-Pardo, M., and Baiget, M. (2004) UGT1A1 gene variations and irinotecan treatment in patients with metastatic colorectal cancer. *Br. J. Cancer*, **91**, 678–682.

127 Rouits, E., Boisdron-Celle, M., Dumont, A., Guerin, O., Morel, A., and Gamelin, E. (2004) Relevance of different UGT1A1 polymorphisms in irinotecan-induced toxicity: a molecular and clinical study of 75 patients. *Clin. Cancer Res.*, **10**, 5151–5159.

128 Carlini, L.E., Meropol, N.J., Bever, J., Andria, M.L., Hill, T., Gold, P., Rogatko, A., Wang, H., and Blanchard, R.L. (2005) UGT1A7 and UGT1A9 polymorphisms predict response and toxicity in colorectal cancer patients treated with capecitabine/irinotecan. *Clin. Cancer Res.*, **11**, 1226–1236.

129 Stewart, C.F., Panetta, J.C., O'Shaughnessy, M.A., Throm, S.L., Fraga, C.H., Owens, T., Liu, T., Billups, C., Rodriguez-Galindo, C., Gajjar, A., *et al.* (2007) UGT1A1 promoter genotype correlates with SN-38 pharmacokinetics, but not severe toxicity in patients receiving low-dose irinotecan. *J. Clin. Oncol.*, **25**, 2594–2600.

130 Ciotti, M., Basu, N., Brangi, M., and Owens, I.S. (1999) Glucuronidation of 7-ethyl-10-hydroxycamptothecin (SN-38) by the human UDP-glucuronosyltransferases encoded at the UGT1 locus. *Biochem. Biophys. Res. Commun.*, **260**, 199–202.

131 Tallman, M.N., Miles, K., Kessler, F., Neilson, J., Tian, X., Ritter, J.K., and Smith, P.C. (2007) The contribution of intestinal UDP-glucuronosyltransferases in modulating 7-ethyl-10-hydroxy-camptothecin (SN-38)-induced gastrointestinal toxicity in rats. *J. Pharmacol. Exp. Ther.*, **320**, 29–37.

132 Ehmer, U., Lankisch, T.O., Erichsen, T.J., Kalthoff, S., Freiberg, N., Wehmeier, M., Manns, M.P., and Strassburg, C.P. (2008) Rapid allelic discrimination by TaqMan PCR for the detection of the Gilbert's syndrome marker UGT1A1*28. *J. Mol. Diagn.*, **10**, 549–552.

133 Kalthoff, S., Ehmer, U., Freiberg, N., Manns, M.P., and Strassburg, C.P. (2010) Coffee induces expression of glucuronosyltransferases via the aryl hydrocarbon receptor and Nrf2 in liver

and stomach. *Gastroenterology*, **139**, 1699–1710.

134 Zhang, D., Chando, T.J., Everett, D.W., Patten, C.J., Dehal, S.S., and Humphreys, W.G. (2005) *In vitro* inhibition of UDP glucuronosyltransferases by atazanavir and other HIV protease inhibitors and the relationship of this property to *in vivo* bilirubin glucuronidation. *Drug Metab. Dispos.*, **33**, 1729–1739.

135 Horsfall, L.J., Zeitlyn, D., Tarekegn, A., Bekele, E., Thomas, M.G., Bradman, N., and Swallow, D.M. (2011) Prevalence of clinically relevant UGT1A alleles and haplotypes in African populations. *Ann. Hum. Genet.*, **75**, 236–246.

136 Cheng, Z., Rios, G.R., King, C.D., Coffman, B.L., Green, M.D., Mojarrabi, B., Mackenzie, P.I., and Tephly, T.R. (1998) Glucuronidation of catechol estrogens by expressed human UDP-glucuronosyltransferases (UGTs) 1A1, 1A3, and 2B7. *Toxicol. Sci.*, **45**, 52–57.

137 Fang, J.L., Beland, F.A., Doerge, D.R., Wiener, D., Guillemette, C., Marques, M.M., and Lazarus, P. (2002) Characterization of benzo(*a*)pyrene-*trans*-7,8-dihydrodiol glucuronidation by human tissue microsomes and overexpressed UDP-glucuronosyltransferase enzymes. *Cancer Res.*, **62**, 1978–1986.

138 Sparks, R., Ulrich, C.M., Bigler, J., Tworoger, S.S., Yasui, Y., Rajan, K.B., Porter, P., Stanczyk, F.Z., Ballard-Barbash, R., Yuan, X., *et al.* (2004) UDP-glucuronosyltransferase and sulfotransferase polymorphisms, sex hormone concentrations, and tumor receptor status in breast cancer patients. *Breast Cancer Res.*, **6**, R488–R498.

139 Mojarrabi, B., Butler, R., and Mackenzie, P.I. (1996) cDNA cloning and characterization of the human UDP glucuronosyltransferase, UGT1A3. *Biochem. Biophys. Res. Commun.*, **225**, 785–790.

140 Green, M.D., King, C.D., Mojarrabi, B., Mackenzie, P.I., and Tephly, T.R. (1998) Glucuronidation of amines and other xenobiotics catalyzed by expressed human UDP-glucuronosyltransferase 1A3. *Drug Metab. Dispos.*, **26**, 507–512.

141 Trottier, J., Verreault, M., Grepper, S., Monte, D., Belanger, J., Kaeding, J., Caron, P., Inaba, T.T., and Barbier, O. (2006) Human UDP-glucuronosyltransferase (UGT)1A3 enzyme conjugates chenodeoxycholic acid in the liver. *Hepatology*, **44**, 1158–1170.

142 Kasai, N., Sakaki, T., Shinkyo, R., Ikushiro, S., Iyanagi, T., Ohta, M., and Inouye, K. (2005) Metabolism of 26,26,26,27,27,27-F6-1 alpha,23*S*,25-trihydroxyvitamin D3 by human UDP-glucuronosyltransferase 1A3. *Drug Metab. Dispos.*, **33**, 102–107.

143 Yan, Z., Caldwell, G.W., Gauthier, D., Leo, G.C., Mei, J., Ho, C.Y., Jones, W.J., Masucci, J.A., Tuman, R.W., Galemmo, R.A., Jr, *et al.* (2006) *N*-glucuronidation of the platelet-derived growth factor receptor tyrosine kinase inhibitor 6,7-(dimethoxy-2,4-dihydroindeno[1,2-*c*] pyrazol-3-yl)-(3-fluoro-phenyl)-amine by human UDP-glucuronosyltransferases. *Drug Metab. Dispos.*, **34**, 748–755.

144 Riedmaier, S., Klein, K., Hofmann, U., Keskitalo, J.E., Neuvonen, P.J., Schwab, M., Niemi, M., and Zanger, U.M. (2010) UDP-glucuronosyltransferase (UGT) polymorphisms affect atorvastatin lactonization *in vitro* and *in vivo*. *Clin. Pharmacol. Ther.*, **87**, 65–73.

145 Ockenga, J., Vogel, A., Teich, N., Keim, V., Manns, M.P., and Strassburg, C.P. (2003) UDP glucuronosyltransferase (UGT1A7) gene polymorphisms increase the risk of chronic pancreatitis and pancreatic cancer. *Gastroenterology*, **124**, 1802–1808.

146 Malfatti, M.A. and Felton, J.S. (2004) Human UDP-glucuronosyltransferase 1A1 is the primary enzyme responsible for the *N*-glucuronidation of *N*-hydroxy-PhIP *in vitro*. *Chem. Res. Toxicol.*, **17**, 1137–1144.

147 La Vecchia, C., D'Avanzo, B., Airoldi, L., Braga, C., and Decarli, A. (1995) Nitrosamine intake and gastric cancer risk. *Eur. J. Cancer Prev.*, **4**, 469–474.

148 Kadlubar, F.F. (1991) Carcinogenic aromatic amine metabolism and DNA adduct detection in humans, in

Xenobiotics and Cancer: Implications for Chemical Carcinogenesis and Cancer Chemotherapy (eds L. Ernster, H. Esumi, Z. Fujii, H.V. Gelboin, R. Kato, and T. Sugimura), Japan Scientific Press, Tokyo, pp. 339–359.

149 Esumi, H., Ohgaki, H., Kohzen, E., Takayama, S., and Sugimura, T. (1989) Induction of lymphoma in CDF1 mice by the food mutagen, 2-amino-1-methyl-6-phenylimidazo[4,5-*b*]pyridine. *Jpn J. Cancer Res.*, **80**, 1176–1178.

150 Wakabayashi, K., Nagao, M., Esumi, H., and Sugimura, T. (1992) Food-derived mutagens and carcinogens. *Cancer Res.*, **52**, 2092s–2098s.

151 Kuper, H., Tzonou, A., Kaklamani, E., Hsieh, C.C., Lagiou, P., Adami, H.O., Trichopoulos, D., and Stuver, S.O. (2000) Tobacco smoking, alcohol consumption and their interaction in the causation of hepatocellular carcinoma. *Int. J. Cancer*, **85**, 498–502.

152 Bock, K.W. (1991) Roles of UDP-glucuronosyltransferases in chemical carcinogenesis. *Crit. Rev. Biochem. Mol. Biol.*, **26**, 129–150.

153 el Mouelhi, M., Didolkar, M.S., Elias, E.G., Guengerich, F.P., and Kauffman, F.C. (1987) Hepatic drug-metabolizing enzymes in primary and secondary tumors of human liver. *Cancer Res.*, **47**, 460–466.

154 Fischer, G., Schauer, A., Hartmann, H., and Bock, K.W. (1985) Increased UDP-glucuronyltransferase in putative preneoplastic foci of human liver after long-term use of oral contraceptives. *Naturwissenschaften*, **72**, 277–278.

155 Hu, Z. and Wells, P.G. (1994) Modulation of benzo[*a*]pyrene bioactivation by glucuronidation in lymphocytes and hepatic microsomes from rats with a hereditary deficiency in bilirubin UDP-glucuronosyltransferase. *Toxicol. Appl. Pharmacol.*, **127**, 306–313.

156 Nowell, S.A., Massengill, J.S., Williams, S., Radominska-Pandya, A., Tephly, T.R., Cheng, Z., Strassburg, C.P., Tukey, R.H., MacLeod, S.L., Lang, N.P., *et al.* (1999) Glucuronidation of 2-hydroxyamino-1-methyl-6-phenylimidazo[4,5-*b*]pyridine by human microsomal UDP-glucuronosyltransferases: identification of specific UGT1A family isoforms involved. *Carcinogenesis*, **20**, 1107–1114.

157 Vienneau, D.S., DeBoni, U., and Wells, P.G. (1995) Potential genoprotective role for UDP-glucuronosyltransferases in chemical carcinogenesis: initiation of micronuclei by benzo(*a*)pyrene and benzo(*e*)pyrene in UDP-glucuronosyltransferase-deficient cultured rat skin fibroblasts. *Cancer Res.*, **55**, 1045–1051.

158 Rothman, N., Garcia-Closas, M., Chatterjee, N., Malats, N., Wu, X., Figueroa, J.D., Real, F.X., Van Den Berg, D., Matullo, G., Baris, D., *et al.* (2010) A multi-stage genome-wide association study of bladder cancer identifies multiple susceptibility loci. *Nat. Genet.*, **42**, 978–984.

159 Saeki, M., Saito, Y., Jinno, H., Sai, K., Hachisuka, A., Kaniwa, N., Ozawa, S., Kawamoto, M., Kamatani, N., Shirao, K., *et al.* (2005) Genetic variations and haplotypes of UGT1A4 in a Japanese population. *Drug Metab. Pharmacokinet.*, **20**, 144–151.

160 Bigler, J., Whitton, J., Lampe, J.W., Fosdick, L., Bostick, R.M., and Potter, J.D. (2001) CYP2C9 and UGT1A6 genotypes modulate the protective effect of aspirin on colon adenoma risk. *Cancer Res.*, **61**, 3566–3569.

161 Chan, A.T., Tranah, G.J., Giovannucci, E.L., Hunter, D.J., and Fuchs, C.S. (2005) Genetic variants in the UGT1A6 enzyme, aspirin use, and the risk of colorectal adenoma. *J. Natl. Cancer Inst.*, **97**, 457–460.

162 McGreavey, L.E., Turner, F., Smith, G., Boylan, K., Timothy Bishop, D., Forman, D., Roland Wolf, C., and Barrett, J.H. (2005) No evidence that polymorphisms in CYP2C8, CYP2C9, UGT1A6, PPARdelta and PPARgamma act as modifiers of the protective effect of regular NSAID use on the risk of colorectal carcinoma. *Pharmacogenet. Genomics*, **15**, 713–721.

163 Hubner, R.A., Muir, K.R., Liu, J.F., Logan, R.F., Grainge, M., Armitage, N., Shepherd, V., Popat, S., and Houlston, R.S. (2006) Genetic variants of UGT1A6 influence risk of colorectal adenoma

recurrence. *Clin. Cancer Res.*, **12**, 6585–6589.

164 Tang, K.S., Lee, C.M., Teng, H.C., Huang, M.J., and Huang, C.S. (2008) UDP-glucuronosyltransferase 1A7 polymorphisms are associated with liver cirrhosis. *Biochem. Biophys. Res. Commun.*, **366**, 643–648.

165 Tseng, C.S., Tang, K.S., Lo, H.W., Ker, C.G., Teng, H.C., and Huang, C.S. (2005) UDP-glucuronosyltransferase 1A7 genetic polymorphisms are associated with hepatocellular carcinoma risk and onset age. *Am. J. Gastroenterol.*, **100**, 1758–1763.

166 Kong, S.Y., Ki, C.S., Yoo, B.C., and Kim, J.W. (2008) UGT1A7 haplotype is associated with an increased risk of hepatocellular carcinoma in hepatitis B carriers. *Cancer Sci.*, **99**, 340–344.

167 Vogel, A., Ockenga, J., Ehmer, U., Barut, A., Kramer, F.-J., Tukey, R.H., Manns, M.P., and Strassburg, C.P. (2002) Polymorphisms of the carcinogen detoxifying UDP-glucuronosyltransferase UGT1A7 in proximal digestive tract cancer. *Z. Gastroenterol.*, **40**, 497–502.

168 Vogel, A., Kneip, S., Barut, S., Ehmer, U., Tukey, R.H., Manns, M.P., and Strassburg, C.P. (2001) Genetic link of hepatocellular carcinoma with polymorphisms of the UDP-glucuronosyltransferase UGT1A7 gene. *Gastroenterology*, **121**, 1136–1144.

169 Vogel, A., Ockenga, J., Tukey, R.H., Manns, M.P., and Strassburg, C.P. (2011) Genotyping of the UDP-glucuronosyltransferase (UGT) 1A7 gene revisited. *Gastroenterology*, **140**, 1692–1693.

170 Stucker, I., Loriot, M.A., N'Koutchou, G., Cenee, S., Bodin, L., Mulot, C., Gelu-Simeon, M., Pelletier, L., Bronowicki, J.P., Degos, F., *et al.* (2007) UDP-glucuronosyltransferase UGT1A7 genetic polymorphisms in hepatocellular carcinoma: a differential impact according to seropositivity of HBV or HCV markers? *BMC Cancer*, **7**, 214.

171 Piepoli, A., Gentile, A., Valvano, M.R., Barana, D., Oliani, C., Cotugno, R., Quitadamo, M., Andriulli, A., and Perri, F. (2006) Lack of association between UGT1A7, UGT1A9, ARP, SPINK1 and CFTR gene polymorphisms and pancreatic cancer in Italian patients. *World J. Gastroenterol.*, **12**, 6343–6348.

172 Araki, J., Kobayashi, Y., Iwasa, M., Urawa, N., Gabazza, E.C., Taguchi, O., Kaito, M., and Adachi, Y. (2005) Polymorphism of UDP-glucuronosyltransferase 1A7 gene: a possible new risk factor for lung cancer. *Eur. J. Cancer*, **41**, 2360–2365.

173 Chen, K., Jin, M., Zhu, Y., Jiang, Q., Yu, W., Ma, X., and Yao, K. (2006) Genetic polymorphisms of the uridine diphosphate glucuronosyltransferase 1A7 and colorectal cancer risk in relation to cigarette smoking and alcohol drinking in a Chinese population. *J. Gastroenterol. Hepatol.*, **21**, 1036–1041.

174 Zheng, Z., Park, J.Y., Guillemette, C., Schantz, S.P., and Lazarus, P. (2001) Tobacco carcinogen-detoxifying enzyme UGT1A7 and its association with orolaryngeal cancer risk. *J. Natl. Cancer Inst.*, **93**, 1411–1418.

175 Butler, L.M., Duguay, Y., Millikan, R.C., Sinha, R., Gagne, J.F., Sandler, R.S., and Guillemette, C. (2005) Joint effects between UDP-glucuronosyltransferase 1A7 genotype and dietary carcinogen exposure on risk of colon cancer. *Cancer Epidemiol. Biomarkers Prev.*, **14**, 1626–1632.

176 Wang, Y., Kato, N., Hoshida, Y., Otsuka, M., Taniguchi, H., Moriyama, M., Shiina, S., Kawabe, T., Ito, Y.M., and Omata, M. (2004) UDP-glucuronosyltransferase 1A7 genetic polymorphisms are associated with hepatocellular carcinoma in Japanese patients with hepatitis C virus infection. *Clin. Cancer Res.*, **10**, 2441–2446.

177 Elahi, A., Bendaly, J., Zheng, Z., Muscat, J.E., Richie, J.P., Jr, Schantz, S.P., and Lazarus, P. (2003) Detection of UGT1A10 polymorphisms and their association with orolaryngeal carcinoma risk. *Cancer*, **98**, 872–880.

178 Strassburg, C.P., Manns, M.P., and Tukey, R.H. (1997) Differential down-regulation of the UDP-glucuronosyltransferase 1A locus is an early event in human liver and biliary cancer. *Cancer Res.*, **57**, 2979–2985.

179 te Morsche, R.H., Drenth, J.P., Truninger, K., Schulz, H.U., Kage, A., Landt, O., Verlaan, M., Rosendahl, J., Macek, M., Jr, Jansen, J.B., *et al.* (2008) UGT1A7 polymorphisms in chronic pancreatitis: an example of genotyping pitfalls. *Pharmacogenomics J.*, **8**, 34–41.

180 Emi, Y., Ikushiro, S., and Iyanagi, T. (1996) Xenobiotic responsive element-mediated transcriptional activation in the UDP-glucuronosyltransferase family 1 gene complex. *J. Biol. Chem.*, **271**, 3952–3958.

181 Munzel, P.A., Lehmkoster, T., Bruck, M., Ritter, J.K., and Bock, K.W. (1998) Aryl hydrocarbon receptor-inducible or constitutive expression of human UDP glucuronosyltransferase UGT1A6. *Arch. Biochem. Biophys.*, **350**, 72–78.

182 Munzel, P.A., Schmohl, S., Buckler, F., Jaehrling, J., Raschko, F.T., Kohle, C., and Bock, K.W. (2003) Contribution of the Ah receptor to the phenolic antioxidant-mediated expression of human and rat UDP-glucuronosyltransferase UGT1A6 in Caco-2 and rat hepatoma 5L cells. *Biochem. Pharmacol.*, **66**, 841–847.

183 Chen, S., Beaton, D., Nguyen, N., Senekeo-Effenberger, K., Brace-Sinnokrak, E., Argikar, U., Remmel, R.P., Trottier, J., Barbier, O., Ritter, J.K., *et al.* (2005) Tissue-specific, inducible, and hormonal control of the human UDP-glucuronosyltransferase-1 (UGT1) locus. *J. Biol. Chem.*, **280**, 37547–37557.

184 Sugatani, J., Yamakawa, K., Tonda, E., Nishitani, S., Yoshinari, K., Degawa, M., Abe, I., Noguchi, H., and Miwa, M. (2004) The induction of human UDP-glucuronosyltransferase 1A1 mediated through a distal enhancer module by flavonoids and xenobiotics. *Biochem. Pharmacol.*, **67**, 989–1000.

185 Auyeung, D.J., Kessler, F.K., and Ritter, J.K. (2003) Mechanism of rat UDP-glucuronosyltransferase 1A6 induction by oltipraz: evidence for a contribution of the aryl hydrocarbon receptor pathway. *Mol. Pharmacol.*, **63**, 119–127.

186 Grams, B., Harms, A., Braun, S., Strassburg, C.P., Manns, M.P., and Obermayer-Straub, P. (2000) Distribution and inducibility by 3-methylcholanthrene of family 1 UDP-glucuronosyltransferases in the rat gastrointestinal tract. *Arch. Biochem. Biophys.*, **377**, 255–265.

187 Chen, Y.H. and Tukey, R.H. (1996) Protein kinase C modulates regulation of the CYP1A1 gene by the aryl hydrocarbon receptor. *J. Biol. Chem.*, **271**, 26261–26266.

188 Zhou, J., Zhang, J., and Xie, W. (2005) Xenobiotic nuclear receptor-mediated regulation of UDP-glucuronosyl-transferases. *Curr. Drug Metab.*, **6**, 289–298.

189 Lankisch, T.O., Gillman, T.C., Erichsen, T.J., Ehmer, U., Kalthoff, S., Freiberg, N., Munzel, P.A., Manns, M.P., and Strassburg, C.P. (2008) Aryl hydrocarbon receptor (AhR)-mediated regulation of the human estrogen and bile acid UDP-glucuronosyltransferase 1A3 gene. *Arch. Toxicol.*, **82**, 573–582.

190 Gardner-Stephen, D.A. and Mackenzie, P.I. (2007) Isolation of the UDP-glucuronosyltransferase 1A3 and 1A4 proximal promoters and characterization of their dependence on the transcription factor hepatocyte nuclear factor 1alpha. *Drug Metab. Dispos.*, **35**, 116–120.

191 Usui, T., Kuno, T., Ueyama, H., Ohkubo, I., and Mizutani, T. (2006) Proximal HNF1 element is essential for the induction of human UDP-glucuronosyltransferase 1A1 by glucocorticoid receptor. *Biochem. Pharmacol.*, **71**, 693–701.

192 Xanthopoulos, K.G., Prezioso, V.R., Chen, W.S., Sladek, F.M., Cortese, R., and Darnell, J.E., Jr (1991) The different tissue transcription patterns of genes for HNF-1, C/EBP, HNF-3, and HNF-4, protein factors that govern liver-specific transcription. *Proc. Natl. Acad. Sci. USA*, **88**, 3807–3811.

193 Sladek, F.M., Zhong, W.M., Lai, E., and Darnell, J.E., Jr (1990) Liver-enriched transcription factor HNF-4 is a novel member of the steroid hormone receptor superfamily. *Genes Dev.*, **4**, 2353–2365.

194 Odom, D.T., Zizlsperger, N., Gordon, D.B., Bell, G.W., Rinaldi, N.J., Murray, H.L., Volkert, T.L., Schreiber, J., Rolfe, P.A., Gifford, D.K., *et al.* (2004) Control

of pancreas and liver gene expression by HNF transcription factors. *Science*, **303**, 1378–1381.

195 Gregory, P.A., Lewinsky, R.H., Gardner-Stephen, D.A., and Mackenzie, P.I. (2004) Coordinate regulation of the human UDP-glucuronosyltransferase 1A8, 1A9, and 1A10 genes by hepatocyte nuclear factor 1alpha and the caudal-related homeodomain protein 2. *Mol. Pharmacol.*, **65**, 953–963.

196 Gardner-Stephen, D.A. and Mackenzie, P.I. (2007) Hepatocyte nuclear factor1 transcription factors are essential for the UDP-glucuronosyltransferase 1A9 promoter response to hepatocyte nuclear factor 4alpha. *Pharmacogenet. Genomics*, **17**, 25–36.

197 Barbier, O., Girard, H., Inoue, Y., Duez, H., Villeneuve, L., Kamiya, A., Fruchart, J.C., Guillemette, C., Gonzalez, F.J., and Staels, B. (2005) Hepatic expression of the UGT1A9 gene is governed by hepatocyte nuclear factor 4alpha. *Mol. Pharmacol.*, **67**, 241–249.

198 Ehmer, U., Kalthoff, S., Lankisch, T.O., Freiberg, N., Manns, M.P., and Strassburg, C.P. (2010) Shared regulation of UGT1A7 by hepatocyte nuclear factor (HNF) 1alpha and HNF-4alpha. *Drug Metab. Dispos.*, **38**, 1246–1257.

199 Metz, R.P., Auyeung, D.J., Kessler, F.K., and Ritter, J.K. (2000) Involvement of hepatocyte nuclear factor 1 in the regulation of the UDP-glucuronosyltransferase 1A7 (UGT1A7) gene in rat hepatocytes. *Mol. Pharmacol.*, **58**, 319–327.

200 Parks, D.J., Blanchard, S.G., Bledsoe, R.K., Chandra, G., Consler, T.G., Kliewer, S.A., Stimmel, J.B., Willson, T.M., Zavacki, A.M., Moore, D.D., *et al.* (1999) Bile acids: natural ligands for an orphan nuclear receptor. *Science*, **284**, 1365–1368.

201 Wang, H., Chen, J., Hollister, K., Sowers, L.C., and Forman, B.M. (1999) Endogenous bile acids are ligands for the nuclear receptor FXR/BAR. *Mol. Cell*, **3**, 543–553.

202 Wang, S., Lai, K., Moy, F.J., Bhat, A., Hartman, H.B., and Evans, M.J. (2006) The nuclear hormone receptor farnesoid X receptor (FXR) is activated by androsterone. *Endocrinology*, **147**, 4025–4033.

203 Watanabe, M., Houten, S.M., Mataki, C., Christoffolete, M.A., Kim, B.W., Sato, H., Messaddeq, N., Harney, J.W., Ezaki, O., Kodama, T., *et al.* (2006) Bile acids induce energy expenditure by promoting intracellular thyroid hormone activation. *Nature*, **439**, 484–489.

204 Downes, M., Verdecia, M.A., Roecker, A.J., Hughes, R., Hogenesch, J.B., Kast-Woelbern, H.R., Bowman, M.E., Ferrer, J.L., Anisfeld, A.M., Edwards, P.A., *et al.* (2003) A chemical, genetic, and structural analysis of the nuclear bile acid receptor FXR. *Mol. Cell*, **11**, 1079–1092.

205 Maloney, P.R., Parks, D.J., Haffner, C.D., Fivush, A.M., Chandra, G., Plunket, K.D., Creech, K.L., Moore, L.B., Wilson, J.G., Lewis, M.C., *et al.* (2000) Identification of a chemical tool for the orphan nuclear receptor FXR. *J. Med. Chem.*, **43**, 2971–2974.

206 Pellicciari, R., Fiorucci, S., Camaioni, E., Clerici, C., Costantino, G., Maloney, P.R., Morelli, A., Parks, D.J., and Willson, T.M. (2002) 6α-Ethyl-chenodeoxycholic acid (6-ECDCA), a potent and selective FXR agonist endowed with anticholestatic activity. *J. Med. Chem.*, **45**, 3569–3572.

207 Dussault, I., Beard, R., Lin, M., Hollister, K., Chen, J., Xiao, J.H., Chandraratna, R., and Forman, B.M. (2003) Identification of gene-selective modulators of the bile acid receptor FXR. *J. Biol. Chem.*, **278**, 7027–7033.

208 Matern, H., Matern, S., Schelzig, C., and Gerok, W. (1980) Bile acid UDP-glucoronyltransferase from human liver. Properties and studies on aglycone substrate specificity. *FEBS Lett.*, **118**, 251–254.

209 Parquet, M., Pessah, M., Sacquet, E., Salvat, C., Raizman, A., and Infante, R. (1985) Glucuronidation of bile acids in human liver, intestine and kidney. An *in vitro* study on hyodeoxycholic acid. *FEBS Lett.*, **189**, 183–187.

210 Barbier, O., Torra, I.P., Sirvent, A., Claudel, T., Blanquart, C., Duran-Sandoval, D., Kuipers, F., Kosykh, V.,

Fruchart, J.C., and Staels, B. (2003) FXR induces the UGT2B4 enzyme in hepatocytes: a potential mechanism of negative feedback control of FXR activity. *Gastroenterology*, **124**, 1926–1940.

211 Gall, W.E., Zawada, G., Mojarrabi, B., Tephly, T.R., Green, M.D., Coffman, B.L., Mackenzie, P.I., and Radominska-Pandya, A. (1999) Differential glucuronidation of bile acids, androgens and estrogens by human UGT1A3 and 2B7. *J. Steroid Biochem. Mol. Biol.*, **70**, 101–108.

212 Forman, B.M., Goode, E., Chen, J., Oro, A.E., Bradley, D.J., Perlmann, T., Noonan, D.J., Burka, L.T., McMorris, T., Lamph, W.W., *et al.* (1995) Identification of a nuclear receptor that is activated by farnesol metabolites. *Cell*, **81**, 687–693.

213 Glass, C.K. (1994) Differential recognition of target genes by nuclear receptor monomers, dimers, and heterodimers. *Endocr. Rev.*, **15**, 391–407.

214 Seol, W., Choi, H.S., and Moore, D.D. (1996) An orphan nuclear hormone receptor that lacks a DNA binding domain and heterodimerizes with other receptors. *Science*, **272**, 1336–1339.

215 Kalthoff, S., Ehmer, U., Freiberg, N., Manns, M.P., and Strassburg, C.P. (2010) Interaction between oxidative stress sensor Nrf2 and xenobiotic-activated aryl hydrocarbon receptor in the regulation of the human phase II detoxifying UDP-glucuronosyltransferase 1A10. *J. Biol. Chem.*, **285**, 5993–6002.

216 Marini, M.G., Chan, K., Casula, L., Kan, Y.W., Cao, A., and Moi, P. (1997) hMAF, a small human transcription factor that heterodimerizes specifically with Nrf1 and Nrf2. *J. Biol. Chem.*, **272**, 16490–16497.

217 Nguyen, T., Sherratt, P.J., and Pickett, C.B. (2003) Regulatory mechanisms controlling gene expression mediated by the antioxidant response element. *Annu. Rev. Pharmacol. Toxicol.*, **43**, 233–260.

218 Venugopal, R. and Jaiswal, A.K. (1998) Nrf2 and Nrf1 in association with Jun proteins regulate antioxidant response element-mediated expression and coordinated induction of genes encoding detoxifying enzymes. *Oncogene*, **17**, 3145–3156.

219 Buckley, D.B. and Klaassen, C.D. (2009) Induction of mouse UDP-glucuronosyltransferase mRNA expression in liver and intestine by activators of aryl-hydrocarbon receptor, constitutive androstane receptor, pregnane X receptor, peroxisome proliferator-activated receptor alpha, and nuclear factor erythroid 2-related factor 2. *Drug Metab. Dispos.*, **37**, 847–856.

220 Yueh, M.F. and Tukey, R.H. (2007) Nrf2–Keap1 signaling pathway regulates human UGT1A1 expression *in vitro* and in transgenic UGT1 mice. *J. Biol. Chem.*, **282**, 8749–8758.

221 Yeager, R.L., Reisman, S.A., Aleksunes, L.M., and Klaassen, C.D. (2009) Introducing the "TCDD-inducible AhR–Nrf2 gene battery". *Toxicol. Sci.*, **111**, 238–246.

222 Girard, H., Levesque, E., Bellemare, J., Journault, K., Caillier, B., and Guillemette, C. (2007) Genetic diversity at the UGT1 locus is amplified by a novel 3′ alternative splicing mechanism leading to nine additional UGT1A proteins that act as regulators of glucuronidation activity. *Pharmacogenet. Genomics*, **17**, 1077–1089.

223 Bellemare, J., Rouleau, M., Girard, H., Harvey, M., and Guillemette, C. (2010) Alternatively spliced products of the UGT1A gene interact with the enzymatically active proteins to inhibit glucuronosyltransferase activity *in vitro*. *Drug Metab. Dispos.*, **38**, 1785–1789.

224 Bellemare, J., Rouleau, M., Harvey, M., Popa, I., Pelletier, G., Tetu, B., and Guillemette, C. (2011) Immunohistochemical expression of conjugating UGT1A-derived isoforms in normal and tumoral drug-metabolizing tissues in humans. *J. Pathol.*, **223**, 425–435.

225 Roy-Chowdhury, J., Huang, T.J., Kesari, K., Lederstein, M., Arias, I.M., and Roy-Chowdhury, N. (1991) Molecular basis for the lack of bilirubin-specific and 3-methylcholanthrene-inducible UDP-glucuronosyltransferase activities in Gunn rats. The two isoforms are encoded by distinct mRNA species that share an identical single base deletion. *J. Biol. Chem.*, **266**, 18294–18298.

226 Crigler, J.F. and Najjar, V.A. (1952) Congenital familial nonhemolytic jaundice with kernicterus. *Pediatrics*, **10**, 169–179.

227 Mackenzie, P.I. and Owens, I.S. (1983) Differences in UDP-glucuronosyltransferase activities in congenic inbred rats homozygous and heterozygous for the jaundice locus. *Biochem. Pharmacol.*, **32**, 3777–3781.

228 Senekeo-Effenberger, K., Chen, S., Brace-Sinnokrak, E., Bonzo, J.A., Yueh, M.F., Argikar, U., Kaeding, J., Trottier, J., Remmel, R.P., Ritter, J.K., *et al.* (2007) Expression of the human UGT1 locus in transgenic mice by 4-chloro-6-(2,3-xylidino)-2-pyrimidinylthioacetic acid (WY-14643) and implications on drug metabolism through peroxisome proliferator-activated receptor alpha activation. *Drug Metab. Dispos.*, **35**, 419–427.

229 Verreault, M., Senekeo-Effenberger, K., Trottier, J., Bonzo, J.A., Belanger, J., Kaeding, J., Staels, B., Caron, P., Tukey, R.H., and Barbier, O. (2006) The liver X-receptor alpha controls hepatic expression of the human bile acid-glucuronidating UGT1A3 enzyme in human cells and transgenic mice. *Hepatology*, **44**, 368–378.

230 Nguyen, N., Bonzo, J.A., Chen, S., Chouinard, S., Kelner, M.J., Hardiman, G., Belanger, A., and Tukey, R.H. (2008) Disruption of the *ugt1* locus in mice resembles human Crigler–Najjar type I disease. *J. Biol. Chem.*, **283**, 7901–7911.

231 Cai, H., Nguyen, N., Peterkin, V., Yang, Y.S., Hotz, K., La Placa, D.B., Chen, S., Tukey, R.H., and Stevens, J.C. (2010) A humanized UGT1 mouse model expressing the UGT1A1*28 allele for assessing drug clearance by UGT1A1-dependent glucuronidation. *Drug Metab. Dispos.*, **38**, 879–886.

232 Ritter, J.K., Kessler, F.K., Thompson, M.T., Grove, A.D., Auyeung, D.J., and Fisher, R.A. (1999) Expression and inducibility of the human bilirubin UDP-glucuronosyltransferase UGT1A1 in liver and cultured primary hepatocytes: evidence for both genetic and environmental influences. *Hepatology*, **30**, 476–484.

233 Sugatani, J., Kojima, H., Ueda, A., Kakizaki, S., Yoshinari, K., Gong, Q.H., Owens, I.S., Negishi, M., and Sueyoshi, T. (2001) The phenobarbital response enhancer module in the human bilirubin UDP-glucuronosyltransferase UGT1A1 gene and regulation by the nuclear receptor CAR. *Hepatology*, **33**, 1232–1238.

234 Ellis, E., Wagner, M., Lammert, F., Nemeth, A., Gumhold, J., Strassburg, C.P., Kylander, C., Katsika, D., Trauner, M., Einarsson, C., *et al.* (2006) Successful treatment of severe unconjugated hyperbilirubinemia via induction of UGT1A1 by rifampicin. *J. Hepatol.*, **44**, 243–245.

235 Gressner, O.A. (2010) In the search of the magic bullet. *Gastroenterology*, **139**, 1453–1457.

4
Sulfotransferases

Michael W.H. Coughtrie

4.1
Introduction

Sulfation is an important pathway for the metabolism of many xenobiotics and important endogenous chemicals. This is generally seen as a detoxification pathway since most sulfate conjugates are devoid of significant biological activity, and they are good substrates for uptake and efflux transporters involved in the elimination of xenobiotics from the body. Paradoxically, for certain compounds such as aromatic amines and benzylic alcohols sulfation is an important step in the bioactivation of many of these promutagens and procarcinogens. Many recent advances have given us insights into the role of sulfation and sulfotransferases (SULTs) in biology.

In humans the SULT superfamily comprises 13 members involved in the sulfation of many drugs and other xenobiotics, steroid hormones, sterols, iodothyronines, and catecholamines. The enzyme reaction utilizes the universal sulfuryl donor 3′-phosphoadenosine-5′-phosphosulfate (PAPS). In the human liver SULT1A1 is the most abundant, and arguably the most important, enzyme from a chemical defense perspective since it is able to sulfate a very wide range of phenols, catechols, and so on, with high affinity. Structural biology studies have identified the molecular basis for the enzymatic reaction. Key conserved amino acids are involved in the binding of PAPS to the enzyme, while specificity seems to be determined by a number of factors, such as specific charged amino acids providing the appropriate environment within the active site in the case of the catecholamine SULT (SULT1A3) or steric hindrance and substrate gating in the case of some of the steroid SULTs.

There is a considerable degree of interindividual (and interethnic) variability in the expression of SULTs within the human population and the genetic basis of this is now becoming clearer, at least for some of the enzymes such as SULT1A1. Common single nucleotide polymorphisms (SNPs) exist, in particular the *SULT1A1*2* allele that has been associated with reduced SULT expression/activity in tissues. Many molecular epidemiological studies have been carried out into the potential association of this allele with susceptibility to a variety of potentially

Metabolism of Drugs and Other Xenobiotics, First Edition. Edited by Pavel Anzenbacher, Ulrich M. Zanger.

chemically induced cancers. On the whole these studies, where they show an association, tend to suggest that the wild-type allele (*SULT1A1*1*) is protective. However, these studies have recently been called into question by the discovery of a common copy number variance polymorphism, where between one and five copies of *SULT1A1* may be observed. This is believed to have the most significant impact over SULT expression/activity levels in tissues; clearly these molecular epidemiology studies should be repeated using the wider range of genetic markers of SULT1A1 function now available.

There are many facets to the role of sulfation and this chapter attempts to capture the more recent and pertinent advances in our understanding of these important enzymes.

4.2 Background

The addition of sulfate, catalyzed by SULT enzymes, is a ubiquitous process in nature, with a vast range of acceptor substrates, including xenobiotics, steroid and thyroid hormones, neurotransmitters, lipids, carbohydrates, and proteins [1, 2]. These reactions are involved in a host of biosynthetic and biotransformation processes, including the biosynthesis of hormones, proteoglycans, sulfolipids, and so on, in addition to detoxification of xenobiotics, that influence a wide range of fundamental biological processes. The vast majority of these reactions utilize the "universal" sulfuryl donor PAPS [3]; however, in bacteria some SULTs (arylsulfate SULTs) catalyze sulfuryl transfer between phenolic xenobiotics in a process independent of PAPS [4]. This is reflected in their structural architecture, which bears no resemblance to PAPS-dependent SULTs [5]. This chapter will focus on the cytosolic PAPS-dependent SULTs (the nomenclature for SULTs used throughout is that described in [6]) involved in the metabolism and elimination of small-molecule xeno- and endobiotics, and in particular their role in the biotransformation of drugs and other xenobiotics in humans. The SULT reaction is summarized in Figure 4.1. In this capacity, sulfation is generally a detoxification reaction, in that sulfate conjugates of xenobiotics tend to be inert (relative to the parent compounds) and are good substrates for the ion transporters, such as members of the multidrug resistance protein family, responsible for the elimination of xenobiotics from the body. This principle also holds for a number of endogenous substrates for sulfation such as estrogens, where sulfation abolishes the ability of, for example, β-estradiol to activate the estrogen receptor. In some cases, however, sulfation can result in an increased biological activity, which has important toxicological implications. The sulfate esters of many benzylic alcohols and hydroxylated aromatic amines are extremely unstable – spontaneously decomposing to form highly reactive electrophiles that can bind to DNA and cause mutations [7].

The original observations that sulfation was involved in the biotransformation of xenobiotics were made in the nineteenth century, when Eugen Baumann isolated the sulfate conjugate of phenol from a patient treated with carbolic acid, having previously identified sulfated phenols in horse urine [8]. A number of

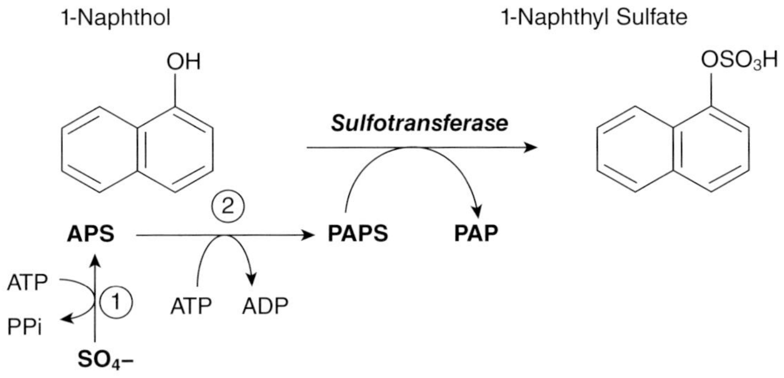

Figure 4.1 SULT reaction. The enzyme reaction utilizes PAPS as sulfuryl donor, which is synthesized in a two-step reaction from inorganic sulfate and ATP. In animals, these two steps are carried out by a single bifunctional enzyme PAPS synthetase, which catalyzes both the ATP sulfurylase (1) and APS kinase (2) reactions.

workers subsequently demonstrated the synthesis of sulfate conjugates of xenobiotics in isolated organs, liver slices, and broken cell preparations (e.g., [9, 10]). The role of PAPS as the sulfuryl donor in these reactions was confirmed by Lipmann in 1956 [11] and it is now clear that it is the cosubstrate for all SULTs with the exception of the bacterial arylsulfate SULTs. It was clear from the early days of SULT research that several forms of the enzyme existed in mammalian liver (e.g., [12, 13]), involved in the sulfation of endogenous (e.g., steroids) and xenobiotic (e.g., phenols, catechols, alcohols) substrates, and (partial) purification of various steroid and phenol SULT enzymes was achieved in the 1960s and 1970s by Adams [14], Barford and Jones [15], McEvoy and Carroll [16], Jakoby [17], and others. Purification and detailed kinetic and molecular characterization of SULTs from various species during the 1980s and 1990s highlighted the extent of the diversity of SULT enzyme family, which was confirmed during the explosion in molecular biology that led to the cloning, expression and characterization of a host of SULTs from many different species. The first SULT cDNA to be cloned was a rat hydroxysteroid SULT of the SULT2A family in 1987 [18], although at the time it was not recognized as a SULT; it was identified as an androgen-repressible protein associated with senescence. The following year, the first identified SULT was cloned – the bovine estrogen SULT1E1 [19]. The completion of genome-sequencing projects for so many species has greatly facilitated phylogenetic analysis of the SULT family; in the human genome there are 13 functional *SULT* genes and a number of pseudogenes.

4.3 PAPS Synthesis

PAPS is the obligate sulfuryl donor for SULTs and is therefore synthesized in all cells where sulfation takes place [3]. PAPS synthesis occurs in a two-step reaction requiring ATP and inorganic sulfate sourced from either the diet/environment or from the sulfoxidation of the sulfur-containing amino acids Cys and Met. The first step in the process results in the formation of adenosine 5′-phosphosulfate (APS) and pyrophosphate, and is catalyzed by ATP sulfurylase. In the tightly coupled second reaction, APS is phosphorylated by APS kinase, requiring a second molecule of ATP. In the vast majority of prokaryotes and lower eukaryotes such as yeast, fungi, and plants, the two stages of PAPS synthesis are catalyzed by separate enzymes; however, in eukaryotes, PAPS synthesis is carried out by a bifunctional enzyme – PAPS synthetase [20, 21]. Some prokaryotes do have fused bifunctional enzymes and in certain cases the order of the fusion is reversed from that seen in metazoans, indicating that two separate gene fusion events have occurred during evolution [22, 23]. This enzyme is therefore a key component of the sulfation system, as are the transporters involved in the uptake of sulfate from the gastrointestinal tract and in the renal reabsorption of sulfate, both of which contribute importantly to sulfate homeostasis and thus sulfation capacity. PAPS concentrations are generally low in tissues such as the liver – much lower than necessary to support sulfation rates observed, indicating that PAPS biosynthesis is rapid and can be accelerated in times of high demand. Depletion of PAPS (either physiologically or genetically) can result in a significantly reduced capacity for sulfation [24, 25].

Most higher metazoans have two isoforms of PAPS synthetase, PAPSS1 and PAPSS2, which can generate two splice variants (PAPSS2a and PAPSS2b) differing by a five-amino-acid sequence in the ATP sulfurylase domain [26]. PAPSS1 is located in the nucleus, whereas PAPSS2 is present in the cytosol [27], and there are distinct differences in the expression patterns of the two proteins, where PAPSS1 is expressed essentially ubiquitously within the body (and is the major isoform) and PAPSS2 expression is more tightly regulated. However, it has recently been shown that the two proteins can heterodimerize [28], although the function (if any) remains to be confirmed. Mutations in *PAPSS* genes are now known to be associated with a variety of diseases. This was first observed in mice, where brachymorphism (short stature associated with undersulfated cartilage proteoglycans) was attributed to a defect in PAPS synthesis [29], which was subsequently shown to be due to a missense mutation leading to a Gly79Arg substitution in the APS kinase domain of PAPSS2 [30]. Brachymorphic mice also show a reduced capacity (by up to 70%) for the sulfation of xenobiotics *in vitro* and *in vivo* [31], and are resistant to the carcinogenic properties of aromatic amines [32]. Mutations in human *PAPSS2* are causative for similar bone growth problems [33] and also for androgen excess disorders in women [34]. PAPSS1 was recently identified as playing a key role in retroviral infection [35] and the *PAPSS1* locus is associated with susceptibility to hepatocellular carcinoma [36]. A number of common polymorphisms in *PAPSS1* and *PAPSS2* have been identified and characterized [37, 38]. Taken together, these studies highlight the breadth of influence of sulfation on biological and physiological processes, and identify PAPS synthesis as a significant source for interindividual variation in sulfation capacity.

4.4
SULT Enzyme Family

The cytosolic SULTs comprise a large superfamily represented in species from bacteria to humans. The genome of *Saccharomyces cerevisiae* does not appear to contain any *SULT* genes or the presence of SULTs, and hence a role for sulfation of small molecules at least in (budding) yeast must be questioned. Yeasts do synthesize PAPS using ATP sulfurylase and APS kinase, but PAPS appears to be used for sulfite production (via PAPS reductase and thioredoxin) rather than as the sulfuryl donor for SULTs [39]. Phylogenetic analysis has identified that SULTs can be classified according to a number of subfamilies that have been described in detail [6], although given the explosion in genome sequencing across the evolutionary spectrum this analysis should be updated accordingly. This classification follows the principle that family members (i.e., SULT1, SULT2, etc.) share at least 45% amino acid sequence identity and subfamily members (i.e., SULT1A, SULT1B, etc.) have a minimum of 60% sequence identity. In vertebrates, there are six distinct SULT families (although not all species express members of each family), with at least an additional five related families found in invertebrates and bacteria (SULTs are particularly abundant in cyanobacteria) and in plants (Figure 4.2). The following summarizes the key known features of each vertebrate SULT family, with a particular focus on the human enzymes where relevant, and Figure 4.3 is a dendrogram illustrating the relationship between the members of the human SULT family. See also Table 4.1.

4.4.1
SULT1 Family

The SULT1 family, which comprises five subfamilies, plays an important role in xenobiotic metabolism as well as in the metabolism (and in regulating the function) of catecholamines, estrogens, thyroid hormones, and eicosanoids. It also contains enzymes capable of bioactivating dietary and environmental procarcinogens. SULT1A enzymes are also called phenol SULTs, since their major substrates contain target phenolic (or catecholic) hydroxyl group(s). SULT1A1 sulfates a very wide range of xenobiotics, usually with low K_m values [42], and as such is generally regarded as the major xenobiotic-metabolizing SULT. In addition, it can sulfate endogenous compounds such as estrogens [43] and iodothyronines [44]; however, the physiological role for this is questionable, particularly given the existence of SULT1E1 that sulfates, for example, 17β-estradiol with extremely high affinity (low K_m) [45] and also sulfates iodothyronines [44]. The SULT1A1 enzyme is widely distributed in human tissues and is the major isoform expressed in the adult liver [46]. A number of common genetic variants of *SULT1A1* have been documented, including a copy number polymorphism and a coding region SNP, both of which have been related to the high degree of variability in expression of this protein [47, 48]. SULT1A1 appears to be found in all mammals; however, unlike a number of other SULT1 family members, there are no orthologs in, for example, fish and

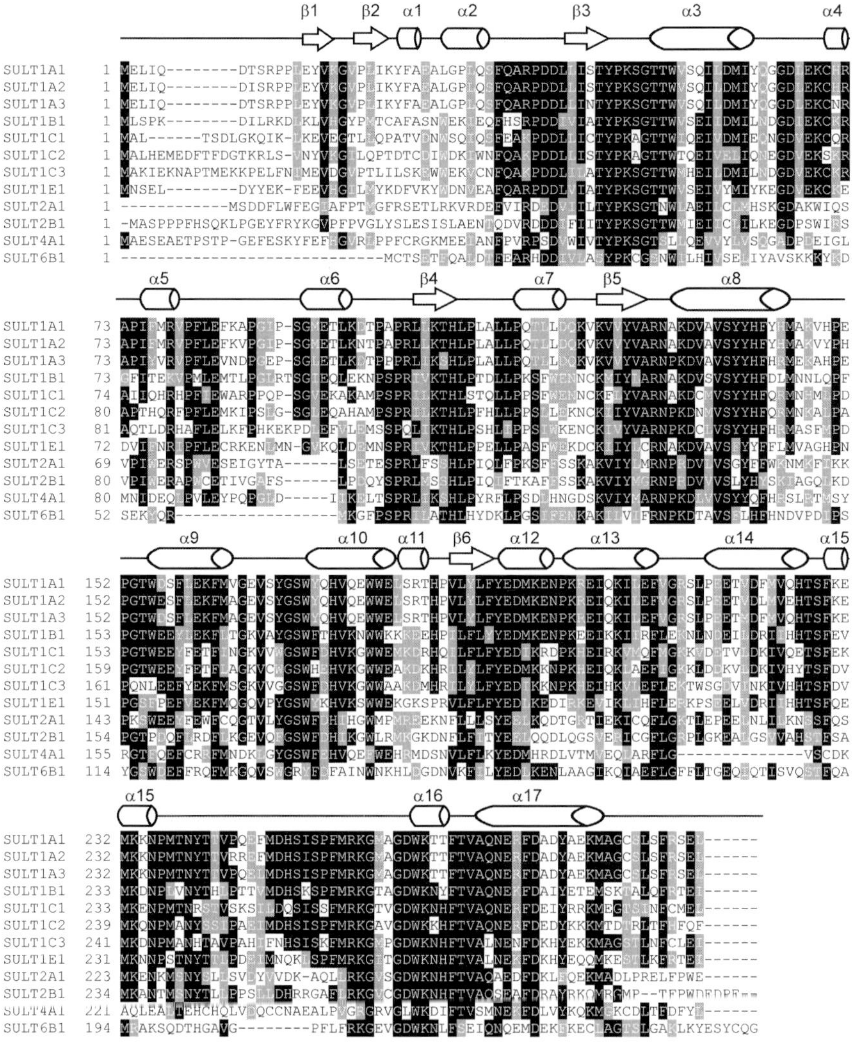

Figure 4.2 Sequence alignment of the human SULT enzyme family. Sequence alignment of the derived amino acid sequences of human SULTs was carried out using ClustalW2 [40] and BoxShade (http://www.ch.embnet.org/software/BOX_form.html). Highly conserved residues are highlighted in white against a black background. The common secondary structure elements of the family are shown above the alignment.

Figure 4.3 Inter-relationships within the SULT enzyme family. Representative SULTs from mammalian and avian species were selected, and their sequences compared using ClustalW2 [40] and the relationships visualized using TREEVIEW [41].

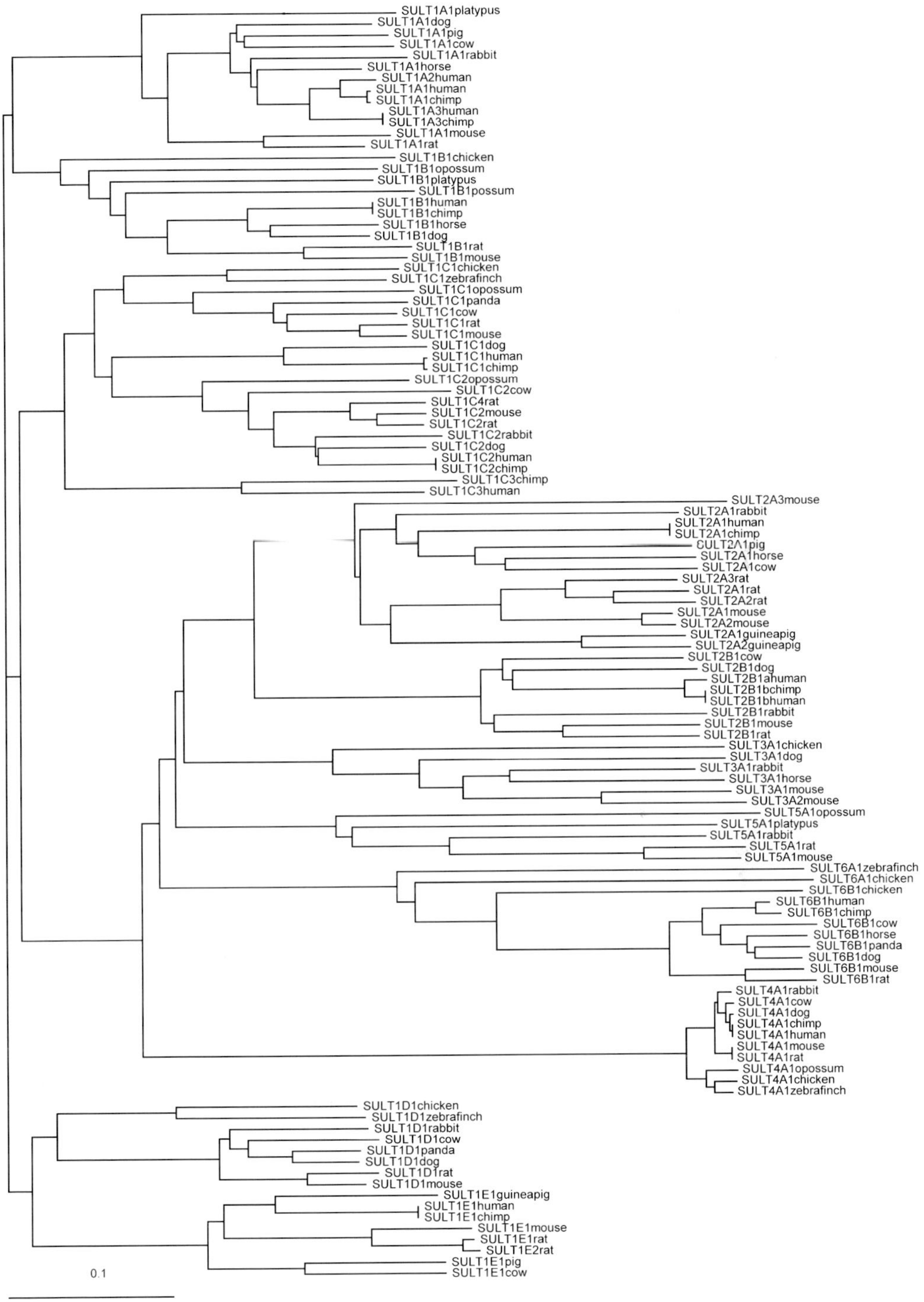
SULT1A1platypus
SULT1A1dog
SULT1A1pig
SULT1A1cow
SULT1A1rabbit
SULT1A1horse
SULT1A2human
SULT1A1human
SULT1A1chimp
SULT1A3human
SULT1A3chimp
SULT1A1mouse
SULT1A1rat
SULT1B1chicken
SULT1B1opossum
SULT1B1platypus
SULT1B1possum
SULT1B1human
SULT1B1chimp
SULT1B1horse
SULT1B1dog
SULT1B1rat
SULT1B1mouse
SULT1C1chicken
SULT1C1zebrafinch
SULT1C1opossum
SULT1C1panda
SULT1C1cow
SULT1C1rat
SULT1C1mouse
SULT1C1dog
SULT1C1human
SULT1C1chimp
SULT1C2opossum
SULT1C2cow
SULT1C4rat
SULT1C2mouse
SULT1C2rat
SULT1C2rabbit
SULT1C2dog
SULT1C2human
SULT1C2chimp
SULT1C3chimp
SULT1C3human
SULT2A3mouse
SULT2A1rabbit
SULT2A1human
SULT2A1chimp
SULT2A1pig
SULT2A1horse
SULT2A1cow
SULT2A3rat
SULT2A1rat
SULT2A2rat
SULT2A1mouse
SULT2A2mouse
SULT2A1guineapig
SULT2A2guineapig
SULT2B1cow
SULT2B1dog
SULT2B1ahuman
SULT2B1bchimp
SULT2B1bhuman
SULT2B1rabbit
SULT2B1mouse
SULT2B1rat
SULT3A1chicken
SULT3A1dog
SULT3A1rabbit
SULT3A1horse
SULT3A1mouse
SULT3A2mouse
SULT5A1opossum
SULT5A1platypus
SULT5A1rabbit
SULT5A1rat
SULT5A1mouse
SULT6A1zebrafinch
SULT6A1chicken
SULT6B1chicken
SULT6B1human
SULT6B1chimp
SULT6B1cow
SULT6B1horse
SULT6B1panda
SULT6B1dog
SULT6B1mouse
SULT6B1rat
SULT4A1rabbit
SULT4A1cow
SULT4A1dog
SULT4A1chimp
SULT4A1human
SULT4A1mouse
SULT4A1rat
SULT4A1opossum
SULT4A1chicken
SULT4A1zebrafinch
SULT1D1chicken
SULT1D1zebrafinch
SULT1D1rabbit
SULT1D1cow
SULT1D1panda
SULT1D1dog
SULT1D1rat
SULT1D1mouse
SULT1E1guineapig
SULT1E1human
SULT1E1chimp
SULT1E1mouse
SULT1E1rat
SULT1E2rat
SULT1E1pig
SULT1E1cow
0.1

Table 4.1 Human SULTs and their substrates.

SULT isoform	Probe substrate	Example drug substrates
SULT1A1	2-aminophenol	acetaminophen, troglitazone, minoxidil, 4-OH-tamoxifen, apomorphine
SULT1A2	no probe substrate known	–
SULT1A3	dopamine	salbutamol, dobutamine
SULT1B1	no probe substrate known	–
SULT1C1	no probe substrate known	–
SULT1C2	no probe substrate known	–
SULT1C3	no probe substrate known	–
SULT1E1	17β-estradiol	17α-ethinylestradiol
SULT2A1	dehydroepiandrosterone	budesonide, dehydroepiandrosterone, pregnenolone
SULT2B1	cholesterol (2B1b), pregnenolone (2B1b)	–
SULT4A1	no substrate known	–
SULT6B1	no probe substrate known	–

birds. SULT1A2 is very closely related (96.3% amino acid sequence identity) to SULT1A1 and the recombinant expressed enzyme is able to sulfate a similar range of compounds, albeit with generally lower affinities and reaction rates [42, 47, 49]. The presence of a *SULT1A2* gene is limited to primate genomes. There has been much debate as to whether SULT1A2 is expressed in human tissues, with suggestions that it is incorrectly spliced [50]. More recently, using an antipeptide antibody specific for SULT1A2, Nowell *et al.* failed to demonstrate expression in any human tissue [51]. However, Glatt's group have demonstrated expression of SULT1A2 in some cell lines [52] and at very low levels in the stomach [53]. It is therefore likely to be of little or no significance in the overall sulfation capacity of a tissue or individual.

The enzyme SULT1A3, or catecholamine SULT, is the product of two very closely related genes, *SULT1A3* and *SULT1A4*, which have been generated by a gene duplication event on chromosome 16 [54]. Although these genes differ in their nucleotide sequence, the predicted amino acid sequences of the protein products are identical. SULT1A3 displays a strong substrate preference (and low micromolar K_m) for dopamine and some other endogenous and xenobiotic catecholamines [42, 55–57], and the *SULT1A3* gene is only found in primates. This presumably represents an evolutionary development driven by the need to produce large amounts of sulfated catecholamines (e.g., dopamine sulfate accounts for almost 100% of the dopamine in the human circulation) [58]. This (and other sulfated catecholamines) are believed to originate primarily from the gastrointestinal tract [59, 60] and this is supported by the fact that the major site of SULT1A3 expression is in the upper gastrointestinal tract [46, 53, 61]. The high degree of specificity displayed by SULT1A3 towards catecholamines (compared with other phenol SULTs such as SULT1A1) is primarily due to the presence, uniquely, of a Glu residue at position 146 (in the human sequence) [56, 57].

SULT1B1 is also a phenol SULT and shares a remarkable similarity in its substrate specificity profile with SULT1A1 [42] – in fact, to date no "probe" substrate has been identified for SULT1B1, although it does generally display much higher K_m values than SULT1A1 for the same substrates [62]. SULT1B1, like SULT1A3, is present at high levels in the gastrointestinal tract, although it is also expressed to a significant extent in the liver [46]. SULT1B1 orthologs are found in birds and mammals. The SULT1C family in humans (and most other mammals) comprises three members – SULTs 1C1, 1C2 and 1C3 – and there are orthologs in fish, birds, and mammals, suggesting that the SULT1C enzymes may be the evolutionary founders of the SULT1 family. In humans the expression of these enzymes does not appear to be particularly high, at least in the adult; however, SULT1C1 is extensively expressed in the developing fetus [63]. There has been considerable interest in the SULT1C enzymes from a toxicological perspective, since in rats the male-specific SULT1C1 mediates the bioactivation of many dietary and environmental procarcinogens such as aromatic and heterocyclic amines, and has high activity towards the hydroxylated metabolites of these compounds [64, 65]. The role of these enzymes in human metabolism and toxicology is less clear, however. In the *Salmonella typhimurium* mutagenicity system used extensively by Glatt's group to study bioactivation by SULTs, SULTs 1C1 and 1C2 did not appear to be particularly strong in bioactivating promutagens [66]. More recently, recombinant SULT1C3 was shown to bioactivate a range of benzylic alcohols from alkylated polycyclic aromatic hydrocarbons [67], although Freimuth *et al.* failed to find expression of SULT1C3 in 20 human tissues [68]. The SULT1D subfamily [69] has not been extensively studied, although it may be that this enzyme sulfates dopamine and other catecholamines in nonprimates – the mouse enzyme has been characterized and in addition to a range of xenobiotics, metabolizes catecholamines [70] and eicosanoids [71]. In humans, *SULT1D* is a pseudogene [72].

SULT1E1, or estrogen SULT, displays a very high affinity (i.e., nanonolar K_m) for endogenous estrogens (in particular β-estradiol), as well as xenobiotic estrogens such as ethinylestradiol [45, 73]. The enzyme will sulfate a range of xenobiotics and also other important endogenous compounds such as iodothyronines [44]. Sulfation of β-estradiol terminates its actions at the estrogen receptors and it is believed that this provides a sensitive mechanism for modulating estrogen action in target (and nontarget) tissues. For example, in the endometrium SULT1E1 expression is tightly regulated during the menstrual cycle, with much higher expression in the luteal phase than in the follicular phase; this expression was suppressed in women taking the oral contraceptive pill and also in early pregnancy [74]. *In vitro* experiments have shown that SULT1E1 is highly regulated by progesterone [75, 76]. In addition to sulfating β-estradiol and other estrogens, SULT1E1 is also an important enzyme involved in the metabolism of iodothyronines [44].

Sulfation is an inactivating pathway since sulfation of active hormone T_3 and prohormone T_4 rapidly and strongly facilitates their breakdown via deiodination by hepatic type 1 iodothyronine deiodinase, thus providing a mechanism for controlling pools of active T_3 [77]. A number of studies have demonstrated that endocrine-disrupting environmental pollutants such as hydroxylated polychlorinated biphenyls and hydroylated polyhalogenated aromatic hydrocarbons are extremely potent inhibitors of β-estradiol sulfation by SULT1E1, and that this may explain the estrogenic properties of these important classes of chemicals [78, 79].

4.4.2
SULT2 Family

The SULT2 family comprises two subfamilies – SULT 2As and SULT2Bs – that sulfate a very wide range of steroids such as dehydroepiandrosterone (DHEA), testosterone, androsterone and pregnenolone, estrogens (to some extent), bile acids, and sterols, in addition to many xenobiotics [80]. This family also appears to be quite closely related to the SULT3 and SULT5 families, which are not present in humans (see below). SULT2A1 has a broad substrate profile, sulfating 3α-, 3β-, and 17β-hydroxyl groups as well as phenolic steroids and xenobiotic alcohols (including benzylic alcohols of polycyclic aromatic hydrocarbons). There are significant interspecies differences in the complement of *SULT2A1* genes, with rats and mice having three each, while humans and other primates have a single gene, *SULT2A1*. DHEAS sulfate (dehydroepiandrosterone sulfate DHEAS) is the major circulating steroid in humans, and is an important precursor for the biosynthesis of estrogens and androgens in extragonadal tissues. This is important, for example, in postmenopausal breast cancer. It is also a key steroid during human fetal development, where it provides the substrate for estrogen biosynthesis by the placenta [81]. The human adrenal gland thus expresses high levels of SULT2A1, especially during fetal development [82]. SULT2A1 is also an important xenobiotic-metabolizing enzyme and may have an important role in the bioactivation of polycyclic benzylic alcohols in particular [83], and is known to metabolize a number of drugs (e.g., [84]).

The *SULT2B1* gene is unique in the SULT family in that it produces two structurally and functionally distinct proteins (SULTs 2B1a and 2B1b), differing in their N-termini, by the use of an alternate exon 1 [85]. SULT2B1 enzymes have little or no activity towards many SULT2A1 substrates including testosterone and bile acids, but they do sulfate pregnenolone. There are dramatic substrate preferences between the two SULT2B enzymes, with SULT2B1a having a pronounced preference for pregnenolone and SULT2B1b displaying a very strong preference for cholesterol [80, 86]. These substrates are poorly sulfated by their respective other enzymes. It has been shown that the differences in substrate specificity between the two SULT2B1 enzymes resides within a short sequence in the unique N-terminus of SULT2B1b [86, 87]. Cholesterol sulfate is an important mediator of keratinocyte differentiation and barrier formation [88], and SULT2B1b is expressed within the skin [89].

4.4.3 SULT3, 4, 5 and 6 Families

The availability of the genome sequences for humans and many other species has led to the identification of a number of other SULT families [68]. In the human genome, the SULT3 family is represented by a single processed pseudogene on chromosome 14 [68]. However, functional *SULT3* genes are found in fish, amphibians, birds, and mammals, and appear related to the steroid SULTs of the SULT2 family and also the SULT5 family. The SULT3 family was first identified in rabbit liver [90] and the rabbit SULT3A1 catalyzed the sulfation of a range of amines, as did the recombinant mouse SULT3A1 and SULT3A2 proteins studied more recently [91].

SULT4A1 was first identified in 2000, isolated from rat and human brain by Falany's group [92]. The predicted amino acid sequences of SULT4A1 proteins from a wide range of species share a remarkable degree of identity (87% from zebrafish to human), and orthologs are present in fish, birds, mammals, and in the sea urchin. SULT4A1 appears to be expressed exclusively in the brain, and in particular brain regions such as the cerebral cortex, cerebellum, brainstem, and pituitary [93]. To date, no substrate has been found for SULT4A1 and sequence analysis combined with X-ray crystallography shows the protein (i) has a shortened PAPS binding domain towards the C-terminus, and (ii) is missing a highly conserved lysine residue that separates the two key PAPS binding residues Arg and Gly (which are at positions 247 and 248 in SULT4A1) in all other SULTs [94]. It is also missing a Trp in the α3-helix (SULT4A1 has a Leu in this position 60) that interacts with the adenine ring of PAPS [94]. Thus, the PAPS binding pocket is predicted to be smaller than for other SULTs and therefore may not readily accommodate the sulfuryl donor. Furthermore, these authors were unable to demonstrate the ability of SULT4A1 to bind PAP. SULT4A1 is therefore not a typical SULT and may be devoid of the ability to catalyze the sulfuryl transfer reaction. An interesting recent observation detailed the interaction of SULT4A1 with the peptidyl prolyl *cis/trans* isomerase Pin1 [95]. This binding was dependent on phosphorylation of SULT4A1 (by Erk1 [96]), and resulted in destabilization and degradation of the protein, although there was no indication as to the physiological function of this interaction (if any).

The SULT5A1 proteins remain uncharacterized, although the genes are present in rodents, rabbits, amphibians, and fish, but not primates. SULT5A1 proteins are related to those of the steroid SULT2 families and the SULT3 family. The first SULT6 family member to be discovered was SULT6B1 from the chicken, the expression of which is high in liver and muscle, and is regulated by growth hormone [97]. The recombinant chicken SULT6B1 catalyzed the sulfation of corticosterone and estradiol *in vitro*. In humans SULT6B1 is expressed predominantly in the testes [68], where a range of alternately spliced products is seen, although neither the function nor the substrate specificity of the enzyme has been determined. SULT6 members are present in many species of mammals, birds, and fish, with distant relatives in sea urchin.

4.5
Assays for SULT Activity

A variety of different methods have been developed to assess SULT enzyme activity, and the availability of a simple and substrate-independent assay has greatly facilitated their study [98]. PAPS is available commercially in a form labeled with ^{35}S, and following incubation with substrate, enzyme, and unlabeled PAPS in an appropriate buffer (normally phosphate) the unreacted PAPS can be precipitated using a combination of barium and zinc salts, leaving the labeled sulfate conjugate in the aqueous layer, which can be quantified by liquid scintillation spectrometry. This PAP^{35}S assay is very useful and applicable to many substrates [42]; however, it is not without its problems. It is not particularly sensitive, with the limit of detection at around 10 pmol reaction product. Secondly, PAP^{35}S is expensive and ^{35}S has a relatively short half-life (87.4 days). We have not found it particularly good for steroid substrates. Other "universal" assays are possible, such as those which measure the formation of 3′-phosphoadenosine-5′-phosphate (PAP) from PAPS by high-performance liquid chromatography [94, 99]. SULT enzyme activity may also be quantified using radioactive acceptor substrates. This is usually used for steroid substrates such as DHEA, 17β-estradiol, and progesterone (e.g., [46, 63]), although xenobiotics such as paracetamol, 4-nitrophenol, and 1-naphthol have also been used [100, 101]. Extraction of the unreacted (and more lipophilic) acceptor substrate into an organic solvent allows rapid separation of the radioactive sulfate.

Working with radioactive material is becoming more burdensome and consequently there is a demand to develop nonradioactive, higher-throughput assays. Another method assays SULT1A activity towards 2-naphthol using microtiter plates [102]. The assay is based on the detection of the formation of 2-naphthylsulfate from 2-naphthol and PAPS; addition of 4-nitrophenylsulfate to the assay provides a PAPS-regenerating system. In contrast to other SULT assays, the second reaction product (PAP, which is a SULT inhibitor) does not accumulate in the reaction mixture; however, the method has a rather limited sensitivity. The widespread availability of mass spectrometers means that assays directly detecting individual sulfate conjugates can be readily devised, with quantitation possible where standards are available. The real challenge is to identify compounds that are able to be used as probe substrates for individual SULT enzymes *in vitro* and *in vivo*, and to date this is an area of the field that is not well advanced.

4.6
Structure and Function of SULT

Most human cytosolic SULTs comprise between 284 and 296 amino acids, resulting in calculated subunit molecular masses between 30 000 and 35 000 Da. An exception is SULT2B1, the a and b variants of which consist of 350 and 365 amino acids, respectively. The SULT enzymes are generally present as dimers in solution with molecular masses between 60 000 and 70 000 Da observed experimentally [45, 103]. The turnover numbers for the enzymes are generally low (in the 1–5 min^{-1} range) [45, 104], although their catalytic power is high, being in the range of 10^{10}–10^{12} over the uncatalyzed reaction [105]. In general, SULTs possess a fairly broad substrate specificity, with considerable overlap in many cases, especially between enzymes of the same subfamily (e.g., [42, 62, 106]). For example, human SULT1A1 sulfates many phenols and catechols with K_m values of less than 5 μM; SULT1B1 sulfates many of the same compounds, although with a reduced affinity. Conversely, several SULT isoenzymes can display remarkable degrees of selectivity, often towards endogenous substrates such as dopamine with SULT1A3 [57] and 17β-estradiol with SULT1E1 [45]. Regioselectivity and stereoselectivity have also been observed with certain substrates and enzymes (e.g., with SULT1A3 and dopamine) [107].

Most SULTs have a conserved sequence (KXXXTVXXE) near the C-terminus of protein, called the KTVE motif. Petrotchenko *et al.* elegantly demonstrated that mutation of a single amino acid in this sequence – Val269Glu in human SULT1E1 and Val260Glu in human SULT2A1 – converts these dimeric enzymes to monomers [108]. Mouse Sult1e1, the first SULT for which an X-ray crystal structure was solved, exists naturally as a monomer in solution [109] and has PE instead of TV in the corresponding sequence; mutation of PE to TV produces a Sult1e1 that is a dimer. Heterodimerization of human SULT2A1 was observed with the wild-type human SULT1E1, but not with the Val269Glu mutant. Thus, the KTVE motif is the common protein–protein interaction motif for both homo- and heterodimerization of SULTs in solution, at least *in vitro* [108]. The function (if any) of heterodimerization of SULTs has not been demonstrated.

The three-dimensional X-ray crystal structures are now available for most of the human SULTs: SULT1A3 [56, 110], SULT2A1 [111–113], SULT1A1 [114, 115], SULT2B1a/b [87], SULT1E1 [116], SULTs 1B1 and 1C1 [117], and SULTs 1C2, 1C3, and 4A1 [94]. The overall protein fold, which is roughly spherical and is remarkably similar to that of uridylate kinase, is conserved across all SULTs, with a core five-stranded parallel β-sheet surrounded by α-helices. PAPS binding is well characterized with structures bound to PAP and PAPS now available, and again is highly conserved. The phosphate–sulfate binding (PSB) loop is formed from a highly conserved region (consensus sequence TYPKSGT) located between strand 3 and helix 3. Absolutely conserved residues in the C-terminal section of the SULT proteins also contribute to PAPS binding – Thr227, Arg257, and Gly259 (in SULT1A3 numbering). Substrate binding regions have also been characterized, but do of course vary between enzymes, reflecting the varying substrate specificities. These are reviewed in [94, 118]. It now appears that the various loops contributing to the active site of the enzyme are somewhat flexible, which may explain the ability to bind such a wide range of chemicals, but also the mechanism of action of some inhibitors (and substrate inhibition in some cases). Binding of PAPS can prime these flexible substrate binding loops (which are often disordered in crystal structures) to interact with the substrate(s) [94]

The sulfonation reaction almost certainly follows a sequential mechanism where a ternary complex is formed followed by the catalytic reaction and product release [119]. The various structures (and other evidence, e.g., [120]) provide evidence for a random bi–bi mechanism; however, they also indicate that substrate and PAPS binding may not be entirely independent [94]. The crystal structure of mouse Sult1e1 in complex with PAP and vanadate indicated that the vanadate ion adopted the expected geometry with the side-chain nitrogens of Lys48, Lys106, and His108 participating in stabilization of the transition state [121]. His108 also hydrogen bonds to the 3-hydroxyl group of estradiol in the mSult1e1–PAP–estradiol complex. This histidine is conserved in all SULTs and mutating it completely abolishes enzyme activity [121, 122], and it is widely accepted to function as a general catalytic base in the sulfonation reaction, activating the reacting hydroxyl by abstraction of the proton. Subsequently, the oxygen anion carries out a nucleophilic attack on the sulfur atom of PAPS. Accumulation of negative charge in the ternary complex then switches the hydrogen bonding of Lys48 from Ser138 to protonate the P–S bridging oxygen of PAPS, thereby completing the sulfuryl transfer.

There are a number of indicators of the structural basis for the substrate specificities of various SULTs. In general, the SULT1 family sulfonate phenolic hydroxyl groups in an aromatic ring, whereas SULT2 family members will preferentially sulfate secondary alcoholic hydroxyls within a saturated ring. Within these families, however, there are striking examples of substrate selectivity. The best studied of these is probably the high degree of selectivity of SULT1A3 for dopamine and other catecholamines compared to phenols, which are preferentially sulfated by SULT1A1 [55]. The human SULT1A family all share a high degree of sequence identity (greater than 93%), and between SULT1A3 and SULT1A1 there are only 20 amino acid differences. Site-directed mutagenesis studies demonstrated that the molecular basis for this specificity for catecholamines resided within a single amino acid–Glu146 in SULT1A3 compared with Ala146 in SULT1A1; in fact, no other SULT has a negatively charged amino acid in this position. Mutating Glu146 in SULT1A3 to Ala resulted in the complete reversal of the specificity of the enzyme for dopamine and 4-nitrophenol [57], and independent verification came from experiments that mutated Ala146 in SULT1A1 to Glu, which showed SULT1A1 gaining selectivity for dopamine and losing it for 4-nitrophenol [123]. This suggested that in SULT1A3 Glu146 forms a salt bridge with the amine nitrogen in dopamine and other catecholamines. The importance of this Glu residue for the specificity of SULT1A3 was subsequently visualized in the SULT1A3 crystal structure [56, 110]. More recently [94], it has been demonstrated that eight of the amino acid differences between SULTs 1A3 and 1A1 reside within the substrate binding pocket/active site of the enzymes. In SULT1A3, which does not readily bind acidic substrates, three of these residues are acidic where they are hydrophobic in SULT1A1, resulting in a much more negatively charged substrate binding pocket for SULT1A3. This would discourage the binding of compounds with negative charge, and favor interaction with catecholamines and other similar compounds carrying a positive charge. See Figure 4.4.

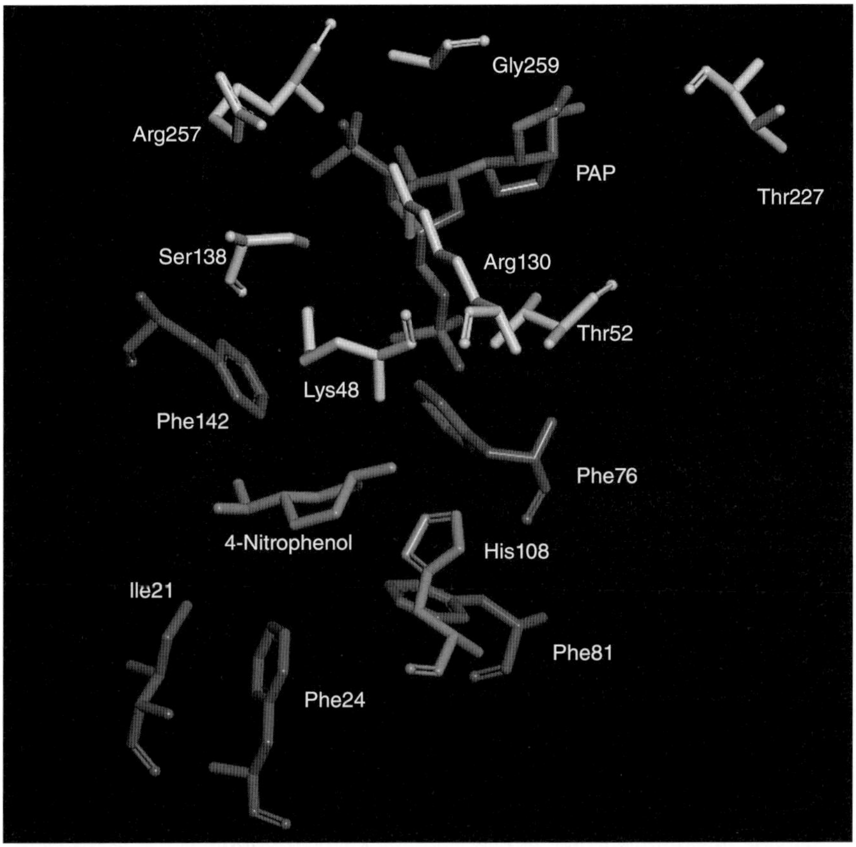

Figure 4.4 Key elements of the SULT active site. Using the X-ray crystal structure data for human SULT1A1 in complex with PAP and 4-nitrophenol (Protein Data Bank ID: 1LS6), the key elements involved in the SULT active site were highlighted. Residues involved in the binding of PAPS are shown in light shading and those forming the hydrophobic substrate binding pocket in dark shading.

For the steroid-sulfating SULTs the mechanistic basis of selectivity relies much more on steric constraint and substrate gating. This was first demonstrated with human SULT1E1 where the lack of binding of other steroids such as DHEA is due to steric hindrance of Tyr81 and the methyl group at C-19 of DHEA. SULT2A1 structures have been solved in complex with substrates DHEA [112] and androsterone [113]. With DHEA, two alternate binding orientations in the active site were observed – one in the position for catalysis and another angled away from the catalytic histidine, which may explain the partial substrate inhibition observed [112]. Androsterone appeared to adopt only the catalytic orientation [113].

The relationship between SULT structure and function is clearly complex, with many factors influencing reaction mechanism, rate, and substrate specificity.

These studies, however, provide a sound basis for predicting the metabolic fate of molecules metabolized by sulfation.

4.7 SULT Pharmacogenetics

The activity of SULTs, and the ability to sulfate xenobiotics and endogenous compounds, varies considerably within the human population. Much early work was conducted on what are now known as SULTs 1A1 and 1A3 using platelets as enzyme source (see [124–126] for reviews). SULT1A1 has received the most intense scrutiny of all the SULTs due to its widespread expression, range of substrates metabolized, and its role in drug metabolism and bioactivation of procarcinogens.

Early molecular studies of SULT1A1 variation, pioneered by Weinshilboum's group, demonstrated that there were a number of SNPs that, *in vitro* at least, were related to altered SULT1A1 expression and activity. Two coding-region SNPs now termed *SULT1A1*2* (G638A; Arg213His) and *SULT1A1*3* (A667G; Met223Val) were identified, with minor allele frequencies of approximately 32 and 1%, respectively, in Caucasians [127, 128]. Two functional promoter polymorphisms were also identified and reported to affect transcription of *SULT1A1* [48]. Individuals homozygous for the *SULT1A1*2* SNP displayed about 15% of the platelet phenol SULT activity of heterozygotes or *1A1*1* homozygotes and that the thermal stability of enzyme activity was associated with *SULT1A1* genotype [47, 127]. Another study confirmed that reduced platelet SULT activity is observed in *1A1*2* homozygotes [129], although the effect was not as pronounced with only a 50% reduction in activity apparent. Further, it was demonstrated *in vitro* that the SULT1A1*2 protein has a reduced half-life relative to the wild-type enzyme and that it was also more extensively ubiquitinated, suggesting increased proteasomal degradation [130]. Recently, SNPs in the 3′-untranslated region of SULT1A1 have been shown to influence gene expression and that a microRNA (miR-631) may also regulate the expression of SULT1A1 dependent upon 3′-untranslated region genotype [131].

Owing to the importance of SULT1A1 in detoxification and bioactivation, a large number of molecular epidemiology studies have been carried out, particularly in relation to cancer susceptibility. A number of these, which have shown positive associations with, for example, breast, lung, colorectal and esophageal cancers, are reviewed in [132]. Recent metadata analyses have suggested that overall there is not a significant association between *SULT1A1*2* and breast cancer susceptibility [133]; however, within particular subgroups statistically significant associations may occur (e.g., in Asian populations) [134].

The genetics of SULT1A1 was revealed to be even more complex when it was discovered that there was a common copy number variation (CNV) in the SULT1A1 gene, where between one and five copies could be present in individuals, and that copy number explained the majority of the variation in SULT1A1 expression in liver [48, 135]. There are striking interethnic differences in the CNV incidence (as there are with the SULT1A1 SNPs); for example, 5% of Caucasians have only one SULT1A1 gene, whereas 25% have at least three copies, while in African-Americans there appear to be very few or no individuals with only one copy, but more than 60% possess three or more. Thus, when conducting molecular genetic studies into the functional sequelae of variation in SULT1A1 coding and noncoding SNPs, CNV and possibly microRNA interactions all need to be taken into consideration.

4.8 Bioactivation and the Role of SULTs in Toxicology

Sulfation is generally accepted to function as predominantly a detoxification pathway, with the presence of enzymes such as SULT1A1 that sulfates a very wide range of substrates with low K_m; however, it has been clear for decades that sulfation is a key step in the bioactivation of many procarcinogens and other compounds [136]. In these situations, the sulfate conjugates are therefore more biologically active than the parent molecules. This is the case not just for dietary and environmental chemicals – in the case of some drugs, sulfation is an essential step in their pharmacology. The best-known example is minoxidil (2,4-diamino-6-piperidinylpyrimidine 3-oxide), which was originally developed as an antihypertensive, but was demonstrated to have significant hypertrichotic properties [137]. The majority of the pharmacological actions of minoxidil, which include smooth muscle relaxation and vasodilation, appear to be dependent on metabolic activation by sulfation [138, 139]. Minoxidil is metabolized by a number of human SULTs, but the most important enzyme is SULT1A1 [140] and sulfation has been shown to occur in the scalp [141, 142]. There are important pharmacogenetics implications here, given the interindividual variability in SULT1A1 expression (see below) and it has been suggested that individuals who do not respond to the hypertrichotic effects of topical minoxidil have low levels of SULT activity in the scalp, whereas responders have higher levels [143].

The role of sulfation and SULTs in the mutagenicity and/or carcinogenicity of many dietary and environmental chemicals has been demonstrated both *in vivo* and *in vitro*, and much of this early work was carried out by the Millers [7, 144]. Some of the best examples are the alkoxy derivatives of allylbenzene such as safrole that, along with related compounds including estragole, are potent rodent hepatocarcinogens. With these chemicals, bioactivation requires metabolism at the 1′-allylic-benzylic position, forming 1′-hydroxy metabolites, which are more potent carcinogens than the parent molecules and are readily sulfated [145]. These metabolites are found in urine of rats, but not humans [146]. The key role of sulfation in the bioactivation and carcinogenicity of such compounds has been elegantly demonstrated *in vivo* in rodents. For example, treating mice with pentachlorophenol (which is a potent inhibitor of SULT activity) prior to administration of 1′-hydroxysafrole resulted in a significant reduction in DNA adduct and tumor formation [32]. Furthermore, these authors demonstrated that the brachymorphic mouse, which carries a genetic mutation causing a significant reduction in the ability to synthesize PAPS [29], is resistant to tumorigenesis when fed 1′-hydroxysafrole [32].

There is also a significant body of evidence from *in vitro* experiments, much of it from the group of Glatt (see [147–149] for reviews), that implicates sulfation in the metabolism and bioactivation of procarcinogens and promutagens. Liver cytosol and purified human SULTs metabolize a number of *N*-hydroxyarylamines, *N*-hydroxy-heterocyclic amines, and arylhydroxamic acids [99, 150, 151], and the metabolism and bioactivation of dietary carcinogens such as *N*-OH-PhIP (PhIP = 2-amino-1-methyl-6-phenylimidazo[4,5-*b*]pyridine) (preferentially by SULT1A1) [152] and benzylic alcohols of polycyclic aromatic hydrocarbons (preferentially by SULT2A1) [153] has been demonstrated using cloned expressed human SULTs.

There has been much debate over the relevance of bioactivation of dietary and environmental carcinogens by sulfation in humans. Clearly, this is important in rodents, as illustrated above. However, there is no conclusive *in vivo* evidence confirming that sulfation plays a key role in the mutagenicity and carcinogenicity of these chemicals in man. The early molecular epidemiology studies involving genetic variants of *SULT1A1* (which is an important enzyme in these reactions, but also detoxifies many metabolites of promutagens/procarcinogens) were driven by the hypothesis that individuals possessing "low" sulfation capacity, as a result of mutations in *SULT1A1* such as *SULT1A1*2*, would be protected against the toxicity of compounds known or suspected to be involved in certain types of cancer and/or that "high" sulfators (e.g., those homozygous for *SULT1A1*1*) would be at increased risk. For most of the studies that have demonstrated any statistically significant associations with *SULT1A1* variants in potentially relevant cancers, such as colorectal or breast, the opposite has been observed, with the *SULT1A1*1* allele being protective (e.g., [154]). It may be that acetylation, an alternate pathway of bioactivation for many of these same chemicals, is more relevant in humans – certainly there are strong associations between mutations in the *N*-acetyltransferase (NAT) genes and certain types of cancer [155, 156]. We also found an increased frequency of SULT1A1*1 associated with old age, suggesting that this allele may confer protection against dietary and/or environmental chemicals. These studies should ideally be carried out again since the discovery of the *SULT1A1* CNV polymorphism calls into question the extent of the influence of *SULT1A1*1* and *SULT1A1*2* on SULT expression and activity [48, 135].

Another important example of the impact of sulfation in toxicology relates to the interaction of hydroxylated metabolites of polyhalogenated aromatic hydrocarbons (PHAHs) with estrogen SULT, SULT1E1. PHAHs such as polychlorinated dibenzo-*p*-dioxins (PCDDs), polychlorinated biphenyls (PCBs), and polychlorinated dibenzfurans (PCDFs) are important environmental pollutants and contaminants that have a range of endocrine disrupting effects, including developmental and reproductive abnormalities [157] in animals, fish, and humans, and an increased risk of endocrine-related cancers such as breast cancer [158, 159]. The estrogenic effects of these compounds are believed to be mediated in significant part by their hydroxylated metabolites [160, 161] in a predominantly estrogen receptor-independent manner [162, 163]. It has been demonstrated that many hydroxylated PHAHs are extremely potent inhibitors of the human estrogen SULT, SULT1E1. For certain OH-PHAHs the effects were seen at nanomolar or subnanomolar concentrations [78, 79], which are consistent with expected localized tissue concentrations. Thus, there is a strong possibility that these compounds can exert their endocrine-disrupting effects by modulating the bioavailability of 17β-estradiol via the major inactivation pathway for this steroid, sulfation. Interestingly, SULT1E1 is also believed to be the main enzyme involved in the sulfation of iodothyronines, including T_4 and the active hormone T_3 [44], and therefore this inhibitory mechanism may also explain the effects of hydroxylated PHAHs on thyroid function for example during fetal development [164].

4.9
Conclusions and Future Perspectives

There have been many significant advances in our understanding of the SULTs and their function in recent years. Insights into the structural features that govern the catalytic activity and specificity, understanding of the genetic basis of interindividual variability in sulfation, and an appreciation of the effects that interfere with sulfation may have all have significant impact beyond the research community. As a major pathway for the elimination of drugs and other xenobiotics such as food additives these advances will provide the relevant industrial sectors with important new information on which to base decisions on molecules in development and on the safety of existing chemicals. A number of significant challenges remain, however – in particular the lack of good *in vivo* (or *in vitro*) probe substrates for following individual SULT isoforms is preventing extensive genotype/phenotype relation and other epidemiological studies involving sulfation. This is an area where significant advances are required and hopefully these will be made in the near future.

References

1 Falany, C.N. (1997) Enzymology of human cytosolic sulfotransferases. *FASEB J.*, **11**, 206–216.

2 Coughtrie, M.W.H. (2002) Sulfation through the looking glass – recent advances in sulfotransferase research for the curious. *Pharmacogenomics J.*, **2**, 297–308.

3 Klaassen, C.D. and Boles, J.W. (1997) The importance of 3′-phosphoadenosine 5′-phosphosulfate (PAPS) in the regulation of sulfation. *FASEB J.*, **11**, 404–418.

4 Kim, D.H., Konishi, L., and Kobashi, K. (1986) Purification, characterization and reaction-mechanism of novel arylsulfotransferase obtained from an anaerobic bacterium of human intestine. *Biochim. Biophys. Acta*, **872**, 33–41.

5 Malojcic, G., Owen, R.L., Grimshaw, J.P.A., Brozzo, M.S., Dreher-Teo, H., and Glockshuber, R. (2008) A structural

and biochemical basis for PAPS-independent sulfuryl transfer by aryl sulfotransferase from uropathogenic *Escherichia coli*. *Proc. Natl. Acad. Sci. USA*, **105**, 19217–19222.
6 Blanchard, R.B., Freimuth, R.R., Buck, J., Weinshilboum, R.M., and Coughtrie, M.W.H. (2004) A proposed nomenclature system for the cytosolic sulfotransferase (SULT) superfamily. *Pharmacogenetics*, **14**, 199–211.
7 Miller, J.A. (1994) Sulfonation in chemical carcinogenesis – history and present status. *Chem. Biol. Interact.*, **92**, 329–341.
8 Baumann, E. (1876) Ueber gepaarte Schwefelsäuren im Harn. *Pflugers Arch.*, **12**, 69–70.
9 DeMeio, R.H. and Arnolt, R.I. (1944) Phenol conjugation: II. The conjugation by rat and cat tissue *in vitro*. *J. Biol. Chem.*, **156**, 577–584.
10 Bernstein, S. and McGilvery, R.W. (1952) The enzymatic conjugation of *m*-aminophenol. *J. Biol. Chem.*, **198**, 195–203.
11 Robbins, P.W. and Lipmann, F. (1956) Identification of enzymatically active sulfate as adenosine-3′-phosphate-5′-phosphosulfate. *J. Am. Chem. Soc.*, **78**, 2652–2653.
12 Nose, Y. and Lipmann, F. (1958) Separation of steroid sulfokinases. *J. Biol. Chem.*, **233**, 1348–1351.
13 Banerjee, R.K. and Roy, A.B. (1966) The sulfotransferases of guinea pig liver. *Mol. Pharmacol.*, **2**, 56–66.
14 Adams, J.B. and Poulos, A. (1967) Enzymic synthesis of steroid sulphates. 3. Isolation and properties of estrogen sulphotransferase of bovine adrenal glands. *Biochim. Biophys. Acta*, **146**, 493–508.
15 Barford, D.J. and Jones, J.G. (1971) Thiol-dependent changes in properties of rat liver sulphotransferases. *Biochem. J.*, **123**, 427–434.
16 McEvoy, F.A. and Carroll, J. (1971) Purification from rat liver of an enzyme that catalyses the sulphurylation of phenols. *Biochem. J.*, **123**, 901–906.
17 Sekura, R.D. and Jakoby, W.B. (1979) Phenol sulfotransferases. *J. Biol. Chem.*, **254**, 5658–5663.
18 Chatterjee, B., Majumdar, D., Ozbilen, O., Murty, C.V.R., and Roy, A.K. (1987) Molecular-cloning and characterization of cDNA for androgen-repressible rat-liver protein, Smp-2. *J. Biol. Chem.*, **262**, 822–825.
19 Nash, A.R., Glenn, W.K., Moore, S.S., Kerr, J., Thompson, A.R., and Thompson, E.O.P. (1988) Oestrogen sulfotransferase: molecular cloning and sequencing of cDNA for the bovine placental enzyme. *Aust. J. Biol. Sci.*, **41**, 507–516.
20 Geller, D.H., Henry, J.G., Belch, J., and Schwartz, N.B. (1987) Copurification and characterization of ATP-sulfurylase and adenosine-5′-phosphosulfate kinase from rat chondrosarcoma. *J. Biol. Chem.*, **262**, 7374–7382.
21 Rosenthal, E. and Leustek, T. (1995) A multifunctional *Urechis caupo* protein, PAPS synthetase, has both ATP sulfurylase and APS kinase activities. *Gene*, **165**, 243–248.
22 Yu, Z.H., Lansdon, E.B., Segel, I.H., and Fisher, A.J. (2007) Crystal structure of the bifunctional ATP sulfurylase – APS kinase from the chemolithotrophic thermophile *Aquifex aeolicus*. *J. Mol. Biol.*, **365**, 732–743.
23 Bradley, M.E., Rest, J.S., Li, W.H., and Schwartz, N.B. (2009) Sulfate activation enzymes: phylogeny and association with pyrophosphatase. *J. Mol. Evol.*, **68**, 1–13.
24 Hjelle, J.J., Hazelton, G.A., and Klaassen, C.D. (1985) Acetaminophen decreases adenosine 3′-phosphate 5′-phosphosulfate and uridine diphosphoglucuronic acid in rat liver. *Drug Metab. Dispos.*, **13**, 35–41.
25 Kim, H.J., Cho, J.H., and Klassen, C.D. (1995) Depletion of hepatic 3′-phosphoadenosine 5′-phosphosulfate (PAPS) and sulfate in rats by xenobiotics that are sulfated. *J. Pharmacol. Exp. Ther.*, **275**, 654–658.
26 Kurima, K., Singh, B., and Schwartz, N.B. (1999) Genomic organization of the mouse and human genes encoding the ATP sulfurylase/adenosine 5′-phosphosulfate kinase isoform SK2. *J. Biol. Chem.*, **274**, 33306–33312.

27 Besset, S., Vincourt, J.B., Amaric, F., and Girard, J.P. (2000) Nuclear localization of PAPS synthetase 1: a sulfate activation pathway in the nucleus of eukaryotic cells. *FASEB J.*, **14**, 345–354.

28 Grum, D., van den Boom, J., Neumann, D., Matena, A., Link, N.M., and Mueller, J.W. (2010) A heterodimer of human 3′-phospho-adenosine-5′-phosphosulphate (PAPS) synthases is a new sulphate activating complex. *Biochem. Biophys. Res. Commun.*, **395**, 420–425.

29 Sugahara, K. and Schwartz, N.B. (1979) Defect in 3′-phosphoadenosine 5′-phosphosulfate formation in brachymorphic mice. *Proc. Natl. Acad. Sci. USA*, **76**, 6615–6618.

30 Kurima, K., Warman, M.L., Krishnan, S., Domowicz, M., Krueger, R.C., Deyrup, A.T., and Schwartz, N.B. (1998) A member of a family of sulfate-activating enzymes causes murine brachymorphism. *Proc. Natl. Acad. Sci. USA*, **95**, 8681–8685.

31 Lyman, S.D. and Poland, A. (1983) Effect of the brachymorphic trait in mice on xenobiotic sulfate ester formation. *Biochem. Pharmacol.*, **32**, 3345–3350.

32 Boberg, E.W., Miller, E.C., Miller, J.A., Poland, A., and Liem, A. (1983) Strong evidence from studies with brachymorphic mice and pentachlorophenol that 1′-sulfooxysafrole is the major ultimate electrophilic and carcinogenic metabolite of 1′-hydroxysafrole in mouse liver. *Cancer Res.*, **43**, 5163–5173.

33 Ul Haque, M.F., King, L.M., Krakow, D., Cantor, R.M., Rusiniak, M.E., Swank, R.T., Superti-Furga, A., Haque, S., Abbas, H., Ahmad, W., Ahmad, M., and Cohn, D.H. (1998) Mutations in orthologous genes in human spondyloepimetaphyseal dysplasia and the brachymorphic mouse. *Nat. Genet.*, **20**, 157–162.

34 Noordam, C., Dhir, V., McNelis, J.C., Schlereth, F., Hanley, N.A., Krone, N., Smeitink, J.A., Smeets, R., Sweep, F.C.G.J., Claahsen-van der Grinten, H.L., and Arlt, W. (2009) Inactivating PAPSS2 mutations in a patient with premature pubarche. *N. Engl. J. Med.*, **360**, 2310–2318.

35 Bruce, J.W., Ahlquist, P., and Young, J.A.T. (2008) The host cell sulfonation pathway contributes to retroviral infection at a step coincident with provirus establishment. *PLoS Pathog.*, **4**, e1000207.

36 Shih, W.L., Yu, M.W., Chen, P.J., Wu, T.W., Lin, C.L., Liu, C.J., Lin, S.M., Tai, D.I., Lee, S.D., and Liaw, Y.F. (2009) Evidence for association with hepatocellular carcinoma at the PAPSS1 locus on chromosome 4q25 in a family-based study. *Eur. J. Hum. Genet.*, **17**, 1250–1259.

37 Xu, Z.H., Freimuth, R.R., Eckloff, B., Wieben, E., and Weinshilboum, R.M. (2002) Human 3′-phosphoadenosine 5′-phosphosulfate synthetase 2 (PAPSS2) pharmacogenetics: gene resequencing, genetic polymorphisms and functional characterization of variant allozymes. *Pharmacogenetics*, **12**, 11–21.

38 Xu, Z.H., Thomae, B.A., Eckloff, B.W., Wieben, E.D., and Weinshilboum, R.M. (2003) Pharmacogenetics of human 3′-phosphoadenosine 5′-phosphosulfate synthetase 1 (PAPSS1): gene resequencing, sequence variation, and functional genomics. *Biochem. Pharmacol.*, **65**, 1787–1796.

39 Schwenn, J.D., Krone, F.A., and Husmann, K. (1988) Yeast PAPS reductase: properties and requirements of the purified enzyme. *Arch. Microbiol.*, **150**, 313–319.

40 Larkin, M.A., Blackshields, G., Brown, N.P., Chenna, R., McGettigan, P.A., McWilliam, H., Valentin, F., Wallace, I.M., Wilm, A., Lopez, R., Thompson, J.D., Gibson, T.J., and Higgins, D.G. (2007) Clustal W and Clustal X version 2.0. *Bioinformatics*, **23**, 2947–2948.

41 Page, R.D.M. (1996) TREEVIEW: an application to display phylogenetic trees on personal computers. *Comput. Appl. Biosci.*, **12**, 357–358.

42 Taskinen, J., Ethell, B.T., Pihlavisto, P., Hood, A.M., Burchell, B., and Coughtrie, M.W.H. (2003) Conjugation of catechols by recombinant human sulfotransferases, UDP-glucuronosyltransferases and soluble

catechol *O*-methyltransferase: structure–conjugation relationships and predictive models. *Drug Metab. Dispos.*, **31**, 1187–1197.

43 Falany, C.N., Wheeler, J., Oh, T.S., and Falany, J.L. (1994) Steroid sulfation by expressed human cytosolic sulfotransferases. *J. Steroid Biochem. Mol. Biol.*, **48**, 369–375.

44 Kester, M.H.A., VanDijk, C.H., Tibboel, D., Hood, A.M., Rose, N.J.M., Meinl, W., Pabel, U., Glatt, H., Falany, C.N., Coughtrie, M.W.H., and Visser, T.J. (1999) Sulfation of thyroid hormone by estrogen sulfotransferase. *J. Clin. Endocrinol. Metab.*, **84**, 2577–2580.

45 Zhang, H.P., Varmalova, O., Vargas, F.M., Falany, C.N., and Leyh, T.S. (1998) Sulfuryl transfer: the catalytic mechanism of human estrogen sulfotransferase. *J. Biol. Chem.*, **273**, 10888–10892.

46 Riches, Z., Stanley, E.L., Bloomer, J.C., and Coughtrie, M.W.H. (2009) Quantitative evaluation of the expression and activity of five major sulfotransferases (SULTs) in human tissues: the SULT "pie". *Drug Metab. Dispos.*, **37**, 2255–2261.

47 Raftogianis, R.B., Wood, T.C., and Weinshilboum, R.M. (1999) Human phenol sulfotransferases SULT1A2 and SULT1A1. Genetic polymorphisms, allozyme properties, and human liver genotype-phenotype correlations. *Biochem. Pharmacol.*, **58**, 605–616.

48 Hebbring, S.J., Adjei, A.A., Baer, J.L., Jenkins, G.D., Zhang, J., Cunningham, J.M., Schaid, D.J., Weinshilboum, R.M., and Thibodeau, S.N. (2007) Human *SULT1A1* gene: copy number differences and functional implications. *Hum. Mol. Genet.*, **16**, 463–470.

49 Ozawa, S., Nagata, K., Shimada, M., Ueda, M., Tsuzuki, T., Yamazoe, Y., and Kato, R. (1995) Primary structures and properties of two related forms of aryl sulfotransferases in human liver. *Pharmacogenetics*, **5**, S135–S140.

50 Dooley, T.P., Haldeman-Cahill, R., Joiner, J., and Wilborn, T.W. (2000) Expression profiling of human sulfotransferase and sulfatase gene superfamilies in epithelial tissues and cultured cells. *Biochem. Biophys. Res. Commun.*, **277**, 236–245.

51 Nowell, S., Green, B., Tang, Y.M., Wiese, R., and Kadlubar, F.F. (2005) Examination of human tissue cytosols for expression of sulfotransferase isoform 1A2 (SULT1A2) using a SULT1A2-specific antibody. *Mol. Pharmacol.*, **67**, 394–399.

52 Meinl, W., Ebert, B., Glatt, H., and Lampen, A. (2008) Sulfotransferase forms expressed in human intestinal Caco-2 and TC7 cells at varying stages of differentiation and role in benzo[*a*]pyrene metabolism. *Drug Metab. Dispos.*, **36**, 276–283.

53 Teubner, W., Meinl, W., Florian, S., Kretzschmar, M., and Glatt, H. (2007) Identification and localization of soluble sulfotransferases in the human gastrointestinal tract. *Biochem. J.*, **404**, 207–215.

54 Hildebrandt, H.A.T., Salavaggione, O.E., Martin, Y.N., Flynn, H.C., Jalal, S., Wieben, E.D., and Weinshilboum, R.M. (2004) Human SULTl A3 pharmacogenetics: gene duplication and functional genomic studies. *Biochem. Biophys. Res. Commun.*, **321**, 870–878.

55 Reiter, C., Mwaluko, G., Dunnette, J., Van Loon, J., and Weinshilboum, R. (1983) Thermolabile and thermostable human platelet phenol sulfotransferase. Substrate specificity and physical separation. *Naunyn Schmiedebergs Arch. Pharmacol.*, **324**, 140–147.

56 Dajani, R., Cleasby, A., Neu, M., Wonacott, A.J., Jhoti, H., Hood, A.M., Modi, S., Hersey, A., Taskinen, J., Cooke, R.M., Manchee, G.R., and Coughtrie, M.W.H. (1999) X-ray crystal structure of human dopamine sulfotransferase, SULT1A3: molecular modelling and QSAR analysis demonstrate a molecular basis for sulfotransferase substrate specificity. *J. Biol. Chem.*, **274**, 37862–37868.

57 Dajani, R., Hood, A.M., and Coughtrie, M.W.H. (1998) A single amino acid, Glu 146, governs the substrate specificity of a human dopamine sulfotransferase, SULT1A3. *Mol. Pharmacol.*, **54**, 942–948.

58 Dousa, M.K. and Tyce, G.M. (1988) Free and conjugated plasma catecholamines,

DOPA and 3-*O*-methyldopa in humans and various animal species. *Proc. Soc. Exp. Biol. Med.*, **188**, 427–434.

59 Eisenhofer, G., Aneman, A., Friberg, P., Hooper, D., Fandriks, L., Lonroth, H., Hunyady, B., and Mezey, E. (1997) Substantial production of dopamine in the human gastrointestinal tract. *J. Clin. Endocrinol. Metab.*, **82**, 3864–3871.

60 Eisenhofer, G., Coughtrie, M.W.H., and Goldstein, D.S. (1999) Dopamine sulphate: an enigma resolved. *Clin. Exp. Pharmacol. Physiol.*, **26**, S41–S53.

61 Rubin, G.L., Sharp, S., Jones, A.L., Glatt, H., Mills, J.A., and Coughtrie, M.W.H. (1996) Design, production and characterisation of antibodies discriminating between the phenol- and monoamine-sulphating forms of human phenol sulphotransferase. *Xenobiotica*, **26**, 1113–1119.

62 Riches, Z., Bloomer, J.C., and Coughtrie, M.W.H. (2007) Comparison of 2-aminophenol and 4-nitrophenol as *in vitro* probe substrates for the major human hepatic sulfotransferase, SULT1A1, demonstrates improved selectivity with 2-aminophenol. *Biochem. Pharmacol.*, **74**, 352–358.

63 Stanley, E.L., Hume, R., and Coughtrie, M.W.H. (2005) Expression profiling of human fetal cytosolic sulfotransferases involved in steroid and thyroid hormone metabolism and in detoxification. *Mol. Cell. Endocrinol.*, **240**, 32–42.

64 Nagata, K., Ozawa, S., Miyata, M., Shimada, M., Gong, D.W., Yamazoe, Y., and Kato, R. (1993) Isolation and expression of a cDNA encoding a male-specific rat sulfotransferase that catalyzes activation of *N*-hydroxy-2-acetylaminofluorene. *J. Biol. Chem.*, **268**, 24720–24725.

65 Glatt, H., Bartsch, I., Christoph, S., Coughtrie, M.W.H., Falany, C.N., Hagen, M., Landsiedel, R., Pabel, U., Phillips, D.H., Seidel, A., and Yamazoe, Y. (1998) Sulfotransferase-mediated activation of mutagens studied using heterologous expression systems. *Chem. Biol. Interact.*, **109**, 195–219.

66 Glatt, H., Boeing, H., Engelke, C.E.H., Kuhlow, L.M.A., Pabel, U., Pomplun, D., Teubner, W., and Meinl, W. (2001) Human cytosolic sulphotransferases: genetics, characteristics, toxicological aspects. *Mutat. Res.*, **482**, 27–40.

67 Meinl, W., Donath, C., Schneider, H., Sommer, Y., and Glatt, H. (2008) SULT1C3, an orphan sequence of the human genome, encodes an enzyme activating various promutagens. *Food Chem. Toxicol.*, **46**, 1249–1256.

68 Freimuth, R.R., Wiepert, M., Chute, C.G., Wieben, E.D., and Weinshilboum, R.M. (2004) Human cytosolic sulfotransferase database mining: identification of seven novel genes and pseudogenes. *Pharmacogenomics J.*, **4**, 54–65.

69 Tsoi, C., Falany, C.N., Morgenstern, R., and Swedmark, S. (2001) Identification of a new subfamily of sulphotransferases: cloning and characterization of canine SULT1D1. *Biochem. J.*, **356**, 891–897.

70 Shimada, M., Terazawa, R., Kamiyama, Y., Honma, W., Nagata, K., and Yamazoe, Y. (2004) Unique properties of a renal sulfotransferase, st1d1, in dopamine metabolism. *J. Pharmacol. Exp. Ther.*, **310**, 808–814.

71 Liu, M.C., Sakakibara, Y., and Liu, C.C. (1999) Bacterial expression, purification, and characterization of a novel mouse sulfotransferase that catalyzes the sulfation of eicosanoids. *Biochem. Biophys. Res. Commun.*, **254**, 65–69.

72 Meinl, W. and Glatt, H. (2001) Structure and localization of the human SULT1B1 gene: neighborhood to SULT1E1 and a SULT1D pseudogene. *Biochem. Biophys. Res. Commun.*, **288**, 855–862.

73 Forbes-Bamforth, K.J. and Coughtrie, M.W.H. (1994) Identification of a new adult human liver sulfotransferase with specificity for endogenous and xenobiotic estrogens. *Biochem. Biophys. Res. Commun.*, **198**, 707–711.

74 Rubin, G.L., Harrold, A.J., Mills, J.A., Falany, C.N., and Coughtrie, M.W.H. (1999) Regulation of sulfotransferase expression in the endometrium during the menstrual cycle, by oral contraceptives and during early pregnancy. *Mol. Hum. Reprod.*, **5**, 995–1002.

75 Tseng, L. and Liu, H.C. (1981) Stimulation of arylsulfotransferase activity by progestins in human endometrium *in vitro*. *J. Clin. Endocrinol. Metab.*, **53**, 418–421.

76 Falany, J.L. and Falany, C.N. (1996) Regulation of estrogen sulfotransferase in human endometrial adenocarcinoma cells by progesterone. *Endocrinology*, **137**, 1395–1401.

77 Visser, T.J. (1994) Role of sulfation in thyroid hormone metabolism. *Chem. Biol. Interact.*, **92**, 293–303.

78 Kester, M.H.A., Bulduk, S., Tibboel, D., Meinl, W., Glatt, H., Falany, C.N., Coughtrie, M.W.H., Bergman, A., Safe, S.H., Kuiper, G.G.J.M., Schuur, A.G., Brouwer, A., and Visser, T.J. (2000) Potent inhibition of estrogen sulfotransferase by hydroxylated PCB metabolites: a novel pathway explaining the estrogenic activity of PCBs. *Endocrinology*, **141**, 1897–1900.

79 Kester, M.H., Bulduk, S., van Toor, H., Tibboel, D., Meinl, W., Glatt, H., Falany, C.N., Coughtrie, M.W.H., Schuur, A.G., Brouwer, A., and Visser, T.J. (2002) Potent inhibition of estrogen sulfotransferase by hydroxylated metabolites of polyhalogenated aromatic hydrocarbons reveals alternative mechanism for estrogenic activity of endocrine disrupters. *J. Clin. Endocrinol. Metab.*, **87**, 1142–1150.

80 Strott, C.A. (2002) Sulfonation and molecular action. *Endocr. Rev.*, **23**, 703–732.

81 Kuss, E. (1994) The fetoplacental unit of primates. *Exp. Clin. Endocrinol.*, **102**, 135–165.

82 Barker, E.V., Hume, R., Hallas, A., and Coughtrie, M.W.H. (1994) Dehydroepiandrosterone sulfotransferase in the developing human fetus – quantitative biochemical and immunological characterization of the hepatic, renal, and adrenal enzymes. *Endocrinology*, **134**, 982–989.

83 Glatt, H.R. (2000) An overview of bioactivation of chemical carcinogens. *Biochem. Soc. Trans.*, **28**, 1–6.

84 Senggunprai, L., Yoshinari, K., and Yamazoe, Y. (2009) Selective role of sulfotransferase 2A1 (SULT2A1) in the *N*-sulfoconjugation of quinolone drugs in humans. *Drug Metab. Dispos.*, **37**, 1711–1717.

85 Her, C., Wood, T.C., Eichler, E.E., Mohrenweiser, H.W., Ramagli, L.S., Sicilaiono, M.J., and Weinshilboum, R.M. (1998) Human hydroxysteroid sulfotransferase SULT2B1: two enzymes encoded by a single chromosome 19 gene. *Genomics*, **53**, 284–295.

86 Fuda, H., Lee, Y.C., Shimizu, C., Javitt, N.B., and Strott, C.A. (2002) Mutational analysis of human hydroxysteroid sulfotransferase SULT2B1 isoforms reveals that exon 1B of the SULT2B1 gene produces cholesterol sulfotransferase, whereas exon 1A yields pregnenolone sulfotransferase. *J. Biol. Chem.*, **277**, 36161–36166.

87 Lee, K.A., Fuda, H., Lee, Y.C., Negishi, M., Strott, C.A., and Pedersen, L.C. (2003) Crystal structure of human cholesterol sulfotransferase (SULT2B1b) in the presence of pregnenolone and 3′-phosphoadenosine 5′-phosphate – rationale for specificity differences between prototypical SULT2A1 and the SULT2B1 isoforms. *J. Biol. Chem.*, **278**, 44593–44599.

88 Jetten, A.M., George, M.A., Nervi, C., Boone, L.R., and Rearick, J.I. (1989) Increased cholesterol sulfate and cholesterol sulfotransferase activity in relation to the multi-step process of differentiation in human epidermal keratinocytes. *J. Invest. Dermatol.*, **92**, 203–209.

89 He, D.N., Meloche, C.A., Dumas, N.A., Frost, A.R., and Falany, C.N. (2004) Different subcellular localization of sulphotransferase 2B1b in human placenta and prostate. *Biochem. J.*, **379**, 533–540.

90 Yoshinari, K., Nagata, K., Ogino, M., Fujita, K., Shiraga, T., Iwasaki, K., Hata, T., and Yamazoe, Y. (1998) Molecular cloning and expression of an amine sulfotransferase cDNA: a new gene family of cytosolic sulfotransferases in mammals. *J. Biochem.*, **123**, 479–486.

91 Takahashi, S., Sakakibara, Y., Mishiro, E., Kouriki, H., Nobe, R., Kurogi, K., Yasuda, S., Liu, M.C., and Suiko, M. (2008) Molecular cloning, expression,

and characterization of mouse amine *N*-sulfotransferases. *Biochem. Biophys. Res. Commun.*, **375**, 531–535.
92 Falany, C.N., Xie, X.W., Wang, J., Ferrer, J., and Falany, J.L. (2000) Molecular cloning and expression of novel sulphotransferase-like cDNAs from human and rat brain. *Biochem. J.*, **346**, 857–864.
93 Liyou, N.E., Buller, K.M., Tresillian, M.J., Elvin, C.M., Scott, H.L., Dodd, P.R., Tannenberg, A.E.G., and McManus, M.E. (2003) Localization of a brain sulfotransferase, SULT4A1, in the human and rat brain: an immunohistochemical study. *J. Histochem. Cytochem.*, **51**, 1655–1664.
94 Allali-Hassani, A., Pan, P.W., Dombrovski, L., Najmanovich, R., Tempel, W., Dong, A.P., Loppnau, P., Martin, F., Thonton, J., Edwards, A.M., Bochkarev, A., Plotnikov, A.N., Vedadi, M., and Arrowsmith, C.H. (2007) Structural and chemical profiling of the human cytosolic sulfotransferases. *PLoS Biol.*, **5**, 1063–1078.
95 Mitchell, D.J. and Minchin, R.F. (2009) Cytosolic aryl sulfotransferase 4A1 interacts with the peptidyl prolyl *cis–trans* isomerase Pin1. *Mol. Pharmacol.*, **76**, 388–395.
96 Mitchell, D.J., Butcher, N.J., and Minchin, R.F. (2011) Phosphorylation/dephosphorylation of human SULT4A1: role of Erk1 and PP2A. *Biochim. Biophys. Acta*, **1813**, 231–237.
97 Cao, H., Agarwal, S.K., and Burnside, J. (1999) Cloning and expression of a novel chicken sulfotransferase cDNA regulated by GH. *J. Endocrinol.*, **160**, 491–500.
98 Foldes, A. and Meek, J.L. (1973) Rat brain phenolsulfotransferase – partial purification and some properties. *Biochim. Biophys. Acta*, **327**, 365–374.
99 Gilissen, R.A.H.J., Bamforth, K.J., Stavenuiter, J.F.C., Coughtrie, M.W.H., and Meerman, J.H.N. (1994) Sulfation of aromatic hydroxamic acids and hydroxylamines by multiple forms of human liver sulfotransferases. *Carcinogenesis*, **15**, 39–45.
100 Coughtrie, M.W.H. and Sharp, S. (1990) Purification and immunochemical characterization of a rat liver sulfotransferase conjugating paracetamol. *Biochem. Pharmacol.*, **40**, 2305–2313.
101 Borthwick, E.B., Burchell, A., and Coughtrie, M.W.H. (1993) Purification and immunochemical characterization of a male-specific rat liver estrogen sulfotransferase. *Biochem. J.*, **289**, 719–725.
102 Frame, L.T., Ozawa, S., Nowell, S.A., Chou, H.C., Delongchamp, R.R., Doerge, D.R., Lang, N.P., and Kadlubar, F.F. (2000) Simple colorimetric assay for phenotyping the major human thermostable phenol sulfotransferase (SULT1A1) using platelet cytosols. *Drug Metab. Dispos.*, **28**, 1063–1068.
103 Dajani, R., Sharp, S., Graham, S., Bethell, S.S., Cooke, R.M., Jamieson, D.J., and Coughtrie, M.W.H. (1999) Kinetic properties of human dopamine sulfotransferase (SULT1A3) expressed in prokaryotic and eukaryotic systems: comparison with the recombinant enzyme purified from *Escherichia coli*. *Protein Expr. Purif.*, **16**, 11–18.
104 Petrotchenko, E.V., Doerflein, M.E., Kakuta, Y., Pedersen, L.C., and Negishi, M. (1999) Substrate gating confers steroid specificity to estrogen sulfotransferase. *J. Biol. Chem.*, **274**, 30019–30022.
105 Bedford, C.T., Kirby, A.J., Logan, C.J., and Drummond, J.N. (1995) Structure–activity studies of sulfate transfer – the hydrolysis and aminolysis of 3-phosphoadenosine 5′-phosphosulfate (PAPS). *Bioorg. Med. Chem.*, **3**, 167–172.
106 Sipila, J., Hood, A.M., Coughtrie, M.W.H., and Taskinen, J. (2003) CoMFA modeling of enzyme kinetics: K_m values for sulfation of diverse phenolic substrates by human catecholamine sulfotransferase SULT1A3. *J. Chem. Inf. Comput. Sci.*, **43**, 1563–1569.
107 Itaaho, K., Alakurtti, S., Yli-Kauhaluoma, J., Taskinen, J., Coughtrie, M.W.H., and Kostiainen, R. (2007) Regioselective sulfonation of dopamine by SULT1A3 *in vitro* provides a molecular explanation for the preponderance of dopamine-3-*O*-sulfate in human blood circulation. *Biochem. Pharmacol.*, **74**, 504–510.

108 Petrotchenko, E.V., Pedersen, L.C., Borchers, C.H., Tomer, K.B., and Negishi, M. (2001) The dimerization motif of cytosolic sulfotransferases. *FEBS Lett.*, **490**, 39–43.

109 Kakuta, Y., Pedersen, L.G., Carter, C.W., Negishi, M., and Pedersen, L.C. (1997) Crystal structure of estrogen sulphotransferase. *Nat. Struct. Biol.*, **4**, 904–908.

110 Bidwell, L.M., McManus, M.E., Gaedigk, A., Kakuta, Y., Negishi, M., Pedersen, L., and Martin, J.L. (1999) Crystal structure of human catecholamine sulfotransferase. *J. Mol. Biol.*, **293**, 521–530.

111 Pedersen, L.C., Petrotchenko, E.V., and Negishi, M. (2000) Crystal structure of SULT2A3, human hydroxysteroid sulfotransferase. *FEBS Lett.*, **475**, 61–64.

112 Rehse, P.H., Zhou, M., and Lin, S.X. (2002) Crystal structure of human dehydroepiandrosterone sulphotransferase in complex with substrate. *Biochem. J.*, **364**, 165–171.

113 Chang, H.J., Shi, R., Rehse, P., and Lin, S.X. (2004) Identifying androsterone (ADT) as a cognate substrate for human dehydroepiandrosterone sulfotransferase (DHEA-ST) important for steroid homeostasis – structure of the enzyme–ADT complex. *J. Biol. Chem.*, **279**, 2689–2696.

114 Gamage, N.U., Duggleby, R.G., Barnett, A.C., Tresillian, M., Latham, C.F., Liyou, N.E., McManus, M.E., and Martin, J.L. (2003) Structure of a human carcinogen-converting enzyme, SULT1A1. Structural and kinetic implications of substrate inhibition. *J. Biol. Chem.*, **278**, 7655.

115 Gamage, N.U., Tsvetanov, S., Duggleby, R.G., McManus, M.E., and Martin, J.L. (2005) The structure of human SULT1A1 crystallized with estradiol – an insight into active site plasticity and substrate inhibition with multi-ring substrates. *J. Biol. Chem.*, **280**, 41482–41486.

116 Pedersen, L.C., Petrotchenko, E., Shevtsov, S., and Negishi, M. (2002) Crystal structure of the human estrogen sulfotransferase–PAPS complex. Evidence for catalytic role of Ser137 in the sulfuryl transfer reaction. *J. Biol. Chem.*, **277**, 17928–17932.

117 Dombrovski, L., Dong, A.P., Bochkarev, A., and Plotnikov, A.N. (2006) Crystal structures of human sulfotransferases SULT1B1 and SULT1C1 complexed with the cofactor product adenosine-3′–5′-diphosphate (PAP). *Proteins*, **64**, 1091–1094.

118 Negishi, M., Pedersen, L.G., Petrotchenko, E., Shevtsov, S., Gorokhov, A., Kakuta, Y., and Pedersen, L.C. (2001) Structure and function of sulfotransferases. *Arch. Biochem. Biophys.*, **390**, 149–157.

119 Chapman, E., Best, M.D., Hanson, S.R., and Wong, C.H. (2004) Sulfotransferases: structure, mechanism, biological activity, inhibition, and synthetic utility. *Angew. Chem. Int. Ed.*, **43**, 3526–3548.

120 Hoff, R.H., Czyryca, P.G., Sun, M.H., Leyh, T.S., and Hengge, A.C. (2006) Transition state of the sulfuryl transfer reaction of estrogen sulfotransferase. *J. Biol. Chem.*, **281**, 30645–30649.

121 Kakuta, Y., Petrotchenko, E.V., Pedersen, L.C., and Negishi, M. (1998) The sulfuryl transfer mechanism: crystal structure of a vanadate complex of estrogen sulfotransferase and mutational analysis. *J. Biol. Chem.*, **273**, 27325–27330.

122 Liu, M.C., Suiko, M., and Sakakibara, Y. (2000) Mutational analysis of the substrate binding/catalytic domains of human M form and P form phenol sulfotransferases. *J. Biol. Chem.*, **275**, 13460–13464.

123 Brix, L.A., Barnett, A.C., Duggleby, R.G., Leggett, B., and McManus, M.E. (1999) Analysis of the substrate specificity of human sulfotransferases SULT1A1 and SULT1A3: site-directed mutagenesis and kinetic studies. *Biochemistry*, **38**, 10474–10479.

124 Weinshilboum, R. (1988) Phenol sulfotransferase inheritance. *Cell. Mol. Neurobiol.*, **8**, 27–33.

125 Weinshilboum, R. (1990) Sulfotransferase pharmacogenetics. *Pharmacol. Ther.*, **45**, 93–107.

126 Weinshilboum, R. and Aksoy, I.A. (1994) Sulfation pharmacogenetics in

humans. *Chem. Biol. Interact.*, **92**, 233–246.

127 Raftogianis, R.B., Wood, T.C., Otterness, D.M., van Loon, J.A., and Weinshilboum, R.M. (1997) Phenol sulfotransferase pharmacogenetics in humans: association of common SULT1A1 alleles with TS PST phenotype. *Biochem. Biophys. Res. Commun.*, **239**, 298–304.

128 Carlini, E.J., Raftogianis, R.B., Wood, T.C., Jin, F., Zheng, W., Rebbeck, T.R., and Weinshilboum, R.M. (2001) Sulfation pharmacogenetics: *SULT1A1* and *SULT1A2* allele frequencies in Caucasian, Chinese and African-American subjects. *Pharmacogenetics*, **11**, 57–68.

129 Nowell, S., Ambrosone, C.B., Ozawa, S., MacLeod, S.L., Mrackova, G., Williams, S., Plaxco, J., Kadlubar, F.F., and Lang, N.P. (2000) Relationship of phenol sulfotransferase activity (SULT1A1) genotype to sulfotransferase phenotype in platelet cytosol. *Pharmacogenetics*, **10**, 789–797.

130 Nagar, S., Walther, S., and Blanchard, R.L. (2006) Sulfotransferase (SULT) 1A1 polymorphic variants *1, *2, and *3 are associated with altered enzymatic activity, cellular phenotype, and protein degradation. *Mol. Pharmacol.*, **69**, 2084–2092.

131 Yu, X.F., Dhakal, I.B., Beggs, M., Edavana, V.K., Williams, S., Zhang, X.M., Mercer, K., Ning, B.T., Lang, N.P., Kadlubar, F.F., and Kadlubar, S. (2010) Functional genetic variants in the 3′-untranslated region of sulfotransferase isoform 1A1 (*SULT1A1*) and their effect on enzymatic activity. *Toxicol. Sci.*, **118**, 391–403.

132 Glatt, H. and Meinl, W. (2004) Pharmacogenetics of soluble sulfotransferases (SULTs). *Naunyn Schmiedebergs Arch. Pharmacol.*, **369**, 55–68.

133 Sun, Y.Y., Zang, Z.H., Xu, X.H., Zhang, Z.L., Zhong, L., Zan, W., Zhao, Y., and Sun, L. (2011) The association of SULT1A1 codon 213 polymorphism and breast cancer susceptibility: meta-analysis from 16 studies involving 23 445 subjects. *Breast Cancer Res. Treat.*, **125**, 215–219.

134 Wang, Z.W., Fu, Y.Y., Tang, C.B., Lu, S., and Chu, W.M. (2010) SULT1A1 R213H polymorphism and breast cancer risk: a meta-analysis based on 8454 cases and 11 800 controls. *Breast Cancer Res. Treat.*, **122**, 193–198.

135 Hebbring, S.J., Moyer, A.M., and Weinshilboum, R.M. (2008) Sulfotransferase gene copy number variation: pharmacogenetics and function. *Cytogenet. Genome Res.*, **123**, 205–210.

136 Miller, J.A. (1970) Carcinogenesis by chemicals: an overview. *Cancer Res.*, **30**, 559–576.

137 Campese, V.M. (1981) Minoxidil: a review of its pharmacological properties and therapeutic use. *Drugs*, **22**, 257–278.

138 Meisheri, K.D., Johnson, G.A., and Puddington, L. (1993) Enzymatic and non-enzymatic sulfation mechanisms in the biological actions of minoxidil. *Biochem. Pharmacol.*, **45**, 271–279.

139 Meisheri, K.D., Cipkus, L.A., and Taylor, C.J. (1988) Mechanism of action of minoxidil sulfate-induced vasodilation: a role for increased K^+ permeability. *J. Pharmacol. Exp. Ther.*, **245**, 751–760.

140 Falany, C.N. and Kerl, E.A. (1990) Sulfation of minoxidil by human liver phenol sulfotransferase. *Biochem. Pharmacol.*, **40**, 1027–1032.

141 Dooley, T.P., Walker, C.J., Hirshey, S.J., Falany, C.N., and Diani, A.R. (1991) Localization of minoxidil sulfotransferase in rat liver and the outer root sheath of anagen pelage and vibrissa follicles. *J. Invest. Dermatol.*, **96**, 65–70.

142 Baker, C.A., Uno, H., and Johnson, G.A. (1994) Minoxidil sulfation in the hair follicle. *Skin Pharmacol.*, **7**, 335–339.

143 Buhl, A.E., Baker, C.A., Dietz, A.J., Murray, F.T., and Johnson, G.A. (1994) Minoxidil sulfotransferase activity influences the efficacy of rogaines topical solution (TS): enzyme studies using scalp and platelets. *J. Invest. Dermatol.*, **102**, 534–534.

144 Miller, J.A. (1994) Research in chemical carcinogenesis with Elizabeth Miller – a

trail of discovery with our associates. *Drug Metab. Rev.*, **26**, 1–36.

145 Wakazono, H., Gardner, I., Eliasson, E., Coughtrie, M.W.H., Kenna, J.G., and Caldwell, J. (1998) Immunochemical identification of hepatic protein adducts derived from estragole. *Chem. Res. Toxicol.*, **11**, 863–872.

146 Benedetti, M.S., Malnoe, A., and Broillet, A.L. (1977) Absorption, metabolism and excretion of safrole in rat and man. *Toxicology*, **7**, 69–83.

147 Glatt, H.R. (1997) Bioactivation of mutagens via sulfation. *FASEB J.*, **11**, 314–321.

148 Glatt, H. (2000) Sulfotransferases in the bioactivation of xenobiotics. *Chem. Biol. Interact.*, **129**, 141–170.

149 Glatt, H., Engelke, C.E.H., Pabel, U., Teubner, W., Jones, A.L., Coughtrie, M.W.H., Andrae, U., Falany, C.N., and Meinl, W. (2000) Sulfotransferases: genetics and role in toxicology. *Toxicol. Lett.*, **112**, 341–348.

150 Gilissen, R.A.H.J., Hume, R., Meerman, J.H.N., and Coughtrie, M.W.H. (1994) Sulfation of *N*-hydroxy-4-aminobiphenyl and *N*-hydroxy-4-acetylaminobiphenyl by human fetal and neonatal sulfotransferase. *Biochem. Pharmacol.*, **48**, 837–840.

151 Meerman, J.H.N., Ringer, D.P., Coughtrie, M.W.H., Bamforth, K.J., and Gilissen, R.A.H.J. (1994) Sulfation of carcinogenic aromatic hydroxylamines and hydroxamic acids by rat and human sulfotransferases – substrate-specificity, developmental aspects and sex-differences. *Chem. Biol. Interact.*, **92**, 321–328.

152 Ozawa, S., Chou, H.C., Kadlubar, F.F., Yamazoe, Y., and Kato, R. (1994) Activation of 2-hydroxyamino-1-methyl-6-phenylimidazo[4,5-*b*]pyridine by cDNA-expressed human and rat arylsulfotransferases. *Jpn. J. Cancer Res.*, **85**, 1220–1228.

153 Glatt, H., Pauly, K., Czich, A., Falany, J.L., and Falany, C.N. (1995) Activation of benzylic alcohols to mutagens by rat and human sulfotransferases expressed in *Escherichia coli*. *Eur. J. Pharmacol.*, **293**, 173–181.

154 Bamber, D.E., Fryer, A.A., Strange, R.C., Elder, J.B., Deakin, M., Rajagopal, R., Fawole, A., Gilissen, R.A.H.J., Campbell, F.C., and Coughtrie, M.W.H. (2001) Phenol sulphotransferase *SULT1A1*1* genotype is associated with reduced risk of colorectal cancer. *Pharmacogenetics*, **11**, 679–685.

155 Hein, D.W., Doll, M.A., Fretland, A.J., Leff, M.A., Webb, S.J., Xiao, G.H., Devanoboyina, U.S., Nangju, N.A., and Feng, Y. (2000) Molecular genetics and epidemiology of the NAT1 and NAT2 acetylation polymorphisms. *Cancer Epidemiol. Biomarkers Prev.*, **9**, 29–42.

156 Hein, D.W. (1988) Acetylator genotype and arylamine-induced carcinogenesis. *Biochim. Biophys. Acta*, **948**, 37–66.

157 Neubert, D. (1997) Vulnerability of the endocrine system to xenobiotic influence. *Regul. Toxicol. Pharmacol.*, **26**, 9–29.

158 Safe, S.H. (1995) Environmental and dietary estrogens and human health: is there a problem. *Environ. Health Perspect.*, **103**, 346–351.

159 Dorgan, J.F., Brock, J.W., Rothman, N., Needham, L.L., Miller, R., Stephenson, H.E., Jr, Schussler, N., and Taylor, P.R. (1999) Serum organochlorine pesticides and PCBs and breast cancer risk: results from a prospective analysis (USA). *Cancer Causes Control*, **10**, 1–11.

160 Safe, S.H. (1994) Polychlorinated biphenyls (PCBs): environmental impact, biochemical and toxic responses, and implications for risk assessment. *Crit. Rev. Toxicol.*, **24**, 87–149.

161 Connor, K., Ramamoorthy, K., Moore, M., Mustain, M., Chen, I., Safe, S., Zacharewski, T., Gillesby, B., Joyeux, A., and Balaguer, P. (1997) Hydroxylated polychlorinated biphenyls (PCBs) as estrogens and antiestrogens: structure–activity relationships. *Toxicol. Appl. Pharmacol.*, **145**, 111–123.

162 Kuiper, G., Lemmen, J.G., Carlsson, B., Corton, J.C., Safe, S.H., van der Saag, P.T., van der Burg, P., and Gustafsson, J.A. (1998) Interaction of estrogenic chemicals and phytoestrogens with estrogen receptor beta. *Endocrinology*, **139**, 4252–4263.

163 Korach, K.S., Sarver, P., Chae, K., McLachlan, J.A., and McKinney, J.D. (1988) Estrogen receptor-binding activity of polychlorinated hydroxybiphenyls: conformationally restricted structural probes. *Mol. Pharmacol.*, **33**, 120–126.

164 Darras, V.M. (2008) Endocrine disrupting polyhalogenated organic pollutants interfere with thyroid hormone signalling in the developing brain. *Cerebellum*, **7**, 26–37.

5
Glutathione *S*-Transferases

Miroslav Dostalek and Anna-Katarina Stark

5.1
Introduction and History

Since their discovery, the glutathione *S*-transferase (GST) enzymes have come to be recognized as one of the most important superfamilies of enzymes involved in the detoxification of endogenous and exogenous electrophilic compounds (for review, also see [1–8]). In 1961, Booth *et al.* [9] described an enzymatic activity in rat liver cytosol catalyzing the conjugation of glutathione (GSH) with 1,2-dichloro-4-nitrobenzene (DCNB). A large number of substrates for GSTs were described in the following years [4]. The first purification concerning GST was reported by Fjellstedt in 1973 [10] using rat liver tissue. Western blotting analysis revealed the existence of homo- and heterodimeric enzymes, and this was the basis for dividing GST into structurally distinct groups [11]. The first three-dimensional structure was reported by Reinemer *et al.* [12] identifying the three-dimensional structure of GST isolated from pig lungs.

Glutathione is composed of glutamate, cysteine, and glycine (γ-Glu–Cys–Gly). It is a member of a superfamily of ubiquitous enzymes, which (i) plays an important role in the cellular detoxification and protection of macromolecules from attack by reactive electrophiles [13]; (ii) is involved in the synthesis of leukotrienes, prostaglandins, testosterone, and progesterone, as well as the degradation of Tyr; and (iii) can modulate protein kinase activity in the nucleus and influence cell proliferation. GST enzymes catalyze a variety of chemical reactions, including, nucleophilic aromatic substitution, isomerization, peroxidase reactions, epoxide ring opening, and reversible Michael additions [4]. However, perhaps the most critical is the conjugation of glutathione with the sulfur atom of Cys into a wide variety of both endogenous and exogenous chemicals with electrophilic functional groups (carcinogens, environmental pollutants, and products of oxidative stress [14, 15]), thereby neutralizing their electrophilic sites to endogenous water-soluble products [13]. Evidence suggest that glutathione exists as the thiolate form (GS^-) at neutral pH when complexed with GST [4]. The stability of thiolate group is provided by Tyr (e.g., α, μ, π, and σ class) or Ser (e.g., θ class) at the N-terminus of cytosolic GSTs [1]. It has been proposed that once a thiolate group is formed,

Metabolism of Drugs and Other Xenobiotics, First Edition. Edited by Pavel Anzenbacher, Ulrich M. Zanger.

it becomes capable of reacting spontaneously by neutrophilic attack with an electrophilic substrate [1]. Glutathione conjugate is converted to the corresponding Cys conjugate following sequential removal of glutathione and Gly. Several transport mechanisms exist for the elimination of the products of glutathione conjugation including P-glycoprotein [16], the multidrug resistance pump [17, 18], the ATP-dependent glutathione conjugate export pump [19], the multispecific organic anion transporter [20], and the broad-specific anion transporter of dinitrophenol *S*-glutathione conjugates [21].

Although the majority of GST-mediated conjugations represent detoxification of electrophilic substrates, GSTs could also result in more reactive compounds than the parent compound (e.g., with halogenated alkenes and alkynes such as hexachlorobutadiene and tetrachloroethene).

5.2 Nomenclature, Structure, and Function

Human GSTs are expressed as three major families: cytosolic, mitochondrial, and microsomal [1]. The cytosolic and mitochondrial GSTs are dimers, while the microsomal forms may exist as monomers, trimers, or higher-order aggregates.

5.2.1 Cytosolic GSTs

The soluble form occurs in bacteria, yeast, molds, fungi, crustaceans, mollusks, worm parasites, frogs, insects, plants, fish, birds, and mammals [4]. In humans, it forms approximately 4% of total soluble protein in the liver [5]. Similarly to cytochrome P450 (CYP) nomenclature, the nomenclature for GSTs has been problematic, as different groups of researchers have developed their own independent nomenclature [22–24]. The proposed nomenclature for human cytosolic GSTs is based on the nomenclature proposed by Mannervik *et al.* [25]. This nomenclature uses lower-case letter processing GST (h, human; r, rat; m, mouse) followed by an upper case Roman letter to indicate the class alpha, mu, pi, theta, zeta, and omega (A, M, P, T, and O) and Arabic numerals to specify the subunit composition on the basis of the chronologic order of discovery (1, 2, 3, 4, etc.) [25]. Allelic variant is represented by lower-case Roman letters [25]. As with CYP, genes are usually denoted in italic, whereas the protein is shown in standard form [25].

Members of the same class generally exhibit greater than 40% amino acid sequence identity with other members in the class, whereas members of a distinct class possess less than 30% similarity (e.g., within the M class, five human enzymes were identified, M1–M5) [5]. Amino acid sequence comparison revealed that the microsomal GST shares no homology with the cytosolic form, suggesting that both groups evolved through independent pathways. However, not only has primary structure comparison been used to classify GSTs [25–29], some other classification criteria have already been published, such as immunoblotting [30–33], kinetic properties [34–37], tertiary structure [2, 3], and quaternary structure [2, 3, 38, 39].

All GSTs are active as dimers containing two subunits of 23–30 kDa (199–244 amino acids in length) – the identity of these subunits determining which GST is present. Each dimer is encoded by independent genes. The subunits are unique to a given class and the diversity of subunits varies from only two (GSTT) to six or more (GSTM) [8]. Each subunit has an active site that appears as a cleft along the domain interface. Each site can be separated into two distinct functional regions – a hydrophilic G-site for binding the physiological structure glutathione and an adjacent hydrophobic H-site for binding structurally diverse electrophilic substrates. Although the active site of GSTs is catalytically independent, the full active site is formed by structural elements from both subunits of the dimer. Most important for this activity is a hydrogen bond between a conserved G-site Tyr residue and the glutathione thiol group. This hydrogen bond stabilizes the thiolate anion of the active site-bound glutathione. The H-site is formed of clusters of nonpolar amino acid side-chains, which provide a highly hydrophobic surface that in the absence of a drug substrate is open to bulk solvent. Binding of substrates to this site has been shown to relate to increased lipophilicity [1, 5].

5.2.1.1 GSTA, GSTM, and GSTP Classes

The major mammalian GST classes are α, μ, and π (e.g., GSTA class accounts for as much as 3% of the soluble protein in human liver). They are considered to be the most highly developed GSTs, as judged by their structural and functional adaptation to the prototypical activity of GSTs (i.e., glutathione conjugation of electrophiles) [40]. The structure of these enzymes differs at two functionally important sites: (i) in the subunit interface, which is conserved within each class but is divergent between classes, and (ii) the relatively open active site in GSTP class enzymes, partially occluded by the μ-loop in proteins belonging to the GSTM class and covered by a mobile C-terminal α-helix in α class enzymes [41].

5.2.1.2 GSTS Class

The σ class is also referred to as human prostaglandin D synthase and catalyzes the isomerization of prostaglandin H_2 to prostaglandin D_2 [42, 43]. In additional to this activity, the enzyme expresses transferase and peroxidase activity. It is closely related to the α/μ/π cluster.

5.2.1.3 GSTT Class

The θ class GSTs are sometimes considered as being a close to an ancestral protein common to all GSTs. In human gastric and colonic mucosa, GST θ class enzymes are present in comparatively high amounts and their expression has been shown to be comparable to that of the α class [44]. Thus, these enzymes may play an important role in the detoxification of electrophilic toxicants, including chemical carcinogens present in the food.

5.2.1.4 GSTO Class

The ω class is newly identified GST subfamily that has some different characteristics in its structure and function from the other members of GSTs. They have a Cys residue in their active sites in contrast to a Ser or Tyr that is in the active sites of other subfamilies. These GSTs have a poor activity with common GST substrates. The GSTO class shows thiol transferase and dehydroascorbate reductase activities [26, 45]; thus, this class plays a role in the defense mechanism against oxidative stress.

5.2.1.5 GSTZ Class

The ζ class catalyzes isomerization of maleylacetoacetate to fumarylacetoacetate and is also referred to as maleylacetoacetate isomerase [29, 46]. Thus, this enzyme is believed to contribute to catabolism of Tyr [29]. In addition, these enzymes catalyze the metabolism of α-haloacids [47]. It has been suggested that ζ class GSTs may be essential for survival under conditions of malnutrition.

5.2.2 Mitochondrial GSTs

The microsomal GSTs were originally thought to belong to the cytosolic GST superfamily. An analysis of their structure indicates that these form their own superfamily [48]. Mitochondria are an important cellular site where reactive oxygen species (ROS) are produced during respiratory coupled oxidative metabolism. Mitochondrial GST is an important defense system against ROS. However, mammalian mitochondria have limited capability to synthesize GST. Thus, the high GST mitochondrial level is approached by ATP-dependent transport of cytosolic GST into mitochondria. In humans, mitochondrial GST is a homodimeric κ class GST (chromosome 7q35). This enzyme has also been found associated with peroxidases, which may play a role in the β-oxidation of fatty acids. Its role in the biotransformation of environmental chemicals remains unclear.

5.2.3 Microsomal GSTs

The microsomal GST and its related membrane-bound proteins are structurally distinct from the soluble form of GSTs [49]. They form a separate superfamily called membrane-associated proteins in eicosanoid and glutathione metabolism (MAPEG). Cytosolic GSTs are active as homo/heterodimers of subunits of 25 kDa, whereas microsomal GST is active as a trimer with a subunit size of 17 kDa [50, 51]. Microsomal GSTs are involved primarily in eicosanoid synthesis; a number of membrane-bound GSTs are known – MGST1, MGST2, MGST3, and leukotriene C_4 synthases. Human microsomal GST1 is observed in large amounts in liver tissue, is distributed in both the microsomal and mitochondrial membrane [3], and is similar to two other membrane-bound GSTs (MGST2 and leukotriene C_4 synthases). These are similar in size, although different in sequence identity

[52]. Prostaglandin E synthase, also called microsomal GST1-like, and 5-lipoxygenase activating protein (FLAP) are also members of the MAPEG superfamily. However, some MAPEG enzymes have detoxicification functions, including high glutathione peroxidase activity. Thus, these enzymes appear to be well suited to protect membranes from the action of lipid hydroperoxides.

5.3 Substrates

Many different compounds, including both endogenous (e.g., amino acids, steroid hormones, eicosanoid) and exogenous compounds, act as GSTs substrates (Table 5.2) [5]. All the substrates are hydrophobic compounds possessing an electrophilic center. These electrophiles range in size from dichloromethane to large aromatic hydrocarbons [53, 54].

Although it is generally believed that glutathione and Cys conjugates of many toxic xenobiotics are nontoxic and eliminated from the body, either as conjugates or mercapturate or methylthio-containing metabolites [35, 55, 56], recent studies [57, 58] show some glutathione and Cys conjugates are of toxicological concern. Two different mechanisms have been described to explain the toxicity of glutathione and Cys conjugates. (i) The conjugates act as direct alkylating agents and their toxic effects are dependent on the sulfur half-mustard moiety of the molecule [57, 58]. (ii) The conversion of glutathione conjugate to its corresponding Cys conjugate, followed by 13-elimination of an electrophilic sulfur-containing fragment from the Cys conjugate [57, 58]. This 13-lyase-mediated reaction can lead to the formation of a reactive species, resulting in toxicity.

5.4 Regulation, Induction, and Inhibition

Regulation of GSTs expression differs between tissues and is often tissue-specific. Table 5.1 shows estimates of the tissue distribution of various GSTs [59]. The regulation of GSTs is of interest because their expression is significantly increased in many cancer diseases, yielding resistance to chemotherapeutic drugs [60–62]. The regulation of cytosolic GSTs is a complex process dependent on both endogenous and exogenous factors, gender [63], tissue-specific factors [64], diet [63], xenobiotics such as polycyclic aromatic hydrocarbons (PAHs), phenolic antioxidants, ROS, organic isothiocyanates, trivalent arsenicals, barbiturates, glucocorticoids, and many others [4, 65]. Most studies on transcriptional regulation have been performed using rodents.

Induction of GSTs is mediated via several transcriptional mechanisms, such as the glucocorticoid-responsive element (GRE) (substrates are glucocorticoids such as dexamethasone), xenobiotic-responsive element (XRE) (substrates are planar aromatic hydrocarbons such as 3-methylcholanthrene, dioxin), and

Table 5.1 Classification and nomenclature of human GSTs [5] (in addition, the σ class (chromosome 4q22.3) is known as a glutathione-dependent prostaglandin D_2 synthase).

	Subunit	Molecular weight (kDa)	Chromosome	Primary tissues	Alleles, nucleotide change
GSTA	A1	25.6	6p12	liver, testis >>> kidney, adrenal > pancreas >> lung, brain > heart	A1*A (–69C)
					A1*B (–69T)
	A2	26.0	6p12	liver, pancreas > testis > kidney > adrenal > brain, lung, heart	A2*A (332C, 335C, 589G, 629A)
					A2*B (332C, 335C, 589G, 629C)
					A2*C (332C, 335G, 589G, 629A)
					A2*E (332T, 335C, 589G, 629A)
	A3	NA	NA	placenta (?)	NA
	A4	25.7	NA	small intestine > spleen	NA
GSTM	M1	26.7	1p13.3	liver >> testis > brain, adrenal, kidney, pancreas > lung, heart	M1*A (519G)
					M1*B (519C)
					M1*0 (deletion)
					M1*A × 2 (duplication)
	M2	26.0	1p13.3	brain > testis > heart > pancreas, kidney > adrenal > lung, liver	NA
	M3	26.3	1p13.3	testis >>> brain, spleen	M3*A (AAGG)
					M3*B (AAG deletion)
	M4	26.0	1p13.3	liver, skeletal muscle > heart, brain >> pancreas > lung, kidney, placenta	M4*A (2517T)
					M4*B (2517C)
	M5	26.0	1p13.3	brain, testis, lung	NA

GSTP	P1	23.0	11q13	brain >> lung, heart, testis > adrenal, kidney, pancreas > liver	four allelic variants:
					*P1*A* (313A, 341C, 555C)
					*P1*B* (313G, 341C, 555T)
					*P1*C* (313G, 341T, 555T)
					*P1*D* (313A, 341T)
GSTT	T1	27.0	22q11.2	kidney, liver > small intestine > brain, spleen, prostate, pancreas, testis > heart, lung	*T1*A* (310A)
					*T1*B* (310C)
					*T1*0* gene deletion
	T2	27.0	22q11.2	liver (?)	*T2*A* (418G)
					*T2*B* (481A)
GSTZ	Z1	24.2	14q24.3	(fetal liver, skeletal mucosa)	*Z1*A* (94A, 124A, 245C)
					*Z1*B* (94A, 124G, 245C)
					*Z1*C* (94G, 124G, 245C)
					*Z1*D* (94G, 124G, 245T)
GSTO	O1		10q24.3	(liver, breast, macrophages, brain)	*O1*A* (419C, 464 + 1 AAG)
					*O1*B* (419C, 464 + 1 del)
					*O1*C* (419A, 464 + 1 AAG)
					*O1*D* (419A, 464 + 1 del)
					*O1*E* (650C)
					*O1*F* (650A)
	O2		10q24.3	(testis, liver, heart, prostate)	*O2*A* (424A)
					*O2*B* (424G)
	O3				O3p (pseudogene)

Table 5.2 Substrates (either directly or as metabolites) for GSTs (modified from Eaton and Bammler [5]).

Environmental carcinogens/toxicants	Pesticides	Drugs	Endogenous molecules
5-Hydroxymethyl-chrysen sulfate	alachlor	adriamycin (doxorubicin)	4-hydroxy-2-nonenal
7-Hydroxymethylbenz[*a*]anthracene sulfate	atrazine	acetaminophen	9-hydroperoxylinoleic acid
4-Nitroquinone oxide	DDT (dichlorodiphenyltrichloroethane)	BCNU (bis-chloromethylnitrosourea)	13-hydroperoxylinoleic acid
Acrolein	lindane	bromosulfophtalein	adenine propenal
Aflatoxin-8,9-epoxide	methyl parathione	cisplatin	aminochrome
AVB-8,9-epoxide	EPN (*O*-ethyl-*O*-4-nitrophenyl phenyl-phosphonothioate)	chlorambucil	androst-5-ene-3,17-dione
Benzo[*a*]pyrene 7,8-dichloromethane		cyclophosphamide	catechol estrogens
Dihydrodiol-9,10-epoxide		ethacrynic acid	cholesterol-5,6-oxide
Butadiene		fosfomycin	dopaminochrome
Ethylene dibromide		menadione (vitamin K_3)	leukotriene A_4
Ethylene oxide		mitozantrone	maleylacetoacetate
Hexachlorobutadiene		nitroglycerine	malondialdehyde
N,*N*-dimethylaminoazobenzene		thiotepa	pregn-5-ene-3,20-dione
Nitropyrene epoxides			prostaglandins
PAH epoxides			
PAH hydroxysulfate esters			
PhIP (2-amino-1-methyl-6-phenylimidazo[4,5-*b*]pyridine)			
Styrene oxide			
Trichloroethylene			

antioxidant-responsive element (ARE) (substrates are phenol antioxidants such as butylated hydroxyanisole, butylated hydroxytoluene) [4, 66]. GSTs could also be induced by oxidative stress; this may be mediated via nuclear factor-κB or activator protein-1 [4]. Post-transcription mechanisms are also involved in the regulation of GSTs [67, 68]. In contrast to the α and π GST subfamily, regulation of the remaining GSTs is still largely unknown and yet to be fully investigated. Owing to the ability of many natural products to induce GST activity there has been an interest in this for explaining the anticancer effect of many fruits and vegetables [5].

Additional interest in GST inhibitors is due to (i) the treatment of parasitic infections (including helminthes, which affect 2 billion people worldwide, and malaria, which causes 300 million acute episodes per year) and (ii) the possible use in cancer therapy. GST enzymes inhibitors can be divided into three main group: (i) nonsubstrate ligands that bind to noncatalytic sites of GSTs, (ii) GST analogs that bind to the G-site of the enzyme, and (iii) hydrophobic compounds that bind to the H-site of the enzyme. A number of inhibitors have been observed *in vitro* (etacrynic acid [69], calvatic acid [70], curcumin [71], disulfiram [72]). However, none of these inhibitors has been clinically approved to date.

5.5 Gene Polymorphism of GSTs

GST enzymes are involved in the detoxification of potentially toxic endogenous and exogenous compounds; numerous epidemiologic studies indicate an association between GST gene polymorphism and increased risk of diseases such as cancer (for reviews, see [5, 73–75]), chronic obstructive pulmonary disease [76], rheumatoid arthritis [77], multiple sclerosis [78], Parkinson's disease [79], and many others. The most extensively studied GST polymorphisms occur in three GST enzymes found in cytosol, μ (GSTM1, 3) [80–85], θ (GSTT1) [86–88], and π (GSTP1) [89, 90], which may lead to a wide interindividual variability in the biotransformation of electrophilic compounds [91, 92].

Due to the strong correlation between phenotype and genotype reported for the GSTs [93, 94], it is reliable to use polymorphic genotypes to identify individuals who lack or have low activity of these enzymes. Compared with CYP or other enzymes like *N*-acetyltransferase type 2 (NAT2), *in vivo* probes to measure GST phenotype are not available. Instead, the GST status of populations has to be evaluated *in vitro* by using cytosols from peripheral blood lymphocytes or erythrocytes [95]. GSTM1 activity is recommended to be determined by *trans*-stilbene oxide; methyl chloride and dichloromethane are generally used to measure the GSTT1 phenotype [96, 97]; and ethacrynic acid is recommended to measure the GSTP1 phenotype [98].

In general, the incidence of lung cancer is higher in individuals lacking the GSTM1 gene compared to individuals expressing the gene [81, 82]. Individuals with the GSTT1-null genotype exhibit decreased ability to detoxify metabolites of several carcinogens, including 1,3-butadiene, methyl bromide, and ethylene oxide

[86, 87]. In contrast, individuals who inherit the GSTT1 gene can produce a mutagenic metabolite of dichloromethane following conjugation with glutathione. Polymorphisms affect the activity of other cytosolic GST such as α, ω, and ζ, but the functional and toxicological implications of these polymorphisms remain unclear [99–101].

5.5.1
GSTA Polymorphism

Five genes (GST1, GST2, GST3, GST4, and GST5) and seven pseudogenes have to date been described. The GSTA1 class genes show significant homology, therefore making SNP design problematic. *GSTT1*0* decreases protein expression [102], *GSTA1*2E* reduces enzymatic activity [103], and no gene polymorphisms have yet been described for GSTA3, GSTA4, and GSTA5.

5.5.2
GSTM Polymorphism

The GSTM1 polymorphism was first described in lymphocyte GST activity by Seidegard *et al.* [104, 105], using *trans*-stilbene oxide as a GSTM substrate. It is recognized that the GSTM1 gene deletion (*GSTM1*0*) is very common in the population, with significant ethnic differences in gene frequency (Table 5.3) [4, 74, 88, 106]. Subjects exhibiting a homozygous deletion of the GSTM1 locus were found to have no enzymatic activity. In addition, the presence of the *GSTM1A* × *2* leads to overexpression and an increase in enzymatic activity [107]. No significant gene polymorphism has been characterized in GSTM2 or GSTM5.

5.5.3
GSTT Polymorphism

This class is considered to be the most ancient of all GSTs and has been described in almost all organisms investigated [27]. A polymorphism for GSTT1 was first

Table 5.3 Frequency of *GSTM1*0* gene polymorphism in various ethnic groups.

Ethnic group	*GSTM1*0/*0* (%) (frequency in population)
Micronesian/Polynesian	64–100
Chinese	35–63
Caucasian	38–67
Japanese	48–51
French national	43
African-American	28–35
Hispanic	49–53
Indian	33
Nigerians	22

Table 5.4 Frequency of *GSTT1*0* gene polymorphism in various ethnic groups.

Ethnic group	*GSTT1*0* genotype (%) (frequency in population)
Caucasian – English, German	12–16
Caucasian – US	15–24
Japanese	45
Chinese	58–62
African-American	24

observed by Pemble *et al.* in 1994 [87]. Like the GSTM1 polymorphism, GSTT1 homozygous GST1*0 genotypes are variable between ethnic groups (Table 5.4) [108, 109]. Although three GSTT2 gene polymorphisms have been previously observed [110], further clinical investigation concerning these alleles is warranted.

5.5.4 GSTP1 Polymorphism

GSTP1 is one of the most extensively studied GST genes. To date, 42 SNPs have been identified in the GSTP1 gene; however, only three alleles have been extensively studied, *GSTP1*A* (Ile105–Ala114), *GSTP1*B* (Val105–Ala114), and *GSTP1*3* (Val105–Val114) [111, 112].

5.5.5 GSTO Polymorphism

Gene polymorphism in both GSTO1 and GSTO2 has been described [113]. Thiotransferase activity was significantly reduced in GSTO1 Asp140 and GSTO1 Asn217, but increased in *GSTO1*B* (del 115) compared to a wild-type GSTO1 [113].

References

1 Armstrong, R.N. (1997) Structure, catalytic mechanism, and evolution of the glutathione transferases. *Chem. Res. Toxicol.*, **10**, 2–18.
2 Dirr, H., Reinemer, P., and Huber, R. (1994) X-ray crystal structures of cytosolic glutathione *S*-transferases. Implications for protein architecture, substrate recognition and catalytic function. *Eur. J. Biochem.*, **220**, 645–661.
3 Wilce, M.C. and Parker, M.W. (1994) Structure and function of glutathione *S*-transferases. *Biochim. Biophys. Acta*, **1205**, 1–18.
4 Hayes, J.D. and Pulford, D.J. (1995) The glutathione *S*-transferase supergene family: regulation of GST and the contribution of the isoenzymes to cancer chemoprotection and drug resistance. *Crit. Rev. Biochem. Mol. Biol.*, **30**, 445–600.
5 Eaton, D.L. and Bammler, T.K. (1999) Concise review of the glutathione *S*-transferases and their significance to toxicology. *Toxicol. Sci.*, **49**, 156–164.

6 Salinas, A.E. and Wong, M.G. (1999) Glutathione *S*-transferases – a review. *Curr. Med. Chem.*, **6**, 279–309.

7 Edwards, R., Dixon, D.P., and Walbot, V. (2000) Plant glutathione *S*-transferases: enzymes with multiple functions in sickness and in health. *Trends Plant Sci.*, **5**, 193–198.

8 Sheehan, D., Meade, G., Foley, V.M., and Dowd, C.A. (2001) Structure, function and evolution of glutathione transferases: implications for classification of non-mammalian members of an ancient enzyme superfamily. *Biochem. J.*, **360**, 1–16.

9 Booth, J., Boyland, E., and Sims, P. (1961) An enzyme from rat liver catalysing conjugations with glutathione. *Biochem. J.*, **79**, 516–524.

10 Fjellstedt, T.A., Allen, R.H., Duncan, B.K., and Jakoby, W.B. (1973) Enzymatic conjugation of epoxides with glutathione. *J. Biol. Chem.*, **248**, 3702–3707.

11 Bass, N.M., Kirsch, R.E., Tuff, S.A., Marks, I., and Saunders, S.J. (1977) Ligandin heterogeneity: evidence that the two non-identical subunits are the monomers of two distinct proteins. *Biochim. Biophys. Acta*, **492**, 163–175.

12 Reinemer, P., Dirr, H.W., Ladenstein, R., Schaffer, J., Gallay, O., and Huber, R. (1991) The three-dimensional structure of class pi glutathione *S*-transferase in complex with glutathione sulfonate at 2.3 A resolution. *EMBO J.*, **10**, 1997–2005.

13 Hayes, J.D. and Strange, R.C. (2000) Glutathione *S*-transferase polymorphisms and their biological consequences. *Pharmacology*, **61**, 154–166.

14 Bolt, H.M. and Thier, R. (2006) Relevance of the deletion polymorphisms of the glutathione *S*-transferases GSTT1 and GSTM1 in pharmacology and toxicology. *Curr. Drug Metab.*, **7**, 613–628.

15 Raimondi, S., Botteri, E., Iodice, S., Lowenfels, A.B., and Maisonneuve, P. (2009) Gene–smoking interaction on colorectal adenoma and cancer risk: review and meta-analysis. *Mutat. Res.*, **670**, 6–14.

16 Gottesman, M.M. and Pastan, I. (1993) Biochemistry of multidrug resistance mediated by the multidrug transporter. *Annu. Rev. Biochem.*, **62**, 385–427.

17 Jedlitschky, G., Leier, I., Buchholz, U., Center, M., and Keppler, D. (1994) ATP-dependent transport of glutathione *S*-conjugates by the multidrug resistance-associated protein. *Cancer Res.*, **54**, 4833–4836.

18 Kavallaris, M. (1997) The role of multidrug resistance-associated protein (MRP) expression in multidrug resistance. *Anticancer Drugs*, **8**, 17–25.

19 Ishikawa, T. (1992) The ATP-dependent glutathione S-conjugate export pump. *Trends Biochem. Sci.*, **17**, 463–468.

20 Heijn, M., Oude Elferink, R.P., and Jansen, P.L. (1992) ATP-dependent multispecific organic anion transport system in rat erythrocyte membrane vesicles. *Am. J. Physiol.*, **262**, C104–C110.

21 Saxena, M., Singhal, S.S., Awasthi, S., Singh, S.V., Labelle, E.F., Zimniak, P., and Awasthi, Y.C. (1992) Dinitrophenyl *S*-glutathione ATPase purified from human muscle catalyzes ATP hydrolysis in the presence of leukotrienes. *Arch. Biochem. Biophys.*, **298**, 231–237.

22 Litwack, G., Ketterer, B., and Arias, I.M. (1971) Ligandin: a hepatic protein which binds steroids, bilirubin, carcinogens and a number of exogenous organic anions. *Nature*, **234**, 466–467.

23 Hayes, J.D. (1986) Purification and physical characterization of glutathione *S*-transferase K. Differential use of *S*-hexylglutathione and glutathione affinity matrices to isolate a novel glutathione *S*-transferase from rat liver. *Biochem. J.*, **233**, 789–798.

24 Kitahara, A., Satoh, K., Nishimura, K., Ishikawa, T., Ruike, K., Sato, K., Tsuda, H., and Ito, N. (1984) Changes in molecular forms of rat hepatic glutathione *S*-transferase during chemical hepatocarcinogenesis. *Cancer Res.*, **44**, 2698–2703.

25 Mannervik, B., Awasthi, Y.C., Board, P.G., Hayes, J.D., Di Ilio, C., Ketterer, B., Listowsky, I., Morgenstern, R., Muramatsu, M., Pearson, W.R., *et al.* (1992) Nomenclature for human

glutathione transferases. *Biochem. J.*, **282**, 305–306.

26 Board, P.G., Coggan, M., Chelvanayagam, G., Easteal, S., Jermiin, L.S., Schulte, G.K., Danley, D.E., Hoth, L.R., Griffor, M.C., Kamath, A.V., Rosner, M.H., Chrunyk, B.A., Perregaux, D.E., Gabel, C.A., Geoghegan, K.F., and Pandit, J. (2000) Identification, characterization, and crystal structure of the Omega class glutathione transferases. *J. Biol. Chem.*, **275**, 24798–24806.

27 Pemble, S.E. and Taylor, J.B. (1992) An evolutionary perspective on glutathione transferases inferred from class-theta glutathione transferase cDNA sequences. *Biochem. J.*, **287**, 957–963.

28 Pemble, S.E., Wardle, A.F., and Taylor, J.B. (1996) Glutathione *S*-transferase class Kappa: characterization by the cloning of rat mitochondrial GST and identification of a human homologue. *Biochem. J.*, **319**, 749–754.

29 Board, P.G., Baker, R.T., Chelvanayagam, G., and Jermiin, L.S. (1997) Zeta, a novel class of glutathione transferases in a range of species from plants to humans. *Biochem. J.*, **328**, 929–935.

30 Hayes, J.D., and Mantle, T.J. (1986) Use of immuno-blot techniques to discriminate between the glutathione *S*-transferase Yf, Yk, Ya, Yn/Yb and Yc subunits and to study their distribution in extrahepatic tissues. Evidence for three immunochemically distinct groups of transferase in the rat. *Biochem. J.*, **233**, 779–788.

31 Blocki, F.A., Ellis, L.B., and Wackett, L.P. (1993) MIF protein are theta-class glutathione *S*-transferase homologs. *Protein Sci.*, **2**, 2095–2102.

32 Fournier, D., Bride, J.M., Poirie, M., Berge, J.B., and Plapp, F.W., Jr (1992) Insect glutathione *S*-transferases. Biochemical characteristics of the major forms from houseflies susceptible and resistant to insecticides. *J. Biol. Chem.*, **267**, 1840–1845.

33 Creaney, J., Wijffels, G.L., Sexton, J.L., Sandeman, R.M., Spithill, T.W., and Parsons, J.C. (1995) *Fasciola hepatica*: localisation of glutathione *S*-transferase isoenzymes in adult and juvenile liver fluke. *Exp. Parasitol.*, **81**, 106–116.

34 Rowe, J.D., Patskovsky, Y.V., Patskovska, L.N., Novikova, E., and Listowsky, I. (1998) Rationale for reclassification of a distinctive subdivision of mammalian class Mu glutathione *S*-transferases that are primarily expressed in testis. *J. Biol. Chem.*, **273**, 9593–9601.

35 Mannervik, B. and Danielson, U.H. (1988) Glutathione transferases – structure and catalytic activity. *CRC Crit. Rev. Biochem.*, **23**, 283–337.

36 Mannervik, B., Alin, P., Guthenberg, C., Jensson, H., Tahir, M.K., Warholm, M., and Jornvall, H. (1985) Identification of three classes of cytosolic glutathione transferase common to several mammalian species: correlation between structural data and enzymatic properties. *Proc. Natl. Acad. Sci. USA*, **82**, 7202–7206.

37 Meyer, D.J. (1993) Significance of an unusually low Km for glutathione in glutathione transferases of the alpha, mu and pi classes. *Xenobiotica*, **23**, 823–834.

38 Hayes, J.D., Strange, R.C., and Percy-Robb, I.W. (1981) A study of the structures of the YaYa and YaYc glutathione *S*-transferases from rat liver cytosol. Evidence that the Ya monomer is responsible for lithocholate-binding activity. *Biochem. J.*, **197**, 491–502.

39 Rossjohn, J., Polekhina, G., Feil, S.C., Allocati, N., Masulli, M., De Illio, C., and Parker, M.W. (1998) A mixed disulfide bond in bacterial glutathione transferase: functional and evolutionary implications. *Structure*, **6**, 721–734.

40 Caccuri, A.M., Antonini, G., Board, P.G., Flanagan, J., Parker, M.W., Paolesse, R., Turella, P., Federici, G., Lo Bello, M., and Ricci, G. (2001) Human glutathione transferase T2-2 discloses some evolutionary strategies for optimization of substrate binding to the active site of glutathione transferases. *J. Biol. Chem.*, **276**, 5427–5431.

41 Armstrong, R.N. (1994) Glutathione *S*-transferases: structure and mechanism of an archetypical detoxication enzyme.

Adv. Enzymol. Relat. Areas Mol. Biol., **69**, 1–44.

42 Jowsey, I.R., Thomson, A.M., Flanagan, J.U., Murdock, P.R., Moore, G.B., Meyer, D.J., Murphy, G.J., Smith, S.A., and Hayes, J.D. (2001) Mammalian class Sigma glutathione *S*-transferases: catalytic properties and tissue-specific expression of human and rat GSH-dependent prostaglandin D_2 synthases. *Biochem. J.*, **359**, 507–516.

43 Meyer, D.J., Muimo, R., Thomas, M., Coates, D., and Isaac, R.E. (1996) Purification and characterization of prostaglandin-H E-isomerase, a sigma-class glutathione *S*-transferase, from *Ascaridia galli*. *Biochem. J.*, **313**, 223–227.

44 de Bruin, W.C., Wagenmans, M.J., Board, P.G., and Peters, W.H. (1999) Expression of glutathione *S*-transferase theta class isoenzymes in human colorectal and gastric cancers. *Carcinogenesis*, **20**, 1453–1457.

45 Yin, Z.L., Dahlstrom, J.E., Le Couteur, D.G., and Board, P.G. (2001) Immunohistochemistry of omega class glutathione *S*-transferase in human tissues. *J. Histochem. Cytochem.*, **49**, 983–987.

46 Board, P.G., Taylor, M.C., Coggan, M., Parker, M.W., Lantum, H.B., and Anders, M.W. (2003) Clarification of the role of key active site residues of glutathione transferase zeta/maleylacetoacetate isomerase by a new spectrophotometric technique. *Biochem. J.*, **374**, 731–737.

47 Tong, Z., Board, P.G., and Anders, M.W. (1998) Glutathione transferase zeta-catalyzed biotransformation of dichloroacetic acid and other alpha-haloacids. *Chem. Res. Toxicol.*, **11**, 1332–1338.

48 Ladner, J.E., Parsons, J.F., Rife, C.L., Gilliland, G.L., and Armstrong, R.N. (2004) Parallel evolutionary pathways for glutathione transferases: structure and mechanism of the mitochondrial class kappa enzyme rGSTK1-1. *Biochemistry*, **43**, 352–361.

49 Morgenstern, R., Guthenberg, C., and Depierre, J.W. (1982) Microsomal glutathione *S*-transferase. Purification, initial characterization and demonstration that it is not identical to the cytosolic glutathione *S*-transferases A, B and C. *Eur. J. Biochem.*, **128**, 243–248.

50 Awasthi, Y.C., Sharma, R., and Singhal, S.S. (1994) Human glutathione *S*-transferases. *Int. J. Biochem.*, **26**, 295–308.

51 Andersson, C., Mosialou, E., Weinander, R., and Morgenstern, R. (1994) Enzymology of microsomal glutathione *S*-transferase. *Adv. Pharmacol.*, **27**, 19–35.

52 Jakobsson, P.J., Mancini, J.A., and Ford-Hutchinson, A.W. (1996) Identification and characterization of a novel human microsomal glutathione *S*-transferase with leukotriene C_4 synthase activity and significant sequence identity to 5-lipoxygenase-activating protein and leukotriene C_4 synthase. *J. Biol. Chem.*, **271**, 22203–22210.

53 Meyer, D.J., Coles, B., Pemble, S.E., Gilmore, K.S., Fraser, G.M., and Ketterer, B. (1991) Theta, a new class of glutathione transferases purified from rat and man. *Biochem. J.*, **274**, 409–414.

54 Ho, D. and Fahl, W.E. (1984) Quantitative significance of glutathione and glutathione-*S*-transferase in regulating benzo[*a*]pyrene anti diol-epoxide level in reconstituted C3H/10T1/2 cell lysates, and comparison to rat liver. *Carcinogenesis*, **5**, 143–148.

55 Chasseaud, L.F. (1979) The role of glutathione and glutathione *S*-transferases in the metabolism of chemical carcinogens and other electrophilic agents. *Adv. Cancer Res.*, **29**, 175–274.

56 Mannervik, B. (1985) The isoenzymes of glutathione transferase. *Adv. Enzymol. Relat. Areas Mol. Biol.*, **57**, 357–417.

57 Anders, M.W., Lash, L., Dekant, W., Elfarra, A.A., and Dohn, D.R. (1988) Biosynthesis and biotransformation of glutathione *S*-conjugates to toxic metabolites. *Crit. Rev. Toxicol.*, **18**, 311–341.

58 Elfarra, A.A. and Anders, M.W. (1984) Renal processing of glutathione

conjugates. Role in nephrotoxicity. *Biochem. Pharmacol.*, **33**, 3729–3732.

59 Sherratt, P.J., Pulford, D.J., Harrison, D.J., Green, T., and Hayes, J.D. (1997) Evidence that human class Theta glutathione *S*-transferase T1-1 can catalyse the activation of dichloromethane, a liver and lung carcinogen in the mouse. Comparison of the tissue distribution of GST T1-1 with that of classes Alpha, Mu and Pi GST in human. *Biochem. J.*, **326**, 837–846.

60 Hudson, C.E., Kelly, M.M., Schwartz, D.A., Schofield, D.A., DeHaven, J.E., Schulte, B.A., and Norris, J.S. (1998) Glutathione *S*-transferase in hormonal carcinogenesis. *Chem. Biol. Interact.*, **111–112**, 343–350.

61 Tew, K.D. (1994) Glutathione-associated enzymes in anticancer drug resistance. *Cancer Res.*, **54**, 4313–4320.

62 O'Brien, M.L. and Tew, K.D. (1996) Glutathione and related enzymes in multidrug resistance. *Eur. J. Cancer*, **32A**, 967–978.

63 Hatayama, I., Satoh, K., and Sato, K. (1986) Developmental and hormonal regulation of the major form of hepatic glutathione *S*-transferase in male mice. *Biochem. Biophys. Res. Commun.*, **140**, 581–588.

64 Rushmore, T.H. and Pickett, C.B. (1990) Transcriptional regulation of the rat glutathione *S*-transferase Ya subunit gene. Characterization of a xenobiotic-responsive element controlling inducible expression by phenolic antioxidants. *J. Biol. Chem.*, **265**, 14648–14653.

65 Daniel, V. (1993) Glutathione *S*-transferases: gene structure and regulation of expression. *Crit. Rev. Biochem. Mol. Biol.*, **28**, 173–207.

66 Kensler, T.W. (1997) Chemoprevention by inducers of carcinogen detoxication enzymes. *Environ. Health Perspect.*, **105** (Suppl. 4), 965–970.

67 Morrow, C.S., Chiu, J., and Cowan, K.H. (1992) Posttranscriptional control of glutathione *S*-transferase pi gene expression in human breast cancer cells. *J. Biol. Chem.*, **267**, 10544–10550.

68 Moffat, G.J., McLaren, A.W., and Wolf, C.R. (1997) Transcriptional and post-transcriptional mechanisms can regulate cell-specific expression of the human Pi-class glutathione *S*-transferase gene. *Biochem. J.*, **324**, 91–95.

69 Ploemen, J.H., van Ommen, B., and van Bladeren, P.J. (1990) Inhibition of rat and human glutathione *S*-transferase isoenzymes by ethacrynic acid and its glutathione conjugate. *Biochem. Pharmacol.*, **40**, 1631–1635.

70 Antonini, G., Pitari, G., Caccuri, A.M., Ricci, G., Boschi, D., Fruttero, R., Gasco, A., and Ascenzi, P. (1997) Inhibition of human placenta glutathione transferase P1-1 by the antibiotic calvatic acid and its diazocyanide analogue – evidence for multiple catalytic intermediates. *Eur. J. Biochem.*, **245**, 663–667.

71 Iersel, M.L., Ploemen, J.P., Struik, I., van Amersfoort, C., Keyzer, A.E., Schefferlie, J.G., and van Bladeren, P.J. (1996) Inhibition of glutathione *S*-transferase activity in human melanoma cells by alpha,beta-unsaturated carbonyl derivatives. Effects of acrolein, cinnamaldehyde, citral, crotonaldehyde, curcumin, ethacrynic acid, and *trans*-2-hexenal. *Chem. Biol. Interact.*, **102**, 117–132.

72 Ploemen, J.P., van Iersel, M.L., Wormhoudt, L.W., Commandeur, J.N., Vermeulen, N.P., and van Bladeren, P.J. (1996) *In vitro* inhibition of rat and human glutathione *S*-transferase isoenzymes by disulfiram and diethyldithiocarbamate. *Biochem. Pharmacol.*, **52**, 197–204.

73 Miller, M.S., McCarver, D.G., Bell, D.A., Eaton, D.L., and Goldstein, J.A. (1997) Genetic polymorphisms in human drug metabolic enzymes. *Fundam. Appl. Toxicol.*, **40**, 1–14.

74 Rebbeck, T.R. (1997) Molecular epidemiology of the human glutathione *S*-transferase genotypes GSTM1 and GSTT1 in cancer susceptibility. *Cancer Epidemiol. Biomarkers Prev.*, **6**, 733–743.

75 Ginsberg, G., Smolenski, S., Hattis, D., Guyton, K.Z., Johns, D.O., and Sonawane, B. (2009) Genetic polymorphism in glutathione transferases (GST): population distribution of GSTM1, T1, and P1

conjugating activity. *J. Toxicol. Environ. Health B*, **12**, 389–439.

76 Ishii, T., Matsuse, T., Teramoto, S., Matsui, H., Miyao, M., Hosoi, T., Takahashi, H., Fukuchi, Y., and Ouchi, Y. (1999) Glutathione *S*-transferase P1 (GSTP1) polymorphism in patients with chronic obstructive pulmonary disease. *Thorax*, **54**, 693–696.

77 Mattey, D.L., Hassell, A.B., Plant, M., Dawes, P.T., Ollier, W.R., Jones, P.W., Fryer, A.A., Alldersea, J.E., and Strange, R.C. (1999) Association of polymorphism in glutathione *S*-transferase loci with susceptibility and outcome in rheumatoid arthritis: comparison with the shared epitope. *Ann. Rheum. Dis.*, **58**, 164–168.

78 Mann, C.L., Davies, M.B., Boggild, M.D., Alldersea, J., Fryer, A.A., Jones, P.W., Ko Ko, C., Young, C., Strange, R.C., and Hawkins, C.P. (2000) Glutathione *S*-transferase polymorphisms in MS: their relationship to disability. *Neurology*, **54**, 552–557.

79 Deng, Y., Newman, B., Dunne, M.P., Silburn, P.A., and Mellick, G.D. (2004) Case-only study of interactions between genetic polymorphisms of GSTM1, P1, T1 and Z1 and smoking in Parkinson's disease. *Neurosci. Lett.*, **366**, 326–331.

80 Seidegard, J., Pero, R.W., Markowitz, M.M., Roush, G., Miller, D.G., and Beattie, E.J. (1990) Isoenzyme(s) of glutathione transferase (class Mu) as a marker for the susceptibility to lung cancer: a follow up study. *Carcinogenesis*, **11**, 33–36.

81 Nazar Stewart, V., Motulsky, A.G., Eaton, D.L., White, E., Hornung, S.K., Leng, Z.T., Stapleton, P., and Weiss, N.S. (1993) The glutathione *S*-transferase mu polymorphism as a marker for susceptibility to lung carcinoma. *Cancer Res.*, **53** (Suppl.), 2313–2318.

82 Hirvonen, A., Husgafvel-Pursiainen, K., Anttila, S., and Vainio, H. (1993) The GSTM1 null genotype as a potential risk modifier for squamous cell carcinoma of the lung. *Carcinogenesis*, **14**, 1479–1481.

83 Yengi, L., Inskip, A., Gilford, J., Alldersea, J., Bailey, L., Smith, A., Lear, J.T., Heagerty, A.H., Bowers, B., Hand, P., Hayes, J.D., Jones, P.W., Strange, R.C., and Fryer, A.A. (1996) Polymorphism at the glutathione *S*-transferase locus GSTM3: interactions with cytochrome P450 and glutathione *S*-transferase genotypes as risk factors for multiple cutaneous basal cell carcinoma. *Cancer Res.*, **56**, 1974–1977.

84 Jourenkova-Mironova, N., Voho, A., Bouchardy, C., Wikman, H., Dayer, P., Benhamou, S., and Hirvonen, A. (1999) Glutathione *S*-transferase GSTM3 and GSTP1 genotypes and larynx cancer risk. *Cancer Epidemiol. Biomarkers Prev.*, **8**, 185–188.

85 Jahnke, V., Matthias, C., Fryer, A., and Strange, R. (1996) Glutathione *S*-transferase and cytochrome-P-450 polymorphism as risk factors for squamous cell carcinoma of the larynx. *Am. J. Surg.*, **172**, 671–673.

86 Wiencke, J.K., Pemble, S., Ketterer, B., and Kelsey, K.T. (1995) Gene deletion of glutathione *S*-transferase theta: correlation with induced genetic damage and potential role in endogenous mutagenesis. *Cancer Epidemiol. Biomarkers Prev.*, **4**, 253–259.

87 Pemble, S., Schroeder, K.R., Spencer, S.R., Meyer, D.J., Hallier, E., Bolt, H.M., Ketterer, B., and Taylor, J.B. (1994) Human glutathione *S*-transferase theta (GSTT1): cDNA cloning and the characterization of a genetic polymorphism. *Biochem. J.*, **300**, 271–276.

88 Chen, H., Sandler, D.P., Taylor, J.A., Shore, D.L., Liu, E., Bloomfield, C.D., and Bell, D.A. (1996) Increased risk for myelodysplastic syndromes in individuals with glutathione transferase theta 1 (GSTT1) gene defect. *Lancet*, **347**, 295–297.

89 Jourenkova-Mironova, N., Voho, A., Bouchardy, C., Wikman, H., Dayer, P., Benhamou, S., and Hirvonen, A. (1999) Glutathione *S*-transferase GSTM1, GSTM3, GSTP1 and GSTT1 genotypes and the risk of smoking-related oral and pharyngeal cancers. *Int. J. Cancer*, **81**, 44–48.

90 Katoh, T., Kaneko, S., Takasawa, S., Nagata, N., Inatomi, H., Ikemura, K., Itoh, H., Matsumoto, T., Kawamoto, T.,

and Bell, D.A. (1999) Human glutathione *S*-transferase P1 polymorphism and susceptibility to smoking related epithelial cancer; oral, lung, gastric, colorectal and urothelial cancer. *Pharmacogenetics*, **9**, 165–169.

91 Harada, S., Abei, M., Tanaka, N., Agarwal, D.P., and Goedde, H.W. (1987) Liver glutathione *S*-transferase polymorphism in Japanese and its pharmacogenetic importance. *Hum. Genet.*, **75**, 322–325.

92 Board, P.G. (1981) Biochemical genetics of glutathione-*S*-transferase in man. *Am. J. Hum. Genet.*, **33**, 36–43.

93 Zhang, F., Qi, L., and Chen, H. (2001) Value of P-glycoprotein and glutathione *S*-transferase-pi as chemo-resistant indicators in ovarian cancers. *Zhonghua Zhong Liu Za Zhi*, **23**, 313–316.

94 Kempkes, M., Golka, K., Reich, S., Reckwitz, T., and Bolt, H.M. (1996) Glutathione *S*-transferase GSTM1 and GSTT1 null genotypes as potential risk factors for urothelial cancer of the bladder. *Arch. Toxicol.*, **71**, 123–126.

95 Soni, M.G., Krishna, T.P., and Krishnaswamy, K. (1995) Human leukocyte glutathione *S*-transferase isozyme (class mu) and susceptibility to smoking-related cancers. *J. Toxicol. Environ. Health*, **46**, 1–8.

96 Casanova, M., Bell, D.A., and Heck, H.D. (1997) Dichloromethane metabolism to formaldehyde and reaction of formaldehyde with nucleic acids in hepatocytes of rodents and humans with and without glutathione *S*-transferase T1 and M1 genes. *Fundam. Appl. Toxicol.*, **37**, 168–180.

97 Guengerich, F.P., Thier, R., Persmark, M., Taylor, J.B., Pemble, S.E., and Ketterer, B. (1995) Conjugation of carcinogens by theta class glutathione *S*-transferases: mechanisms and relevance to variations in human risk. *Pharmacogenetics*, **5**, S103–S107.

98 Henderson, C.J., Smith, A.G., Ure, J., Brown, K., Bacon, E.J., and Wolf, C.R. (1998) Increased skin tumorigenesis in mice lacking pi class glutathione *S*-transferases. *Proc. Natl. Acad. Sci. USA*, **95**, 5275–5280.

99 Coles, B.F. and Kadlubar, F.F. (2005) Human alpha class glutathione *S*-transferases: genetic polymorphism, expression, and susceptibility to disease. *Methods Enzymol.*, **401**, 9–42.

100 Whitbread, A.K., Masoumi, A., Tetlow, N., Schmuck, E., Coggan, M., and Board, P.G. (2005) Characterization of the omega class of glutathione transferases. *Methods Enzymol.*, **401**, 78–99.

101 Board, P.G. and Anders, M.W. (2005) Human glutathione transferase zeta. *Methods Enzymol.*, **401**, 61–77.

102 Morel, F., Rauch, C., Coles, B., Le Ferrec, E., and Guillouzo, A. (2002) The human glutathione transferase alpha locus: genomic organization of the gene cluster and functional characterization of the genetic polymorphism in the hGSTA1 promoter. *Pharmacogenetics*, **12**, 277–286.

103 Ning, B., Wang, C., Morel, F., Nowell, S., Ratnasinghe, D.L., Carter, W., Kadlubar, F.F., and Coles, B. (2004) Human glutathione *S*-transferase A2 polymorphisms: variant expression, distribution in prostate cancer cases/controls and a novel form. *Pharmacogenetics*, **14**, 35–44.

104 Seidegard, J. and Pero, R.W. (1985) The hereditary transmission of high glutathione transferase activity towards *trans*-stilbene oxide in human mononuclear leukocytes. *Hum. Genet.*, **69**, 66–68.

105 Seidegard, J., DePierre, J.W., and Pero, R.W. (1985) Hereditary interindividual differences in the glutathione transferase activity towards *trans*-stilbene oxide in resting human mononuclear leukocytes are due to a particular isozyme(s). *Carcinogenesis*, **6**, 1211–1216.

106 Zhao, B., Lee, E.J., Wong, J.Y., Yeoh, P.N., and Gong, N.H. (1995) Frequency of mutant CYP1A1, NAT2 and GSTM1 alleles in normal Indians and Malays. *Pharmacogenetics*, **5**, 275–280.

107 McLellan, R.A., Oscarson, M., Alexandrie, A.K., Seidegard, J., Evans, D.A., Rannug, A., and Ingelman-Sundberg, M. (1997) Characterization of a human glutathione *S*-transferase mu cluster containing a duplicated GSTM1 gene that causes ultrarapid enzyme activity. *Mol. Pharmacol.*, **52**, 958–965.

108 Nelson, H.H., Wiencke, J.K., Christiani, D.C., Cheng, T.J., Zuo, Z.F., Schwartz, B.S., Lee, B.K., Spitz, M.R., Wang, M., Xu, X., *et al.* (1995) Ethnic differences in the prevalence of the homozygous deleted genotype of glutathione *S*-transferase theta. *Carcinogenesis*, **16**, 1243–1245.

109 Lee, E.J., Wong, J.Y., Yeoh, P.N., and Gong, N.H. (1995) Glutathione *S* transferase-theta (GSTT1) genetic polymorphism among Chinese, Malays and Indians in Singapore. *Pharmacogenetics*, **5**, 332–334.

110 Coggan, M., Whitbread, L., Whittington, A., and Board, P. (1998) Structure and organization of the human theta-class glutathione *S*-transferase and D-dopachrome tautomerase gene complex. *Biochem. J.*, **334**, 617–623.

111 Ali-Osman, F., Akande, O., Antoun, G., Mao, J.X., and Buolamwini, J. (1997) Molecular cloning, characterization, and expression in *Escherichia coli* of full-length cDNAs of three human glutathione *S*-transferase Pi gene variants. Evidence for differential catalytic activity of the encoded proteins. *J. Biol. Chem.*, **272**, 10004–10012.

112 Harries, L.W., Stubbins, M.J., Forman, D., Howard, G.C., and Wolf, C.R. (1997) Identification of genetic polymorphisms at the glutathione *S*-transferase Pi locus and association with susceptibility to bladder, testicular and prostate cancer. *Carcinogenesis*, **18**, 641–644.

113 Whitbread, A.K., Tetlow, N., Eyre, H.J., Sutherland, G.R., and Board, P.G. (2003) Characterization of the human Omega class glutathione transferase genes and associated polymorphisms. *Pharmacogenetics*, **13**, 131–144.

6
Hydrolytic Enzymes

Bingfang Yan

6.1
Carboxylesterases

6.1.1
Overview

The primary functions of carboxylesterases rest in two modes of action – catalytic and interacting proteins [1–3]. As enzymes, carboxylesterases catalyze both hydrolytic and synthetic reactions, with hydrolysis being the predominant type [1–5]. They hydrolyze carboxylic acid esters, thioesters, and amides (Figure 6.1). Typical examples of synthetic reactions catalyzed by carboxylesterases are transesterification and the formation of fatty acid ethyl esters (Figure 6.1). Hydrolysis of drugs usually leads to drastic changes in structure and charges, and thus has profound pharmacokinetic and pharmacodynamic consequences [1–3]. In addition to therapeutic agents, carboxylesterases hydrolyze lipids such as triglycerides and cholesterol esters [1–3, 6]. During the mobilization of lipids, hydrolysis and re-esterification are coupled, and constitute a so-called re-esterification–hydrolysis cycle [7]. Carboxylesterases are known to protect against a large array of insecticides, such as organophosphates and pyrethroids [8, 9]. The mechanisms for the detoxification vary depending on the type of insecticides. Pyrethroids, for example, are detoxified by hydrolysis. In contrast, organophosphates are detoxified by forming irreversible complexes, commonly referred to as the scavenging mechanism. While carboxylesterases act as catalytic proteins, not all of the functions result directly from catalysis. For example, β-glucuronidase is normally targeted to the lysosome. However, a significant amount of this enzyme is retained in the endoplasmic reticulum by interacting with microsomal carboxylesterases. The microsomal β-glucuronidase has been shown to hydrolyze glucuronidated hormones (e.g., steroids), thus providing an effective mechanism that recycles physiologically important molecules [10].

Metabolism of Drugs and Other Xenobiotics, First Edition. Edited by Pavel Anzenbacher, Ulrich M. Zanger.

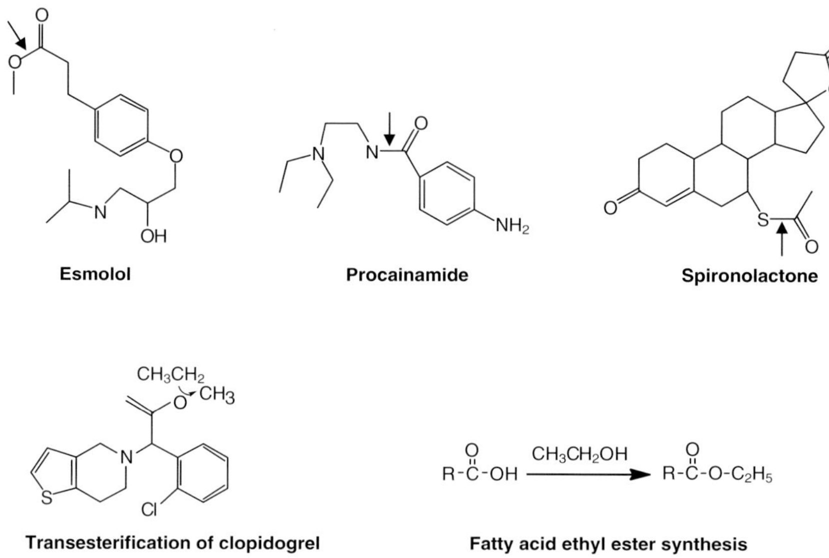

Figure 6.1 Chemical structure of representative drugs metabolized by carboxylesterases. The chemical bonds hydrolyzed by carboxylesterases are marked with an arrow.

6.1.2
Classification and Structural Features

Without exception, all mammalian species studied express multiple forms of carboxylesterases. Previously, classification of carboxylesterases was made according to substrate specificity and isoelectrophoretic points [11]. These approaches soon became unsatisfactory because these enzymes have overlapping substrate specificity or the same carboxylesterase has different isoelectrophoretic points due to aggregation or differential glycosylation. Currently, sequence identity is used to classify carboxylesterases. In this system, all mammalian carboxylesterases (e.g., human and rodents) are taken into consideration [2]. Members in the same family have a sequence identity of 60% or higher; otherwise, a different family is assigned. According to this method, six families are created: CES1, CES2, CES3, CES4, CES5, and CES6. The CES1 family contains the largest number of carboxylesterases and has eight subfamilies [2].

6.1.2.1 Human Carboxylesterases

Based on molecular cloning and bioinformatics studies, there are seven distinct carboxylesterase genes in the human genome [1, 12, 13]. These genes are assigned to the CES1, CES2, CES3, CES5, and CES6 families, respectively (Table 6.1). All human carboxylesterases show a sequence identity of 39–44% [12, 13]. The CES1 family has three members, including CES1A1, CES1A2, and CES1A3. CES1A2 is an alternative form of CES1A3, thus humans may express CES1A2 or CES1A3,

Table 6.1 Comparison of human carboxylesterases.

Property	CES1	CES2	CES3	CES5	CES6
Residues	567	559	571	575	567
Multigenes	yes	no	no	no	no
Endoplasmic reticulum retention	yes	yes	yes	no	no
Cys residues	5	4	5	6	4
N-glycosylation sites	1	2	1	3	3
Secretory	no	no	no	yes	yes

but not both. Among three CES1 members, only the CES1A1 and CES1A2 genes encode functional proteins [14, 15]. The CES1A3 gene, formerly termed CES1A4, has a premature stop codon and thus is considered a pseudogene [16]. The CES1A1 and CES1A2 proteins differ by only four amino acids, and these residues are located in the signal peptide. Therefore, these genes actually encode identical mature carboxylesterases. In contrast to the CES1 family, humans have only a single member in the CES2 family [1]. The CES2 gene uses three alternative promoters for transcriptions and the relative activities of these promoters differ depending on a tissue [17]. Likewise, humans have a single member in the CES3, CES5, and CES6 family, respectively. CES3 is much less active toward commonly used substrates [18]. Human CES5 is a secretory protein [12]. Human CES6 is a putative carboxylesterase based on the sequence alignment analyses against the human genome. The hydrolytic activity of CES5 and CES6 remains to be determined.

6.1.2.2 Salient Features of Carboxylesterases

Mammalian carboxylesterases have several salient structural features. These enzymes are synthesized as a large precursor with an N-terminal cleavable signal peptide [19–21]. Normally, this peptide directs newly translated proteins into the lumen of the endoplasmic reticulum for secretion. However, many carboxylesterases are retained in the endoplasmic reticulum. These endoplasmic reticulum carboxylesterases all have a C-terminal tetrapeptide HXEL, keeping carboxylesterases from being secreted [19–21]. In addition, carboxylesterases are glycoproteins and secretory carboxylesterases (e.g., CES5) are glycosylated to a much greater extent [20, 21]. The extensive glycosylation of serum carboxylesterases suggests that glycosylation facilitates the secretory process and increases solubility. Another important post-translational modification of carboxylesterases is the formation of disulfide bonds. Folding and refolding studies suggest that disulfide bonds play roles in the formation of the catalytically active conformation [22].

6.1.2.3 Secondary and Crystal Structure

In additional to many salient structural features, carboxylesterases exhibit a unique assembly on the secondary structure. The core segments of carboxylesterases are arranged as alternate α-helix and β-sheets connected by loops with a varying length [23]. Such unique arrangements place carboxylesterases into the superfamily of proteins commonly referred to as the α/β-hydrolase-fold proteins. Consistent with the similarity of the secondary structure, carboxylesterases share a crystal structure with members of the α/β-fold enzymes such as acetylcholinesterase [24, 25]. Overall, carboxylesterases have three functional domains – the catalytic domain surrounded by the αβ domain and the regulatory domain. Like other members, carboxylesterases have the catalytic triad located at the base of the deep catalytic gorge. However, carboxylesterases show some important differences. For example, human carboxylesterase CES1 has two substrate binding pockets: one is small and rigid, and the other is large and flexible [24]. The small/rigid pocket likely provides selectivity, whereas the large/flexible pocket is promiscuous. Even among carboxylesterases, notable differences exist. For example, an *N*-linked glycosylation chain is located at the product exit in a rabbit carboxylesterase, but not in human CES1 [24, 26]. This carbohydrate chain presumably enhances catalysis by facilitating product exit. Furthermore, human CES1 exists as trimer or hexamer, whereas the rabbit enzyme exists as a monomer [26].

6.1.3
Catalytic Mechanism, Substrate Specificity, and Activators and Inhibitors

Like many other α/β-fold enzymes, carboxylesterases use a two-step reaction mechanism for the catalysis [1–3]. In the past decade, tremendous progress has been made on the substrate specificity of carboxylesterases, particularly CES1 and CES2 [1–3, 27]. The catalytic activity of carboxylesterases can be enhanced by activators such as pinacolone [28], and inhibited by compounds such as benzil and trifluoromethyl ketone derivatives [29–31].

6.1.3.1 Catalytic Mechanism

The catalytic triad of carboxylesterases is made of the nucleophile (Ser), the base (His), and the acid (Glu) [2, 24–26]. As shown in Figure 6.2, the first step of the reaction involves the attack by the nucleophile Ser on the carbonyl carbon of a substrate, resulting in the release of the alcohol moiety from the substrate, and simultaneously forming a covalent linkage between the enzyme and the remaining acid moiety of the substrate. Subsequently, the covalent linkage is cleaved through a water molecule activated by the base His, leading to the release of the acyl moiety of the substrate accompanied by the regeneration of the enzyme (Figure 6.2). The two-step hydrolysis mechanism, however, provides a molecular explanation for the toxicity of organophosphorus compounds. These insecticides, usually called hemisubstrates, interact similarly as true substrates. However, the resultant organophosphate–enzyme complex creates a steric exclusion, which prevents the second nucleophilic attack by the activated water molecule [32] (Figure 6.2). Interaction with acetylcholinesterase represents toxicity, whereas interaction with carboxylesterases is considered detoxification against these insecticides.

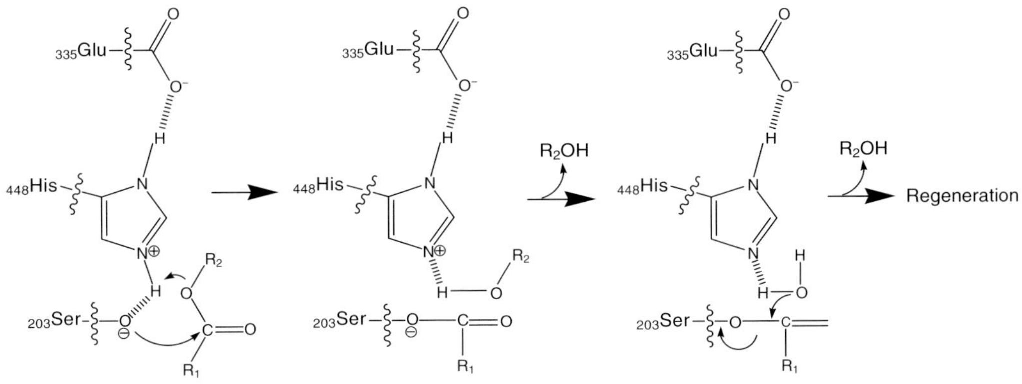

Figure 6.2 Catalytic cycle of carboxylesterases.

6.1.3.2 **Substrate Specificity**

It is well established that carboxylesterases hydrolyze compounds containing such functional groups as carboxylic acid ester (e.g., esmolol), amide (e.g., procainamide), and thioester (e.g., spironolactone). The hydrolysis of carboxylic acid esters, however, usually proceeds faster than that of other hydrolytic bonds. For example, procaine is hydrolyzed much faster than its amide counterpart procainamide [33]. Thus, procaine is used as a local anesthetic and has no systemic application. In contrast, procainamide reaches the systematic circulation and is used to treat cardiac arrhythmia. Consistent with the hydrolysis of amide bonds, carboxylesterases catalyze deamination, which is responsible for the metabolism of rufinamide–a recently approved compound for Lennox–Gastaut syndrome (a special type of seizure) [34].

Carboxylesterases generally exhibit broad and overlapping substrate specificity. However, certain carboxylesterases exhibit apparent preference for certain substrates. Human CES1 and CES2 have been well characterized for their substrate specificity [1, 2, 4, 27]. CES1 preferably hydrolyzes carboxylic esters with a bigger acyl moiety, whereas the opposite is true with CES2 (Figure 6.3). For example, the acyl moiety (oseltamivir carboxylate) of oseltamivir is much bigger than the alcohol moiety (ethanol); therefore, this anti-influenza viral agent is hydrolyzed by CES1, but not CES2 (Figure 6.3). Conversely, the acyl moiety of prasugrel is much smaller than the alcohol moiety, thus this anticancer agent is predominately hydrolyzed by CES2. The alcohol/acid size-based preference also applies to compounds with multiple ester bonds as well. The psychomotor stimulant cocaine, for example, contains two ester bonds, and complete hydrolysis produces ecgonine, methanol, and benzoic acid. Among these products, ecgonine is the largest and acts as the acid moiety relative to methanol, but as the alcohol moiety relative to benzoic acid. Consistent with the alcohol/acid size-based preference, CES1 hydrolyzes ecgonine-methyl ester, whereas CES2 hydrolyzes benzoate-ecgoninyl ester (Figure 6.3). However, this rule has notable exceptions. For example, illicit heroine

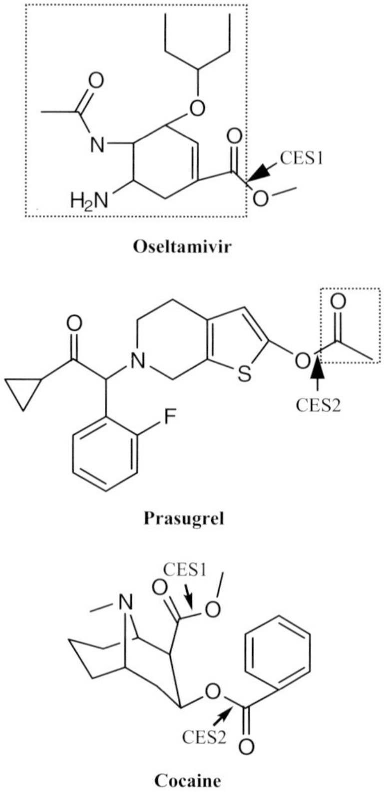

Figure 6.3 Substrate preference between human carboxylesterases CES1 and CES2. The acid moieties of oseltamivir and prasugrel are boxed. Bonds undergoing hydrolysis are marked with an arrow and the carboxylesterases involved in the hydrolysis are specified.

contains two ester bonds, both sharing the alcohol moiety [24]. This alcohol moiety is much bigger than the acids in both cases. Interestingly, both ester bonds are preferably hydrolyzed by CES1, but not CES2 [8].

6.1.3.3 Activators and Inhibitors

Like many other enzyme systems, the activity of carboxylesterases can be enhanced or inhibited. While inhibition has been extensively studied, activation of carboxylesterase activity is not well understood. Several chemicals such as pinacolone have been shown to increase the hydrolytic activity of carboxylesterases. Increased activity has been observed *in vitro* and *in vivo* by these chemicals [28]. They are metabolites of soman – a potent and irreversible inhibitor of Ser enzymes, including carboxylesterases. The precise mechanism remains to be elucidated for the enhanced hydrolytic activity. Interestingly, the commonly used solvent acetone also enhances the hydrolytic activity of carboxylesterases [28], pointing to a possible mechanism of improving the accessibility of enzymes to a substrate.

In contrast to activation, several types of inhibitions are synthesized and well characterized. Ester drugs hydrolyzed by the same carboxylesterases may function as competitive inhibitors toward each other. For example, clopidogrel and oseltamivir are both substrates of CES1, with the former being kinetically favorable [27]. As a result, clopidogrel inhibits the hydrolysis of oseltamivir by as much as 90% when the same concentrations are used. The first-pass hydrolysis accounts for 90% of total oseltamivir activation [35–37], presumably due to the initial high concentration in the liver. Coadministration of clopidogrel inhibits the first-pass activation of oseltamivir and likely attenuates the activation of oseltamivir.

The second type of inhibition is achieved by chemicals that irreversibly modify the active-site Ser residues – so-called Ser enzyme inhibitors. In addition to organophosphorus insecticides, several irreversible inhibitors of Ser enzymes are well characterized, including phenylmethylsulfonyl fluoride (PMSF) and inorganic salts such as sodium fluoride [38]. While these inhibitors generally act nonspecifically among Ser enzymes, the IC_{50} values can vary markedly from one carboxylesterase to another. For example, rat carboxylesterase hydrolase A is around 1000 times more sensitive than hydrolase B based on the IC_{50} values (100 nM versus 100 μM) [38]. Some chemicals such as malathion can function as inhibitors and substrates. This organophosphorothioate (OPT) contains a P=S bond and two carboxylic acid bonds. Oxidative desulfuration of OPTs results in the formation of a P=O bond – the corresponding oxon. The oxon is an irreversible inhibitor of carboxylesterases. The carboxylic acid bonds, however, are subjected to hydrolysis by carboxylesterases. Hydrolytic metabolism of malathion represents detoxification (inactivation) and is correlated well with the abundance of CES1 in humans [39].

Two classes of compounds, with a potential of clinical use, are well characterized for the inhibition of carboxylesterases [27–31, 40] (Figure 6.4). Benzil derivatives belong to one of the classes and trifluoromethyl ketone (TFK)-containing analogs belong to the other. Both benzil and TFK compounds inhibit catalysis of carboxylesterases by acting on the active-site residue Ser. Compounds with this type of inhibition are called transitional analog inhibitors and the inhibition is reversible. Among TFK compounds, thioether analogs are more potent than their sulfinyl or sulfonyl counterparts [41]. This is more evident with prolonged preincubation. The precise mechanism of their different potency remains to be determined. It has been postulated that these substitution moieties may vary in supporting the equilibrium between the ketone and *gem*-diol forms of a TKF compound, and the ketone form is more inhibitory. Another interesting phenomenon with TFK compounds is their selectivity on acetylcholinesterase and butyrylcholinesterase. Many TFK compounds efficaciously inhibit carboxylesterases, but surprisingly have little inhibition against cholinesterases. This is interesting because carboxylesterases are highly related to cholinesterases in terms of the overall crystal structures and the sequence identity. However, TFK compounds show only some selectivity in inhibiting various carboxylesterases. For example, human CES1 and CES2 are comparably inhibited by a panel of TFK compounds [41]. Dofcylthiotrifluoropropane – the highest selectivity in this panel – exhibits

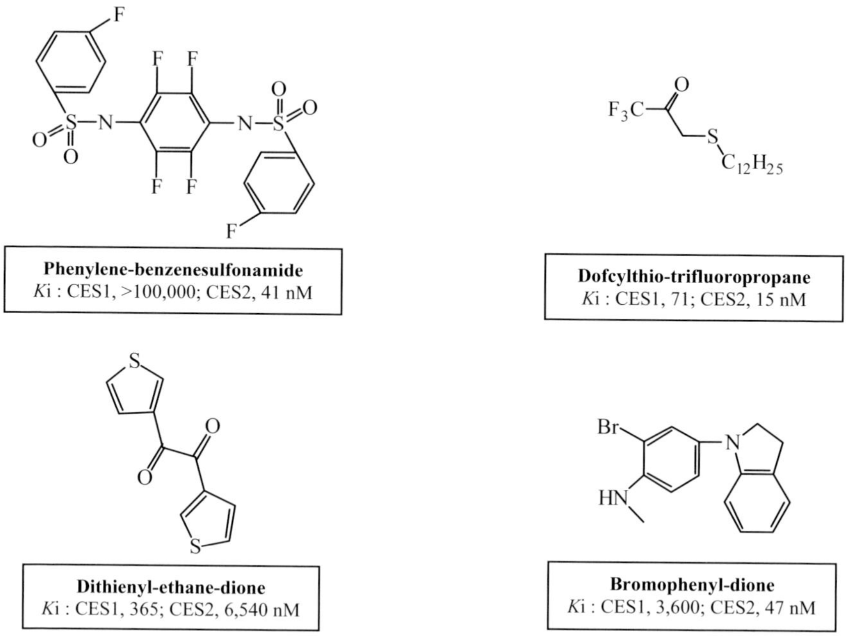

Figure 6.4 Selective inhibitors of CES1 and CES2 with K_i values.

only a 5-fold difference in the inhibitory potency between CES1 and CES2 based on the K_i values (Figure 6.4).

Benzil derivatives and their related compounds, in contrast, show much higher selectivity on the inhibition of various carboxylesterases [30, 31]. For example, dithienyl ethane-dione is around 20 times more potent for the inhibition of CES1 than CES2 (Figure 6.4). Conversely, phenylene-chlorobenzenesulfonamide inhibits CES2 with a K_i value of 41 nM – three magnitudes lower than that of CES1 (Figure 6.4). Actually, a panel of benzene sulfonamides tested shows little inhibition on CES1, although they all inhibit CES2 [30]. The highly selective inhibitors are bulky in shape and such bulky structure likely presents a greater steric effect than TFK compounds. Apparently, the combination of a steric bulky structure with TFK compounds will likely produce more selective and potent inhibitors [31]. As described above, these compounds are transitional analog inhibitors, and thus they have hypothetic sizes of the alcohol and acyl moieties as seen in the substrates.

6.1.4
Pharmacogenomics of Carboxylesterases

The pharmacogenomics of carboxylesterases deals with several issues from altered hydrolysis to potential interactions with other systems that eliminate drugs and other xenobiotics. Single nucleotide polymorphisms (SNPs) are increasingly identified in carboxylesterase genes [1] and some of them have been linked to poor clinical outcomes [41–46]. However, hydrolysis of carboxylic acid esters by carboxylesterases leads to the formation of products with an alcohol and a carboxylic acid. These functional groups can undergo further metabolism, notably conjugation reactions [47]. In addition, the carboxylic acid is negatively charged and elimination of the acid is likely achieved by transporters, presenting other interactions [48, 49].

6.1.4.1 Polymorphisms

It has been shown that carboxylesterase-based hydrolysis exhibits a large interindividual variability, particularly when populations of various ages are considered. Many factors such as hormones and xenobiotic exposure may alter the expression and contribute to individual variation in hydrolysis. However, genetic variation is increasingly recognized as an important contributor to the large interindividual variability. The National Center for Biotechnology Information SNP database lists a large number of SNPs in the CES1, CES2, and CES3 genes. In addition, several investigators reported the existence of CES SNPs [41–46]. Generally, the CES1 gene has the most and the CES3 gene has the least reported SNPs [1]. SNPs can occur in the regulatory region, intron, and exon. Some exon SNPs result in the substitution of amino acids. Several SNPs have been linked directly to altered pharmacokinetics of ester drugs [41–46]. For example, a patient carrying a CES1 Gly143Glu and Asp260 frameshift shows a profound defect in the hydrolytic elimination of methylphenidate–a widely used psychostimulant [50]. Likewise, patients carrying the R34W heterozygous genotype of CES2 have a profound alteration in the pharmacokinetics of irinotecan with a decreased area under the concentration–time curve (AUC) ratio (hydrolytic species/parent drug) by as much as 40% [43].

6.1.4.2 Interaction with the Cytochrome P450 Enzyme System

Many drugs metabolized by carboxylesterases are also metabolized by other enzyme systems, particularly the cytochrome P450 (CYP) system. Hydrolysis generally proceeds faster than oxidation, therefore hydrolysis usually determines the fate of the parent drug [51–55]. In some cases, hydrolysis and oxidation compete for the metabolism of a drug, and the relative activity has profound clinical consequences. For example, the antiplatelet agent clopidogrel undergoes both hydrolysis and oxidation [4, 52–55] (Figure 6.5). Hydrolysis represents inactivation, whereas oxidation represents activation. The hydrolysis is catalyzed by CES1 [4], whereas the oxidation is catalyzed by several CYPs, such as CYP2C19 and CYP3A4 [52–55]. In other cases, hydrolysis and oxidation occur sequentially, and both are involved in the activation. For example, prasugrel–another antiplatelet agent–undergoes both hydrolysis and oxidation [4, 52–55] (Figure 6.5). Importantly, both hydrolysis and oxidation are required for the production of the final active metabolite. The hydrolysis is catalyzed by CES2 and the oxidation is catalyzed by multiple CYP enzymes.

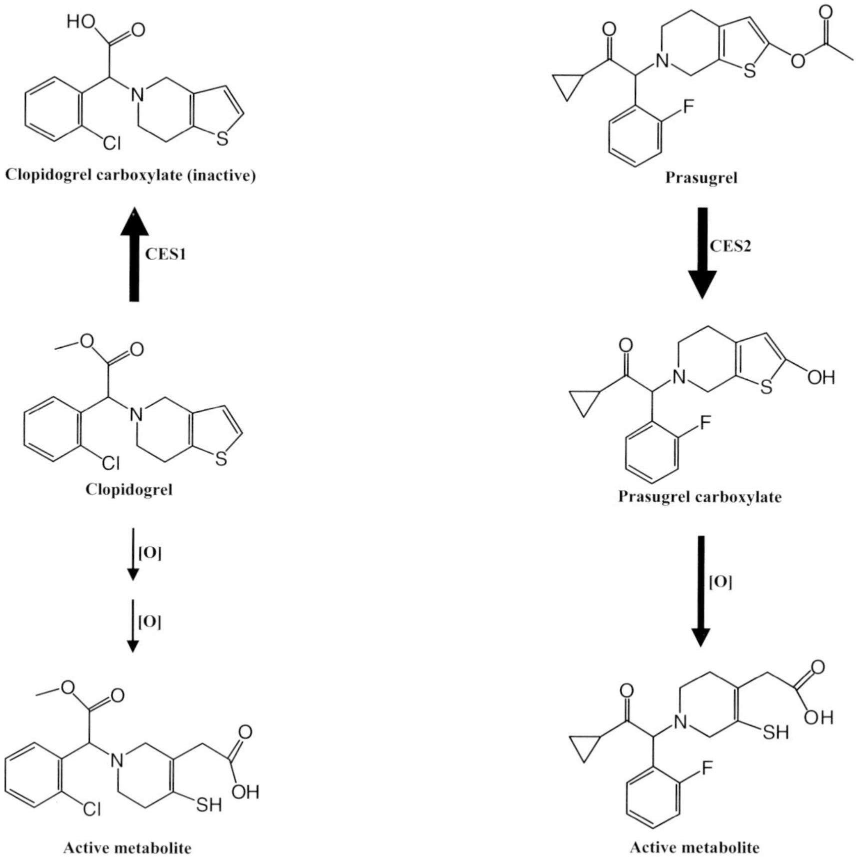

Figure 6.5 Hydrolysis–oxidation coupled reactions. Both clopidogrel and prasugrel are antiplatelet agents and undergo metabolic activation.

6.1.4.3 Interaction with UDP-Glucuronosyltransferases

In addition to phase I enzymes, in many cases the action of carboxylesterases is directly associated with the action of phase II enzymes, notably UDP-glucuronosyltransferases (UGTs) [47, 56, 57]. These conjugation enzymes use the cofactor uridine diphosphate-glucuronic acid (UDPG), and add sugars to lipids and other nonpolar xenobiotics. Conjugation with a sugar moiety drastically increases the hydrophilicity, thus favoring elimination. While the site of glucuronidation in a compound usually occurs at an electron-rich nucleophilic heteroatom such as O, N and S, the majority of drugs for glucuronidation contain such functional groups as an alcohol/phenol or carboxylic acid. These groups are produced by hydrolysis. In many cases, the hydrolysis/glucuronidation cycle has direct clinical consequences.

The hydrolysis–glucuronidation interaction is nicely illustrated by the anticancer prodrug irinotecan [56]. This prodrug undergoes hydrolytic activation by CES2 to the cytotoxic metabolite 7-ethyl-10-hydroxycamptothecin (SN-38), which is a potent inhibitor of DNA topoisomerase I. However, SN-38 is also a substrate of UGTs, notably UGT1A1. Glucuronidated SN-38 no longer has therapeutic activity. As a result, an unbalanced hydrolysis over glucuronidation may increase systematic toxicity such as neutropenia. It has been demonstrated that increased SN-38 exposure is directly related to the severity of neutropenia [58]. Patients carrying the UGT1A1*28 polymorphism, particularly the homozygous genotype, show a higher SN-38 AUC value and increased risk for the development of neutropenia [58].

6.1.4.4 **Interactions with Drug Transporters**

A third type of interaction as a result of the action of carboxylesterases occurs during the process of drug uptake and effluxing. Hydrolysis leads to the production of carboxylic acids, which are normally negatively charged. Charged molecules have poor membrane penetration activity and are usually transported by drug transporters. Therefore, carboxylesterase-coupled transporter activity is another major determinant of the efficacy and toxicity of ester drugs [59–61]. For example, transporters such as multidrug resistance protein-4 (MRP4) have been shown to efflux the various types of irinotecan metabolites and overexpression of this transporter increases the resistance toward this chemotherapeutic drug [62]. We recently tested whether MRP4 interplays with CES2. Cells stably transfected with MRP4 or the corresponding vector were transfected again to overexpress CES2 and then exposed to irinotecan. MRP4 stable line markedly decreased the cytotoxicity when exposed to irinotecan.

6.1.4.5 **Drug–Insecticide Interactions**

Carboxylesterases are known to play critical roles in detoxification of several major types of organophosphorus, carbamate, and pyrethroid insecticides [9, 63]. These hydrolytic enzymes detoxify organophosphates by acting as scavenging proteins. In contrast, carboxylesterases detoxify carbamates and pyrethroids by hydrolysis. Therefore, in all these cases, the metabolism of ester drugs should decrease. However, lower hydrolysis of certain insecticides may alter the metabolism of drugs by other enzyme systems. For example, many pyrethroids are potent inducers of multiple nuclear receptors such as the pregnane X receptor (PXR). Activation of this receptor leads to the induction of many metabolizing enzymes, such as CYP3A4. A recent study has demonstrated that the activation of PXR is significantly decreased in cells transfected with a carboxylesterase [8]. It is therefore expected that coexposure to organophosphorus and pyrethroid insecticides likely increases the expression of genes regulated by PXR. It should be emphasized that the precise nature of drug–insecticide interactions remains largely unknown.

6.1.5
Comparison between Human and Animal Carboxylesterases

Mammalian carboxylesterases exhibit many similarities and differences [2]. Without exception, all mammalian species studied express multiple forms of carboxylesterases and the highest carboxylesterase activity is present in the liver [24, 38]. In many cases, compounds such as aspirin are comparably hydrolyzed by human and rodent carboxylesterases [4]. However, there are notable differences between human carboxylesterases and those from other mammalian species. For example, high levels of carboxylesterases are present in rodents, but not humans [4, 21]. Likewise, several major rat carboxylesterases are suppressed by glucocorticoids such as dexamethasone; conversely, this steroid causes slight induction of human carboxylesterases [51, 64]. The local anesthetic procaine is hydrolyzed much faster by rat microsomes than their human counterparts [65]. These differences raise concerns regarding the relevance of animal models to the human situation.

6.1.5.1 Tissue Distribution

While the liver contains the highest overall carboxylesterase activity [24], abundant expression of certain carboxylesterases is detected in the gastrointestinal track, lung, and kidney [1, 4, 21]. Interestingly, rodents have high levels of carboxylesterases in the testis [20, 22]. In contrast, human testes contain less carboxylesterase activity. In addition, rodents but not humans contain abundant serum carboxylesterases. Actually, none of the well-characterized human carboxylesterases (i.e., CES1, CES2, and CES3) have been detected by Western blots in normal serum [4, 21]. However, a low level of carboxylesterases is expressed in leukocytes [66]. Certain liver diseases may increase the presence of liver carboxylesterases in the blood [67]. Nevertheless, the abundant presence of serum carboxylesterases in rodents may contribute to species differences in the metabolism of ester drugs. For example, rodents are relatively resistant to liver toxicity in response to oseltamivir [68]. One explanation is that rodents hydrolyze this antiviral agent in the blood and only intracellular hydrolysis in hepatocytes has toxicity [27].

6.1.5.2 Species-Specific Hydrolysis

Like the tissue distribution, carboxylesterase-based hydrolysis exhibits both similarities and differences among various species. Liver microsomes from human, monkey, dog, guinea pig, hamster, mouse, and rat all contain two kinetically distinct hydrolytic activities toward *p*-nitrophenylacetate with K_m values of 25–55 and 300–800 μM, respectively [38, 69]. Significantly, the relative activity between low and high K_m carboxylesterases is comparable, ranging from 40 to 60% with the single exception of the guinea pig [38, 69]. Microsomes from guinea pig contain predominately low K_m activity (80%). In both the human and rat, the low K_m carboxylesterase is responsible for the hydrolysis of clopidogrel, whereas the high K_m enzyme is responsible for the hydrolysis of aspirin [4]. Although there is remarkable similarity in the hydrolysis of certain esters among various species, there are equally remarkable species differences in terms of hydrolyzing other esters [70–72]. For example, meperidine – the first synthetic opioid – is rapidly hydrolyzed by dog, but not human liver microsomes [71]. Deltamethrin and esfenvalerate are both pyrethroid types of insecticides. Based on the specific activity, human liver microsomes are 6 times as active as rat microsomes in hydrolyzing deltamethrin.

In contrast, rat liver microsomes are twice as active as rat microsomes in hydrolyzing esfenvalerate [70].

6.1.5.3 Ontogenic Expression

There is a remarkable similarity between human and rodent carboxylesterases in terms of ontogenic expression. Rat carboxylesterases are extremely low and suddenly increased 3 weeks after birth [69]. Likewise, the expression of CES1 and CES2 shows an age-dependent expression. Overall, adults express the highest levels of CES1 and CES2 mRNA, pediatric donors express less CES1 and CES2, but fetal donors express the lowest levels for both enzymes [73]. Based on the values of the means, the adult group has CES1 at levels 319-fold higher than the fetal group and around 50% higher than the child group [73]. Likewise, the adult group expresses CES2 at levels 55-fold higher than the fetal group and around 40% higher than the child group. In addition to the large difference among various age groups (intergroup), there is a large interindividual variability within a group. Interestingly, interindividual variability is inversely correlated with age. The fetal group, for example, has a 431-fold difference (ratio between the maximum and the minimum) in CES1 mRNA with a coefficient of variation of as high as 172%. The pediatric and adult groups, however, vary less in CES1 mRNA with a 218- and 12-fold difference, respectively.

6.1.5.4 Regulated Expression

Many factors have been shown to regulate the expression of carboxylesterases, including age, hormones, drugs, insecticides, and other chemicals [51, 64, 69, 73–76]. Some of the factors regulate the expression of these enzymes similarly across species. For example, the anticonvulsant agent phenobarbital causes slight or moderate induction in rodents and humans [64, 69]. Other chemicals, such as dexamethasone, exert profound species-dependent regulatory effects. This synthetic glucocorticoid has been shown to slightly increase the expression of human carboxylesterases [64]. In contrast, dexamethasone decreases the expression of multiple rat carboxylesterases and a significant decrease occurs even at nanomolar dexamethasone [51].

In addition, structurally related compounds may have different effects on carboxylesterase expression. For example, pregnenolone 16α-carbonitrile is structurally related to dexamethasone and surprisingly causes a moderate induction of hydrolase S – a rat carboxylesterase [21]. In contrast, dexamethasone suppresses the expression of this enzyme [51]. Furthermore, chemicals with the same or similar effects on the expression of CYP enzymes may differentially regulate the expression of carboxylesterases. For example, expression of hydrolase S is significantly suppressed by isoniazid, but slightly increased by streptozotocin; both of them are CYP2E1 inducers [21, 77]. The CYP1A enzyme inducers β-naphthoflavone and 3-methylcholanthrene have opposing effects – the former suppresses the expression of hydrolase S, whereas the latter slightly induces it [21, 77]. The differential response of carboxylesterase genes to the same type of CYP inducers suggests that these chemicals use multiple signaling pathways to exert their biological effects.

6.2
Epoxide Hydrolases

6.2.1
Overview

Epoxide hydrolases (EH) constitute another major class of hydrolytic enzymes [78–81]. Like other hydrolases, EHs use water as the cofactor. However, EHs catalyze addition of water into a substrate instead of breaking the substrate apart. An epoxide is a cyclic ether with three ring atoms and the catalytic addition of water leads to the production of a diol. Epoxide-containing compounds, although sharing the epoxide moiety, are structurally diverse, ranging from small-size compounds such as epoxyethane to large bulky molecules such as benzo[*a*]pyrene-7,8-epoxide (Figure 6.6). Epoxide-containing compounds are formed through oxidation of carbon–carbon double bonds in aliphatic chains or aromatic rings. The oxidation is primarily catalyzed by the CYP system. An aromatic epoxide is commonly referred to as an arene oxide or an oxirane. Figure 6.6 shows some examples of epoxides.

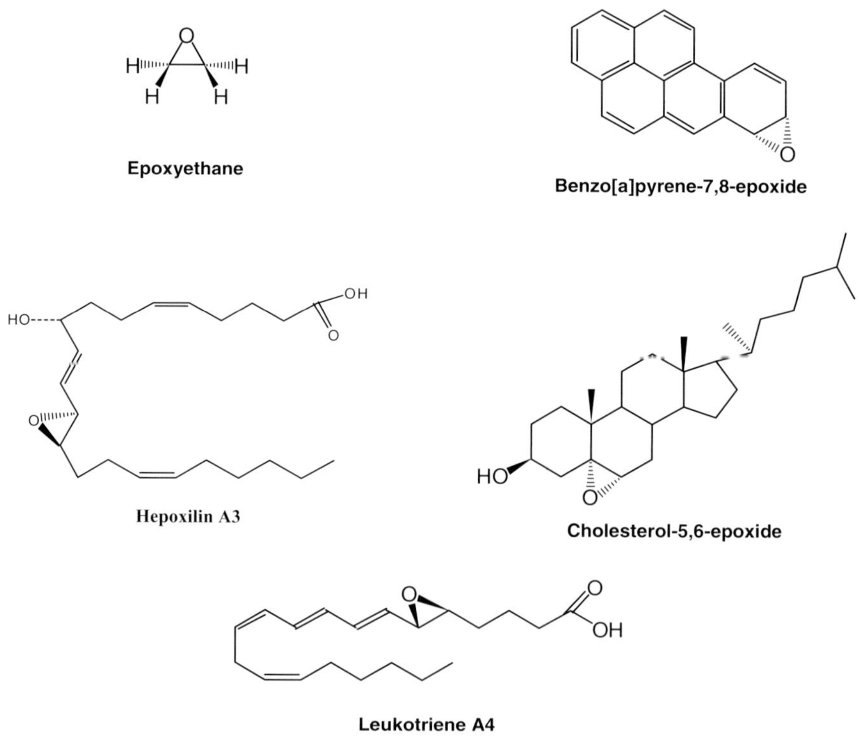

Figure 6.6 Examples of substrates of EHs.

Epoxides are structurally strained and the oxygen–carbon bonds in epoxides are polarized. As a result, epoxides are usually more reactive than other ethers. Certain oxiranes are among the most reactive species toward macromolecules such as DNA. Compared with epoxides, the corresponding diols are much less reactive. Therefore, it is generally accepted that the action of EHs represents detoxification. Indeed, many studies in animal models have documented that deletion of the microsomal EH (mEH) gene markedly increases the mutagenic effect and the incidence of cancer when exposed to compounds whose intermediate epoxides are substrates of this enzyme [82]. In addition to oncologic risk, dysfunction of the mEH gene is linked to the risk of drug-induced toxicity, such as with phenytoin–an antiepileptic that is metabolized into toxic epoxide [83]. Hydrolysis of certain epoxides may, however, lead to increased toxicity. For example, leukotoxin–a linoleic acid oxide produced by leukocytes–has been associated with the development of adult respiratory distress syndrome [84]. *In vitro* study has established that leukotoxin is rapidly converted into the corresponding diols and it is the diol metabolite that exerts severe cytotoxicity.

In addition to toxicological significance, hydrolysis of epoxides has important implications in molecular signaling [80, 81]. Many unsaturated long-chain fatty acids undergo epoxidation, and the epoxides and their corresponding diols differ markedly in conferring signal transduction. The role of EHs in the lipid signaling is nicely illustrated by one of the metabolic pathways of arachidonic acid. This fatty acid is epoxided by CYP expoxygenase enzymes to epoxyeicosatrienoic acids (EETs) and the epoxided compounds are substrates of EHs. EETs have a wide range of cardiovascular effects, including vasorelaxation, anti-inflammation, and profibrinolysis [80, 81, 85]. These activities are critical for the normal function of the cardiovascular system. However, the hydrolytic metabolites of these epoxide species produced by EHs either lack these activities or have much reduced potency. Therefore, there is an increasing interest in developing chemical inhibitors to block the hydrolysis of these epoxides by EHs [85, 86].

6.2.2
Classification and Structural Features

The classification of human EHs was historically based on the substrate specificity in conjunction with subcellular localization [78–81]. While recommendation has been made to classify these enzymes based on sequence identity, not all EHs have been characterized at the sequence level. There are five distinct forms of human EHs, including mEH, soluble EH (sEH), leukotriene A_4 hydrolase (LTA4H), cholesterol EH (CEH), and hepoxilin hydrolase (HH). As their names imply, the last three EHs have narrow substrate specificity. In contrast, mEH and sEH hydrolyze a large number of structurally diverse epoxide-containing compounds. These two EHs as well as LTA4H have been cloned and surprisingly they share little sequence identity. It should be noted that the human genome contains two other EH genes. They share a sequence identity of 45%, but their proteins remain to be characterized [87].

Table 6.2 Comparison of EHs.

Property	mEH	sEH	LTA4H	HH	CEH
Subcellular	microsome	cytosol/microsome	nucleus/cytosol	cytosol	microsome
Chromosome	1	8	12	?	?
Substrate	broad	broad	narrow	narrow	narrow
Catalysis	triad	triad	zinc metal	?	?
Phosphatase	no	yes	no	no	no
Peptidase	no	no	yes	no	no
Dimeric	no	yes	no	no	yes

chromosome 16. Some EHs such as sEH are abundantly present in the cytosolic fractions, whereas others such as mEH are primarily present in the microsomal fraction. mEH is anchored through the membrane of the endoplasmic reticulum and its catalytic machinery faces the cytosolic compartment. Such a topological arrangement resembles that of CYPs–an enzyme system that catalyzes epoxidation of xenobiotics. Therefore, the primary role of mEH is to hydrolyze epoxides formed by CYP-based catalysis. Interestingly, high levels of LTA4H are present in the nucleus, although the significance of such presence remains to be determined.

It is well established that mEH and sEH have broad substrate specificity, and thus play major roles in the metabolism of drugs and other xenobiotics. Other EHs have narrower substrate specificity and fulfill particular functions. Indeed, the action of HH is related to inflammation, whereas the action of LTA4H is associated with the development of cardiovascular diseases. As described above, various EHs differ in their catalytic machinery. mEH and sEH use the catalytic triad, whereas LTA4H uses the metal zinc for catalysis. In addition to EH activity, several EHs catalyze other type of hydrolysis. sEH has a phosphatase domain and LTA4H has peptidase activity. While the bifunctional activity in sEH is achieved by different catalytic sites, it appears that LTA4H uses the same catalytic site for both EH and peptidase activities. Nevertheless, the physiological significance for the bifunctional catalysis remains to be established. Some EHs form dimers for catalysis. For example, sEH is a homodimeric enzyme with two monomers interacting in an opposite manner. Namely, the N-terminal phosphatase domain is in close proximity to the C-terminal EH domain. It is tempting to speculate that these two catalytic machineries share a catalytic requirement (e.g., activated water) and the approximate interaction strengthens respective activity. It has been recently reported that CEH activity is a result of a functional dimerization of 3β-hydroxysterol-Δ^7-reductase and 3β-hydroxysterol-Δ^8-Δ^7-isomerase. In support of this notion, coexpression of both enzymes leads to robust increases in the hydrolysis of cholesterol-5,6-epoxide [91].

6.3 Paraoxonases

6.3.1 Overview

Paraoxonases (PONs) constitute another major class of hydrolases [92–95]. They are called PONs not based on their functionality, but rather for historical reasons. The PON activity was first described six decades ago based on the hydrolysis of the organophosphate paraoxon. Serum esterase(s) hydrolyzing paraoxon was referred to as A-esterase (i.e., PON). Esterases inhibited by organophosphates were referred to as B-esterases (i.e., carboxylesterases). Many decades later, it has become clear that the so-called serum PON is one of the enzymes involved in the hydrolysis and formation of lactones. The PON activity of a PON, however, represents a promiscuous effect as seen with many other xenobiotic enzymes. Figure 6.8 shows representative examples of substrates metabolized by PONs.

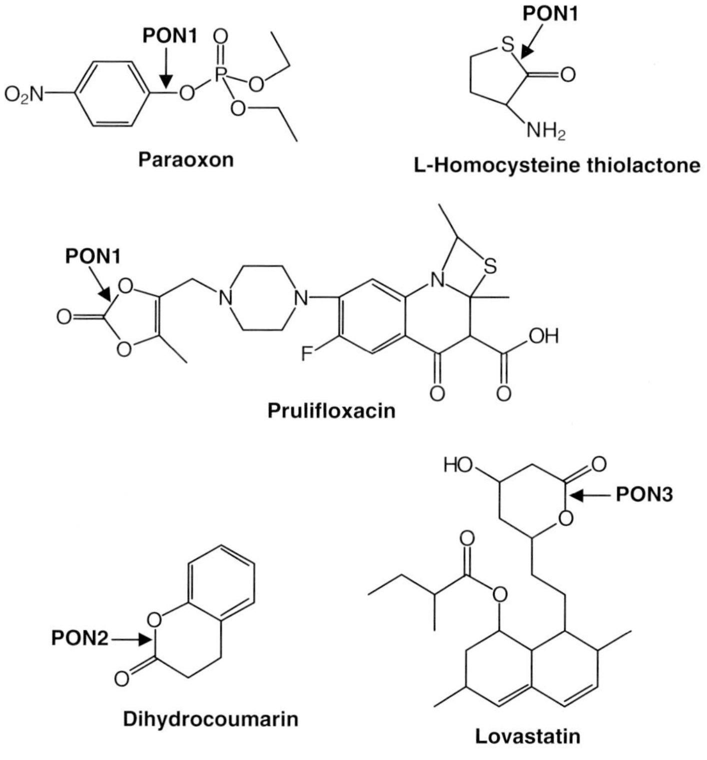

Figure 6.8 Examples of substrates of PONs.

PONs have three major functions: to protect against lipid peroxidation, to metabolize therapeutic agents, and to detoxify organophosphorus insecticides [92–95]. As described below, not all PONs have these functions nor are they equally effective if they share the functions. It has been shown that PON activity in the plasma is associated with high-density lipoproteins (HDLs) and the PON status has been linked to the development of an array of diseases, notably the process of atherogenesis [92, 96]. In support of its antiatherogenic role, PON knockout mice exhibit increases in lipoprotein oxidation and atherosclerosis, and transgenic expression of human PONs has the opposite effect [96–98]. It has been proposed that their antiatherogenic activity is achieved by removing oxidized cholesteryl esters and phospholipids in lipoproteins (e.g., low-density lipoproteins (LDLs) and HDL). The enzymatic degradation involves initial lactonization and subsequent hydrolysis of the formed lactone, leading to the removal of oxidized fatty acid chain from the LDL or HDL particles.

The robustness of the lactonase activity has implicated that PONs play critical roles in the metabolism of therapeutic agents with a lactone moiety [94, 99]. Lactone prodrugs require hydrolysis to exert pharmacological activity. Prulifloxacin – an antibiotic with a lactone moiety – is hydrolytically activated in the blood and its overall antibiotic activity correlates well with the plasma PON activity. Plasma PON status is also inversely related to organophosphate toxicity [100]. The detoxification of organophosphorus insecticides is nicely illustrated by genetically modified mice. Mice lacking PON1 all died within 2 h upon exposure to the organophosphate chlorpyrifos oxon [101], whereas wild-type mice receiving the same dose all survived. The potentiated toxicity by chlorpyrifos oxon was much less in mice transgenically expressing human Q192 than R192 PON, as the mutant R192 has lower hydrolytic activity toward chlorpyrifos oxon [102].

6.3.2
Classification and Structural Features

Humans have three PONs: PON1, PON2 and PON3 [92–95, 103, 104]. Like the carboxylesterase genes, the PON genes are clustered on a single chromosome – chromosome 17. The PON3 gene is flanked by the PON1 and PON2 genes. The PON1 and PON2 genes each span a total of 17 kb, and the PON3 gene spans 21 kb. They share a sequence identity of around 60% at the protein level and around 70% at the nucleotide level. All PONs are comparable in terms of molecular mass (43 kDa). PON1 and PON3 are expressed primarily in the liver and the kidney. However, they are secreted into the blood and associated with HDL particles. In contrast, PON2 is expressed ubiquitously. Based on phyletic analysis, the PON2 gene is the ancestral gene for other PON genes.

X-ray crystallographic study has revealed that PON1 is structurally configured like a propeller [96]. This propeller structure consists of six blades and each blade contains four β-sheets. These sheets line the propeller peripherally from the center. There is a central tunnel of the propeller that functions as the catalytic gorge. This tunnel has two calcium atoms – one is located at the bottom and the other in the center of the tunnel. The one at the bottom is involved in catalysis and the one in the center is critical in maintaining the structural integrity. On the top of the tunnel is a structure made of three helices. Two of the these helices form a unique lid over the active site, and are involved in anchoring PON1 to cell membranes and HDL particles in serum. The third helix is assumed to position substrates for hydrolysis and thus plays role in substrate specificity. This catalytic gorge supports the hydrolysis of lactones and esters as well as phosphotriesters in the case of PON1.

Like other hydrolases, the expression of PONs is altered by many factors, such as disease conditions and therapeutic agents. It is generally accepted that one of the major functions of PONs is to protect against the atherosclerotic process. Therefore, studies on the regulated expression of PONs have focused largely on disease mediators such as hyperglycemia and cytokines. It is relatively consistent that stimuli with increased secretion of proinflammatory cytokines and oxidative stress all decrease the activity of plasma PON activity [105, 106], which is highly related to the assembly of HDL. Conversely, antioxidant compounds such as polyphenols induce PONs [107]. Diabetic patients show lower PON activity in the plasma, but interestingly, hepatoma cells cultured in hyperglycemic conditions express higher levels of PON1, pointing to a possibility of a compensatory mechanism in diabetes.

The regulated expression of PONs by various factors is achieved largely by transcription and multiple transcriptional factors have been identified to play roles in the regulation. For example, pomegranate juice – rich in polyphenol antioxidants – induces PON2 with an involvement of the activation of activator protein-1 and peroxisome proliferator-activated receptor-γ [108]. It appears that these two transcription factors operate independently and have an additive effect in the induction. Pitavastatin, however, induces PONs by activating protein kinase Cζ, leading to the increased binding of transcription factor specificity protein-1 (Sp-1) to the PON1 promoter [109]. Interestingly, several other statins, including simvastatin, fluvastatin, and pravastatin, were found to repress the PON1 promoter [110]. It appears that the repression is mediated by the liver X receptor. In addition to the altered regulation, the association of PON1 with HDL seems impaired in disease conditions such as diabetes and antioxidants enhance the association [111].

6.3.3
Catalytic Mechanism

While the various catalytic activities share the gorge, the amino acids involved vary depending on the type of substrates [93, 96, 112]. It appears that lactonase and esterase, but not phosphatase, activity use the same catalytic machinery (Figure 6.9). For both lactonase and esterase activities, the dyad formed by His115–His134 is critical and substitution of either His residue abolishes the hydrolytic activity toward lactones or esters. In contrast, this dyad seem to have no effect on the hydrolysis of phosphatase activity. As a matter of fact, substitution of His115 with Trp (H115W) leads to increased activity toward paraoxon. However, Phe222 is

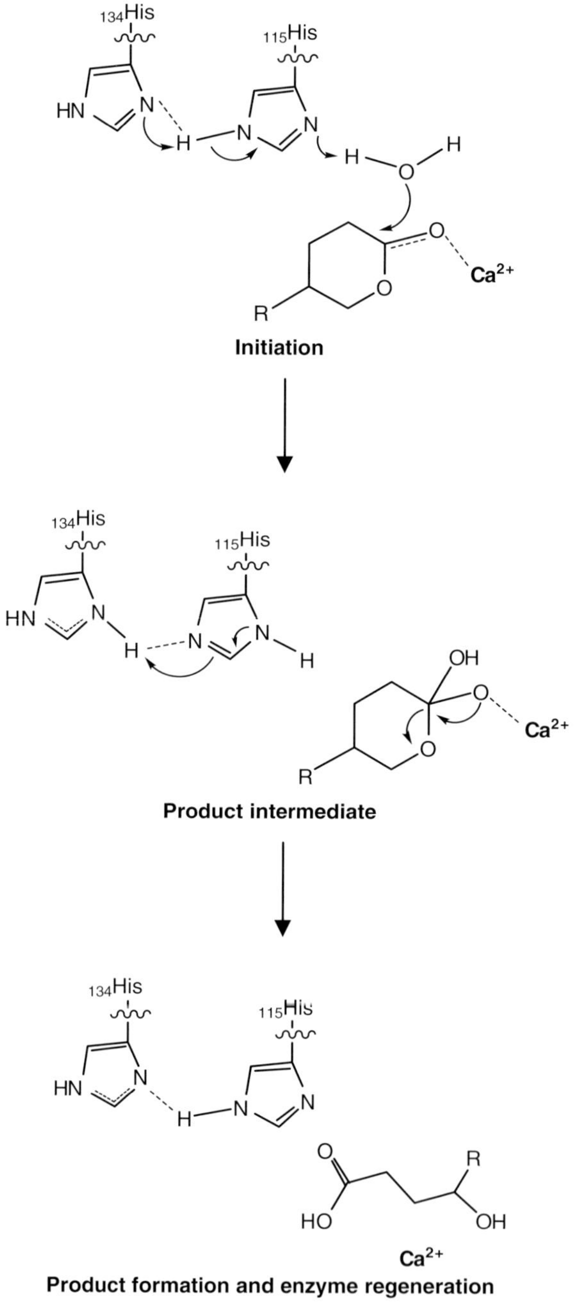

Figure 6.9 Catalytic mechanism of PONs.

critical for phosphatase activity, but not for lactonase or esterase activity. In addition, residues far from the catalytic pocket, particularly some in the β-sheets of the propeller, are found to profoundly alter catalysis – presumably this is their critical role in maintaining the integrity of the overall structure.

Unlike carboxylesterases and EHs, PONs catalyze hydrolysis without the formation of an acyl-enzyme complex. However, it appears that a modified catalytic triad is involved as well. In PONs, a hydroxyl ion, instead of an amino acid nucleophile, attacks the carbonyl of the lactone/ester substrates. His115 of the His115–His134 dyad acts as a general base, deprotonates a water molecule, and generates the hydroxyl ion (Figure 6.9). The strength of His115 as the general base is coordinated by His134 through proton shuttling. The attack by the hydroxyl ion leads to the formation of a negative intermediate of the substrate and this intermediate is temporarily stabilized by the catalytic calcium – a function of the oxyanion hole seen in carboxylesterases and EHs. As mentioned above, the catalytic mechanism by the His115–His134 dyad does not apply to the hydrolysis of organophosphates such as paraoxon. The catalytic machinery in the phosphatase activity remains to be elucidated.

Among PONs, PON1 has the broadest spectrum of substrate specificity [112] (Figure 6.8). While all PONs hydrolyze esters and lactones, PON1, but not PON2 or PON3, hydrolyzes phosphotriesters (Table 6.3). Structure–reactivity studies with recombinant PON1 have revealed several important findings regarding substrate specificity. Based on catalytic efficiency, lactones are the best substrates, followed by esters and phosphotriesters. Aryl esters are better substrates than aliphatic esters. Steric factors, but not the pK_a of the leaving group, play a determinant role in the hydrolysis of aryl esters, whereas the hydrolysis of aliphatic esters shows some dependence on the pK_a of the leaving group. However, the hydrolysis of lactones shows almost no dependence on the pK_a of the leaving group. PON1 is also shown to hydrolyze thiolactones such as L-homocysteine thiolactone (LHT) (Figure 6.8). LHT is known to promote atherothrombosis [113]. In addition to hydrolysis of lactones, all PONs have been shown to catalyze the formation of lactones – so-called lactonizing activity [114].

The activity of PONs can also be inhibited by many therapeutic agents at pharmacological concentrations. For example, the antibiotic cefazolin inhibits PON1 with an IC_{50} value of 8.4 μM [115]. Likewise, many cardiovascular therapeutics such

Table 6.3 Comparison of PONs.

Property	PON1	PON2	PON3
Lactonase activity	yes	yes	yes
Esterase activity	high	moderate	low
PON activity	yes	no	no
HDL association	yes	unknown	yes
Cellular stress	unknown	antagonism	unknown

as digoxin and verapamil inhibit PON1 with IC_{50} values of 0.012 and 0.672 μM, respectively [116]. The mode of inhibition varies depending on the inhibitor. Cefazolin is a competitive inhibitor, whereas digoxin acts noncompetitively. Interestingly, certain phospholipids differentially modulate the activities of PON1 between PON and arylesterase. For example, lysophosphatidylinositol inhibits PON activity, but enhances arylesterase activity [117]. It has been suggested that the inhibition is likely due to direct interaction with the noncatalytic site, whereas the enhancement is due to modulated micelle formation [117]. PONs are shown to protect against oxidative stress through a mechanism of scavenging, and therefore are sensitive to oxidized lipids and free radicals [118]. It appears that inhibition of PON activity involves the loss of functional Cys284.

6.4
Other Hydrolases

6.4.1
Carbonic Anhydrases

There are at least five distinct carbonic anhydrase families (α, β, γ, δ, and ε) and they are ambiguously expressed with a broad subcellular distribution [119]. These enzymes catalyze the formation of bicarbonate from carbon dioxide and water. Several members in this family have been found to catalyze hydrolysis of esters and their esterase activity can be enhanced through site-directed mutagenesis. While no direct evidence links these enzymes to drug metabolism, they are targets of many therapeutic agents. For example, acetazolamide – an antiglaucoma agent – is an inhibitor of carbonic anhydrase. Methazolamide – another carbonic anhydrase inhibitor – is also used to treat glaucoma. Methazolamide has a longer half-life than acetazolamide with less adverse effects in the kidney [119].

6.4.2
Cholinesterases

There are two cholinesterases – acetylcholinesterase and butyrylcholinesterase (or pseudocholinesterase) [120, 121]. As their names imply, the former hydrolyzes acetylcholine (a neurotransmitter) with higher efficiency, whereas the later hydrolyzes butyrylcholine faster. As a matter of fact, hydrolysis of acetylcholine by acetylcholinesterase is so efficient that the hydrolysis of acetylcholine is limited only by the diffusion rate. Such a high efficiency fits well with the primary functionality of this enzyme – termination of neurotransmission of acetylcholine. Acetylcholinesterase and butyrylcholinesterase differ in their relative abundance among various tissues. Acetylcholinesterase is abundantly present in the neural synapses, whereas butyrylcholinesterase is abundantly present in the plasma. Like carboxylesterases and certain EHs, both cholinesterases belong to the α/β-hydrolase-fold superfamily. Cholinesterases use the Ser–His–Glu triad for catalysis. Acetylcho-

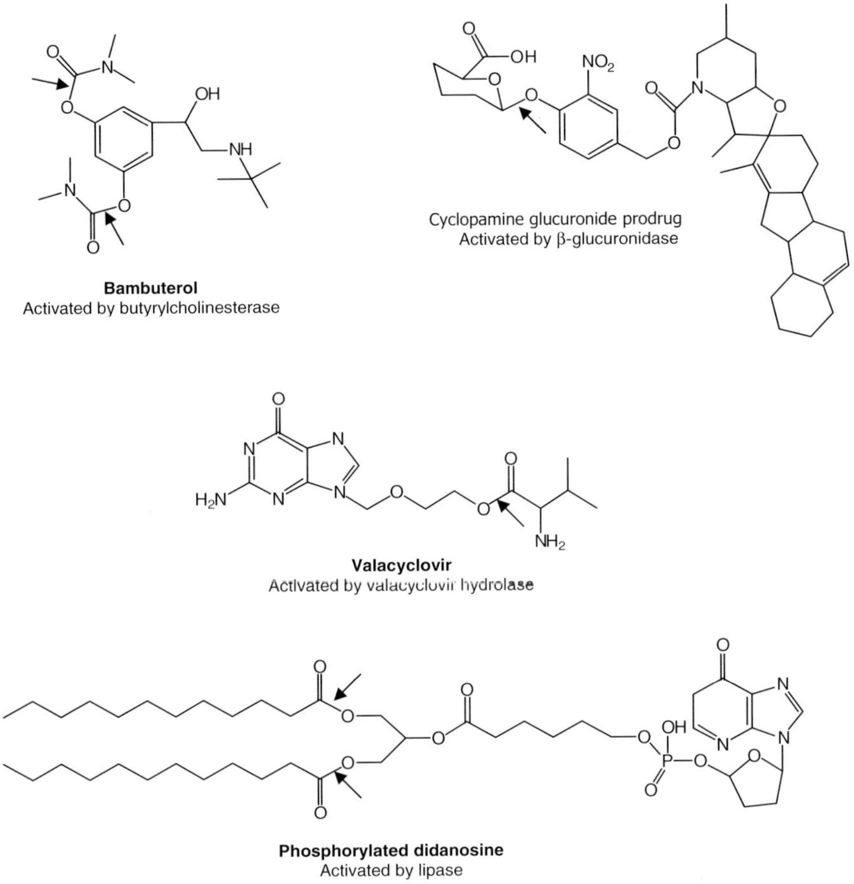

Figure 6.10 Examples of drugs metabolized by other hydrolases.

linesterase has a narrower catalytic gorge with high substrate selectivity. In contrast, butyrylcholinesterase has a larger catalytic gorge and thus is more promiscuous. There are many drugs targeting cholinesterases, particularly acetylcholinesterase. In contrast, butyrylcholinesterase is commonly used for prodrug activation [121] (Figure 6.10). Genetic variation of butyrylcholinesterase is associated with the prolonged effect of muscle relaxants such as succinylcholine.

6.4.3
β-Glucuronidase

β-Glucuronidase belongs to the protein family of glycosidases and hydrolyzes glycosidic bonds. Humans express a single β-glucuronidase gene and the encoded protein has a molecular weight of around 80 kDa. However, this enzyme normally exists as homotetramer and is targeted to two major subcellular compartments – the endoplasmic reticulum and the lysosome. As described above, the endoplasmic reticulum-targeted β-glucuronidase represents the portion of those that interact with carboxylesterases. The microsomal β-glucuronidase has been shown to hydrolyze glucuronidated hormones (e.g., steroids), thus providing an effective mechanism that recycles physiologically important molecules [10]. Biologically, β-glucuronidase exists as a 332-kDa homotetramer. β-Glucuronidase is increasingly used for the development of glucuronide prodrugs [122] (Figure 6.10).

6.4.4 Lipases

Lipolytic enzymes constitute a superfamily of proteins and involve a wide range of biological activities from nutrient processing to the production of signal molecules. Some of them, such as pancreatic lipase, tend to have broad substrate specificity, whereas others, such as cholesterol esterase, have a much narrower spectrum of substrates. The hydrolytic activity of these enzymes is much enhanced at the lipid/water interface – commonly referred as to interfacial activation. Lipases, like carboxylesterases, can also hydrolyze soluble substrates. It is therefore assumed that they are involved in drug metabolism as well. Nonetheless, lipase-based hydrolysis has been used for lipid prodrug activation [123] (Figure 6.10).

6.4.5 Peptidases/Proteases

These enzymes represent a superfamily of proteins that hydrolyze proteins. Majority of these enzymes use Ser as the nucleophile. They hydrolyze standard ester substrates such as *p*-nitrophenylacetate, but their participation in the hydrolysis of small drugs is very limited. Nevertheless, peptide and protein drugs are increasingly used for treating various diseases [124], and specification of individual peptidase in the elimination of these drugs will soon become an important area of study.

6.4.6 Valacylovirase

This enzyme was originally named valacyclovir hydrolase as it is highly active toward the antiviral agent valacyclovir [125] (Figure 6.10). It soon became clear that this enzyme hydrolyzes many anticancer and viral nucleosides, such as floxuridine, gemcitabine, valganciclovir, and zidovudine. Valacylovirase has a structure of β-sheets spaced by α-helices at various lengths. Like other members of the α/β-fold hydrolases, valacylovirase uses a nucleophile-based triad for the catalysis. The catalytic triad of valacylovirase is made of Ser122, His255, and Asp227. Such relative location among these three residues is identical to that seen in the α/β-fold hydrolase members that have a relatively large size (more than 400 residues). Interestingly, human valacylovirase has only 274 residues – a length of typical proteases. Nevertheless, valacylovirase does not have protease activity [125].

References

1 Sanghani, S.P., Sanghani, P.C., Schiel, M.A., and Bosron, W.F. (2009) Human carboxylesterases: an update on CES1, CES2 and CES3. *Protein Pept. Lett.*, **16**, 1207–1214.

2 Satoh, T. and Hosokawa, M. (2006) Structure, function and regulation of carboxylesterases. *Chem. Biol. Interact.*, **162**, 195–211.

3 Imai, T. (2006) Human carboxylesterase isozymes: catalytic properties and rational drug design. *Drug Metab. Pharmacokinet.*, **21**, 173–185.

4 Tang, M., Mukundan, M., Yang, J., Charpentier, N., LeCluyse, E.L., Black, C., Yang, D., Shi, D., and Yan, B. (2006) Antiplatelet agents aspirin and clopidogrel are hydrolyzed by distinct carboxylesterases, and clopidogrel is transesterificated in the presence of ethyl alcohol. *J. Pharmacol. Exp. Ther.*, **319**, 1467–1476.

5 Bora, P.S., Guruge, B.L., and Bora, N.S. (2003) Molecular characterization of human eye and heart fatty acid ethyl ester synthase/carboxylesterase by site-directed mutagenesis. *Biochem. Biophys. Res. Commun.*, **312**, 1094–1098.

6 Zhao, B., Natarajan, R., and Ghosh, S. (2005) Human liver cholesteryl ester hydrolase: cloning, molecular characterization, and role in cellular cholesterol homeostasis. *Physiol. Genomics*, **23**, 304–310.

7 Wei, E., Alam, M., Sun, F., Agellon, L.B., Vance, D.E., and Lehner, R. (2007) Apolipoprotein B and triacylglycerol secretion in human triacylglycerol hydrolase transgenic mice. *J. Lipid Res.*, **48**, 2597–2606.

8 Yang, D., Wang, X., Yang, D., and Yan, B. (2009) Pyrethroid insecticides: isoform-dependent hydrolysis, induction of cytochrome P450 3A4 and evidence on the involvement of the pregnane X receptor. *Toxicol. Appl. Pharmacol.*, **237**, 49–58.

9 Maxwell, D.M., Lieske, C.N., and Brecht, K.M. (1994) Oxime-induced reactivation of carboxylesterase inhibited by organophosphorus compounds. *Chem. Res. Toxicol.*, **7**, 428–433.

10 Zhu, B.T., Evaristus, E.N., Antoniak, S.K., Sarabia, S.F., Ricci, M.J., and Liehr, J.G. (1996) Metabolic deglucuronidation and demethylation of estrogen conjugates as a source of parent estrogens and catecholestrogen metabolites in Syrian hamster kidney, a target organ of estrogen-induced tumorigenesis. *Toxicol. Appl. Pharmacol.*, **136**, 186–193.

11 Junge, W. and Krisch, K. (1973) Current problems on the structure and classification of mammalian liver carboxylesterases (EC 3.1.1.1). *Mol. Cell. Biochem.*, **1**, 41–52.

12 Holmes, R.S., Cox, L.A., and Vandeberg, J.L. (2008) Mammalian carboxylesterase 5: comparative biochemistry and genomics. *Comp. Biochem. Physiol. D*, **3**, 195–204.

13 Holmes, R.S., Cox, L.A., and Vandeberg, J.L. (2009) A new class of mammalian carboxylesterase CES6. *Comp. Biochem. Physiol. D*, **4**, 209–217.

14 Hosokawa, M., Furihata, T., Yaginuma, Y., Yamamoto, N., Watanabe, N., Tsukada, E., Ohhata, Y., Kobayashi, K., Satoh, T., and Chiba, K. (2008) Structural organization and characterization of the regulatory element of the human carboxylesterase (CES1A1 and CES1A2) genes. *Drug Metab. Pharmacokinet.*, **23**, 73–84.

15 Yan, B., Matoney, L., and Yang, D. (1999) Human placental carboxylesterases: enzymatic characterization, molecular cloning, and evidence for the existence of multiple forms. *Placenta*, **20**, 599–607.

16 Kroetz, D.L., McBride, O.W., and Gonzalez, F.J. (1993) Glycosylation-

dependent activity of baculovirus-expressed human liver carboxylesterases: cDNA cloning and characterization of two highly similar enzyme forms. *Biochemistry*, **32**, 11606–11617.
17 Wu, M.H., Chen, P., Remo, B.F., Cook, E.H., Jr, Das, S., and Dolan, M.E. (2003) Characterization of multiple promoters in the human carboxylesterase 2 gene. *Pharmacogenetics*, **13**, 425–435.
18 Sanghani, S.P., Quinney, S.K., Fredenburg, T.B., Davis, W.I., Murry, D.J., and Bosron, W.F. (2004) Hydrolysis of irinotecan and its oxidative metabolites, 7-ethyl-10-[4-*N*-(5-aminopentanoic acid)-1-piperidino] carbonyloxycamptothecin and 7-ethyl-10-[4-(1-piperidino)-1-amino]-carbonyloxycamptothecin, by human carboxylesterases CES1A1, CES2, and a newly expressed carboxylesterase isoenzyme, CES3. *Drug Metab. Dispos.*, **32**, 505–511.
19 Yan, B., Yang, D., Brady, M., and Parkinson, A. (1994) Rat kidney carboxylesterase: cloning, sequencing, cellular localization and relationship to liver hydrolase B. *J. Biol. Chem.*, **269**, 29688–29696.
20 Yan, B., Yang, D., Brady, M., and Parkinson, A. (1995) Rat testicular carboxylesterase: cloning, sequencing, cellular localization and relationship to liver hydrolase A. *Arch. Biochem. Biophys.*, **316**, 899–908.
21 Yan, B., Yang, D., Bolluck, P., and Parkinson, A. (1996) Rat serum carboxylesterase: cloning, expression, regulation and evidence of secretion from liver. *J. Biol. Chem.*, **270**, 19128–19134.
22 Song, X., Gragen, S., Li, Y., Ma, Y., Liu, J., Yang, D., Matoney, L., and Yan, B. (2004) Intramolecular disulfide bonds are required for folding hydrolase B into a catalytically active conformation but not for maintaining it during catalysis. *Biochem. Biophys. Res. Commun.*, **319**, 1072–1080.
23 Ollis, D.L., Cheah, E., Cygler, M., Dijkstra, B., Frolow, F., Franken, S.M., Harel, M., Remington, S.J., Silman, I., Schrag, J., Sussman, J.L., Verschueren, K.H.G., and Goldman, A. (1992) The α/β hydrolase fold. *Protein Eng.*, **5**, 197–211.
24 Bencharit, S., Morton, C.L., Xue, Y., Potter, P.M., and Redinbo, M.R. (2003) Structural basis of heroin and cocaine metabolism by a promiscuous human drug-processing enzyme. *Nat. Struct. Biol.*, **10**, 349–356.
25 Sussman, J.L., Harel, M., Frolow, F., Oefner, C., Goldman, A., Toker, L., and Silman, I. (1991) Atomic structure of acetylcholinesterase from *Torpedo californica*: a prototypic acetylcholine-binding protein. *Science*, **253**, 872–879.
26 Bencharit, S., Morton, C.L., Howard-Williams, E.L., Danks, M.K., Potter, P.M., and Redinbo, M.R. (2002) Structural insights into CPT-11 activation by mammalian carboxylesterases. *Nat. Struct. Biol.*, **9**, 337–342.
27 Shi, D., Yang, J., Yang, D., LeCluyse, E.L., Black, C., You, L., Akhlaghi, F., and Yan, B. (2006) Anti-influenza prodrug oseltamivir is activated by carboxylesterase HCE1 and the activation is inhibited by anti-platelet agent clopidogrel. *J. Pharmacol. Exp. Ther.*, **319**, 1477–1484.
28 Luttrell, W.E. and Castle, M.C. (1993) Enhancement of hepatic microsomal esterase activity following soman pretreatment in guinea pigs. *Biochem. Pharmacol.*, **46**, 2083–2092.
29 Wheelock, C.E., Nishi, K., Ying, A., Jones, P.D., Colvin, M.E., Olmstead, M.M., and Hammock, B.D. (2008) Influence of sulfur oxidation state and steric bulk upon trifluoromethyl ketone (TFK) binding kinetics to carboxylesterases and fatty acid amide hydrolase (FAAH). *Bioorg. Med. Chem.*, **16**, 2114–2130.
30 Hicks, L.D., Hyatt, J.L., Stoddard, S., Tsurkan, L., Edwards, C.C., Wadkins, R.M., and Potter, P.M. (2009) Improved, selective, human intestinal carboxylesterase inhibitors designed to modulate 7-ethyl-10-[4-(1-piperidino)-1-piperidino]carbonyloxycamptothecin (irinotecan; CPT-11) toxicity. *J. Med. Chem.*, **52**, 3742–3752.
31 Harada, T., Nakagawa, Y., Wadkins, R.M., Potter, P.M., and Wheelock, C.E.

(2009) Comparison of benzil and trifluoromethyl ketone (TFK)-mediated carboxylesterase inhibition using classical and 3D-quantitative structure–activity relationship analysis. *Bioorg. Med. Chem.*, **17**, 149–164.

32 Taylor, P. and Radic, Z. (1994) The cholinesterases: from genes to proteins. *Annu. Rev. Pharmacol. Toxicol.*, **34**, 281–320.

33 Alvares, A.P. and Pratt, W.B. (1990) Pathways of drug metabolism, in *Principle of Drug Action*, 2nd edn (eds W.B. Pratt and P. Taylor), Churchill Livingstone, London, pp. 383–384.

34 Perucca, E., Cloyd, J., Critchley, D., and Fuseau, E. (2008) Rufinamide: clinical pharmacokinetics and concentration–response relationships in patients with epilepsy. *Epilepsia*, **49**, 1123–1141.

35 Pindel, E.V., Kedishvili, N.Y., Abraham, T.L., Brzezinski, M.R., Zhang, J., Dean, R.A., and Bosron, W.F. (1997) Purification and cloning of a broad substrate specificity human liver carboxylesterase that catalyzes the hydrolysis of cocaine and heroin. *J. Biol. Chem.*, **272**, 14769–14775.

36 Schentag, J.J., Hill, G., Chu, T., and Rayner, C.R. (2007) Similarity in pharmacokinetics of oseltamivir and oseltamivir carboxylate in Japanese and Caucasian subjects. *J. Clin. Pharmacol.*, **47**, 689–696.

37 Abe, M., Smith, J., Urae, A., Barrett, J., Kinoshita, H., and Rayner, C.R. (2006) Pharmacokinetics of oseltamivir in young and very elderly subjects. *Ann. Pharmacother.*, **40**, 1724–1730.

38 Morgan, E.W., Yan, B., Petersen, D., Greenway, D., and Parkinson, A. (1994) Purification and characterization of two rat liver microsomal carboxylesterases (hydrolase A and B). *Arch. Biochem. Biophys.*, **315**, 494–513.

39 Hosokawa, M., Endo, T., Fujisawa, M., Hara, S., Iwata, N., Sato, Y., and Satoh, T. (1995) Interindividual variation in carboxylesterase levels in human liver microsomes. *Drug Metab. Dispos.*, **23**, 1022–1027.

40 Wadkins, R.M., Hyatt, J.L., Edwards, C.C., Tsurkan, L., Redinbo, M.R., Wheelock, C.E., Jones, P.D., Hammock, B.D., and Potter, P.M. (2007) Analysis of mammalian carboxylesterase inhibition by trifluoromethylketone-containing compounds. *Mol. Pharmacol.*, **71**, 713–723.

41 Nemoda, Z., Angyal, N., Tarnok, Z., Gadoros, J., and Sasvari-Szekely, M. (2009) Carboxylesterase 1 gene polymorphism and methylphenidate response in ADHD. *Neuropharmacology*, **57**, 731–733.

42 Ribelles, N., López-Siles, J., Sánchez, A., González, E., Sánchez, M.J., Carabantes, F., Sánchez-Rovira, P., Márquez, A., Dueñas, R., Sevilla, I., and Alba, E. (2008) A carboxylesterase 2 gene polymorphism as predictor of capecitabine on response and time to progression. *Curr. Drug Metab.*, **9**, 336–343.

43 Kim, S.R., Sai, K., Tanaka-Kagawa, T., Jinno, H., Ozawa, S., Kaniwa, N., Saito, Y., Akasawa, A., Matsumoto, K., Saito, H., Kamatani, N., Shirao, K., Yamamoto, N., Yoshida, T., Minami, H., Ohtsu, A., Saijo, N., and Sawada, J. (2007) Haplotypes and a novel defective allele of CES2 found in a Japanese population. *Drug Metab. Dispos.*, **35**, 1865–1872.

44 Bellott, R., Le Morvan, V., Charasson, V., Laurand, A., Colotte, M., Zanger, U.M., Klein, K., Smith, D., Bonnet, J., and Robert, J. (2008) Functional study of the 830C>G polymorphism of the human carboxylesterase 2 gene. *Cancer Chemother. Pharmacol.*, **61**, 481–488.

45 Geshi, E., Kimura, T., Yoshimura, M., Suzuki, H., Koba, S., Sakai, T., Saito, T., Koga, A., Muramatsu, M., and Katagiri, T. (2005) A single nucleotide polymorphism in the carboxylesterase gene is associated with the responsiveness to imidapril medication and the promoter activity. *Hypertens. Res.*, **28**, 719–725.

46 Kubo, T., Kim, S.R., Sai, K., Saito, Y., Nakajima, T., Matsumoto, K., Saito, H., Shirao, K., Yamamoto, N., Minami, H., Ohtsu, A., Yoshida, T., Saijo, N., Ohno, Y., Ozawa, S., and Sawada, J. (2005) Functional characterization of three naturally occurring single nucleotide polymorphisms in the CES2 gene

encoding carboxylesterase 2 (HCE-2). *Drug Metab. Dispos.*, **33**, 1482–1487.
47 Guillemette, C. (2003) Pharmacogenomics of human UDP-glucuronosyltransferase enzymes. *Pharmacogenomics J.*, **3**, 136–158.
48 Muntané, J. (2009) Regulation of drug metabolism and transporters. *Curr. Drug Metab.*, **10**, 932–945.
49 Russel, F.G., Koenderink, J.B., and Masereeuw, R. (2008) Multidrug resistance protein 4 (MRP4/ABCC4): a versatile efflux transporter for drugs and signalling molecules. *Trends Pharmacol. Sci.*, **29**, 200–207.
50 Zhu, H.J., Patrick, K.S., Yuan, H.J., Wang, J.S., Donovan, J.L., DeVane, C.L., Malcolm, R., Johnson, J.A., Youngblood, G.L., Sweet, D.H., Langaee, T.Y., and Markowitz, J.S. (2008) Two CES1 gene mutations lead to dysfunctional carboxylesterase 1 activity in man: clinical significance and molecular basis. *Am. J. Hum. Genet.*, **82**, 1241–1248.
51 Shi, D., Yang, J., Yang, D., You, L., and Yan, B. (2008) Dexamethasone suppresses the expression of multiple rat carboxylesterases through transcriptional repression: evidence for an involvement of the glucocorticoid receptor. *Toxicology*, **254**, 97–105.
52 Williams, E.T., Jones, K.O., Ponsler, G.D., Lowery, S.M., Perkins, E.J., Wrighton, S.A., Ruterbories, K.J., Kazui, M., and Farid, N.A. (2008) The biotransformation of prasugrel, a new thienopyridine prodrug, by the human carboxylesterases 1 and 2. *Drug Metab. Dispos.*, **36**, 1227–1232.
53 Farid, N.A., Payne, C.D., Small, D.S., Winters, K.J., Ernest, C.S., 2nd, Brandt, J.T., Darstein, C., Jakubowski, J.A., and Salazar, D.E. (2007) Cytochrome P450 3A inhibition by ketoconazole affects prasugrel and clopidogrel pharmacokinetics and pharmacodynamics differently. *Clin. Pharmacol. Ther.*, **81**, 735–741.
54 Clarke, T.A. and Waskell, L.A. (2003) The metabolism of clopidogrel is catalyzed by human cytochrome P450 3A and is inhibited by atorvastatin. *Drug Metab. Dispos.*, **31**, 53–59.
55 Lau, W.C., Gurbel, P.A., Watkins, P.B., Neer, C.J., Hopp, A.S., Carville, D.G., Guyer, K.E., Tait, A.R., and Bates, E.R. (2004) Contribution of hepatic cytochrome P450 3A4 metabolic activity to the phenomenon of clopidogrel resistance. *Circulation*, **109**, 166–171.
56 Charasson, V., Haaz, M.C., and Robert, J. (2002) Determination of drug interactions occurring with the metabolic pathways of irinotecan. *Drug Metab. Dispos.*, **30**, 731–733.
57 Schulz, C., Boeck, S., Heinemann, V., and Stemmler, H.J. (2009) UGT1A1 genotyping: a predictor of irinotecan-associated side effects and drug efficacy? *Anticancer Drugs*, **20**, 867–879.
58 Ramchandani, R.P., Wang, Y., Booth, B.P., Ibrahim, A., Johnson, J.R., Rahman, A., Mehta, M., Innocenti, F., Ratain, M.J., and Gobburu, J.V. (2007) The role of SN-38 exposure, UGT1A1*28 polymorphism, and baseline bilirubin level in predicting severe irinotecan toxicity. *J. Clin. Pharmacol.*, **47**, 78–86.
59 Ose, A., Ito, M., Kusuhara, H., Yamatsugu, K., Kanai, M., Shibasaki, M., Hosokawa, M., Schuetz, J.D., and Sugiyama, Y. (2009) Limited brain distribution of [3*R*,4*R*,5*S*]-4-acetamido-5-amino-3-(1-ethylpropoxy)-1-cyclohexene-1-carboxylate phosphate (Ro 64-0802), a pharmacologically active form of oseltamivir, by active efflux across the blood-brain barrier mediated by organic anion transporter 3 (Oat3/Slc22a8) and multidrug resistance-associated protein 4 (Mrp4/Abcc4). *Drug Metab. Dispos.*, **37**, 315–321.
60 Ose, A., Kusuhara, H., Yamatsugu, K., Kanai, M., Shibasaki, M., Fujita, T., Yamamoto, A., and Sugiyama, Y. (2008) P-glycoprotein restricts the penetration of oseltamivir across the blood–brain barrier. *Drug Metab. Dispos.*, **36**, 427–434.
61 Ogihara, T., Kano, T., Wagatsuma, T., Wada, S., Yabuuchi, H., Enomoto, S., Morimoto, K., Shirasaka, Y., Kobayashi, S., and Tamai, I. (2009) Oseltamivir (tamiflu) is a substrate of peptide transporter 1. *Drug Metab. Dispos.*, **37**, 1676–1681.

62 Tian, Q., Zhang, J., Tan, T.M., Chan, E., Duan, W., Chan, S.Y., Boelsterli, U.A., Ho, P.C., Yang, H., Bian, J.S., Huang, M., Zhu, Y.Z., Xiong, W., Li, X., and Zhou, S. (2005) Human multidrug resistance associated protein 4 confers resistance to camptothecins. *Pharm. Res.*, **22**, 1837–1853.
63 Dettbarn, W.D., Yang, Z.P., and Milatovic, D. (1999) Different role of carboxylesterases in toxicity and tolerance to paraoxon and DFP. *Chem. Biol. Interact.*, **119–120**, 445–454.
64 Zhu, W., Song, L., Matoney, L., LeCluyse, E., and Yan, B. (2000) Dexamethasone differentially regulates the expression of carboxylesterase genes in humans and rats. *Drug Metab. Dispos.*, **28**, 186–191.
65 Jewell, C., Ackermann, C., Payne, N.A., Fate, G., Voorman, R., and Williams, F.M. (2007) Specificity of procaine and ester hydrolysis by human, minipig, and rat skin and liver. *Drug Metab. Dispos.*, **35**, 2015–2022.
66 Cecchin, E., Corona, G., Masier, S., Biason, P., Cattarossi, G., Frustaci, S., Buonadonna, A., Colussi, A., and Toffoli, G. (2005) Carboxylesterase isoform 2 mRNA expression in peripheral blood mononuclear cells is a predictive marker of the irinotecan to SN38 activation step in colorectal cancer patients. *Clin. Cancer Res.*, **11**, 6901–6907.
67 Na, K., Lee, E.Y., Lee, H.J., Kim, K.Y., Lee, H., Jeong, S.K., Jeong, A.S., Cho, S.Y., Kim, S.A., Song, S.Y., Kim, K.S., Cho, S.W., Kim, H., and Paik, Y.K. (2009) Human plasma carboxylesterase 1, a novel serologic biomarker candidate for hepatocellular carcinoma. *Proteomics*, **9**, 3989–3999.
68 Fowler, S., Lennon, S.M., Hoffmann, G., and Rayner, C.R. (2007) Comments on "Anti-influenza prodrug oseltamivir is activated by carboxylesterase human carboxylesterase 1, and the activation is inhibited by antiplatelet agent clopidogrel". *J. Pharmacol. Exp. Ther.*, **322**, 422–423.
69 Morgan, E.W., Yan, B., Greenway, D., and Parkinson, A. (1994) Regulation of two rat liver microsomal carboxylesterase isozymes: species differences, tissue distribution and the effects of age, sex and xenobiotic treatment of rats. *Arch. Biochem. Biophys.*, **315**, 514–526.
70 Godin, S.J., Scollon, E.J., Hughes, M.F., Potter, P.M., DeVito, M.J., and Ross, M.K. (2006) Species differences in the *in vitro* metabolism of deltamethrin and esfenvalerate: differential oxidative and hydrolytic metabolism by humans and rats. *Drug Metab. Dispos.*, **34**, 1764–1771.
71 Luttrell, W.E. and Castle, M.C. (1988) Species differences in the hydrolysis of meperidine and its inhibition by organophosphate compounds. *Fundam. Appl. Toxicol.*, **11**, 323–332.
72 Liu, K., Guengerich, F.P., and Yang, S.K. (1991) Enantioselective hydrolysis of lorazepam 3-acetate by esterases in human and rat liver microsomes and rat brain S9 fraction. *Drug Metab. Dispos.*, **19**, 609–613.
73 Yang, D., Pearce, R., Wang, X., Gaedigk, R., Wan, Y.J.Y., and Yan, B. (2009) Human carboxylesterases HCE1 and HCE2: ontogenic expression, inter-individual variability and differential hydrolysis of oseltamivir, aspirin, deltamethrin and permethrin. *Biochem. Pharmacol.*, **77**, 238–247.
74 Yang, D., Li, Y., Yuan, X., Matoney, L., and Yan, B. (2001) Regulation of rat carboxylesterase expression by 2,3,7,8-tetrachlorodibenzo-*p*-dioxin (TCDD) involves multiple signaling pathways. *Toxicol. Sci.*, **64**, 20–27.
75 Yang, J., Shi, D., Yang, D., Song, X., and Yan, B. (2007) Interleukin-6 suppresses the expression of carboxylesterases HCE1 and HCE2 through transcriptional repression. *Mol. Pharmacol.*, **72**, 686–694.
76 Zhu, H.J., Appel, D.I., Jiang, Y., and Markowitz, J.S. (2009) Age- and sex-related expression and activity of carboxylesterase 1 and 2 in mouse and human liver. *Drug Metab. Dispos.*, **37**, 1819–1825.
77 Lake, B.G., Renwick, A.B., Cunninghame, M.E., Price, R.J., Surry, D., and Evans, D.C. (1998) Comparison of the effects of some CYP3A and other enzyme inducers on replicative DNA

synthesis and cytochrome P450 isoforms in rat liver. *Toxicology*, **131**, 9–20.

78 Barth, S., Fischer, M., Schmid, R.D., and Pleiss, J. (2004) Sequence and structure of epoxide hydrolases: a systematic analysis. *Proteins*, **55**, 846–855.

79 Oguro, A., Sakamoto, K., Suzuki, S., and Imaoka, S. (2009) Contribution of hydrolase and phosphatase domains in soluble epoxide hydrolase to vascular endothelial growth factor expression and cell growth. *Biol. Pharm. Bull.*, **32**, 1962–1967.

80 Marino, J.P., Jr (2009) Soluble epoxide hydrolase, a target with multiple opportunities for cardiovascular drug discovery. *Curr. Top. Med. Chem.*, **9**, 452–463.

81 Morisseau, C. and Hammock, B.D. (2005) Epoxide hydrolases: mechanisms, inhibitor designs, and biological roles. *Annu. Rev. Pharmacol. Toxicol.*, **45**, 311–333.

82 Wickliffe, J.K., Herring, S.M., Hallberg, L.M., Galbert, L.A., Masters, O.E., 3rd, Ammenheuser, M.M., Xie, J., Friedberg, E.C., Lloyd, R.S., Abdel-Rahman, S.Z., and Ward, J.B., Jr (2007) Detoxification of olefinic epoxides and nucleotide excision repair of epoxide-mediated DNA damage: insights from animal models examining human sensitivity to 1,3-butadiene. *Chem. Biol. Interact.*, **166**, 226–231.

83 Azzato, E.M., Chen, R.A., Wacholder, S., Chanock, S.J., Klebanoff, M.A., and Caporaso, N.E. (2010) Maternal EPHX1 polymorphisms and risk of phenytoin-induced congenital malformations. *Pharmacogenet. Genomics*, **20**, 58–63.

84 Zheng, J., Plopper, C.G., Lakritz, J., Storms, D.H., and Hammock, B.D. (2001) Leukotoxin-diol: a putative toxic mediator involved in acute respiratory distress syndrome. *Am. J. Respir. Cell Mol. Biol.*, **25**, 434–438.

85 Imig, J.D. and Hammock, B.D. (2009) Soluble epoxide hydrolase as a therapeutic target for cardiovascular diseases. *Nat. Rev. Drug Discov.*, **8**, 794–805.

86 Imig, J.D. (2010) Targeting epoxides for organ damage in hypertension. *J. Cardiovasc. Pharmacol.*, **56**, 329–335.

87 Decker, M., Arand, M., and Cronin, A. (2009) Mammalian epoxide hydrolases in xenobiotic metabolism and signalling. *Arch. Toxicol.*, **83**, 297–318.

88 Carr, P.D. and Ollis, D.L. (2009) Alpha/beta hydrolase fold: an update. *Protein Pept. Lett.*, **16**, 1137–1148.

89 Haeggström, J.Z., Tholander, F., and Wetterholm, A. (2007) Structure and catalytic mechanisms of leukotriene A4 hydrolase. *Prostaglandins Other Lipid Mediat.*, **83**, 198–202.

90 Tholander, F., Muroya, A., Roques, B.P., Fournié-Zaluski, M.C., Thunnissen, M.M., and Haeggström, J.Z. (2008) Structure-based dissection of the active site chemistry of leukotriene A4 hydrolase: implications for M1 aminopeptidases and inhibitor design. *Chem. Biol.*, **15**, 920–929.

91 de Medina, P., Paillasse, M.R., Segala, G., Poirot, M., and Silvente-Poirot, S. (2010) Identification and pharmacological characterization of cholesterol-5,6-epoxide hydrolase as a target for tamoxifen and AEBS ligands. *Proc. Natl. Acad. Sci. USA*, **107**, 13520–13525.

92 Camps, J., Marsillach, J., and Joven, J. (2009) The paraoxonases: role in human diseases and methodological difficulties in measurement. *Crit. Rev. Clin. Lab. Sci.*, **46**, 83–106.

93 Khersonsky, O. and Tawfik, D.S. (2006) The histidine 115–histidine 134 dyad mediates the lactonase activity of mammalian serum paraoxonases. *J. Biol. Chem.*, **281**, 7649–7656.

94 Draganov, D.I. (2010) Lactonases with organophosphatase activity: structural and evolutionary perspectives. *Chem. Biol. Interact.*, **187**, 370–372.

95 Gupta, N., Gill, K., and Singh, S. (2009) Paraoxonases: structure, gene polymorphism and role in coronary artery disease. *Indian J. Med. Res.*, **130**, 361–368.

96 Harel, M., Aharoni, A., Gaidukov, L., Brumshtein, B., Khersonsky, O., Meged, R., Dvir, H., Ravelli, R.B., McCarthy, A., Toker, L., Silman, I., Sussman, J.L., and Tawfik, D.S. (2004) Structure and

evolution of the serum paraoxonase family of detoxifying and anti-atherosclerotic enzymes. *Nat. Struct. Mol. Biol.*, **11**, 412–419.

97 Rozenberg, O., Rosenblat, M., Coleman, R., Shih, D.M., and Aviram, M. (2003) Paraoxonase (PON1) deficiency is associated with increased macrophage oxidative stress: studies in PON1-knockout mice. *Free Radic. Biol. Med.*, **34**, 774–784.

98 Shih, D.M., Xia, Y.R., Wang, X.P., Wang, S.S., Bourquard, N., Fogelman, A.M., Lusis, A.J., and Reddy, S.T. (2007) Decreased obesity and atherosclerosis in human paraoxonase 3 transgenic mice. *Circ. Res.*, **100**, 1200–1207.

99 Tougou, K., Nakamura, A., Watanabe, S., Okuyama, Y., and Morino, A. (1998) Paraoxonase has a major role in the hydrolysis of prulifloxacin (NM441), a prodrug of a new antibacterial agent. *Drug Metab. Dispos.*, **26**, 355–359.

100 Mackenzie Ross, S.J., Brewin, C.R., Curran, H.V., Furlong, C.E., Abraham-Smith, K.M., and Harrison, V. (2010) Neuropsychological and psychiatric functioning in sheep farmers exposed to low levels of organophosphate pesticides. *Neurotoxicol. Teratol.*, **32**, 452–459.

101 Shih, D.M., Gu, L., Xia, Y.R., Navab, M., Li, W.F., Hama, S., Castellani, L.W., Furlong, C.E., Costa, L.G., Fogelman, A.M., and Lusis, A.J. (1998) Mice lacking serum paraoxonase are susceptible to organophosphate toxicity and atherosclerosis. *Nature*, **394**, 284–287.

102 Jansen, K.L., Cole, T.B., Park, S.S., Furlong, C.E., and Costa, L.G. (2009) Paraoxonase 1 (PON1) modulates the toxicity of mixed organophosphorus compounds. *Toxicol. Appl. Pharmacol.*, **236**, 142–153.

103 Primo-Parmo, S.L., Sorenson, R.C., Teiber, J., and La Du, B.N. (1996) The human serum paraoxonase/arylesterase gene (PON1) is one member of a multigene family. *Genomics*, **33**, 498–507.

104 Draganov, D.I. and La Du, B.N. (2004) Pharmacogenetics of paraoxonases: a brief review. *Naunyn Schmiedebergs Arch. Pharmacol.*, **369**, 78–88.

105 bin Ali, A., Zhang, Q., Lim, Y.K., Fang, D., Retnam, L., and Lim, S.K. (2003) Expression of major HDL-associated antioxidant PON-1 is gender dependent and regulated during inflammation. *Free Radic. Biol. Med.*, **34**, 824–829.

106 Precourt, L.P., Seidman, E., Delvin, E., Amre, D., Deslandres, C., Dominguez, M., Sinnett, D., and Levy, E. (2009) Comparative expression analysis reveals differences in the regulation of intestinal paraoxonase family members. *Int. J. Biochem. Cell Biol.*, **41**, 1628–1637.

107 Gouédard, C., Barouki, R., and Morel, Y. (2004) Dietary polyphenols increase paraoxonase 1 gene expression by an aryl hydrocarbon receptor-dependent mechanism. *Mol. Cell. Biol.*, **24**, 5209–5222.

108 Shiner, M., Fuhrman, B., and Aviram, M. (2007) Macrophage paraoxonase 2 (PON2) expression is up-regulated by pomegranate juice phenolic anti-oxidants via PPAR gamma and AP-1 pathway activation. *Atherosclerosis*, **195**, 313–321.

109 Arii, K., Suehiro, T., Ikeda, Y., Kumon, Y., Inoue, M., Inada, S., Takata, H., Ishibashi, A., Hashimoto, K., and Terada, Y. (2010) Role of protein kinase C in pitavastatin-induced human paraoxonase I expression in Huh7 cells. *Metabolism*, **59**, 1287–1293.

110 Gouédard, C., Koum-Besson, N., Barouki, R., and Morel, Y. (2003) Opposite regulation of the human paraoxonase-1 gene PON-1 by fenofibrate and statins. *Mol. Pharmacol.*, **63**, 945–956.

111 Fuhrman, B., Gantman, A., and Aviram, M. (2010) Paraoxonase 1 (PON1) deficiency in mice is associated with reduced expression of macrophage SR-BI and consequently the loss of HDL cytoprotection against apoptosis. *Atherosclerosis*, **211**, 61–68.

112 Khersonsky, O. and Tawfik, D.S. (2005) Structure–reactivity studies of serum paraoxonase PON1 suggest that its native activity is lactonase. *Biochemistry*, **44**, 6371–6382.

113 Jakubowski, H. (2010) The role of paraoxonase 1 in the detoxification of homocysteine thiolactone. *Adv. Exp. Med. Biol.*, **660**, 113–127.

114 Teiber, J.F., Draganov, D.I., and La Du, B.N. (2003) Lactonase and lactonizing activities of human serum paraoxonase (PON1) and rabbit serum PON3. *Biochem. Pharmacol.*, **66**, 887–896.

115 Sinan, S., Kockar, F., Gencer, N., Yildirim, H., and Arslan, O. (2006) Effects of some antibiotics on paraoxonase from human serum *in vitro* and from mouse serum and liver *in vivo*. *Biol. Pharm. Bull.*, **29**, 1559–1563.

116 Işgör, M.M. and Beydemir, S. (2010) Some cardiovascular therapeutics inhibit paraoxonase 1 (PON1) from human serum. *Eur. J. Pharmacol.*, **645**, 135–142.

117 Park, C.H., Nguyen, S.D., Kim, M.R., Jeong, T.S., and Sok, D.E. (2006) Differential effect of lysophospholipids on activities of human plasma paraoxonase1, either soluble or lipid-bound. *Lipids*, **41**, 371–380.

118 Nguyen, S.D., Hung, N.D., Cheon-Ho, P., Ree, K.M., and Dai-Eun, S. (2009) Oxidative inactivation of lactonase activity of purified human paraoxonase 1 (PON1). *Biochim. Biophys. Acta*, **1790**, 155–160.

119 Isik, S., Kockar, F., Aydin, M., Arslan, O., Guler, O.O., Innocenti, A., Scozzafava, A., and Supuran, C.T. (2009) Carbonic anhydrase inhibitors: inhibition of the beta-class enzyme from the yeast *Saccharomyces cerevisiae* with sulfonamides and sulfamates. *Bioorg. Med. Chem.*, **17**, 1158–1163.

120 Darreh-Shori, T. and Soininen, H. (2010) Effects of cholinesterase inhibitors on the activities and protein levels of cholinesterases in the cerebrospinal fluid of patients with Alzheimer's disease: a review of recent clinical studies. *Curr. Alzheimer Res.*, **7**, 67–73.

121 Moriarty, L.M., Lally, M.N., Carolan, C.G., Jones, M., Clancy, J.M., and Gilmer, J.F. (2008) Discovery of a "true" aspirin prodrug. *J. Med. Chem.*, **51**, 7991–7999.

122 Hamon, F., Renoux, B., Chadéneau, C., Muller, J.M., and Papot, S. (2010) Study of a cyclopamine glucuronide prodrug for the selective chemotherapy of glioblastoma. *Eur. J. Med. Chem.*, **45**, 1678–1682.

123 Lalanne, M., Khoury, H., Deroussent, A., Bosquet, N., Benech, H., Clayette, P., Couvreur, P., Vassal, G., Paci, A., and Andrieux, K. (2009) Metabolism evaluation of biomimetic prodrugs by *in vitro* models and mass spectrometry. *Int. J. Pharm.*, **379**, 235–243.

124 Cattaneo, A. (2010) Tanezumab, a recombinant humanized mAb against nerve growth factor for the treatment of acute and chronic pain. *Curr. Opin. Mol. Ther.*, **12**, 94–106.

125 Lai, L., Xu, Z., Zhou, J., Lee, K.D., and Amidon, G.L. (2008) Molecular basis of prodrug activation by human valacyclovirase, an alpha-amino acid ester hydrolase. *J. Biol. Chem.*, **283**, 9318–9327.

7
Transporting Systems

Anne T. Nies, Claudia Resch, and Tadashi Namisaki

7.1
Introduction

Membrane transport proteins are embedded in the lipid bilayer of biological membranes where they govern the movement of solutes or the solvent from one side to the other. In particular, transporters in the plasma membrane determine which substances enter or leave a cell, because it is virtually impossible for ions and most small molecules to cross biological membranes at a sufficient rate by simple diffusion [1, 2]. Plasma membrane transporters thereby control (i) the influx of essential nutrients or endogenous substrates (e.g., sugars, amino acids, nucleotides, vitamins, inorganic ions), (ii) the efflux of dietary and environmental toxins, of other xenobiotics, and of end products of metabolism, and (iii) the establishment of electrochemical gradients. Since a number of membrane transporters also accept drugs as substrates, they may play important roles in processes affecting drug pharmacokinetics (absorption, distribution, elimination) and in the development of cellular drug resistance through altered uptake or efflux. These topics will be discussed in the present chapter.

It is of interest to note that membrane transporters are of interest in other areas of pharmacology as well. Transporters may serve as drug targets. For example, the serotonin transporter protein SERT (encoded by *SLC6A4*) is the target of several selective serotonin reuptake inhibitors, which are very effective for the treatment of depression [3]. In parasitic protozoa, transporters may either be used for drug delivery or serve as drug targets. This could open up novel treatment options, for example, for malaria, African sleeping sickness, and leishmaniasis [4, 5].

7.2
Classification of Drug Transporters and Transport Mechanisms

Membrane transport proteins can be grouped into various classes, the most common ones being ion channels, water channels (aquaporins), ATP-binding cassette (ABC) transporters, ion transport ATPases, and solute carriers (SLCs). In

Metabolism of Drugs and Other Xenobiotics, First Edition. Edited by Pavel Anzenbacher, Ulrich M. Zanger.

the initial draft of the human genome, at least 1200 genes (more than 4% of the total genes) were assigned to be membrane proteins with transport function [6, 7]. These genes and their encoded proteins may be collectively considered as the "transportome" [8].

Membrane proteins with transport function typically have several transmembrane segments, each consisting of a stretch of 20–25 hydrophobic amino acids that spans the lipid bilayer. However, they largely differ in transport mechanisms. Channels form pores in biological membranes of rather limited specificity. Substance flow through channels follows the concentration gradient of the transported ion or small molecule and is controlled by the channels' open probability. By this, high transport rates of 10^7–10^9 molecules/s may be achieved. Transporters (also designated as "carriers"), however, are able to specifically bind a substrate, but this high precision is traded in for slow transport rates of about 10^3–10^5 molecules/s. Of note, no sugar channels have evolved, but different sugar transporters exist in eukaryotes that can discriminate between sugars of the same size and are able to selectively transport, for example, glucose, but not fructose.

Considering drug transport, pharmacologists generally focus on two transporter superfamilies – the SLC superfamily (Section 7.3) and the ABC transporters (Section 7.4) [9]. ABC transporters as well as ion transport ATPases are primary-active transporters that build up ion or solute gradients across membranes by directly utilizing the energy released during ATP hydrolysis. ABC family members transport a large variety of small molecules including peptides, lipids, and endogenous and xenobiotic organic anions and organic cations, including drugs. Ion transport ATPases contribute to maintain ion gradients (e.g., Na^+, K^+, H^+, Ca^{2+}, Cu^{2+}) across biological membranes, which may be used by secondary-active transporters. Of interest, the copper ATPases ATP7A and ATP7B not only efflux Cu^{2+} but also platinum drugs and may, therefore, contribute to drug resistance [10]. The SLC superfamily comprises at least 370 transporters grouped in 50 families ([11–15] and updates at http://www.bioparadigms.org/slc/menu.asp). They include passive transporters (uniporters = facilitative transporters), which move one type of molecule down its concentration gradient, and secondary-active transporters (cotransporters), which couple the movement of one type of molecule against its concentration gradient with movement of another type of molecule down its concentration gradient.

7.3
Drug Transporters of the SLC Superfamily

Table 7.1 gives an overview of all known SLC families. Many families comprise mitochondrial or vesicular transporters or transporters for physiological compounds. Relevant drug-transporting family members are indicated, as well as selected drug substrates. Particularly, members of the *SLC15*, *SLC16*, *SLCO*, *SLC22*, *SLC28*, *SLC29*, and *SLC47* family may play important roles in the pharmacokinetics of drugs.

Table 7.1 List of currently known solute carrier families, selected drug-transporting members, and selected drug substrates.

Gene family	Family name	Number of family members	Predominant physiological substrates	Drug-transporting family member (gene name)	Drug-transporting family member (protein name)	Selected drug substrates
SLC1	high-affinity glutamate and neutral amino acid transporter	7	glutamate, neutral amino acids			
SLC2	facilitative GLUT transporter	14	glucose, fructose, galactose, urate			
SLC3	heavy subunits of the heteromeric amino acid transporters	2				
SLC4	bicarbonate transporter	11	Cl^-, HCO_3^-			
SLC5	Na^+ glucose cotransporter	12	glucose, galactose, short-chain fatty acids			
SLC6	Na^+- and Cl^--dependent neurotransmitter transporter	21	γ-aminobutyric acid, dopamine, serotonin, noradrenalin, amino acids			
SLC7	cationic amino acid transporter/ glycoprotein-associated	14	cationic amino acids			
SLC8	Na^+/Ca^{2+} exchanger	3	Na^+, Ca^{2+}			
SLC9	Na^+/H^+ exchanger	13	Na^+, H^+, Li^+, NH_4^+			

(*Continued*)

Table 7.1 (*Continued*)

Gene family	Family name	Number of family members	Predominant physiological substrates	Drug-transporting family member (gene name)	Drug-transporting family member (protein name)	Selected drug substrates
SLC10	Na^+ bile salt cotransporter	7	bile salts			
SLC11	H^+-coupled metal ion transporter	2	Fe^{2+}, Cd^{2+}, Co^{2+}, Cu^+, Mn^{2+}, Ni^{2+}, Pb^{2+}, Zn^{2+}			
SLC12	electroneutral cation-coupled Cl^- cotransporter	9	Na^+/K^+ (or NH_4^+)/2 Cl^-			
SLC13	human Na^+-sulfate/carboxylate cotransporter	5	Na^+, SO_4^{2-}, $S_2O_3^{2-}$, SeO_4^{2-}, succinate, citrate			
SLC14	urea transporter	2	urea			
SLC15	proton oligopeptide cotransporter	4	di-, tripeptides	*SLC15A1*	PEPT1	β-lactam antibiotics
SLC16	monocarboxylate transporter	14	lactate, pyruvate, ketone bodies	*SLC16A1*	MCT1	salicylate, statins
SLC17	vesicular glutamate transporter	8	glutamate			
SLC18	vesicular amine transporter	3	serotonin, dopamine, epinephrine, norepinephrine, histamine			
SLC19	folate/thiamine transporter	3	folate, thiamine			
SLC20	type III Na^+-phosphate cotransporter	2	Na^+, phosphate			

SLCO	organic anion transporter	11	bile salts, organic anions, thyroid hormones, steroid sulfates	*SLCO1A2*	OATP1A2	fexofenadine, fluoroquinolones, saquinavir, statins
				SLCO1B1	OATP1B1	benzylpenicillin, methotrexate, rifampicin, statins, troglitazone, valsartan
				SLCO1B3	OATP1B3	digoxin, enalapril, fexofenadine, methotrexate, paclitaxel, statins, valsartan
				SLCO2B1	OATP2B1	bosentan, statins, glibenclamide
				SLCO3A1	OATP3A1	benzylpenicillin
SLC22	organic cation/anion/zwitterion transporter	26	large variety of organic cations, anions, zwitterions	*SLC22A1*	OCT1	aciclovir, disopyramide, lamivudine, metformin, platinum compounds
				SLC22A2	OCT2	cimetidine, metformin, platinum compounds, ranitidine
				SLC22A3	OCT3	lidocaine, metformin, platinum compounds, quinidine
				SLC22A4	OCTN1	pyrilamine, quinidine, verapamil
				SLC22A5	OCTN2	pyrilamine, quinidine, verapamil

(*Continued*)

Table 7.1 (*Continued*)

Gene family	Family name	Number of family members	Predominant physiological substrates	Drug-transporting family member (gene name)	Drug-transporting family member (protein name)	Selected drug substrates
				SLC22A6	OAT1	aciclovir, bumetanide, captopril, cimetidine, furosemide, indomethacin, salicylate
				SLC22A7	OAT2	cimetidine, erythromycin, 5-fluorouracil, methotrexate, taxol, tetracycline
				SLC22A8	OAT3	benzylpenicillin, bumetanide, cimetidine, furosemide, methotrexate, olmesartan, pravastatin, quinaprilat, salicylate, statins, topotecan
SLC23	Na^+-dependent ascorbic acid transporter	4	Na^+, ascorbic acid			
SLC24	$Na^+/(Ca^{2+}$-$K^+)$ exchanger	6	Na^+, Ca^{2+}, K^+			
SLC25	mitochondrial carriers	46	various metabolites			
SLC26	multifunctional anion exchanger	11	HCO_3^-, Cl^-, SO_4^{2-}, oxalate			
SLC27	fatty acid transporter	6	(very) long-chain fatty acids			

SLC28	Na^+-coupled nucleoside transporter	3	Na^+, purine and pyrimidine nucleosides	*SLC28A1*	CNT1	5-azacytidine, cytarabine, 5-fluoro-5′-deoxyuridine, gemcitabine, zalcitabine, zidovudine
				SLC28A2	CNT2	5-azacytidine, 5-fluoro-5′-deoxyuridine
				SLC28A3	CNT3	cytarabine, 5-fluoro-5′ -deoxyuridine, gemcitabine, 6-mercaptopurine, 6-thioguanine,zalcitabine, zidovudine
SLC29	facilitative nucleoside transporter	4	purine and pyrimidine nucleosides, some nucleobases	*SLC29A1*	ENT1	5-azacytidine, cytarabine, 5-fluoro-5′-deoxyuridine, gemcitabine, lamivudine, zalcitabine, zidovudine
				SLC29A2	ENT2	cytarabine, 5-fluoro-5′ -deoxyuridine, gemcitabine, 6-mercaptopurine, 6-thioguanine, zalcitabine, zidovudine
SLC30	zinc efflux transporter	10	zinc			
SLC31	copper transporter	2	copper	*SLC31A1*	CTR1	platinum compounds
				SLC31A2	CTR2	platinum compounds
SLC32	vesicular inhibitory amino acid transporter	1	γ-aminobutyric acid, glycine			
SLC33	acetyl-CoA transporter	1	acetyl-CoA			

(*Continued*)

Table 7.1 (*Continued*)

Gene family	Family name	Number of family members	Predominant physiological substrates	Drug-transporting family member (gene name)	Drug-transporting family member (protein name)	Selected drug substrates
SLC34	type II Na^+-phosphate cotransporter	3	Na^+, HPO^{4-}			
SLC35	nucleotide-sugar transporter	23	UDP-sugars			
SLC36	proton-coupled amino acid transporter	4	H^+, amino acids			
SLC37	sugar-phosphate/ phosphate exchanger	4	glycerol 3-phosphate, glucose 6- phosphate			
SLC38	system A and system N Na^+-coupled neutral amino acid transporters	11	H^+, Na^+, amino acids			
SLC39	metal ion transporter	14	zinc, manganese			
SLC40	basolateral iron transporter	1	ferrous iron			
SLC41	MgtE-like magnesium transporter	3	Mg^{2+} (Sr^{2+}, Zn^{2+}, Cu^{2+}, Fe^{2+}, Co^{2+}, Ba^{2+}, Cd^{2+})			
SLC42	Rh ammonium transporter	3	NH_4^+, H^+			
SLC43	Na^+-independent, system-L-like amino acid transporter	3	neutral amino acids			

SLC44	choline-like transporter	5	choline			
SLC45	putative sugar transporter	4	glucose, galactose			
SLC46	folate transporter	3	folate			
SLC47	Multidrug and toxin extrusion (MATE)	2	organic cations	*SLC47A1*	MATE1	aciclovir, cimetidine, cisplatin, fexofenadine, metformin, procainamide, quinine, salicylate, topotecan
				SLC47A2	MATE2-K	aciclovir, captopril, cisplatin, metformin, procainamide, quinine, tetracycline, topotecan, verapamil
SLC48	heme transporter	1	heme			
SLC50	sugar efflux transporter	1	glucose			
SLC51	transporters of steroid-derived molecules (OSTα–OSTβ)	2	glycine- and taurine-conjugated bile acids			

Modified and compiled from http://www.bioparadigms.org/slc/menu.asp and [2, 9, 16–28].

7.4
ABC Drug Transporters

The 48 known human ABC transporters are divided on the basis of their amino acid sequence similarity and phylogeny into seven subfamilies designated A–G [29]. Members of three ABC subfamilies have been recognized to play key roles in drug efflux from cells: MDR1 P-glycoprotein (MDR1 P-gp, encoded by *ABCB1*), the breast cancer resistance protein BCRP (encoded by *ABCG2*), and the multidrug resistance proteins (MRPs) of the ABCC subfamily (Table 7.2). The recently identified *ABCC13* gene is now considered a pseudogene incapable of encoding a functional ABCC/MRP transporter (Entrez Gene ID: 150000). Table 7.2 summarizes relevant characteristics of these drug-transporting ABC members.

7.5
Drug Transporters and Disease

Genetic variants in transporter genes causing lack of transporter function have been recognized as the molecular basis of several inherited diseases displaying Mendelian inheritance (Table 7.3). Analysis of the phenotypic consequences of these disease-associated variants has importantly contributed to the knowledge on substrates and function of transporters. A few examples are given. (i) Cystic fibrosis is an autosomal-recessive disease affecting ion and fluid homeostasis of epithelia [36]. Cystic fibrosis is caused by nonsynonymous variants of the cystic fibrosis transmembrane conductance regulator glycoprotein (CFTR, encoded by *ABCC7*), which is a cAMP-activated chloride channel. Of interest, many of the more than 800 known variants lead to a misfolded and misprocessed protein. Small molecules ("pharmacological chaperones") that rescue misfolded CFTR *in vitro* or potentiate CFTR function may become important therapeutic drugs for the treatment of cystic fibrosis [37, 38]. (ii) Other examples are inherited liver diseases that are due to lack-of-function variants in genes encoding transporters localized in the canalicular membrane of hepatocytes [30, 39–41].

In addition, large numbers of genetic transporter variants, commonly referred to as single nucleotide polymorphisms (SNPs), have been associated with susceptibility to complex disease. A well-studied example among the ABC drug transporters is P-gp, which typically effluxes a variety of neutral or cationic compounds with bulky structure [42]. The localization of P-gp in the apical membrane of bronchial, renal, and intestinal epithelial cells, of hepatocytes, and at blood–tissue barriers supports the notion that it plays a central role in tissue defense against chemically diverse toxicants (Figure 7.1, Table 7.2, and [42, 43]). Accordingly, certain P-gp SNPs have been associated with susceptibility to, for example, inflammatory bowel disease, both Crohn's disease and ulcerative colitis [44–46], and development of renal cancer [47]. BCRP, whose localization is in part overlapping with that of MDR1 [48] and which is also supposed to be involved in tissue defense [43], may likewise be a candidate gene for development of renal cell carcinoma [49].

Table 7.2 ABC transporters involved in drug absorption, distribution, and excretion.

ABC gene	Transporter name	Tissues/cells	Physiological substrates	Resistance profile to anticancer drug	Selected other drugs
ABCB1	MDR1 P-gp	intestinal enterocytes (luminal), kidney proximal tubule (luminal), hepatocytes (canalicular), brain endothelia (luminal)		anthracyclines, camptothecins, epipodophyllotoxins, imatinib, methotrexate, mitoxantrone, taxanes, vinca alkaloids	cyclosporine, digoxin, indinavir, loperamide, tacrolimus, verapamil
ABCC1	MRP1	ubiquitous, mainly blood–tissue barriers	bilirubin glucuronides, folate, GSH, GSSG, leukotriene C_4, sulfated steroids	anthracyclines, camptothecins, epipodophyllotoxins, imatinib, methotrexate, mitoxantrone, vinca alkaloids	saquinavir, grepafloxacin
ABCC2	MRP2	hepatocytes (canalicular), kidney (proximal tubule, luminal), enterocytes (luminal)	bilirubin glucuronides, GSH, GSSG, leukotriene C_4, sulfated steroids	anthracyclines, camptothecins, cisplatin, epipodophyllotoxins, methotrexate, mitoxantrone, taxanes, vinca alkaloids	enalapril, fexofenadine, rifampicin, ritonavir, statins, valsartan
ABCC3	MRP3	hepatocytes (sinusoidal), intestinal enterocytes (basolateral), kidney distal tubule	bilirubin glucuronides, leukotriene C_4, sulfated steroids	etoposide, methotrexate	fexofenadine, morphine glucuronide
ABCC4	MRP4	kidney proximal tubule (luminal), choroid plexus, hepatocytes (sinusoidal), platelets, brain endothelia (luminal)	bile salts + GSH, cAMP, cGMP, folate, leukotriene C_4, prostanoids, sulfated steroids, urate	6-mercaptopurine, 6-thioguanine, methotrexate, topotecan	ceftizoxime, enalapril, furosemide, olmesartan, pravastatin
ABCG2	BCRP	hepatocytes (canalicular), brain endothelia (luminal), placenta, stem cells, mammary glands (lactating)	sulfated steroids	anthracyclines, epipodophyllotoxins, imatinib, methotrexate, mitoxantrone, topotecan	statins

Data compiled from [2, 9, 30–35].

Table 7.3 Examples of human genetic diseases linked to loss-of-function variants in ABC or SLC transporters.

Gene	Chromosomal location	Mendelian disorder	MIM
ABCA1	9q31.1	Tangier disease	205400
ABCA3	16p13.3	surfactant metabolism dysfunction	610921
ABCA4	1p22	Stargardt disease	248200
ABCA12	2q34	lamellar ichthyosis, type 2	601277
ABCB2/TAP1	6p21.3	bare lymphocyte syndrome, type 1	604571
ABCB3/TAP2	6p21.3	bare lymphocyte syndrome, type 1	604571
ABCB4	7q21.1	progressive familial intrahepatic cholestasis, type 3	602347
ABCB7	Xq13.3	X-linked sideroblastosis and anemia	301310
ABCB11	2q24	progressive familial intrahepatic cholestasis, type 2	601847
ABCC2	10q24	Dubin–Johnson syndrome	237500
ABCC6	16p13.1	pseudoxanthoma elasticum	264800
ABCC7/CFTR	7q31.2	cystic fibrosis	219700
ABCC8/SUR1	11p15.1	familial hyperinsulinemic hypoglycemia, type 1	265450
ABCC9	12p12.1	dilated cardiomyopathy with ventricular tachycardia	608569
ABCD1	Xq28	adrenoleukodystrophy	300100
ABCG5	2p21	sitosterolemia	210250
ABCG8	2p21	sitosterolemia	210250
SLC2A2	3q26.1–q26.2	Fanconi–Bickel syndrome	227810
SLC2A9	4p16–p15.3	hypouricemia, renal 2	612076
SLC3A1	2p16.3	cystinuria	220100
SLC5A1	22q12.3	glucose/galactose malabsorption	606824
SLC6A8	Xq28	X-linked creatine deficiency syndrome	300352
SLC10A2	13q33	bile acid malabsorption, primary	613291
SLC11A2	12q13	anemia, hypochromic microcytic	206100
SLC12A3	16q13	Gitelman syndrome	263800
SLC19A2	1q23.3	thiamine-responsive megaloblastic anemia syndrome	249270
SLC22A5	5q31.1	carnitine deficiency, systemic primary	212140
SLC22A12	11q13.1	hypouricemia, renal 1	220150
SLC26A3	7q31	congenital chloride diarrhea	126650
SLC34A3	9q34	hypophosphatemic rickets with hypercalciuria	241530
SLC35A1	6q15	congenital disorder of glycosylation, type IIf	603585
SLC37A4	11q23.3	glycogen storage disease Ib	232220
SLC40A1	2q32	autosomal dominant hemochromatosis	606069
SLC42A1/RHAG	6p21.1–p11	anemia, hemolytic, Rh-null, regulator type	268150
SLC46A1	17q11.2	folate malabsorption, hereditary	229050

Modified from [9, 29]. Chromosomal location and MIM (Mendelian Inheritance in Man) according to "Gene" and "OMIM" database, respectively, at www.ncbi.nlm.nih.gov.

Moreover, some genetic variants in hepatocanalicular ABC transporter genes increase the risk for intrahepatic cholestasis of pregnancy [50–52], acquired and drug-induced forms of cholestasis [53, 54], or cholangiocarcinoma [55].

Genome-wide association studies have become valuable tools to unravel the involvement of transporters in the development of complex disease. By this tech-

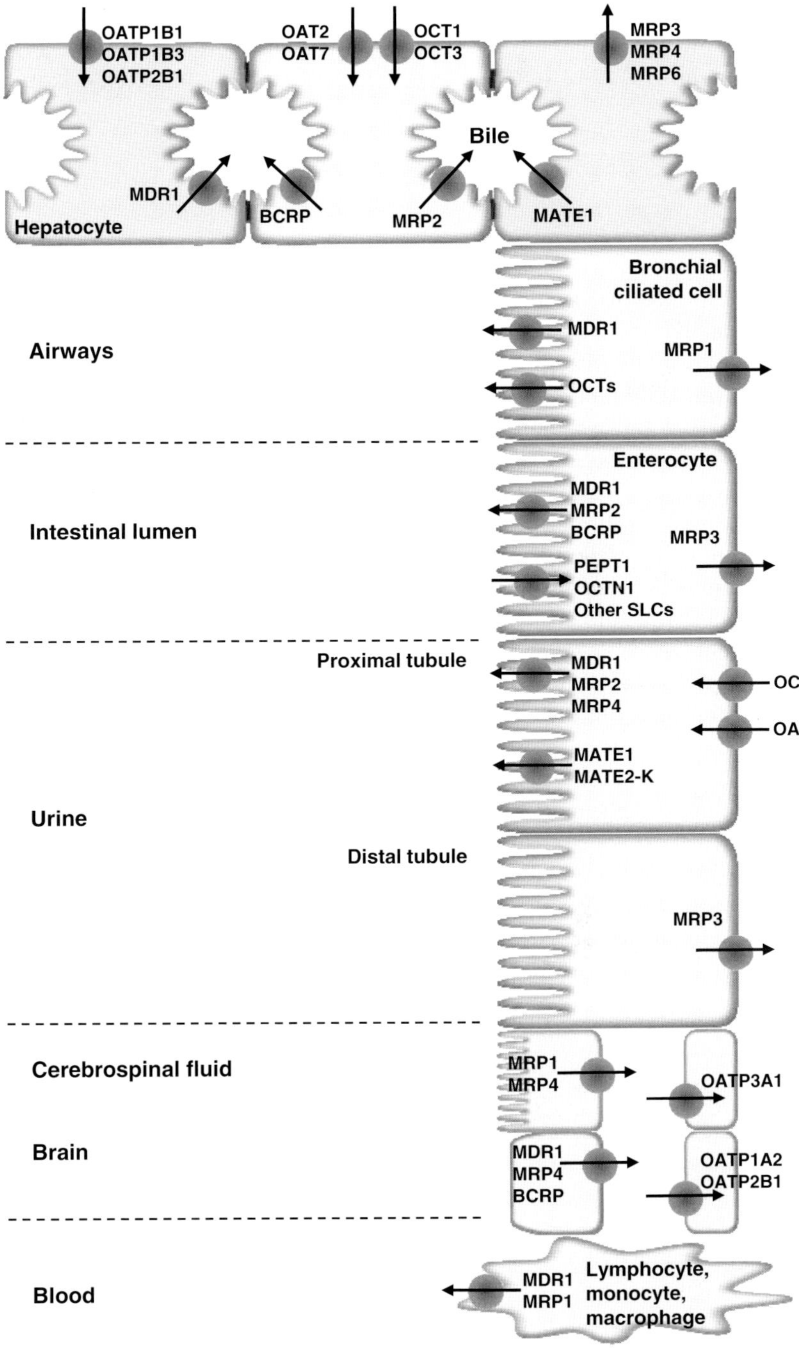

Figure 7.1 The absorption, distribution, and elimination of drugs require multiple and distinct ABC drug efflux pumps and SLC drug transporters at different tissues and organs. The most relevant ones are depicted and further discussed in the text.

nology, certain genetic variants in the *SLC22A3* (*OCT3*) gene were identified to be associated with susceptibility to prostate cancer [56] or coronary artery disease [57] and in the *SLC22A2* (*OCT2*) gene with susceptibility to chronic kidney disease [58].

7.6
Drug Transporters and Pharmacokinetics

Comprehensive microarray analyses of drug transporter expression identified a large number of human tissues expressing drug transporters [59, 60]. In the focus of research are transporters in the absorptive and secretory cells of the small intestine, liver, and kidney, because these are the major organs of drug absorption, metabolism, and excretion (Figure 7.1) [31], where they work in concert with drug-metabolizing enzymes. The combined action of uptake and efflux transporters being localized either on the apical or basolateral membrane of polarized cells thus results in transcellular substrate movement in the small intestine, liver, and kidney. Moreover, different transporters with overlapping substrate specificities are often simultaneously expressed in the same cell type. This may serve as a protective mechanism to ensure elimination of potentially harmful compounds. Mice deficient in two or more ABC transporters are a powerful tool to study the individual and combined roles of multiple transport systems [61]. In addition to localization in organs of drug absorption and elimination, transporters are also present in blood–tissue barriers where they reduce drug disposition to sanctuary tissues such as the brain, the testis, and the fetus [43]. However, these barriers may pose a great challenge for drug delivery (e.g., to brain tumors) or to treat epilepsy [62, 63]. The analysis of expression and localization of transporters in the skin or lung, for example, is of increasing interest to understand the pharmacokinetics of topically applied or inhaled drugs, respectively [2]. Moreover, knowledge of transporter expression in blood cells is of great relevance, for example, for the pharmacotherapy of hematological malignancies and of HIV infection [64].

Transporter expression can be regulated on different levels. The work by Klaassen and Aleksunes [65] gives an excellent comprehensive overview on the current knowledge of regulatory factors that influence transporter expression, including transcriptional regulation by nuclear receptors, post-translational modifications, and developmental stage.

7.6.1
Intestinal Transporters

The brush border (luminal) membrane of small intestinal enterocytes is the principal barrier that orally administered drugs as well as dietary constituents need to pass for being taken up into the body [66, 67]. Among the different transporters present in the luminal membrane is P-gp, which is the best-characterized drug-efflux pump. P-gp mainly transports neutral and cationic organic compounds (Table 7.2, [42]). Its localization in the brush border membrane of enterocytes [68] supports the notion that P-gp actively effluxes drugs back into the intestinal lumen, thereby limiting absorption and oral bioavailability of many drugs. The key role of P-gp for drug absorption was initially shown in *Mdr1a* knockout mice. For example, the oral bioavailability of paclitaxel, digoxin, and HIV protease inhibitors is markedly increased in *Mdr1a* knockout mice compared to wild-type mice [69–71]. The importance of P-gp for oral bioavailability was also demonstrated in humans (e.g., for cyclosporin and digoxin) [72, 73]. The contribution of other ABC efflux pumps such as MRP2 and BCRP, which are also localized in the brush border membrane of human enterocytes [48, 74, 75], as well as drug-metabolizing enzymes to oral bioavailability has been shown with different knockout mouse models [76, 77].

In addition to ABC efflux pumps, transcripts from several SLC transporters from different families have been detected, including *SLC15A1, SLCO1A2, SLCO2B1, SLC22A4,* and *SLC28A1* mRNA [16, 66, 67]. Luminal localization has been demonstrated, for example, for PEPT1/SLC15A1 [78] and OCTN1/SLC22A4 [79], and is discussed for SLCO transporters as well [80, 81].

7.6.2
Hepatic Transporters

Excretion into bile is a major route of elimination for many drugs and drug metabolites. Hepatobiliary elimination can be considered as a vectorial process involving several steps. The initial step is mediated by uptake transporters in the sinusoidal (basolateral) membrane of the hepatocytes. These include members of the OATP (organic anion-transporting polypeptide) family (i.e., OATP1B1, OATP1B3, OATP2B1 [32]) and of the SLC22 family (i.e., OCT1, OCT3, OAT2, OAT7 [17, 18]). Many drugs taken up by hepatocytes require a phase I cytochrome P450 (CYP)-dependent oxidation [82] (see also Chapter 2) and/or phase II conjugation (see also Chapter 3–6) before they can be excreted into bile [83], whereas other drugs remain unchanged. Several ABC transporters in the canalicular (apical) membrane mediate the final step of hepatobiliary elimination (i.e., drug or drug metabolite transport into bile). As for the enterocytes, these include P-gp, MRP2, and BCRP. Of interest, MATE1 (encoded by *SLC47A1*) was recently identified in the canalicular membrane where it may mediate the excretion of organic cations into bile in exchange for protons [84].

7.6.3
Renal Transporters

Drug secretion via the kidney may also be considered as vectorial transport involving the coordinate function of uptake transporters in the basolateral and of efflux transporters in the apical membrane of proximal tubule epithelial cells. Uptake of organic anions and organic cations from blood may be mediated by OATs and particularly OCT2, respectively, whereas drug efflux transporters in the apical membrane, such as P-gp, MRP2, MRP4, MATE1, and MATE2-K, allow for drug excretion into urine [85].

7.6.4
Transporters at the Blood–Brain Barrier

The domain-specific localization of transporters in the brain capillary endothelial cells (BCECs) is important for maintenance of the blood–brain barrier function. BCECs are not fenestrated, but closely sealed by tight junctions that prevent a paracellular exchange of solutes between blood and brain [86]. Transport of substances destined for the brain parenchymal cells hence requires their uptake across the luminal (blood-facing) membrane into the endothelial cells, their transcellular transport, and finally their efflux across the abluminal (brain-facing) membrane into the interstitial fluid. Brain uptake of essential nutrients such as glucose, amino acids, and nucleosides is ensured by several luminal uptake transporters. However, the presence of the ABC transporters P-gp, MRP4, MRP5, and BCRP, likewise located in the luminal membrane of BCECs [87–89], may limit brain penetration and efficacy of drugs for the treatment, for example, of brain tumors or epilepsy [62, 63]. The functional relevance of these ABC transporters is supported by studies with *Mdr1a*, *Mrp4*, or *Bcrp* knockout mice that have a highly increased brain penetration of drugs typically transported by these ABC efflux pumps [90–92].

7.7
Role of Drug Transporters in Chemotherapy Resistance

Cancer cells are often resistant against a large variety of structurally diverse anticancer drugs. This multidrug resistance phenotype may be caused by several different mechanisms, including the presence of drug transporters that prevent anticancer drugs from reaching target intracellular concentrations [93, 94]. An enhanced drug efflux is most often mediated by ABC transporters such as P-gp, the MRPs of the ABCC subfamily, and BCRP (Table 7.2 and [33–35, 95, 96]). Drug substrates include methotrexate, vinca alkaloids, anthracyclines (e.g., adriamycin), podophyllotoxins, taxanes (e.g., paclitaxel), inhibitors of receptor tyrosine kinases (e.g., imatinib), and camptothecins (e.g., irinotecan). As the presence of these drug efflux pumps has been shown in clinical samples from many human cancers, ABC drug transporters may indeed contribute to clinical drug resistance, although their precise role in establishing clinical drug resistance is still under investigation. Small molecules functioning as inhibitors of ABC efflux pumps may be employed to reverse and thereby overcome multidrug resistance. Third-generation reversal agents currently used in clinical trials show promising results compared to earlier-generation agents [97]. Reasons for the frequently observed failure of reversal agents are, for example, the overlapping substrate specificities of several ABC drug transporters and toxicity, which may be caused by inhibiting important physiological functions of the ABC efflux pumps [98].

Uptake transporters of the SLC superfamily that transport nutrients as physiological substrates may also accept drugs as substrates and may therefore contribute to cellular drug sensitivity (Table 7.1 and [8, 99]). For example, nucleoside transporters of the SLC28 and SLC29 family sensitize cells to nucleoside analogs (e.g., cladribine, fludarabine, gemcitabine) [19, 100] and folate transporters of the SLC19 family sensitize to methotrexate [101]. Cellular uptake of platinum drugs may be mediated by copper transporters of the SLC31 family [20] and of organic cation transporters of the SLC22 family [17, 102]. The relevance of uptake transporters for the sensitivity of cells to other anticancer drugs is not yet clear and is currently under investigation.

7.8
Pharmacogenomics of Drug Transporters: Implications for Clinical Drug Response

While inherited disorders of membrane transport have been known for many years (Section 7.5), the impact of SNPs in drug transporter genes on interindividual variability of drug response has only been recently studied and the field is growing rapidly [103, 104]. From the large number of naturally occurring genetic variants in all transporter genes, the following transporter genes are at present discussed intensively: *ABCB1*, *SLCO1B1*, *SLC22A1*, and *SLC22A2*. For more detailed discussions on pharmacogenomics of these transporters the reader is referred to recent reviews (e.g., [16, 17, 105–110]).

Only one example should be mentioned here: from the more than 100 genetic variants occurring in the *ABCB1* gene, one synonymous SNP (*c.3435C > T*, rs1045642) has received considerable attention because it was associated with altered P-gp activity and function [111]. *ABCB1 c.3435C > T* is part of a common haplotype with *c.1236C > T* and *c.2677G > T* [112]. Despite discordant results, numerous studies reported that *c.3435C > T* (alone or in combination) is associated with altered mRNA expression, *in vitro* substrate efflux from lymphocytes, pharmacokinetics of P-gp drug substrates in clinical studies, and drug response in HIV or epilepsy patients [106, 113]. The synonymous variant apparently alters kinetics of protein translation leading to a change in protein folding and function [114].

Acknowledgments

The authors' work on the importance of transporters in drug therapy is supported by the Robert-Bosch Foundation Stuttgart, IZEPHA grants **6-0-0/672** and **8-0-0/674**, the Federal Ministry for Education and Research (Berlin, Germany) grant **03 IS 2061C**, EU-ITN grant (**PITN-GA-2009-238132**), and the Sander-Stiftung (no. **2010.059.1**). We thank Dr Matthias Schwab and Dr Elke Schaeffeler for helpful discussions and valuable suggestions.

References

1 van Winkle, L.J. (1999) *Biomembrane Transport*, Academic Press, San Diego, CA.

2 Dobson, P.D. and Kell, D.B. (2008) Carrier-mediated cellular uptake of pharmaceutical drugs: an exception or the rule? *Nat. Rev. Drug Discov.*, **7**, 205–220.

3 Murphy, D.L., Fox, M.A., Timpano, K.R., Moya, P.R., Ren-Patterson, R., Andrews, A.M., Holmes, A., Lesch, K.P., and Wendland, J.R. (2008) How the serotonin story is being rewritten by new gene-based discoveries principally related to SLC6A4, the serotonin transporter gene, which functions to influence all cellular serotonin systems. *Neuropharmacology*, **55**, 932–960.

4 Landfear, S.M. (2010) Transporters for drug delivery and as drug targets in parasitic protozoa. *Clin. Pharmacol. Ther.*, **87**, 122–125.

5 Kerb, R., Fux, R., Morike, K., Kremsner, P.G., Gil, J.P., Gleiter, C.H., and Schwab, M. (2009) Pharmacogenetics of antimalarial drugs: effect on metabolism and transport. *Lancet Infect. Dis.*, **9**, 760–774.

6 Lander, E.S., Linton, L.M., Birren, B., Nusbaum, C., Zody, M.C., Baldwin, J., Devon, K., Dewar, K., Doyle, M., FitzHugh, W., Funke, R., Gage, D., Harris, K., Heaford, A., Howland, J., *et al.* (2001) Initial sequencing and analysis of the human genome. *Nature*, **409**, 860–921.

7 Venter, J.C., Adams, M.D., Myers, E.W., Li, P.W., Mural, R.J., Sutton, G.G., Smith, H.O., Yandell, M., Evans, C.A., Holt, R.A., Gocayne, J.D., Amanatides, P., Ballew, R.M., Huson, D.H., Wortman, J.R., *et al.* (2001) The sequence of the human genome. *Science*, **291**, 1304–1351.

8 Huang, Y., Anderle, P., Bussey, K.J., Barbacioru, C., Shankavaram, U., Dai, Z., Reinhold, W.C., Papp, A., Weinstein, J.N., and Sadee, W. (2004) Membrane transporters and channels: role of the transportome in cancer chemosensitivity and chemoresistance. *Cancer Res.*, **64**, 4294–4301.

9 Giacomini, K.M. and Sugiyama, Y. (2006) Membrane transporters and drug response, in *Goodman & Gilman's The Pharmacological Basis of Therapeutics* (eds L.L. Brunton, J.S. Lazo, and R.L. Parker), McGraw Hill, New York, pp. 41–70.

10 Kelland, L. (2007) The resurgence of platinum-based cancer chemotherapy. *Nat. Rev. Cancer*, **7**, 573–584.

11 Saier, M.H., Jr (2000) A functional-phylogenetic classification system for transmembrane solute transporters. *Microbiol. Mol. Biol. Rev.*, **64**, 354–411.

12 Hediger, M.A., Romero, M.F., Peng, J.B., Rolfs, A., Takanaga, H., and Bruford, E.A. (2004) The ABCs of solute carriers: physiological, pathological and therapeutic implications of human membrane transport proteins. Introduction. *Pflugers Arch.*, **447**, 465–468.

13 Fredriksson, R., Nordstrom, K.J., Stephansson, O., Hagglund, M.G., and Schioth, H.B. (2008) The solute carrier (SLC) complement of the human genome: phylogenetic classification reveals four major families. *FEBS Lett.*, **582**, 3811–3816.

14 He, L., Vasiliou, K., and Nebert, D.W. (2009) Analysis and update of the human solute carrier (SLC) gene superfamily. *Hum. Genomics*, **3**, 195–206.

15 Schlessinger, A., Matsson, P., Shima, J.E., Pieper, U., Yee, S.W., Kelly, L., Apeltsin, L., Stroud, R.M., Ferrin, T.E., Giacomini, K.M., and Sali, A. (2010) Comparison of human solute carriers. *Protein Sci.*, **19**, 412–428.

16 Zair, Z.M., Eloranta, J.J., Stieger, B., and Kullak-Ublick, G.A. (2008) Pharmacogenetics of OATP (SLC21/SLCO), OAT and OCT (SLC22) and PEPT (SLC15) transporters in the intestine, liver and kidney. *Pharmacogenomics*, **9**, 597–624.

17 Nies, A.T., Koepsell, H., Damme, K., and Schwab, M. (2011) Organic cation transporters (OCTs, MATEs), *in vitro*

and *in vivo* evidence for the importance in drug therapy, in *Drug Transporters* (eds M.F. Fromm and R.B. Kim), Springer, Berlin, pp. 105–167.

18 Burckhardt, G. and Burckhardt, B.C. (2011) *In vitro* and *in vivo* evidence of the importance of organic anion transporters (OATs) in drug therapy, in *Drug Transporters* (eds M.F. Fromm and R.B. Kim), Springer, Berlin, pp. 29–104.

19 Errasti-Murugarren, E. and Pastor-Anglada, M. (2010) Drug transporter pharmacogenetics in nucleoside-based therapies. *Pharmacogenomics*, **11**, 809–841.

20 Howell, S.B., Safaei, R., Larson, C.A., and Sailor, M.J. (2010) Copper transporters and the cellular pharmacology of the platinum-containing cancer drugs. *Mol. Pharmacol.*, **77**, 887 891.

21 Baldwin, S.A., Beal, P.R., Yao, S.Y., King, A.E., Cass, C.E., and Young, J.D. (2004) The equilibrative nucleoside transporter family, SLC29. *Pflugers Arch.*, **447**, 735–743.

22 Omote, H., Hiasa, M., Matsumoto, T., Otsuka, M., and Moriyama, Y. (2006) The MATE proteins as fundamental transporters of metabolic and xenobiotic organic cations. *Trends Pharmacol. Sci.*, **27**, 587–593.

23 Koepsell, H., Lips, K., and Volk, C. (2007) Polyspecific organic cation transporters: structure, function, physiological roles, and biopharmaceutical implications. *Pharm. Res.*, **24**, 1227–1251.

24 Morris, M.E. and Felmlee, M.A. (2008) Overview of the proton-coupled MCT (SLC16A) family of transporters: characterization, function and role in the transport of the drug of abuse gamma-hydroxybutyric acid. *AAPS J.*, **10**, 311–321.

25 Hagenbuch, B. and Gui, C. (2008) Xenobiotic transporters of the human organic anion transporting polypeptides (OATP) family. *Xenobiotica*, **38**, 778–801.

26 Rubio-Aliaga, I. and Daniel, H. (2008) Peptide transporters and their roles in physiological processes and drug disposition. *Xenobiotica*, **38**, 1022–1042.

27 Terada, T. and Inui, K.I. (2008) Physiological and pharmacokinetic roles of H^+/organic cation antiporters (MATE/SLC47A). *Biochem. Pharmacol.*, **75**, 1689–1696.

28 Merezhinskaya, N. and Fishbein, W.N. (2009) Monocarboxylate transporters: past, present, and future. *Histol. Histopathol.*, **24**, 243–264.

29 Dean, M. and Annilo, T. (2005) Evolution of the ATP-binding cassette (ABC) transporter superfamily in vertebrates. *Annu. Rev. Genomics Hum. Genet.*, **6**, 123–142.

30 Nies, A.T. and Keppler, D. (2007) The apical conjugate efflux pump ABCC2 (MRP2). *Pflugers Arch.*, **453**, 643–659.

31 Giacomini, K.M., Huang, S.M., Tweedie, D.J., Benet, L.Z., Brouwer, K.L., Chu, X., Dahlin, A., Evers, R., Fischer, V., Hillgren, K.M., Hoffmaster, K.A., Ishikawa, T., Keppler, D., Kim, R.B., Lee, C.A., *et al.* (2010) Membrane transporters in drug development. *Nat. Rev. Drug Discov.*, **9**, 215–236.

32 Nies, A.T., Schwab, M., and Keppler, D. (2008) Interplay of conjugating enzymes with OATP uptake transporters and ABCC/MRP efflux pumps in the elimination of drugs. *Expert Opin. Drug Metab. Toxicol.*, **4**, 545–568.

33 Deeley, R.G., Westlake, C., and Cole, S.P. (2006) Transmembrane transport of endo- and xenobiotics by mammalian ATP-binding cassette multidrug resistance proteins. *Physiol. Rev.*, **86**, 849–899.

34 Szakacs, G., Paterson, J.K., Ludwig, J.A., Booth-Genthe, C., and Gottesman, M.M. (2006) Targeting multidrug resistance in cancer. *Nat. Rev. Drug Discov.*, **5**, 219–234.

35 Keppler, D. (2011) Multidrug resistance proteins (MRPs, ABCCs): importance for pathophysiology and drug therapy, in *Drug Transporters* (eds M.F. Fromm and R.B. Kim), Springer, Berlin, pp. 299–323.

36 Riordan, J.R. (2008) CFTR function and prospects for therapy. *Annu. Rev. Biochem.*, **77**, 701–726.

37 Loo, T.W., Bartlett, M.C., and Clarke, D.M. (2005) Rescue of folding defects in ABC transporters using pharmacological

chaperones. *J. Bioenerg. Biomembr.*, **37**, 501–507.

38 Welsh, M.J. (2010) Targeting the basic defect in cystic fibrosis. *N. Engl. J. Med.*, **363**, 2056–2057.

39 Stapelbroek, J.M., van Erpecum, K.J., Klomp, L.W., and Houwen, R.H. (2010) Liver disease associated with canalicular transport defects: current and future therapies. *J. Hepatol.*, **52**, 258–271.

40 Davit-Spraul, A., Gonzales, E., Baussan, C., and Jacquemin, E. (2010) The spectrum of liver diseases related to ABCB4 gene mutations: pathophysiology and clinical aspects. *Semin. Liver Dis.*, **30**, 134–146.

41 Stieger, B. (2011) The role of the sodium-taurocholate cotransporting polypeptide (NTCP) and of the bile salt export pump (BSEP) in physiology and pathophysiology of bile formation, in *Drug Transporters* (eds M.F. Fromm and R.B. Kim), Springer, Berlin, pp. 205–259.

42 Ambudkar, S.V., Kimchi-Sarfaty, C., Sauna, Z.E., and Gottesman, M.M. (2003) P-glycoprotein: from genomics to mechanism. *Oncogene*, **22**, 7468–7485.

43 Leslie, E.M., Deeley, R.G., and Cole, S.P. (2005) Multidrug resistance proteins: role of P-glycoprotein, MRP1, MRP2, and BCRP (ABCG2) in tissue defense. *Toxicol. Appl. Pharmacol.*, **204**, 216–237.

44 Brant, S.R., Panhuysen, C.I., Nicolae, D., Reddy, D.M., Bonen, D.K., Karaliukas, R., Zhang, L., Swanson, E., Datta, L.W., Moran, T., Ravenhill, G., Duerr, R.H., Achkar, J.P., Karban, A.S., and Cho, J.H. (2003) MDR1 Ala893 polymorphism is associated with inflammatory bowel disease. *Am. J. Hum. Genet.*, **73**, 1282–1292.

45 Schwab, M., Schaeffeler, E., Marx, C., Fromm, M.F., Kaskas, B., Metzler, J., Stange, E., Herfarth, H., Schoelmerich, J., Gregor, M., Walker, S., Cascorbi, I., Roots, I., Brinkmann, U., Zanger, U.M., *et al.* (2003) Association between the C3435T MDR1 gene polymorphism and susceptibility for ulcerative colitis. *Gastroenterology*, **124**, 26–33.

46 Potocnik, U., Ferkolj, I., Glavac, D., and Dean, M. (2004) Polymorphisms in multidrug resistance 1 (MDR1) gene are associated with refractory Crohn disease and ulcerative colitis. *Genes Immun.*, **5**, 530–539.

47 Siegsmund, M., Brinkmann, U., Schaffeler, E., Weirich, G., Schwab, M., Eichelbaum, M., Fritz, P., Burk, O., Decker, J., Alken, P., Rothenpieler, U., Kerb, R., Hoffmeyer, S., and Brauch, H. (2002) Association of the P-glycoprotein transporter MDR1(C3435T) polymorphism with the susceptibility to renal epithelial tumors. *J. Am. Soc. Nephrol.*, **13**, 1847–1854.

48 Maliepaard, M., Scheffer, G.L., Faneyte, I.F., van Gastelen, M.A., Pijnenborg, A.C., Schinkel, A.H., van de Vijver, M.J., Scheper, R.J., and Schellens, J.H. (2001) Subcellular localization and distribution of the breast cancer resistance protein transporter in normal human tissues. *Cancer Res.*, **61**, 3458–3464.

49 Korenaga, Y., Naito, K., Okayama, N., Hirata, H., Suehiro, Y., Hamanaka, Y., Matsuyama, H., and Hinoda, Y. (2005) Association of the BCRP C421A polymorphism with nonpapillary renal cell carcinoma. *Int. J. Cancer*, **117**, 431–434.

50 Savander, M., Ropponen, A., Avela, K., Weerasekera, N., Cormand, B., Hirvioja, M.L., Riikonen, S., Ylikorkala, O., Lehesjoki, A.E., Williamson, C., and Aittomaki, K. (2003) Genetic evidence of heterogeneity in intrahepatic cholestasis of pregnancy. *Gut*, **52**, 1025–1029.

51 Pauli-Magnus, C., Lang, T., Meier, Y., Zodan-Marin, T., Jung, D., Breymann, C., Zimmermann, R., Kenngott, S., Beuers, U., Reichel, C., Kerb, R., Penger, A., Meier, P.J., and Kullak-Ublick, G.A. (2004) Sequence analysis of bile salt export pump (ABCB11) and multidrug resistance P-glycoprotein 3 (ABCB4, MDR3) in patients with intrahepatic cholestasis of pregnancy. *Pharmacogenetics*, **14**, 91–102.

52 Dixon, P.H., van Mil, S.W., Chambers, J., Strautnieks, S., Thompson, R.J., Lammert, F., Kubitz, R., Keitel, V., Glantz, A., Mattsson, L.A., Marschall, H.U., Molokhia, M., Moore, G.E., Linton, K.J., and Williamson, C. (2009) Contribution of variant alleles of ABCB11 to susceptibility to intrahepatic

cholestasis of pregnancy. *Gut*, **58**, 537–544.
53 Meier, Y., Pauli-Magnus, C., Zanger, U.M., Klein, K., Schaeffeler, E., Nussler, A.K., Nussler, N., Eichelbaum, M., Meier, P.J., and Stieger, B. (2006) Interindividual variability of canalicular ATP-binding-cassette (ABC)-transporter expression in human liver. *Hepatology*, **44**, 62–74.
54 Lang, C., Meier, Y., Stieger, B., Beuers, U., Lang, T., Kerb, R., Kullak-Ublick, G.A., Meier, P.J., and Pauli-Magnus, C. (2007) Mutations and polymorphisms in the bile salt export pump and the multidrug resistance protein 3 associated with drug-induced liver injury. *Pharmacogenet. Genomics*, **17**, 47–60.
55 Hoblinger, A., Grunhage, F., Sauerbruch, T., and Lammert, F. (2009) Association of the c.3972C>T variant of the multidrug resistance-associated protein 2 gene (MRP2/ABCC2) with susceptibility to bile duct cancer. *Digestion*, **80**, 36–39.
56 Eeles, R.A., Kote-Jarai, Z., Giles, G.G., Olama, A.A., Guy, M., Jugurnauth, S.K., Mulholland, S., Leongamornlert, D.A., Edwards, S.M., Morrison, J., Field, H.I., Southey, M.C., Severi, G., Donovan, J.L., Hamdy, F.C., *et al.* (2008) Multiple newly identified loci associated with prostate cancer susceptibility. *Nat. Genet.*, **40**, 316–321.
57 Tregouet, D.A., Konig, I.R., Erdmann, J., Munteanu, A., Braund, P.S., Hall, A.S., Grosshennig, A., Linsel-Nitschke, P., Perret, C., DeSuremain, M., Meitinger, T., Wright, B.J., Preuss, M., Balmforth, A.J., Ball, S.G., *et al.* (2009) Genome-wide haplotype association study identifies the SLC22A3–LPAL2–LPA gene cluster as a risk locus for coronary artery disease. *Nat. Genet.*, **41**, 283–285.
58 Kottgen, A., Pattaro, C., Boger, C.A., Fuchsberger, C., Olden, M., Glazer, N.L., Parsa, A., Gao, X., Yang, Q., Smith, A.V., O'Connell, J.R., Li, M., Schmidt, H., Tanaka, T., Isaacs, A., *et al.* (2010) New loci associated with kidney function and chronic kidney disease. *Nat. Genet.*, **42**, 376–384.
59 Nishimura, M. and Naito, S. (2005) Tissue-specific mRNA expression profiles of human ATP-binding cassette and solute carrier transporter superfamilies. *Drug Metab. Pharmacokinet.*, **20**, 452–477.
60 Bleasby, K., Castle, J.C., Roberts, C.J., Cheng, C., Bailey, W.J., Sina, J.F., Kulkarni, A.V., Hafey, M.J., Evers, R., Johnson, J.M., Ulrich, R.G., and Slatter, J.G. (2006) Expression profiles of 50 xenobiotic transporter genes in humans and pre-clinical species: a resource for investigations into drug disposition. *Xenobiotica*, **36**, 963–988.
61 Lagas, J.S., Vlaming, M.L., and Schinkel, A.H. (2009) Pharmacokinetic assessment of multiple ATP-binding cassette transporters: the power of combination knockout mice. *Mol. Interv.*, **9**, 136–145.
62 Nies, A.T. (2007) The role of membrane transporters in drug delivery to brain tumors. *Cancer Lett.*, **254**, 11–29.
63 Potschka, H. (2010) Transporter hypothesis of drug-resistant epilepsy: challenges for pharmacogenetic approaches. *Pharmacogenomics*, **11**, 1427–1438.
64 Köck, K., Grube, M., Jedlitschky, G., Oevermann, L., Siegmund, W., Ritter, C.A., and Kroemer, H.K. (2007) Expression of adenosine triphosphate-binding cassette (ABC) drug transporters in peripheral blood cells: relevance for physiology and pharmacotherapy. *Clin. Pharmacokinet.*, **46**, 449–470.
65 Klaassen, C.D. and Aleksunes, L.M. (2010) Xenobiotic, bile acid, and cholesterol transporters: function and regulation. *Pharmacol. Rev.*, **62**, 1–96.
66 Oostendorp, R.L., Beijnen, J.H., and Schellens, J.H. (2009) The biological and clinical role of drug transporters at the intestinal barrier. *Cancer Treat. Rev.*, **35**, 137–147.
67 Shugarts, S. and Benet, L.Z. (2009) The role of transporters in the pharmacokinetics of orally administered drugs. *Pharm. Res.*, **26**, 2039–2054.
68 Cordon-Cardo, C., O'Brien, J.P., Boccia, J., Casals, D., Bertino, J.R., and Melamed, M.R. (1990) Expression of the multidrug resistance gene product

(P-glycoprotein) in human normal and tumor tissues. *J. Histochem. Cytochem.*, **38**, 1277–1287.

69 Sparreboom, A., van Asperen, J., Mayer, U., Schinkel, A.H., Smit, J.W., Meijer, D.K., Borst, P., Nooijen, W.J., Beijnen, J.H., and van Tellingen, O. (1997) Limited oral bioavailability and active epithelial excretion of paclitaxel (Taxol) caused by P-glycoprotein in the intestine. *Proc. Natl. Acad. Sci. USA*, **94**, 2031–2035.

70 Schinkel, A.H., Wagenaar, E., van Deemter, L., Mol, C.A., and Borst, P. (1995) Absence of the mdr1a P-Glycoprotein in mice affects tissue distribution and pharmacokinetics of dexamethasone, digoxin, and cyclosporin A. *J. Clin. Invest.*, **96**, 1698–1705.

71 Kim, R.B., Fromm, M.F., Wandel, C., Leake, B., Wood, A.J., Roden, D.M., and Wilkinson, G.R. (1998) The drug transporter P-glycoprotein limits oral absorption and brain entry of HIV-1 protease inhibitors. *J. Clin. Invest.*, **101**, 289–294.

72 Drescher, S., Glaeser, H., Murdter, T., Hitzl, M., Eichelbaum, M., and Fromm, M.F. (2003) P-glycoprotein-mediated intestinal and biliary digoxin transport in humans. *Clin. Pharmacol. Ther.*, **73**, 223–231.

73 Lown, K.S., Mayo, R.R., Leichtman, A.B., Hsiao, H.L., Turgeon, D.K., Schmiedlin-Ren, P., Brown, M.B., Guo, W., Rossi, S.J., Benet, L.Z., and Watkins, P.B. (1997) Role of intestinal P-glycoprotein (mdr1) in interpatient variation in the oral bioavailability of cyclosporine. *Clin. Pharmacol. Ther.*, **62**, 248–260.

74 Fromm, M.F., Kauffmann, H.M., Fritz, P., Burk, O., Kroemer, H.K., Warzok, R.W., Eichelbaum, M., Siegmund, W., and Schrenk, D. (2000) The effect of rifampin treatment on intestinal expression of human MRP transporters. *Am. J. Pathol.*, **157**, 1575–1580.

75 Sandusky, G.E., Mintze, K.S., Pratt, S.E., and Dantzig, A.H. (2002) Expression of multidrug resistance-associated protein 2 (MRP2) in normal human tissues and carcinomas using tissue microarrays. *Histopathology*, **41**, 65–74.

76 Marchetti, S., de Vries, N.A., Buckle, T., Bolijn, M.J., van Eijndhoven, M.A., Beijnen, J.H., Mazzanti, R., van Tellingen, O., and Schellens, J.H. (2008) Effect of the ATP-binding cassette drug transporters ABCB1, ABCG2, and ABCC2 on erlotinib hydrochloride (Tarceva) disposition in *in vitro* and *in vivo* pharmacokinetic studies employing Bcrp1$^{-/-}$/Mdr1a/1b$^{-/-}$ (triple-knockout) and wild-type mice. *Mol. Cancer Ther.*, **7**, 2280–2287.

77 van Waterschoot, R.A., Lagas, J.S., Wagenaar, E., Rosing, H., Beijnen, J.H., and Schinkel, A.H. (2010) Individual and combined roles of CYP3A, P-glycoprotein (MDR1/ABCB1) and MRP2 (ABCC2) in the pharmacokinetics of docetaxel. *Int. J. Cancer*, **127**, 2959–2964.

78 Groneberg, D.A., Doring, F., Eynott, P.R., Fischer, A., and Daniel, H. (2001) Intestinal peptide transport: *ex vivo* uptake studies and localization of peptide carrier PEPT1. *Am. J. Physiol. Gastrointest. Liver Physiol.*, **281**, G697–G704.

79 Sugiura, T., Kato, S., Shimizu, T., Wakayama, T., Nakamichi, N., Kubo, Y., Iwata, D., Suzuki, K., Soga, T., Asano, M., Iseki, S., Tamai, I., Tsuji, A., and Kato, Y. (2010) Functional expression of carnitine/organic cation transporter OCTN1/SLC22A4 in mouse small intestine and liver. *Drug Metab. Dispos.*, **38**, 1665–1672.

80 Kobayashi, D., Nozawa, T., Imai, K., Nezu, J., Tsuji, A., and Tamai, I. (2003) Involvement of human organic anion transporting polypeptide OATP-B (SLC21A9) in pH-dependent transport across intestinal apical membrane. *J. Pharmacol. Exp. Ther.*, **306**, 703–708.

81 Glaeser, H., Bailey, D.G., Dresser, G.K., Gregor, J.C., Schwarz, U.I., McGrath, J.S., Jolicoeur, E., Lee, W., Leake, B.F., Tirona, R.G., and Kim, R.B. (2007) Intestinal drug transporter expression and the impact of grapefruit juice in humans. *Clin. Pharmacol. Ther.*, **81**, 362–370.

82 Zanger, U.M., Turpeinen, M., Klein, K., and Schwab, M. (2008) Functional pharmacogenetics/genomics of human

cytochromes P450 involved in drug biotransformation. *Anal. Bioanal. Chem.*, **392**, 1093–1108.

83 Keppler, D. (2005) Uptake and efflux transporters for conjugates in human hepatocytes. *Methods Enzymol.*, **400**, 531–542.

84 Otsuka, M., Matsumoto, T., Morimoto, R., Arioka, S., Omote, H., and Moriyama, Y. (2005) A human transporter protein that mediates the final excretion step for toxic organic cations. *Proc. Natl. Acad. Sci. USA*, **102**, 17923–17928.

85 Feng, B., LaPerle, J.L., Chang, G., and Varma, M.V. (2010) Renal clearance in drug discovery and development: molecular descriptors, drug transporters and disease state. *Expert Opin. Drug Metab. Toxicol.*, **6**, 939–952.

86 Rubin, L.L. and Staddon, J.M. (1999) The cell biology of the blood–brain barrier. *Annu. Rev. Neurosci.*, **22**, 11–28.

87 Cordon-Cardo, C., O'Brien, J.P., Casals, D., Rittman-Grauer, L., Biedler, J.L., Melamed, M.R., and Bertino, J.R. (1989) Multidrug-resistance gene (P-glycoprotein) is expressed by endothelial cells at blood–brain barrier sites. *Proc. Natl. Acad. Sci. USA*, **86**, 695–698.

88 Nies, A.T., Jedlitschky, G., König, J., Herold-Mende, C., Steiner, H.H., Schmitt, H.P., and Keppler, D. (2004) Expression and immunolocalization of the multidrug resistance proteins, MRP1–MRP6 (ABCC1–ABCC6), in human brain. *Neuroscience*, **129**, 349–360.

89 Cooray, H.C., Blackmore, C.G., Maskell, L., and Barrand, M.A. (2002) Localisation of breast cancer resistance protein in microvessel endothelium of human brain. *Neuroreport*, **13**, 2059–2063.

90 Schinkel, A.H. (1999) P-glycoprotein, a gatekeeper in the blood–brain barrier. *Adv. Drug Deliv. Rev.*, **36**, 179–194.

91 Leggas, M., Adachi, M., Scheffer, G.L., Sun, D., Wielinga, P., Du, G., Mercer, K.E., Zhuang, Y., Panetta, J.C., Johnston, B., Scheper, R.J., Stewart, C.F., and Schuetz, J.D. (2004) Mrp4 confers resistance to topotecan and protects the brain from chemotherapy. *Mol. Cell. Biol.*, **24**, 7612–7621.

92 de Vries, N.A., Zhao, J., Kroon, E., Buckle, T., Beijnen, J.H., and van Tellingen, O. (2007) P-glycoprotein and breast cancer resistance protein: two dominant transporters working together in limiting the brain penetration of topotecan. *Clin. Cancer Res.*, **13**, 6440–6449.

93 Gottesman, M.M. (2002) Mechanisms of cancer drug resistance. *Annu. Rev. Med.*, **53**, 615–627.

94 Baguley, B.C. (2010) Multidrug resistance in cancer. *Methods Mol. Biol.*, **596**, 1–14.

95 Nies, A.T., Rius, M., and Keppler, D. (2007) Multidrug resistance proteins of the ABCC subfamily, in *Drug Transporters: Molecular Characterization and Role in Drug Disposition* (eds G. You and M.E. Morris), John Wiley & Sons, Inc, Hoboken, NJ, pp. 263–318.

96 Robey, R.W., To, K.K., Polgar, O., Dohse, M., Fetsch, P., Dean, M., and Bates, S.E. (2009) ABCG2: a perspective. *Adv. Drug Deliv. Rev.*, **61**, 3–13.

97 Lee, C.H. (2010) Reversing agents for ATP-binding cassette drug transporters. *Methods Mol. Biol.*, **596**, 325–340.

98 Sharom, F.J. (2008) ABC multidrug transporters: structure, function and role in chemoresistance. *Pharmacogenomics*, **9**, 105–127.

99 Okabe, M., Szakacs, G., Reimers, M.A., Suzuki, T., Hall, M.D., Abe, T., Weinstein, J.N., and Gottesman, M.M. (2008) Profiling SLCO and SLC22 genes in the NCI-60 cancer cell lines to identify drug uptake transporters. *Mol. Cancer Ther.*, **7**, 3081–3091.

100 Damaraju, V.L., Sawyer, M.B., Mackey, J.R., Young, J.D., and Cass, C.E. (2009) Human nucleoside transporters: biomarkers for response to nucleoside drugs. *Nucleosides Nucleotides Nucleic Acids*, **28**, 450–463.

101 Ganapathy, V., Smith, S.B., and Prasad, P.D. (2004) SLC19: the folate/thiamine transporter family. *Pflugers Arch.*, **447**, 641–646.

102 More, S.S., Li, S., Yee, S.W., Chen, L., Xu, Z., Jablons, D.M., and Giacomini, K.M. (2010) Organic cation transporters

modulate the uptake and cytotoxicity of picoplatin, a third-generation platinum analogue. *Mol. Cancer Ther.*, **9**, 1058–1069.

103 Kroetz, D.L., Yee, S.W., and Giacomini, K.M. (2010) The pharmacogenomics of membrane transporters project: research at the interface of genomics and transporter pharmacology. *Clin. Pharmacol. Ther.*, **87**, 109–116.

104 Yee, S.W., Chen, L., and Giacomini, K.M. (2010) Pharmacogenomics of membrane transporters: past, present and future. *Pharmacogenomics*, **11**, 475–479.

105 Kerb, R. (2006) Implications of genetic polymorphisms in drug transporters for pharmacotherapy. *Cancer Lett.*, **234**, 4–33.

106 Chinn, L.W. and Kroetz, D.L. (2007) ABCB1 pharmacogenetics: progress, pitfalls, and promise. *Clin. Pharmacol. Ther.*, **81**, 265–269.

107 Kalliokoski, A. and Niemi, M. (2009) Impact of OATP transporters on pharmacokinetics. *Br. J. Pharmacol.*, **158**, 693–705.

108 Franke, R.M., Gardner, E.R., and Sparreboom, A. (2010) Pharmacogenetics of drug transporters. *Curr. Pharm. Des.*, **16**, 220–230.

109 Cascorbi, I. (2011) P-glycoprotein: tissue distribution, substrates, and functional consequences of genetic variations, in *Drug Transporters* (eds M.F. Fromm and R.B. Kim), Springer, Berlin, pp. 261–283.

110 König, J. (2011) Uptake transporters of the human OATP family: molecular characteristics, substrates, their role in drug–drug interactions, and functional consequences of polymorphisms, in *Drug Transporters* (eds M.F. Fromm and R.B. Kim), Springer, Berlin, pp. 1–28.

111 Hoffmeyer, S., Burk, O., von Richter, O., Arnold, H.P., Brockmöller, J., Johne, A., Cascorbi, I., Gerloff, T., Roots, I., Eichelbaum, M., and Brinkmann, U. (2000) Functional polymorphisms of the human multidrug-resistance gene: multiple sequence variations and correlation of one allele with P-glycoprotein expression and activity *in vivo*. *Proc. Natl. Acad. Sci. USA*, **97**, 3473–3478.

112 Kim, R.B., Leake, B.F., Choo, E.F., Dresser, G.K., Kubba, S.V., Schwarz, U.I., Taylor, A., Xie, H.G., McKinsey, J., Zhou, S., Lan, L.B., Schuetz, J.D., Schuetz, E.G., and Wilkinson, G.R. (2001) Identification of functionally variant MDR1 alleles among European Americans and African Americans. *Clin. Pharmacol. Ther.*, **70**, 189–199.

113 Kerb, R. and Schwab, M. (2010) ADME pharmacogenetics and its impact on drug–drug interactions, in *Enzyme- and Transporter-Based Drug–Drug Interactions: Progress and Future Challenges* (eds K.S. Pang, A.D. Rodrigues, and R.M. Peter), Springer, New York, pp. 51–74.

114 Kimchi-Sarfaty, C., Oh, J.M., Kim, I.W., Sauna, Z.E., Calcagno, A.M., Ambudkar, S.V., and Gottesman, M.M. (2007) A "silent" polymorphism in the MDR1 gene changes substrate specificity. *Science*, **315**, 525–528.

8
Transcriptional Regulation of Human Drug-Metabolizing Cytochrome P450 Enzymes

Zdenek Dvorak

8.1
Factors Affecting Drug-Metabolizing Cytochromes P450

Human drug-metabolizing cytochromes P450 (cytochrome P450CYPs) comprise the CYP1, CYP2, and CYP3 families. The activities of CYPs are regulated by several mechanisms, determined by various factors and/or influenced by many stimuli. The expression and activity of CYPs is influenced by environmental and genetic factors, and depends also on the physiological and pathophysiological status of the organism. The resulting activity of individual CYP isoforms is therefore a combination of all of the different factors and mechanism, and it is often difficult to predict the real and effective CYP activity *in vivo* in every individual. The aim of this chapter is to summarize our knowledge on the transcriptional regulation of drug-metabolizing CYP expression in man.

8.1.1
Genetic Polymorphism

An important genetic factor influencing the activity of drug-metabolizing CYPs is gene polymorphism [1]. The most prominent and clinically important is polymorphism of CYP2D6, formerly called spartein-debrisoquine polymorphism [2, 3]. The impact of this polymorphism is altered pharmacokinetics of the drugs metabolized by CYP2D6 and we distinguish so-called ultrarapid metabolizers (duplicated gene) or slow metabolizers (mutated gene). Similarly, gene polymorphism of CYP2C19 is responsible for diminished capability of the body to metabolize CYP2C19 substrates such as *S*-mephenytoin. The main CYP2C19 polymorphisms are mutations CYP2C19m1 (in exon 5) and CYP2C19m2 (in exon 4), leading to the absence of the protein or truncated inactive protein, respectively [4, 5]. While it was though in the past that polymorphism of CYP3A5 does not have any significant clinical or epidemiological impact, since its substrate specificity is identical to that of CYP3A4, recent studies show that CYP3A5 polymorphism is responsible for altered pharmacokinetics of several drugs (e.g., tacrolimus) [6, 7]. Another example of CYP gene polymorphism is the CYP1A1 mutation in the 3′-noncoding region

Metabolism of Drugs and Other Xenobiotics, First Edition. Edited by Pavel Anzenbacher, Ulrich M. Zanger.

and in exon 7 that increases the activity of the enzyme after induction. This polymorphism represents an increased risk of lung cancer for Japanese, but not Caucasian populations [8, 9]. Overall, genetic polymorphism of CYPs varies between different races and also within races, representing a great challenge for personalized and rationalized pharmacotherapy.

8.1.2
Physiological and Pathophysiological Factors

The expression and activity of drug-metabolizing enzymes is affected by a variety of physiological factors, such as age [10], sex [11, 12], pregnancy [13], and menstrual cycle [14]. Many pathophysiological states such as inflammation [15, 16], infection [17–19], cancer [20–22], and diabetes [23, 24] also drastically alter the expression of drug-metabolizing CYPs. For detailed reviews, see the cited references.

8.1.3
Environmental Factors

The effects of environmental chemicals, physical factors (UV light, radiation), and microbial agents (viruses, bacteria, parasites) may ultimately affect the expression and activity of biotransformation enzymes. The molecular basis of the influence of environmental factors on CYP gene expression comprises common mechanisms and studying environmental factors as a whole is rather an epidemiological discipline [25].

The majority of drug–drug interactions are caused by inhibition of one or several CYPs by xenobiotics (drug, food constituent, toxin, etc.). There are plenty of reviews on CYP inhibition in the literature [26–28] and this is not the primary focus of the current chapter.

8.2
Transcriptional Regulation of CYP

Gene induction is a complex process that begins usually by binding of a small molecule, a ligand (drug, hormone), to a receptor (regulatory protein), which ultimately results in the expression functional protein (CYP enzyme). The whole process also comprises receptor conformation change, dissociation of multiprotein complexes, receptor translocation from the cytosol to nucleus, recruitment of coactivators, binding to DNA, mRNA synthesis, post-transcriptional modifications, translation of mRNA to protein, post-translational processing, and sometimes receptor protein degradation by the proteasome–ubiquitin system. These processes are differentially involved in the regulation of drug-metabolizing CYPs. For example, proteasome-mediated degradation of CYP1B1 [29], CYP2B [30], CYP2E1 [31, 32], and CYP3A4 [33, 34] proteins, post-translational regulation of

CYP2E1 [35, 36], or post-transcriptional regulation of CYP1A1 [37–39], CYP1A2 [40–42], and CYP2E1 [43] have described.

8.2.1
Xenoreceptors, and Steroid and Nuclear Receptors

A breakpoint in the understanding of the regulation of drug-metabolizing enzymes was the discovery of so-called xenoreceptors (xenobiotic sensors or xenosensors), initially considered as orphan receptors.

8.2.1.1 Aryl Hydrocarbon Receptor

The aryl hydrocarbon receptor (AhR) was the first xenoreceptor discovered [44]. It is also called the dioxin receptor, since it is activated by both polyaromatic hydrocarbons (polycyclic aromatic hydrocarbons (PAHs)) and dioxin compounds [45]. Based on the classical endocrinology concept, AhR is not a receptor, but a ligand-activated transcriptional factor. A variety of xenobiotics are exogenous ligands of AhR, including synthetic organic compounds such as polyaromatic amines, PAHs, polychlorinated aromatic compounds, dioxins [46], SP600125 [47–49], and U0126 [50], natural compounds such as resveratrol [47, 48, 51], berberine [52], and flavonoids [53–56], and drugs such as omeprazole [57–59], lansoprazole [60, 61], and TSU-16 [62]. While AhR was considered for many years as an orphan, a number of endogenous AhR ligands have been identified to date and AhR has been "deorphanized" [46, 63]. Endogenous AhR ligands include bilirubin [64], biliverdin [65], indirubin [66], indole and tryptophan derivatives [67, 68], and arachidonic acid derivatives [69–72]. Until the identification of endogenous ligands, AhR was believed to be only responsible for the induction of biotransformation enzymes such as CYP1A1, CYP1A2, CYP1B1, glutathione *S*-transferases (GSTs), UDP-glucuronosyltransferases (UGTs), and NADHP reductase [73]. Recognition of endogenous AhR ligands helped to understand the physiological roles of AhR. Indeed, it is now clear that AhR plays various endogenous functions [74], such as regulating the cell cycle and proliferation [75, 76], immune response [77–79], circadian rhythm [80], tumor promotion [81, 82], expression of lipid metabolism genes [83, 84], and so on. Examples of AhR-driven genes other than drug-metabolizing genes include the AhR repressor, transforming growth factor-β, p27, interleukin-1β, Jun, and Bax. Surprisingly, AhR was shown to be a ubiquitin-E3 ligase involved in the process of protein degradation, including AhR itself [85, 86]. Regarding molecular functions of AhR, in its resting state it is sequestered in the cytosol in a multiprotein complex with the heat shock protein hsp90 and other proteins. When the lipophilic ligand penetrates the cell membrane, it binds to AhR, which in turn translocates to the nucleus, where it forms a heterodimer with the AhR nuclear translocator (aryl hydrocarbon receptor nuclear translocatorARNT) [87–91]. The AhR/ARNT heterodimer then binds to a specific DNA sequence called the dioxin-responsive element (DRE) or xenobiotic-responsive element (XRE) (consensus sequence 5′-T/GNGCGTGA/CG/CA-3′; core sequence 5′-GCGTG-3′) in the promoter and triggers the expression of target genes [45, 87].

Finally, AhR undergoes nuclear export followed by proteasome–5′-ubiquitin-dependent degradation, serving as a negative feedback [92–94].

8.2.1.2 Pregnane X Receptor

The role of the pregnane X receptor (PXR; NR1I2) in the expression of drug-metabolizing enzymes was first determined in 1998 by Kliewer and Lehmann [95, 96], who were followed by others [97–100]. Soon after, the crystal structure of PXR alone or in complex with several ligands was elucidated and the PXR boom began [101, 102]. PXR is a nuclear receptor that is transcriptionally active in the form of a heterodimer with retinoic X receptor (RXR)-α (NR2B1), PXR/RXR-α, that binds to a core AGGTCA-like sequence having various structural motives (DR-3, DR-4, ER-6, IR-6) [103–105]. Specific interaction between ligands and PXR is promoted by steroid receptor coactivator (SRC)-1 [45, 106]. Activators (ligands) of PXR are diverse xenochemicals [107, 108], including drugs, herbal medicines [109], antiestrogens [110], and environmental pollutants such as phthalates [111, 112]. Activation of PXR by drugs is often a cause of drug–drug interactions. Examples of drugs that activate PXR are the antibiotic rifampicin [97], azole antimycotics [113], anticonvulsives carbamazepine, phenytoin [114] or valproic acid [115], benzodiazepines midazolam and medazepam [116], calcium channel blocker nifedipine [117], and so on. PXR controls the expression of the CYP2A6, CYP2B6, CYP2C, and CYP3A subfamilies [104], as well as the expression of some phase II enzymes [118–121] and transporters [122–126]. PXR also has many endogenous functions; it regulates metabolism of lipids, carbohydrates, cholesterol, and bile acids [127–133]. Apart from detoxification genes, PXR regulates the expression of apolipoprotein A1 or high-density lipoprotein [134, 135]. There are also some consistent findings on putative PXR endogenous ligands such as vitamin E [136, 137], vitamin K [138], β-carotene [139], or bile acids [140, 141].

8.2.1.3 Constitutive Androstane Receptor

The Constitutive androstane receptor (CAR; NR1I3, sometimes referred as the constitutively activated receptor) was recognized as a regulator of expression of drug-metabolizing enzymes at the same time as PXR [142, 143]. Unlike PXR, CAR is located in the cytosol in complex with hsp90 [144] and it undergoes cytosol-to-nucleus translocation upon activation by activators such as phenobarbital [145]. The majority of activators activate CAR indirectly and the mechanism of CAR activation is not yet fully understood [146]. It probably involves several protein phosphatases [144, 147]. Transcriptionally active CAR binds its DNA sequences (similar or identical to that of PXR) [148] in the form of a CAR/RXR heterodimer [149]. While SRC-1 promotes CAR transcriptional activity, another transcription factor SHP represses CAR [150]. There are only isolated reports on true ligands of CAR. It is well known that various androstanes act as inverse agonists of CAR [151]. 1,4-Bis-(2-(3,5-dichloropyridyloxy))benzene (TCPOBOP) was identified as the first agonist of mouse CAR [152]. The first agonist of human CAR – 6-(4-Chlorophenyl)imidazo[2,1-*b*][1,3]thiazole-5-carbaldehyde *O*-(3,4-dichlorobenzyl) oxime (CITCO) – was described in 2003 by Maglich *et al.* [153]. Other human CAR ligands are di(2-ethylhexyl) phthalate (DEHP) [154] and valproic acid [115]. CAR and PXR share the majority of xenobiotic activators [155, 156]. A candidate endogenous CAR ligand is farnesol [157]. Target genes of CAR greatly overlap with PXR target genes for both drug-metabolizing enzymes and other endogenous genes. An example of a CAR-driven gene is that for amino levulinate synthase-1 [158].

8.2.1.4 **Steroid and Nuclear Receptors**

The xenoreceptors AhR, PXR, and CAR, apart from their role in the regulation of drug-metabolizing enzymes, are involved in various endogenous functions. Therefore, it is not surprising that steroid and nuclear receptors, not yet associated with drug metabolism, were found to play a role in regulating drug-metabolizing enzymes [159]. In particular, estrogen receptor (ER-α; NR3A1, ER-β; NR3A2) [160], glucocorticoid receptor (GR; NR3C1) [161], thyroid receptor (TR-α, NR1A1; TR-β, NR1A2) [159, 162], retinoic acid receptor (RAR-α, NR1B1; RAR-β, NR1B2; RAR-γ, NR1B3) [163, 164], peroxisome proliferator-activated receptor (PPAR-α, NR1C1; PPAR-β, NR1C2; PPAR-γ, NR1C3) [165, 166], and vitamin D receptor (VDR, NR1I1) [167–170] are involved in the regulation of drug-metabolizing enzymes.

8.2.2
Transcriptional Mechanisms

Nuclear and steroid receptors, including xenoreceptors, function at the molecular level via at least three distinct mechanisms.

8.2.2.1 **Direct Binding to the Gene Promoter**

The classical mechanism, also referred as *cis*-regulation, is based on the direct interaction of the ligand–receptor complex with a specific sequence in DNA in the promoter of the target gene. Active receptor (with bound ligand) recruits usually transcriptional coactivators, corepressors, and other proteins, and the binding of such as structure to the promoter triggers the expression of target genes. It is a common mechanism for all xenoreceptors, and steroid and nuclear receptors involved in the regulation of drug-metabolizing CYPs. The sequences in DNA are then named according to the receptor bound (e.g., "glucocorticoid response element" for the binding of the GR/GR homodimer, etc.).

8.2.2.2 **Indirect Binding to the Gene Promoter**

The activated transcriptional factor or receptor binds to its cognate DNA sequence in complex with other proteins. It may occur that the receptor is not in direct contact with DNA, while it is integral and indispensable for the correct transcriptional function. This type of regulation is called *trans*-regulation. While it is not, *a priori*, functionally different from *cis*-regulation, it may be experienced failure of *in silico* modeling, when searching for receptor-responsive genes based on the presence of its responsive elements in DNA. An example is GR-mediated regulation of CYP2A6 expression [171].

8.2.2.3 Regulating the Regulator

Biochemical and physiological processes often occur in cascades. Some nuclear receptors are subordinated to another receptor in the way that receptor X transcriptionally regulates receptor Y. Consequently, activation of receptor X leads to triggering of expression of target genes for receptor Y (*vide infra*).

8.2.3 Receptor Cross-Talk

There exist mutual interactions between xenoreceptors, steroid receptors, and nuclear receptors by several mechanisms, usually called cross-talk. Cross-interaction or cross-talk between signaling pathways for two or more receptors results in functional molecular and physiological consequences. Examples of mechanisms of cross-talk are given below (see also www.hepatologyinvitro.com).

8.2.3.1 Ligand Sharing

Conventionally, ligand L_x and L_y bind to their receptors R_x and R_y, respectively. In the case of ligand sharing, one ligand may activate two different receptors, such that L_x binds and activates both R_x and R_y. The final cellular response is then mixed by the effects of both activated receptors by one molecule. Examples are activation of PXR/CAR by bile acids and valproate [115] or PXR/GR by rifampicin [172]. In addition, one molecule can be at the same time an agonist for R_x and an antagonist for R_y. Several azole antimycotics are agonists of PXR [113] and antagonists of GR [173].

8.2.3.2 Response Element Sharing

Some receptors bind not only to their specific receptor response elements (RREs) in gene promoters, but also to gene promoters for another receptor. While R_x and R_y binds normally to RRE_x and RRE_y, respectively, binding of R_x to RRE_y represents cross-talk based on response element sharing. For instance, PXR and CAR share several response elements in the CYP3A4 promoter [174]. Response element sharing may result in cross-gene expression (e.g., activation of VDR-responsive genes such as CYP24 by PXR or CAR that binds to VDRE) [175, 176].

8.2.3.3 Receptor Cascade

There exists a certain transcriptional hierarchy among nuclear and steroid receptors, when receptor R_x regulates the expression (level, amount) of receptor R_y. Since receptors are transcriptional regulators, this type of cross-talk is also referred to as "regulating the regulator." One example is upregulation of PXR, CAR, and RXR by GR. Therefore, the inducibility of CYP genes via PXR and CAR is enhanced in the presence of glucocorticoids that maintain higher levels of PXR and CAR [177–180]. On the contrary, antiglucocorticoid stimuli such as perturbation of microtubules [181], inflammation [182], or ketoconazole [173] impair inducibility of CYP genes.

8.2.3.4 Coactivator Sharing

Steroid and nuclear receptors share transcriptional coactivators (e.g., SRC-1) or corepressors (e.g., the nuclear receptor corepressor NCoR1, SMRT (silencing mediator for retinoic acid and thyroid hormone receptors)). Hence, given by intracellular stoichiometry, the amount of coactivators or corepressors and their affinity to individual receptors modulate the transcriptional activity of receptors. Moreover, receptor R_x may serve as a transcriptional coactivator of R_y. This is a case of AhR that is the transcriptional coactivator of ER [183].

8.2.3.5 Metabolic Cross-Talk

This is a common regulatory negative (positive) feedback mechanism in enzymatic metabolic pathways, where the end product modulates the catalytic activity of the first enzyme in the cascade. Similarly, in receptor cascades, the target gene G_x of receptor R_x that is activated by ligand L_x may metabolize ligand L_y, and consequently alter the activity of receptor R_y and expression of gene G_y. For instance, CAR upregulates UGT1A1 [184], which in turn inactivates TR ligands T3 and T4 [185].

The above-mentioned cross-talk may combine in many ways. For instance, in CAR it may share a ligand and responsive elements with PXR, it is transcriptionally controlled by GR, and it transcriptionally controls enzymes involved in TR ligand metabolism.

8.2.4 Ligands – Agonists and Antagonists

Nuclear receptors, steroid receptors, and xenoreceptors become transcriptionally active upon a binding of a ligand. From the functional point of view, there is no principal difference between this type of receptor and ligand-activated transcriptional factors. Indeed, while GR, ER, or TR are typical receptors having their own glands secreting hormones that activate these receptors, AhR, RAR, or RXR are rather ligand-activated transcriptional factors.

Two basic properties of the receptors are recognition and transduction. Recognition means that the receptor exists in the state that enables recognition and binding of a ligand. For this purpose the receptor must meet several criteria, including saturation, reversibility of binding, stereo-specificity, specificity towards the ligands, and tissue specificity. Transduction means that binding of an agonist to the receptor must lead to a functional response. Receptors are coupled with different effectors and amplification systems. For steroid and nuclear receptors, the effector is DNA promoter. Receptors bind structurally related compounds with different affinity, which is usually the highest for natural ligands or hormones. The measure of the affinity of a ligand for a receptor is the equilibrium dissociation constant K_D. The affinity defines the relation between the concentration of a ligand and the fractional occupancy of the receptor. In clinical pharmacology and toxicology, we often examine the relation between dose (concentration of a ligand) and response (functional response). According to the Clark theory, the effect of a drug is proportional to the fractional occupancy of a receptor and the maximal response is attained when all receptors are occupied. This is not true for so-called spare receptors, when the maximal response is reached even with only a portion of receptors occupied with a ligand [186]. The ability of a drug (agonist) to bind a receptor and to attain maximal effect is called the efficacy or intrinsic efficacy. A measure of efficacy is the maximal effective concentration EC_{MAX} or half maximal effective concentration EC_{50} that refers to the ability of a drug to attain 50% of the maximal effect. The ability of a drug to elicit measurable functional change is called potency. It compares the concentrations of two different drugs that elicit the maximal response.

The relative maximal effect of a drug in certain tissues in comparison with the natural ligand is called the activity or intrinsic activity (IA). According to activity, we distinguish several types of ligands, including superagonists ($IA > 1$), full agonists ($IA = 1$), partial agonists ($IA = 0$–1), antagonists ($IA = 0$), and inverse agonist ($IA < 0$) [187–189]. Of particular interest are partial agonists that represent the majority of xenobiotic ligands for nuclear and steroid receptors. There is a lot of confusion in the scientific literature when partial agonists are referred to as antagonists; in fact, pure antagonists are very rare, if any (often given by methodology limitations). In comparison with the endogenous ligand, partial agonists never elicit maximal response, even if all receptors are occupied by the partial agonist. While partial agonists have a similar potency as full agonists (EC_{50}), the efficacy of a partial agonist is lower than that of a full agonist. Therefore, partial agonists elicit very low measurable functional responses even when the major portion of the receptors is occupied. Importantly, partial agonists behave as functional antagonists – when combining a full agonist with a partial agonist, the effect of the full agonist is diminished by the partial agonist, hence displaying antagonistic behavior.

8.3 Regulation of Drug-Metabolizing CYPs

8.3.1 CYP1A Subfamily

The CYP1A subfamily comprises two members – CYP1A1 and CYP1A2. These two enzymes metabolize a variety of environmental pollutants such as PAHs or polyaromatic amines [190], several drugs including antidepressants, caffeine, theophyline, clozapine, and so on [191, 192], and endogenous compounds such as eicosanoids [69] and retinoids [193]. Biotransformation of organic pollutants by CYP1A enzymes often leads to metabolic activation of procarcinogens to ultimate carcinogens. Therefore, induction of CYP1A enzymes by xenobiotics is considered as a risk factor in terms of chemically induced carcinogenesis. While CYP1A2 is expressed exclusively in the liver (some reports showed CYP1A2 also in lung [194]), CYP1A1 is expressed mainly in extrahepatic tissues, including the intestine, lungs, placenta, and skin [45]. A key transcriptional regulator of CYP1A genes is AhR, which is ubiquitously expressed in human tissues. Both CYP1A1 and CYP1A2 are highly inducible by xenobiotics; the activators of AhR are thus CYP1A inducers. Activation of AhR by exogenous ligands such as PAHs or dioxins leads to endocrine disruption and many toxic effects. However, activation of AhR by endogenous ligands is necessary for many cellular functions, including immune response, cell cycle control, and differentiation [195]. From this point of view, AhR resembles the Dr Jekyll and Mr Hyde story [196]. Since AhR is continuously exposed to endogenous ligands, the final cellular response to exogenous ligand depends on the nature of the AhR ligand in terms of receptor agonism or antagonism [48]. Activated AhR binds in the form of an AhR/ARNT heterodimer to XRE in the enhancer upstream of the CYP1A genes. The transactivation domain of AhR can facilitate the binding of the transcription factors, TATA-box binding protein (TBP) and nuclear factor (NF)-1, to the CYP1A1 promoter [159]. In the recognition sites for the AhR/ARNT heterodimer, the consensus XRE sequences are present in multiple copies in the CYP1A1 promoter [197]. In parallel, coactivator proteins SRC-1, NCoA-2, or p/CIP associate with the CYP1A1 gene, and function as a bridge between AhR/ARNT bound to the XREs and the core transcription initiation complex at the TATA-box of the promoter. The interaction of AhR/ARNT with the coactivators and with other transcription factors (NF-1, TBP, TFIIF, PolII) results in the bending of upstream region of CYP1A1 gene, bringing the enhancer and promoter into close proximity [159]. Apart from AhR, other nuclear and steroid receptors transcriptionally regulate CYP1A gene expression. Recently, it was demonstrated that CAR transcriptionally activates CYP1A1 and CYP1A2 genes through a common regulatory region in the 5′-flanking region [198].

Androgens determine sexually dimorphic constitutive and xenobiotic-inducible expression of CYP1As in rats, mice and pigs. There is evidence for the androgen-mediated downregulation of CYP1As by mechanisms not yet known [199, 200]. There exists cross-talk between progesterone receptor (PR) and AhR having an impact on the expression of CYP1A genes [201]. Some studies showed repressive effects of PR on AhR functions [201], whereas others demonstrated induction of CYP1A1 protein, mRNA, and catalytic activity by progesterone [202]. It is speculated that the steroid structure of gestagens is able to induce CYP1A1 in an AhR-dependent manner [203]. Several studies reported cross-talk between the AhR and ER signaling pathways by various mechanisms, therefore ER is an important regulator of CYP1A genes. (i) Activated AhR redirects liganded ER from estrogen target genes to AhR target genes [204]. Both AF-1 and AF-2 domains are important in mediating ER-dependent increases in AhR activity [205]. (ii) The AhR complex directly interacts with the inhibitory dioxin-responsive elements (iXREs) present in the promoter regions of estrogen-responsive genes [206, 207]. (iii) AhR also functions as a ubiquitin-E3 ligase and it also directs ER to proteasome–ubiquitin degradation [85, 86]. (iv) AhR downregulates the ER levels via binding to six partial and two full-length repressor XRE sites in the promoter of the ER gene [208]. (v) ER and AhR share several coactivator proteins, such as SRC-1 and RIP140. The similarities in molecular mechanisms of ER and AhR action cause the receptors to compete in the recruitment of common coactivators [209, 210]. There are numerous reports on the involvement of GR in the modulation of AhR functions and CYP1A gene expression. The effects of GR are species- and cell-type-dependent. There are intronic GR-responsive element (glucocorticoid-responsive element-GRE) sequences conserved between the human, rat, and mouse CYP1A1. In human liver cells, synthetic glucocorticoid dexamethasone inhibits CYP1A1 induction at the enzyme protein level, but it does not influence the expression of CYP1A1 mRNA [211, 212]. In human hepatoma HepG2 cells and in primary human hepatocytes, the expression of AhR is suppressed by dexamethasone [213, 214]. In contrast to CYP1A1, dexamethasone synergistically enhances the induction of CYP1A2 by AhR ligands, such as β-naphthoflavone, 2,3,7,8-tetrachlorodibenzo-*p*-dioxin (TCDD), or 3-methylcholanthrene, in human hepatocytes [213, 215].

Signaling pathways of AhR and TR share several coactivators, thus there exists AhR–TR cross-talk and TR modulates the expression of CYP1A genes. Interaction of AhR/ARNT with SMRT leads to inhibition of AhR/ARNT binding to XREs [216]. Two other factors that are common for the proper functioning of AhR and TR are TRIP230 [162] and XAP2 cochaperone protein [217]; however, their exact role in AhR–TR cross-talk is not yet clear. Similarly, retinoids via RAR share the SMRT coactivator with AhR, giving a tentative link for transcriptional cross-talk between AhR and RAR [218, 219]. It was confirmed that the formation of the AhR/SMRT complex is responsible for transcriptional repression of the AhR pathway by retinoids [164]. However, the presence of a retinoic acid-responsive element that is transactivated by the liganded RAR-α1 was found in the 5′-regulatory region of the CYP1A1 gene [220]. The involvement of PPAR-α in CYP1A1 gene regulation was demonstrated and two peroxisome proliferator response elements (PPREs) that bind PPAR-α/RXR have been identified at positions −931/−919 and −531/−519 of the CYP1A1 promoter. Therefore, AhR and PPAR-α agonists cooperate for CYP1A1 induction [165, 166].

Finally, hypoxic conditions modulate the AhR–CYP1A signaling pathway. Hypoxia induces the production of reactive oxygen species that in turn activate NF-κB, which represses AhR, and downregulates CYP1A1 and CYP1A2 [221]. Cells adapt to hypoxia by upregulating the transcription of multiple genes, the majority of which are induced by hypoxia-inducible factor (HIF)-1 [222]. HIF-1α translocates to the nucleus, and dimerizes with HIF-1β or ARNT to form HIF-1. Since ARNT is also a heterodimerization partner of AhR, hypoxia decreases the availability of ARNT, thus causing a downregulation of CYP1A1 and CYP1A2 [223].

Regarding hormones not acting via steroid and nuclear receptors, it seems that insulin negatively modulates CYP1A inducibility [224–226] while glucagon has no effect on the AhR–CYP1A signaling pathway [227, 228].

8.3.2
CYP1B1

In adults, CYP1B1 mRNA is expressed in the liver, lymphocytes, and uterine endometrium, but not in lung [229]. The regulation of CYP1B1 involves a variety of both transcriptional and post-transcriptional mechanisms [230]. CYP1B1 protein undergoes proteasome-mediated degradation that varies with the polymorphic forms of CYP1B1 [29]. Estradiol 4-hydroxylation is a characteristic reaction catalyzed by human CYP1B1. In humans CYP1B1 is overexpressed in tumor cells [231], and this has important implications for tumor development and progression, and the development of anticancer drugs specifically activated by CYP1B1 [232]. The main regulator of CYP1B1 is AhR; however, there are striking differences in CYP1B1 regulation in comparison to CYP1A genes. Potential enhancer elements for TCDD induction are located from −1022 to −852, including three XREs; XRE3 at −853, XRE4 at −940, and XRE5 at −989. AhR/ARNT heterodimer binds to XRE2 at −834, XRE3 at −853, XRE6 at −1024, and XRE7 at −1490. In addition, nuclear transcriptional factor specificity protein-1 (Sp-1) binds near XRE2 and XRE8. Mutual interaction of XRE2 and XRE3 is important for transcriptional regulation and the Sp-1 binding to the Sp-1-like motif (−824), which enhances both the constitutive and inducible transcriptional activities of the human CYP1B1 gene [233]. CYP1B1 is constitutively expressed and TCDD- and 3-methylcholanthrene-inducible in several cancer cell lines, including human colon carcinoma cell line LS180, breast cancer MCF-7 cells, human hepatoma HepG2 cells, human choriocarcinoma cell line JEG-3, and the squamous cell carcinoma line A431 [234]. Significant induction of CYP1B1 mRNA, protein, and catalytic activity by TCDD was observed in human renal adenocarcinoma ACHN cells [235] and human mammary stromal fibroblasts [236]. CYP1B1 is inducible also by natural compounds such as indole-3-carbinol [237] or endogenous AhR ligands such as indirubin [238]. Interestingly, resveratrol – a partial agonist of AhR – downregulated CYP1B1 in human medulloblastoma cells [239]. The expression and induction of CYP1B1 in human liver and renal cells is cell-specific, and is due to transcriptional mechanisms [240, 241]. It was suggested that AhR-mediated cell-specific differences in CYP1B1 constitutive expression are due to inaccessibility of the 5′-enhancer region in HepG2 cells to transcriptional activators due to a higher-order chromatin structure that does not involve histone acetylation or due to the action of a repressor protein at *cis* elements located outside of the −2296 to +25 region of the CYP1B1 promoter [242]. Dioxin-mediated induction of CYP1B1 comprises recruitment of the transcriptional coactivators SRC-1, SRC-2, p300, and Brahma (BRM)/Switch 2-related gene 1 [243]. Many authors demonstrated differential regulation of CYP1A1 and CYP1B1 by AhR ligands (e.g., in MCF-7 cells) [244, 245]. The role in CYP1B1 expression could be also played by ER [246]. Prostaglandin E_2 induces CYP1B1 expression by a mechanism involving ligand-independent activation of the ER as a result of the activation of extracellular regulated kinase, Akt, and protein kinase A in breast cancer cells [247]. Since CYP1B1 mRNA is upregulated by all-*trans*-retinoic acid in human leukemic cells, the involvement of RAR is likely [248].

8.3.3 CYP2A6

The human CYP2A gene subfamily comprises three members – CYP2A6, CYP2A7, and CYP2A13. The most important is CYP2A6 that plays roles in the metabolism of nicotine and some clinically used drugs. It is expressed mainly in the liver. Two mutant alleles of the CYP2A6 gene have been identified – CYP2A6*2 and CYP2A6*3. Gene polymorphism affects *in vivo* catalytic activity of CYP2A6 when homozygosity for both mutated alleles confers a "poor metabolizer" [249]. Unfortunately, only little is known about transcriptional regulation of CYP2A6. Dexamethasone induced CYP2A6 catalytic activity in 49 primary cultures of human hepatocytes, indicating involvement of GR in the process [250]. A recent study revealed the nonclassical mechanism of dexamethasone-mediated upregulation of CYP2A6 involving GR and increased binding of hepatocyte nuclear factor (HNF)-4α to the proximal promoter [171]. Further analyses of the CYP2A6 promoter showed that maximal promoter activity is harbored in the sequence spanning from −112 to −61. The constitutive hepatic expression of CYP2A6 is governed by an interplay between the transcription factors HNF-4α, CCAAT-box/enhancer binding protein (C/EBP)-α, C/EBP-β, and octamer transcription factor (Oct)-1 [251]. Since rifampicin, phenobarbital, and CITCO induced CYP2A6 in human hepatocytes, it was anticipated that PXR and CAR could be the regulators of CYP2A6. Itoh *et al.* found that CYP2A6 is induced via PXR and proliferator-activated receptor-γ coactivator (PGC)-1α through binding of PXR/PGC-1α to two DR-4-like elements at the distal response region at −5476 and −4618 [252]. An ongoing study confirmed the involvement of PXR in CYP2A6 expression, when silencing of PXR mRNA in human hepatocytes infected with PXR/small interfering RNA adenoviral vector decreased the basal and ligand-activated CYP2A6 mRNA [253].

8.3.4
CYP2B6

CYP2B6 protein is expressed in human liver, brain, intestine, and kidney, and at a lower level in the lung. CYP2B6 mRNA was detected in human liver, kidney, lung, trachea, and intestine [254, 255]. Human CYP2B6 is inducible by variety of xenobiotics via activation of PXR and CAR xenoreceptors [256], such as 3-hydroxy-3-methyl-glutaryl (HMG)-CoA reductase inhibitors (lovastatin, simvastatin, fluvastatin, atorvastatin) [257], metamizol [258], ritonavir [259], oltipraz [260, 261], artemisin drugs [262], histone deacetylase inhibitors (valproic acid, phenylbutyrate, trichostatin A) [263], and so on. Basal expression of CYP2B6 is correlated with the expression of PXR and CAR [264]. The relative contribution of PXR and CAR to CYP2B6 differs among the individual xenobiotics – some of them being dual activators while others are selective activators of PXR and CAR. An asymmetrical cross-regulation of CYP2B6 and CYP3A4 by CAR, but not PXR, has been suggested, where CAR exhibits preferential induction of CYP2B6 relative to CYP3A4 because of its weak binding and functional activation of the CYP3A4 ER-6 [265]. Induction of CYP2B6 selectively via CAR occurs with phenytoin [266], dehydroepiandrosterone [267], carbamazepine, efavirenz, and nevirapine [268]. A typical CYP2B6 inducer via CAR is phenobarbital; the induction is regulated by a conserved 51-bp element called the phenobarbital-responsive enhancer module (PBREM) that is located between −1733 and −1683 bp in the gene's 5′-flanking region [143]. Selective PXR activators and CYP2B6 inducers are endosulfan [269] and calcium channel modulators (nifedipine, nicardipine, isradipine, BK8644) [117].Also, PXR activated by ligands such as rifampicin and hyperforin was shown to be capable of activating the PBREM region of the CYP2B6 gene [270]. In addition, a distal xenobiotic-responsive enhancer module containing one DR-4 motif binding PXR and CAR located −8.5 kb upstream from the CYP2B6 encoding region was described [271]. Finally, so-called okadaic acid-responsive element (OARE) was identified in the proximal CYP2B6 promoter (−256/−233). CAR binds indirectly binds to the OARE, which enhances CYP2B6 inducibility by xenobiotics [272].

An important regulator of CYP2B6 is GR since it upregulates PXR, RXR [178], and CAR [180]. Therefore, inducibility of CYP2B6 by xenobiotics is enhanced in the presence of glucocorticoids. Conversely, antiglucocorticoid stimuli such as inflammatory cytokines [182, 273], microtubule disruptors [181], and GR antagonists [173] downregulate CYP2B6. In addition, GR-enhanced expression of CYP2B6 is mediated through an indirect mechanism that does not require increased expression of nuclear receptors [274]. Nuclear receptor VDR binds and transactivates those XREs (ER-6, DR-3, and DR-4) previously identified in the CYP2B6 (but also in CYP3A4 and CYP2C9) promoter, and shown to be targeted by PXR and/or CAR. Therefore, VDR– PXR/CAR functional cross-talk results in CYP2B6 induction by vitamin D [168]. The agonists of liver X receptor (LXR) [275] and inhibitors of 2,3-oxidosqualene : lanosterol cyclase [276] upregulate CYP2B6. Multiple ER-α-bound regions were detected in the upstream regulatory sequences of the CYP2B gene cluster. ER-α and ER-β increase CYP2B6-regulated gene expression through a functional ERE located at −1669 to −1657 in the upstream regulatory region of CYP2B6 [277].

Several transcription factors, including C/EBP-α [278], HNF-4 [279], hepatocyte growth factor (HGF), and activating transcription factor (ATF)-5 [280], were described to be involved in hepatic expression of CYP2B6. Transcriptional factor early growth response (EGR1)-1 directly binds to the proximal promoter of CYP2B6 and coordinates the nearby HNF-4α with CAR at the distal enhancer element to activate the promoter. Thus, synergy of drug activation and the stimulation of cellular signals are necessary for CAR to activate the CYP2B6 gene [281]. In addition, synergistic cooperation between C/EBP-α and HNF-4α with CAR was demonstrated to be needed for maximal CYP2B6 induction [282]. There is an indication that AMP-dependent protein kinase is involved in the process of phenobarbital-mediated CYP2B6 induction [283].

8.3.5
CYP2C Subfamily

The human CYP2C subfamily comprises four members–CYP2C8, CYP2C9, CYP2C18, and CYP2C19. CYP2C enzymes are expressed predominantly in the liver, and they are responsible for the metabolism of therapeutically used drugs such as warfarin, mephenytoin, omeprazole, and anti-inflammatory drugs, but also for the metabolism of endogenous compounds. CYP2C genes (except CYP2C18) are inducible by variety of xenobiotics and drugs, including rifampicin, dexamethasone, phenobarbital, dehydroepiandrostenole, and so on [117, 284–286]. The master transcriptional regulators of CYP2C expression and xenobiotic-mediated induction are xenoreceptors CAR and PXR (i.e., the activators of CAR and PXR are usually inducers of CYP2C genes) [287].

Early investigations revealed the roles of hepatocyte proliferation factor and HNF-4 in the expression of CYP2C9 and CYP2C18 [288]. There exists cross-talk between CAR and PXR in terms of sharing response elements in the CYP2C9 promoter. Xenobiotic-mediated induction of CYP2C9 involves the binding of PXR/CAR to PXR-RE/CAR-RE (RE = responsive element) located at −1839/−1824 bp and CAR binding to CAR-RE located at −2899/−2883 in the CYP2C9 upstream promoter [289]. A distal CAR/PXR binding site constitutively regulating transcription of CYP2C9 was identified in the CYP2C9 promoter [290]. It is a PBREM-like enhancer module, located between −2900 and −2841 bp, consisting of two DR-5 nuclear receptor binding motifs capable of binding human CAR and, to a lesser extent, human PXR. A *cis*-acting 27-bp regulatory element within the protein-coding region immediately after the translation start codon in the human CYP2C9 gene is involved in the negative regulation of CYP2C9 by a yet-unknown protein of 100 kDa size [291]. Several transcriptional factors including C/EBP-α [278], HNF-4α [279, 292–296], HNF-3 [297], GATA-4 [298], NCoA-6 [299], PGC-1, and SRC-1 [294] were found to play a role in the expression and induction of CYP2C9. Similar to the case of CYP2B6, VDR binds and transactivates those XREs (ER-6, DR-3, and DR-4) previously identified in the CYP2C9 promoter, and shown to be targeted by PXR and/or CAR [168].

There is a PXR/CAR-binding site in the CYP2C8 distal promoter that confers inducibility of CYP2C8 via the PXR agonist/ligand rifampicin and the CAR agonist/ligand CITCO. A HNF-4α binding site within the CYP2C8 basal promoter region was identified [296, 300].

The CYP2C19 promoter contains a functional CAR binding site (CAR-RE; −1891/−1876 bp) that binds also PXR and a GRE at −1750/−1736 bp [301]. The expression of CYP2C19 is controlled also by transcription factor GATA-4 [302] and HNF-4α [295, 296].

Interestingly, GR plays a dual role in the regulation of CYP2C genes. (i) GR upregulates PXR, RXR, and CAR receptors, and therefore CYP2C gene inducibility by xenobiotics is enhanced in the presence of glucocorticoids [178, 180]. (ii) Functional GRE sequences were identified in the promoters of CYP2C8 [300], CYP2C9 [303], and CYP2C19 [301]; hence, GR also plays a direct role in the induction of CYP2C genes by glucocorticoids. Additionally, antiglucocorticoid stimuli negatively influence the expression and induction of CYP2C genes [173, 181, 182, 273].

8.3.6
CYP3A Subfamily

The CYP3A subfamily contains three members – CYP3A4, CYP3A5, and CYP3A7. While CYP3A4 and CYP3A5 are adult forms, CYP3A7 is a fetal form and is not discussed in the current chapter. The enzymes CYP3A4 and CYP3A5 account for the metabolism of approximately 60% of all known drugs, and are responsible for the majority of drug–drug interactions. They overlap in their substrate specificities and mechanisms of regulation. The major hepatic form is CYP3A4, whereas CYP3A5 is the dominant CYP3A form in extrahepatic tissues. Hepatic CYP3A5 is polymorphic. Numerous structurally unrelated compounds are CYP3A4 inducers [265, 268], such as benzodiazepines [116], calcium channel modulators [117], statins [257, 304], paclitaxel [305], flavonoids [306], vitamin E [137], carotenoids [139, 307], organochlorine pesticides [308], forskolin [309], artemisin [262], valproic acid [115], azole antimycotics [113], and so on.

The regulation of CYP3A4 was a subject of extensive research since the discovery of CYP3A4. The breakpoint was the discovery of xenoreceptors PXR and CAR [310]. Indeed, the master regulators of human CYP3A4 are PXR and CAR. In proximal CYP3A4 promoter (pPXRE), a PXR/CAR binding site having the ER-6 motif was identified (−172/−149) [96]. One year later, a potent enhancer module (XREM), containing two PXR/CAR binding sites −7738/−7715 and −7698/−7682, having DR-3 and ER-6 motifs was identified [311]. Furthermore, the cooperation between proximal and distal PXR/CAR binding modules was demonstrated [312]. Several putative binding sites for C/EBP and HNF-3 were found by computer analysis of the CYP3A4 promoter. C/EBP-β-liver inhibitory protein (LIP) antagonizes constitutive C/EBP transactivators (C/EBP-α and C/EBP-β-liver activating protein (LAP)). Analysis of the −3557 to −6954 bp region of the CYP3A4 promoter demonstrated the presence of four functional C/EBP-β-responsive motifs within this distal flanking region. Within this distal enhancer site in the CYP3A4 gene, C/EBP-β-LAP binds and activates transcription, whereas the truncated form, C/EBP-β-LIP, antagonizes LAP activity and causes gene repression [313]. In addition, C/EBP-α regulates hepatic CYP3A4 expression cooperatively with HNF-3γ by a mechanism that involves chromatin remodeling [174, 314, 315]. The latest findings revealed the presence of a region from −11.4 to −10.5 kb upstream in the CYP3A4 promoter, designated as the constitutive liver enhancer module of CYP3A4 (CLEM4), which is important for the constitutive activation of the CYP3A4 gene and which is responsible for the interindividual variability of CYP3A4 expression. The distal enhancer module CLEM4 binds HNF-1α, HNF-4α, upstream stimulatory factor (USF)-1, and activator protein-1 (AP-1) [316]. The importance of HNF-4 together with PGC-1 for CYP3A4 expression was confirmed also by other authors [317, 318].

Similar to CYP2B6 and CYP2C9, the expression of hepatic CYP3A4 is regulated by VDR that binds in the form of a VDR/RXR heterodimer to both the proximal ER-6 and the distal DR-3 motifs as PXR/RXR and CAR/RXR [168, 319]. In addition, VDR regulates the expression of intestinal CYP3A4 [167, 320, 321]. Since PXR, CAR, and VDR act in the form of heterodimers with RXR, it makes sense that retinoids are inducers of CYP3A4. Indeed, retinoids recruit CAR/RXR-α and VDR/RXR-α to the proximal ER-6 and distal XREM nuclear receptor response elements of the CYP3A4 gene promoter [169, 322]. Two binding sites for the bile acid receptor (farnesoid X receptor (FXR)) were identified in the CYP3A4 promoter, implying that secondary bile acids induce CYP3A4 via PXR, while primary bile acids induce CYP3A4 via FXR [323]. Induction of CYP3A4 occurs also through LXR [275]. The roles of other factors including HIF-1 [324], SMRT [325], transcription factor 1 family [326], HGF [327], small heterodimer partner (NR1I0, repressor of PXR) [328], and molecular chaperone HDJ-1 [329] in CYP3A4 regulation were also demonstrated.

Important regulators of CYP3A4 expression are glucocorticoids via GR by multiple mechanisms. (i) Similar to the case of the CYP2B6 and CYP2C subfamily, GR upregulates xenoreceptors PXR and CAR; hence, the inducibility of CYP3A4 by xenobiotics is enhanced in the presence of glucocorticoids [178, 180]. Logically, the factors inhibiting GR functions also diminish the expression and induction of CYP3A4 [173, 181, 182, 273]. (ii) Synthetic glucocorticoid dexamethasone is a ligand for both GR and PXR. It has a sequential effect on CYP3A4 induction kinetics; at submicromolar concentrations (0.1 μM) dexamethasone fully activates GR, while at supramicromolar concentrations (above10 μM) dexamethasone activates PXR [179, 330]. (iii) CYP3A5 – a glucocorticoid-inducible gene [331] – contains a dexamethasone-responsive enhancer module in its promoter (–891/–1109) in the form of two GRE half-sites [332]. (iv) Similar to the case of CYP2A6, indirect binding of the GR/GR homodimer to the promoter of CYP3A4 through HNF-4, HNF-3, or C/EBP was described [292, 333]. Recently, the roles for microRNA in post-transcriptional and post-translational regulation of PXR and CYP3A4 were revealed [334, 335].

Expression of CYP3A5 is regulated similar to that of CYP3A4. In addition, the transcription of the CYP3A5 gene is cooperatively regulated by NF-Y, Sp-1, and Sp-3 [336]. Androgen response element was identified in the CYP3A5 proximal promoter [337].

Acknowledgments

Our laboratory is supported by the grants from the Czech Scientific Agency **GACR503/10/0579** and **GACR304/10/0149**, and GACR303/12/G163 – Center of Excellence.

References

1 Zhou, S.F., Liu, J.P., and Chowbay, B. (2009) Polymorphism of human cytochrome P450 enzymes and its clinical impact. *Drug Metab. Rev.*, **41**, 89–295.

2 Zhou, S.F. (2009) Polymorphism of human cytochrome P450 2D6 and its clinical significance: part I. *Clin. Pharmacokinet.*, **48**, 689–723.

3 Zhou, S.F. (2009) Polymorphism of human cytochrome P450 2D6 and its clinical significance: part II. *Clin. Pharmacokinet.*, **48**, 761–804.

4 Klotz, U. (2006) Clinical impact of CYP2C19 polymorphism on the action of proton pump inhibitors: a review of a special problem. *Int. J. Clin. Pharmacol. Ther.*, **44**, 297–302.

5 Klotz, U. (2009) Impact of CYP2C19 polymorphisms on the clinical action of proton pump inhibitors (PPIs). *Eur. J. Clin. Pharmacol.*, **65**, 1–2.

6 Wojnowski, L. and Kamdem, L.K. (2006) Clinical implications of CYP3A polymorphisms. *Expert Opin. Drug Metab. Toxicol.*, **2**, 171–182.

7 Wang, J. (2009) CYP3A polymorphisms and immunosuppressive drugs in solid-organ transplantation. *Expert Rev. Mol. Diagn.*, **9**, 383–390.

8 Agundez, J.A. (2004) Cytochrome P450 gene polymorphism and cancer. *Curr. Drug Metab.*, **5**, 211–224.

9 Shi, X., Zhou, S., Wang, Z., Zhou, Z., and Wang, Z. (2008) CYP1A1 and GSTM1 polymorphisms and lung cancer risk in Chinese populations: a meta-analysis. *Lung Cancer*, **59**, 155–163.

10 Klotz, U. (2009) Pharmacokinetics and drug metabolism in the elderly. *Drug Metab. Rev.*, **41**, 67–76.

11 Scandlyn, M.J., Stuart, E.C., and Rosengren, R.J. (2008) Sex-specific differences in CYP450 isoforms in humans. *Expert Opin. Drug Metab. Toxicol.*, **4**, 413–424.

12 Waxman, D.J. and O'Connor, C. (2006) Growth hormone regulation of sex-dependent liver gene expression. *Mol. Endocrinol.*, **20**, 2613–2629.

13 Pavek, P., Ceckova, M., and Staud, F. (2009) Variation of drug kinetics in pregnancy. *Curr. Drug Metab.*, **10**, 520–529.

14 Mitchell, S.C., Smith, R.L., and Waring, R.H. (2009) The menstrual cycle and drug metabolism. *Curr. Drug Metab.*, **10**, 499–507.

15 Aitken, A.E., Richardson, T.A., and Morgan, E.T. (2006) Regulation of drug-metabolizing enzymes and transporters in inflammation. *Annu. Rev. Pharmacol. Toxicol.*, **46**, 123–149.

16 Zordoky, B.N. and El-Kadi, A.O. (2009) Role of NF-kappaB in the regulation of cytochrome P450 enzymes. *Curr. Drug Metab.*, **10**, 164–178.

17 Renton, K.W. (2005) Regulation of drug metabolism and disposition during inflammation and infection. *Expert Opin. Drug Metab. Toxicol.*, **1**, 629–640.

18 Morgan, E.T. (2009) Impact of infectious and inflammatory disease on cytochrome P450-mediated drug metabolism and pharmacokinetics. *Clin. Pharmacol. Ther.*, **85**, 434–438.

19 Croyle, M.A. (2009) Long-term virus-induced alterations of CYP3A-mediated drug metabolism: a look at the virology, immunology and molecular biology of a multi-faceted problem. *Expert Opin. Drug Metab. Toxicol.*, **5**, 1189–1211.

20 Robertson, G.R., Liddle, C., and Clarke, S.J. (2008) Inflammation and altered drug clearance in cancer: transcriptional repression of a human CYP3A4 transgene in tumor-bearing mice. *Clin. Pharmacol. Ther.*, **83**, 894–897.

21 Kacevska, M., Robertson, G.R., Clarke, S.J., and Liddle, C. (2008) Inflammation and CYP3A4-mediated drug metabolism in advanced cancer: impact and implications for chemotherapeutic drug dosing. *Expert Opin. Drug Metab. Toxicol.*, **4**, 137–149.

22 Assenat, E., Gerbal-chaloin, S., Maurel, P., Vilarem, M.J., and Pascussi, J.M. (2006) Is nuclear factor kappa-B the missing link between inflammation, cancer and alteration in hepatic drug metabolism in patients with cancer? *Eur. J. Cancer*, **42**, 785–792.

23 Pearson, E.R. (2009) Pharmacogenetics in diabetes. *Curr. Diab. Rep.*, **9**, 172–181.

24 Cheng, P.Y. and Morgan, E.T. (2001) Hepatic cytochrome P450 regulation in disease states. *Curr. Drug Metab.*, **2**, 165–183.

25 Nebert, D.W. and Dalton, T.P. (2006) The role of cytochrome P450 enzymes in endogenous signalling pathways and environmental carcinogenesis. *Nat. Rev. Cancer*, **6**, 947–960.

26 Zhou, S.F. (2008) Potential strategies for minimizing mechanism-based inhibition of cytochrome P450 3A4. *Curr. Pharm. Des.*, **14**, 990–1000.

27 Zhou, S.F. (2008) Drugs behave as substrates, inhibitors and inducers of human cytochrome P450 3A4. *Curr. Drug Metab.*, **9**, 310–322.

28 Masubuchi, Y. and Horie, T. (2007) Toxicological significance of mechanism-based inactivation of cytochrome p450 enzymes by drugs. *Crit. Rev. Toxicol.*, **37**, 389–412.

29 Bandiera, S., Weidlich, S., Harth, V., Broede, P., Ko, Y., and Friedberg, T. (2005) Proteasomal degradation of

human CYP1B1: effect of the Asn453Ser polymorphism on the post-translational regulation of CYP1B1 expression. *Mol. Pharmacol.*, **67**, 435–443.

30 Lee, C.M., Kim, B.Y., Li, L., and Morgan, E.T. (2008) Nitric oxide-dependent proteasomal degradation of cytochrome P450 2B proteins. *J. Biol. Chem.*, **283**, 889–898.

31 Morishima, Y., Peng, H.M., Lin, H.L., Hollenberg, P.F., Sunahara, R.K., Osawa, Y., and Pratt, W.B. (2005) Regulation of cytochrome P450 2E1 by heat shock protein 90-dependent stabilization and CHIP-dependent proteasomal degradation. *Biochemistry*, **44**, 16333–16340.

32 Huan, J.Y., Streicher, J.M., Bleyle, L.A., and Koop, D.R. (2004) Proteasome-dependent degradation of cytochromes P450 2E1 and 2B1 expressed in tetracycline-regulated HeLa cells. *Toxicol. Appl. Pharmacol.*, **199**, 332–343.

33 Zangar, R.C., Kimzey, A.L., Okita, J.R., Wunschel, D.S., Edwards, R.J., Kim, H., and Okita, R.T. (2002) Cytochrome P450 3A conjugation to ubiquitin in a process distinct from classical ubiquitination pathway. *Mol. Pharmacol.*, **61**, 892–904.

34 Zangar, R.C., Bollinger, N., Verma, S., Karin, N.J., and Lu, Y. (2008) The nuclear factor-kappa B pathway regulates cytochrome P450 3A4 protein stability. *Mol. Pharmacol.*, **73**, 1652–1658.

35 Freeman, J.E. and Wolf, C.R. (1994) Evidence against a role for serine 129 in determining murine cytochrome P450 Cyp2e-1 protein levels. *Biochemistry*, **33**, 13963–13966.

36 Martini, R., Ingelman-Sundberg, M., and Murray, M. (1997) Pretranslational and posttranslational regulation of rat hepatic CYPs 3A2 and 2E1 by disulfiram. *Biochem. Pharmacol.*, **54**, 1323–1329.

37 Lekas, P., Tin, K.L., Lee, C., and Prokipcak, R.D. (2000) The human cytochrome P450 1A1 mRNA is rapidly degraded in HepG2 cells. *Arch. Biochem. Biophys.*, **384**, 311–318.

38 Mattingly, C.J. and Toscano, W.A. (2001) Posttranscriptional silencing of cytochrome P4501A1 (CYP1A1) during zebrafish (*Danio rerio*) development. *Dev. Dyn.*, **222**, 645–654.

39 Elbekai, R.H. and El-Kadi, A.O. (2007) Transcriptional activation and posttranscriptional modification of Cyp1a1 by arsenite, cadmium, and chromium. *Toxicol. Lett.*, **172**, 106–119.

40 Raffalli-Mathieu, F., Geneste, O., and Lang, M.A. (1997) Characterization of two nuclear proteins that interact with cytochrome P-450 1A2 mRNA. Regulation of RNA binding and possible role in the expression of the Cyp1a2 gene. *Eur. J. Biochem.*, **245**, 17–24.

41 Delaporte, E. and Renton, K.W. (1997) Cytochrome P4501A1 and cytochrome P4501A2 are downregulated at both transcriptional and post-transcriptional levels by conditions resulting in interferon-alpha/beta induction. *Life Sci.*, **60**, 787–796.

42 Daujat, M., Clair, P., Astier, C., Fabre, I., Pineau, T., Yerle, M., Gellin, J., and Maurel, P. (1991) Induction, regulation and messenger half-life of cytochromes P450 IA1, IA2 and IIIA6 in primary cultures of rabbit hepatocytes. CYP 1A1, 1A2 and 3A6 chromosome location in the rabbit and evidence that post-transcriptional control of gene IA2 does not involve mRNA stabilization. *Eur. J. Biochem.*, **200**, 501–510.

43 Pan, J., Hong, J.Y., and Yang, C.S. (1992) Post-transcriptional regulation of mouse renal cytochrome P450 2E1 by testosterone. *Arch. Biochem. Biophys.*, **299**, 110–115.

44 Guenthner, T.M. and Nebert, D.W, (1977) Cytosolic receptor for aryl hydrocarbon hydroxylase induction by polycyclic aromatic compounds. Evidence for structural and regulatory variants among established cell cultured lines. *J. Biol. Chem.*, **252**, 8981–8989.

45 Pavek, P. and Dvorak, Z. (2008) Xenobiotic-induced transcriptional regulation of xenobiotic metabolizing enzymes of the cytochrome P450 superfamily in human extrahepatic tissues. *Curr. Drug Metab.*, **9**, 129–143.

46 Denison, M.S. and Nagy, S.R. (2003) Activation of the aryl hydrocarbon receptor by structurally diverse

exogenous and endogenous chemicals. *Annu. Rev. Pharmacol. Toxicol.*, **43**, 309–334.

47 Bachleda, P. and Dvorak, Z. (2008) Pharmacological inhibitors of JNK and ERK kinases SP600125 and U0126 are not appropriate tools for studies of drug metabolism because they activate aryl hydrocarbon receptor. *Gen. Physiol. Biophys.*, **27**, 143–145.

48 Dvorak, Z., Vrzal, R., Henklova, P., Jancova, P., Anzenbacherova, E., Maurel, P., Svecova, L., Pavek, P., Ehrmann, J., Havlik, R., Bednar, P., Lemr, K., and Ulrichova, J. (2008) JNK inhibitor SP600125 is a partial agonist of human aryl hydrocarbon receptor and induces CYP1A1 and CYP1A2 genes in primary human hepatocytes. *Biochem. Pharmacol.*, **75**, 580–588.

49 Joiakim, A., Mathieu, P.A., Palermo, C., Gasiewicz, T.A., and Reiners, J.J., Jr (2003) The Jun N-terminal kinase inhibitor SP600125 is a ligand and antagonist of the aryl hydrocarbon receptor. *Drug Metab.Dispos.* **31**, 1279–1282.

50 Andrieux, L., Langouet, S., Fautrel, A., Ezan, F., Krauser, J.A., Savouret, J.F., Guengerich, F.P., Baffet, G., and Guillouzo, A. (2004) Aryl hydrocarbon receptor activation and cytochrome P450 1A induction by the mitogen-activated protein kinase inhibitor U0126 in hepatocytes. *Mol. Pharmacol.*, **65**, 934–943.

51 Revel, A., Raanani, H., Younglai, E., Xu, J., Rogers, I., Han, R., Savouret, J.F., and Casper, R.F. (2003) Resveratrol, a natural aryl hydrocarbon receptor antagonist, protects lung from DNA damage and apoptosis caused by benzo[*a*]pyrene. *J. Appl. Toxicol.*, **23**, 255–261.

52 Vrzal, R., Zdarilova, A., Ulrichova, J., Blaha, L., Giesy, J.P., and Dvorak, Z. (2005) Activation of the aryl hydrocarbon receptor by berberine in HepG2 and H4IIE cells: biphasic effect on CYP1A1. *Biochem. Pharmacol.*, **70**, 925–936.

53 Fukuda, I., Mukai, R., Kawase, M., Yoshida, K., and Ashida, H. (2007) Interaction between the aryl hydrocarbon receptor and its antagonists, flavonoids. *Biochem. Biophys. Res. Commun.*, **359**, 822–827.

54 Amakura, Y., Tsutsumi, T., Sasaki, K., Nakamura, M., Yoshida, T., and Maitani, T. (2008) Influence of food polyphenols on aryl hydrocarbon receptor-signaling pathway estimated by *in vitro* bioassay. *Phytochemistry*, **69**, 3117–3130.

55 Ashida, H., Nishiumi, S., and Fukuda, I. (2008) An update on the dietary ligands of the AhR. *Expert Opin. Drug Metab. Toxicol.*, **4**, 1429–1447.

56 Moon, Y.J., Wang, X., and Morris, M.E. (2006) Dietary flavonoids: effects on xenobiotic and carcinogen metabolism. *Toxicol. In Vitro*, **20**, 187–210.

57 Daujat, M., Peryt, B., Lesca, P., Fourtanier, G., Domergue, J., and Maurel, P. (1992) Omeprazole, an inducer of human CYP1A1 and 1A2, is not a ligand for the Ah receptor. *Biochem. Biophys. Res. Commun.*, **188**, 820–825.

58 Murray, I.A. and Perdew, G.H. (2008) Omeprazole stimulates the induction of human insulin-like growth factor binding protein-1 through aryl hydrocarbon receptor activation. *J. Pharmacol. Exp. Ther.*, **324**, 1102–1110.

59 Yoshinari, K., Ueda, R., Kusano, K., Yoshimura, T., Nagata, K., and Yamazoe, Y. (2008) Omeprazole transactivates human CYP1A1 and CYP1A2 expression through the common regulatory region containing multiple xenobiotic-responsive elements. *Biochem. Pharmacol.*, **76**, 139–145.

60 Curi-Pedrosa, R., Daujat, M., Pichard, L., Ourlin, J.C., Clair, P., Gervot, L., Lesca, P., Domergue, J., Joyeux, H., Fourtanier, G., *et al.* (1994) Omeprazole and lansoprazole are mixed inducers of CYP1A and CYP3A in human hepatocytes in primary culture. *J. Pharmacol. Exp. Ther.*, **269**, 384–392.

61 Daujat, M., Charrasse, S., Fabre, I., Lesca, P., Jounaidi, Y., Larroque, C., Poellinger, L., and Maurel, P. (1996) Induction of CYP1A1 gene by benzimidazole derivatives during Caco-2 cell differentiation. Evidence for an aryl-hydrocarbon receptor-mediated mechanism. *Eur. J. Biochem.*, **237**, 642–652.

62 Matsuoka-Kawano, K., Yoshinari, K., Nagayama, S., and Yamazoe, Y. (2010) TSU-16, (*Z*)-3-[(2,4-dimethylpyrrol-5-yl) methylidenyl]-2-indolinone, is a potent activator of aryl hydrocarbon receptor and increases CYP1A1 and CYP1A2 expression in human hepatocytes. *Chem. Biol. Interact.*, **185**, 33–41.

63 Nguyen, L.P. and Bradfield, C.A. (2008) The search for endogenous activators of the aryl hydrocarbon receptor. *Chem. Res. Toxicol.*, **21**, 102–116.

64 Sinal, C.J. and Bend, J.R. (1997) Aryl hydrocarbon receptor-dependent induction of cyp1a1 by bilirubin in mouse hepatoma Hepa 1c1c7 cells. *Mol. Pharmacol.*, **52**, 590–599.

65 Phelan, D., Winter, G.M., Rogers, W.J., Lam, J.C., and Denison, M.S. (1998) Activation of the Ah receptor signal transduction pathway by bilirubin and biliverdin. *Arch. Biochem. Biophys.*, **357**, 155–163.

66 Adachi, J., Mori, Y., Matsui, S., Takigami, H., Fujino, J., Kitagawa, H., Miller, C.A., 3rd, Kato, T., Saeki, K., and Matsuda, T. (2001) Indirubin and indigo are potent aryl hydrocarbon receptor ligands present in human urine. *J. Biol. Chem.*, **276**, 31475–31478.

67 Wincent, E., Amini, N., Luecke, S., Glatt, H., Bergman, J., Crescenzi, C., Rannug, A., and Rannug, U. (2009) The suggested physiologic aryl hydrocarbon receptor activator and cytochrome P4501 substrate 6-formylindolo[3,2-*b*]carbazole is present in humans. *J. Biol. Chem.*, **284**, 2690–2696.

68 Wincent, E., Shirani, H., Bergman, J., Rannug, U., and Janosik, T. (2009) Synthesis and biological evaluation of fused thio- and selenopyrans as new indolocarbazole analogues with aryl hydrocarbon receptor affinity. *Bioorg. Med. Chem.*, **17**, 1648–1653.

69 Rifkind, A.B. (2006) CYP1A in TCDD toxicity and in physiology–with particular reference to CYP dependent arachidonic acid metabolism and other endogenous substrates. *Drug Metab. Rev.*, **38**, 291–335.

70 Chiaro, C.R., Morales, J.L., Prabhu, K.S., and Perdew, G.H. (2008) Leukotriene A4 metabolites are endogenous ligands for the Ah receptor. *Biochemistry*, **47**, 8445–8455.

71 Chiaro, C.R., Patel, R.D., and Perdew, G.H. (2008) 12(*R*)-Hydroxy-5(*Z*),8(*Z*),10(*E*),14(*Z*)-eicosatetraenoic acid [12(*R*)-HETE], an arachidonic acid derivative, is an activator of the aryl hydrocarbon receptor. *Mol. Pharmacol.*, **74**, 1649–1656.

72 Seidel, S.D., Winters, G.M., Rogers, W.J., Ziccardi, M.H., Li, V., Keser, B., and Denison, M.S. (2001) Activation of the Ah receptor signaling pathway by prostaglandins. *J. Biochem. Mol. Toxicol.*, **15**, 187–196.

73 Harper, P.A., Riddick, D.S., and Okey, A.B. (2006) Regulating the regulator: factors that control levels and activity of the aryl hydrocarbon receptor. *Biochem. Pharmacol.*, **72**, 267–279.

74 Puga, A., Ma, C., and Marlowe, J.L. (2009) The aryl hydrocarbon receptor cross-talks with multiple signal transduction pathways. *Biochem. Pharmacol.*, **77**, 713–722.

75 Marlowe, J.L. and Puga, A. (2005) Aryl hydrocarbon receptor, cell cycle regulation, toxicity, and tumorigenesis. *J. Cell. Biochem.*, **96**, 1174–1184.

76 Bock, K.W. and Kohle, C. (2005) Ah receptor- and TCDD-mediated liver tumor promotion: clonal selection and expansion of cells evading growth arrest and apoptosis. *Biochem. Pharmacol.*, **69**, 1403–1408.

77 Esser, C. (2009) The immune phenotype of AhR null mouse mutants: not a simple mirror of xenobiotic receptor over-activation. *Biochem. Pharmacol.*, **77**, 597–607.

78 Esser, C., Rannug, A., and Stockinger, B. (2009) The aryl hydrocarbon receptor in immunity. *Trends Immunol.*, **30**, 447–454.

79 Head, J.L. and Lawrence, B.P. (2009) The aryl hydrocarbon receptor is a modulator of anti-viral immunity. *Biochem. Pharmacol.*, **77**, 642–653.

80 Shimba, S. and Watabe, Y. (2009) Crosstalk between the AHR signaling pathway and circadian rhythm. *Biochem. Pharmacol.*, **77**, 560–565.

81 Gasiewicz, T.A., Henry, E.C., and Collins, L.L. (2008) Expression and

activity of aryl hydrocarbon receptors in development and cancer. *Crit. Rev. Eukaryot. Gene Expr.*, **18**, 279–321.

82 Ray, S. and Swanson, H.I. (2009) Activation of the aryl hydrocarbon receptor by TCDD inhibits senescence: a tumor promoting event? *Biochem. Pharmacol.*, **77**, 681–688.

83 Gouedard, C., Barouki, R. and Morel, Y. (2004) Induction of the paraoxonase-1 gene expression by resveratrol. *Arterioscler. Thromb. Vasc. Biol.*, **24**, 2378–2383.

84 Gouedard, C., Barouki, R., and Morel, Y. (2004) Dietary polyphenols increase paraoxonase 1 gene expression by an aryl hydrocarbon receptor-dependent mechanism. *Mol. Cell. Biol.*, **24**, 5209–5222.

85 Ohtake, F., Fujii-Kuriyama, Y., and Kato, S. (2009) AhR acts as an E3 ubiquitin ligase to modulate steroid receptor functions. *Biochem. Pharmacol.*, **77**, 474–484.

86 Ohtake, F., Baba, A., Takada, I., Okada, M., Iwasaki, K., Miki, H., Takahashi, S., Kouzmenko, A., Nohara, K., Chiba, T., Fujii-Kuriyama, Y., and Kato, S. (2007) Dioxin receptor is a ligand-dependent E3 ubiquitin ligase. *Nature*, **446**, 562–566.

87 Henklova, P., Vrzal, R., Ulrichova, J., and Dvorak, Z. (2008) Role of mitogen-activated protein kinases in aryl hydrocarbon receptor signaling. *Chem. Biol. Interact.*, **172**, 93–104.

88 McGuire, J., Whitelaw, M.L., Pongratz, I., Gustafsson, J.A., and Poellinger, L. (1994) A cellular factor stimulates ligand-dependent release of hsp90 from the basic helix–loop–helix dioxin receptor. *Mol. Cell. Biol.*, **14**, 2438–2446.

89 Lees, M.J. and Whitelaw, M.L. (1999) Multiple roles of ligand in transforming the dioxin receptor to an active basic helix–loop–helix/PAS transcription factor complex with the nuclear protein Arnt. *Mol. Cell. Biol.*, **19**, 5811–5822.

90 Heid, S.E., Pollenz, R.S., and Swanson, H.I. (2000) Role of heat shock protein 90 dissociation in mediating agonist-induced activation of the aryl hydrocarbon receptor. *Mol. Pharmacol.*, **57**, 82–92.

91 Pollenz, R.S., Sattler, C.A., and Poland, A. (1994) The aryl hydrocarbon receptor and aryl hydrocarbon receptor nuclear translocator protein show distinct subcellular localizations in Hepa 1c1c7 cells by immunofluorescence microscopy. *Mol. Pharmacol.*, **45**, 428–438.

92 Pollenz, R.S. (2007) Specific blockage of ligand-induced degradation of the Ah receptor by proteasome but not calpain inhibitors in cell culture lines from different species. *Biochem. Pharmacol.*, **74**, 131–143.

93 Pollenz, R.S. and Buggy, C. (2006) Ligand-dependent and -independent degradation of the human aryl hydrocarbon receptor (hAHR) in cell culture models. *Chem. Biol. Interact.*, **164**, 49–59.

94 Pollenz, R.S., Popat, J., and Dougherty, E.J. (2005) Role of the carboxy-terminal transactivation domain and active transcription in the ligand-induced and ligand-independent degradation of the mouse Ahb-1 receptor. *Biochem. Pharmacol.*, **70**, 1623–1633.

95 Kliewer, S.A., Moore, J.T., Wade, L., Staudinger, J.L., Watson, M.A., Jones, S.A., McKee, D.D., Oliver, B.B., Willson, T.M., Zetterstrom, R.H., Perlmann, T., and Lehmann, J.M. (1998) An orphan nuclear receptor activated by pregnanes defines a novel steroid signaling pathway. *Cell*, **92**, 73–82.

96 Lehmann, J.M., McKee, D.D., Watson, M.A., Willson, T.M., Moore, J.T., and Kliewer, S.A. (1998) The human orphan nuclear receptor PXR is activated by compounds that regulate CYP3A4 gene expression and cause drug interactions. *J. Clin. Invest.*, **102**, 1016–1023.

97 Bertilsson, G., Heidrich, J., Svensson, K., Asman, M., Jendeberg, L., Sydow-Backman, M., Ohlsson, R., Postlind, H., Blomquist, P., and Berkenstam, A. (1998) Identification of a human nuclear receptor defines a new signaling pathway for CYP3A induction. *Proc. Natl. Acad. Sci. USA*, **95**, 12208–12213.

98 Schuetz, E.G., Brimer, C., and Schuetz, J.D. (1998) Environmental xenobiotics and the antihormones cyproterone acetate and spironolactone use the

nuclear hormone pregnenolone X receptor to activate the CYP3A23 hormone response element. *Mol. Pharmacol.*, **54**, 1113–1117.

99 Pascussi, J.M., Jounaidi, Y., Drocourt, L., Domergue, J., Balabaud, C., Maurel, P., and Vilarem, M.J. (1999) Evidence for the presence of a functional pregnane X receptor response element in the CYP3A7 promoter gene. *Biochem. Biophys. Res. Commun.*, **260**, 377–381.

100 Jones, S.A., Moore, L.B., Shenk, J.L., Wisely, G.B., Hamilton, G.A., McKee, D.D., Tomkinson, N.C., LeCluyse, E.L., Lambert, M.H., Willson, T.M., Kliewer, S.A., and Moore, J.T. (2000) The pregnane X receptor: a promiscuous xenobiotic receptor that has diverged during evolution. *Mol. Endocrinol.*, **14**, 27–39.

101 Watkins, R.E., Wisely, G.B., Moore, L.B., Collins, J.L., Lambert, M.H., Williams, S.P., Willson, T.M., Kliewer, S.A., and Redinbo, M.R. (2001) The human nuclear xenobiotic receptor PXR: structural determinants of directed promiscuity. *Science*, **292**, 2329–2333.

102 Watkins, R.E., Maglich, J.M., Moore, L.B., Wisely, G.B., Noble, S.M., Davis-Searles, P.R., Lambert, M.H., Kliewer, S.A., and Redinbo, M.R. (2003) 2.1 A crystal structure of human PXR in complex with the St. John's wort compound hyperforin. *Biochemistry*, **42**, 1430–1438.

103 Pascussi, J.M., Gerbal-Chaloin, S., Drocourt, L., Maurel, P., and Vilarem, M.J. (2003) The expression of CYP2B6, CYP2C9 and CYP3A4 genes: a tangle of networks of nuclear and steroid receptors. *Biochim. Biophys. Acta*, **1619**, 243–253.

104 Pascussi, J.M., Gerbal-Chaloin, S., Duret, C., Daujat-Chavanieu, M., Vilarem, M.J., and Maurel, P. (2008) The tangle of nuclear receptors that controls xenobiotic metabolism and transport: crosstalk and consequences. *Annu. Rev. Pharmacol. Toxicol.*, **48**, 1–32.

105 Wan, Y.J., An, D., Cai, Y., Repa, J.J., Hung-Po Chen, T., Flores, M., Postic, C., Magnuson, M.A., Chen, J., Chien, K.R., French, S., Mangelsdorf, D.J., and Sucov, H.M. (2000) Hepatocyte-specific mutation establishes retinoid X receptor alpha as a heterodimeric integrator of multiple physiological processes in the liver. *Mol. Cell. Biol.*, **20**, 4436–4444.

106 Watkins, R.E., Davis-Searles, P.R., Lambert, M.H., and Redinbo, M.R. (2003) Coactivator binding promotes the specific interaction between ligand and the pregnane X receptor. *J. Mol. Biol.*, **331**, 815–828.

107 Waxman, D.J. (1999) P450 gene induction by structurally diverse xenochemicals: central role of nuclear receptors CAR, PXR, and PPAR. *Arch. Biochem. Biophys.*, **369**, 11–23.

108 Ngan, C.H., Beglov, D., Rudnitskaya, A.N., Kozakov, D., Waxman, D.J., and Vajda, S. (2009) The structural basis of pregnane X receptor binding promiscuity. *Biochemistry*, **48**, 11572–11581.

109 Chang, T.K. (2009) Activation of pregnane X receptor (PXR) and constitutive androstane receptor (CAR) by herbal medicines. *AAPS J.*, **11**, 590–601.

110 Mnif, W., Pascussi, J.M., Pillon, A., Escande, A., Bartegi, A., Nicolas, J.C., Cavailles, V., Duchesne, M.J., and Balaguer, P. (2007) Estrogens and antiestrogens activate hPXR. *Toxicol. Lett.*, **170**, 19–29.

111 Hurst, C.H. and Waxman, D.J. (2004) Environmental phthalate monoesters activate pregnane X receptor-mediated transcription. *Toxicol. Appl. Pharmacol.*, **199**, 266–274.

112 Wyde, M.E., Kirwan, S.E., Zhang, F., Laughter, A., Hoffman, H.B., Bartolucci-Page, E., Gaido, K.W., Yan, B., and You, L. (2005) Di-*n*-butyl phthalate activates constitutive androstane receptor and pregnane X receptor and enhances the expression of steroid-metabolizing enzymes in the liver of rat fetuses. *Toxicol. Sci.*, **86**, 281–290.

113 Svecova, L., Vrzal, R., Burysek, L., Anzenbacherova, E., Cerveny, L., Grim, J., Trejtnar, F., Kunes, J., Pour, M., Staud, F., Anzenbacher, P., Dvorak, Z., and Pavek, P. (2008) Azole antimycotics differentially affect rifampicin-induced pregnane X receptor-mediated CYP3A4 gene expression. *Drug Metab. Dispos.*, **36**, 339–348.

114 Luo, G., Cunningham, M., Kim, S., Burn, T., Lin, J., Sinz, M., Hamilton, G., Rizzo, C., Jolley, S., Gilbert, D., Downey, A., Mudra, D., Graham, R., Carroll, K., Xie, J., Madan, A., Parkinson, A., Christ, D., Selling, B., LeCluyse, E., and Gan, L.S. (2002) CYP3A4 induction by drugs: correlation between a pregnane X receptor reporter gene assay and CYP3A4 expression in human hepatocytes. *Drug Metab. Dispos.*, **30**, 795–804.

115 Cerveny, L., Svecova, L., Anzenbacherova, E., Vrzal, R., Staud, F., Dvorak, Z., Ulrichova, J., Anzenbacher, P., and Pavek, P. (2007) Valproic acid induces CYP3A4 and MDR1 gene expression by activation of constitutive androstane receptor and pregnane X receptor pathways. *Drug Metab. Dispos.*, **35**, 1032–1041.

116 Vrzal, R., Kubesova, K., Pavek, P., and Dvorak, Z. (2010) Benzodiazepines medazepam and midazolam are activators of pregnane X receptor and weak inducers of CYP3A4: investigation in primary cultures of human hepatocytes and hepatocarcinoma cell lines. *Toxicol. Lett.*, **193**, 183–188.

117 Drocourt, L., Pascussi, J.M., Assenat, E., Fabre, J.M., Maurel, P., and Vilarem, M.J. (2001) Calcium channel modulators of the dihydropyridine family are human pregnane X receptor activators and inducers of CYP3A, CYP2B, and CYP2C in human hepatocytes. *Drug Metab. Dispos.*, **29**, 1325–1331.

118 Rushmore, T.H. and Kong, A.N. (2002) Pharmacogenomics, regulation and signaling pathways of phase I and II drug metabolizing enzymes. *Curr. Drug Metab.*, **3**, 481–490.

119 Zhou, J., Zhang, J., and Xie, W. (2005) Xenobiotic nuclear receptor-mediated regulation of UDP-glucuronosyl-transferases. *Curr. Drug Metab.*, **6**, 289–298.

120 Dixit, S.G., Tirona, R.G., and Kim, R.B. (2005) Beyond CAR and PXR. *Curr. Drug Metab.*, **6**, 385–397.

121 Runge-Morris, M. and Kocarek, T.A. (2005) Regulation of sulfotransferases by xenobiotic receptors. *Curr. Drug Metab.*, **6**, 299–307.

122 Klaassen, C.D. and Slitt, A.L. (2005) Regulation of hepatic transporters by xenobiotic receptors. *Curr. Drug Metab.*, **6**, 309–328.

123 Xu, C., Li, C.Y., and Kong, A.N. (2005) Induction of phase I, II and III drug metabolism/transport by xenobiotics. *Arch. Pharm. Res.*, **28**, 249–268.

124 Bock, K.W. and Bock-Hennig, B.S. (2010) UDP-glucuronosyltransferases (UGTs): from purification of Ah-receptor-inducible UGT1A6 to coordinate regulation of subsets of CYPs, UGTs, and ABC transporters by nuclear receptors. *Drug Metab. Rev.*, **42**, 6–13.

125 Kohle, C. and Bock, K.W. (2009) Coordinate regulation of human drug-metabolizing enzymes, and conjugate transporters by the Ah receptor, pregnane X receptor and constitutive androstane receptor. *Biochem. Pharmacol.*, **77**, 689–699.

126 Urquhart, B.L., Tirona, R.G., and Kim, R.B. (2007) Nuclear receptors and the regulation of drug-metabolizing enzymes and drug transporters: implications for interindividual variability in response to drugs. *J. Clin. Pharmacol.*, **47**, 566–578.

127 Konno, Y., Negishi, M., and Kodama, S. (2008) The roles of nuclear receptors CAR and PXR in hepatic energy metabolism. *Drug Metab. Pharmacokinet.*, **23**, 8–13.

128 di Masi, A., Marinis, E.D., Ascenzi, P., and Marino, M. (2009) Nuclear receptors CAR and PXR: molecular, functional, and biomedical aspects. *Mol. Aspects Med.*, **30**, 297–343.

129 Moreau, A., Vilarem, M.J., Maurel, P., and Pascussi, J.M. (2008) Xenoreceptors CAR and PXR activation and consequences on lipid metabolism, glucose homeostasis, and inflammatory response. *Mol. Pharm.*, **5**, 35–41.

130 Wada, T., Gao, J., and Xie, W. (2009) PXR and CAR in energy metabolism. *Trends Endocrinol. Metab.*, **20**, 273–279.

131 Kakizaki, S., Yamazaki, Y., Takizawa, D., and Negishi, M. (2008) New insights on the xenobiotic-sensing nuclear receptors

in liver diseases–CAR and PXR. *Curr. Drug Metab.*, **9**, 614–621.

132 Roth, A., Looser, R., Kaufmann, M., Blattler, S.M., Rencurel, F., Huang, W., Moore, D.D., and Meyer, U.A. (2008) Regulatory cross-talk between drug metabolism and lipid homeostasis: constitutive androstane receptor and pregnane X receptor increase Insig-1 expression. *Mol. Pharmacol.*, **73**, 1282–1289.

133 Moreau, A., Teruel, C., Beylot, M., Albalea, V., Tamasi, V., Umbdenstock, T., Parmentier, Y., Sa-Cunha, A., Suc, B., Fabre, J.M., Navarro, F., Ramos, J., Meyer, U., Maurel, P., Vilarem, M.J., and Pascussi, J.M. (2009) A novel pregnane X receptor and S14-mediated lipogenic pathway in human hepatocyte. *Hepatology*, **49**, 2068–2079.

134 Bachmann, K., Patel, H., Batayneh, Z., Slama, J., White, D., Posey, J., Ekins, S., Gold, D., and Sambucetti, L. (2004) PXR and the regulation of apoA1 and HDL-cholesterol in rodents. *Pharmacol. Res.*, **50**, 237–246.

135 de Haan, W., de Vries-van der Weij, J., Mol, I.M., Hoekstra, M., Romijn, J.A., Jukema, J.W., Havekes, L.M., Princen, H.M., and Rensen, P.C. (2009) PXR agonism decreases plasma HDL levels in ApoE3-Leiden.CETP mice. *Biochim. Biophys. Acta*, **1791**, 191–197.

136 Traber, M.G. (2004) Vitamin E, nuclear receptors and xenobiotic metabolism. *Arch. Biochem. Biophys.*, **423**, 6–11.

137 Landes, N., Pfluger, P., Kluth, D., Birringer, M., Ruhl, R., Bol, G.F., Glatt, H., and Brigelius-Flohe, R. (2003) Vitamin E activates gene expression via the pregnane X receptor. *Biochem. Pharmacol.*, **65**, 269–273.

138 Igarashi, M., Yogiashi, Y., Mihara, M., Takada, I., Kitagawa, H., and Kato, S. (2007) Vitamin K induces osteoblast differentiation through pregnane X receptor-mediated transcriptional control of the Msx2 gene. *Mol. Cell. Biol.*, **27**, 7947–7954.

139 Ruhl, R. (2005) Induction of PXR-mediated metabolism by beta-carotene. *Biochim. Biophys. Acta*, **1740**, 162–169.

140 Zollner, G., Marschall, H.U., Wagner, M., and Trauner, M. (2006) Role of nuclear receptors in the adaptive response to bile acids and cholestasis: pathogenetic and therapeutic considerations. *Mol. Pharm.*, **3**, 231–251.

141 Barbier, O., Trottier, J., Kaeding, J., Caron, P., and Verreault, M. (2009) Lipid-activated transcription factors control bile acid glucuronidation. *Mol. Cell. Biochem.*, **326**, 3–8.

142 Honkakoski, P., Zelko, I., Sueyoshi, T., and Negishi, M. (1998) The nuclear orphan receptor CAR-retinoid X receptor heterodimer activates the phenobarbital-responsive enhancer module of the CYP2B gene. *Mol. Cell. Biol.*, **18**, 5652–5658.

143 Sueyoshi, T., Kawamoto, T., Zelko, I., Honkakoski, P., and Negishi, M. (1999) The repressed nuclear receptor CAR responds to phenobarbital in activating the human CYP2B6 gene. *J. Biol. Chem.*, **274**, 6043–6046.

144 Yoshinari, K., Kobayashi, K., Moore, R., Kawamoto, T., and Negishi, M. (2003) Identification of the nuclear receptor CAR:HSP90 complex in mouse liver and recruitment of protein phosphatase 2A in response to phenobarbital. *FEBS Lett.*, **548**, 17–20.

145 Kawamoto, T., Sueyoshi, T., Zelko, I., Moore, R., Washburn, K., and Negishi, M. (1999) Phenobarbital-responsive nuclear translocation of the receptor CAR in induction of the CYP2B gene. *Mol. Cell. Biol.*, **19**, 6318–6322.

146 Zelko, I., Sueyoshi, T., Kawamoto, T., Moore, R., and Negishi, M. (2001) The peptide near the C terminus regulates receptor CAR nuclear translocation induced by xenochemicals in mouse liver. *Mol. Cell. Biol.*, **21**, 2838–2846.

147 Sueyoshi, T., Moore, R., Sugatani, J., Matsumura, Y., and Negishi, M. (2008) PPP1R16A, the membrane subunit of protein phosphatase 1beta, signals nuclear translocation of the nuclear receptor constitutive active/androstane receptor. *Mol. Pharmacol.*, **73**, 1113–1121.

148 Sueyoshi, T. and Negishi, M. (2001) Phenobarbital response elements of cytochrome P450 genes and nuclear receptors. *Annu. Rev. Pharmacol. Toxicol.*, **41**, 123–143.

149 Auerbach, S.S., Stoner, M.A., Su, S., and Omiecinski, C.J. (2005) Retinoid X receptor-alpha-dependent transactivation by a naturally occurring structural variant of human constitutive androstane receptor (NR1I3). *Mol. Pharmacol.*, **68**, 1239–1253.

150 Bae, Y., Kemper, J.K., and Kemper, B. (2004) Repression of CAR-mediated transactivation of CYP2B genes by the orphan nuclear receptor, short heterodimer partner (SHP). *DNA Cell Biol.*, **23**, 81–91.

151 Forman, B.M., Tzameli, I., Choi, H.S., Chen, J., Simha, D., Seol, W., Evans, R.M., and Moore, D.D. (1998) Androstane metabolites bind to and deactivate the nuclear receptor CAR-beta. *Nature*, **395**, 612–615.

152 Tzameli, I., Pissios, P., Schuetz, E.G., and Moore, D.D. (2000) The xenobiotic compound 1,4-bis[2-(3,5-dichloropyridyloxy)]benzene is an agonist ligand for the nuclear receptor CAR. *Mol. Cell. Biol.*, **20**, 2951–2958.

153 Maglich, J.M., Parks, D.J., Moore, L.B., Collins, J.L., Goodwin, B., Billin, A.N., Stoltz, C.A., Kliewer, S.A., Lambert, M.H., Willson, T.M., and Moore, J.T. (2003) Identification of a novel human constitutive androstane receptor (CAR) agonist and its use in the identification of CAR target genes. *J. Biol. Chem.*, **278**, 17277–17283.

154 DeKeyser, J.G., Stagliano, M.C., Auerbach, S.S., Prabhu, K.S., Jones, A.D., and Omiecinski, C.J. (2009) Di(2-ethylhexyl) phthalate is a highly potent agonist for the human constitutive androstane receptor splice variant CAR2. *Mol. Pharmacol.*, **75**, 1005–1013.

155 Chang, T.K. and Waxman, D.J. (2006) Synthetic drugs and natural products as modulators of constitutive androstane receptor (CAR) and pregnane X receptor (PXR). *Drug Metab. Rev.*, **38**, 51–73.

156 Willson, T.M. and Kliewer, S.A. (2002) PXR, CAR and drug metabolism. *Nat. Rev. Drug Discov.*, **1**, 259–266.

157 Kocarek, T.A. and Mercer-Haines, N.A. (2002) Squalestatin 1-inducible expression of rat CYP2B: evidence that an endogenous isoprenoid is an activator of the constitutive androstane receptor. *Mol. Pharmacol.*, **62**, 1177–1186.

158 Kakizaki, S., Yamamoto, Y., Ueda, A., Moore, R., Sueyoshi, T., and Negishi, M. (2003) Phenobarbital induction of drug/steroid-metabolizing enzymes and nuclear receptor CAR. *Biochim. Biophys. Acta*, **1619**, 239–242.

159 Monostory, K., Pascussi, J.M., Kobori, L., and Dvorak, Z. (2009) Hormonal regulation of CYP1A expression. *Drug Metab. Rev.*, **41**, 547–572.

160 Safe, S. and Wormke, M. (2003) Inhibitory aryl hydrocarbon receptor-estrogen receptor alpha cross-talk and mechanisms of action. *Chem. Res. Toxicol.*, **16**, 807–816.

161 Dvorak, Z. and Pavek, P. (2010) Regulation of drug-metabolizing cytochrome P450 enzymes by glucocorticoids. *Drug Metab. Rev.*, **42**, 621–635.

162 Beischlag, T.V., Taylor, R.T., Rose, D.W., Yoon, D., Chen, Y., Lee, W.H., Rosenfeld, M.G., and Hankinson, O. (2004) Recruitment of thyroid hormone receptor/retinoblastoma-interacting protein 230 by the aryl hydrocarbon receptor nuclear translocator is required for the transcriptional response to both dioxin and hypoxia. *J. Biol. Chem.*, **279**, 54620–54628.

163 Murphy, K.A., Quadro, L., and White, L.A. (2007) The intersection between the aryl hydrocarbon receptor (AhR)- and retinoic acid-signaling pathways. *Vitam. Horm.*, **75**, 33–67.

164 Fallone, F., Villard, P.H., Seree, E., Rimet, O., Nguyen, Q.B., Bourgarel-Rey, V., Fouchier, F., Barra, Y., Durand, A., and Lacarelle, B. (2004) Retinoids repress Ah receptor CYP1A1 induction pathway through the SMRT corepressor. *Biochem. Biophys. Res. Commun.*, **322**, 551–556.

165 Seree, E., Villard, P.H., Pascussi, J.M., Pineau, T., Maurel, P., Nguyen, Q.B., Fallone, F., Martin, P.M., Champion, S., Lacarelle, B., Savouret, J.F., and Barra, Y. (2004) Evidence for a new human CYP1A1 regulation pathway involving PPAR-alpha and 2 PPRE sites. *Gastroenterology*, **127**, 1436–1445.

166 Fallone, F., Villard, P.H., Decome, L., Seree, E., Meo, M., Chacon, C., Durand, A., Barra, Y., and Lacarelle, B. (2005) PPARalpha activation potentiates AhR-induced CYP1A1 expression. *Toxicology*, **216**, 122–128.

167 Pavek, P., Pospechova, K., Svecova, L., Syrova, Z., Stejskalova, L., Blazkova, J., Dvorak, Z., and Blahos, J. (2010) Intestinal cell-specific vitamin D receptor (VDR)-mediated transcriptional regulation of CYP3A4 gene. *Biochem. Pharmacol.*, **79**, 277–287.

168 Drocourt, L., Ourlin, J.C., Pascussi, J.M., Maurel, P., and Vilarem, M.J. (2002) Expression of CYP3A4, CYP2B6, and CYP2C9 is regulated by the vitamin D receptor pathway in primary human hepatocytes. *J. Biol. Chem.*, **277**, 25125–25132.

169 Wang, K., Chen, S., Xie, W., and Wan, Y.J. (2008) Retinoids induce cytochrome P450 3A4 through RXR/VDR-mediated pathway. *Biochem. Pharmacol.*, **75**, 2204–2213.

170 Matsubara, T., Yoshinari, K., Aoyama, K., Sugawara, M., Sekiya, Y., Nagata, K., and Yamazoe, Y. (2008) Role of vitamin D receptor in the lithocholic acid-mediated CYP3A induction *in vitro* and *in vivo*. *Drug Metab. Dispos.*, **36**, 2058–2063.

171 Onica, T., Nichols, K., Larin, M., Ng, L., Maslen, A., Dvorak, Z., Pascussi, J.M., Vilarem, M.J., Maurel, P., and Kirby, G.M. (2008) Dexamethasone-mediated up regulation of human CYP2A6 involves the glucocorticoid receptor and increased binding of hepatic nuclear factor 4α to the proximal promoter. *Mol. Pharmacol.*, **73**, 451–460.

172 Calleja, C., Pascussi, J.M., Mani, J.C., Maurel, P., and Vilarem, M.J. (1998) The antibiotic rifampicin is a nonsteroidal ligand and activator of the human glucocorticoid receptor. *Nat. Med.*, **4**, 92–96.

173 Duret, C., Daujat-Chavanieu, M., Pascussi, J.M., Pichard-Garcia, L., Balaguer, P., Fabre, J.M., Vilarem, M.J., Maurel, P., and Gerbal-Chaloin, S. (2006) Ketoconazole and miconazole are antagonists of the human glucocorticoid receptor: consequences on the expression and function of the constitutive androstane receptor and the pregnane X receptor. *Mol. Pharmacol.*, **70**, 329–339.

174 Martinez-Jimenez, C.P., Jover, R., Donato, M.T., Castell, J.V., and Gomez-Lechon, M.J. (2007) Transcriptional regulation and expression of CYP3A4 in hepatocytes. *Curr. Drug Metab.*, **8**, 185–194.

175 Pascussi, J.M., Robert, A., Nguyen, M., Walrant-Debray, O., Garabedian, M., Martin, P., Pineau, T., Saric, J., Navarro, F., Maurel, P., and Vilarem, M.J. (2005) Possible involvement of pregnane X receptor-enhanced CYP24 expression in drug-induced osteomalacia. *J. Clin. Invest.*, **115**, 177–186.

176 Moreau, A., Maurel, P., Vilarem, M.J., and Pascussi, J.M. (2007) Constitutive androstane receptor–vitamin D receptor crosstalk: consequence on CYP24 gene expression. *Biochem. Biophys. Res. Commun.*, **360**, 76–82.

177 Pascussi, J.M., Busson-Le Coniat, M., Maurel, P., and Vilarem, M.J. (2003) Transcriptional analysis of the orphan nuclear receptor constitutive androstane receptor (NR1I3) gene promoter: identification of a distal glucocorticoid response element. *Mol. Endocrinol.*, **17**, 42–55.

178 Pascussi, J.M., Drocourt, L., Fabre, J.M., Maurel, P., and Vilarem, M.J. (2000) Dexamethasone induces pregnane X receptor and retinoid X receptor-alpha expression in human hepatocytes: synergistic increase of CYP3A4 induction by pregnane X receptor activators. *Mol. Pharmacol.*, **58**, 361–372.

179 Pascussi, J.M., Drocourt, L., Gerbal-Chaloin, S., Fabre, J.M., Maurel, P., and Vilarem, M.J. (2001) Dual effect of dexamethasone on CYP3A4 gene expression in human hepatocytes. Sequential role of glucocorticoid receptor and pregnane X receptor. *Eur. J. Biochem.*, **268**, 6346–6358.

180 Pascussi, J.M., Gerbal-Chaloin, S., Fabre, J.M., Maurel, P., and Vilarem, M.J. (2000) Dexamethasone enhances constitutive androstane receptor expression in human hepatocytes:

consequences on cytochrome P450 gene regulation. *Mol. Pharmacol.*, **58**, 1441–1450.

181 Dvorak, Z., Modriansky, M., Pichard-Garcia, L., Balaguer, P., Vilarem, M.J., Ulrichova, J., Maurel, P., and Pascussi, J.M. (2003) Colchicine down-regulates cytochrome P450 2B6, 2C8, 2C9, and 3A4 in human hepatocytes by affecting their glucocorticoid receptor-mediated regulation. *Mol. Pharmacol.*, **64**, 160–169.

182 Assenat, E., Gerbal-Chaloin, S., Larrey, D., Saric, J., Fabre, J.M., Maurel, P., Vilarem, M.J., and Pascussi, J.M. (2004) Interleukin 1beta inhibits CAR-induced expression of hepatic genes involved in drug and bilirubin clearance. *Hepatology*, **40**, 951–960.

183 Ohtake, F., Takeyama, K., Matsumoto, T., Kitagawa, H., Yamamoto, Y., Nohara, K., Tohyama, C., Krust, A., Mimura, J., Chambon, P., Yanagisawa, J., Fujii-Kuriyama, Y., and Kato, S. (2003) Modulation of oestrogen receptor signalling by association with the activated dioxin receptor. *Nature*, **423**, 545–550.

184 Sugatani, J., Kojima, H., Ueda, A., Kakizaki, S., Yoshinari, K., Gong, Q.H., Owens, I.S., Negishi, M., and Sueyoshi, T. (2001) The phenobarbital response enhancer module in the human bilirubin UDP-glucuronosyltransferase UGT1A1 gene and regulation by the nuclear receptor CAR. *Hepatology*, **33**, 1232–1238.

185 Tong, Z., Li, H., Goljer, I., McConnell, O., and Chandrasekaran, A. (2007) *In vitro* glucuronidation of thyroxine and triiodothyronine by liver microsomes and recombinant human UDP-glucuronosyltransferases. *Drug Metab. Dispos.*, **35**, 2203–2210.

186 Marunaka, Y., Niisato, N., and Miyazaki, H. (2005) New concept of spare receptors and effectors. *J. Membr. Biol.*, **203**, 31–39.

187 Leff, P. (1995) Inverse agonism: theory and practice. *Trends Pharmacol. Sci.*, **16**, 256.

188 Leff, P. (1995) The two-state model of receptor activation. *Trends Pharmacol. Sci.*, **16**, 89–97.

189 Carlier, P.R., Chow, E.S., Barlow, R.L., and Bloomquist, J.R. (2002) Discovery of non-zwitterionic GABA(A) receptor full agonists and a superagonist. *Bioorg. Med. Chem. Lett.*, **12**, 1985–1988.

190 Shimada, T. (2006) Xenobiotic-metabolizing enzymes involved in activation and detoxification of carcinogenic polycyclic aromatic hydrocarbons. *Drug Metab. Pharmacokinet.*, **21**, 257–276.

191 Zhou, S.F., Wang, B., Yang, L.P., and Liu, J.P. (2010) Structure, function, regulation and polymorphism and the clinical significance of human cytochrome P450 1A2. *Drug Metab. Rev.*, **42**, 268–354.

192 Wojcikowski, J., Boksa, J., and Daniel, W.A. (2010) Main contribution of the cytochrome P450 isoenzyme 1A2 (CYP1A2) to *N*-demethylation and 5-sulfoxidation of the phenothiazine neuroleptic chlorpromazine in human liver – a comparison with other phenothiazines. *Biochem. Pharmacol.*, **80**, 1252–1259.

193 Roberts, E.S., Vaz, A.D., and Coon, M.J. (1992) Role of isozymes of rabbit microsomal cytochrome P-450 in the metabolism of retinoic acid, retinol, and retinal. *Mol. Pharmacol.*, **41**, 427–433.

194 Wei, C., Caccavale, R.J., Kehoe, J.J., Thomas, P.E., and Iba, M.M. (2001) CYP1A2 is expressed along with CYP1A1 in the human lung. *Cancer Lett.*, **171**, 113–120.

195 Barouki, R., Coumoul, X., and Fernandez-Salguero, P.M. (2007) The aryl hydrocarbon receptor, more than a xenobiotic-interacting protein. *FEBS Lett.*, **581**, 3608–3615.

196 Bradshaw, T.D., Trapani, V., Vasselin, D.A., and Westwell, A.D. (2002) The aryl hydrocarbon receptor in anticancer drug discovery: friend or foe? *Curr. Pharm. Des.*, **8**, 2475–2490.

197 Swanson, H.I., Chan, W.K., and Bradfield, C.A. (1995) DNA binding specificities and pairing rules of the Ah receptor, ARNT, and SIM proteins. *J. Biol. Chem.*, **270**, 26292–26302.

198 Yoshinari, K., Yoda, N., Toriyabe, T., and Yamazoe, Y. (2010) Constitutive androstane receptor transcriptionally

activates human CYP1A1 and CYP1A2 genes through a common regulatory element in the 5′-flanking region. *Biochem. Pharmacol.*, **79**, 261–269.

199 Degawa, M., Hishinuma, T., Yoshida, H., and Hashimoto, Y. (1987) Species, sex and organ differences in induction of a cytochrome P-450 isozyme responsible for carcinogen activation: effects of dietary hepatocarcinogenic tryptophan pyrolysate components in mice and rats. *Carcinogenesis*, **8**, 1913–1918.

200 Kojima, M., Sekimoto, M., and Degawa, M. (2008) A novel gender-related difference in the constitutive expression of hepatic cytochrome P4501A subfamily enzymes in Meishan pigs. *Biochem. Pharmacol.*, **75**, 1076–1082.

201 Kuil, C.W., Brouwer, A., van der Saag, P.T., and van der Burg, B. (1998) Interference between progesterone and dioxin signal transduction pathways. Different mechanisms are involved in repression by the progesterone receptor A and B isoforms. *J. Biol. Chem.*, **273**, 8829–8834.

202 Lee, S.S., Jeong, H.G., and Yang, K.H. (1998) Effects of estradiol and progesterone on cytochrome P4501A1 expression in Hepa 1c1c7 cells. *Biochem. Mol. Biol. Int.*, **45**, 775–781.

203 Eugster, H.P., Probst, M., Wurgler, F.E., and Sengstag, C. (1993) Caffeine, estradiol, and progesterone interact with human CYP1A1 and CYP1A2. Evidence from cDNA-directed expression in *Saccharomyces cerevisiae*. *Drug Metab. Dispos.*, **21**, 43–49.

204 Matthews, J., Wihlen, B., Thomsen, J., and Gustafsson, J.A. (2005) Aryl hydrocarbon receptor-mediated transcription: ligand-dependent recruitment of estrogen receptor alpha to 2,3,7,8-tetrachlorodibenzo-*p*-dioxin-responsive promoters. *Mol. Cell. Biol.*, **25**, 5317–5328.

205 MacPherson, L., Lo, R., Ahmed, S., Pansoy, A., and Matthews, J. (2009) Activation function 2 mediates dioxin-induced recruitment of estrogen receptor alpha to CYP1A1 and CYP1B1. *Biochem. Biophys. Res. Commun.*, **385**, 263–268.

206 Porter, W., Wang, F., Duan, R., Qin, C., Castro-Rivera, E., Kim, K., and Safe, S. (2001) Transcriptional activation of heat shock protein 27 gene expression by 17beta-estradiol and modulation by antiestrogens and aryl hydrocarbon receptor agonists. *J. Mol. Endocrinol.*, **26**, 31–42.

207 Duan, R., Porter, W., Samudio, I., Vyhlidal, C., Kladde, M., and Safe, S. (1999) Transcriptional activation of c-*fos* protooncogene by 17beta-estradiol: mechanism of aryl hydrocarbon receptor-mediated inhibition. *Mol. Endocrinol.*, **13**, 1511–1521.

208 White, T.E. and Gasiewicz, T.A. (1993) The human estrogen receptor structural gene contains a DNA sequence that binds activated mouse and human Ah receptors: a possible mechanism of estrogen receptor regulation by 2,3,7,8-tetrachlorodibenzo-*p*-dioxin. *Biochem. Biophys. Res. Commun.*, **193**, 956–962.

209 Kumar, M.B. and Perdew, G.H. (1999) Nuclear receptor coactivator SRC-1 interacts with the Q-rich subdomain of the AhR and modulates its transactivation potential. *Gene Expr.*, **8**, 273–286.

210 Kumar, M.B., Tarpey, R.W., and Perdew, G.H. (1999) Differential recruitment of coactivator RIP140 by Ah and estrogen receptors. Absence of a role for LXXLL motifs. *J. Biol. Chem.*, **274**, 22155–22164.

211 Monostory, K., Kohalmy, K., Prough, R.A., Kobori, L., and Vereczkey, L. (2005) The effect of synthetic glucocorticoid, dexamethasone on CYP1A1 inducibility in adult rat and human hepatocytes. *FEBS Lett.*, **579**, 229–235.

212 Sonneveld, E., Jonas, A., Meijer, O.C., Brouwer, A., and van der Burg, B. (2007) Glucocorticoid-enhanced expression of dioxin target genes through regulation of the rat aryl hydrocarbon receptor. *Toxicol. Sci.*, **99**, 455–469.

213 Vrzal, R., Stejskalova, L., Monostory, K., Maurel, P., Bachleda, P., Pavek, P., and Dvorak, Z. (2009) Dexamethasone controls aryl hydrocarbon receptor (AhR)-mediated CYP1A1 and CYP1A2

expression and activity in primary cultures of human hepatocytes. *Chem. Biol. Interact.*, **179**, 288–296.

214 Dvorak, Z., Vrzal, R., Pavek, P., and Ulrichova, J. (2008) An evidence for regulatory cross-talk between aryl hydrocarbon receptor and glucocorticoid receptor in HepG2 cells. *Physiol. Res.*, **57**, 427–435.

215 Vrzal, R., Daujat-Chavanieu, M., Pascussi, J.M., Ulrichova, J., Maurel, P., and Dvorak, Z. (2008) Microtubules-interfering agents restrict aryl hydrocarbon receptor-mediated CYP1A2 induction in primary cultures of human hepatocytes via c-jun-N-terminal kinase and glucocorticoid receptor. *Eur. J. Pharmacol.*, **581**, 244–254.

216 Nguyen, T.A., Hoivik, D., Lee, J.E., and Safe, S. (1999) Interactions of nuclear receptor coactivator/corepressor proteins with the aryl hydrocarbon receptor complex. *Arch. Biochem. Biophys.*, **367**, 250–257.

217 Froidevaux, M.S., Berg, P., Seugnet, I., Decherf, S., Becker, N., Sachs, L.M., Bilesimo, P., Nygard, M., Pongratz, I., and Demeneix, B.A. (2006) The co-chaperone XAP2 is required for activation of hypothalamic thyrotropin-releasing hormone transcription *in vivo*. *EMBO Rep.*, **7**, 1035–1039.

218 Rushing, S.R. and Denison, M.S. (2002) The silencing mediator of retinoic acid and thyroid hormone receptors can interact with the aryl hydrocarbon (Ah) receptor but fails to repress Ah receptor-dependent gene expression. *Arch. Biochem. Biophys.*, **403**, 189–201.

219 Gambone, C.J., Hutcheson, J.M., Gabriel, J.L., Beard, R.L., Chandraratna, R.A., Soprano, K.J., and Soprano, D.R. (2002) Unique property of some synthetic retinoids: activation of the aryl hydrocarbon receptor pathway. *Mol. Pharmacol.*, **61**, 334–342.

220 Vecchini, F., Lenoir-Viale, M.C., Cathelineau, C., Magdalou, J., Bernard, B.A., and Shroot, B. (1994) Presence of a retinoid responsive element in the promoter region of the human cytochrome P4501A1 gene. *Biochem. Biophys. Res. Commun.*, **201**, 1205–1212.

221 Tian, Y., Ke, S., Denison, M.S., Rabson, A.B., and Gallo, M.A. (1999) Ah receptor and NF-kappaB interactions, a potential mechanism for dioxin toxicity. *J. Biol. Chem.*, **274**, 510–515.

222 Aragones, J., Jones, D.R., Martin, S., San Juan, M.A., Alfranca, A., Vidal, F., Vara, A., Merida, I., and Landazuri, M.O. (2001) Evidence for the involvement of diacylglycerol kinase in the activation of hypoxia-inducible transcription factor 1 by low oxygen tension. *J. Biol. Chem.*, **276**, 10548–10555.

223 Chan, W.K., Yao, G., Gu, Y.Z., and Bradfield, C.A. (1999) Cross-talk between the aryl hydrocarbon receptor and hypoxia inducible factor signaling pathways. Demonstration of competition and compensation. *J. Biol. Chem.*, **274**, 12115–12123.

224 Backlund, M., Johansson, I., Mkrtchian, S., and Ingelman-Sundberg, M. (1997) Signal transduction-mediated activation of the aryl hydrocarbon receptor in rat hepatoma H4IIE cells. *J. Biol. Chem.*, **272**, 31755–31763.

225 Polzer, R.J., Coffing, S.L., Marcus, C.B., Park, S.S., Gelboin, H.V., and Baird, W.M. (1995) Inhibition of benzo[*a*]pyrene metabolism by insulin, FITC–insulin and an FITC–insulin–antibody conjugate in the human hepatoma cell line HepG2. *Chem. Biol. Interact.*, **97**, 307–318.

226 Sidhu, J.S. and Omiecinski, C.J. (1999) Insulin-mediated modulation of cytochrome P450 gene induction profiles in primary rat hepatocyte cultures. *J. Biochem. Mol. Toxicol.*, **13**, 1–9.

227 Sidhu, J.S. and Omiecinski, C.J. (1995) cAMP-associated inhibition of phenobarbital-inducible cytochrome P450 gene expression in primary rat hepatocyte cultures. *J. Biol. Chem.*, **270**, 12762–12773.

228 Viitala, P., Posti, K., Lindfors, A., Pelkonen, O., and Raunio, H. (2001) cAMP mediated upregulation of CYP2A5 in mouse hepatocytes. *Biochem. Biophys. Res. Commun.*, **280**, 761–767.

229 Hakkola, J., Pasanen, M., Pelkonen, O., Hukkanen, J., Evisalmi, S., Anttila, S.,

Rane, A., Mantyla, M., Purkunen, R., Saarikoski, S., Tooming, M., and Raunio, H. (1997) Expression of CYP1B1 in human adult and fetal tissues and differential inducibility of CYP1B1 and CYP1A1 by Ah receptor ligands in human placenta and cultured cells. *Carcinogenesis*, **18**, 391–397.

230 McFadyen, M.C., Rooney, P.H., Melvin, W.T., and Murray, G.I. (2003) Quantitative analysis of the Ah receptor/cytochrome P450 CYP1B1/CYP1A1 signalling pathway. *Biochem. Pharmacol.*, **65**, 1663–1674.

231 Lin, P., Chang, H., Ho, W.L., Wu, M.H., and Su, J.M. (2003) Association of aryl hydrocarbon receptor and cytochrome P4501B1 expressions in human non-small cell lung cancers. *Lung Cancer*, **42**, 255–261.

232 Murray, G.I., Melvin, W.T., Greenlee, W.F., and Burke, M.D. (2001) Regulation, function, and tissue-specific expression of cytochrome P450 CYP1B1. *Annu. Rev. Pharmacol. Toxicol.*, **41**, 297–316.

233 Tsuchiya, Y., Nakajima, M., and Yokoi, T. (2003) Critical enhancer region to which AhR/ARNT and Sp1 bind in the human CYP1B1 gene. *J. Biochem.*, **133**, 583–592.

234 Li, W., Harper, P.A., Tang, B.K., and Okey, A.B. (1998) Regulation of cytochrome P450 enzymes by aryl hydrocarbon receptor in human cells: CYP1A2 expression in the LS180 colon carcinoma cell line after treatment with 2,3,7,8-tetrachlorodibenzo-*p*-dioxin or 3-methylcholanthrene. *Biochem. Pharmacol.*, **56**, 599–612.

235 Spink, D.C., Spink, B.C., Cao, J.Q., Gierthy, J.F., Hayes, C.L., Li, Y., and Sutter, T.R. (1997) Induction of cytochrome P450 1B1 and catechol estrogen metabolism in ACHN human renal adenocarcinoma cells. *J. Steroid Biochem. Mol. Biol.*, **62**, 223–232.

236 Eltom, S.E., Larsen, M.C., and Jefcoate, C.R. (1998) Expression of CYP1B1 but not CYP1A1 by primary cultured human mammary stromal fibroblasts constitutively and in response to dioxin exposure: role of the Ah receptor. *Carcinogenesis*, **19**, 1437–1444.

237 Ociepa-Zawal, M., Rubis, B., Lacinski, M., and Trzeciak, W.H. (2007) The effect of indole-3-carbinol on the expression of CYP1A1, CYP1B1 and AhR genes and proliferation of MCF-7 cells. *Acta Biochim. Pol.*, **54**, 113–117.

238 Spink, B.C., Hussain, M.M., Katz, B.H., Eisele, L., and Spink, D.C. (2003) Transient induction of cytochromes P450 1A1 and 1B1 in MCF-7 human breast cancer cells by indirubin. *Biochem. Pharmacol.*, **66**, 2313–2321.

239 Liu, J., Wang, Q., Wu, D.C., Wang, X.W., Sun, Y., Chen, X.Y., Zhang, K.L., and Li, H. (2004) Differential regulation of CYP1A1 and CYP1B1 expression in resveratrol-treated human medulloblastoma cells. *Neurosci. Lett.*, **363**, 257–261.

240 Kress, S. and Greenlee, W.F. (1997) Cell-specific regulation of human CYP1A1 and CYP1B1 genes. *Cancer Res.*, **57**, 1264–1269.

241 Spink, D.C., Spink, B.C., Cao, J.Q., DePasquale, J.A., Pentecost, B.T., Fasco, M.J., Li, Y., and Sutter, T.R. (1998) Differential expression of CYP1A1 and CYP1B1 in human breast epithelial cells and breast tumor cells. *Carcinogenesis*, **19**, 291–298.

242 Shehin, S.E., Stephenson, R.O., and Greenlee, W.F. (2000) Transcriptional regulation of the human CYP1B1 gene. Evidence for involvement of an aryl hydrocarbon receptor response element in constitutive expression. *J. Biol. Chem.*, **275**, 6770–6776.

243 Taylor, R.T., Wang, F., Hsu, E.L., and Hankinson, O. (2009) Roles of coactivator proteins in dioxin induction of CYP1A1 and CYP1B1 in human breast cancer cells. *Toxicol. Sci.*, **107**, 1–8.

244 Spink, B.C., Fasco, M.J., Gierthy, J.F., and Spink, D.C. (1998) 12-*O*-tetradecanoylphorbol-13-acetate upregulates the Ah receptor and differentially alters CYP1B1 and CYP1A1 expression in MCF-7 breast cancer cells. *J. Cell. Biochem.*, **70**, 289–296.

245 Coumoul, X., Diry, M., Robillot, C., and Barouki, R. (2001) Differential regulation of cytochrome P450 1A1 and

1B1 by a combination of dioxin and pesticides in the breast tumor cell line MCF-7. *Cancer Res.*, **61**, 3942–3948.

246 Angus, W.G., Larsen, M.C., and Jefcoate, C.R. (1999) Expression of CYP1A1 and CYP1B1 depends on cell-specific factors in human breast cancer cell lines: role of estrogen receptor status. *Carcinogenesis*, **20**, 947–955.

247 Han, E.H., Kim, H.G., Hwang, Y.P., Song, G.Y., and Jeong, H.G. (2010) Prostaglandin E_2 induces CYP1B1 expression via ligand-independent activation of the ERalpha pathway in human breast cancer cells. *Toxicol. Sci.*, **114**, 204–216.

248 Kawai, M., Chen, J., Cheung, C.Y., and Chang, T.K. (2003) Transcript profiling of cytochrome P450 genes in HL-60 human leukemic cells: upregulation of CYP1B1 by all-*trans*-retinoic acid. *Mol. Cell. Biochem.*, **248**, 57–65.

249 Raunio, H., Rautio, A., and Pelkonen, O. (1999) The CYP2A subfamily: function, expression and genetic polymorphism. *IARC Sci. Publ.*, **148**, 197–207.

250 Meunier, V., Bourrie, M., Julian, B., Marti, E., Guillou, F., Berger, Y., and Fabre, G. (2000) Expression and induction of CYP1A1/1A2, CYP2A6 and CYP3A4 in primary cultures of human hepatocytes: a 10-year follow-up. *Xenobiotica*, **30**, 589–607.

251 Pitarque, M., Rodriguez-Antona, C., Oscarson, M., and Ingelman-Sundberg, M. (2005) Transcriptional regulation of the human CYP2A6 gene. *J. Pharmacol. Exp. Ther.*, **313**, 814–822.

252 Itoh, M., Nakajima, M., Higashi, E., Yoshida, R., Nagata, K., Yamazoe, Y., and Yokoi, T. (2006) Induction of human CYP2A6 is mediated by the pregnane X receptor with peroxisome proliferator-activated receptor-gamma coactivator 1alpha. *J. Pharmacol. Exp. Ther.*, **319**, 693–702.

253 Kojima, K., Nagata, K., Matsubara, T., and Yamazoe, Y. (2007) Broad but distinct role of pregnane X receptor on the expression of individual cytochrome p450s in human hepatocytes. *Drug Metab. Pharmacokinet.*, **22**, 276–286.

254 Gervot, L., Rochat, B., Gautier, J.C., Bohnenstengel, F., Kroemer, H., de Berardinis, V., Martin, H., Beaune, P., and de Waziers, I. (1999) Human CYP2B6: expression, inducibility and catalytic activities. *Pharmacogenetics*, **9**, 295–306.

255 Code, E.L., Crespi, C.L., Penman, B.W., Gonzalez, F.J., Chang, T.K., and Waxman, D.J. (1997) Human cytochrome P4502B6: interindividual hepatic expression, substrate specificity, and role in procarcinogen activation. *Drug Metab. Dispos.*, **25**, 985–993.

256 Wang, H. and Negishi, M. (2003) Transcriptional regulation of cytochrome p450 2B genes by nuclear receptors. *Curr. Drug Metab.*, **4**, 515–525.

257 Kocarek, T.A., Dahn, M.S., Cai, H., Strom, S.C., and Mercer-Haines, N.A. (2002) Regulation of CYP2B6 and CYP3A expression by hydroxymethylglutaryl coenzyme A inhibitors in primary cultured human hepatocytes. *Drug Metab. Dispos.*, **30**, 1400–1405.

258 Saussele, T., Burk, O., Blievernicht, J.K., Klein, K., Nussler, A., Nussler, N., Hengstler, J.G., Eichelbaum, M., Schwab, M., and Zanger, U.M. (2007) Selective induction of human hepatic cytochromes P450 2B6 and 3A4 by metamizole. *Clin. Pharmacol. Ther.*, **82**, 265–274.

259 Kharasch, E.D., Mitchell, D., Coles, R., and Blanco, R. (2008) Rapid clinical induction of hepatic cytochrome P4502B6 activity by ritonavir. *Antimicrob. Agents Chemother.*, **52**, 1663–1669.

260 Piton, A., Rauch, C., Langouet, S., Guillouzo, A., and Morel, F. (2010) Involvement of pregnane X receptor in the regulation of CYP2B6 gene expression by oltipraz in human hepatocytes. *Toxicol. In Vitro*, **24**, 452–459.

261 Merrell, M.D., Jackson, J.P., Augustine, L.M., Fisher, C.D., Slitt, A.L., Maher, J.M., Huang, W., Moore, D.D., Zhang, Y., Klaassen, C.D., and Cherrington, N.J. (2008) The Nrf2 activator oltipraz also activates the constitutive androstane

receptor. *Drug Metab. Dispos.*, **36**, 1716–1721.

262 Burk, O., Arnold, K.A., Nussler, A.K., Schaeffeler, E., Efimova, E., Avery, B.A., Avery, M.A., Fromm, M.F., and Eichelbaum, M. (2005) Antimalarial artemisinin drugs induce cytochrome P450 and MDR1 expression by activation of xenosensors pregnane X receptor and constitutive androstane receptor. *Mol. Pharmacol.*, **67**, 1954–1965.

263 Takizawa, D., Kakizaki, S., Horiguchi, N., Tojima, H., Yamazaki, Y., Ichikawa, T., Sato, K., and Mori, M. (2010) Histone deacetylase inhibitors induce cytochrome P450 2B by activating nuclear receptor CAR. *Drug Metab. Dispos.*, **38**, 1493–1498.

264 Chang, T.K., Bandiera, S.M., and Chen, J. (2003) Constitutive androstane receptor and pregnane X receptor gene expression in human liver: interindividual variability and correlation with CYP2B6 mRNA levels. *Drug Metab. Dispos.*, **31**, 7–10.

265 Faucette, S.R., Sueyoshi, T., Smith, C.M., Negishi, M., Lecluyse, E.L., and Wang, H. (2006) Differential regulation of hepatic CYP2B6 and CYP3A4 genes by constitutive androstane receptor but not pregnane X receptor. *J. Pharmacol. Exp. Ther.*, **317**, 1200–1209.

266 Wang, H., Faucette, S., Moore, R., Sueyoshi, T., Negishi, M., and LeCluyse, E. (2004) Human constitutive androstane receptor mediates induction of CYP2B6 gene expression by phenytoin. *J. Biol. Chem.*, **279**, 29295–29301.

267 Kohalmy, K., Tamasi, V., Kobori, L., Sarvary, E., Pascussi, J.M., Porrogi, P., Rozman, D., Prough, R.A., Meyer, U.A., and Monostory, K. (2007) Dehydroepiandrosterone induces human CYP2B6 through the constitutive androstane receptor. *Drug Metab. Dispos.*, **35**, 1495–1501.

268 Faucette, S.R., Zhang, T.C., Moore, R., Sueyoshi, T., Omiecinski, C.J., LeCluyse, E.L., Negishi, M., and Wang, H. (2007) Relative activation of human pregnane X receptor versus constitutive androstane receptor defines distinct classes of CYP2B6 and CYP3A4 inducers. *J. Pharmacol. Exp. Ther.*, **320**, 72–80.

269 Casabar, R.C., Das, P.C., Dekrey, G.K., Gardiner, C.S., Cao, Y., Rose, R.L., and Wallace, A.D. (2010) Endosulfan induces CYP2B6 and CYP3A4 by activating the pregnane X receptor. *Toxicol. Appl. Pharmacol.*, **245**, 335–343.

270 Goodwin, B., Moore, L.B., Stoltz, C.M., McKee, D.D., and Kliewer, S.A. (2001) Regulation of the human CYP2B6 gene by the nuclear pregnane X receptor. *Mol. Pharmacol.*, **60**, 427–431.

271 Wang, H., Faucette, S., Sueyoshi, T., Moore, R., Ferguson, S., Negishi, M., and LeCluyse, E.L. (2003) A novel distal enhancer module regulated by pregnane X receptor/constitutive androstane receptor is essential for the maximal induction of CYP2B6 gene expression. *J. Biol. Chem.*, **278**, 14146–14152.

272 Swales, K., Kakizaki, S., Yamamoto, Y., Inoue, K., Kobayashi, K., and Negishi, M. (2005) Novel CAR-mediated mechanism for synergistic activation of two distinct elements within the human cytochrome P450 2B6 gene in HepG2 cells. *J. Biol. Chem.*, **280**, 3458–3466.

273 Pascussi, J.M., Gerbal-Chaloin, S., Pichard-Garcia, L., Daujat, M., Fabre, J.M., Maurel, P., and Vilarem, M.J. (2000) Interleukin-6 negatively regulates the expression of pregnane X receptor and constitutively activated receptor in primary human hepatocytes. *Biochem. Biophys. Res. Commun.*, **274**, 707–713.

274 Wang, H., Faucette, S.R., Gilbert, D., Jolley, S.L., Sueyoshi, T., Negishi, M., and LeCluyse, E.L. (2003) Glucocorticoid receptor enhancement of pregnane X receptor-mediated CYP2B6 regulation in primary human hepatocytes. *Drug Metab. Dispos.*, **31**, 620–630.

275 Duniec-Dmuchowski, Z., Ellis, E., Strom, S.C., and Kocarek, T.A. (2007) Regulation of CYP3A4 and CYP2B6 expression by liver X receptor agonists. *Biochem. Pharmacol.*, **74**, 1535–1540.

276 Duniec-Dmuchowski, Z., Fang, H.L., Strom, S.C., Ellis, E., Runge-Morris, M., and Kocarek, T.A. (2009) Human pregnane X receptor activation and CYP3A4/CYP2B6 induction by 2,3-oxidosqualene:lanosterol cyclase

inhibition. *Drug Metab. Dispos.*, **37**, 900–908.
277 Lo, R., Burgoon, L., Macpherson, L., Ahmed, S., and Matthews, J. (2010) Estrogen receptor-dependent regulation of CYP2B6 in human breast cancer cells. *Biochim. Biophys. Acta*, **1799**, 469–479.
278 Jover, R., Bort, R., Gomez-Lechon, M.J., and Castell, J.V. (1998) Re-expression of C/EBP alpha induces CYP2B6, CYP2C9 and CYP2D6 genes in HepG2 cells. *FEBS Lett.*, **431**, 227–230.
279 Jover, R., Bort, R., Gomez-Lechon, M.J., and Castell, J.V. (2001) Cytochrome P450 regulation by hepatocyte nuclear factor 4 in human hepatocytes: a study using adenovirus-mediated antisense targeting. *Hepatology*, **33**, 668–675.
280 Pascual, M., Gomez-Lechon, M.J., Castell, J.V., and Jover, R. (2008) ATF5 is a highly abundant liver-enriched transcription factor that cooperates with constitutive androstane receptor in the transactivation of CYP2B6: implications in hepatic stress responses. *Drug Metab. Dispos.*, **36**, 1063–1072.
281 Inoue, K. and Negishi, M. (2008) Nuclear receptor CAR requires early growth response 1 to activate the human cytochrome P450 2B6 gene. *J. Biol. Chem.*, **283**, 10425–10432.
282 Benet, M., Lahoz, A., Guzman, C., Castell, J.V., and Jover, R. (2010) CCAAT/enhancer-binding protein alpha (C/EBPalpha) and hepatocyte nuclear factor 4alpha (HNF4alpha) synergistically cooperate with constitutive androstane receptor to transactivate the human cytochrome P450 2B6 (CYP2B6) gene: application to the development of a metabolically competent human hepatic cell model. *J. Biol. Chem.*, **285**, 28457–28471.
283 Rencurel, F., Stenhouse, A., Hawley, S.A., Friedberg, T., Hardie, D.G., Sutherland, C., and Wolf, C.R. (2005) AMP-activated protein kinase mediates phenobarbital induction of CYP2B gene expression in hepatocytes and a newly derived human hepatoma cell line. *J. Biol. Chem.*, **280**, 4367–4373.
284 Gerbal-Chaloin, S., Pascussi, J.M., Pichard-Garcia, L., Daujat, M., Waechter, F., Fabre, J.M., Carrere, N., and Maurel, P. (2001) Induction of CYP2C genes in human hepatocytes in primary culture. *Drug Metab. Dispos.*, **29**, 242–251.
285 Raucy, J.L., Mueller, L., Duan, K., Allen, S.W., Strom, S., and Lasker, J.M. (2002) Expression and induction of CYP2C P450 enzymes in primary cultures of human hepatocytes. *J. Pharmacol. Exp. Ther.*, **302**, 475–482.
286 Belic, A., Temesvari, M., Kohalmy, K., Vrzal, R., Dvorak, Z., Rozman, D., and Monostory, K. (2009) Investigation of the CYP2C9 induction profile in human hepatocytes by combining experimental and modelling approaches. *Curr. Drug Metab.*, **10**, 1066–1074.
287 Sahi, J., Shord, S.S., Lindley, C., Ferguson, S., and LeCluyse, E.L. (2009) Regulation of cytochrome P450 2C9 expression in primary cultures of human hepatocytes. *J. Biochem. Mol. Toxicol.*, **23**, 43–58.
288 Ibeanu, G.C. and Goldstein, J.A. (1995) Transcriptional regulation of human CYP2C genes: functional comparison of CYP2C9 and CYP2C18 promoter regions. *Biochemistry*, **34**, 8028–8036.
289 Chen, Y., Ferguson, S.S., Negishi, M., and Goldstein, J.A. (2004) Induction of human CYP2C9 by rifampicin, hyperforin, and phenobarbital is mediated by the pregnane X receptor. *J. Pharmacol. Exp. Ther.*, **308**, 495–501.
290 Ferguson, S.S., LeCluyse, E.L., Negishi, M., and Goldstein, J.A. (2002) Regulation of human CYP2C9 by the constitutive androstane receptor: discovery of a new distal binding site. *Mol. Pharmacol.*, **62**, 737–746.
291 Xiang, S., Parsons, H.K., and Murray, M. (1998) Identification of a novel transcriptional silencer in the protein-coding region of the human CYP2C9 gene. *Gene*, **209**, 123–129.
292 Pavek, P., Cerveny, L., Svecova, L., Brysch, M., Libra, A., Vrzal, R., Nachtigal, P., Staud, F., Ulrichova, J., Fendrich, Z., and Dvorak, Z. (2007) Examination of glucocorticoid receptor alpha-mediated transcriptional regulation of P-glycoprotein, CYP3A4, and CYP2C9 genes in placental

trophoblast cell lines. *Placenta*, **28**, 1004–1011.

293 Chen, Y., Kissling, G., Negishi, M., and Goldstein, J.A. (2005) The nuclear receptors constitutive androstane receptor and pregnane X receptor cross-talk with hepatic nuclear factor 4alpha to synergistically activate the human CYP2C9 promoter. *J. Pharmacol. Exp. Ther.*, **314**, 1125–1133.

294 Martinez-Jimenez, C.P., Castell, J.V., Gomez-Lechon, M.J., and Jover, R. (2006) Transcriptional activation of CYP2C9, CYP1A1, and CYP1A2 by hepatocyte nuclear factor 4alpha requires coactivators peroxisomal proliferator activated receptor-gamma coactivator 1alpha and steroid receptor coactivator 1. *Mol. Pharmacol.*, **70**, 1681–1692.

295 Kawashima, S., Kobayashi, K., Takama, K., Higuchi, T., Furihata, T., Hosokawa, M., and Chiba, K. (2006) Involvement of hepatocyte nuclear factor 4alpha in the different expression level between CYP2C9 and CYP2C19 in the human liver. *Drug Metab. Dispos.*, **34**, 1012–1018.

296 Rana, R., Chen, Y., Ferguson, S.S., Kissling, G.E., Surapureddi, S., and Goldstein, J.A. (2010) Hepatocyte nuclear factor 4α regulates rifampicin-mediated induction of CYP2C genes in primary cultures of human hepatocytes. *Drug Metab. Dispos.*, **38**, 591–599.

297 Bort, R., Gomez-Lechon, M.J., Castell, J.V., and Jover, R. (2004) Role of hepatocyte nuclear factor 3 gamma in the expression of human CYP2C genes. *Arch. Biochem. Biophys.*, **426**, 63–72.

298 Mwinyi, J., Nekvindova, J., Cavaco, I., Hofmann, Y., Pedersen, R.S., Landman, E., Mkrtchian, S., and Ingelman-Sundberg, M. (2010) New insights into the regulation of CYP2C9 gene expression: the role of the transcription factor GATA-4. *Drug Metab. Dispos.*, **38**, 415–421.

299 Surapureddi, S., Rana, R., Reddy, J.K., and Goldstein, J.A. (2008) Nuclear receptor coactivator 6 mediates the synergistic activation of human cytochrome P-450 2C9 by the constitutive androstane receptor and hepatic nuclear factor-4alpha. *Mol. Pharmacol.*, **74**, 913–923.

300 Ferguson, S.S., Chen, Y., LeCluyse, E.L., Negishi, M., and Goldstein, J.A. (2005) Human CYP2C8 is transcriptionally regulated by the nuclear receptors constitutive androstane receptor, pregnane X receptor, glucocorticoid receptor, and hepatic nuclear factor 4alpha. *Mol. Pharmacol.*, **68**, 747–757.

301 Chen, Y., Ferguson, S.S., Negishi, M., and Goldstein, J.A. (2003) Identification of constitutive androstane receptor and glucocorticoid receptor binding sites in the CYP2C19 promoter. *Mol. Pharmacol.*, **64**, 316–324.

302 Mwinyi, J., Hofmann, Y., Pedersen, R.S., Nekvindova, J., Cavaco, I., Mkrtchian, S., and Ingelman-Sundberg, M. (2010) The transcription factor GATA-4 regulates cytochrome P4502C19 gene expression. *Life Sci.*, **86**, 699–706.

303 Gerbal-Chaloin, S., Daujat, M., Pascussi, J.M., Pichard-Garcia, L., Vilarem, M.J., and Maurel, P. (2002) Transcriptional regulation of CYP2C9 gene. Role of glucocorticoid receptor and constitutive androstane receptor. *J. Biol. Chem.*, **277**, 209–217.

304 Willrich, M.A., Hirata, M.H., and Hirata, R.D. (2009) Statin regulation of CYP3A4 and CYP3A5 expression. *Pharmacogenomics*, **10**, 1017–1024.

305 Nallani, S.C., Goodwin, B., Buckley, A.R., Buckley, D.J., and Desai, P.B. (2004) Differences in the induction of cytochrome P450 3A4 by taxane anticancer drugs, docetaxel and paclitaxel, assessed employing primary human hepatocytes. *Cancer Chemother. Pharmacol.*, **54**, 219–229.

306 Raucy, J.L. (2003) Regulation of CYP3A4 expression in human hepatocytes by pharmaceuticals and natural products. *Drug Metab. Dispos.*, **31**, 533–539.

307 Ruhl, R., Sczech, R., Landes, N., Pfluger, P., Kluth, D., and Schweigert, F.J. (2004) Carotenoids and their metabolites are naturally occurring activators of gene expression via the pregnane X receptor. *Eur. J. Nutr.*, **43**, 336–343.

308 Coumoul, X., Diry, M., and Barouki, R. (2002) PXR-dependent induction of human CYP3A4 gene expression by

organochlorine pesticides. *Biochem. Pharmacol.*, **64**, 1513–1519.
309 Dowless, M.S., Barbee, J.L., Borchert, K.M., Bocchinfuso, W.P., and Houck, K.A. (2005) Cyclic AMP-independent activation of CYP3A4 gene expression by forskolin. *Eur. J. Pharmacol.*, **512**, 9–13.
310 Goodwin, B., Redinbo, M.R., and Kliewer, S.A. (2002) Regulation of cyp3a gene transcription by the pregnane X receptor. *Annu. Rev. Pharmacol. Toxicol.*, **42**, 1–23.
311 Goodwin, B., Hodgson, E., and Liddle, C. (1999) The orphan human pregnane X receptor mediates the transcriptional activation of CYP3A4 by rifampicin through a distal enhancer module. *Mol. Pharmacol.*, **56**, 1329–1339.
312 Goodwin, B., Hodgson, E., D'Costa, D.J., Robertson, G.R., and Liddle, C. (2002) Transcriptional regulation of the human CYP3A4 gene by the constitutive androstane receptor. *Mol. Pharmacol.*, **62**, 359–365.
313 Martinez-Jimenez, C.P., Gomez-Lechon, M.J., Castell, J.V., and Jover, R. (2005) Transcriptional regulation of the human hepatic CYP3A4: identification of a new distal enhancer region responsive to CCAAT/enhancer-binding protein beta isoforms (liver activating protein and liver inhibitory protein). *Mol. Pharmacol.*, **67**, 2088–2101.
314 Rodriguez-Antona, C., Bort, R., Jover, R., Tindberg, N., Ingelman-Sundberg, M., Gomez-Lechon, M.J., and Castell, J.V. (2003) Transcriptional regulation of human CYP3A4 basal expression by CCAAT enhancer-binding protein alpha and hepatocyte nuclear factor-3 gamma. *Mol. Pharmacol.*, **63**, 1180–1189.
315 Bombail, V., Taylor, K., Gibson, G.G., and Plant, N. (2004) Role of Sp1, C/EBP alpha, HNF3, and PXR in the basal- and xenobiotic-mediated regulation of the CYP3A4 gene. *Drug Metab. Dispos.*, **32**, 525–535.
316 Matsumura, K., Saito, T., Takahashi, Y., Ozeki, T., Kiyotani, K., Fujieda, M., Yamazaki, H., Kunitoh, H., and Kamataki, T. (2004) Identification of a novel polymorphic enhancer of the human CYP3A4 gene. *Mol. Pharmacol.*, **65**, 326–334.
317 Tegude, H., Schnabel, A., Zanger, U.M., Klein, K., Eichelbaum, M., and Burk, O. (2007) Molecular mechanism of basal CYP3A4 regulation by hepatocyte nuclear factor 4alpha: evidence for direct regulation in the intestine. *Drug Metab. Dispos.*, **35**, 946–954.
318 Bhalla, S., Ozalp, C., Fang, S., Xiang, L., and Kemper, J.K. (2004) Ligand-activated pregnane X receptor interferes with HNF-4 signaling by targeting a common coactivator PGC-1alpha. Functional implications in hepatic cholesterol and glucose metabolism. *J. Biol. Chem.*, **279**, 45139–45147.
319 Elizondo, G. and Medina-Diaz, I.M. (2003) Induction of CYP3A4 by 1alpha,25-dyhydroxyvitamin D3 in HepG2 cells. *Life Sci.*, **73**, 141–149.
320 Thompson, P.D., Jurutka, P.W., Whitfield, G.K., Myskowski, S.M., Eichhorst, K.R., Dominguez, C.E., Haussler, C.A., and Haussler, M.R. (2002) Liganded VDR induces CYP3A4 in small intestinal and colon cancer cells via DR3 and ER6 vitamin D responsive elements. *Biochem. Biophys. Res. Commun.*, **299**, 730–738.
321 Yasunami, Y., Hara, H., Iwamura, T., Kataoka, T., and Adachi, T. (2004) c-jun N-terminal kinase modulates 1,25-dihydroxyvitamin D3-induced cytochrome P450 3A4 gene expression. *Drug Metab. Dispos.*, **32**, 685–688.
322 Chen, S., Wang, K., and Wan, Y.J. (2010) Retinoids activate RXR/CAR-mediated pathway and induce CYP3A. *Biochem. Pharmacol.*, **79**, 270–276.
323 Gnerre, C., Blattler, S., Kaufmann, M.R., Looser, R., and Meyer, U.A. (2004) Regulation of CYP3A4 by the bile acid receptor FXR: evidence for functional binding sites in the CYP3A4 gene. *Pharmacogenetics*, **14**, 635–645.
324 Legendre, C., Hori, T., Loyer, P., Aninat, C., Ishida, S., Glaise, D., Lucas-Clerc, C., Boudjema, K., Guguen-Guillouzo, C., Corlu, A., and Morel, F. (2009) Drug-metabolising enzymes are down-regulated by hypoxia in differentiated human hepatoma HepaRG cells: HIF-1alpha involvement

in CYP3A4 repression. *Eur. J. Cancer*, **45**, 2882–2892.

325 Johnson, D.R., Li, C.W., Chen, L.Y., Ghosh, J.C., and Chen, J.D. (2006) Regulation and binding of pregnane X receptor by nuclear receptor corepressor silencing mediator of retinoid and thyroid hormone receptors (SMRT). *Mol. Pharmacol.*, **69**, 99–108.

326 Riffel, A.K., Schuenemann, E., and Vyhlidal, C.A. (2009) Regulation of the CYP3A4 and CYP3A7 promoters by members of the nuclear factor I transcription factor family. *Mol. Pharmacol.*, **76**, 1104–1114.

327 Donato, M.T., Gomez-Lechon, M.J., Jover, R., Nakamura, T., and Castell, J.V. (1998) Human hepatocyte growth factor down-regulates the expression of cytochrome P450 isozymes in human hepatocytes in primary culture. *J. Pharmacol. Exp. Ther.*, **284**, 760–767.

328 Ourlin, J.C., Lasserre, F., Pineau, T., Fabre, J.M., Sa-Cunha, A., Maurel, P., Vilarem, M.J., and Pascussi, J.M. (2003) The small heterodimer partner interacts with the pregnane X receptor and represses its transcriptional activity. *Mol. Endocrinol.*, **17**, 1693–1703.

329 Ahn, T., and Yun, C.H. (2004) High-level expression of human cytochrome P450 3A4 by co-expression with human molecular chaperone HDJ-1 (Hsp40). *Arch. Pharm. Res.*, **27**, 319–323.

330 El-Sankary, W., Plant, N.J., Gibson, G.G., and Moore, D.J. (2000) Regulation of the CYP3A4 gene by hydrocortisone and xenobiotics: role of the glucocorticoid and pregnane X receptors. *Drug Metab. Dispos.*, **28**, 493–496.

331 Hukkanen, J., Vaisanen, T., Lassila, A., Piipari, R., Anttila, S., Pelkonen, O., Raunio, H., and Hakkola, J. (2003) Regulation of CYP3A5 by glucocorticoids and cigarette smoke in human lung-derived cells. *J. Pharmacol. Exp. Ther.*, **304**, 745–752.

332 Schuetz, J.D., Schuetz, E.G., Thottassery, J.V., Guzelian, P.S., Strom, S., and Sun, D. (1996) Identification of a novel dexamethasone responsive enhancer in the human CYP3A5 gene and its activation in human and rat liver cells. *Mol. Pharmacol.*, **49**, 63–72.

333 El-Sankary, W., Bombail, V., Gibson, G.G., and Plant, N. (2002) Glucocorticoid-mediated induction of CYP3A4 is decreased by disruption of a protein:DNA interaction distinct from the pregnane X receptor response element. *Drug Metab. Dispos.*, **30**, 1029–1034.

334 Pan, Y.Z., Gao, W., and Yu, A.M. (2009) MicroRNAs regulate CYP3A4 expression via direct and indirect targeting. *Drug Metab. Dispos.*, **37**, 2112–2117.

335 Takagi, S., Nakajima, M., Mohri, T., and Yokoi, T. (2008) Post-transcriptional regulation of human pregnane X receptor by micro-RNA affects the expression of cytochrome P450 3A4. *J. Biol. Chem.*, **283**, 9674–9680.

336 Iwano, S., Saito, T., Takahashi, Y., Fujita, K., and Kamataki, T. (2001) Cooperative regulation of CYP3A5 gene transcription by NF-Y and Sp family members. *Biochem. Biophys. Res. Commun.*, **286**, 55–60.

337 Moilanen, A.M., Hakkola, J., Vaarala, M.H., Kauppila, S., Hirvikoski, P., Vuoristo, J.T., Edwards, R.J., and Paavonen, T.K. (2007) Characterization of androgen-regulated expression of CYP3A5 in human prostate. *Carcinogenesis*, **28**, 916–921.

9
Importance of Pharmacogenomics

Ulrich M. Zanger, Kathrin Klein, and Jessica Rieger

9.1
Introduction

Drugs administered to treat a disease or ailment do not work satisfactorily in every patient and they may lead to unexpected or toxic effects (adverse drug reactions (ADRs)) in some treated patients. Variability in drug response is not rare, but is widespread and occurs despite (or because) patients are usually treated with standard doses [1–3]. Unexpected drug response – due to lack of efficacy or side-effects – may lead to patient noncompliance, which further magnifies the problem [4]. Recent data on the epidemiology of ADRs in the United Kingdom showed that the burden on the healthcare systems is high, and accounts for considerable morbidity, mortality, and extra costs [5]. Drug response variability also affects drug discovery and development processes. Thus, serious ADRs have accounted for most of the drug withdrawals in recent years and for a significant fraction of investigational drugs that failed due to toxicity during clinical trials [6, 7].

The familiar quotation "What is food to one man is bitter poison to others" by the Roman philosopher Lucretius Cato (96–55 BC) documents that a personal perspective of medicine is by no means new, but has always guided medical thinking. However, while the personal approach in older times was mainly left to the intuition of the physician, we can now take advantage of an exponentially growing amount of "personal" molecular biological information. In 1959, the German geneticist Friedrich Vogel coined the term "pharmacogenetics" to describe inherited differences in drug response. During the past six decades numerous observations have been made on how genes and gene variants affect drug metabolism, pharmacokinetics, drug efficacy, and adverse side-effects [8].

However, despite extensive progress in understanding the basis for individuality, translation of this knowledge into clinical practice has been slow and not on a broad front [9–11]. A major reason for this is the multifactorial nature of both the pharmacokinetics and pharmacodynamics aspects of drug responses. Only in rare cases will a single gene of major impact be alone responsible, whereas in most cases multiple genetic together with nongenetic factors contribute to variability. The term pharmacogenomics indicates, as an extension of pharmacogenetics,

Metabolism of Drugs and Other Xenobiotics, First Edition. Edited by Pavel Anzenbacher, Ulrich M. Zanger.

the inclusion of multigenic and genome-wide approaches, as well as other genomics and epigenomics approaches to develop complex biomarkers for drug response. These will hopefully allow more specific drug therapy tailored to genetically defined subsets of patients and diseases classified at the molecular level. In this chapter we review the most important pharmacogenetic polymorphisms, and we discuss the opportunities and challenges of pharmacogenomics.

9.2 Pharmacogenetic Polymorphisms

Most drug-metabolizing enzymes exhibit extremely large interindividual variability in expression and function, which influences the bioavailability of many drugs. This can in part be explained by genetic polymorphisms creating a spectrum of variants with different activities. Several inherited pharmacogenetic traits were discovered approximately 50–60 years ago by following up on individual observations of side-effects or abnormal metabolite patterns [3, 8, 12]. Extensive research including family and twin studies, population studies, and basic biochemical and molecular genetic studies uncovered numerous genes and gene polymorphisms that have a significant impact on drug responses (Table 9.1). These monogenically inherited variations form the cornerstones of pharmacogenetics and they illustrate many general principles.

9.2.1 Lessons from Early Examples

Chemical individuality in metabolic enzymes was discovered in the early 1900s by Sir Archibald Garrod [13], who later developed the new concept of inherited disorders of metabolism, already foreseeing the basic principles of pharmacogenetics [8]. During World War II it was observed that approximately 10% of African-American soldiers, but only very few white soldiers, suffered from hemolysis following treatment with primaquine or some other antimalarials [14]. A deficiency of G6PDH (see Table 9.1 for further details and abbreviations/definitions), which affects erythrocyte metabolism, was identified as the underlying cause. Today we know that G6PDH deficiency in its heterozygous form confers partial protection against malaria. The *G6PDH* locus on the X-chromosome is one of the most polymorphic sites in the human genome and the distribution *G6PDH* low-activity alleles matches the prevalence of malaria.

Around the same time it was discovered that biotransformation of the antituberculosis drug isoniazid to acetylisoniazid differs widely between individuals, which could be roughly distinguished into either *rapid* or *slow acetylators*. The latter phenotype was associated with peripheral neuropathy as a result of isoniazid toxicity. Family studies showed that the slow acetylator phenotype was inherited as an autosomal recessive trait, but it took four decades until allele variants of the gene encoding the responsible enzyme, NAT2, were identified (Table 9.1). The

Table 9.1 Selected genetic polymorphisms of ADME genes.

Polymorphic gene	Common loss-of-function alleles[a)]	Gain-of-function alleles	Prevalence of slow metabolizer phenotype	Affected drugs (examples)	Clinical relevance
ALDH (aldehyde dehydrogenase)	*ALDH1A1*2, *3* *ALDH2*2 (E504K)*	not known	0.02 –0 (Caucasian) 0 (Caucasian) 0.4 (Asian)	mivacurium, procaine, succinylcholine, cyclophosphamide	alcohol flush reaction; nitroglycerin bioactivation
BCHE (butyrylcholine esterase)	*BCHE*K* (Ala539Thr) *BCHE*A* (Asp70Gly)	not known	0.17 (Caucasian)	mivacurium, procaine, succinylcholine	muscular paralysis, postanesthetic apnea, hypocholinesterasemia
FV (coagulation factor V)	*FVL=F5* (R506Q)	not known	0.02 (Caucasian)	heparin, oral contraceptives, estrogens, selective estrogen receptor modulators	↑ venous thromboembolism
CYP2B6 (cytochrome P450 2B6)	*CYP2B6*6, *11,*12, . . . , *18*	*CYP2B6*4,*22*	0.06–0.25 (Asian, Caucasian, African)	efavirenz	PM: ↑ AUC and CNS side-effects, ↓ patient compliance
CYP2C9 (cytochrome P450 2C9)	*CYP2C9*2, *3*	not known	0–0.17	NSAIDs, warfarin, acenocoumarol	PM: ↑ anticoagulation effects of warfarin, gastrointestinal bleeding
CYP2C19 (cytochrome P450 2C19)	*CYP2C19*2, *3*	*CYP2C19*17*	0.03 (Caucasian)–0.3 (Asian)	omeprazole, mephenytoin (probe drug), clopidogrel	PM: ↑ eradication rate PM: ↓ efficacy EM: ↑ bleeding
CYP2D6 (cytochrome P450 2D6)	*CYP2D6*4, *41, *10, *17, . . .*	*CYP2D6*N x n*	0.01 (Asian, African)–0.1 (Caucasian)	antidepressants, codeine, tamoxifen	PM: ↑ antidepressant toxicity PM: ↓ codeine analgesia PM: ↑ breast cancer relapse
CYP3A5 (cytochrome P450 3A5)	*CYP3A5*3*	not known	0.5 (African), 0.7 (Asian), 0.85(Caucasian)	tacrolimus	↓ efficacy of tacrolimus in organ transplantation
DPYD (dihydropyrimidine dehydrogenase)	*DPYD*2A*	not known	0.01 (Caucasian)	5-FU, capecitabine	↑ neurotoxicity

(Continued)

Table 9.1 (*Continued*)

Polymorphic gene	Common loss-of-function alleles[a)]	Gain-of-function alleles	Prevalence of slow metabolizer phenotype	Affected drugs (examples)	Clinical relevance
G6PDH (glucose-6-phosphate dehydrogenase)	G6PD202G>A (A–)	not known	0 (Caucasian), 0.06 (African)	many drugs generating electrophilic reactive metabolites in human cells	severe anemia after antimalarial treatment
MDR1 (multidrug resistance protein 1)	2677 (T>G/A), 3435 (T>C)	not known	0.43 (Caucasian), 0.89 (African)	digoxin, HIV protease inhibitors	↓ CD4 response; ↓ digoxin bioavailability
NAT2 (*N*-acetyltransferase type2)	*NAT2*5, *6, *7*	not known	0.01–0.46	isoniazid, sulfonamides, dapsone, phenelzine, hydralazine, procainamide	slow acetylation phenotype; ↑ antibacterial efficacy; ↑ adverse effects
SLCO1B1 *(OATP1B1)* (organic anion transporting polypeptide1)	*OATP1B1*5* *(V174A)*	not known	0.12–0.2 (Caucasian)	methotrexate, repaglinide, rifampin, statins, torsemide	myopathy on statin treatment
TPMT (thiopurine *S*-methyltransferase)	*TPMT*2, *3A, *3B, *3C*	$(GCC)_5$, $(GCC)_7$ trinucleotide promoter repeats; *V4, *V5 (VNTR repeats)	0.002–0.044 (Caucasian)	6-mercaptopurine, 6-thioguanine, azathioprine	↑ hematopoietic toxicity and secondary cancers; ↑ myelosuppression on thiopurine treatment
UGT1A1 (UDP-glucurosyltransferase 1A1)	*UGT1A1*28*	*UGT1A1*36*	0.31 (Caucasian)	bilirubin, irinotecan	Gilbert–Meulengracht syndrome (benign jaundice); neutropenia (irinotecan); dose reduction is recommended (US Food and Drug Administration)
VKORC1 (vitamin K epoxide reductase)	"A alleles" (−1639G>A or 1173C>T)	not known	0.1 (African), 0.38 (Caucasian), 0.91 (Asian)	warfarin, acenocoumarol, phenprocoumon	PM: ↓ warfarin maintenance dose

a) See Table 9.2 for web sites providing further information.

incidence of NAT2 slow acetylators in different ethnicities varies dramatically from 5 to 70% [12].

Lessons learned from these and other early examples included the existence of large interethnic variability, the absence of a clinical phenotype in some (e.g., NAT2), but not all (e.g., G6PDH, UGT1A1) pharmacogenetic polymorphisms, and later the existence of multiple alleles coding for the polymorphic enzyme with different impact on function and different allele frequencies.

9.2.2 Cytochrome P450 Polymorphisms

The majority of drugs and other xenobiotics undergo oxidative biotransformations catalyzed by cytochrome P450 (CYP) enzymes. Approximately a dozen isoforms of the CYP families 1, 2, and 3 are mainly responsible for this task. Functionally relevant polymorphisms affect CYPs 2D6, 2C19, 2C9, 2B6, and 3A5. Although genetic variations exist also in the other CYPs, their clinical penetrance is lower due to limited functional effect, rarity of occurrence, or absence of clinically relevant substrates. Information on allele nomenclature, functional properties, and many other aspects can be found in a number of database resources, which are listed in Table 9.2.

CYP2D6 was originally discovered through its genetic polymorphism, namely though studies on phenotypically deficient debrisoquine 4-hydroxylation [15] and sparteine *N*-oxidation [16], which were soon later shown to be due to the same metabolic deficiency. This enzyme metabolizes a large number of drugs from virtually all therapeutic classes, including analgesics, antiarrhythmics, antidepressants, antipsychotics, β-blockers, anticancer drugs, and others. Liver expression ranges from undetectable up to at least around 70 pmol/mg of microsomal protein [17]. Most of this expression variation is due to genetic polymorphism, whereas environmental and nongenetic factors have little influence (except for inhibitory drug–drug interactions). CYP2D6 is also expressed in several extrahepatic tissues, most notably in the gastrointestinal tract and in different areas of the human brain.

Polymorphic drug oxidation by CYP2D6 results from a multiplicity of allelic variants that cover a continuum of activity phenotypes. Poor metabolizers (PMs) carry two nonfunctional alleles (e.g., **3, *4, *5, *6, *7* (i.e., total number of functional gene copies = 0)), which results in absent enzyme protein in the liver; intermediate metabolizers (IMs) carry one nonfunctional and one partially deficient allele (e.g., **10, *17, *41*), which corresponds to less than one functional gene copy; extensive metabolizers (EMs) carry one or two fully functional copies (e.g., **1* or **2*); and ultrarapid metabolizers (UMs) have three or more functional gene copies. Genotype predicts phenotype rather well as shown in several large studies of *in vivo* phenotyped volunteers [18–21]. Interestingly, most of the phenotypic variability can be explained by hepatic expression differences, rather than coding variants, due to aberrant splicing (e.g., alleles *CYP2D6*4* and *CYP2D6*41*) or overexpression by increased copy number [22, 23]. As in other polymorphisms, allele frequencies vary considerably between different ethnicities (Table 9.1). For

Table 9.2 Selected web sites providing data for pharmacogenomics and personalized medicine.

Project	Contents	URL
PharmaADME	core list of standardized evidence-based drug-metabolizing (ADME) genetic biomarkers	http://www.pharmaadme.org/joomla
PharmGKB	curated database on knowledge about impact of human genetic variations on drug response	http://www.pharmgkb.org
Aldehyde Dehydrogenase Gene Superfamily Database	overview on ALDH genes, variants, and function	http://www.aldh.org
CYP-allele database	CYP allele nomenclature and function	http://www.cypalleles.ki.se
Cytochrome P450 interaction table	overview of known substrates, inhibitors, and inducers of CYP isozymes	http://medicine.iupui.edu/clinpharm/ddis
Super CYP	database containing drugs, CYP–drug interactions, and alleles	http://bioinformatics.charite.de/supercyp/index.php?site=home
NAT-allele database	NAT allele nomenclature and function	http://louisville.edu/medschool/pharmacology/consensus-human-arylamine-n-acetyltransferase-gene-nomenclature
UGT-allele database	UGT allele nomenclature and function	http://www.pharmacogenomics.pha.ulaval.ca/sgc/ugt_alleles
	homepage of the committee for naming UGTs	http://www.flinders.edu.au/medicine/sites/clinical-pharmacology/ugt-homepage.cfm
PMT database	pharmacogenetics of membrane transporters	http://pharmacogenetics.ucsf.edu

TP-search database	drug transporter database	http://125.206.112.67/tp-search/index.html
US Food and Drug Administration transporter database	information on transporters important in drug discovery process	http://bts.ucsf.edu/fdatransportal
SLC tables	latest updates on solute carrier families and members	http://www.bioparadigms.org/slc/intro.htm
1000 Genomes Project	catalog of human genetic variation (next-generation sequencing)	http://www.1000genomes.org/page.php
The Centre of Applied Genomics Database of Genomic Variants	curated catalog of structural variation in the human genome	http://projects.tcag.ca/variation/?source=hg18
NCBI dbSNP	database of short genetic variations	http://www.ncbi.nlm.nih.gov/projects/SNP
National Human Genome Research Institute (NHGRI) GWAS Catalog	catalog of published GWAS	http://www.genome.gov/gwastudies
HuGE navigator	integrated, searchable knowledge base of genetic associations and human genome epidemiology	http://hugenavigator.net/HuGENavigator/gWAHitStartPage.do?
eQTL resources	web browser of eQTL throughout the human genome and other tools	http://eqtl.uchicago.edu/Home.html
National Institute of Environmental Health Sciences (NIEHS) Environmental Genome SNPs Project	environmental exposures related to interindividual sequence variation in human genes	http://egp.gs.washington.edu/finished_genes.html
HUGO Gene Nomenclature Committee (HGNC)	curated online repository including links to genomic, proteomic, phenotypic information, and gene family pages	http://www.genenames.org
Genetics home reference on genetic conditions	guide to understanding genetic conditions and related genes/chromosomes	http://ghr.nlm.nih.gov
dbGaP (Database of Genotypes and Phenotypes)	archive of genotype–phenotype interaction studies	http://preview.ncbi.nlm.nih.gov/gap

example, the two most frequent deficient alleles in Caucasians (**4* and **41*) are practically absent in Asians and Africans, where other partially defective alleles (**17* and **10*, respectively) dominate [24].

Evidence for the impact of the *CYP2D6* genotype on drug response exists for many of the drugs inactivated by the enzyme as well as for a number of produgs. In the first case, PMs have been shown to be at risk of overdosing or side-effects (e.g., for antiarrhythmics [25, 26] and antidepressants [27–29]). One example of the second scenario is biotransformation of codeine to morphine. Increased effectiveness of codeine with sometimes life-threatening opioid intoxication was reported in patients with multiple *CYP2D6* gene copies [30, 31]. A second example is the selective estrogen receptor modulator tamoxifen. Two metabolites formed by CYP2D6–4-hydroxytamoxifen and the secondary metabolite endoxifen [32]–have higher affinity to the estrogen receptor. Recent retrospective and prospective studies demonstrated that the CYP2D6 genotype influences plasma concentrations of these active metabolites and treatment outcome [33, 34]. Genotype-based tamoxifen dosing to determine optimal tamoxifen dose resulted in successfully elevated endoxifen levels in IMs, whereas in PMs the concentration was still lower, suggesting that tamoxifen may not be a useful treatment for CYP2D6 PMs [35].

CYP2C19 was discovered by its marked genetic polymorphism, resulting in PM and EM phenotypes of the antiepileptic *S*-mephenytoin [36]. About 3–5% of white and black populations, but up to 20% of Asians are CYP2C19 PMs [12]. The two most common null alleles are *CYP2C19*2*, encoding a cryptic splice variant resulting in no activity *in vivo*, which occurs with higher frequency in Africans and Asians (around 20–30%) compared to Caucasians (around 15%), and *CYP2C19*3*, which occurs primarily in Asians. A further promoter variant *CYP2C19*17* is associated with increased substrate turnover [37].

CYP2C19 is the major enzyme for inactivation of proton pump inhibitors (PPI) including omeprazole and pantoprazole. The common *Heliobacter pylori* eradication strategy involves application of two antibiotics (e.g., amoxicillin and clarithromycin), together with a PPI, which elevates intragastric pH to increase the stability of the antibiotics, leading to a higher success rate of therapy in *CYP2C19* PMs, due to their lower rate of PPI metabolism [38]. The CYP2C19 genotype also has an impact on the metabolism of and response to several antidepressants including amitriptyline [27] and citalopram [39], as well as the bioactivated anticoagulant clopidogrel [40]. Lower anticoagulation effect of clopidogrel in CYP2C19 PMs is associated with increased risk of major adverse cardiovascular events, whereas presence of the gain-of-function allele *CYP2C19*17* was associated with a lower risk of cardiovascular events, but higher risk of bleeding [41].

CYP2C9 differs from the afore-mentioned polymorphic CYPs in that its main variants lead to amino acid changes that can have differential effects on different substrates, which are usually weakly acidic substances like the anticoagulant warfarin, the anticonvulsants phenytoin and valproic acid, cardiovascular drugs like rosuvastatin and losartan, sulfonylurea antidiabetics like tolbutamide, and several nonsteroidal anti-inflammatory drugs (NSAIDs) [42]. Many of these drugs have a narrow therapeutic index and variations in CYP2C9 activity are thus among the recognized factors for drug response.

The CYP-allele web site (Table 9.2) lists 35 alleles, of which the initially discovered alleles **2* (Arg144Cys) and **3* (Ile359Leu) are the most investigated. These variants are present at around 10 and 8%, respectively, in Caucasians, but very rare in Africans and Asians. *In vitro* and *in vivo* these variants confer reductions in substrate clearance of around 70% in **3* homozygotes and around 50% heterozygotes, whereas the **2* variant is less severely affected. Numerous studies demonstrated the clinical significance of the *CYP2C9* polymorphism, such as for hypoglycemic drugs, NSAIDs, and warfarin, where it explains some of the variation in anticoagulant response next to vitamin K epoxide reductase polymorphisms [43].

CYP2B6 is a minor P450 in human liver, but it metabolizes several clinically used drugs including the prodrug cyclophosphamide, the antiretroviral drugs efavirenz and nevirapine, the antidepressant and smoking cessation agent bupropion, the benzodiazepine diazepam, the antimalarial artemisinin, anesthetics like propofol and ketamine, the synthetic opioid methadone, as well as including MDMA (3,4-methylenedioxymethamphetamine) and nicotine, and environmental chemicals like insecticides [44, 45]. Although CYP2B6 is highly inducible by ligands of the xenosensors constitutive androstane receptor (CAR) and pregnane X receptor (PXR), including, for example, rifampin, barbiturates, cyclophosphamide, artemisinin, efavirenz, metamizole, and statins [46–48], *CYP2B6* polymorphisms turned out to be of clinical significance for certain drugs, in particular the anti-HIV drug efavirenz.

The CYP-allele web site (Table 9.2) currently lists 29 distinct alleles with proven functional effect. The most common variant, *CYP2B6*6*, harbors two amino acid changes – Gln172His and Lys262Arg – that occur in various haplotype combinations with other single nucleotide polymorphisms (SNPs) and frequencies between 15 and 60% across different populations. *CYP2B6*6* is associated with 50–75% decreased hepatic protein expression [44]. The causal variant for decreased expression was identified as the c.516G>T (Gln172His) polymorphism, which prevents correct splicing of the CYP2B6 pre-mRNA and leads to a shorter mRNA that lacks exons 4–6 [49]. Another important deficient allele is *CYP2B6*18* (c.983C>T (Ile328Thr)), which is more frequent in black African populations (Table 9.1). An allele associated with increased transcription *in vitro* was also identified (*CYP2B6*22* [50]). The −82T>C change was shown to alter the TATA-box into a functional CCAAT/enhancer-binding protein-binding site that changes transcription start and inducibility [50, 51].

CYP2B6 is mainly responsible for metabolism of the non-nucleosidic reverse transcriptase inhibitor efavirenz into 8-hydroxy and 8,14-dihydroxylated metabolites [52]. Patients with subtherapeutic plasma concentrations can develop resistance and treatment failure, whereas those with too high plasma concentrations are at increased risk of central nervous system (CNS) side-effects. The partially deficient CYP2B6*6 allele and other deficient alleles were correlated in several studies to higher median area under the concentration–time curve (AUC) values

[53, 54]. In a prospective, genotype-based dose adjustment study the therapeutic dose of efavirenz could be successfully reduced and CNS-related side-effects decreased [55]. CYP2B6 and CAR polymorphisms were shown, in addition to nongenetic factors, to be associated with efavirenz treatment discontinuation because of side-effects – a common problem in therapeutic HIV management [56].

The important CYP3A subfamily comprises four functional genes: the most abundant and highly drug-inducible CYP3A4, and the minor forms CYP3A5, CYP3A7, and CYP3A43. CYP3A4 and CYP3A5 have broad, strongly overlapping substrate specificity including substances from most therapeutic categories; and due to high expression of CYP3A4 in liver and gut this enzyme is responsible for large first-pass metabolism of many drugs [57, 58]. In contrast to CYP3A4, which will be discussed later, expression of CYP3A5 in liver is polymorphic [59, 60] in that only a fraction of about 5–10% of Caucasians, but 60% or more of Africans or African-Americans express the active enzyme. CYP3A5 is on average expressed at less than 10% of CYP3A4; its contribution to drug metabolism is in some cases high enough to result in significant associations between the major splice site variant *CYP3A5*3* [59, 60] and reduced metabolism, in particular for the immunosuppressant tacrolimus [61, 62] and several HIV protease inhibitors [63].

9.2.3
Polymorphisms in Further Drug-Metabolizing Enzymes

TPMT (Table 9.1) is a cytosolic enzyme that catalyzes the inactivating methylation of a number of thiopurine drugs, in particular 6-mercaptopurine, 6-thioguanine, and azathioprine, which are used to treat leukemia, autoimmune diseases, and inflammatory bowel diseases, and as immunosuppressants after organ transplantation. Mercaptopurine pharmacogenetics is based on monogenic inheritance of TPMT activity, which was found to be a major determinant of the efficacy and toxicity of these drugs [64–66]. The most common TPMT variant alleles (Table 9.1) harbor nonsynonymous coding SNPs and explain most of the phenotypic variation, which can in this case be easily determined in Caucasians populations. Their identification is clinically very important to avoid the potentially fatal myelosuppression by these dangerous drugs, which is also mentioned in the drug labels. However, even such convincing circumstances has so far not resulted in wide clinical acceptance, as most of oncology, hematology, and pediatrics departments in the European Union do not regularly perform TPMT genotyping or phenotyping before administrating thiopurine drugs [10].

DPD is the ubiquitous rate-limiting enzyme for the catabolism of uracil and thymine. It also converts 5-fluorouracil (5-FU) to the inactive dihydrofluorouracil and more than 80% of administered 5-FU is catabolized via DPD. Inherited complete *DPYD* deficiency leading to thymine-uraciluria, which is associated with a variety of neurological symptoms, was shown to be caused by defective splicing due to a consensus splice site variant [67]. Heterozygous DPD deficiency, which occurs in approximately 1% of the normal population, plays a limited role in determining 5-FU toxicity as shown in several studies, including one prospective study with 683 patients on 5-FU monotherapy [68]. However, other factors including mode of administration, sex, and other factors are also important.

The UGT isoform UGT1A1 is exclusively responsible for the glucuronidation of bilirubin – the cytotoxic and water-insoluble major product of heme degradation. A large number of diverse *UGT1A1* genetic variants influence its expression/activity to various degrees. The more severe ones are associated with Crigler–Najjar type I and II diseases. Benign hereditary hyperbilirubinemia – also known as Gilbert–Meulengracht syndrome – results in most cases from a TA-repeat polymorphism in the TATA-box of the UGT1A1 promoter. Compared to the normal $A(TA)_6TAA$ genotype, the $A(TA)_7TAA$ variant (*UGT1A1*28*) expresses at lower levels and affects drug glucuronidation in about 10% of Caucasians who are homozygous for this allele [69].

Among several other endogenous and exogenous substrates, the topoisomerase 1 inhibitor irinotecan used to treat metastatic colorectal cancer has gained attention in recent years. The drug is bioactivated by carboxylesterase-2 to yield the chemotherapeutic metabolite 7-ethyl-10-hydroxycamptothecin (SN-38), which depends on UGT1A1 for inactivation and excretion. Carriers of the *UGT1A1*28/*28* genotype are at increased risk of hematotoxicity [70]. Consideration of genotype, but not mandatory genetic testing has been, included in the irinotecan drug label [71]. Another polymorphically expressed UGT1A enzyme is UGT1A3, which was recently shown to play a role in statin lactonization [72].

Additional examples of polymorphisms in drug-metabolizing enzymes are discussed in several other chapters of this book.

9.2.4
Polymorphic Drug Transporters

As described in Chapter 7, many genetic variants in transporter genes causing lack of transporter function are associated with clinical phenotypes. This fact indicates an important function of these genes for the transport and distribution of endogenous substances. The importance of transporter polymorphisms for pharmacogenetics/genomics is best illustrated by the *MDR1* gene, which has so far received the most attention. *MDR1* encodes the ATP-binding cassette (ABC) transporter ABCB1 (P-glycoprotein (P-gp)) – a transmembrane transporter that catalyzes typically the efflux of bulky substances, which are often also substrates of CYP3A4, into the extracellular space. ABCB1 is localized in the apical membrane of bronchial, renal, and intestinal epithelial cells, of hepatocytes, and in the endothelial cells at the blood–tissue barrier, where it plays a central role in tissue defense against chemically diverse toxicants [73]. *MDR1* was one of the earliest transporter genes systematically investigated for polymorphic expression and in pharmacogenetics. Substrates of P-gp include many important drugs with a narrow therapeutic range, including chemotherapeutic agents, cyclosporin A, verapamil, terfenadine, fexofenadin, and most HIV-1 protease inhibitors. Despite many initially controversial results, ABCB1 pharmacogenetics has helped tremendously to define the role of transporters in the uptake, excretion, and distribution of foreign substances, and to understand the particular difficulties in transporter pharmacogenomics [74–76]. The most frequently studied synonymous 3435C>T polymorphism in exon 26, which was initially shown to be associated with decreased P-gp expression in intestinal epithelia [77], led to an increased interest in potential mechanisms of silent mutations [78–80].

Further important examples of polymorphic drug transporters include OATP1B1, which was identified as a determinant of statin-related myopathy (see below), and the bile acid transporter breast cancer resistance protein (BCRP), which are discussed in Chapter 7. Considering the large number of transporter genes in the human genome, which exceeds the number of CYP enzyme genes and the fact that transporter pharmacogenomics started less than 15 years ago, an increased recognition of the importance of transporter pharmacogenomics may be expected in the future. Owing to the more complex nature of transport phenomena in various organs of the body, more sophisticated study designs, better definition of phenotypes, and larger sample numbers will be necessary to translate knowledge from this area into clinics [81, 82].

9.3 Polygenic and Multifactorial Aspects of Drug Metabolism Phenotype

The pharmacogenetic polymorphisms described above are mostly examples of monogenic inheritance, where polymorphisms within the gene itself (*cis*-acting) dominate any other influences. However, these are exceptional cases, whereas expression and functional variability of most genes as well as drug response in general will usually depend on multifactorial influences, which include multigenic as well as nongenetic factors. Multigenic influences may reside, for example, in other genes that affect transcription, splicing, translation, mRNA and protein stability, cofactor supply, or interaction with various electron donators in the case of CYPs (*trans*-acting genetic polymorphisms). A rather new area of research concerns various aspects of epigenetics, in particular DNA methylation and the regulation of gene expression by microRNAs (miRNAs). Also of great importance in pharmacogenomics, but not discussed here in detail, is the consideration of nongenetic factors such as drug–drug interactions and other environmental factors (e.g., circadian rhythm [83], physiological and pathophysiological conditions [84], as well as sex- and age-related differences [85, 86]).

9.3.1 Polygenic Inheritance: CYP1A2 and CYP3A4 Conundrums

While numerous alleles coding for protein variants of CYP1A2 and CYP3A4 are known (CYP-allele web site, Table 9.2) and new functionally relevant polymorphisms continue to be discovered [87, 88], genetic prediction remained unsatisfactory, despite the several resequencing and genotyping studies that have been performed [89–93]. The intensely studied CYP3A4*1B promoter variant, which occurs in white populations at around 2–9%, but at higher frequencies in Africans, is still controversially discussed [94–96]. Taken together, the known variants of these two genes cannot explain their variability on a population level.

There is nevertheless evidence that the activity of these two genes is also mainly controlled by genetic factors. Thus, by measuring the caffeine metabolic ratio as a CYP1A2 activity marker in a large cohort ($n = 378$) of mono- and dizygotic twins selected to exclude the influence of smoking, oral contraceptives, and gender, Brøsen *et al.* found a strong overall heritability of 0.725 [97]. Similarly, antipyrine 4-hydroxylation rate, which is mainly catalyzed by CYP3A4, appears to be largely inherited (88%), as shown in twin studies [98]. Kalow *et al.* furthermore argued in favor of a genetic basis for the variability in CYP3A4 drug oxidation capacity based on repeated drug administration data [99].

Primary candidates for influential *trans*-acting genes are the constitutive and ligand-dependent transcription factors involved in CYP1A2 and CYP3A4 transcriptional regulation. Initial studies that investigated the relevance of SNPs in various nuclear receptor genes, including the aryl hydrocarbon receptor (AhR), CAR, and PXR [100–102], revealed variants with limited impact on their targets. Recently, systematic candidate gene studies were carried out, where several genes of potential impact were studied with respect to their influence on CYP expression and function in human liver cohorts. In one study, Klein *et al.* [103] investigated expression of CYP1A2 at the mRNA, protein, and activity level in 150 liver samples in relation to 169 SNPs in 17 candidate genes, including the CYP1A locus. SNPs in various regulator genes including the AhR pathway showed consistent changes, and multivariate analysis indicated that polymorphisms and nongenetic factors together explained 42, 38, and 33% of CYP1A2 variation at the activity, protein, and mRNA levels, respectively.

A similar candidate gene approach to identify genetic markers of CYP3A4 by Lamba *et al.* [104] identified sex and polymorphisms in FoxA2, hepatocyte nuclear factor (HNF)-4α, FoxA3, PXR, ABCB1, and the CYP3A4 promoter, together explaining approximately one-fourth of the variation in hepatic CYP3A4 expression at the RNA level. Klein *et al.* [105] analyzed CYP3A4 variation at the mRNA, protein, and functional level, and identified several polymorphisms in transcriptional regulators and other influential genes not previously implicated in the regulation of CYP3A4. Additional studies in volunteers and gene silencing experiments in primary human hepatocytes confirmed a strong impact of peroxisome proliferator-activated receptor (PPAR)-α on CYP3A4 expression and function [105].

Other well-established influential transgenes for CYP-dependent drug metabolism function are the electron donator proteins CYP oxidoreductase (POR) and cytochrome b_5. Whereas rare mutations in POR were recently shown to result in severe clinical phenotypes [106], more common polymorphisms could explain in part CYP functional variability [107–109]. While these and other new findings of polymorphisms in *trans*-acting genes are highly interesting in terms of understanding the regulation of CYP expression and function, it remains to be established how useful they will be in clinical pharmacogenomics.

9.3.2 Epigenetic Influences on Drug Metabolism

Some heritable changes in gene function are not based on DNA sequence variations and the term epigenetics has been coined to describe such phenomena. Two important mechanisms known to have profound effects on gene expression are DNA methylation and histone protein modifications. Whereas DNA methylation is involved in normal cellular control of gene expression, histone modifications affect the accessibility and transcriptional activity of the chromatin within the cell. In addition to these processes, epigenetics also comprises gene regulation by miRNAs. Epigenetic patterns are principally reversible and may thus be influenced by environmental factors. They can furthermore change with age and differ from tissue to tissue. The influence of epigenetic processes on pharmacologically relevant genes and drug response is a rather new area of research that has recently been summarized [110, 111].

For example, differential gene expression analysis in the human HepG2 hepatoma cell line using 5-aza-2′-deoxycytidine to inhibit DNA methylation and trichostatin A to inhibit histone deacetylation demonstrated widespread effects on more than 1500 and 500 genes, respectively, including induction of CYP3A genes and other CYPs, as well as several transcription factors [112]. Dynamic patterns of histone methylation are also associated with ontogenic expression of CYP2E1 in the human liver [113]. Importantly, CYP1A1 promoter methylation in human lung tissue was found to be lowest in heavy tobacco smokers and highest in nonsmokers, providing an example of environmental influence on DNA methylation patterns [114]. Another study showed an inverse correlation between CYP1A2 mRNA and extent of methylation at two CpG sites near the transcription start site in human liver samples [115]. These and other examples illustrate the potential impact of DNA methylation on gene expression patterns of pharmacogenes, which could even influence that of future generations, as epigenetic changes can principally be transmitted to offspring.

A newer area where recent advances suggest future impact on pharmacogenomics is regulation of gene expression by noncoding RNAs, in particular miRNAs. miRNAs are single-stranded, noncoding RNA molecules consisting of about 22 nucleotides, which play an important role mainly in post-transcriptional gene regulation by targeting seed sequences in the 3′-untranslated region of target mRNAs [116]. However, miRNAs not only modulate expression of probably more than half of all genes, but they can also be master regulators in differentiation, development, and apoptosis, and differential miRNA expression is associated with disease stage, such as in certain cancers, where miRNAs function as oncogenes or tumor suppressors. A current problem of miRNA information management relates to the large number of miRNAs, estimated at over 1000 different molecules per mammalian species and their poorly defined binding specificities, which allows for a vast number of potential miRNA–target gene interactions [117]. Various databases have been developed, using different algorithms to predict potential binding sites [118]. Specialized databases (e.g., miRecords [119], miRò [120]) and dedicated software programs (e.g., MIRNA-DISTILLER [121]) allow us to compile miRNA predictions from different databases to facilitate data management.

Several examples demonstrate that miRNAs can influence expression of genes relevant for drug absorption, distribution, metabolism, and excretion (ADME genes), thus providing an additional layer of variability that may help to explain drug failure or adverse events. Some metabolic enzymes were shown to be directly regulated by miRNAs, such as CYP1B1 and CYP3A4 by miR-27b [122, 123], and CYP2E1 by miR-378 [124]. The influence of miRNAs on nuclear receptor expression appears to have an even larger impact on the regulation of drug metabolism, because one receptor usually regulates several or many target genes. In some instances miRNAs may thus be regarded as the "regulators of the regulators."

Thus, the xenosensor PXR (NR1I2), which regulates transcription of at least 40 target genes in response to xenobiotic inducers, was shown to be under control of miR-148a, thereby influencing CYP3A4 and CYP2B6 expression levels, and the metabolism of xenobiotic drug substrates of these enzymes [125]. Further, HNF-4α is regulated by miR-24 and miR-34a. Overexpression of these miRNAs results in a decrease of HNF-4α and concurrent downregulation of its target genes. As HNF-4α is a master regulator of hepatic gene expression, these miRNAs may also contribute to liver pathology and drug response [126]. The vitamin D receptor (VDR), another transcriptional regulator of CYP3A4, is also regulated by the CYP3A4-targeting miR-27b, resulting in an indirect and a direct mechanism for miRNA regulation of CYP3A4 [123]. An additional validated target of miR-27b is PPAR-γ [127, 128] and liver X receptor (LXR) was shown to be regulated by miR-613 [129], further supporting an important role of miRNAs in hepatic gene regulation.

Of special interest for pharmacogenetic aspects are SNPs in miRNAs and miRNA binding sites, as well as miRNA copy number variations, which have been found to affect gene expression. An interesting question is therefore whether "miRNA pharmacogenetics" could be of relevance. A genome-wide study found a low level of DNA variation in functional miRNA regions, whereas higher levels of variation are present in predicted target sites, where SNPs may stabilize or destabilize miRNA binding [130]. For example, the dihydrofolate reductase (DHFR) gene harbors a so-called miRSNP in its 3′-untranslated region, which was found to cause loss of miR-24 binding leading to DHFR overexpression and association with methotrexate resistance [131].

Thus, although the field of epigenetic regulation of drug metabolism and drug response genes is probably still in its infancy, these examples demonstrate an important impact of this level of gene regulation.

9.4 Genomics Technologies and Approaches

Modern technology has revolutionized the speed and output of molecular discovery. The completion of the human genome sequence in 2003 catalyzed the development of next-generation sequencing and genome-wide microarray technology to study SNPs, structural genomic variants, the entire transcriptome, as well as new databases and *in silico* tools that facilitate analysis of this new wave of information. Two powerful approaches will be briefly discussed – genome-wide association studies (GWAS) and the expression quantitative trait loci (eQTL) approach.

9.4.1
GWAS – A Matured Tool in Pharmacogenomics

Genome-wide SNP arrays that reliably determine 500 000 or more genotypes are now a commonly used tool to test association with disease susceptibility, severity of disease, or any qualitative or quantitative phenotype. A fundamental conceptual advantage of GWAS over analysis of candidate genes is the unbiased approach, which permits discovery of entirely new relationships between genes and phenotypes. The biggest disadvantage, however, is the large number of tests that have to be performed, which requires appropriate corrections for multiple testing, thus severely limiting statistical power – a particular concern in pharmacogenomic applications [132, 133]. More than 1200 published GWAS, which provide tremendous new insight into the relationship between genetic variants, biochemical pathways, and inheritable traits, have been cataloged on the dedicated NHGRI (National Human Genome Research Institute) web site (Table 9.2) [134].

Despite controversial initial discussion, GWAS turned out to be a powerful approach to identify genetic variants associated with drug effect and ADRs. Illustrative examples for the first category include the confirmation of strong association of variants in VKORC1 and CYP2C9 for stable warfarin dosing. Although this association was been established before, the GWAS ruled out important contributions by other loci – a prerequisite for large clinical trials. Similarly, the highly heritable platelet response to clopidogrel could be attributed to *CYP2C19* as the major gene [40].

Application of GWAS to ADRs includes a study on rare statin-induced myopathy using DNA samples from only 85 cases that identified common variants in the statin transporter SLCO1B1, demonstrating that GWAS can be successful with rather small sample sizes [135]. Additional GWAS identified determinants of severe drug hypersensitivity reactions, which cannot be predicted based on the drug's pharmacology. Cholestatic hepatitis induced by flucloxacillin, used to treat staphylococcal infections, has been associated with the HLA-B*5701 allele [136], which had previously been shown to be also strongly associated to hypersensitivity against the anti-HIV agent abacavir [137]. Another recently identified HLA allele (A*3101) was significantly associated with carbamazepine-induced hypersensitivity syndrome in GWAS including only 22 affected subjects [138]. It should finally be noted that numerous GWAS did not result in any significant finding [133].

In the near future, we will see many more GWAS to identify genetic drug effects and ADR determinants in almost all areas of drug treatment. The 1000 Genomes Project (Table 9.2) will uncover most or all variants present in the major human populations and this will soon allow the development of microarrays with 5 million or more encoded SNPs, including many rare variants. Their importance was recognized when the early microarray studies failed to identify common SNPs (frequency greater than 5%) explaining common diseases, also known as the missing heritability problem [139]. Common variants usually have a weak effect, whereas rare variants can have large effects, however, until now they have consistently been blinded out from most pharmacogenomics studies. The CYP-allele nomenclature web site (Table 9.2) consists to a large part of such variants and many more are currently being identified among ADME genes in the course of the 1000 Genomes Project [140]. However, the future challenge will not be to detect them, but to predict their functionality and impact on drug response. Additional problems that need to be addressed in current pharmacogenomics include, for example, better standardization of disease phenotypes, the collection of larger cohorts of well-phenotyped patients, and pooling biological samples through international collaborations.

9.4.2 Genetical Genomics: Identifying Novel Polymorphic ADME Genes

Over 300 ADME and ADME-related genes and even more drug target genes have been identified in the human genome (PharmaADME and PharmGKB web sites, see Table 9.2). Only a few of these have so far been systematically investigated with respect to genetic and other factors of variability. A relatively new approach to identify unknown functional genetic variants that modulate gene expression, also termed genetical genomics, is the mapping of eQTL by using genome-wide association methods in cohorts of unrelated individuals [141, 142]. In this strategy, individual transcript levels are determined in a selected tissue or cell type by using microarrays. In genomic DNA of the same individuals, of the order of 10^5–10^6 SNPs are genotyped in parallel. By considering each individual gene transcript as a quantitative trait, association analysis identifies SNPs that are significantly associated to expression. The eQTL strategy thus differs from the above-mentioned GWAS, which typically focus on a single or only a few complex phenotypes. A limitation of this approach is that only very strong genotype–phenotype relationships survive stringent statistical correction for multiple testing. Schadt *et al.* [143] used this approach to compare more than 39 000 transcripts and 782 476 unique SNPs in 427 human liver samples, revealing more than 6000 relationships between SNP genotypes and liver gene expression traits, of which around 1350 remained significant after multiple testing correction. Remarkably, the number of identified *trans*-eQTL was much smaller compared to *cis*-eQTL, which was explained by the lack of statistical power to detect relatively weak *trans* effects.

Two independent similar studies by Innocenti *et al.* [144] and Schroeder *et al.* [145] compared their results to the former one, both noting an astounding lack of reproducibility of eQTL results. It was suggested that tissue sampling procedures, clinical descriptors, drug exposure, and unknown factors may contribute to expression variability, and failure to control for such covariates may result in lack of reproducibility. The study by Schroeder *et al.* [145] verified a subset of 95 associations related to ADME of drugs. Of these, 21 were true replications, and 74 were newly discovered associations in enzymes, transporters, transcriptional regulators, and other pharmacologically relevant genes.

In a focused analysis on liver-expressed CYPs, Yang *et al.* [85] used data from one of the former studies [143] for genome-wide coexpression network analysis. They identified gene modules (subnetworks) relevant for CYP expression and enriched for certain functional pathways (e.g., comprising nuclear receptor or inflammation-related genes). In addition, they performed eQTL analysis on 10 liver CYP activities. Surprisingly few genotype–phenotype relationships were discovered in this study. Of 54 SNPs significantly associated with CYP activities, 30 mapped to the CYP2D6 locus, whereas all others represented *trans*-eQTLs. Thus, while no *cis*-eQTL were detected for CYP1A2, CYP3A4, or other CYP genes, the *trans*-eQTL identified did not agree with any of the results of the above-mentioned candidate gene approaches. This apparent contradiction may be related to the different approaches and the general difficulty in reproducing *trans*-acting relationships. It should also be kept in mind that the much lower number of SNPs tested in candidate gene approaches leads to higher statistical power compared to genome-wide associations. Taken together, these studies extended the knowledge about the genetics of interindividual variability of liver gene expression considerably, but they also emphasize current limitations and challenges.

9.5 Conclusions

Pharmacogenomics is nurtured by two major streams of research – a basic research stream that aims to discover genetic variation and to understand mechanisms of biological genotype–phenotype correlation, and a clinically oriented stream that builds upon basic knowledge to investigate genetic factors in relation to drug response phenotypes and to apply novel diagnostic tools to translate this into clinical care. Modern technology has revolutionized the speed and output of molecular discovery, providing us with a new armament for research. This will open up many opportunities for interesting discoveries in basic research. However, many challenges remain in order to apply this knowledge clinically.

References

1 Meyer, U.A. (2000) Pharmacogenetics and adverse drug reactions. *Lancet*, **356**, 1667–1671.

2 Wilkinson, G.R. (2005) Drug metabolism and variability among patients in drug response. *N. Engl. J. Med*, **352**, 2211–2221.

3 Eichelbaum, M., Ingelman-Sundberg, M., and Evans, W.E. (2006) Pharmacogenomics and individualized drug therapy. *Annu. Rev. Med*, **57**, 119–137.

4 Lubomirov, R., Colombo, S., di Iulio, J., Ledergerber, B., Martinez, R., Cavassini,

M., *et al.* (2011) Association of pharmacogenetic markers with premature discontinuation of first-line anti-HIV therapy: an observational cohort study. *J. Infect. Dis.*, **203**, 246–257.

5 Pirmohamed, M., James, S., Meakin, S., Green, C., Scott, A.K., Walley, T.J., *et al.* (2004) Adverse drug reactions as cause of admission to hospital: prospective analysis of 18 820 patients. *Br. Med. J.*, **329**, 15–19.

6 Wienkers, L.C. and Heath, T.G. (2005) Predicting *in vivo* drug interactions from *in vitro* drug discovery data. *Nat. Rev. Drug Discov.*, **4**, 825–833.

7 Roses, A.D. (2008) Pharmacogenetics in drug discovery and development: a translational perspective. *Nat. Rev. Drug Discov.*, **7**, 807–817.

8 Meyer, U.A. (2004) Pharmacogenetics – five decades of therapeutic lessons from genetic diversity. *Nat. Rev. Genet.*, **5**, 669–676.

9 Frueh, F.W. and Gurwitz, D. (2004) From pharmacogenetics to personalized medicine: a vital need for educating health professionals and the community. *Pharmacogenomics*, **5**, 571–579.

10 Woelderink, A., Ibarreta, D., Hopkins, M.M., and Rodriguez-Cerezo, E. (2006) The current clinical practice of pharmacogenetic testing in Europe: TPMT and HER2 as case studies. *Pharmacogenomics J.*, **6**, 3–7.

11 Pirmohamed, M. (2009) The applications of pharmacogenetics to prescribing: what is currently practicable? *Clin. Med.*, **9**, 493–495.

12 Meyer, U.A. and Zanger, U.M. (1997) Molecular mechanisms of genetic polymorphisms of drug metabolism. *Annu. Rev. Pharmacol. Toxicol.*, **37**, 269–296.

13 Garrod, A.E. (2002) The incidence of alkaptonuria: a study in chemical individuality. 1902 [classical article]. *Yale J. Biol. Med.*, **75**, 221–231.

14 Earle, D.P., Jr and Bigelow, F.S. (1948) Studies on the chemotherapy of the human malarias; effect of pamaquine on the blood cells of man. *J. Clin. Invest.*, **27**, 121–129.

15 Mahgoub, A., Idle, J.R., Dring, L.G., Lancaster, R., and Smith, R.L. (1977) Polymorphic hydroxylation of debrisoquine in man. *Lancet*, **2**, 584–586.

16 Eichelbaum, M., Spannbrucker, N., Steincke, B., and Dengler, H.J. (1979) Defective *N*-oxidation of sparteine in man: a new pharmacogenetic defect. *Eur. J. Clin. Pharmacol.*, **16**, 183–187.

17 Langenfeld, E., Zanger, U.M., Jung, K., Meyer, H.E., and Marcus, K. (2009) Mass spectrometry-based absolute quantification of microsomal cytochrome P450 2D6 in human liver. *Proteomics*, **9**, 2313–2323.

18 Sachse, C., Brockmöller, J., Bauer, S., and Roots, I. (1997) Cytochrome P450 2D6 variants in a Caucasian population: allele frequencies and phenotypic consequences. *Am. J. Hum. Genet.*, **60**, 284–295.

19 Griese, E.U., Zanger, U.M., Brudermanns, U., Gaedigk, A., Mikus, G., Mörike, K., *et al.* (1998) Assessment of the predictive power of genotypes for the in-vivo catalytic function of CYP2D6 in a German population. *Pharmacogenetics*, **8**, 15–26.

20 Schaeffeler, E., Schwab, M., Eichelbaum, M., and Zanger, U.M. (2003) CYP2D6 genotyping strategy based on gene copy number determination by TaqMan real-time PCR. *Hum. Mutat.*, **22**, 476–485.

21 Raimundo, S., Toscano, C., Klein, K., Fischer, J., Griese, E.-U., Eichelbaum, M., *et al.* (2004) A novel intronic mutation, 2988G>A, with high predictivity for impaired function of cytochrome P450 2D6 in white subjects. *Clin. Pharmacol. Ther.*, **76**, 128–138.

22 Zanger, U.M., Fischer, J., Raimundo, S., Stüven, T., Evert, B.O., Schwab, M., *et al.* (2001) Comprehensive analysis of the genetic factors determining expression and function of hepatic CYP2D6. *Pharmacogenetics*, **11**, 573–585.

23 Toscano, C., Klein, K., Blievernicht, J., Schaeffeler, E., Saussele, T., Raimundo, S., *et al.* (2006) Impaired expression of CYP2D6 in intermediate metabolizers carrying the *41 allele caused by the intronic SNP 2988G>A: evidence for

modulation of splicing events. *Pharmacogenet. Genomics*, **16**, 755–766.

24 Gaedigk, A. (2000) Interethnic differences of drug-metabolizing enzymes. *Int. J. Clin. Pharmacol. Ther.*, **38**, 61–68.

25 Darbar, D. and Roden, D.M. (2006) Pharmacogenetics of antiarrhythmic therapy. *Expert Opin. Pharmacother.*, **7**, 1583–1590.

26 Rau, T., Wuttke, H., Michels, L.M., Werner, U., Bergmann, K., Kreft, M., *et al.* (2009) Impact of the CYP2D6 genotype on the clinical effects of metoprolol: a prospective longitudinal study. *Clin. Pharmacol. Ther.*, **85**, 269–272.

27 Steimer, W., Zöpf, K., von Amelunxen, S., Pfeiffer, H., Bachofer, J., Popp, J., *et al.* (2005) Amitriptyline or not, that is the question: pharmacogenetic testing of CYP2D6 and CYP2C19 identifies patients with low or high risk for side-effects in amitriptyline therapy. *Clin. Chem.*, **51**, 376–385.

28 Laika, B., Leucht, S., Heres, S., and Steimer, W. (2009) Intermediate metabolizer: increased side-effects in psychoactive drug therapy. The key to cost-effectiveness of pretreatment CYP2D6 screening? *Pharmacogenomics J.*, **9**, 395–403.

29 Crisafulli, C., Fabbri, C., Porcelli, S., Drago, A., Spina, E., De Ronchi, D., *et al.* (2011) Pharmacogenetics of antidepressants. *Front. Pharmacol.*, **2**, 6.

30 Gasche, Y., Daali, Y., Fathi, M., Chiappe, A., Cottini, S., Dayer, P., *et al.* (2004) Codeine intoxication associated with ultrarapid CYP2D6 metabolism. *N. Engl. J. Med.*, **351**, 2827–2831.

31 Madadi, P., Ross, C.J.D., Hayden, M.R., Carleton, B.C., Gaedigk, A., Leeder, J.S., *et al.* (2009) Pharmacogenetics of neonatal opioid toxicity following maternal use of codeine during breastfeeding: a case-control study. *Clin. Pharmacol. Ther.*, **85**, 31–35.

32 Johnson, M.D., Zuo, H., Lee, K.-H., Trebley, J.P., Rae, J.M., Weatherman, R.V., *et al.* (2004) Pharmacological characterization of 4-hydroxy-*N*-desmethyl tamoxifen, a novel active metabolite of tamoxifen. *Breast Cancer Res.*, **85**, 151–159.

33 Goetz, M.P., Rae, J.M., Suman, V.J., Safgren, S.L., Ames, M.M., Visscher, D.W., *et al.* (2005) Pharmacogenetics of tamoxifen biotransformation is associated with clinical outcomes of efficacy and hot flashes. *J. Clin. Oncol.*, **23**, 9312–9318.

34 Schroth, W., Goetz, M.P., Hamann, U., Fasching, P.A., Schmidt, M., Winter, S., *et al.* (2009) Association between CYP2D6 polymorphisms and outcomes among women with early stage breast cancer treated with tamoxifen. *JAMA*, **302**, 1429–1436.

35 Irvin, W.J., Jr, Walko, C.M., Weck, K.E., Ibrahim, J.G., Chiu, W.K., Dees, E.C., *et al.* (2011) Genotype-guided tamoxifen dosing increases active metabolite exposure in women with reduced CYP2D6 metabolism: a multicenter study. *J. Clin. Oncol.*, **29**, 3232–3239.

36 Küpfer, A. and Preisig, R. (1984) Pharmacogenetics of mephenytoin: a new drug hydroxylation polymorphism in man. *Eur. J. Clin. Pharmacol.*, **26**, 753–759.

37 Sim, S.C., Risinger, C., Dahl, M.-L., Aklillu, E., Christensen, M., Bertilsson, L., *et al.* (2006) A common novel CYP2C19 gene variant causes ultrarapid drug metabolism relevant for the drug response to proton pump inhibitors and antidepressants. *Clin. Pharmacol. Ther.*, **79**, 103–113.

38 Yang J.-C. and Lin C.-J. (2010) CYP2C19 genotypes in the pharmacokinetics/pharmacodynamics of proton pump inhibitor-based therapy of *Helicobacter pylori* infection. *Expert Opin. Drug Metab. Toxicol.*, **6**, 29–41.

39 Rudberg, I., Mohebi, B., Hermann, M., Refsum, H., and Molden, E. (2008) Impact of the ultrarapid CYP2C19*17 allele on serum concentration of escitalopram in psychiatric patients. *Clin. Pharmacol. Ther.*, **83**, 322–327.

40 Shuldiner, A.R., O'Connell, J.R., Bliden, K.P., Gandhi, A., Ryan, K., Horenstein, R.B., *et al.* (2009) Association of cytochrome P450 2C19 genotype with the antiplatelet effect and clinical

efficacy of clopidogrel therapy. *JAMA*, **302**, 849–857.

41 Zabalza, M., Subirana, I., Sala, J., Lluis-Ganella, C., Lucas, G., Tomás, M., *et al.* (2012) Meta-analyses of the association between cytochrome CYP2C19 loss- and gain-of-function polymorphisms and cardiovascular outcomes in patients with coronary artery disease treated with clopidogrel. *Heart*, **98**, 100–108.

42 Kirchheiner, J. and Brockmöller, J. (2005) Clinical consequences of cytochrome P450 2C9 polymorphisms. *Clin. Pharmacol. Ther.*, **77**, 1–16.

43 Li, J., Wang, S., Barone, J., and Malone, B. (2009) Warfarin pharmacogenomics. *P T*, **34**, 422–427.

44 Zanger, U.M., Klein, K., Saussele, T., Blievernicht, J., Hofmann, M.H., and Schwab, M. (2007) Polymorphic CYP2B6: molecular mechanisms and emerging clinical significance. *Pharmacogenomics*, **8**, 743–759.

45 Hodgson, E. and Rose, R.L. (2007) The importance of cytochrome P450 2B6 in the human metabolism of environmental chemicals. *Pharmacol. Ther.*, **113**, 420–428.

46 Faucette, S.R., Wang, H., Hamilton, G.A., Jolley, S.L., Gilbert, D., Lindley, C., *et al.* (2004) Regulation of CYP2B6 in primary human hepatocytes by prototypical inducers. *Drug Metab. Dispos.*, **32**, 348–358.

47 Saussele, T., Burk, O., Blievernicht, J.K., Klein, K., Nussler, A., Nussler, N., *et al.* (2007) Selective induction of human hepatic cytochromes P450 2B6 and 3A4 by metamizole. *Clin. Pharmacol. Ther.*, **82**, 265–274.

48 Feidt, D.M., Klein, K., Hofmann, U., Riedmaier, S., Knobeloch, D., Thasler, W.E., *et al.* (2010) Profiling induction of cytochrome p450 enzyme activity by statins using a new liquid chromatography-tandem mass spectrometry cocktail assay in human hepatocytes. *Drug Metab. Dispos.*, **38**, 1589–1597.

49 Hofmann, M.H., Blievernicht, J.K., Klein, K., Saussele, T., Schaeffeler, E., Schwab, M., *et al.* (2008) Aberrant splicing caused by single nucleotide polymorphism c.516G>T [Q172H], a marker of CYP2B6*6, is responsible for decreased expression and activity of CYP2B6 in liver. *J. Pharmacol. Exp. Ther.*, **325**, 284–292.

50 Zukunft, J., Lang, T., Richter, T., Hirsch-Ernst, K.I., Nussler, A.K., Klein, K., *et al.* (2005) A natural CYP2B6 TATA box polymorphism (–82T→C) leading to enhanced transcription and relocation of the transcriptional start site. *Mol. Pharmacol.*, **67**, 1772–1782.

51 Li, H., Ferguson, S.S., and Wang, H. (2010) Synergistically enhanced CYP2B6 inducibility between a polymorphic mutation in CYP2B6 promoter and pregnane X receptor activation. *Mol. Pharmacol.*, **78**, 704–713.

52 Ward, B.A., Gorski, J.C., Jones, D.R., Hall, S.D., Flockhart, D.A., and Desta, Z. (2003) The cytochrome P450 2B6 (CYP2B6) is the main catalyst of efavirenz primary and secondary metabolism: implication for HIV/AIDS therapy and utility of efavirenz as a substrate marker of CYP2B6 catalytic activity. *J. Pharmacol. Exp. Ther.*, **306**, 287–300.

53 Rotger, M., Tegude, H., Colombo, S., Cavassini, M., Furrer, H., Décosterd, L., *et al.* (2007) Predictive value of known and novel alleles of CYP2B6 for efavirenz plasma concentrations in HIV-infected individuals. *Clin. Pharmacol. Ther.*, **81**, 557–566.

54 Telenti, A. and Zanger, U.M. (2008) Pharmacogenetics of anti-HIV drugs. *Annu. Rev. Pharmacol. Toxicol.*, **48**, 227–256.

55 Gatanaga, H., Hayashida, T., Tsuchiya, K., Yoshino, M., Kuwahara, T., Tsukada, H., *et al.* (2007) Successful efavirenz dose reduction in HIV type 1-infected individuals with cytochrome P450 2B6 *6 and *26. *Clin. Infect. Dis.*, **45**, 1230–1237.

56 Wyen, C., Hendra, H., Siccardi, M., Platten, M., Jaeger, H., Harrer, T., *et al.* (2011) Cytochrome P450 2B6 (CYP2B6) and constitutive androstane receptor (CAR) polymorphisms are associated with early discontinuation of efavirenz-containing regimens. *J. Antimicrob. Chemother.*, **66**, 2092–2098.

57 Wrighton, S.A., Schuetz, E.G., Thummel, K.E., Shen, D.D., Korzekwa, K.R., and Watkins, P.B. (2000) The human CYP3A subfamily: practical considerations. *Drug Metab. Rev.*, **32**, 339–361.
58 Rendic, S. (2002) Summary of information on human CYP enzymes: human P450 metabolism data. *Drug Metab. Rev.*, **34**, 83–448.
59 Kuehl, P., Zhang, J., Lin, Y., Lamba, J., Assem, M., Schuetz, J., *et al.* (2001) Sequence diversity in CYP3A promoters and characterization of the genetic basis of polymorphic CYP3A5 expression. *Nat. Genet.*, **27**, 383–391.
60 Hustert, E., Haberl, M., Burk, O., Wolbold, R., He, Y.Q., Klein, K., *et al.* (2001) The genetic determinants of the CYP3A5 polymorphism. *Pharmacogenetics*, **11**, 773–779.
61 Kamdem, L.K., Streit, F., Zanger, U.M., Brockmöller, J., Oellerich, M., Armstrong, V.W., *et al.* (2005) Contribution of CYP3A5 to the *in vitro* hepatic clearance of tacrolimus. *Clin. Chem.*, **51**, 1374–1381.
62 Anglicheau, D., Legendre, C., Beaune, P., and Thervet, E. (2007) Cytochrome P450 3A polymorphisms and immunosuppressive drugs: an update. *Pharmacogenomics*, **8**, 835–849.
63 Mouly, S.J., Matheny, C., Paine, M.F., Smith, G., Lamba, J., Lamba, V., *et al.* (2005) Variation in oral clearance of saquinavir is predicted by CYP3A5*1 genotype but not by enterocyte content of cytochrome P450 3A5. *Clin. Pharmacol. Ther.*, **78**, 605–618.
64 Weinshilboum, R.M. and Sladek, S.L. (1980) Mercaptopurine pharmacogenetics: monogenic inheritance of erythrocyte thiopurine methyltransferase activity. *Am. J. Hum. Genet.*, **32**, 651–662.
65 Schwab, M., Schäffeler, E., Marx, C., Fischer, C., Lang, T., Behrens, C., *et al.* (2002) Azathioprine therapy and adverse drug reactions in patients with inflammatory bowel disease: impact of thiopurine *S*-methyltransferase polymorphism. *Pharmacogenetics*, **12**, 429–436.
66 Stanulla, M., Schaeffeler, E., Flohr, T., Cario, G., Schrauder, A., Zimmermann, M., *et al.* (2005) Thiopurine methyltransferase (TPMT) genotype and early treatment response to mercaptopurine in childhood acute lymphoblastic leukemia. *JAMA*, **293**, 1485–1489.
67 Wei, X., McLeod, H.L., McMurrough, J., Gonzalez, F.J., and Fernandez-Salguero, P. (1996) Molecular basis of the human dihydropyrimidine dehydrogenase deficiency and 5-fluorouracil toxicity. *J. Clin. Invest.*, **98**, 610–615.
68 Schwab, M., Zanger, U.M., Marx, C., Schaeffeler, E., Klein, K., Dippon, J., *et al.* (2008) Role of genetic and nongenetic factors for fluorouracil treatment-related severe toxicity: a prospective clinical trial by the German 5-FU Toxicity Study Group. *J. Clin. Oncol.*, **26**, 2131–2138.
69 Bosma, P.J., Chowdhury, J.R., Bakker, C., Gantla, S., de Boer, A., Oostra, B.A., *et al.* (1995) The genetic basis of the reduced expression of bilirubin UDP-glucuronosyltransferase 1 in Gilbert's syndrome. *N. Engl. J. Med.*, **333**, 1171–1175.
70 Innocenti, F., Undevia, S.D., Iyer, L., Chen, P.X., Das, S., Kocherginsky, M., *et al.* (2004) Genetic variants in the UDP-glucuronosyltransferase 1A1 gene predict the risk of severe neutropenia of irinotecan. *J. Clin. Oncol.*, **22**, 1382–1388.
71 Maitland, M.L., Vasisht, K., and Ratain, M.J. (2006) TPMT, UGT1A1 and DPYD: genotyping to ensure safer cancer therapy? *Trends Pharmacol. Sci.*, **27**, 432–437.
72 Riedmaier, S., Klein, K., Hofmann, U., Keskitalo, J.E., Neuvonen, P.J., Schwab, M., *et al.* (2010) UDP-glucuronosyltransferase (UGT) polymorphisms affect atorvastatin lactonization *in vitro* and *in vivo*. *Clin. Pharmacol. Ther.*, **87**, 65–73.
73 van Waterschoot, R.A.B., Lagas, J.S., Wagenaar, E., van der Kruijssen, C.M.M., van Herwaarden, A.E., Song, J.-Y., *et al.* (2009) Absence of both cytochrome P450 3A and P-glycoprotein dramatically increases docetaxel oral

bioavailability and risk of intestinal toxicity. *Cancer Res.*, **69**, 8996–9002.

74 Chinn, L.W. and Kroetz, D.L. (2007) ABCB1 pharmacogenetics: progress, pitfalls, and promise. *Clin. Pharmacol. Ther.*, **81**, 265–269.

75 Leschziner, G.D., Andrew, T., Pirmohamed, M., and Johnson, M.R. (2007) ABCB1 genotype and PGP expression, function and therapeutic drug response: a critical review and recommendations for future research. *Pharmacogenomics J.*, **7**, 154–179.

76 Stieger, B. and Meier, P.J. (2011) Pharmacogenetics of drug transporters in the enterohepatic circulation. *Pharmacogenomics*, **12**, 611–631.

77 Hoffmeyer, S., Burk, O., von Richter, O., Arnold, H.P., Brockmöller, J., Johne, A., *et al.* (2000) Functional polymorphisms of the human multidrug-resistance gene: multiple sequence variations and correlation of one allele with P-glycoprotein expression and activity *in vivo*. *Proc. Natl. Acad. Sci. USA*, **97**, 3473–3478.

78 Wang, D., Johnson, A.D., Papp, A.C., Kroetz, D.L., and Sadée, W. (2005) Multidrug resistance polypeptide 1 (MDR1, ABCB1) variant 3435C>T affects mRNA stability. *Pharmacogenet. Genomics*, **15**, 693–704.

79 Kimchi-Sarfaty, C., Oh, J.M., Kim, I.-W., Sauna, Z.E., Calcagno, A.M., Ambudkar, S.V., *et al.* (2007) A "silent" polymorphism in the MDR1 gene changes substrate specificity. *Science*, **315**, 525–528.

80 Sauna, Z.E., Kimchi-Sarfaty, C., Ambudkar, S.V., and Gottesman, M.M. (2007) Silent polymorphisms speak: how they affect pharmacogenomics and the treatment of cancer. *Cancer Res.*, **67**, 9609–9612.

81 Nies, A.T., Schwab, M., and Keppler, D. (2008) Interplay of conjugating enzymes with OATP uptake transporters and ABCC/MRP efflux pumps in the elimination of drugs. *Expert Opin. Drug Metab. Toxicol.*, **4**, 545–568.

82 Zaïr, Z.M., Eloranta, J.J., Stieger, B., and Kullak-Ublick, G.A. (2008) Pharmacogenetics of OATP (SLC21/SLCO), OAT and OCT (SLC22) and PEPT (SLC15) transporters in the intestine, liver and kidney. *Pharmacogenomics*, **9**, 597–624.

83 Levi, F. and Schibler, U. (2007) Circadian rhythms: mechanisms and therapeutic implications. *Annu. Rev. Pharmacol. Toxicol.*, **47**, 593–628.

84 Morgan, E.T., Goralski, K.B., Piquette-Miller, M., Renton, K.W., Robertson, G.R., Chaluvadi, M.R., *et al.* (2008) Regulation of drug-metabolizing enzymes and transporters in infection, inflammation, and cancer. *Drug Metab. Dispos.*, **36**, 205–216.

85 Yang, X., Zhang, B., Molony, C., Chudin, E., Hao, K., Zhu, J., *et al.* (2010) Systematic genetic and genomic analysis of cytochrome P450 enzyme activities in human liver. *Genome Res.*, **20**, 1020–1036.

86 Zhang, Y., Klein, K., Sugathan, A., Nassery, N., Dombkowski, A.A., Zanger, U.M., *et al.* (2011) Transcriptional profiling of human liver identifies sex-biased genes associated with polygenic dyslipidemia and coronary artery disease. *PLoS ONE*, **6**, e23506.

87 Wang, D., Guo, Y., Wrighton, S.A., Cooke, G.E., and Sadee, W. (2011) Intronic polymorphism in CYP3A4 affects hepatic expression and response to statin drugs. *Pharmacogenomics J.*, **11**, 274–286.

88 Palma, B.B., Silva E Sousa, M., Vosmeer, C.R., Lastdrager, J., Rueff, J., Vermeulen, N.P.E., *et al.* (2010) Functional characterization of eight human cytochrome P450 1A2 gene variants by recombinant protein expression. *Pharmacogenomics J.*, **10**, 478–488.

89 Schirmer, M., Rosenberger, A., Klein, K., Kulle, B., Toliat, M.R., Nürnberg, P., *et al.* (2007) Sex-dependent genetic markers of CYP3A4 expression and activity in human liver microsomes. *Pharmacogenomics*, **8**, 443–453.

90 Perera, M.A., Thirumaran, R.K., Cox, N.J., Hanauer, S., Das, S., Brimer-Cline, C., *et al.* (2009) Prediction of CYP3A4 enzyme activity using haplotype tag SNPs in African Americans. *Pharmacogenomics J.*, **9**, 49–60.

91 Chen, X., Wang, H., Zhou, G., Zhang, X., Dong, X., Zhi, L., *et al.* (2009) Molecular population genetics of human CYP3A locus: signatures of positive selection and implications for evolutionary environmental medicine. *Environ. Health Perspect.*, **117**, 1541–1548.

92 Jorge-Nebert, L.F., Jiang, Z., Chakraborty, R., Watson, J., Jin, L., McGarvey, S.T., *et al.* (2010) Analysis of human CYP1A1 and CYP1A2 genes and their shared bidirectional promoter in eight world populations. *Hum. Mutat.*, **31**, 27–40.

93 Eiselt, R., Domanski, T.L., Zibat, A., Mueller, R., Presecan-Siedel, E., Hustert, E., *et al.* (2001) Identification and functional characterization of eight CYP3A4 protein variants. *Pharmacogenetics*, **11**, 447–458.

94 Wojnowski, L. and Kamdem, L.K. (2006) Clinical implications of CYP3A polymorphisms. *Expert Opin. Drug Metab. Toxicol.*, **2**, 171–182.

95 Keshava, C., McCanlies, E.C., and Weston, A. (2004) CYP3A4 polymorphisms – potential risk factors for breast and prostate cancer: a HuGE review. *Am. J. Epidemiol.*, **160**, 825–841.

96 Perera, M.A. (2010) The missing linkage: what pharmacogenetic associations are left to find in CYP3A? *Expert Opin. Drug Metab. Toxicol.*, **6**, 17–28.

97 Rasmussen, B.B., Brix, T.H., Kyvik, K.O., and Brøsen, K. (2002) The interindividual differences in the 3-demthylation of caffeine alias CYP1A2 is determined by both genetic and environmental factors. *Pharmacogenetics*, **12**, 473–478.

98 Penno, M.B., Dvorchik, B.H., and Vesell, E.S. (1981) Genetic variation in rates of antipyrine metabolite formation: a study in uninduced twins. *Proc. Natl. Acad. Sci. USA*, **78**, 5193–5196.

99 Ozdemir, V., Kalow, W., Tang, B.K., Paterson, A.D., Walker, S.E., Endrenyi, L., *et al.* (2000) Evaluation of the genetic component of variability in CYP3A4 activity: a repeated drug administration method. *Pharmacogenetics*, **10**, 373–388.

100 Okey, A.B., Franc, M.A., Moffat, I.D., Tijet, N., Boutros, P.C., Korkalainen, M., *et al.* (2005) Toxicological implications of polymorphisms in receptors for xenobiotic chemicals: the case of the aryl hydrocarbon receptor. *Toxicol. Appl. Pharmacol.*, **207** (Suppl.), 43–51.

101 Lamba, J., Lamba, V., and Schuetz, E. (2005) Genetic variants of PXR (NR1I2) and CAR (NR1I3) and their implications in drug metabolism and pharmacogenetics. *Curr. Drug Metab.*, **6**, 369–383.

102 Lamba, J., Lamba, V., Strom, S., Venkataramanan, R., and Schuetz, E. (2008) Novel single nucleotide polymorphisms in the promoter and intron 1 of human pregnane X receptor/NR1I2 and their association with CYP3A4 expression. *Drug Metab. Dispos.*, **36**, 169–181.

103 Klein, K., Winter, S., Turpeinen, M., Schwab, M., and Zanger, U.M. (2010) Pathway-targeted pharmacogenomics of CYP1A2 in human liver. *Front. Pharmacol.*, **1**, 129.

104 Lamba, V., Panetta, J.C., Strom, S., and Schuetz, E.G. (2010) Genetic predictors of interindividual variability in hepatic CYP3A4 expression. *J. Pharmacol. Exp. Ther.*, **332**, 1088–1099.

105 Klein, K., Thomas, M., Winter, S., Nuessler, A.K., Niemi, M., Schwab, M., *et al.* (2012) PPARalpha is a novel genetic determinant of CYP3A4 *in vitro* and *in vivo*. *Clin. Pharmacol. Ther.*, in press.

106 Flück, C.E., Pandey, A.V., Huang, N., Agrawal, V., and Miller, W.L. (2008) P450 oxidoreductase deficiency – a new form of congenital adrenal hyperplasia. *Endocr. Dev.*, **13**, 67–81.

107 Hart, S.N. and Zhong, X.-B. (2008) P450 oxidoreductase: genetic polymorphisms and implications for drug metabolism and toxicity. *Expert Opin. Drug Metab. Toxicol.*, **4**, 439–452.

108 Gomes, A.M., Winter, S., Klein, K., Turpeinen, M., Schaeffeler, E., Schwab, M., *et al.* (2009) Pharmacogenomics of human liver cytochrome P450 oxidoreductase: multifactorial analysis and impact on microsomal drug oxidation. *Pharmacogenomics*, **10**, 579–599.

109 Oneda, B., Crettol, S., Sirot, E.J., Bochud, M., Ansermot, N., and Eap, C.B. (2009) The P450 oxidoreductase genotype is associated with CYP3A activity *in vivo* as measured by the midazolam phenotyping test. *Pharmacogenet. Genomics*, **19**, 877–883.

110 Gomez, A. and Ingelman-Sundberg, M. (2009) Epigenetic and microRNA-dependent control of cytochrome P450 expression: a gap between DNA and protein. *Pharmacogenomics*, **10**, 1067–1076.

111 Baer-Dubowska, W., Majchrzak-Celińska, A., and Cichocki, M. (2011) Pharmocoepigenetics: a new approach to predicting individual drug responses and targeting new drugs. *Pharmacol. Rep.*, **63**, 293–304.

112 Dannenberg, L.O. and Edenberg, H.J. (2006) Epigenetics of gene expression in human hepatoma cells: expression profiling the response to inhibition of DNA methylation and histone deacetylation. *BMC Genomics*, **7**, 181.

113 Vieira, I., Sonnier, M., and Cresteil, T. (1996) Developmental expression of CYP2E1 in the human liver. Hypermethylation control of gene expression during the neonatal period. *Eur. J. Biochem.*, **238**, 476–483.

114 Anttila, S., Hakkola, J., Tuominen, P., Elovaara, E., Husgafvel-Pursiainen, K., Karjalainen, A., *et al.* (2003) Methylation of cytochrome P4501A1 promoter in the lung is associated with tobacco smoking. *Cancer Res.*, **63**, 8623–8628.

115 Ghotbi, R., Gomez, A., Milani, L., Tybring, G., Syvänen, A.-C., Bertilsson, L., *et al.* (2009) Allele-specific expression and gene methylation in the control of CYP1A2 mRNA level in human livers. *Pharmacogenomics J.*, **9**, 208–217.

116 Bartel, D.P. (2009) MicroRNAs: target recognition and regulatory functions. *Cell*, **136**, 215–233.

117 Friedman, R.C., Farh, K.K.-H., Burge, C.B., and Bartel, D.P. (2009) Most mammalian mRNAs are conserved targets of microRNAs. *Genome Res.*, **19**, 92–105.

118 Sethupathy, P., Megraw, M., and Hatzigeorgiou, A.G. (2006) A guide through present computational approaches for the identification of mammalian microRNA targets. *Nat. Methods*, **3**, 881–886.

119 Xiao, F., Zuo, Z., Cai, G., Kang, S., Gao, X., and Li, T. (2009) miRecords: an integrated resource for microRNA–target interactions. *Nucleic Acids Res.*, **37**, D105–D110.

120 Laganà, A., Forte, S., Giudice, A., Arena, M.R., Puglisi, P.L., Giugno, R., *et al.* (2009) miRò: a miRNA knowledge base. *Database (Oxford)*, **2009**, bap008.

121 Rieger, J.K. and Zanger, U.M. (2011) MIRNA-DISTILLER: a stand-alone application to compile microRNA data from databases. *Front. Gene.*, **2**, 39.

122 Tsuchiya, Y., Nakajima, M., Takagi, S., Taniya, T., and Yokoi, T. (2006) MicroRNA regulates the expression of human cytochrome P450 1B1. *Cancer Res.*, **66**, 9090–9098.

123 Pan, Y.-Z., Gao, W., and Yu, A.-M. (2009) MicroRNAs regulate CYP3A4 expression via direct and indirect targeting. *Drug Metab. Dispos.*, **37**, 2112–2117.

124 Mohri, T., Nakajima, M., Fukami, T., Takamiya, M., Aoki, Y., and Yokoi, T. (2010) Human CYP2E1 is regulated by miR-378. *Biochem. Pharmacol.*, **79**, 1045–1052.

125 Takagi, S., Nakajima, M., Mohri, T., and Yokoi, T. (2008) Post-transcriptional regulation of human pregnane X receptor by micro-RNA affects the expression of cytochrome P450 3A4. *J. Biol. Chem.*, **283**, 9674–9680.

126 Takagi, S., Nakajima, M., Kida, K., Yamaura, Y., Fukami, T., and Yokoi, T. (2010) MicroRNAs regulate human hepatocyte nuclear factor 4alpha, modulating the expression of metabolic enzymes and cell cycle. *J. Biol. Chem.*, **285**, 4415–4422.

127 Karbiener, M., Fischer, C., Nowitsch, S., Opriessnig, P., Papak, C., Ailhaud, G., *et al.* (2009) microRNA miR-27b impairs human adipocyte differentiation and targets PPARgamma. *Biochem. Biophys. Res. Commun.*, **390**, 247–251.

128 Jennewein, C., von Knethen, A., Schmid, T., and Brüne, B. (2010) MicroRNA-27b contributes to lipopolysaccharide-mediated peroxisome

proliferator-activated receptor gamma (PPARgamma) mRNA destabilization. *J. Biol. Chem.*, **285**, 11846–11853.

129 Ou, Z., Wada, T., Gramignoli, R., Li, S., Strom, S.C., Huang, M., *et al.* (2011) MicroRNA hsa-miR-613 targets the human LXRα gene and mediates a feedback loop of LXRα autoregulation. *Mol. Endocrinol.*, **25**, 584–596.

130 Saunders, M.A., Liang, H., and Li, W.-H. (2007) Human polymorphism at microRNAs and microRNA target sites. *Proc. Natl. Acad. Sci. USA*, **104**, 3300–3305.

131 Mishra, P.J., Humeniuk, R., Mishra, P.J., Longo-Sorbello, G.S.A., Banerjee, D., and Bertino, J.R. (2007) A miR-24 microRNA binding-site polymorphism in dihydrofolate reductase gene leads to methotrexate resistance. *Proc. Natl. Acad. Sci. USA*, **104**, 13513–13518.

132 Motsinger-Reif, A.A., Jorgenson, E., Relling, M.V., Kroetz, D.L., Weinshilboum, R., Cox, N.J., *et al.* (2010) Genome-wide association studies in pharmacogenomics: successes and lessons. *Pharmacogenet. Genomics*, doi:10.1097/FPC.0b013e32833d7b45.

133 Daly, A.K. (2010) Genome-wide association studies in pharmacogenomics. *Nat. Rev. Genet.*, **11**, 241–246.

134 Hindorff, L.A., Sethupathy, P., Junkins, H.A., Ramos, E.M., Mehta, J.P., Collins, F.S., *et al.* (2009) Potential etiologic and functional implications of genome-wide association loci for human diseases and traits. *Proc. Natl. Acad. Sci. USA*, **106**, 9362–9367.

135 SEARCH Collaboratorive Group (2008) SLCO1B1 variants and statin-induced myopathy–a genomewide study. *N. Engl. J. Med.*, **359**, 789–799.

136 Daly, A.K., Donaldson, P.T., Bhatnagar, P., Shen, Y., Pe'er, I., Floratos, A., *et al.* (2009) HLA-B*5701 genotype is a major determinant of drug-induced liver injury due to flucloxacillin. *Nat. Genet.*, **41**, 816–819.

137 Mallal, S., Phillips, E., Carosi, G., Molina, J.-M., Workman, C., Tomazic, J., *et al.* (2008) HLA-B*5701 screening for hypersensitivity to abacavir. *N. Engl. J. Med.*, **358**, 568–579.

138 McCormack, M., Alfirevic, A., Bourgeois, S., Farrell, J.J., Kasperavičiūte, D., Carrington, M., *et al.* (2011) HLA-A*3101 and carbamazepine-induced hypersensitivity reactions in Europeans. *N. Engl. J. Med.*, **364**, 1134–1143.

139 Manolio, T.A., Collins, F.S., Cox, N.J., Goldstein, D.B., Hindorff, L.A., Hunter, D.J., *et al.* (2009) Finding the missing heritability of complex diseases. *Nature*, **461**, 747–753.

140 Gamazon, E.R., Zhang, W., Huang, R.S., Dolan, M.E., and Cox, N.J. (2009) A pharmacogene database enhanced by the 1000 Genomes Project. *Pharmacogenet. Genomics*, **19**, 829–832.

141 Gilad, Y., Rifkin, S.A., and Pritchard, J.K. (2008) Revealing the architecture of gene regulation: the promise of eQTL studies. *Trends Genet.*, **24**, 408–415.

142 Cheung, V.G. and Spielman, R.S. (2009) Genetics of human gene expression: mapping DNA variants that influence gene expression. *Nat. Rev. Genet.*, **10**, 595–604.

143 Schadt, E.E., Molony, C., Chudin, E., Hao, K., Yang, X., Lum, P.Y., *et al.* (2008) Mapping the genetic architecture of gene expression in human liver. *PLoS Biol.*, **6**, e107.

144 Innocenti, F., Cooper, G.M., Stanaway, I.B., Gamazon, E.R., Smith, J.D., Mirkov, S., *et al.* (2011) Identification, replication, and functional fine-mapping of expression quantitative trait Loci in primary human liver tissue. *PLoS Genet.*, **7**, e1002078.

145 Schroeder, A., Klein, K., Winter, S., Schwab, M., Bonin, M., Zell, A., *et al.* (2011) Genomics of ADME gene expression: mapping expression quantitative trait loci relevant for absorption, distribution, metabolism and excretion of drugs in human liver. *Pharmacogenomics J.*, doi:10.1038/tpj.2011.44.

Part Two
Metabolism of Drugs

10
Introduction to Drug Metabolism

Ulrich M. Zanger

10.1
Introduction

Most drugs in clinical use, but also many drugs used for recreational purposes and other foreign substances, have lipophilic properties, because otherwise they would not be sufficiently absorbed. Once in the system, lipophilic substances are difficult to eliminate by the kidneys, and their continuous uptake over longer periods would lead to their accumulation in cell membranes and fat deposits of the body. In fact, without conversion into more hydrophilic products, the elimination half-life of very lipophilic chemicals can be of the order of several years. It is thus the major function of drug metabolism, also referred to as xenobiotic biotransformation, to increase the hydrophilicity of foreign substances that have entered the body, in order to enable their efficient elimination through the kidneys or the intestine (Figure 10.1). Often, but not always, this process goes in parallel with a loss of pharmacological activity; hence, the term detoxification is in use as another synonym. However, drug metabolism can also lead to toxic metabolites, referred to as biotoxification. In drug therapy, it is important to balance out positive and negative effects by reaching a steady-state plasma concentration within the so-called therapeutic window – a concentration range where the drug has proven pharmacological effect without being "overdosed" or "underdosed."

10.2
Historical Aspects

During the early nineteenth century it was already observed that drugs leave the body not unchanged, but chemically altered by a variety of metabolic processes. It is quite remarkable that the major pathways of drug metabolism had already been elucidated by the end of the 19th century, including oxidation and reduction, hydrolysis, conjugation with glycine, sulfuric acid, and glucuronic acid, acetylation, and others. Since the development of more sensitive analytical techniques, especially chromatographic and mass spectrometric methods, the field of drug

Metabolism of Drugs and Other Xenobiotics, First Edition. Edited by Pavel Anzenbacher, Ulrich M. Zanger.

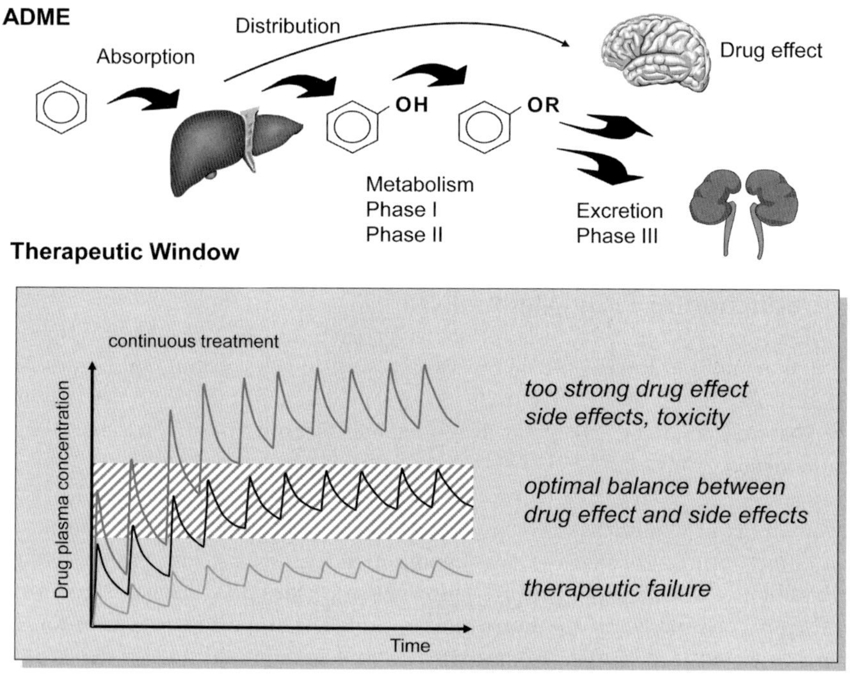

Figure 10.1 Absorption, distribution, metabolism, and excretion (ADME) processes determine the fate of drugs and other xenobiotics in the human body. Optimal drug therapy requires that the steady-state plasma concentration lies within the therapeutic window. Higher or lower drug concentrations can result in adverse drug responses as indicated.

metabolism has developed rapidly since about 1950 as a subspecialty of biochemistry and pharmacology, and many discoveries in biochemistry, including enzyme systems and reaction types, were actually made through drug metabolism studies. Detailed historical accounts of the drug metabolism field have been presented earlier [1, 2]. Today, knowledge about the metabolism of newly developed drugs is a world-wide regulatory requirement because of its importance for drug safety, pharmacokinetics, and pharmacodynamics [3].

10.3
Diversity of Drug Metabolic Pathways

A common reaction sequence comprises an initial functionalization reaction (traditionally termed phase I), followed by conjugation of the newly created or exposed functional group to a hydrophilic moiety (phase II). It should be realized, however, that this scheme is not generally applicable as there are many drugs that are cleared via only phase I or only phase II reactions, or sometimes even via pathways in the opposite order. A more detailed discussion of classification concepts and of the reactions and their requirements is presented in Chapter 1 and the following chapters in the first part of the book.

Phase I pathways comprise numerous functionalization reactions including various types of oxidations primarily catalyzed by multiple microsomal cytochrome P450 (CYP) monooxygenases and several other enzyme systems, but also reductions, as well as reactions that unmask existing functional groups, often catalyzed by hydrolytic enzymes. Phase I reactions fulfill a 2-fold purpose – while introducing a hydrophilic group, this step also prepares the substrate for the following phase II reactions. These include a plethora of conjugation reactions that add sugars, sulfates, acetyl or methyl groups, amino acids, glutathione, fatty acids, and others to one or more of the functional groups available in the substrate molecule. The term phase III was coined more recently and refers to a battery of efflux transporters that help to extrude the polar drug metabolites from the cells into interstitial fluid, bloodstream, or bile canaliculi.

Owing to the bewildering diversity of metabolic pathways, a foreign compound that enters the body can be metabolized along several biotransformation pathways, leading to many different metabolites, each of which can be a substrate for further biotransformation reactions. For example, the antiarrhythmic drug verapamil (Chapter 12) is converted to at least 21 phase I and 16 phase II metabolites [4], and the selective estrogen receptor modulator tamoxifen (Chapter 13) is transformed into at least 22 metabolites [5]. It is probably so that more or less all chemically possible metabolites of a drug are formed at least to a minor extent, depending on the chemical reactivity of the substance and the availability of enzymes and cofactors with adequate catalytic properties. While identification of the major metabolites and the pathways leading to them, usually accomplished during very early phases of drug development, is of primary importance for pharmacokinetics and pharmacodynamics, minor metabolites can cause toxicity unrelated to the pharmacological action of the drug.

10.4 Influence of Drug Metabolism on Pharmacological Activity

Biotransformation usually has the additional effect that it converts active drugs to inactive drug metabolites (detoxification), although in many cases metabolites are also pharmacologically active. For example, whereas hydroxylated metabolites of statins still possess their characteristic 3-hydroxy-3-methyl-glutaryl (HMG)-CoA-like dihydroxy heptanoic acid moiety and are thus pharmacologically active, the corresponding cyclic lactones are not (see Chapter 12). The converse scenario that is sometimes intentionally used in drug development is the biotransformation of an inactive drug to an active metabolite (prodrug concept [6]). Some examples are the lactone statins lovastatin and simvastatin, which are activated by paraoxonases (PONs) [7]; the camptothecin derivative irinotecan (see Chapter 13), which is activated by carboxylesterases to the potent topoisomerase

I inhibitor 7-ethyl-10-hydroxycamptothecin (SN-38) [8]; codeine (see Chapter 15), which is transformed into the potent antipain drug morphine by the polymorphic CYP2D6 enzyme [9]; or the platelet aggregation inhibitor clopidogrel (see Chapter 12), which is activated into a thiol metabolite by the hydrolytic PON1 enzyme [10]. In the case of tamoxifen (see Chapter 13), the hydroxylated derivatives 4-hydroxytamoxifen and endoxifen exhibit approximately 100-fold stronger binding to the estrogen receptor than the mother drug, and are believed to be mainly responsible for its pharmacological effects [5].

10.5 Biotoxification

In contrast to the usually reversible drug effects and dose-related side-effects, a further possibility and general danger is the biotoxification of a nontoxic compound into toxic or carcinogenic metabolite(s). Toxicities generated in this manner, which includes mainly irreversible necrotic and immunological reactions, are usually unrelated to the pharmacological drug effects and can be extremely dangerous because they may occur with low drug doses or be unrelated to drug dose, and are often unexpected and unpredictable [11, 12]. With its large capacity for drug biotransformation, the liver represents a major site of drug-induced toxicity. In fact, a wide range of therapeutic agents have been withdrawn from the market because of hepatotoxicity. Mechanistically, formation of chemically reactive metabolites plays a central role in most cases of hepatotoxic drugs. One of the best-studied examples is the biotoxification of paracetamol (acetaminophen; see Chapters 1 and 15). A small percentage of the dose undergoes oxidative metabolism to the hepatotoxic metabolite *N*-acetyl-*p*-benzoquinone imine (NAPQI). If overdosed, this metabolite first uses up the cellular glutathione stores and then binds covalently to hepatic proteins, which leads to multiple perturbations, finally causing a characteristic centrilobular hepatic necrosis [12]. Other examples of biotoxification are also presented in later chapters dealing with xenobiotics other than drugs (e.g., the sequence of multiple metabolic steps that lead to the carcinogenic metabolites of polycyclic aromatic hydrocarbons (Chapter 22)).

10.6 Extrahepatic Drug Metabolism

While the liver is the primary organ for biotransformation, because it has most of the drug-metabolizing enzymes available at high concentrations, many other tissues have at least some capabilities to metabolize drugs. Pharmacokinetically, most important next to the liver is the gut, which contains an array of phase I and phase II enzymes in the enterocytes along the intestine that are not regulated coordinately with the liver enzymes [13, 14]. The marked contribution of the gut to first-pass metabolism of orally administered drugs has also been shown *in vivo* in numerous studies that compared drug clearance after administration of the same dose either intraorally or intravenously [15]. More limited, but still significant, drug metabolism capacity is present in the lungs, heart, blood, skin, kidney, placenta, adrenal gland, pancreas, mammary gland, uterus, ovary, testes, prostate, and brain [16–23]. As the biochemical machinery as well as their regulation differs between tissues, their contribution to systemic or local drug metabolism depends on both the tissue and the drug, as well as on environmental conditions.

10.7 Factors Affecting Drug Metabolism Activity

Optimal drug therapy, at least in the sense of achieving a steady-state plasma concentration that lies within the therapeutic window (Figure 10.1), would be much easier to achieve if there was not the extraordinarily large variability of drug metabolism among humans. Although much progress has been made in identifying factors and mechanisms that affect the metabolism of drugs and other xenobiotics, accurate prediction of the fate of a drug in a particular patient is still a vision and far away from application in routine clinical practice. Often the terms *interindividual* versus *intraindividual* variability are used in this context. However, from a mechanistic point of view another classification of variability is more appropriate – the distinction between *temporally constant (static) factors* and those that change over time (i.e., *temporally variable factors*). The first category comprises mainly the germline genotype, particularly drug-metabolizing enzyme polymorphisms, and sex, both of which contribute mainly to interindividual variability. The second category includes age, hormonal and disease states, circadian rhythm, environmental factors such as drug–drug and drug–food interactions, and others, all of which contribute to both inter- and intraindividual variability.

Understanding the factors that influence drug-metabolizing enzymes and their activities under different healthy and diseased conditions can help to improve drug treatment so as to avoid failures in drug development. Thus, in early drug development it is desirable to predict the *in vivo* clearance of new drug candidates as reliably as possible. General strategies to study drug metabolism and pharmacokinetics by *in vitro* methods have been established [24]. Moreover, an early appraisal of drug metabolism factors affecting the likely success of drug candidates has become routinely implemented into early phases of drug development [25, 26]. In the following sections, the most important factors causing variable drug metabolic activity in humans are discussed.

10.7.1 Genetic Polymorphism

The influence of genetic polymorphisms in genes encoding drug-metabolizing enzymes has been studied for over 50 years [27]. The degree of drug metabolism variability conferred by genetic polymorphism is enormous, both in terms of the number of affected enzymes and pathways as well as in terms of quantitative variability. Functional polymorphisms exist in practically all drug-metabolizing enzyme genes, although not all of them are clinically relevant, due to low frequency or lack of penetrance. Clinically relevant polymorphisms include those of CYPs 2D6, 2C19, 2C9, 2B6, and 3A5, as well as the UDP-glucurosyltransferase *UGT*1A1*, thiopurine *S*-methyltransferase (TPMT), and *N*-acetyltransferase type 2 (NAT2) (for details, see Chapter 9 and the chapters covering the respective enzyme families). Germline genetic polymorphisms affect primarily baseline drug metabolism capacity, which can vary 1000-fold in the case of complete enzyme deficiency. This is possible if null alleles exist, as, for example, in CYPs 2C19 and 2D6 [28], as well as in TPMT [29] and NAT2 [30]. Less pronounced differences, which can still be clinically relevant, are caused by variants that lead to a relative loss or gain of expression and/or activity.

The consequences of polymorphic drug metabolism for drug therapy need to be considered in pharmacological context as described above. Loss-of-function variants will lead to reduced clearance and increased plasma concentrations of the drug itself, while gain-of-function variants will lead to increased clearance and lower drug concentrations. If the drug itself is pharmacologically active, this results in a higher and lower drug effect, and potentially drug-related toxicity due to overdosing. In the case of a prodrug, the opposite consequences are to be expected. An example for the latter is the increased formation of morphine from codeine by CYP2D6 ultrarapid metabolizers [31].

Examples of polymorphisms that affect the inducibility of drug metabolic pathways were also found, but at surprisingly low frequency, and they seem to be more difficult to reproduce. For example, the *CYP1A2*1C* and *CYP1A2*1F* alleles have been associated with decreased [32] and increased [33] caffeine 3-demethylation, respectively, in smokers only, indicating that the two alleles may influence CYP1A2 inducibility in opposite manner. A recent example is the *CYP2B6*22* variant –82T>C, which leads to increased baseline expression and synergistically increased pregnane X receptor (PXR)-mediated inducibility due to a rearrangement of transcription factor binding sites in the CYP2B6 promoter [34, 35].

10.7.2 Sex

It should be noted that the English language differs between biological (sex) and social (gender) differences between men and women, and that both can affect drug response. As far as pharmacokinetics and drug metabolism are concerned, the relevant term is sex, which influences a number of physiologically important parameters, including body weight, fat distribution, liver blood flow, and expression of drug-metabolizing enzymes and transporters [36–38]. The influence of sex on drug metabolism is very pronounced in some animals, including rats and mice, which express some CYP isoforms in a strictly sex-dependent manner, which was shown to be due to temporally different plasma profiles of growth hormone in female versus male animals [39]. In humans the differences are more subtle and their relevance for drug treatment is a matter of continuous debate. This is in part also due to the lack of systematic data because only since 1998 has the US Food and Drug Administration (FDA) requires that new drug applications include safety and effectiveness data separated by sex.

Most reported differences in drug metabolism indicate that women metabolize drugs more quickly than men. This is particularly the case for substrates of the major drug-metabolizing CYP, CYP3A4 (e.g., antipyrine, alfentanil, erythromycin, midazolam, verapamil), although studies often lead to contradictory results [40]. Analyses in human liver have indeed shown a pronounced difference in hepatic CYP3A4 with up to approximately 2-fold higher levels of protein in female compared to male liver tissue [41–44]. For unclear reasons this relatively pronounced difference in gene expression is apparently not fully translated into pharmacokinetic differences, which are often only of the order of 20–50% and substrate-dependent. There are also some drugs that are metabolized more rapidly by men. Faster conversion in males compared to females of caffeine to paraxanthine, which is catalyzed by CYP1A2, was found in Americans [45] as well as in Chinese [46]. Glucuronidation of paracetamol also proceeds more rapidly in men than in women [47].

A recent genome-wide gene expression profiling study in a large number of human livers (112 male and 112 female) identified more than 1300 genes whose expression was significantly affected by sex, with 75% of them showing higher expression in females [48]. Among these were 40 ADME/ADME-related genes, including CYP1A2, CYP3A4, and CYP7A1 showing female bias, and CYP3A5, CYP27B1, and UGT2B15 showing male bias. These data confirmed that some human drug-metabolizing enzymes show modest sex-biased expression differences, but several discrepancies and questions remain unexplained.

10.7.3 Age

It is now well established that drug metabolism capacity is also influenced by age. Particularly at the extremes of life (i.e., in neonates and in the elderly) drug metabolism capacity can be substantially lower. In neonates, this is due to immaturity of several enzyme systems including CYPs [49–51] and UGTs [52], which fully develop only during the first year of life. In addition, there are some peculiarities in the expression of specific isoforms (e.g., CYP3A7 is a fetally expressed form of the CYP3A subfamily) [53]. In the elderly population, the ability to clear drugs is clearly decreased. This is particularly relevant for drugs with a narrow therapeutic window, including antipsychotics and antidepressants, anticoagulants (warfarin), and β-blockers. Clearance of paracetamol and benzodiazepines is also lower in older people. However, this does not seem to be a consequence of lower expression or activity of drug-metabolizing enzyme systems. Studies in human liver have found an increase in CYP expression and activity, which affects most CYPs, although the increase with age is rather minor and sometimes also depends on sex [44]. Other reasons for limited drug clearance in the elderly are polypharmacy (i.e., inhibition of enzymes due to the intake of sometimes eight or more drugs daily) as well as reduced liver blood flow and renal function [40].

10.7.4
Influence of Diseases and Pathophysiological Factors

Disease states generally have a negative effect on drug metabolism capacity. In severe liver cirrhosis a major effect is due to reduction in blood flow, resulting in reduced clearance and increased plasma concentration of the unchanged drug. The loss of functional hepatocytes furthermore contributes not only by loss of drug metabolic capacity, but also by a decreased ability of the liver to synthesize serum proteins such as albumin, which leads to decreased protein binding of drugs and consequently increased unbound drug levels.

During infection, inflammation, and cancer the expression of many drug-metabolizing enzymes and drug transporters is severely downregulated [54–56]. The common pathophysiological factors in these disease states are circulating proinflammatory cytokines such as interleukin-1β and -6, and tumor necrosis factor-α, which act as signaling molecules to elicit marked changes in liver gene expression profiles, including the upregulation of acute-phase proteins such as C-reactive protein, and concomitant downregulation of many, but not all, drug-metabolizing enzymes and drug transporters. Particularly affected are the CYPs 1A2, 2B6, 2C8, 2C9, 2C19, 2D6, and 3A4, but differences occur with respect to the degree of downregulation and cytokine-specific responses. The mechanism of these effects has been shown to be at least in part due to transcriptional suppression [55, 57, 58]. Altered levels of drug-metabolizing enzymes and transporters during inflammation were also found in extrahepatic tissues (e.g., in brain, intestine, and placenta) with implications for drug treatment in diverse clinical settings.

Alcoholic and nonalcoholic fatty liver disease (NAFLD), or hepatic steatosis, is a reversible condition characterized by the abnormal retention of large amounts of triglycerides that are accumulated in fat vesicles. NAFLD is associated with diabetes, obesity, and metabolic syndrome, and in severe cases proceeds to non-alcoholic steatohepatitis. Most studies of drug-metabolizing enzymes in NAFLD have concentrated on CYPs in diet-induced overweight rats or genetically obese *db/db* mice, whereas human studies are rare. Available data show moderately reduced expression for most but not all CYP1–3 subfamilies, while CYP2E1 and fatty acid-metabolizing CYP4A proteins are upregulated [59]. These findings have, however, not yet been reproduced in a human primary hepatocyte model of NAFLD [60]. Organic anion transporting polypeptide (OATP) uptake transporters and ATP-binding cassette (ABC) transporters also appear to be downregulated in these conditions. These data suggest that drug metabolism may be only moderately affected by NAFLD, but in nonalcoholic steatohepatitis it may be comparably downregulated as in other inflammatory conditions.

10.7.5
Environmental Influences

Only a short overview of the almost unlimited exogenous sources of drug metabolism variability can be given here. Among the most important environmental factors are drug–drug and drug–food interactions, and alcohol drinking and smoking habits.

The three major types of drug–drug interactions (which also apply to drug–food interactions) that can be distinguished are reversible (competitive or noncompetitive) inhibition, irreversible (mechanism-based) inactivation, and induction of enzyme activity. Owing to the great importance of drug–drug interactions in clinical practice, various *in vitro* methods have been developed to predict drug interaction potential of a given substance, which are based on experimental models such as liver microsomes, human primary hepatocytes, or recombinant enzyme systems [61]. Application of these tools has become standard practice in the early phase of drug development to assess drug interaction potential [62]. CYPs are prone to irreversible inhibition via mechanism-based inactivation, which usually involves bioactivation of the metabolized drug or xenobiotic to a reactive intermediate, which then covalently binds to and inactivates the P450 enzyme with irreversible loss of enzyme activity [63]. Clinically important mechanism-based inhibitors of CYP3A4 include antibacterials (clarithromycin, erythromycin), anticancer agents (tamoxifen, irinotecan), anti-HIV agents (ritonavir), antihypertensives (dihydralazine, verapamil), sex steroids (gestodene), and several herbal constituents (e.g., bergamottin and glabridin). Enzymatic activity can then only be restored by *de novo* protein synthesis, which can have direct implications for drug treatment. A further consequence can be the formation of neoantigens and the triggering of an autoimmune response, resulting in autoantibodies and toxicological consequences [64]. Examples are tienilic acid and dihydralazine. Tienilic acid is activated by CYP2C9 and covalent binding to the enzyme results in formation of an autoantibody directed against CYP2C9, termed anti-liver/kidney microsomal autoantibody type 2 [65]. The toxicological significance of the autoimmune response for drug-induced liver toxicity remains unclear, however. Many drugs and xenobiotics lead to the third kind of drug–drug interactions, which are based on enzyme induction. In contrast to inhibitory drug–drug interactions this kind of interaction results in faster metabolism. Inducers bind to "xenosensors" – ligand-activated transcription factors (e.g., nuclear receptors CAR and PXR, and the aryl hydrocarbon receptor (AhR)) that lead to a marked and coordinated transcriptional upregulation of drug-metabolizing enzymes, transporters, and some additional genes. As a consequence, more enzyme protein is synthesized, resulting in faster biotransformation and leading either to subtherapeutic drug levels or to increased bioactivation of a prodrug [66]. The mechanisms of transcriptional regulation of drug-metabolizing enzymes are discussed in Chapter 8.

The influence of alcohol and cigarette smoking on drug metabolism has been extensively studied. Both of these recreational drugs are regularly consumed at unhealthy doses by very large proportions of the populations of most developed countries. The influence of these agents on drug metabolism should therefore be known by medical doctors, pharmacists, and patients. In Chapters 17 and 18, the metabolism of these two drugs and many more aspects are discussed in detail. Here, it suffices to mention that ethanol is metabolized mainly via alcohol dehydrogenase (ADH). Chronic alcohol consumption leads to induction of CYP2E1, which then also contributes to metabolism. Consequently, ethanol interacts with numerous drugs that are metabolized or toxicologically activated via CYP2E1 and ADH. In addition, the long-term hepatic effects of ethanol consumption mentioned above have to be considered.

Regular cigarette smoking also has long known effects on drug and xenobiotics metabolism. Thus, CYPs 1A1/1A2 and 2E1 are induced by nicotine, and smokers express high levels of CYP1A1 in their lungs, where it can convert polycyclic aromatic hydrocarbons into reactive and potentially carcinogenic epoxides. Detailed summaries on the influence of smoking on the metabolism of psychotropic and other medications can be found in specialized reviews [67, 68].

10.8
Conclusions

The complexity of human drug metabolism arises from several specific features of the xenobiotic biotransformation system, which differs in some aspects from that of endogenous pathways. Both genetic and nongenetic factors have to be considered in order to understand why the biotransformation of a drug or xenobiotic can differ dramatically both between different individuals as well as within an individual over time. Genetic polymorphism is widespread among drug-metabolizing enzymes and transporters, and acts as a temporally constant factor to limit the possible activity range of a certain enzyme or pathway, with sometimes fairly predictable effects on drug or metabolite plasma concentrations. Similarly, sex also contributes to baseline drug metabolism capacity, although differences appear to be of modest clinical relevance. Many temporally variable factors change drug metabolism activity over time, including age, hormonal and disease states, circadian rhythm, and environmental factors, such as drug–drug and drug–food interactions, which are often specific for a particular drug, enzyme, or pathway. Optimal drug therapy therefore requires detailed knowledge about the involved metabolic pathways, the responsible enzymes, and their properties and variability. The following Chapters 11–18 summarize our current knowledge about the metabolism of drugs from five major therapeutic classes, as well as of most recreational drugs consumed in Western countries, including illicit ones as well as the two major social drugs – alcohol and nicotine. It is hoped that this compilation of actual knowledge on drug metabolism provides a valuable resource for everyone interested in this fascinating field.

References

1 Conti, A. and Bickel, M.H. (1977) History of drug metabolism: discoveries of the major pathways in the 19th century. *Drug Metab. Rev.*, **6**, 1–50.

2 Bachmann, C. and Bickel, M.H. (1985) History of drug metabolism: the first half of the 20th century. *Drug Metab. Rev.*, **16**, 185–253.

3 Huang, S.-M., Strong, J.M., Zhang, L., Reynolds, K.S., Nallani, S., and Temple, R. (2008) New era in drug interaction evaluation: US Food and Drug Administration update on CYP enzymes, transporters, and the guidance process. *J. Clin. Pharmacol.*, **48**, 662–670.

4 Borlak, J., Walles, M., Elend, M., Thum, T., Preiss, A., and Levsen, K. (2003) Verapamil: identification of novel metabolites in cultures of primary human hepatocytes and human urine by LC-MS^n and LC-NMR. *Xenobiotica*, **33**, 655–676.

5 Mürdter, T.E., Schroth, W., Bacchus-Gerybadze, L., Winter, S., Heinkele, G., and Simon, W. (2011) Activity levels of tamoxifen metabolites at the estrogen receptor and the impact of genetic polymorphisms of phase I and II enzymes on their concentration levels in plasma. *Clin. Pharmacol. Ther.*, **89**, 708–717.

6 Testa, B. and Mayer, J.M. (2003) *Hydrolysis in Drug and Prodrug Metabolism: Chemistry, Biochemistry, and Enzymology*, VHCA, Zurich.

7 Billecke, S., Draganov, D., Counsell, R., Stetson, P., Watson, C., and Hsu, C. (2000) Human serum paraoxonase (PON1) isozymes Q and R hydrolyze lactones and cyclic carbonate esters. *Drug Metab. Dispos.*, **28**, 1335–1342.

8 Kawato, Y., Aonuma, M., Hirota, Y., Kuga, H., and Sato, K. (1991) Intracellular roles of SN-38, a metabolite of the camptothecin derivative CPT-11, in the antitumor effect of CPT-11. *Cancer Res.*, **51**, 4187–4191.

9 Leppert, W. (2011) CYP2D6 in the metabolism of opioids for mild to moderate pain. *Pharmacology*, **87**, 274–285.

10 Bouman, H.J., Schömig, E., van Werkum, J.W., Velder, J., Hackeng, C.M., and Hirschhäuser, C. (2011) Paraoxonase-1 is a major determinant of clopidogrel efficacy. *Nat. Med.*, **17**, 110–116.

11 Guengerich, F.P. (2006) Cytochrome P450s and other enzymes in drug metabolism and toxicity. *AAPS J.*, **8**, E101–E111.

12 Baillie, T.A. and Rettie, A.E. (2011) Role of biotransformation in drug-induced toxicity: influence of intra- and inter-species differences in drug metabolism. *Drug Metab. Pharmacokinet*, **26**, 15–29.

13 von Richter, O., Burk, O., Fromm, M.F., Thon, K.P., Eichelbaum, M., and Kivistö, K.T. (2004) Cytochrome P450 3A4 and P-glycoprotein expression in human small intestinal enterocytes and hepatocytes: a comparative analysis in paired tissue specimens. *Clin. Pharmacol. Ther.*, **75**, 172–183.

14 Pavek, P. and Dvorak, Z. (2008) Xenobiotic-induced transcriptional regulation of xenobiotic metabolizing enzymes of the cytochrome P450 superfamily in human extrahepatic tissues. *Curr. Drug Metab.*, **9**, 129–143.

15 von Richter, O., Greiner, B., Fromm, M.F., Fraser, R., Omari, T., and Barclay, M.L. (2001) Determination of *in vivo* absorption, metabolism, and transport of drugs by the human intestinal wall and liver with a novel perfusion technique. *Clin. Pharmacol. Ther.*, **70**, 217–227.

16 Buters, J.T., Sakai, S., Richter, T., Pineau, T., Alexander, D.L., and Savas, U. (1999) Cytochrome P450 CYP1B1 determines susceptibility to 7,12-dimethylbenz[*a*]anthracene-induced lymphomas. *Proc. Natl. Acad. Sci. USA*, **96**, 1977–1982.

17 Ding, X. and Kaminsky, L.S. (2003) Human extrahepatic cytochromes P450: function in xenobiotic metabolism and tissue-selective chemical toxicity in the respiratory and gastrointestinal tracts. *Annu. Rev. Pharmacol. Toxicol.*, **43**, 149–173.

18 Siegle, I., Fritz, P., Eckhardt, K., Zanger, U.M., and Eichelbaum, M. (2001) Cellular localization and regional distribution of CYP2D6 mRNA and protein expression in human brain. *Pharmacogenetics*, **11**, 237–245.

19 Haining, R.L. and Nichols-Haining, M. (2007) Cytochrome P450-catalyzed pathways in human brain: metabolism meets pharmacology or old drugs with new mechanism of action? *Pharmacol. Ther.*, **113**, 537–545.

20 Nakamura, A., Nakajima, M., Yamanaka, H., Fujiwara, R., and Yokoi, T. (2008) Expression of UGT1A and UGT2B

mRNA in human normal tissues and various cell lines. *Drug Metab. Dispos.*, **36**, 1461–1464.

21 Chaudhary, K.R., Batchu, S.N., and Seubert, J.M. (2009) Cytochrome P450 enzymes and the heart. *IUBMB Life*, **61**, 954–960.

22 Dutheil, F., Dauchy, S., Diry, M., Sazdovitch, V., Cloarec, O., and Mellottée, L. (2009) Xenobiotic-metabolizing enzymes and transporters in the normal human brain: regional and cellular mapping as a basis for putative roles in cerebral function. *Drug Metab. Dispos.*, **37**, 1528–1538.

23 Miksys, S. and Tyndale, R.F. (2009) Brain drug-metabolizing cytochrome P450 enzymes are active *in vivo*, demonstrated by mechanism-based enzyme inhibition. *Neuropsychopharmacology*, **34**, 634–640.

24 Pelkonen, O. and Turpeinen, M. (2007) *In vitro–in vivo* extrapolation of hepatic clearance: biological tools, scaling factors, model assumptions and correct concentrations. *Xenobiotica*, **37**, 1066–1089.

25 Rostami-Hodjegan, A. and Tucker, G.T. (2007) Simulation and prediction of *in vivo* drug metabolism in human populations from *in vitro* data. *Nat. Rev. Drug Discov.*, **6**, 140–148.

26 Eissing, T., Kuepfer, L., Becker, C., Block, M., Coboeken, K., and Gaub, T. (2011) A computational systems biology software platform for multiscale modeling and simulation: integrating whole-body physiology, disease biology, and molecular reaction networks. *Front. Physiol.*, **2**, 4.

27 Meyer, U.A. (2004) Pharmacogenetics – five decades of therapeutic lessons from genetic diversity. *Nat. Rev. Genet.*, **5**, 669–676.

28 Zanger, U.M., Turpeinen, M., Klein, K., and Schwab, M. (2008) Functional pharmacogenetics/genomics of human cytochromes P450 involved in drug biotransformation. *Anal. Bioanal. Chem.*, **392**, 1093–1108.

29 Schaeffeler, E., Zanger, U.M., Eichelbaum, M., Asante-Poku, S., Shin, J.-G., and Schwab, M. (2008) Highly multiplexed genotyping of thiopurine *S*-methyltransferase variants using MALD-TOF mass spectrometry: reliable genotyping in different ethnic groups. *Clin. Chem.*, **54**, 1637–1647.

30 Hein, D.W. (2009) *N*-acetyltransferase SNPs: emerging concepts serve as a paradigm for understanding complexities of personalized medicine. *Expert Opin. Drug Metab. Toxicol.*, **5**, 353–366.

31 Gasche, Y., Daali, Y., Fathi, M., Chiappe, A., Cottini, S., and Dayer, P. (2004) Codeine intoxication associated with ultrarapid CYP2D6 metabolism. *N. Engl. J. Med.*, **351**, 2827–2831.

32 Nakajima, M., Yokoi, T., Mizutani, M., Kinoshita, M., Funayama, M., and Kamataki, T. (1999) Genetic polymorphism in the 5′-flanking region of human CYP1A2 gene: effect on the CYP1A2 inducibility in humans. *J. Biochem.*, **125**, 803–808.

33 Sachse, C., Brockmöller, J., Bauer, S., and Roots, I. (1999) Functional significance of a C→A polymorphism in intron 1 of the cytochrome P450 CYP1A2 gene tested with caffeine. *Br. J. Clin. Pharmacol.*, **47**, 445–449.

34 Zukunft, J., Lang, T., Richter, T., Hirsch-Ernst, K.I., Nussler, A.K., and Klein, K. (2005) A natural CYP2B6 TATA box polymorphism (–82T→C) leading to enhanced transcription and relocation of the transcriptional start site. *Mol. Pharmacol.*, **67**, 1772–1782.

35 Li, H., Ferguson, S.S., and Wang, H. (2010) Synergistically enhanced CYP2B6 inducibility between a polymorphic mutation in CYP2B6 promoter and pregnane X receptor activation. *Mol. Pharmacol.*, **78**, 704–713.

36 Beierle, I., Meibohm, B., and Derendorf, H. (1999) Gender differences in pharmacokinetics and pharmacodynamics. *Int. J. Clin. Pharmacol. Ther.*, **37**, 529–547.

37 Gandhi, M., Aweeka, F., Greenblatt, R.M., and Blaschke, T.F. (2004) Sex differences in pharmacokinetics and pharmacodynamics. *Annu. Rev. Pharmacol. Toxicol.*, **44**, 499–523.

38 Scandlyn, M.J., Stuart, E.C., and Rosengren, R.J. (2008) Sex-specific differences in CYP450 isoforms in humans. *Expert Opin. Drug Metab. Toxicol.*, **4**, 413–424.

39 Waxman, D.J. and Holloway, M.G. (2009) Sex differences in the expression of hepatic drug metabolizing enzymes. *Mol. Pharmacol.*, **76**, 215–228.

40 Cotreau, M.M., von Moltke, L.L., and Greenblatt, D.J. (2005) The influence of age and sex on the clearance of cytochrome P450 3A substrates. *Clin. Pharmacokinet.*, **44**, 33–60.

41 Schmidt, R., Baumann, F., Hanschmann, H., Geissler, F., and Preiss, R. (2001) Gender difference in ifosfamide metabolism by human liver microsomes. *Eur. J. Drug Metab. Pharmacokinet.*, **26**, 193–200.

42 Wolbold, R., Klein, K., Burk, O., Nüssler, A.K., Neuhaus, P., and Eichelbaum, M. (2003) Sex is a major determinant of CYP3A4 expression in human liver. *Hepatology*, **38**, 978–988.

43 Lamba, V., Panetta, J.C., Strom, S., and Schuetz, E.G. (2010) Genetic predictors of interindividual variability in hepatic CYP3A4 expression. *J. Pharmacol. Exp. Ther.*, **332**, 1088–1099.

44 Yang, X., Zhang, B., Molony, C., Chudin, E., Hao, K., and Zhu, J. (2010) Systematic genetic and genomic analysis of cytochrome P450 enzyme activities in human liver. *Genome Res.*, **20**, 1020–1036.

45 Relling, M.V., Lin, J.S., Ayers, G.D., and Evans, W.E. (1992) Racial and gender differences in *N*-acetyltransferase, xanthine oxidase, and CYP1A2 activities. *Clin. Pharmacol. Ther.*, **52**, 643–658.

46 Ou-Yang, D.S., Huang, S.L., Wang, W., Xie, H.G., Xu, Z.H., and Shu, Y. (2000) Phenotypic polymorphism and gender-related differences of CYP1A2 activity in a Chinese population. *Br. J. Clin. Pharmacol.*, **49**, 145–151.

47 Bock, K.W., Schrenk, D., Forster, A., Griese, E.U., Mörike, K., and Brockmeier, D. (1994) The influence of environmental and genetic factors on CYP2D6, CYP1A2 and UDP-glucuronosyltransferases in man using sparteine, caffeine, and paracetamol as probes. *Pharmacogenetics*, **4**, 209–218.

48 Zhang, Y., Klein, K., Sugathan, A., Nassery, N., Dombkowski, A., and Zanger, U.M. (2011) Transcriptional profiling of human liver identifies sex-biased genes associated with polygenic dyslipidemia and coronary artery disease. *PLoS ONE*, **6**, e23506.

49 Kinirons, M.T. and O'Mahony, M.S. (2004) Drug metabolism and ageing. *Br. J. Clin. Pharmacol.*, **57**, 540–544.

50 Koukouritaki, S.B., Manro, J.R., Marsh, S.A., Stevens, J.C., Rettie, A.E., and McCarver, D.G. (2004) Developmental expression of human hepatic CYP2C9 and CYP2C19. *J. Pharmacol. Exp. Ther.*, **308**, 965–974.

51 Stevens, J.C., Marsh, S.A., Zaya, M.J., Regina, K.J., Divakaran, K., and Le, M. (2008) Developmental changes in human liver CYP2D6 expression. *Drug Metab. Dispos.*, **36**, 1587–1593.

52 Court, M.H. (2010) Interindividual variability in hepatic drug glucuronidation: studies into the role of age, sex, enzyme inducers, and genetic polymorphism using the human liver bank as a model system. *Drug Metab. Rev.*, **42**, 209–224.

53 Leeder, J.S., Gaedigk, R., Marcucci, K.A., Gaedigk, A., Vyhlidal, C.A., and Schindel, B.P. (2005) Variability of CYP3A7 expression in human fetal liver. *J. Pharmacol. Exp. Ther.*, **314**, 626–635.

54 Slaviero, K.A., Clarke, S.J., and Rivory, L.P. (2003) Inflammatory response: an unrecognised source of variability in the pharmacokinetics and pharmacodynamics of cancer chemotherapy. *Lancet Oncol.*, **4**, 224–232.

55 Aitken, A.E., Richardson, T.A., and Morgan, E.T. (2006) Regulation of drug-metabolizing enzymes and transporters in inflammation. *Annu. Rev. Pharmacol. Toxicol.*, **46**, 123–149.

56 Le Vee, M., Gripon, P., Stieger, B., and Fardel, O. (2008) Down-regulation of organic anion transporter expression in human hepatocytes exposed to the proinflammatory cytokine interleukin 1beta. *Drug Metab. Dispos.*, **36**, 217–222.

57 Jover, R., Bort, R., Gómez-Lechón, M.J., and Castell, J.V. (2002) Down-regulation of human CYP3A4 by the inflammatory signal interleukin-6: molecular mechanism and transcription factors involved. *FASEB J.*, **16**, 1799–1801.

58 Aitken, A.E. and Morgan, E.T. (2007) Gene-specific effects of inflammatory cytokines on cytochrome P450 2C, 2B6

and 3A4 mRNA levels in human hepatocytes. *Drug Metab. Dispos.*, **35**, 1687–1693.

59 Buechler, C. and Weiss, T.S. (2011) Does hepatic steatosis affect drug metabolizing enzymes in the liver? *Curr. Drug Metab.*, **12**, 24–34.

60 Gómez-Lechón, M.J., Donato, M.T., Martínez-Romero, A., Jiménez, N., Castell, J.V., and O'Connor, J.-E. (2007) A human hepatocellular *in vitro* model to investigate steatosis. *Chem. Biol. Interact.*, **165**, 106–116.

61 Pelkonen, O., Turpeinen, M., Uusitalo, J., Rautio, A., and Raunio, H. (2005) Prediction of drug metabolism and interactions on the basis of *in vitro* investigations *Basic Clin. Pharmacol. Toxicol.*, **96**, 167–175.

62 Zhang, L., Zhang, Y.D., Zhao, P., and Huang, S.-M. (2009) Predicting drug–drug interactions: an FDA perspective. *AAPS J.*, **11**, 300–306.

63 Kalgutkar, A.S., Obach, R.S., and Maurer, T.S. (2007) Mechanism-based inactivation of cytochrome P450 enzymes: chemical mechanisms, structure–activity relationships and relationship to clinical drug–drug interactions and idiosyncratic adverse drug reactions. *Curr. Drug Metab.*, **8**, 407–447.

64 Masubuchi, Y. and Horie, T. (2007) Toxicological significance of mechanism-based inactivation of cytochrome p450 enzymes by drugs. *Crit. Rev. Toxicol.*, **37**, 389–412.

65 Beaune, P., Dansette, P.M., Mansuy, D., Kiffel, L., and Finck, M. (1987) Human anti-endoplasmic reticulum autoantibodies appearing in a drug-induced hepatitis are directed against a human liver cytochrome P-450 that hydroxylates the drug. *Proc. Natl. Acad. Sci. USA*, **84**, 551–555.

66 Pelkonen, O., Turpeinen, M., Hakkola, J., Honkakoski, P., Hukkanen, J., and Raunio, H. (2008) Inhibition and induction of human cytochrome P450 enzymes: current status. *Arch. Toxicol.*, **82**, 667–715.

67 Zevin, S. and Benowitz, N.L. (1999) Drug interactions with tobacco smoking. An update. *Clin Pharmacokinet.*, **36**, 425–438.

68 Desai, H.D., Seabolt, J., and Jann, M.W. (2001) Smoking in patients receiving psychotropic medications: a pharmacokinetic perspective. *CNS Drugs*, **15**, 469–494.

11
Central Nervous System Drugs

Pierre Baumann and Christoph Hiemke

11.1
Introduction

Central nervous system drugs comprise many classes of drugs such as anesthetics, anticonvulsants, psychotropic drugs (including antidepressants, antipsychotics, hypnotics and anxiolytics, drugs of abuse, opioids, and others), antimigraine drugs, cognitive enhancers, and others. Knowledge about the metabolism of these drugs is of high clinical interest as, depending on the metabolic pathway, active metabolites may be formed that contribute to the overall pharmacological profile. This is particularly considered in studies about the relationship between drug plasma concentrations and their clinical effectiveness. They yield the basis for therapeutic drug monitoring (TDM) – an instrument widely used in psychiatry [1, 2] and in neurology [3]. Moreover, during the past 30 years, the importance of a genetic control of the metabolism of drugs is increasingly recognized. Most central nervous system drugs are metabolized by one or several forms of cytochrome P450 (CYP), many of which present a genetic polymorphism [4–7]. Therefore, pharmacogenetic tests are also a useful tool for optimizing pharmacotherapy, alone or in combination with TDM. Finally, knowledge about the mechanisms implicated in drug metabolism helps to interpret pharmacokinetic interactions. However, the role of other enzymatic systems, especially phase II enzymes that also play an important role, is less clear and their contribution will therefore only be marginally described. Due to limited space available, not all categories of central nervous system drugs will be considered in this chapter.

11.2
Antidepressants

Tricyclic antidepressants and structurally related agents as well as monoamine oxidase (MAO) inhibitors are still considered to be effective antidepressant agents,

Metabolism of Drugs and Other Xenobiotics, First Edition. Edited by Pavel Anzenbacher, Ulrich M. Zanger.

but SSRIs (selective serotonin reuptake inhibitors), SNRIs (serotonin and norepinephrine reuptake inhibitors; dual reuptake inhibitors), and other recently introduced drugs are now more commonly used, mainly because of their better clinical effectiveness (comparable efficacy, but better tolerance and safety). Antidepressants were shown to be effective in the treatment of anxiety disorders and, among them, serotonergic agents appeared to be effective agents for the treatment of obsessive compulsive disorder. In contrast, noradrenergic rather than serotonergic antidepressants show efficacy for the treatment of pain (see Chapter 15). The metabolism and pharmacogenetics of antidepressants and the usefulness of TDM were recently presented in a number of reviews [8–10].

11.2.1
Tricyclic Antidepressants and Structurally Related Compounds

Generally, tricyclic antidepressants of the tertiary amine type (amitriptyline, imipramine, clomipramine, doxepin, dothiepin, and trimipramine) undergo *N*-demethylation to the corresponding secondary amines by several CYP isoforms (CYP1A2, CYP2D6, CYP2C19, and CYP3A4; their relative contribution may vary considerably, depending on the compound), and both the tertiary (amitriptyline, imipramine, clomipramine, trimipramine) and secondary amines (nortriptyline, desipramine, desmethylclomipramine) are hydroxylated mainly by CYP2D6 [11–15]. Lofepramine – an acetylated derivative from desipramine – and amitriptyline *N*-oxide and imipramine *N*-oxide may be considered as prodrugs, which are "activated" by biotransformation to desipramine, amitriptyline, and imipramine, respectively. While from the above-mentioned tricyclic drugs, only trimipramine is a chiral compound, hydroxylation of amitriptyline and nortriptyline yields altogether stereoselectively eight 8-OH-derivatives, which are also reuptake inhibitors of biogenic amines: the (–)-*E*-10-OH, (+)-*E*-10-OH, (–)-*Z*-10-OH, and (+)-*Z*-10-OH metabolites. The formation of *E*-10-OH-nortriptyline and, in particular, that of (–)-*E*-10-OH-nortriptyline (but not that of *Z*-10-OH-nortriptyline) from nortriptyline is performed by CYP2D6 [16, 17]). Hydroxylation of nortriptyline depends on the number of functional *CYP2D6* genes [18].

Trimipramine is stereoselectively metabolized, in that CYP2D6 is preferentially implicated in the formation of L-2-OH-trimipramine and CYP2C19 in that of *N*-desmethyltrimipramine. CYP3A4 also contributes to its metabolism [19, 20].

Conflicting results were obtained in studies about maprotiline, which is metabolized to numerous hydroxylated metabolites [21, 22], but *in vitro*, CYP2D6 and, to a minor extent, CYP1A2 *N*-demethylate this antidepressant [23].

Mianserin and mirtazapine differ only by a substitution of a C-atom by a N-atom. Regarding mianserin, its *S*-eutomer is more readily 8-hydroxylated and oxidized to its *N*-oxide than the distomer *R*-mianserin, which is preferentially *N*-demethylated [24, 25]. CYP2D6, CYP2B6, CYP3A4, and CYP1A2 contribute to 8-hydroxylation of mianserin, while CYP2B6, CYP2C19, CYP1A2, CYP3A4, and CYP2D6 show *N*-demethylating activity of mianserin [25]. *In vivo* studies suggest that CYP2D6 preferentially oxidizes *S*-(+)-mianserin in contrast to *R*-(–)-mianserin

[26, 27]. CYP2D6 hydroxylates mirtazapine (*S*-(+)-mirtazapine is considered the eutomer) preferentially to *S*-(+)-8-OH-mirtazapine, but CYP1A2 is also implicated. *N*(2)-demethylation and *N*(2)-oxidation is carried out by CYP3A4 [28]. *S*-(+)-mirtazapine is mainly metabolized by 8-hydroxylation, while *R*-(−)-mirtazapine is preferentially and reversibly *N*-glucuronidated as a quaternary ammonium glucuronide [29]. Recently, the contribution of CYP2B6 in the stereoselective metabolism of mirtazapine could be demonstrated (Jaquenoud Sirot *et al.*, revised manuscript).

Opipramol, despite its tricyclic structure, is a weak reuptake inhibitor of biogenic amines, but a σ-receptor agonist. As a substrate of CYP2D6, its main metabolite is deshydroxyethylopipramol [30, 31].

Doxepin and dothiepin differ from amitriptyline by substitution of its C-atom at position 11 by an atom of O or S, respectively; this explains the presence of geometric isomers in these molecules. The geometric *Z*-isomer is considered to be responsible for the antidepressant effect of doxepin, which is a mixture of 85% *E*-(*trans*)- and 15% *Z*-(*cis*)-isomers. Formation of the pharmacologically active metabolite *Z*-*N*-desmethyldoxepin is important [32]. CYP2D6 is mainly involved in the formation of (*E*)-2-OH-doxepin and 2-OH-desmethyldoxepin, while CYP2C19, CYP3A4, and CYP2C9 contribute to its *N*-demethylation [33–35]. For dothiepin, actually introduced as its (pharmacologically active) *E*-isomer, the mechanisms responsible for the formation of its main metabolites – northiaden, dothiepin sulfoxide, and northiaden sulfoxide – remain to be studied [36, 37], but CYP1A2 seems to be involved [9].

Finally, many antidepressants (e.g., tertiary amines such as imipramine [38]) and their hydroxy metabolites are readily glucuronidated [39, 40].

11.2.2
SSRIs

Escitalopram (*S*-citalopram) has to be considered as the clinically active enantiomer of citalopram, while the distomer *R*-citalopram allosterically impairs the binding of escitalopram to the serotonin transporter [41]. In citalopram-treated patients, *S*-citalopram only reaches about 50–70% of the plasma concentrations of *R*-citalopram [42]. CYP2C19, CYP3A4, and, to some extent, CYP2D6 control the stereoselective *N*-demethylation of racemic citalopram to *N*-demethylcitalopram, but CYP2C19 preferentially *N*-demethylates escitalopram rather than the opposite enantiomer [43–47]. Recent studies showed that CYP2C19 is also involved in the biotransformation of escitalopram to its propionic acid derivative [48] (Figure 11.1). There is also a stereoselective deamination of citalopram to a propionic acid derivative by MAO-A and MAO-B [49, 50]. In human blood, where only MAO-B is present in platelets, only escitalopram but not *R*-citalopram is metabolized to the propionic acid derivative [51]. Due to low levels of CYP activity in the human brain, citalopram is preferentially metabolized by CYP in the periphery, but by MAO-A and MAO-B in the brain.

S- and *R*-fluoxetine, and *S*-norfluoxetine, in contrast to *R*-norfluoxetine, are the pharmacologically active enantiomers of fluoxetine. CYP2C19, CYP3A, CYP2C9,

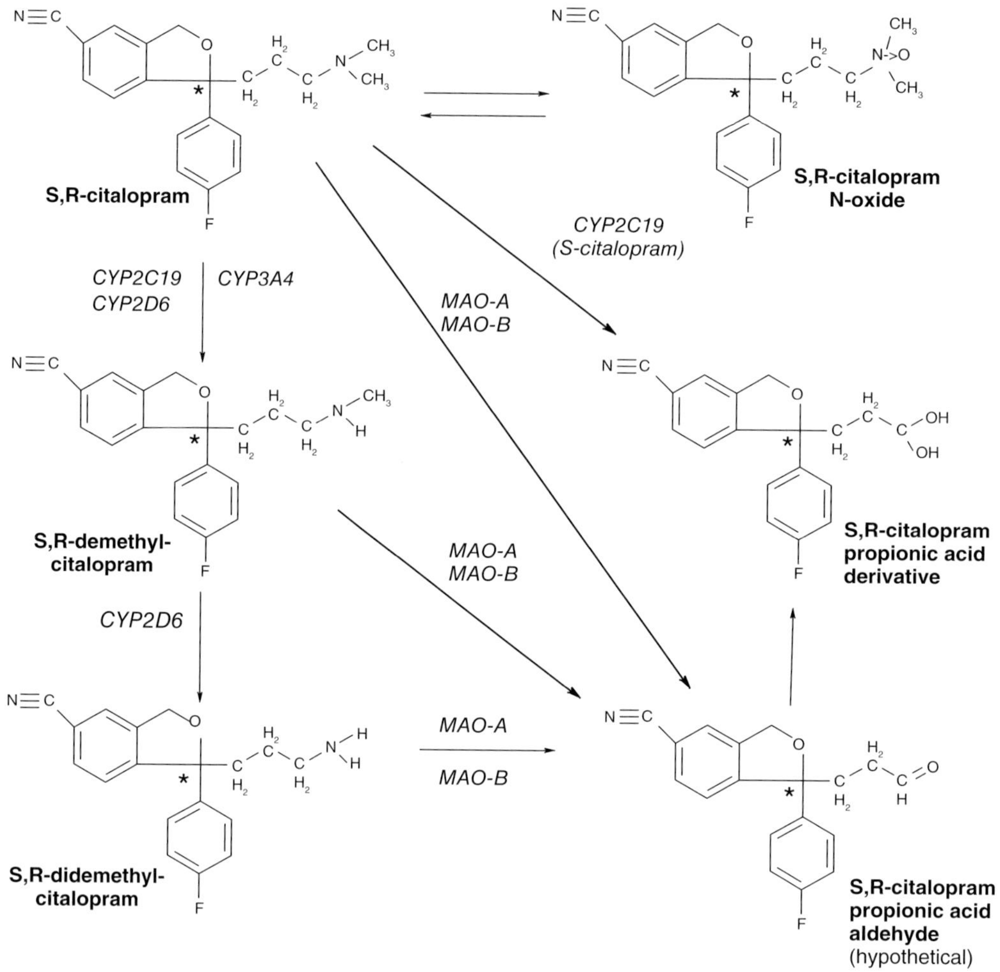

Figure 11.1 Metabolism of citalopram by CYP, MAO-A, and MAO B. *Asymmetric center.

and CYP2D6 are responsible for *N*-demethylation of fluoxetine [52–55]. In healthy volunteers, the pharmacokinetics of *S*- and *R*-fluoxetine, and *S*-norfluoxetine, but not *R*-norfluoxetine, depend on their CYP2D6 genotype, after a single dose of fluoxetine [56].

The metabolic pathways of fluvoxamine are poorly understood. CYP1A2–an isozyme induced in smokers–contributes to its biotransformation. Its activity may mask that of CYP2D6 [57–59], which yields a carboxylic acid metabolite [60]. CYP2C19, which is inhibited by fluvoxamine, is probably not involved in its biotransformation [61].

Paroxetine is submitted to demethylenation by CYP2D6 [62, 63]. The pharmacokinetics of paroxetine are not linear, due to a mechanism-based inhibition of CYP2D6 by a metabolite [64].

In vitro studies allowed calculating the relative contribution of CYP isoforms in the *N*-demethylation of sertraline to its main metabolite *N*-demethylsertraline (norsertraline): CYP2D6 (35%), CYP2C9 (29%), CYP2B6 (14%), CYP2C19 (13%), and CYP3A4 (9%) [65–67], but a clinical pharmacogenetic study could not confirm this important role of CYP2D6 [53]. Sertraline is also deaminated by MAO-B, probably to a ketone [68, 69].

11.2.3
Other Recent Antidepressants

Nefazodone is hydroxylated by CYP3A4 (but not by CYP2D6) to the active metabolite (side-chain) OH-nefazodone and to a lesser extent to *p*-OH-nefazodone, and dealkylated by CYP3A4 (but not by CYP2D6) to *m*-chlorophenylpiperazine (mCPP)—a common active metabolite of nefazodone and trazodone. Hydroxylation of mCPP to OH-mCPP is carried out by CYP2D6 [70]. In CYP2D6-genotyped subjects treated with nefazodone, plasma concentrations of mCPP are higher in subjects presenting a genetic deficiency of this enzyme (poor metabolizers (PMs)) than in extensive metabolizers (EMs) (see Chapter 1) [71]. CYP3A4 controls the biotransformation of trazodone to mCPP [72].

Duloxetine and venlafaxine are both dual (norepinephrine and serotonin) uptake inhibitor antidepressants. The main metabolites of the chiral compound duloxetine introduced as a single isomer [73] are 4-OH-, 6-OH-5-methoxy-, and 4,6-dihydroxyduloxetine. It is a substrate and an inhibitor of CYP2D6 [74]. CYP2D6, and to a lesser extent CYP2C9 and CYP2C19 mediate, *in vitro*, the formation of the active metabolite *O*-demethylvenlafaxine from venlafaxine. CYP2C19, CYP2C9, and CYP3A4 *N*-demethylate venlafaxine to the minor metabolite *N*-demethylvenlafaxine [75]. Pharmacogenetic studies confirmed the importance of CYP2D6 in the elimination of venlafaxine [76, 77]. The racemic drug is dose dependently and stereoselectively *O*- and *N*-demethylated [78–81]. *N,O*-didesmethylvenlafaxine, mainly metabolized by conjugation, is a common metabolite of the recently introduced antidepressant desvenlafaxine (*O*-demethylvenlafaxine) [82] and of venlafaxine.

Apparently, CYP2D6 does not metabolize bupropion and its metabolites erythrohydrobupropion and threohydrobupropion, which in fact are amino alcohols [83]. CYP2B6 oxidizes bupropion to the pharmacologically active 4-OH-bupropion [84–86].

CYP is probably not involved in the metabolism of the racemic drug milnacipran introduced as its *Z*-isomer [87, 88]. Preliminary observations suggest that the metabolism of minaprine may be impaired in subjects presenting a genetic deficiency of CYP2D6 [89]. CYP3A4, in contrast to CYP2D6 and other forms of CYP, contributes to the biotransformation of the chiral drug reboxetine [90].

Agomelatine S20098 (*N*-[2-(7-methoxy-1-naphtyl)-ethyl]acetamide) acts as an agonist of melatonin receptors (MT_1, MT_2) and as an antagonist of 5-HT_{2c} receptors [91]. Seven metabolites were identified; the major metabolism (90%) is epoxide formation via CYP1A2 [92]. Moreover, CYP2C9 seems to be involved in its *O*-demethylation and hydroxylation.

Finally, St John's Wort is also introduced as an antidepressant. Several components may contribute to its overall pharmacological activity profile, including hyperforin, hypericin, pseudohypericin, quercetine, amentoflavone, and biapigenine [93] (see Chapter 21).

11.2.4
MAO Inhibitors

The metabolism of the MAO inhibitors phenelzine, tranylcypromine, pargyline, and deprenyl has been poorly investigated [94]. *R*-deprenyl rather than *S*-deprenyl seems to be metabolized by CYP2D6. Phenelzine and its metabolite phenethylamine are metabolized by MAO [95].

CYP2C19 [96, 97] rather than CYP2D6 [98] is involved in the metabolism of the MAO-A inhibitor moclobemide [99] to a morphine lactam derivative (Ro 12-8095). Morpholine *N*-oxide (Ro 12-5637) is formed by flavin-containing monooxygenase (FMO) [100].

11.3
Antipsychotics

Phenothiazines, butyrophenones, and thioxanthenes were the first groups of antipsychotic (or neuroleptic or typical antipsychotic) drugs introduced for the treatment of schizophrenia and other psychotic states. The more recently introduced atypical antipsychotics (or second-generation antipsychotics) are not a homogeneous group with regard to their chemical constitution. Some of them are now also available for the treatment of bipolar diseases (mania, bipolar depression). Many antipsychotics are substrates of CYP2D6. They may induce adverse effects of the extrapyramidal type, especially at higher doses or at higher plasma concentrations, as they may be observed in patients with a genetic CYP2D6 deficiency. TDM and pharmacogenetic tests may be considered useful tools for guiding pharmacotherapy with antipsychotics [10, 101, 102].

11.3.1
Phenothiazines and Thioxanthenes

The metabolism of chlorpromazine, which was the first antipsychotic drug introduced on the market is complex, as dozens of metabolites are formed by *N*-demethylation, sulfoxidation, and hydroxylation [103]. CYP2D6 and to a lesser extent CYP1A2 are the major enzymes responsible for the formation of 7-OH-chlorpromazine [4, 104].

In a study with healthy volunteers, there was no evidence for differences in the pharmacokinetics of levomepromazine between CYP2D6 EMs and PMs [105].

The elimination kinetics of perphenazine in plasma differs between EMs compared to PMs (CYP2D6) [106]. In genotyped patients, its dose-corrected steady-state levels were significantly higher in PMs [107].

A second asymmetric center is introduced in the chiral drug thioridazine by its sulfoxidation to the active metabolite mesoridazine. The latter compound is then further oxidized to therapeutically active sulfone sulforidazine. Thioridazine and the sulfoxidized metabolites are also *N*-demethylated. The formation of mesoridazine and partly that of the cardiotoxic thioridazine-ring sulfoxide appear to be controlled by CYP2D6 [108–110]. CYP1A2 and CYP3A4 play a major role in the 5-sulfoxidation and *N*-demethylation of thioridazine [111]. The data collected by stereoselective high-performance liquid chromatography suggest that CYP2D6 is involved in the formation of *S*-thioridazine 2-SO (FE ("fast eluting")) and *R*-thioridazine 2-SO (SE ("slow eluting")) and probably also in that of *S*-thioridazine 5-SO (FE) and *R*-thioridazine 5-SO (SE) (ring oxide). CYP2C19 also contributes to the metabolism of thioridazine [110].

Perazine is *N*-demethylated by CYP2C19, and oxidized by CYP1A2 and CYP3A4 to its 5-sulfoxide, but other CYP forms are also involved in its biotransformation [112].

A pharmacogenetic study demonstrated the implication of CYP2D6 in the pharmacokinetics of zuclopenthixol [113].

11.3.2
Butyrophenones and Related Compounds

Haloperidol is metabolized to the chiral compound "reduced haloperidol," which is then partly back-oxidized [114]. Important pathways include glucuroconjugation and hydroxylation. CYP2D6 and CYP3A4 control dealkylation of both compounds [115]. In PMs (CYP2D6) treated with haloperidol, its plasma half-life was significantly longer and its clearance lower [116, 117], and plasma concentrations of reduced haloperidol were higher than in EMs [118]. In patients who experienced extrapyramidal side-effects while treated with haloperidol, reduced haloperidol plasma concentrations and reduced haloperidol/haloperidol ratios were higher than in other patients [119]. In Japanese patients carrying a CYP2D6*10 allele, which is frequent (50%) in this ethnic group, significantly higher plasma concentrations of haloperidol and reduced haloperidol were observed [120].

In vitro, CYP3A4 and CYP1A2 are implicated in the dealkylation of pimozide [121], and clinical studies showed the contribution of CYP2D6 [122].

11.3.3
Atypical Antipsychotics

In vitro studies suggest the formation by CYP2D6 of some unknown minor metabolites from clozapine [123]. CYP2C19, CYP3A4, CYP2D6, CYP1A2, and CYP2C9,

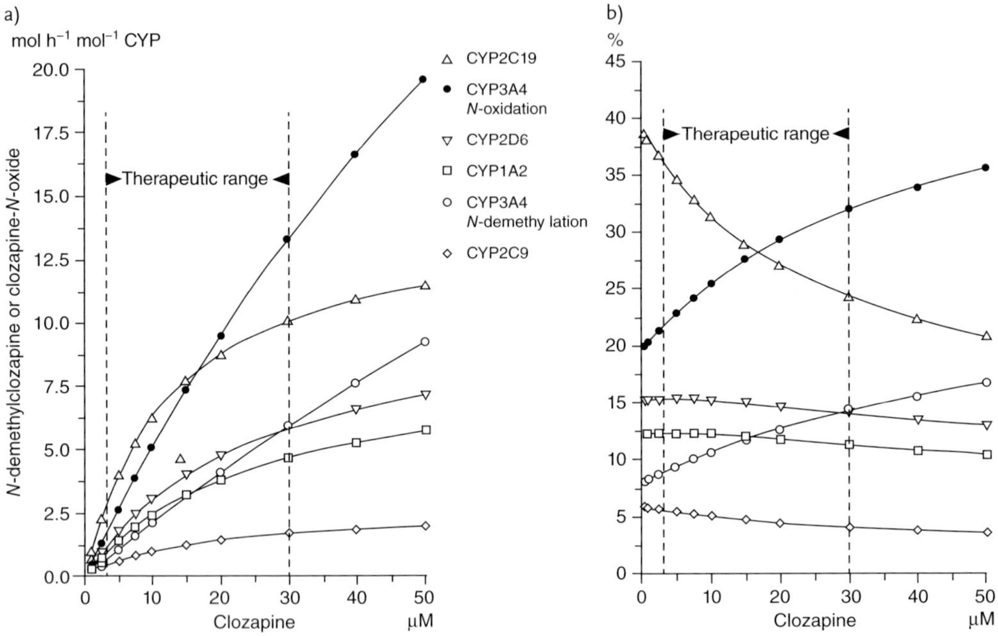

Figure 11.2 Biotransformation of clozapine to *N*-demethylclozapine and clozapine *N*-oxide. (a) Reaction rate per mole of CYP isoform. (b) Percentage contributions simulated for an "average" liver; relative distribution of 10 : 30 : 5 : 5 : 1.5 for CYP1A2, 3A4, 2C9, 2C19, and 2D6. (From [126]. Reproduced with permission of the publisher.)

in decreasing order, are implicated in its *N*-demethylation [124–126]. CYP3A4 is involved in the formation of clozapine *N*-oxide [126]. No evidence was found for the formation of the *N*-oxide of clozapine and of demethylclozapine by CYP2D6 [125, 127]. A panel study with CYP2D6- and CYP2C19-phenotyped subjects could not confirm the implication of these enzymes in the metabolism of clozapine [128], but in a recent clinical study, CYP1A2 was found to be the most important CYP isoform contributing to the metabolism of clozapine, while CYP2C19 and CYP3A4 contributed moderately. CYP2B6, CYP2C9, CYP2D6, CYP3A5, and CYP3A7 polymorphisms did not influence clozapine kinetics [129]. However, Figure 11.2 shows that the role of different isoforms of CYP in the *N*-demethylation of clozapine and formation of its *N*-oxide depends on the clozapine dose, but also on the relative distribution of CYP isoforms in the individuals [126]. A similar situation was also described for sertraline [66].

Olanzapine is metabolized by glucuronidation, FMO3, and CYP1A2, which is mainly implicated in its *N*-demethylation. CYP2D6 catalyzes its biotransformation to the minor metabolite 2-hydroxymethylolanzapine [130–132].

In vitro, risperidone is metabolized by CYP2D6, but also by CYP3A4, to the active and chiral metabolite 9-OH-risperidone (paliperidone) [133–135]: CYP2D6 contributes mainly to the formation of (+)-9-OH-risperidone, while CYP3A4 forms preferentially the opposite enantiomer [136]. The sum of risperidone and 9-OH-risperidone is considered to constitute the "active moiety" [137]. Both compounds are dealkylated [138] by CYP3A [139]. CYP2D6 deficiency may represent a risk for an impaired tolerance of a risperidone treatment [140, 141]. Generally, in steady-state conditions, the risperidone/9-OH-risperidone ratio in plasma is higher in CYP2D6 PMs than in EMs [135, 141]. Paliperidone is not considerably metabolized, and, especially, CYP2D6 and CYP3A4 are only marginally involved [138]. This drug is also available as its palmitate (i.e., as an ester) in a unique extended-release delivery system [142].

In vitro, CYP3A4 controls biotransformation of ziprasidone to its sulfoxide and sulfone, and to a dealkylation product [143]. CYP2C19 activity, in contrast to that of CYP2D6, correlated with the *in vitro* formation of the sulfone and the sulfoxide in human liver microsomes, but no significant formation of metabolites by CYP2D6, CYP2C9, CYP2C19, and CYP1A2 could be observed using recombinant enzymes [144]. The major pathway is claimed to occur via reduction by aldehyde oxidation, but this remains to be fully described [145, 146].

CYP3A4 is the main CYP form contributing to the formation of *N*-demethylzotepine and zotepine *S*-sulfoxide from zotepine, *in vitro*, while its 2- and 3-hydroxylations are carried out by CYP1A2 and CYP2D6, respectively [147]. It is apparently not a substrate of CYP2C19 [148].

CYP3A4 is the main enzyme responsible for the *N*-dealkylation of quetiapine to norquetiapine [149]–a potent norepinephrine transport inhibitor [150]. CYP2D6 is implicated in quetiapine 7-hydroxylation [149, 151]. *O*-dealkylation and sulfoxidation are also observed [152].

Sertindole is metabolized by CYP3A4 and CYP2D6. In PMs (CYP2D6), its clearance and the area under the concentration–time curve (AUC) ratio dehydrosertindole/sertindole is lower than in EMs [153].

Sulpiride and amisulpride are almost not metabolized [154].

Aripiprazole is mainly metabolized by CYP3A4 and CYP2D6. Dehydroaripiprazole (OPC-14857) is its main and active metabolite, which is also a substrate of CYP3A4 [155].

Asenapine carries two asymmetric centers, but it is introduced as a single enantiomer, which is metabolized to its *N*-oxide and its *N*-demethylated product. This biotransformation occurs by glucuroconjugation and CYP (seemingly by CYP3A4 and CYP1A2) [156].

Iloperidone is metabolized by hydroxylation, and *O*- and *N*-dealkylation, involving mainly CYP2D6 and CYP3A4, and one of its main metabolites–an alcohol–is produced by its reduction [157, 158].

11.4
Tranquillizers and Hypnotic Agents

Among the (minor) tranquillizers (or anxiolytics) and hypnotic agents, benzodiazepines and related compounds are the most widely introduced therapeutic agents. By their mechanism of action, imidazopyridines and pyrrolones can also be considered to be part of this group. Barbiturates–the classical hypnotic agents–have only historical significance due to their unfavorable adverse effects profile. Finally, buspirone, introduced for the treatment of anxiety disorders, is a serotonergic agent. Together with other anxiolytic anticonvulsants, they will be described below (Section 11.6).

Several benzodiazepines are substrates of CYP2C19, as shown for diazepam [159, 160], while CYP2D6 plays only a minor, if any, role. In a panel study with Caucasian subjects, the pharmacokinetics of diazepam and of its metabolite demethyldiazepam were found to differ between CYP2C19, but not between CYP2D6 PMs and EMs [161]. Mean plasma half-lives of diazepam (nordiazepam) were 88 h (128 h) and 41 h (59 h) in PMs and EMs (CYP2C19), respectively. In contrast, in Chinese subjects, the kinetics of diazepam did not differ between EMs and PMs of mephenytoin (the plasma half-life was similar to that measured in Caucasian PMs!), but the plasma half-life of demethyldiazepam was longer in PMs than in EMs [162]. CYP3A4 is involved in the hydroxylation of diazepam to temazepam [160, 163]. *In vitro* experiments showed that the metabolism of flunitrazepam to 3′-OH-flunitrazepam and demethylflunitrazepam is mediated by CYP2C19, CYP3A4, and CYP1A2 [164, 165]. Clobazam is probably a substrate of CYP2C19 [166].

The chiral drug oxazepam is readily used in patients suffering from hepatic problems as it is mainly glucuronidated (UDP-glucurosyltransferases UGT2B15, UGT1A9, and UGT2B7). However, its metabolism is complicated by the fact that there is mesomerization between *S*- and *R*-oxazepam [167]. CYP3A4 is the main CYP form implicated in the metabolism of midazolam, triazolam, and alprazolam [168–170]. Pharmacogenetic studies suggest that CYP2C19 is implicated in the metabolism of quazepam [171], but also in that of alprazolam [172]. Midazolam, which is metabolized to 1′-OH- and 4′-OH-midazolam, is used as a probe for CYP3A phenotyping [173]. In Japanese subjects, CYP2C19 does not seem to contribute notably to the elimination of triazolam [174] and alprazolam [175]. CYP3A4 catalyzes biotransformation of alprazolam to the main metabolite 4-OH-alprazolam [169], while the minor α-hydroxy metabolite is formed by CYP3A4, CYP2C9, and CYP2C19 [176]. The role of CYP in the metabolism of estazolam to 4′-OH-4-OH and 1-oxo-estazolam remains to be elucidated as a group of authors [177] did not find any evidence for CYP2C19, CYP1A2, and CYP3A4 to be involved.

CYP3A4 is the main enzyme responsible for the metabolism of zolpidem [178, 179], zopiclone [180], and zaleplon [181], in contrast to CYP2D6, CYP1A2, and other CYP forms. Zopiclone is metabolized stereoselectively to its *N*-oxide, to *N*-desmethylzopiclone, and it is also decarboxylated [182]. Eszopiclone (*S*-zopiclone) is now also available as a hypnotic agent. 5-Oxo-zaleplon is the main metabolite of zaleplon [183].

CYP3A4, CYP1A2, and CYP2C19 may be implicated in the metabolism of the serotonergic buspirone as its plasma concentrations are increased by grapefruit juice, itraconazole, erythromycin [184], and fluvoxamine [185]. *In vitro*, buspirone is dealkylated, *N*-oxidized, and hydroxylated, mainly by CYP3A4, CYP3A5, and, to a minor extent, also by CYP2D6 [186].

Melatonin – an endogenous indoleamine – has also been introduced as a sleep-inducing drug, the metabolism of which is partly carried out by CYP1A2 [187].

11.5 Psychostimulants

Among the psychostimulants, several compounds were introduced for the treatment of attention-deficit hyperactivity disorder (ADHD) [188].

Methylphenidate (MPH) – an inhibitor but not a substrate of CYP2D6 – is metabolized to ritalinic acid, ethylphenidate, *p*-OH-MPH, and a lactam [189, 190]. Recently, dexmethylphenidate (*d-threo*-MPH; *R,R*-(+)-MPH) was introduced as a single enantiomer.

Atomoxetine (formerly known as tomoxatone) was initially proposed as an antidepressant, but clinical studies could not confirm its clinical effectiveness. Now available for the treatment of ADHD, it is metabolized mainly by CYP2D6 to the major metabolite 4-OH-atomoxetine, while CYP2C19 demethylates it to *N*-desmethylatomoxetine. Other CYP forms play a minor role [191–193].

The metabolism of the anorectic drug dexfenfluramine is impaired in CYP2D6 PMs in comparison to EMs [194]. The role of CYP2D6 in the metabolism of amphetamine derivatives has recently been discussed [190, 195]. Some ring 4-methoxylated amphetamine derivatives such as 4-methoxyamphetamine are *O*-demethylated by CYP2D6, *in vitro* [196].

11.6 Anticonvulsants and Mood Stabilizers

Anticonvulsants represent a group of agents available for the treatment of epilepsy, but some of them were also introduced as mood stabilizers and/or anxiolytic agents. Mood stabilizers form a very inhomogeneous group as besides their classical representatives, lithium salts, some anticonvulsants, and antipsychotics are used for the treatment or prophylaxis of bipolar depression and mania [197].

Several authors published reviews about the metabolism of anticonvulsants [163, 198, 199]. Only oxcarbazepine, but not felbamate, gabapentin, lamotrigine, levetiracetam, tiagabine, topiramate, vigabatrin, and zonisamide among the recent anticonvulsants seem to have an active metabolite [199].

Phenobarbital (phenobarbitone) is stereoselectively metabolized [200]. Pharmacogenetic studies confirmed that racemic phenobarbital is partly metabolized to *p*-OH-phenobarbital by CYP2C19 [201, 202]. The 4′-hydroxylation of mephobarbital is stereoselectively mediated by CYP2C19 [203]. Its *S*-enantiomer is mainly *N*-demethylated to phenobarbital, at least partly by CYP2B6.

CYP3A4 metabolizes carbamazepine to the active metabolite 10,11-epoxy carbamazepine (autoinduction!). CYP2C8 contributes to a minor extent to this biotransformation. The epoxide is then hydrolyzed to a diol (*trans*-10,11-dihydroxy-10,11-dihydro-carbamazepine) [204]. Other metabolic pathways for carbamazepine include formation of hydroxylated carbamazepine by CYP1A2 and conjugation by UGT.

Conjugation of valproate (VPA) is responsible for about 50% of its metabolism [198]. Mitochondrial β-oxidation to 2-ene-VPA accounts for another 40%. The control of the metabolism of VPA by CYP2C9 is genetically polymorphic and it includes the formation of the possibly toxic metabolite 4-ene-VPA, and the inactive products 4- and 5-OH-VPA [205, 206]. CYP2A6 is at least partly involved in 3-OH-VPA formation, while CYP2B6 plays a minor role in the VPA biotransformation to 4-ene-VPA, 4-OH-VPA, and 5-OH-VPA [206].

Felbamate is to a large extent excreted without metabolism, but also as conjugated products. Nevertheless, by oxidative metabolism, *p*-OH and 2-OH metabolites are formed [199].

The anticonvulsants pregabalin ((*S*)-3-aminomethyl-5-methylhexanoic acid) and gabapentin have also been introduced for the treatment of anxiety disorders and pain. They display structural similarities with leucine and γ-aminobutyric acid, respectively, and they are excreted almost without metabolism [207].

Lamotrigine is eliminated mainly by conjugation with glucuronic acid [208].

Levetiracetam ((*S*)-α-ethyl-2-oxo-1-pyrrolidine) is an amide largely (one-third of the overall elimination process, almost two-thirds being excreted unchanged in urine) submitted to enzymatic (type B esterase) hydrolysis to the carboxylic acid (L057) [209].

The prodrug oxcarbazepine is extensively reduced by cytosol arylketone reductase to the clinically relevant (*S*)-(+)- and (*R*)-(−)-10-hydroxy-10,11-dihydrocarbazepine (monohydroxy derivative), which is then also conjugated by UGT. Both enantiomers display similar anticonvulsive activity, but the *S*-enantiomer is preferentially formed [210].

Phenytoin (5,5-diphenylhydantoin) is stereoselectively metabolized to 4′-OH-phenyl-5-phenylhydantoin (HPPH), with CYP2C9 mainly implicated in the formation of (*S*)-HPPH [211]. CYP2C19 contributes to the formation of this metabolite, and to that of 3′-HPPH and 3′,4′-diHPPH [163]. Mephenytoin represents the classical probe for CYP2C19 phenotyping. This enzyme stereoselectively hydroxylates *S*-mephenytoin to *S*-4-OH′-mephenytoin [212], while CYP2B6 is implicated in the *N*-demethylation of mephenytoin to 5-phenyl-5-ethylhydantoin (nirvanol) [213, 214].

CYP3A4 controls the metabolism of tiagabine to 5-oxo-tiagabine, but glucuronides are also extensively formed [198].

Topiramate – introduced as an anticonvulsant and for migraine prophylaxis [215] – is mainly eliminated unchanged by the kidneys, but there is the formation of a dozen metabolites, including phase II metabolites [216], by poorly elucidated mechanisms regarding the enzymes involved [199]. Topiramate metabolism is induced by drugs such as phenytoin [217].

Vigabatrin is almost eliminated without metabolism [198].

Zonisamide (3-sulphamoyl 1,2-benzisoxazole) is reduced by CYP3A to 2-sulfamoylacetylphenmol, but also *N*-acetylated and glucuronidated [198, 218].

11.7 Agents for Dementia and Cognitive Enhancers

Dementia is not a homogeneous pathological entity, but its origin and clinical manifestations may be multiple: Alzheimer's disease, vascular dementia, Lewy body-type dementia, but also BPSD/BPSSD (behavioral and psychological symptoms (and signs) of dementia) are included. The availability and usefulness of the few agents for dementia depend on the diagnosis and on the symptoms observed in the individual patient. Four agents have so far been introduced for the treatment of dementia: three inhibitors of cholinesterase (donepezil, galantamine, and rivastigmine) and a *N*-methyl-D-aspartate (NMDA) receptor antagonist (memantine), but data about their metabolism are relatively scarce [219]. Tacrine – a substrate of CYP1A2 – has to be mentioned for historical reasons, but is no longer available [220].

Donepezil is a dimethylated catechol derivative that may be demethylated at both sites, but other dealkylation and conjugation products are also described [221]. CYP3A4 and, to some extent, CYP2D6 are involved in the biotransformation of this drug [222, 223]. Preliminary observations suggest that the CYP2D6 genetic polymorphism may have an impact on the clinical outcome of the patients [223].

Galantamine is submitted to several metabolic pathways – it is metabolized by CYP2D6 and CYP3A4 to *O*-desmethylgalantamine and galantamine-*N*-oxide, respectively [224, 225], and it is also glucuronidated.

Almost 50% of administered memantine is excreted unchanged in urine. Metabolites are a *N*-glucuronide, 6-hydroxymemantine, and 1-nitroso-deaminated memantine [226]. Interestingly, CYPs seem to play a minor role in its metabolism (more studies are needed!), but it is a strong inhibitor of CYP2B6 [227].

Finally, rivastigmine – an ester – is submitted to hydrolysis by cholinesterase to a phenolic compound (ZNS 114-666; NAP 226-90) [219, 228].

11.8 Antimigraine Drugs

The group of triptans used for the treatment of migraine comprises more than half a dozen compounds [229]. The metabolism of eletriptan is managed by CYP3A4 and only partly by CYP2D6; the *N*-demethylated metabolite does not add to the overall clinical activity [230]. The dimethylamino side-chain of sumatriptan is oxidized mainly by MAO-A to an indole acetic derivative [231], but the sulfonamide group is also deaminated.

11.9
Other Drugs

Disulfiram is an agent used for the treatment of alcoholism and metabolized to methyl-diethyldithiocarbamate, which may then be esterified to its methyl ester, but also to diethylthiocarbamic acid methyl ester [232]. Acamprosate is apparently not submitted to biotransformation [233].

L-DOPA – the classical anti-Parkinson's drug – has to be considered as a prodrug to dopamine, but it is also an endogenously occurring neutral amino acid formed from L-tyrosine by tyrosine hydroxylase. As such, it is hardly measurable as it is rapidly metabolized by aromatic amino acid decarboxylase to dopamine. Benserazide only peripherally inhibits this enzyme. Catecholamine-*O*-methyltransferase (COMT) methylates both L-DOPA and dopamine, which together with its methylated product is also metabolized by MAO – the final products are 3,4-dihydroxyphenylacetic acid, 3,4-dihydroxyphenyl glycol, and homovanillic acid [234].

COMT inhibitors are used as comedications with L-DOPA in order to increase its availability as a precursor of dopamine. They include the catechol derivatives entacapone and tolcapone, also used for the treatment of Parkinson's disease. They are mainly excreted as glucuronides 70 and 30%, respectively. Entacapone (*E*-isomer) is partly mesomerized to *Z*-entacapone. To a minor extent, only tolcapone, but not entacapone, is *O*-methylated by COMT, and metabolized by CYP3A4 and CYP2A6 to the corresponding alcohol and carboxylic acid metabolites [234].

Some MAO-B inhibitors were also introduced for the treatment of Parkinson's disease. CYP2B6 is the main enzyme responsible for the biotransformation of selegiline (L-deprenyl) – a selective and nonreversible MAO-B inhibitor – to L-(–)-methamphetamine and L-(–)-desmethylselegiline; CYP1A2 is also involved in selegiline *N*-demethylation, while CYP3A4 and CYP2C19 play a role in both pathways. The demethylated metabolite is further metabolized to L-amphetamine. The amphetamines are then *p*-hydroxylated at the benzene ring [235–238].

Rasagiline – the *R*-enantiomer of a racemic mixture and a selective MAO-B inhibitor – is *N*-dealkylated and hydroxylated by mainly CYP1A2 to 1(*R*)-aminoindan, and 3-OH-propargyl-1-aminoindan and 3-OH-1-aminoindan, respectively [239].

11.10
Conclusions

During recent years, there has been considerable development in our knowledge about the enzymes implicated in the biotransformation of central nervous system drugs, due to an increased awareness about the clinical relevance of pharmacogenetics and to progress in technological instruments facilitating drug analysis in the clinical context. Unfortunately, however, the metabolism of many classical central nervous system drugs was mainly studied before the individual CYP isoforms were known and their precise role remains to be elucidated. For newer drugs, important metabolites are not always available ubiquitously for comprehensive drug metabolism studies. Nevertheless, present knowledge about the metabolism of central nervous system drugs is of considerable clinical value, such as for the interpretation of drug–drug interactions and for nonresponse or adverse effects determined by a pharmacogenetic particularity in drug metabolism.

References

1 Baumann, P., Hiemke, C., Ulrich, S., Eckermann, G., Gaertner, I., Kuss, H.J., Laux, G., Müller-Oerlinghausen, B., Rao, M.L., Riederer, P., and Zernig, G. (2004) The AGNP-TDM expert group consensus guidelines: therapeutic drug monitoring in psychiatry. *Pharmacopsychiatry*, **37**, 243–265.

2 Hiemke, C., Baumann, P., Bergemann, N., Conca, A., Dietmaier, O., Egberts, K., Fric, M., Gerlach, M., Greiner, C., Gründer, G., Haen, E., Havemann-Reinecke, U., Jaquenoud Sirot, E., Kirchherr, H., Laux, G., Lutz, U.C., Messer, T., Müller, M.J., Pfuhlmann, B., Rambeck, B., Riederer, P., Schoppek, B., Stingl, J., Uhr, M., Ulrich, S., Waschgler, R., Zernig, G., and The TDM group of the AGNP (2011) AGNP consensus guidelines for therapeutic drug monitoring in psychiatry: update 2011. *Pharmacopsychiatry*, **44**, 195–235.

3 Johannessen, S.I. (2005) Can pharmacokinetic variability be controlled for the patient's benefit? The place of TDM for new AEDs. *Ther. Drug Monit.*, **27**, 710–713.

4 Zhou, S.F. (2009) Polymorphism of human cytochrome P450 2D6 and its clinical significance: part I. *Clin. Pharmacokinet.* **48**, 689–723.

5 Gardiner, S.J. and Begg, E.J. (2006) Pharmacogenetics, drug-metabolizing enzymes, and clinical practice. *Pharmacol. Rev.* **58**, 521–590.

6 Anzenbacher, P. and Anzenbacherova, E. (2001) Cytochromes P450 and metabolism of xenobiotics. *Cell. Mol. Life Sci.*, **58**, 737–747.

7 Desta, Z., Zhao, X., Shin, J.G., and Flockhart, D.A. (2002) Clinical significance of the cytochrome P450 2C19 genetic polymorphism. *Clin. Pharmacokinet.*, **41**, 913–958.

8 Wille, S.M., Cooreman, S.G., Neels, H.M., and Lambert, W.E. (2008) Relevant issues in the monitoring and the toxicology of antidepressants. *Crit. Rev. Clin. Lab. Sci.*, **45**, 25–89.

9 Pilgrim, J.L., Gerostamoulos, D., and Drummer, O.H. (2011) Review: pharmacogenetic aspects of the effect of cytochrome P450 polymorphisms on serotonergic drug metabolism, response, interactions, and adverse effects. *Forensic Sci. Med. Pathol.*, **7**, 162–184.

10 Kirchheiner, J., Nickchen, K., Bauer, M., Wong, M.L., Licinio, J., Roots, I., and Brockmöller, J. (2004) Pharmacogenetics of antidepressants and antipsychotics: the contribution of allelic variations to the phenotype of drug response. *Mol. Psychiatry*, **9**, 442–473.

11 Coutts, R.T., Su, P., and Baker, G.B. (1994) Involvement of CYP2D6, CYP3A4, and other cytochrome P-450 isozymes in *N*-dealkylation reactions. *J. Pharmacol. Toxicol. Methods*, **31**, 177–186.

12 Koyama, E., Tanaka, T., Chiba, K., Kawakatsu, S., Morinobu, S., Totsuka, S., and Ishizaki, T. (1996) Steady-state plasma concentrations of imipramine and desipramine in relation to *S*-mephenytoin 4′-hydroxylation status in Japanese depressive patients. *J. Clin. Psychopharmacol.*, **16**, 286–293.

13 Koyama, E., Chiba, K., Tani, M., and Ishizaki, T. (1997) Reappraisal of human CYP isoforms involved in imipramine *N*- demethylation and 2-hydroxylation: a study using microsomes obtained from putative extensive and poor metabolizers of *S*-mephenytoin and eleven

recombinant human CYPs. *J. Pharmacol. Exp. Ther.*, **281**, 1199–1210.

14 Koyama, E., Sohn, D.R., Shin, S.G., Chiba, K., Shin, J.G., Kim, Y.H., Echizen, H., and Ishizaki, T. (1994) Metabolic disposition of imipramine in oriental subjects: relation to metoprolol alpha-hydroxylation and *S*- mephenytoin 4′-hydroxylation phenotypes. *J. Pharmacol. Exp. Ther.*, **271**, 860–867.

15 Dahl, M.L., Bertilsson, L., and Nordin, C. (1996) Steady-state plasma levels of nortriptyline and its 10-hydroxy metabolite: relationship to the CYP2D6 genotype. *Psychopharmacology*, **123**, 315–319.

16 Breyer-Pfaff, U., Pfandl, B., Nill, K., Nusser, E., Monney, C., Jonzier-Perey, M., Baettig, D., and Baumann, P. (1992) Enantioselective amitriptyline metabolism in patients phenotyped for two cytochrome P450 isozymes. *Clin. Pharmacol. Ther.*, **52**, 350–358.

17 Breyer-Pfaff, U. (2004) The metabolic fate of amitriptyline, nortriptyline and amitriptylinoxide in man. *Drug Metab. Rev.*, **36**, 723–746.

18 Dalén, P., Dahl, M.L., Bernal Ruiz, M.L., Nordin, J., and Bertilsson, L. (1998) 10-Hydroxylation of nortriptyline in white persons with o, 1, 2, 3, and 13 functional CYP2D6 genes. *Clin. Pharmacol. Ther.*, **63**, 444–452.

19 Eap, C.B., Laurian, S., Souche, A., Koeb, L., Reymond, P., Buclin, T., and Baumann, P. (1992) Influence of quinidine on the pharmacokinetics of trimipramine and on its effect on the waking EEG of healthy volunteers – a pilot study on two subjects. *Neuropsychobiology*, **25**, 214–220.

20 Eap, C.B., Bender, S., Gastpar, M., Fischer, W., Haarmann, C., Powell, K., Jonzier-Perey, M., Cochard, N., and Baumann, P. (2000) Steady state plasma levels of the enantiomers of trimipramine and of its metabolites in CYP2D6-, CYP2C19- and CYP3A4/5-phenotyped patients. *Ther. Drug Monit.*, **22**, 209–214.

21 Gabris, G., Baumann, P., Jonzier-Perey, M., Bosshart, P., Woggon, B., and Küpfer, A. (1985) *N*-methylation of maprotiline in debrisoquine/mephenitoin-phenotyped depressive patients. *Biochem. Pharmacol.*, **34**, 409–410.

22 Firkusny, L. and Gleiter, C.H. (1994) Maprotiline metabolism appears to co-segregate with the genetically-determined CYP2D6 polymorphic hydroxylation of debrisoquine. *Br. J. Clin. Pharmacol.*, **37**, 383–388.

23 Brachtendorf, L., Jetter, A., Beckurts, K.T., Holscher, A.H., and Fuhr, U. (2002) Cytochrome P-450 enzymes contributing to demethylation of maprotiline in man. *Pharmacol. Toxicol.*, **90**, 144–149.

24 Chow, T., Hiroi, T., Imaoka, S., Chiba, K., and Funae, Y. (1999) Isoform-selective metabolism of mianserin by cytochrome p-450 2D. *Drug Metab. Dispos.*, **27**, 1200–1204.

25 Koyama, E., Chiba, K., Tani, M., and Ishizaki, T. (1996) Identification of human cytochrome P450 isoforms involved in the stereoselective metabolism of mianserin enantiomers. *J. Pharmacol. Exp. Ther.*, **278**, 21–30.

26 Dahl, M.L., Tybring, G., Elwin, C.E., Alm, C., Andreasson, K., Gyllenpalm, M., and Bertilsson, L. (1994) Stereoselective disposition of mianserin is related to debrisoquin hydroxylation polymorphism. *Clin. Pharmacol. Ther.*, **56**, 176–183.

27 Eap, C.B., de Mendonça Lima, C.A., Macciardi, F., Woggon, B., Powell, K., and Baumann, P. (1998) Steady state concentrations of the enantiomers of mianserin and desmethylmianserin in poor and in homozygous and heterozygous extensive metabolizers of debrisoquine. *Ther. Drug Monit.*, **20**, 7–13.

28 Dahl, M.L., Voortman, G., Alm, C., Elwin, C.E., Delbressine, L., Vos, R., Bogaards, J.J.P., and Bertilsson, L. (1997) *In vitro* and *in vivo* studies on the disposition of mirtazapine in humans. *Clin. Drug Invest.*, **13**, 37–46.

29 Timmer, C.J., Sitsen, J.M.A., and Delbressine, L.P. (2000) Clinical pharmacokinetics of mirtazapine. *Clin. Pharmacokinet.*, **38**, 461–474.

30 Lappenberg-Pelzer, M. (1998) Identification and determination of

opipramol metabolites in plasma and urine. *J. Anal. Toxicol.*, **22**, 215–219.

31 Muller, W.E. and Siebert, B. (1998) Opipramol im Vergleich zu anderen Therapeutika – Neue pharmakologische Daten. *Fortschr. Neurol. Psychiatry*, **66** (Suppl. 1), S9–S12.

32 Midha, K.K., Hubbard, J.W., McKay, G., Hawes, E.M., Korchinski, E.D., Gurnsey, T., Cooper, J.K., and Schwede, R. (1992) Stereoselective pharmacokinetics of doxepin isomers. *Eur. J. Clin. Pharmacol.*, **42**, 539–544.

33 Härtter, S., Tybring, G., Friedberg, T., Weigmann, H., and Hiemke, C. (2002) The *N*-demethylation of the doxepin isomers is mainly catalyzed by the polymorphic CYP2C19. *Pharm. Res.*, **19**, 1034–1037.

34 Kirchheiner, J., Meineke, I., Muller, G., Roots, I., and Brockmöller, J. (2002) Contributions of CYP2D6, CYP2C9 and CYP2C19 to the biotransformation of *E*- and *Z*-doxepin in healthy volunteers. *Pharmacogenetics*, **12**, 571–580.

35 Haritos, V.S., Ghabrial, H., Ahokas, J.T., and Ching, M.S. (2000) Role of cytochrome P450 2D6 (CYP2D6) in the stereospecific metabolism of *E*- and *Z*-doxepin. *Pharmacogenetics*, **10**, 591–603.

36 Heal, D., Cheetham, S., Martin, K., Browning, J., Luscombe, G., and Buckett, R. (1992) Comparative pharmacology of dothiepin, its metabolites, and other antidepressant drugs. *Drug Dev. Res.*, **27**, 121–136.

37 Maguire, K.P., Burrows, G.D., Norman, T.R., and Scoggins, B.A. (1981) Metabolism and pharmacokinetics of dothiepin. *Br. J. Clin. Pharmacol.*, **12**, 405–409.

38 Nakajima, M., Tanaka, E., Kobayashi, T., Ohashi, N., Kume, T., and Yokoi, T. (2002) Imipramine *N*-glucuronidation in human liver microsomes: biphasic kinetics and characterization of UDP-glucuronosyltransferase isoforms. *Drug Metab. Dispos.*, **30**, 636–642.

39 Liston, H.L., Markowitz, J.S., and DeVane, C.L. (2001) Drug glucuronidation in clinical psychopharmacology. *J. Clin. Psychopharmacol.*, **21**, 500–515.

40 Burchell, B. (1999) Transformation reactions: glucuronidation, in *Handbook of Drug Metabolism* (ed. T.F. Woolf), Dekker, New York, pp. 153–173.

41 Sanchez, C. (2006) The pharmacology of citalopram enantiomers: the antagonism by *R*-citalopram on the effect of *S*-citalopram. *Basic Clin. Pharmacol. Toxicol.*, **99**, 91–95.

42 Steinacher, L., Vandel, P., Zullino, D.F., Eap, C.B., Brawand-Amey, M., and Baumann, P. (2002) Carbamazepine augmentation in depressive patients non-responding to citalopram: a pharmacokinetic and clinical pilot study. *Eur. Neuropsychopharmacol.*, **12**, 255–260.

43 Kobayashi, K., Chiba, K., Yagi, T., Shimada, N., Taniguchi, T., Horie, T., Tani, M., Yamamoto, T., Ishizaki, T., and Kuroiwa, Y. (1997) Identification of cytochrome P450 isoforms involved in citalopram *N*-demethylation by human liver microsomes. *J. Pharmacol. Exp. Ther.*, **280**, 927–933.

44 Rochat, B., Amey, M., Gillet, M., Meyer, U.A., and Baumann, P. (1997) Identification of three cytochrome P450 isozymes involved in *N*-demethylation of citalopram enantiomers in human liver microsomes. *Pharmacogenetics*, **7**, 1–10.

45 Olesen, O.V. and Linnet, K. (1999) Studies on the stereoselective metabolism of citalopram by human liver microsomes and cDNA-expressed cytochrome P450 enzymes. *Pharmacology*, **59**, 298–309.

46 Sindrup, S.H., Brøsen, K., Hansen, M.G.J., Aaes-Jørgensen, T., Fredricson Overø, K., and Gram, L.F. (1993) Pharmacokinetics of citalopram in relation to the sparteine and the mephenytoin oxidation polymorphisms. *Ther. Drug Monit.*, **15**, 11–17.

47 Herrlin, K., Yasui-Furukori, N., Tybring, G., Widen, J., Gustafsson, L.L., and Bertilsson, L. (2003) Metabolism of citalopram enantiomers in CYP2C19/CYP2D6 phenotyped panels of healthy Swedes. *Br. J. Clin. Pharmacol.*, **56**, 415–421.

48 Rudberg, I., Reubsaet, J.L., Hermann, M., Refsum, H., and Molden, E. (2009)

Identification of a novel CYP2C19-mediated metabolic pathway of S-citalopram *in vitro*. *Drug Metab. Dispos.*, **37**, 2340–2348.

49 Kosel, M., Gnerre, C., Voirol, P., Amey, M., Rochat, B., Bouras, C., Testa, B., and Baumann, P. (2002) *In vitro* biotransformation of the selective serotonin reuptake inhibitor citalopram, its enantiomers and demethylated metabolites by monoamine oxidase in rat and human brain preparations. *Mol. Psychiatry*, **7**, 181–188.

50 Rochat, B., Kosel, M., Boss, G., Testa, B., Gillet, M., and Baumann, P. (1998) Stereoselective biotransformation of the selective serotonin reuptake inhibitor, citalopram, and its demethylated metabolites by monoamine oxidases in human liver. *Biochem. Pharmacol.*, **56**, 15–23.

51 Kosel, M., Amey, M., Aubert, A.C., and Baumann, P. (2001) *In vitro* metabolism of citalopram by monoamine oxidase B in human blood. *Eur. Neuropsychopharmacol.*, **11**, 75–78.

52 Von Moltke, L.L., Greenblatt, D.J., Duan, S.X., Schmider, J., Wright, C.E., Harmatz, J.S., and Shader, R.I. (1997) Human cytochromes mediating *N*-demethylation of fluoxetine *in vitro*. *Psychopharmacology*, **132**, 402–407.

53 Hamelin, B.A., Turgeon, J., Vallée, F., Bélanger, P.M., Paquet, F., and Lebel, M. (1996) The disposition of fluoxetine but not sertraline is altered in poor metabolizers of debrisoquin. *Clin. Pharmacol. Ther.*, **60**, 512–521.

54 Liu, Z.Q., Shu, Y., Huang, S.L., Wang, L.S., He, N., and Zhou, H.H. (2001) Effects of CYP2C19 genotype and CYP2C9 on fluoxetine *N*-demethylation in human liver macrosomes. *Acta Pharmacol. Sin.*, **22**, 85–90.

55 Scordo, M.G., Spina, E., Dahl, M.L., Gatti, G., and Perucca, E. (2005) Influence of CYP2C9, 2C19 and 2D6 genetic polymorphisms on the steady-state plasma concentrations of the enantiomers of fluoxetine and norfluoxetine. *Basic Clin. Pharmacol. Toxicol.*, **97**, 296–301.

56 Fjordside, L., Jeppesen, U., Eap, C.B., Powell, K., Baumann, P., and Brøsen, K. (1999) The stereoselective metabolism of fluoxetine in poor and extensive metabolizers of sparteine. *Pharmacogenetics*, **9**, 55–60.

57 Spigset, O., Granberg, K., Hägg, S., Söderström, E., and Dahlqvist, R. (1998) Non-linear fluvoxamine disposition. *Br. J. Clin. Pharmacol.*, **45**, 257–263.

58 Carrillo, J.A., Dahl, M.L., Svensson, J.O., Alm, C., Rodriguez, I., and Bertilsson, L. (1996) Disposition of fluvoxamine in humans is determined by the polymorphic CYP2D6 and also by the CYP1A2 activity. *Clin. Pharmacol. Ther.*, **60**, 183–190.

59 Spigset, O., Hägg, S., Söderström, E., and Dahlqvist, R. (1999) Lack of correlation between fluvoxamine clearance and CYP1A2 activity as measured by systemic caffeine clearance. *Eur. J. Clin. Pharmacol.*, **54**, 943–946.

60 Spigset, O., Axelsson, S., Norstrom, A., Hagg, S., and Dahlqvist, R. (2001) The major fluvoxamine metabolite in urine is formed by CYP2D6. *Eur. J. Clin. Pharmacol.*, **57**, 653–658.

61 Jann, M.W., Zumbrunnen, T.L., Kazmi, Y.R., VanDenBerg, C.M., Desai, H.D., Weidler, D.J., and Flockhart, D.A. (2002) Pharmacokinetics of fluvoxamine in relation to CYP2C19 phenotype and genotype. *Drug Metab. Drug Interact.*, **19**, 1–11.

62 Sindrup, S.H., Brøsen, K., Gram, L.F., Hallas, J., Skjelbo, E., Allen, A., Allen, G.D., Cooper, S.M., Mellows, G., Tasker, T.C.G., and Zussman, B.D. (1992) The relationship between paroxetine and the sparteine oxidation polymorphism. *Clin. Pharmacol. Ther.*, **51**, 278–287.

63 Bloomer, J.C., Woods, F.R., Haddock, R.E., Lennard, M.S., and Tucker, G.T. (1992) The role of cytochrome P4502D6 in the metabolism of paroxetine by human liver microsomes. *Br. J. Clin. Pharmacol.*, **33**, 521–523.

64 Bertelsen, K.M., Venkatakrishnan, K., Von Moltke, L.L., Obach, R.S., and Greenblatt, D.J. (2003) Apparent mechanism-based inhibition of human CYP2D6 *in vitro* by paroxetine: comparison with fluoxetine and

quinidine. *Drug Metab. Dispos.*, **31**, 289–293.

65 Kobayashi, K., Ishizuka, T., Shimada, N., Yoshimura, Y., Kamijima, K., and Chiba, K. (1999) Sertraline *N*-demethylation is catalyzed by multiple isoforms of human cytochrome P-450 *in vitro*. *Drug Metab. Dispos.*, **27**, 763–766.

66 Greenblatt, D.J., Von Moltke, L.L., Harmatz, J.S., and Shader, R.I. (1999) Human cytochromes mediating sertraline biotransformation: seeking attribution. *J. Clin. Psychopharmacol.*, **19**, 489–493.

67 Xu, Z.H., Wang, W., Zhao, X.J., Huang, S.L., Zhu, B., He, N., Shu, Y., Liu, Z.Q., and Zhou, H.H. (1999) Evidence for involvement of polymorphic CYP2C19 and 2C9 in the *N*-demethylation of sertraline in human liver microsomes. *Br. J. Clin. Pharmacol.*, **48**, 416–423.

68 Obach, R.S., Cox, L.M., and Tremaine, L.M. (2005) Sertraline is metabolized by multiple cytochrome P450 enzymes, monoamine oxidases, and glucuronyl transferases in human: an *in vitro* study. *Drug Metab. Dispos.*, **33**, 262–270.

69 DeVane, C.L., Liston, H.L., and Markowitz, J.S. (2002) Clinical pharmacokinetics of sertraline. *Clin. Pharmacokinet.*, **41**, 1247–1266.

70 Von Moltke, L.L., Greenblatt, D.J., Granda, B.W., Grassi, J.M., Schmider, J., Harmatz, J.S., and Shader, R.I. (1999) Nefazodone, meta-chlorophenylpiperazine, and their metabolites *in vitro*: cytochromes mediating transformation, and P450-3A4 inhibitory actions. *Psychopharmacology*, **145**, 113–122.

71 Barbhaiya, R.H., Buch, A.B., and Greene, D.S. (1996) Single and multiple dose pharmacokinetics of nefazodone in subjects classified as extensive and poor metabolizers of dextromethorphan. *Br. J. Clin. Pharmacol.*, **42**, 573–581.

72 Zalma, A., Von Moltke, L.L., Granda, B.W., Harmatz, J.S., Shader, R.I., and Greenblatt, D.J. (2000) *In vitro* metabolism of trazodone by CYP3A: inhibition by ketoconazole and human immunodeficiency viral protease inhibitors. *Biol. Psychiatry*, **47**, 655–661.

73 Lantz, R.J., Gillespie, T.A., Rash, T.J., Kuo, F., Skinner, M., Kuan, H.Y., and Knadler, M.P. (2003) Metabolism, excretion, and pharmacokinetics of duloxetine in healthy human subjects. *Drug Metab. Dispos.*, **31**, 1142–1150.

74 Skinner, M.H., Kuan, H.Y., Pan, A., Sathirakul, K., Knadler, M.P., Gonzales, C.R., Yeo, K.P., Reddy, S., Lim, M., Ayan-Oshodi, M., and Wise, S.D. (2003) Duloxetine is both an inhibitor and a substrate of cytochrome P4502D6 in healthy volunteers. *Clin. Pharmacol. Ther.*, **73**, 170–177.

75 Fogelman, S.M., Schmider, J., Venkatakrishnan, K., Von Moltke, L.L., Harmatz, J.S., Shader, R.I., and Greenblatt, D.J. (1999) *O*- and *N*-demethylation of venlafaxine *in vitro* by human liver microsomes and by microsomes from cDNA-transfected cells: effect of metabolic inhibitors and SSRI antidepressants. *Neuropsychopharmacology*, **20**, 480–490.

76 Lessard, E., Yessine, M.A., Hamelin, B.A., O'Hara, G., LeBlanc, J., and Turgeon, J. (1999) Influence of CYP2D6 activity on the disposition and cardiovascular toxicity of the antidepressant agent venlafaxine in humans. *Pharmacogenetics*, **9**, 435–443.

77 Veefkind, A.H., Haffmans, P.M.J., and Hoencamp, E. (2000) Venlafaxine serum levels and CYP2D6 genotype. *Ther. Drug Monit.*, **22**, 202–208.

78 Otton, S.V., Ball, S.E., Cheung, S.W., Inaba, T., Rudolph, R.L., and Sellers, E.M. (1996) Venlafaxine oxidation *in vitro* is catalysed by CYP2D6. *Br. J. Clin. Pharmacol.*, **41**, 149–156.

79 Eap, C.B., Bertel-Laubscher, R., Zullino, D., Amey, M., and Baumann, P. (2000) Marked increase of venlafaxine enantiomer concentrations as a consequence of metabolic interactions: a case report. *Pharmacopsychiatry*, **33**, 112–115.

80 Eap, C.B., Lessard, E., Baumann, P., Brawand-Amey, M., Yessine, M.A., O'Hara, G., and Turgeon, J. (2003) Role of CYP2D6 in the stereoselective

disposition of venlafaxine in humans. *Pharmacogenetics*, **13**, 39–47.

81 Fukuda, T., Yamamoto, I., Nishida, Y., Zhou, Q., Ohno, M., Takada, K., and Azuma, J. (1999) Effect of the CYP2D6*10 genotype on venlafaxine pharmacokinetics in healthy adult volunteers. *Br. J. Clin. Pharmacol.*, **47**, 450–453.

82 Sopko, M.A., Jr, Ehret, M.J., and Grgas, M. (2008) Desvenlafaxine: another "me too" drug? *Ann. Pharmacother.*, **42**, 1439–1446.

83 Pollock, B.G., Sweet, R.A., Kirshner, M., and Reynolds, C.F., III (1996) Bupropion plasma levels and CYP2D6 phenotype. *Ther. Drug Monit.*, **18**, 581–585.

84 Hesse, L.M., Venkatakrishnan, K., Court, M.H., Von Moltke, L.L., Duan, S.X., Shader, R.I., and Greenblatt, D.J. (2000) CYP2B6 mediates the *in vitro* hydroxylation of bupropion: potential drug interactions with other antidepressants. *Drug Metab. Dispos.*, **28**, 1176–1183.

85 Kirchheiner, J., Klein, C., Meineke, I., Sasse, J., Zanger, U.M., Murdter, T.E., Roots, I., and Brockmöller, J. (2003) Bupropion and 4-OH-bupropion pharmacokinetics in relation to genetic polymorphisms in CYP2B6. *Pharmacogenetics*, **13**, 619–626.

86 Golden, R.N., De Vane, C.L., Laizure, S.C., Rudorfer, M.V., Sherer, M.A., and Potter, W.Z. (1988) Bupropion in depression. II. The role of metabolites in clinical outcome. *Arch. Gen. Psychiatry*, **45**, 145–149.

87 Spencer, C.M. and Wilde, M.I. (1998) Milnacipran – a review of its use in depression. *Drugs*, **56**, 405–427.

88 Puozzo, C., Lens, S., Reh, C., Michaelis, K., Rosillon, D., Deroubaix, X., and Deprez, D. (2005) Lack of interaction of milnacipran with the cytochrome p450 isoenzymes frequently involved in the metabolism of antidepressants. *Clin. Pharmacokinet.*, **44**, 977–988.

89 Davi, H., Bonnet, J.M., and Berger, Y. (1992) Disposition of minaprine in animals and in human extensive and limited debrisoquine hydroxylators. *Xenobiotica*, **22**, 171–184.

90 Herman, B.D., Fleishaker, J.C., and Brown, M.T. (1999) Ketoconazole inhibits the clearance of the enantiomers of the antidepressant reboxetine in humans. *Clin. Pharmacol. Ther.*, **66**, 374–379.

91 de Bodinat, C., Guardiola-Lemaitre, B., Mocaer, E., Renard, P., Munoz, C., and Millan, M.J. (2010) Agomelatine, the first melatonergic antidepressant: discovery, characterization and development. *Nat. Rev. Drug Discov.*, **9**, 628–642.

92 Bogaards, J.J., *et al.* (2000) Prediction of interindividual variation in drug plasma levels in vivo from individual enzyme kinetic data and physiologically based pharmacokinetic modeling. *Eur. J. Pharm. Sci.*, **12**, 117–124.

93 Gurley, B.J., Swain, A., Hubbard, M.A., Williams, D.K., Barone, G., Hartsfield, F., Tong, Y., Carrier, D.J., Cheboyina, S., and Battu, S.K. (2008) Clinical assessment of CYP2D6-mediated herb–drug interactions in humans: effects of milk thistle, black cohosh, goldenseal, kava kava, St. John's wort, and Echinacea. *Mol. Nutr. Food Res.*, **52**, 755–763.

94 Baker, G.B., Urichuk, L.J., McKenna, K.F., and Kennedy, S.H. (1999) Metabolism of monoamine oxidase inhibitors. *Cell. Mol. Neurobiol.*, **19**, 411–426.

95 Malllinger, A.G. and Smith, E. (1991) Pharmacokinetics of monoamine oxidase inhibitors. *Psychopharmacol. Bull.*, **27**, 493–502.

96 Schoerlin, M.P., Blouin, R.A., Pfefen, J.P., and Guentert, T.W. (1990) Comparison of the pharmacokinetics of moclobemide in poor and efficient metabolizers of debrisoquine. *Acta Psychiatr. Scand.*, **360** (Suppl.), 98–100.

97 Gram, L.F., Guentert, T.W., Grange, S., Vistisen, K., and Brøsen, K. (1995) Moclobemide, a substrate of CYP2C19 and an inhibitor of CYP2C19, CYP2D6, and CYP1A2: a panel study. *Clin. Pharmacol. Ther.*, **57**, 670–677.

98 Härtter, S., Dingemanse, J., Baier, D., Ziegler, G., and Hiemke, C. (1996) The role of cytochrome P450 2D6 in the

metabolism of moclobemide. *Eur. Neuropsychopharmacol.*, **6**, 225–230.

99 Mayersohn, M. and Guentert, T.W. (1995) Clinical pharmacokinetics of the monoamine oxidase-A inhibitor moclobemide. *Clin. Pharmacokinet.*, **29**, 292–332.

100 Hoskins, J., Shenfield, G., Murray, M., and Gross, A. (2001) Characterization of moclobemide *N*-oxidation in human liver microsomes. *Xenobiotica*, **31**, 387–397.

101 Mauri, M.C., Volonteri, L.S., Colasanti, A., Fiorentini, A., De Gaspari, I.F., and Bareggi, S.R. (2007) Clinical pharmacokinetics of atypical antipsychotics: a critical review of the relationship between plasma concentrations and clinical response. *Clin. Pharmacokinet.*, **46**, 359–388.

102 Caccia, S. (2002) New antipsychotic agents for schizophrenia: pharmacokinetics and metabolism update. *Curr. Opin. Investig. Drugs*, **3**, 1073–1080.

103 Yeung, P.K.F., Hubbard, J.W., Korchinski, E.D., and Midha, K.K. (1993) Pharmacokinetics of chlorpromazine and key metabolites. *Eur. J. Clin. Pharmacol.*, **45**, 563–569.

104 Muralidharan, G., Cooper, J.K., Hawes, E.M., Korchinski, E.D., and Midha, K.K. (1996) Quinidine inhibits the 7-hydroxylation of chlorpromazine in extensive metabolisers of debrisoquine. *Eur. J. Clin. Pharmacol.*, **50**, 121–128.

105 Bagli, M., Höflich, G., Rao, M.L., Langer, M., Baumann, P., Kolbinger, M., Barlage, U., Kasper, S., and Möller, H.J. (1995) Bioequivalence and absolute bioavailability of oblong and coated levomepromazine tablets in CYP2D6 phenotyped subjects. *Int. J. Clin. Pharmacol. Ther.*, **33**, 646–652.

106 Dahl-Puustinen, M.L., Lidén, A., Alm, C., Nordin, C., and Bertilsson, L. (1989) Disposition of perphenazine is related to polymorphic debrisoquin hydroxylation in human beings. *Clin. Pharmacol. Ther.*, **46**, 78–81.

107 Linnet, K. and Wiborg, O. (1996) Steady-state serum concentrations of the neuroleptic perphenazine in relation to CYP2D6 genetic polymorphism. *Clin. Pharmacol. Ther.*, **60**, 41–47.

108 von Bahr, C., Movin, G., Nordin, C., Lidén, A., Hammarlund-Udenaes, M., Hedberg, A., Ring, H., and Sjöqvist, F. (1991) Plasma levels of thioridazine and metabolites are influenced by the debrisoquin hydroxylation phenotype. *Clin. Pharmacol. Ther.*, **49**, 234–240.

109 Meyer, J.W., Woggon, B., Baumann, P., and Meyer, U.A. (1990) Clinical implication of slow sulphoxidation of thioridazine in a poor metabolizer of the debrisoquine type. *Eur. J. Clin. Pharmacol.*, **39**, 613–614.

110 Eap, C.B., Guentert, T.W., Schäublin-Loidl, M., Stabl, M., Koeb, L., Powell, K., and Baumann, P. (1996) Plasma levels of the enantiomers of thioridazine, thioridazine 2-sulfoxide, thioridazine 2-sulfone, and thioridazine 5-sulfoxide in poor and extensive metabolizers of dextromethorphan and mephenytoin. *Clin. Pharmacol. Ther.*, **59**, 322–331.

111 Wojcikowski, J., Maurel, P., and Daniel, W.A. (2006) Characterization of human cytochrome p450 enzymes involved in the metabolism of the piperidine-type phenothiazine neuroleptic thioridazine. *Drug Metab. Dispos.*, **34**, 471–476.

112 Wojcikowski, J., Pichard-Garcia, L., Maurel, P., and Daniel, W.A. (2004) The metabolism of the piperazine-type phenothiazine neuroleptic perazine by the human cytochrome P-450 isoenzymes. *Eur. Neuropsychopharmacol.*, **14**, 199–208.

113 Dahl, M.L., Ekqvist, B., Widén, J., and Bertilsson, L. (1991) Disposition of the neuroleptic zuclopenthixol cosegregates with the polymorphic hydroxylation of debrisoquine in humans. *Acta Psychiatr. Scand.*, **84**, 99–102.

114 Eyles, D.W., McGrath, J.J., Stedman, T.J., and Pond, S.M. (1998) Chirality of reduced haloperidol in humans. *Eur. Neuropsychopharmacol.*, **8**, 127–129.

115 Kudo, S. and Ishizaki, T. (1999) Pharmacokinetics of haloperidol – an update. *Clin. Pharmacokinet.*, **37**, 435–456.

116 Llerena, A., Alm, C., Dahl, M.L., Ekqvist, B., and Bertilsson, L. (1992) Haloperidol disposition is dependent on

debrisoquine hydroxylation phenotype. *Ther. Drug Monit.*, **14**, 92–97.

117 Desai, M., Tanus-Santos, J.E., Li, L., Gorski, J.C., Arefayene, M., Liu, Y., Desta, Z., and Flockhart, D.A. (2003) Pharmacokinetics and QT interval pharmacodynamics of oral haloperidol in poor and extensive metabolizers of CYP2D6. *Pharmacogenomics J.*, **3**, 105–113.

118 Llerena, A., Dahl, M.L., Ekqvist, B., and Bertilsson, L. (1992) Haloperidol disposition is dependent on the debrisoquine hydroxylation phenotype–increased plasma levels of the reduced metabolite in poor metabolizers. *Ther. Drug Monit.*, **14**, 261–264.

119 Lane, H.Y., Hu, O.Y.P., Jann, M.W., Deng, H.C., Lin, H.N., and Chang, W.H. (1997) Dextromethorphan phenotyping and haloperidol disposition in schizophrenic patients. *Psychiatry Res.*, **69**, 105–111.

120 Mihara, K., Suzuki, A., Kondo, T., Yasui, N., Furukori, H., Nagashima, U., Otani, K., Kaneko, S., and Inoue, Y. (1999) Effects of the CYP2D6*10 allele on the steady-state plasma concentrations of haloperidol and reduced haloperidol in Japanese patients with schizophrenia. *Clin. Pharmacol. Ther.*, **65**, 291–294.

121 Desta, Z., Kerbusch, T., Soukhova, N., Richard, E., Ko, J.W., and Flockhart, D.A. (1998) Identification and characterization of human cytochrome P450 isoforms interacting with pimozide. *J. Pharmacol. Exp. Ther.*, **285**, 428–437.

122 Desta, Z., Kerbusch, T., and Flockhart, D.A. (1999) Effect of clarithromycin on the pharmacokinetics and pharmacodynamics of pimozide in healthy poor and extensive metabolizers of cytochrome P450 2D6 (CYP2D6). *Clin. Pharmacol. Ther.*, **65**, 10–20.

123 Fischer, V., Vogels, B., Maurer, G., and Tynes, R.E. (1992) The antipsychotic clozapine is metabolized by the polymorphic human microsomal and recombinant cytochrome P450 2D6. *J. Pharmacol. Exp. Ther.*, **260**, 1355–1360.

124 Olesen, O.V. and Linnet, K. (2000) Fluvoxamine–clozapine drug interaction: inhibition *in vitro* of five cytochrome P450 isoforms involved in clozapine metabolism. *J. Clin. Psychopharmacol.*, **20**, 35–42.

125 Eiermann, B., Engel, G., Johansson, I., Zanger, U.M., and Bertilsson, L. (1997) The involvement of CYP1A2 and CYP3A4 in the metabolism of clozapine. *Br. J. Clin. Pharmacol.*, **44**, 439–446.

126 Linnet, K. and Olesen, O.V. (1997) Metabolism of clozapine by cDNA-expressed human cytochrome P450 enzymes. *Drug Metab. Dispos.*, **25**, 1379–1382.

127 Wetzel, H., Anghelescu, I., Szegedi, A., Wiesner, J., Weigmann, H., Härtter, S., and Hiemke, C. (1998) Pharmacokinetic interactions of clozapine with selective serotonin reuptake inhibitors: differential effects of fluvoxamine and paroxetine in a prospective study. *J. Clin. Psychopharmacol.*, **18**, 2–9.

128 Dahl, M.L., Llerena, A., Bondesson, U., Lindström, L., and Bertilsson, L. (1994) Disposition of clozapine in man–lack of association with debrisoquine and *S*-mephenytoin hydroxylation polymorphisms. *Br. J. Clin. Pharmacol.*, **37**, 71–74.

129 Jaquenoud Sirot, E., Knezevic, B., Morena, G.P., Harenberg, S., Oneda, B., Crettol, S., Ansermot, N., Baumann, P., and Eap, C.B. (2009) ABCB1 and cytochrome P450 polymorphisms: clinical pharmacogenetics of clozapine. *J. Clin. Psychopharmacol.*, **29**, 319–326

130 Ring, B.J., Catlow, J., Lindsay, T.J., Gillespie, T., Roskos, L.K., Cerimele, B.J., Swanson, S.P., Hamman, M.A., and Wrighton, S.A. (1996) Identification of the human cytochromes P450 responsible for the *in vitro* formation of the major oxidative metabolites of the antipsychotic agent olanzapine. *J. Pharmacol. Exp. Ther.*, **276**, 658–666.

131 Shirley, K.L., Hon, Y.Y., Penzak, S.R., Lam, Y.W., Spratlin, V., and Jann, M.W. (2003) Correlation of cytochrome P450 (CYP) 1A2 activity using caffeine phenotyping and olanzapine disposition in healthy volunteers. *Neuropsychopharmacology*, **28**, 961–966.

132 Carrillo, J.A., Herraiz, A.G., Ramos, S.I., Gervasini, G., Vizcaino, S., and Benitez, J. (2003) Role of the smoking-induced cytochrome P450 (CYP)1A2 and polymorphic CYP2D6 in steady-state concentration of olanzapine. *J. Clin. Psychopharmacol.*, **23**, 119–127.

133 Huang, M.L., Van Peer, A., Woestenborghs, R., De Coster, R., Heykants, J., Jansen, A.A.I., Zylicz, Z., Visscher, H.W., and Jonkman, J.H.G. (1993) Pharmacokinetics of the novel antipsychotic agent risperidone and the prolactin response in healthy subjects. *Clin. Pharmacol. Ther.*, **54**, 257–268.

134 Fang, J., Bourin, M., and Baker, G.B. (1999) Metabolism of risperidone to 9-hydroxyrisperidone by human cytochromes P450 2D6 and 3A4. *Naunyn Schmiedebergs Arch. Pharmacol.*, **359**, 147–151.

135 Scordo, M.G., Spina, E., Facciolà, G., Avenoso, A., Johansson, I., and Dahl, M.L. (1999) Cytochrome P450 2D6 genotype and steady state plasma levels of risperidone and 9-hydroxyrisperidone. *Psychopharmacology*, **147**, 300–305.

136 Yasui-Furukori, N., Hidestrand, M., Spina, E., Facciolà, G., Scordo, M.G., and Tybring, G. (2001) Different enantioselective 9-hydroxylation of risperidone by the two human CYP2D6 and CYP3A4 enzymes. *Drug Metab. Dispos.*, **29**, 1263–1268.

137 Nyberg, S., Dahl, M.L., and Halldin, C. (1995) A PET study of D_2 and 5-HT_2 receptor occupancy induced by risperidone in poor metabolizers of debrisoquin and risperidone. *Psychopharmacology*, **119**, 345–348.

138 Vermeir, M., Naessens, I., Remmerie, B., Mannens, G., Hendrickx, J., Sterkens, P., Talluri, K., Boom, S., Eerdekens, M., van Osselaer, N., and Cleton, A. (2008) Absorption, metabolism, and excretion of paliperidone, a new monoaminergic antagonist, in humans. *Drug Metab. Dispos.*, **36**, 769–779.

139 Jung, S.M., Kim, K.A., Cho, H.K., Jung, I.G., Park, P.W., Byun, W.T., and Park, J.Y. (2005) Cytochrome P450 3A inhibitor itraconazole affects plasma concentrations of risperidone and 9-hydroxyrisperidone in schizophrenic patients. *Clin. Pharmacol. Ther.*, **78**, 520–528.

140 Bork, J.A., Rogers, T., Wedlund, P.J., and De Leon, J. (1999) A pilot study on risperidone metabolism: the role of cytochromes P450 2D6 and 3A. *J. Clin. Psychiatry*, **60**, 469–476.

141 Olesen, O.V., Licht, R.W., Thomsen, E., Bruun, T., Viftrup, J.E., and Linnet, K. (1998) Serum concentrations and side effects in psychiatric patients during risperidone therapy. *Ther. Drug Monit.*, **20**, 380–384.

142 Dlugosz, H., Nasrallah, H.A., Dlugosz, H., and Nasrallah, H.A. (2007) Paliperidone: a new extended-release oral atypical antipsychotic. *Expert Opin. Pharmacother.*, **8**, 2307–2313.

143 Prakash, C., Kamel, A., Cui, D., Whalen, R.D., Miceli, J.J., and Tweedie, D. (2000) Identification of the major human liver cytochrome P450 isoform(s) responsible for the formation of the primary metabolites of ziprasidone and prediction of possible drug interactions. *Br. J. Clin. Pharmacol.*, **49** (Suppl. 1), 35S–42S.

144 Prakash, C., Kamel, A., Gummerus, J., and Wilner, K. (1997) Metabolism and excretion of a new antipsychotic drug, ziprasidone, in humans. *Drug Metab. Dispos.*, **25**, 863–872.

145 Gunasekara, N.S., Spencer, C.M., and Keating, G.M. (2002) Ziprasidone: a review of its use in schizophrenia and schizoaffective disorder. *Drugs*, **62**, 1217–1251.

146 Beedham, C., Miceli, J.J., and Obach, R.S. (2003) Ziprasidone metabolism, aldehyde oxidase, and clinical implications. *J. Clin. Psychopharmacol.*, **23**, 229–232.

147 Shiraga, T., Kaneko, H., Iwasaki, K., Tozuka, Z., Suzuki, A., and Hata, T. (1999) Identification of cytochrome P450 enzymes involved in the metabolism of zotepine, an antipsychotic drug, in human liver microsomes. *Xenobiotica*, **29**, 217–229.

148 Kondo, T., Tanaka, O., Otani, K., Mihara, K., Tokinaga, N., Kaneko, S.,

Chiba, K., and Ishizaki, T. (1996) Possible inhibitory effect of diazepam on the metabolism of zotepine, an antipsychotic drug. *Psychopharmacology*, **127**, 311–314.

149 Gunasekara, N.S. and Spencer, C.M. (1998) Quetiapine – a review of its use in schizophrenia. *CNS Drugs*, **9**, 325–340.

150 Jensen, N.H., Rodriguiz, R.M., Caron, M.G., Wetsel, W.C., Rothman, R.B., and Roth, B.L. (2008) *N*-desalkylquetiapine, a potent norepinephrine reuptake inhibitor and partial 5-HT_{1A} agonist, as a putative mediator of quetiapine's antidepressant activity. *Neuropsychopharmacology*, **33**, 2303–2312.

151 DeVane, C.L. and Nemeroff, C.B. (2001) Clinical pharmacokinetics of quetiapine – an atypical antipsychotic. *Clin. Pharmacokinet.*, **40**, 509–522.

152 Grimm, S.W., Richtand, N.M., Winter, H.R., Stams, K.R., and Reele, S.B. (2005) Effects of cytochrome P450 3A modulators ketoconazole and carbamazepine on quetiapine pharmacokinetics. *Br. J. Clin. Pharmacol.*, **61**, 58–69.

153 Wong, S.L., Menacherry, S., Mulford, D., Schmitz, P.J., Locke, C., and Granneman, G.R. (1997) Pharmacokinetics of sertindole and dehydrosertindole in volunteers with normal or impaired renal function. *Eur. J. Clin. Pharmacol.*, **52**, 223–227.

154 Coukell, A.J., Spencer, C.M., and Benfield, P. (1996) Amisulpride – a review of its pharmacodynamic and pharmacokinetic properties and therapeutic efficacy in the management of schizophrenia. *CNS Drugs*, **6**, 237–256.

155 Kubo, M., Koue, T., Inaba, A., Takeda, H., Maune, H., Fukuda, T., and Azuma, J. (2005) Influence of itraconazole co-administration and CYP2D6 genotype on the pharmacokinetics of the new antipsychotic ARIPIPRAZOLE. *Drug Metab. Pharmacokinet.*, **20**, 55–64.

156 Weber, J. and McCormack, P.L. (2009) Asenapine. *CNS Drugs*, **23**, 781–792.

157 Mutlib, A.E., Strupczewski, J.T., and Chesson, S.M. (1995) Application of hyphenated LC/NMR and LC/MS techniques in rapid identification of *in vitro* and *in vivo* metabolites of iloperidone. *Drug Metab. Dispos.*, **23**, 951–964.

158 Citrome, L. (2010) Iloperidone: chemistry, pharmacodynamics, pharmacokinetics and metabolism, clinical efficacy, safety and tolerability, regulatory affairs, and an opinion. *Expert Opin. Drug Metab. Toxicol.*, **6**, 1551–1564.

159 Bertilsson, L. and Dahl, M.L. (1996) Polymorphic drug oxidation – relevance to the treatment of psychiatric disorders. *CNS Drugs*, **5**, 200–223.

160 Inomata, S., Nagashima, A., Itagaki, F., Homma, M., Nishimura, M., Osaka, Y., Okuyama, K., Tanaka, E., Nakamura, T., Kohda, Y., Naito, S., Miyabe, M., and Toyooka, H. (2005) CYP2C19 genotype affects diazepam pharmacokinetics and emergence from general anesthesia. *Clin. Pharmacol. Ther.*, **78**, 647–655.

161 Bertilsson, L., Henthorn, T.K., Sanz, E., Tybring, G., Säwe, J., and Villén, T. (1989) Importance of genetic factors in the regulation of diazepam metabolism: relationship to *S*-mephenytoin, but not debrisoquin, hydroxylation phenotype. *Clin. Pharmacol. Ther.*, **45**, 348–355.

162 Zhang, Y., Reviriego, J., Lou, Y.Q., Sjöqvist, F., and Bertilsson, L. (1990) Diazepam metabolism in native Chinese poor and extensive hydroxylators of *S*-mephenytoin: interethnic differences in comparison with white subjects. *Pharmacol. Ther.*, **48**, 496–502.

163 Klotz, U. (2007) The role of pharmacogenetics in the metabolism of antiepileptic drugs: pharmacokinetic and therapeutic implications. *Clin. Pharmacokinet.*, **46**, 271–279.

164 Griebel, G. (1999) Is there a future for neuropeptide receptor ligands in the treatment of anxiety disorders? *Pharmacol. Ther.*, **82**, 1–61.

165 Gafni, I., Busto, U.E., Tyndale, R.F., Kaplan, H.L., and Sellers, E.M. (2003) The role of cytochrome P450 2C19 activity in flunitrazepam metabolism *in vivo*. *J. Clin. Psychopharmacol.*, **23**, 169–175.

166 Parmeggiani, A., Posar, A., Sangiorgi, S., and Giovanardi-Rossi, P. (2004) Unusual side-effects due to clobazam: a case report with genetic study of CYP2C19. *Brain Dev.*, **26**, 63–66.

167 Court, M.H., Hao, Q., Krishnaswamy, S., Bekaii-Saab, T., Al Rohaimi, A., Von Moltke, L.L., and Greenblatt, D.J. (2004) UDP-glucuronosyltransferase (UGT) 2B15 pharmacogenetics: UGT2B15 D85Y genotype and gender are major determinants of oxazepam glucuronidation by human liver. *J. Pharmacol. Exp. Ther.*, **310**, 656–665.

168 Kronbach, T., Mathys, D., Umeno, M., Gonzalez, F.J., and Meyer, U.A. (1989) Oxidation of midazolam and triazolam by human liver cytochrome P450IIIA4. *Mol. Pharmacol.*, **36**, 89–96.

169 Greenblatt, D.J., Von Moltke, L.L., Harmatz, J.S., Ciraulo, D.A., and Shader, R.I. (1993) Alprazolam pharmacokinetics, metabolism, and plasma levels: clinical implications. *J. Clin. Psychiatry*, **54**, 4–14.

170 Gorski, J.C., Jones, D.R., Hamman, M.A., Wrighton, S.A., and Hall, S.D. (1999) Biotransformation of alprazolam by members of the human cytochrome P4503A subfamily. *Xenobiotica*, **29**, 931–944.

171 Fukasawa, T., Yasui-Furukori, N., Aoshima, T., Suzuki, A., Tateishi, T., and Otani, K. (2004) Single oral dose pharmacokinetics of quazepam is influenced by CYP2C19 activity. *Ther. Drug Monit.*, **26**, 529–533.

172 Suzuki, Y., Shioiri, T., Muratake, T., Kawashima, Y., Sato, S., Hagiwara, M., Inoue, Y., Shimoda, K., and Someya, T. (2003) Effects of concomitant fluvoxamine on the metabolism of alprazolam in Japanese psychiatric patients: interaction with CYP2C19 mutated alleles. *Eur. J. Clin. Pharmacol.*, **58**, 829–833.

173 Eap, C.B., Buclin, T., Hustert, E., Bleiber, G., Powell Golay, K., Aubert, A.C., Baumann, P., Telenti, A., and Kerb, R. (2004) Pharmacokinetics of midazolam in CYP3A4–and CYP3A5-genotyped subjects. *Eur. J. Clin. Pharmacol.*, **60**, 231–236.

174 Yasui, N., Otani, K., Ohkubo, T., Osanai, T., Sugawara, K., Chiba, K., Ishizaki, T., and Kaneko, S. (1997) Single-dose pharmacokinetics and pharmacodynamics of oral triazolam in relation to cytochrome P450C19 (CYP2C19) activity. *Ther. Drug Monit.*, **19**, 371–374.

175 Otani, K., Yasui, N., Kaneko, S., Ohkubo, T., Osanai, T., Sugawara, K., Hayashi, K., Chiba, K., and Ishizaki, T. (1997) Effects of genetically determined *S*-mephenytoin 4-hydroxylation status and cigarette smoking on the single-dose pharmacokinetics of oral alprazolam. *Neuropsychopharmacology*, **16**, 8–14.

176 Mizugaki, M., Hiratsuka, M., Agatsuma, Y., Matsubara, Y., Fujii, K., Kure, S., and Narisawa, K. (2000) Rapid detection of CYP2C18 genotypes by real-time fluorescence polymerase chain reaction. *J. Pharm. Pharmacol.*, **52**, 199–205.

177 Aoshima, T., Fukasawa, T., Otsuji, Y., Okuyama, N., Gerstenberg, G., Miura, M., Ohkubo, T., Sugawara, K., and Otani, K. (2003) Effects of the CYP2C19 genotype and cigarette smoking on the single oral dose pharmacokinetics and pharmacodynamics of estazolam. *Prog. Neuropsychopharmacol. Biol. Psychiatry*, **27**, 535–538.

178 Venkatakrishnan, K., Greenblatt, D.J., Von Moltke, L.L., and Shader, R.I. (1998) Alprazolam is another substrate for human cytochrome P450-3A isoforms. *J. Clin. Psychopharmacol.*, **18**, 256.

179 Holm, K.J. and Goa, K.L. (2000) Zolpidem–an update of its pharmacology, therapeutic efficacy and tolerability in the treatment of insomnia. *Drugs*, **59**, 865–889.

180 Haffen, E., Vandel, P., Bonin, B., and Vandel, S. (1999) Citalopram pharmacokinetic interaction with clomipramine. UDP-glucuronosyltransferase inhibition? A case report. *Therapie*, **54**, 768–770.

181 Renwick, A.B., Mistry, H., Ball, S.E., Walters, D.G., Kao, J., and Lake, B.G. (1998) Metabolism of zaleplon by human hepatic microsomal cytochrome P450 isoforms. *Xenobiotica*, **28**, 337–348.

182 Noble, S., Langtry, H.D., and Lamb, H.M. (1998) Zopiclone–an update of its pharmacology, clinical efficacy and tolerability in the treatment of insomnia. *Drugs*, **55**, 277–302.

183 Drover, D.R. (2004) Comparative pharmacokinetics and pharmacodynamics of short-acting hypnosedatives–Zaleplon, Zolpidem and Zopiclone. *Clin. Pharmacokinet.*, **42**, 227–238.

184 Lilja, J.J., Kivistö, K.T., Backman, J.T., Lamberg, T.S., and Neuvonen, P.J. (1998) Grapefruit juice substantially increases plasma concentrations of buspirone. *Clin. Pharmacol. Ther.*, **64**, 655–660.

185 Lamberg, T.S., Kivistö, K.T., Laitila, J., Mårtensson, K., and Neuvonen, P.J. (1998) The effect of fluvoxamine on the pharmacokinetics and pharmacodynamics of buspirone. *Eur. J. Clin. Pharmacol.*, **54**, 761–766.

186 Zhu, M., Zhao, W., Jimenez, H., Zhang, D., Yeola, S., Dai, R., Vachharajani, N., and Mitroka, J. (2005) Cytochrome P450 3A-mediated metabolism of buspirone in human liver microsomes. *Drug Metab. Dispos.*, **33**, 500–507.

187 Härtter, S., Nordmark, A., Rose, D.M., Bertilsson, L., Tybring, G., and Laine, K. (2003) Effects of caffeine intake on the pharmacokinetics of melatonin, a probe drug for CYP1A2 activity. *Br. J. Clin. Pharmacol.*, **56**, 679–682.

188 May, D.E. and Kratochvil, C.J. (2010) Attention-deficit hyperactivity disorder: recent advances in paediatric pharmacotherapy. *Drugs*, **70**, 15–40.

189 DeVane, C.L., Markowitz, J.S., Carson, S.W., Boulton, D.W., Gill, H.S., Nahas, Z., and Risch, S.C. (2000) Single-dose pharmacokinetics of methylphenidate in CYP2D6 extensive and poor metabolizers. *J. Clin. Psychopharmacol.*, **20**, 347–349.

190 Markowitz, J.S. and Patrick, K.S. (2001) Pharmacokinetic and pharmacodynamic drug interactions in the treatment of attention-deficit hyperactivity disorder. *Clin. Pharmacokinet.*, **40**, 753–772.

191 Ring, B.J., Gillespie, J.S., Eckstein, J.A., and Wrighton, S.A. (2002) Identification of the human cytochromes P450 responsible for atomoxetine metabolism. *Drug Metab. Dispos.*, **30**, 319–323.

192 Sauer, J.M., Ponsler, G.D., Mattiuz, E.L., Long, A.J., Witcher, J.W., Thomasson, H.R., and Desante, K.A. (2003) Disposition and metabolic fate of atomoxetine hydrochloride: the role of CYP2D6 in human disposition and metabolism. *Drug Metab. Dispos.*, **31**, 98–107.

193 Sauer, J.M., Ring, B.J., and Witcher, J.W. (2005) Clinical pharmacokinetics of atomoxetine. *Clin. Pharmacokinet.*, **44**, 571–590.

194 Gross, A.S., Phillips, A.C., Rieutord, A., and Shenfield, G.M. (1996) The influence of the sparteine/debrisoquine genetic polymorphism on the disposition of dexfenfluramine. *Br. J. Clin. Pharmacol.*, **41**, 311–317.

195 Quinn, D.I., Wodak, A., and Day, R.O. (1997) Pharmacokinetic and pharmacodynamic principles of illicit druf use and treatment of illicit drug users. *Clin. Pharmacokinet.*, **33**, 344–400.

196 Bach, M.V., Coutts, R.T., and Baker, G.B. (1999) Involvement of CYP2D6 in the *in vitro* metabolism of amphetamine, two *N*-alkylamphetamines and their 4-methoxylated derivatives. *Xenobiotica*, **29**, 719–732.

197 Yatham, L.N., Kennedy, S.H., Schaffer, A., Parikh, S.V., Beaulieu, S., O'Donovan, C., MacQueen, G., McIntyre, R.S., Sharma, V., Ravindran, A., Young, L.T., Young, A.H., Alda, M., Milev, R., Vieta, E., Calabrese, J.R., Berk, M., Ha, K., and Kapczinski, F. (2009) Canadian Network for Mood and Anxiety Treatments (CANMAT) and International Society for Bipolar Disorders (ISBD) collaborative update of CANMAT guidelines for the management of patients with bipolar disorder: update 2009. *Bipolar. Disord.*, **11**, 225–255.

198 Ketter, T.A., Frye, M.A., Corà-Locatelli, G., Kimbrell, T.A., and Post, R.M. (1999) Metabolism and excretion of mood stabilizers and new anticonvulsants. *Cell. Mol. Neurobiol.*, **19**, 511–532.

199 Johannessen, S.I., Battino, D., Berry, D.J., Bialer, M., Kramer, G., Tomson, T.,

and Patsalos, P.N. (2003) Therapeutic drug monitoring of the newer antiepileptic drugs. *Ther. Drug Monit.*, **25**, 347–363.

200 Küpfer, A. and Branch, R.A. (1985) Stereoselective mephobarbital hydroxylation cosegregates with mephenytoin hydroxylation. *Clin. Pharmacol. Ther.*, **38**, 414–418.

201 Hadama, A., Ieiri, I., Morita, T., Kimura, M., Urae, A., Irie, S., Kaneda, T., Mamiya, K., Tashiro, N., Higuchi, S., and Otsubo, K. (2001) *p*-Hydroxylation of phenobarbital: relationship to (*S*)-mephenytoin hydroxylation (CYP2C19) polymorphism. *Ther. Drug Monit.*, **23**, 115–118.

202 Mamiya, K., Hadama, A., Yukawa, E., Ieiri, I., Otsubo, K., Ninomiya, H., Tashiro, N., and Higuchi, S. (2000) CYP2C19 polymorphism effect on phenobarbitone–pharmacokinetics in Japanese patients with epilepsy: analysis by population pharmacokinetics. *Eur. J. Clin. Pharmacol.*, **55**, 821–825.

203 Kobayashi, K., Morita, J., Chiba, K., Wanibuchi, A., Kimura, M., Irie, S., Urae, A., and Ishizaki, T. (2004) Pharmacogenetic roles of CYP2C19 and CYP2B6 in the metabolism of *R*- and *S*-mephobarbital in humans. *Pharmacogenetics*, **14**, 549–556.

204 Bertilsson, L. and Tomson, T. (1986) Clinical pharmacokinetics and pharmacological effects of carnbamazepine and carbamazepine-10,11-epoxide–an update. *Clin. Pharmacokinet.*, **11**, 177–198.

205 Ho, P.C., Abbott, F.S., Zanger, U.M., and Chang, T.K. (2003) Influence of CYP2C9 genotypes on the formation of a hepatotoxic metabolite of valproic acid in human liver microsomes. *Pharmacogenomics J.*, **3**, 335–342.

206 Kiang, T.K., Ho, P.C., Anari, M.R., Tong, V., Abbott, F.S., and Chang, T.K. (2006) Contribution of CYP2C9, CYP2A6, and CYP2B6 to valproic acid metabolism in hepatic microsomes from individuals with the CYP2C9*1/*1 genotype. *Toxicol. Sci.*, **94**, 261–271.

207 Bockbrader, H.N., Wesche, D., Miller, R., Chapel, S., Janiczek, N., and Burger, P. (2010) A comparison of the pharmacokinetics and pharmacodynamics of pregabalin and gabapentin. *Clin. Pharmacokinet.*, **49**, 661–669.

208 Christensen, J., Petrenaite, V., Atterman, J., Sidenius, P., Ohman, I., Tomson, T., and Sabers, A. (2007) Oral contraceptives induce lamotrigine metabolism: evidence from a double-blind, placebo-controlled trial. *Epilepsia*, **48**, 484–489.

209 Patsalos, P.N. (2004) Clinical pharmacokinetics of levetiracetam. *Clin. Pharmacokinet.*, **43**, 707–724.

210 May, T.W., Korn-Merker, E., and Rambeck, B. (2003) Clinical pharmacokinetics of oxcarbazepine. *Clin. Pharmacokinet.*, **42**, 1023–1042.

211 Lee, C.R. (2004) CYP2C9 genotype as a predictor of drug disposition in humans. *Methods Find. Exp. Clin. Pharmacol.*, **26**, 463–472.

212 Küpfer, A. and Preisig, R. (1984) Pharmacogenetics of mephenytoin: a new drug hydroxylation polymorphism in man. *Eur. J. Clin. Pharmacol.*, **26**, 753–759.

213 Heyn, H., White, R.B., and Stevens, J.C. (1996) Catalytic role of cytochrome P4502B6 in the *N*-demethylation of *S*-mephenytoin. *Drug Metab. Dispos.*, **24**, 948–954.

214 Guttendorf, R.J. and Wedlund, P.J. (1992) Genetic aspects of drug disposition and therapeutics. *J. Clin. Pharmacol.*, **32**, 107–117.

215 Shank, R.P. and Maryanoff, B.E. (2008) Molecular pharmacodynamics, clinical therapeutics, and pharmacokinetics of topiramate. *CNS Neurosci. Ther.*, **14**, 120–142.

216 Caldwell, G.W., Wu, W.N., Masucci, J.A., McKown, L.A., Gauthier, D., Jones, W.J., Leo, G.C., and Maryanoff, B.E. (2005) Metabolism and excretion of the antiepileptic/antimigraine drug, Topiramate in animals and humans. *Eur. J. Drug Metab. Pharmacokinet.*, **30**, 151–164.

217 Sachdeo, R.C., Sachdeo, S.K., Levy, R.H., Streeter, A.J., Bishop, F.E., Kunze, K.L., Mather, G.G., Roskos, L.K., Shen, D.D., Thummel, K.E., Trager, W.F.,

Curtin, C.R., Doose, D.R., Gisclon, L.G., and Bialer, M. (2002) Topiramate and phenytoin pharmacokinetics during repetitive monotherapy and combination therapy to epileptic patients. *Epilepsia*, **43**, 691–696.

218 Leppik, I.E. (2004) Zonisamide: chemistry, mechanism of action, and pharmacokinetics. *Seizure*, **13** (Suppl. 1), S5–S9.

219 Farlow, M.R. (2001) Pharmacokinetic profiles of current therapies for Alzheimer's disease: implications for switching to galantamine. *Clin. Ther.*, **23** (Suppl. A), A13–A24.

220 Larsen, J.T., Hansen, L.L., and Brøsen, K. (1999) Tacrine is not an ideal probe drug for measuring CYP1A2 activity *in vivo*. *Br. J. Clin. Pharmacol.*, **48**, 663–668.

221 Tiseo, P.J., Perdomo, C.A., and Friedhoff, L.T. (1998) Metabolism and elimination of ^{14}C-donepezil in healthy volunteers: a single-dose study. *Br. J. Clin. Pharmacol.*, **46** (Suppl. 1), 19–24.

222 Tiseo, P.J., Perdomo, C.A., and Friedhoff, L.T. (1998) Concurrent administration of donepezil HCl and ketoconazole: assessment of pharmacokinetic changes following single and multiple doses. *Br. J. Clin. Pharmacol.*, **46** (Suppl. 1), 30–34.

223 Varsaldi, F., Miglio, G., Scordo, M.G., Dahl, M.L., Villa, L.M., Biolcati, A., Lombardi, G., Varsaldi, F., Miglio, G., Scordo, M.G., Dahl, M.L., Villa, L.M., Biolcati, A., and Lombardi, G. (2006) Impact of the CYP2D6 polymorphism on steady-state plasma concentrations and clinical outcome of donepezil in Alzheimer's disease patients. *Eur. J. Clin. Pharmacol.*, **62**, 721–726.

224 Farlow, M.R. (2003) Clinical pharmacokinetics of galantamine. *Clin. Pharmacokinet.*, **42**, 1383–1392.

225 Lilienfeld, S. (2002) Galantamine – a novel cholinergic drug with a unique dual mode of action for the treatment of patients with Alzheimer's disease. *CNS Drug. Rev.*, **8**, 159–176.

226 Jarvis, B. and Figgitt, D.P. (2003) Memantine. *Drugs Aging*, **20**, 465–476.

227 Micuda, S., Mundlova, L., Anzenbacherova, E., Anzenbacher, P., Chladek, J., Fuksa, L., and Martinkova, J. (2004) Inhibitory effects of memantine on human cytochrome P450 activities: prediction of *in vivo* drug interactions. *Eur. J. Clin. Pharmacol.*, **60**, 583–589.

228 Gobburu, J.V.S., Tammara, V., Lesko, L., Jhee, S.S., Sramek, J.J., Cutler, N.R., and Yuan, R. (2001) Pharmacokinetic–pharmacodynamic modeling of rivastigmine, a cholinesterase inhibitor, in patients with Alzheimer's disease. *J. Clin. Pharmacol.*, **41**, 1082–1090.

229 Johnston, M.M. and Rapoport, A.M. (2010) Triptans for the management of migraine. *Drugs*, **70**, 1505–1518.

230 Sandrini, G., Perrotta, A., Tassorelli, C., and Nappi, G. (2009) Eletriptan. *Expert Opin. Drug Metab. Toxicol.*, **5**, 1587–1598.

231 Dixon, C.M., Park, G.R., and Tarbit, M.H. (1994) Characterization of the enzyme responsible for the metabolism of sumatriptan in human liver. *Biochem. Pharmacol.*, **47**, 1253–1257.

232 Johansson, B. (1992) A review of the pharmacokinetics and pharmacodynamics of disulfiram and its metabolites. *Acta Psychiatr. Scand. Suppl.*, **369**, 15–26.

233 Saivin, S., Hulot, T., Chabac, S., Potgieter, A., Durbin, P., and Houin, G. (1998) Clinical pharmacokinetics of acamprosate. *Clin. Pharmacokinet.*, **35**, 331–345.

234 Kaakkola, S. (2000) Clinical pharmacology, therapeutic use and potential of COMT inhibitors in Parkinson's disease. *Drugs*, **59**, 1233–1250.

235 Heinonen, E.H., Anttila, M.I., and Lammintausta, R.A.S. (1994) Pharmacokinetic aspects of L-deprenyl (selegiline) and its metabolites. *Clin. Pharmacol. Ther.*, **56**, 742–749.

236 Kivistö, K.T., Wang, J.S., Backman, J.T., Nyman, L., Taavitsainen, P., Anttila, M., and Neuvonen, P.J. (2001) Selegiline pharmacokinetics are unaffected by the CYP3A4 inhibitor itraconazole. *Eur. J. Clin. Pharmacol.*, **57**, 37–42.

237 Laine, K., Anttila, M., Nyman, L., Wahlberg, A., and Bertilsson, L. (2001) CYP2C19 polymorphism is not important for the *in vivo* metabolism of selegiline. *Eur. J. Clin. Pharmacol.*, **57**, 137–142.

238 Hidestrand, M., Oscarson, M., Salonen, J.S., Nyman, L., Pelkonen, O., Turpeinen, M., and Ingelman-Sundberg, M. (2001) CYP2B6 and CYP2C19 as the major enzymes responsible for the metabolism of selegiline, a drug used in the treatment of Parkinson's disease, as revealed from experiments with recombinant enzymes. *Drug Metab. Dispos.*, **29**, 1480–1484.

239 Guay, D.R. (2006) Rasagiline (TVP-1012): a new selective monoamine oxidase inhibitor for Parkinson's disease. *Am. J. Geriatr. Pharmacother.*, **4**, 330–346.

12
Cardiovascular Drugs

Stephan Riedmaier and Ulrich M. Zanger

12.1
Introduction

A large number of drugs from different groups are used for the treatment of various cardiovascular diseases. Here, we review how these drugs are metabolized in humans. This chapter starts with a focus on drugs to treat hypertension – the most common cardiovascular disease, which also causes many pathological changes of the heart and the vasculature. These drugs target the body's regulatory network to control blood pressure and water balance – the renin–angiotensin–aldosterone system (RAAS).

Treatment of congestive heart failure (CHF) also involves the management of hypertension, as well as drug-based interference with the sympathetic nervous system. Drugs of this class are agonists or antagonists of α- or β-adrenergic receptors influencing vasoconstriction or vasodilation and cardiac filling or output. Furthermore, diuretics can be used to adjust ion and water retention, and are therefore of high importance in managing congestive symptoms of CHF.

Arrhythmias may range from asymptomatic clinical findings to life-threatening diseases. Therefore, calcium channel blockers are important drugs to treat these diseases. They are also used to treat hypertension due to their vasodilatory effects.

Anticoagulants are included in this chapter due to their importance in the prevention of thrombosis. Finally, lipid-lowering drugs are presented, used for the treatment of hyperlipidemias and dyslipidemias – the major causes of atherosclerosis and atherosclerosis-induced diseases like coronary heart disease as well as cerebrovascular and peripheral vascular disease.

12.2
RAAS as a Target for Angiotensin-Converting Enzyme Inhibitors and AT_1 Receptor Blockers

The blood pressure is under the central control of the RAAS (Figure 12.1). Most important in this pathway is the conversion of angiotensinogen to angiotensin I

Metabolism of Drugs and Other Xenobiotics, First Edition. Edited by Pavel Anzenbacher, Ulrich M. Zanger.

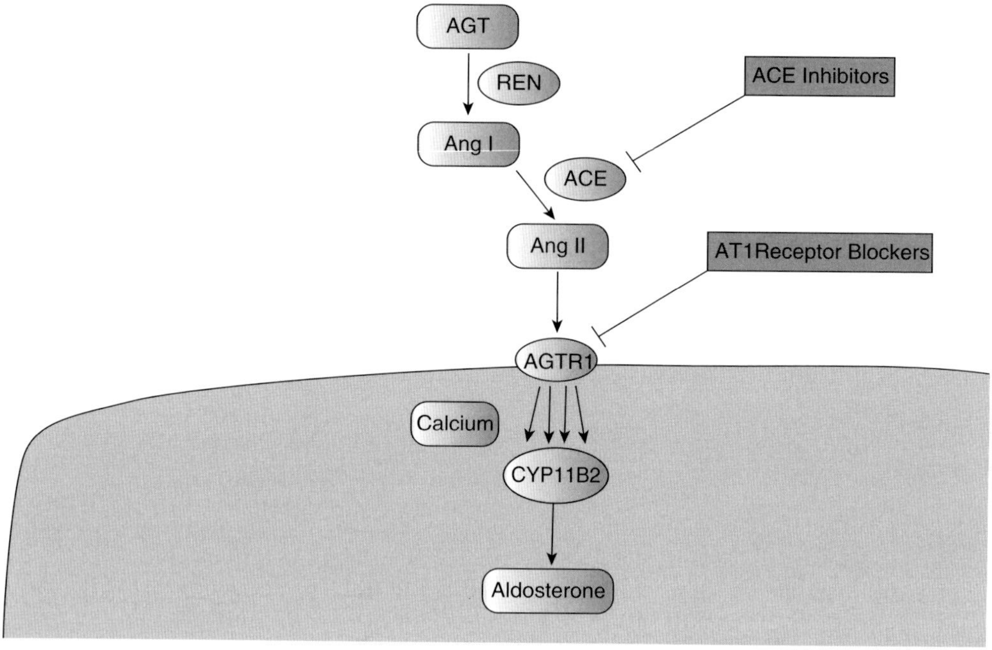

Figure 12.1 RAAS. Arrows show the classical pathway, starting with angiotensinogen (AGT), which is converted to angiotensin I (Ang I) and later to angiotensin II (Ang II), which in the end activates angiotensin receptor 1 (AGTR1). Important enzymes are renin (REN), ACE, and CYP11B2.

by renin followed by its conversion to angiotensin II by angiotensin-converting enzyme (ACE). Subsequent binding of angiotensin II to angiotensin II receptor type 1 induces the synthesis of aldosterone, leading to increased water and salt resorption, and potassium excretion by the kidneys, and in this way to higher blood pressure. RAAS is the target of two important types of antihypertensive drugs – ACE inhibitors and angiotensin II receptor type 1 blockers (ARBs).

12.2.1 ACE Inhibitors

ACE inhibitors can be classified into three groups according to their chemical structure (Table 12.1): (i) dicarboxyl-containing substances (ramipril, enalapril, lisinopril, benazepril, quinapril, moexipril, spirapril, perindopril, pentopril, cilazapril), (ii) sulfhydryl-containing substances (captopril, fentiapril, pivalopril, zofenopril, alacepril), and (iii) phosphorus-containing substances (fosinopril). Many of them are prodrugs containing ester groups to increase their oral bioavailability. All of them have similar therapeutic indications, effectiveness in blocking angiotensin II production, and adverse effects [1].

Table 12.1 Pharmacokinetics, metabolism, and transport of ACE inhibitors [1–4].

	Ramipril (A)	**Captopril (B)**	**Fosinopril (C)**
	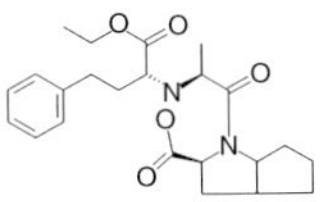	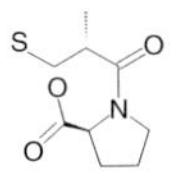	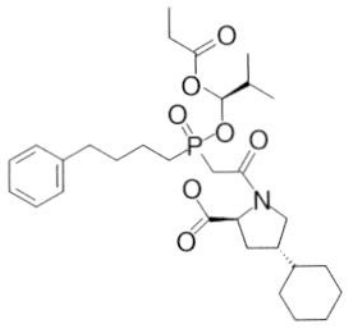
Bioavailability	28%; ramiprilat: 44%		
Half-life	initial: 2–4 h (tissue distribution) apparent elimination: 9–18 h terminal elimination: >50 h (due to ACE binding)	2 h	12 h
Absorption	50–60%	60–75%; decreased by food	36%; decreased by food
Excretion	2/3 renal	40–50% unchanged metabolized to captopril cysteine disulfide 95% renal	ester prodrug hepatic to fosinoprilat *p*-OH-fosinopril (1–5%); fosinoprilat-acyl-β-glucuronide (20–30%)
Metabolizing enzymes	esterases		
Transporters	PEPT1/2		PEPT1/2

The prodrug ramipril is converted to its active metabolite ramiprilat by cleavage of its ester moiety (Figure 12.2). It is rapidly absorbed and ramiprilat peak concentrations are achieved in 3 h [1]. Compared to other members of this group, ramipril is a highly lipophilic ACE inhibitor that is extensively metabolized. A single-dose study in eight patients revealed that one-third of total circulating ramipril and ramiprilat is biliary excreted, and two-thirds are excreted via the kidney. Main metabolites after 24 h excreted via urine were diketopiperazine acid (around 13% of total dose) and ramiprilat (around 4.5%); main metabolites in bile were diketopiperazine acid (around 9%), ramiprilat glucuronide (around 3.5%), and diketopiperazine (2%). Only a negligible fraction of the given dose was excreted as unchanged drug [3].

Interestingly, subgroups could be identified, with 50% showing a "fast" ramiprilat elimination of 80 h and 50% showing a variable elimination of much longer half-lifes (up to 166 h). One possible explanation may be variation in binding constants to its target ACE due to polymorph ACE genes. Due to immediate and

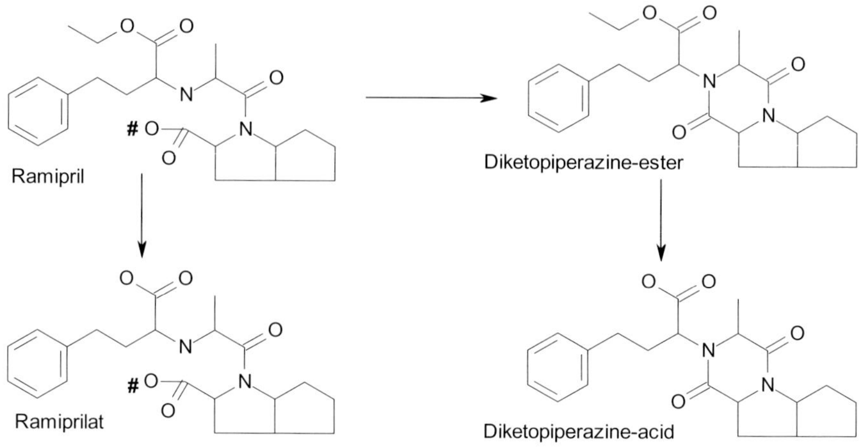

Figure 12.2 Metabolism of ramipril. The prodrug ramipril is metabolized by hepatic esterases to the active diacid ramiprilat, to the inactive metabolites diketopiperazine-ester and acid, and to glucuronides of ramipril and ramiprilat (glucuronidation site marked by the hash symbol (#)).

saturable binding to ACE, which is partly circulating and partly noncirculating (vessel endothelium bound), their elimination is highly dependent on dissociation from ACE. This is also the reason why ACE inhibitors show unconventional pharmacokinetics/pharmacodynamics properties as their absorption and elimination phases not only depend on the corresponding absorption or elimination constants, but also on total ACE binding capacity and ACE inhibitor affinity [2].

Variation in ramipril hydrolysis may also be influenced by plasma/hepatic or tissue esterases [5]. Important plasma esterases are butyrylcholinesterase (BChE), paraoxonase PON1, and albumin [6], whereas carboxylesterases CES1, 2, and 4 [7] and PON1, 2, and 3 are liver-expressed esterases [8].

Transport of ACE inhibitors was described to be mediated by the jejunal peptide carriers PEPT1/2, which transport nutrients and other peptide-like drugs like β-lactam antibiotics [2].

12.2.2
ARBs

ARBs are more effective in reducing the activation of AT_1 receptors, but do not influence alternative non-ACE–angiotensin II pathways. Levels of numerous substrates of ACE are not affected by ARBs. Both ACEs and ARBs increase renin release, but ARBs also increase angiotensin II formation leading to indirectly stimulated AT_2 receptors. Whether these facts result in differences in therapeutic outcome is not clear.

Table 12.2 Pharmacokinetics, metabolism, and transport of AT_1 receptor blockers [1, 9–12, 13].

	Losartan	**Candesartan**	**Irbesartan**
	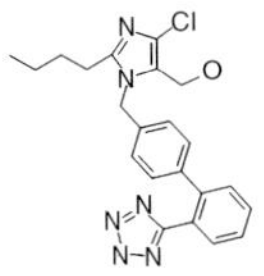	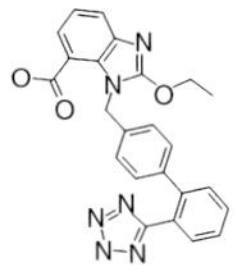	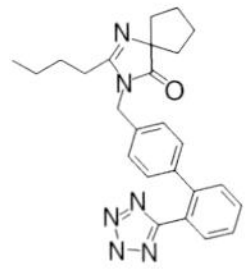
Bioavailability	33–35%	15%	60–80%
Half-life	1.5–2.5 h; E-3174: 6–9 h	9 h	11–15 h
Absorption	high		rapid and complete
Excretion	12% renal (4% unchanged, 6% as E-3174) 14% converted to E-3174 *N*1-glucuronidation by UGT1A10 *N*2-glucuronidation by UGT1A1/3/10 and UGT2B7/17	33% renal ester prodrug; complete hydrolysis in intestinal wall 75% excreted unchanged <20% CYP2C9 (*O*-de-ethylation); *N*2-glucuronidation by UGT1A3 and UGT2B7 *O*-glucuronidation by UGT1A7/8/9/10 and UGT2B7	20% renal *N*2-glucuronidation (probably UGT1A3)
Metabolizing enzymes	CYP2C9 (CYP3A4)	CYP2C9	CYP2C9
Transporters	P-gp, URAT1 OATs, inhibitor of OAT1		

Losartan was the first orally available, nonpeptide angiotensin II receptor antagonist being highly selective for the AT_1 receptor. The selectivity rank order of ARBs to AT_1 is candesartan > irbesartan > telmisartan = valsartan > losartan [1]. Basic pharmacokinetic parameters of losartan are summarized in Table 12.2.

The biotransformation of losartan (Figure 12.3) involves three major steps: oxidation, hydroxylation, and glucuronidation. It involves the formation of an aldehyde intermediate (E-3179) followed either by its oxidation to the major metabolite E-3174 or by hydroxylation to P1. Additionally minor metabolites are formed via hydroxylation of losartan (M1, M2, and M5). Finally *N*-glucuronides at the tetrazole ring have been identified for losartan and E-3174 [11, 12, 14].

Phase I enzymes responsible for the oxidation/hydroxylation reactions are cytochrome P450 CYP2C9 and CYP3A4. Early studies with recombinant human liver CYPs, isoform-specific inhibitors as well as isoform-specific antibodies suggested an important role for CYP3A4 in these reactions [11, 15]. However, later *in vitro* studies at physiological concentrations in yeast and human liver microsomes identified CYP2C9 as the dominant isozyme, with CYP3A4 being only relevant at higher drug concentrations [16]. *In vivo* studies supported these findings as

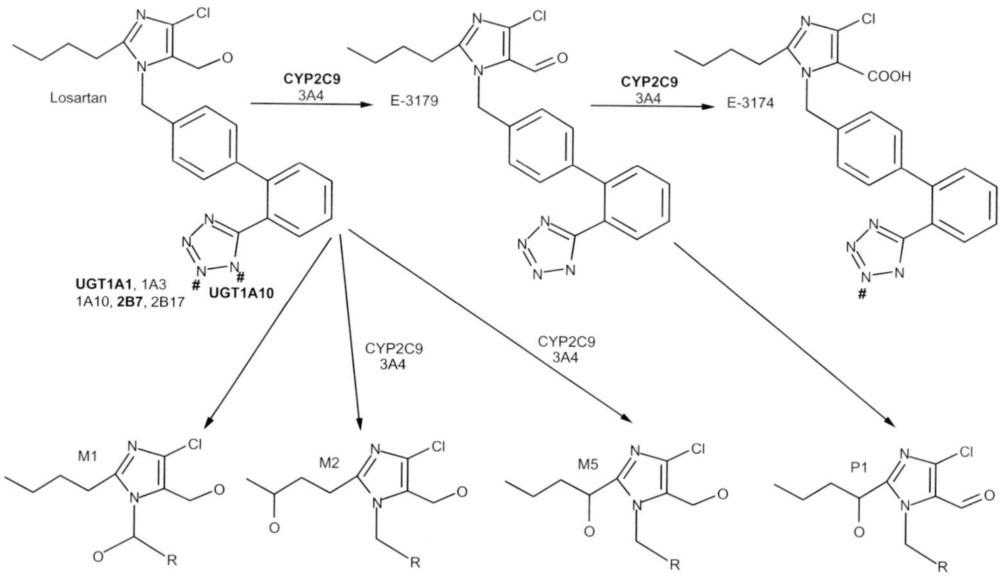

Figure 12.3 Metabolism of losartan and responsible CYPs enzymes. Enzymes with a major contribution are given in bold. In metabolites M1, M2, M5 and P1, the tetrazol-biphenyl chain is represented by R. Sites for *N*-glucuronidation are marked by the hash symbols (#).

the CYP3A4 inhibitors ketokonazole, erythromycin, and itraconazole resulted in no significant differences in the area under the concentration–time curve (AUC) or half-life of losartan [17, 18]. Another study with the CYP2C9 inhibitor fluvastatin, however, also showed no significant AUC or half-life change, suggesting that both CYP isozymes are important in this reaction [19]. An important role of CYP2D6 or CYP2C19 in E-3174 formation was ruled out by a study using extensive and poor metabolizers of debrisoquine (CYP2D6) or mephenytoin (CYP2C19) [20].

Phase II products have been found in the form of *N*-glucuronides of losartan (but not *O*-glucuronides) mainly at the N2 position (and to a small part also at N1) of the tetrazole ring. A significant and equal contribution to N2 glucuronidation was observed for UDP-glucurosyltransferase UGT1A1 and 2B7 (with minor a contribution of UGT1A3, 1A10, and 2B17) and to N1 glucuronidation for UGT1A10 [14].

Losartan, but not its major metabolite E-3174, was shown to be a substrate of the intestinal uptake transporter P-glycoprotein. Additional transporters may be involved in losartan uptake, but an influence of MRP1 or MRP2 was ruled out [21]. Although some sartans resemble peptide derivatives and have high affinity for PEPT1 or PEPT2, intestinal uptake via these transporters was not found [22]. Hepatic excretion via OATP1B1, OATP1B3, OAT1 and OAT3, as well as MRP2 was shown for olmesartan and valsartan [24, 25]. Kidney proximal tubule transporters URAT1 [13] and rabbit OATs [23] were identified to interact with losartan.

12.3
Adrenergic Receptor Agonists

Many important cardiovascular drugs are working by interference with the function of the sympathetic nervous system, thereby influencing sympathetically innervated organs. Most synthetic agonists are structural analogs of the catecholamines and have therapeutic advantages compared to epinephrine.

12.3.1
α_1-Selective Adrenergic Receptor Agonists

These drugs exert their clinical effect mainly in vascular smooth muscles, which leads to an increase of peripheral vascular resistance and maintenance or increase of blood pressure. Clinical utility is limited, and examples of these types are the relatively specific α_1-receptor agonists methoxamine and phenylephrine (Table 12.3), which at high concentrations also activate β-adrenergic receptors.

Table 12.3 Pharmacokinetics, metabolism, and transport of the α_1-selective adrenergic receptor agonist phenylephrine [26, 27].

	Phenylephrine (PE)
	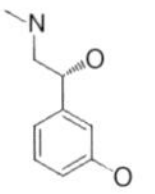
Bioavailability	38%
Half-life	2.1–3.4 h
Absorption	
Excretion	renal: 46% PE-*O*-sulfate 30% 3-OH-mandelic acid 3-OH-phenylglycol PE-3-*O*-glucuronide phenylglycol-3-*O*-sulfate (glucuronide and sulfate conjugates formed presystemically in small intestine)
Metabolizing enzymes	MAO, sulfotransferases
Transporters	

Table 12.4 Pharmacokinetics, metabolism, and transport of α_2-selective adrenergic receptor agonists [1, 9, 10, 28].

	Clonidine	Guanfacine	Methyldopa
	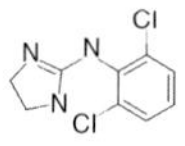	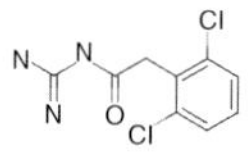	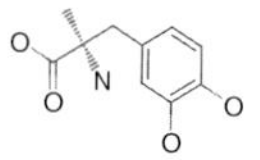
Bioavailability	~100%		25%
Half-life	6–24 h	12–24 h	2 h
Absorption	high	rapid and complete	50%
Excretion	50% unchanged, renal 20% biliary 10% as *p*-OH-clonidine	mainly renal 50% unchanged	metabolized to active α-methylnorepinephrine mainly: methyldopa-*O*-sulfate
Metabolizing enzymes	CYP2D6		
Transporters	P-gp inhibitor of: OCT1, OCT3, OCTN1, OCTN2		active amino acid transporter

12.3.2
α_2-Selective Adrenergic Receptor Agonists

These are important drugs for the treatment of hypertension (Table 12.4). Their method of action results from activating α_2-adrenergic receptors in the cardiovascular control center of the central nervous system (nucleus tractus solitarii in medulla oblongata). Similarly acting drugs are guanfacine and methyldopa.

The imidazoline clonidine was developed in the 1960s. Its major pharmacological effects are changes in blood pressure and heart rate. The hypotensive response of this drug results from decreased central outflow of impulses in the sympathetic nervous system, but the exact mechanism of action is not completely understood. The existence of noradrenergic imidazoline preferring binding sites in this area of the brain has been suggested and the activation of these receptors might be the way in which clonidine exerts its hypotensive effects [29].

Two-thirds of *p*-OH-clonidine are produced by CYP2D6, but CYP1A2, CYP3A4, CYP1A1, and CYP3A5 are also involved in clonidine metabolism (Figure 12.4) [30].

Clonidine is a substrate of P-gp [31] and of a previously undescribed clonidine/H^+ exchanger in the mouse blood–brain barrier (K_m = 0.62 mM). Additionally, clonidine was reported to be an efficient inhibitor of organic cation transporters (OCT1 [32], the kidney transporter OCT3 [33], OCTN1 [34], and OCTN2 [35].

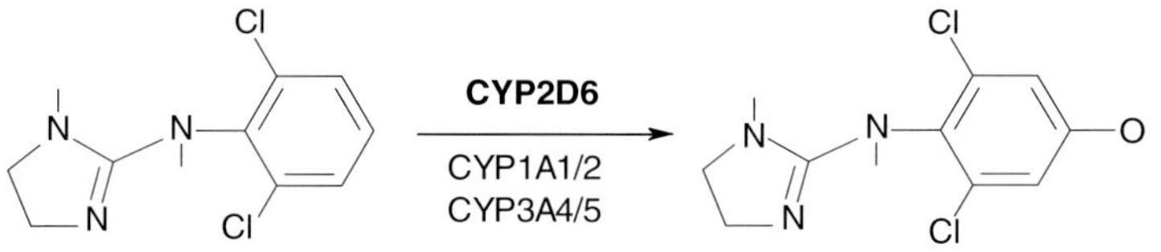

Figure 12.4 Metabolism of clonidine. CYP2D6 is given in bold, as it is the major metabolizing enzyme.

12.3.3
β-Selective Adrenergic Receptor Agonists

Today, β-adrenergic receptor agonists have a major role in the treatment of asthma or chronic obstructive pulmonary disease, only. One of the important adverse effects of β-adrenergic agonists in treating asthma results from stimulating β_1-adrenergic receptors in the heart. Strategies to avoid these were the development of drugs specifically targeting β_2-adrenergic receptors, of drugs with lower rates of metabolism and increased bioavailability via structural modifications, and administration of these drugs by inhalation in the form of an aerosol to keep systemic drug concentrations low. Drugs of this group include metaproterenol, fenoterol, or ritodrine.

12.4
Adrenergic Receptor Antagonists

Most drugs in the group of adrenergic receptor antagonists inhibit the interference of norepinephrine and epinephrine with α- or β-adrenergic receptors in a competitive way. Important structural differences between the various types of adrenergic receptors made it possible to interfere selectively with responses to the sympathetic nervous system. For example, selective β_1-adrenergic receptor blockers like metoprolol can inhibit effectively the epinephrine/norepinephrine activity on the heart with only low interference with β_2-adrenergic receptors (bronchial smooth muscles) or α_1- or α_2-adrenergic receptors.

12.4.1
α_1-Selective Adrenergic Receptor Antagonists

Drugs of this class inhibit vasoconstriction resulting from endogenous catecholamines. This leads to vasodilation in arteriolar resistance veins and vessels, and a fall in blood pressure. Baroreceptor reflexes oppose this fall of blood pressure by increased rate and output of the heart as well as fluid retention.

Prazosin (Table 12.5) is the prototype of α_1-selective adrenergic receptor antagonists containing a piperazinyl quinazoline nucleus and has a 1000-fold higher affinity for α_1- than for α_2-receptors, with similar potencies at receptor subtypes α_{1A}, α_{1B}, and α_{1D}. Prazosin blocks specifically α_1-adrenergic receptors in arterioles

Table 12.5 Pharmacokinetics, metabolism, and transport of α_1-selective adrenergic receptor antagonists [1, 9, 10, 36, 37].

	Prazosin	Terazosin	Doxazosin
	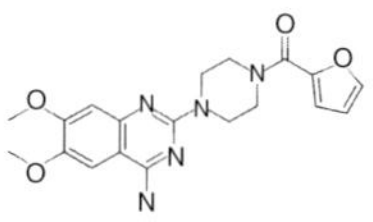	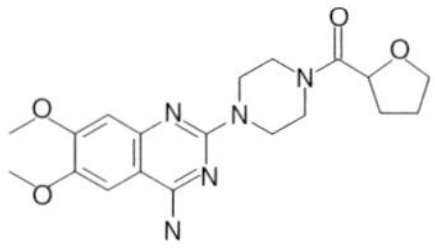	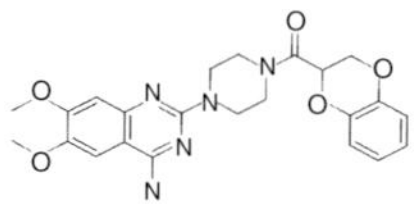
Bioavailability	50–70%	>90%	65%
Half-life	in plasma 2–3 h	12 h	22 h
Absorption	high		
Excretion	renal: minimally unchanged hepatic: extensively metabolized	renal: 10% unchanged hepatic: 20% unchanged metabolized to: piperazine-, 6-*O*-demethyl-, 7-*O*-demethyl-, diamine-terazosin	63% hepatic; 9% renal 4.8% unchanged metabolized: 23% *O*-demethylation (quinazoline nucleus) 12% hydroxylation (benzodioxan moiety)
Metabolizing enzymes			
Transporters	OCT1, OCT2, OCT3, P-gp, BCRP		

and veins, leading to a lowered peripheral vascular resistance and venous return to the heart. It decreases cardiac preload and does not increase cardiac output or rate.

Several metabolites have been identified in humans and animals (6-*O*-demethyl-, 7-*O*-demethyl-prazosin, 21-piperazinyl-4-amino-6,7-dimethoxyquinazoline, 2,4-diamino-6,7-dimethoxyquinazoline; Figure 12.5). *N*- and *O*-glucuronidation occurs in prazosin metabolism. The *N*-glucuronides of the parent drug (M13) and of M1 are the most common metabolites in hepatocytes. Three glutathione-conjugated metabolites were detected (M9, M12, and M14) with M9 being the most common one in humans. Prazosin is a substrate of the ATP-binding cassette (ABC) transporters breast cancer resistance protein (BCRP; ABCG2) [38] and P-gp ($K_m = 20\,\mu M$ [39]), as well as of OCT1 ($IC_{50} = 1.8\,\mu M$), OCT2 ($IC_{50} > 100\,\mu M$) and OCT3 ($IC_{50} = 12.6\,\mu M$) [40].

12.4.2
α_2-Selective Adrenergic Receptor Antagonists

Drugs such as yohimbine (Table 12.6) act predominantly in the central nervous system, and increase the sympathetic outflow and release of norepinephrine from

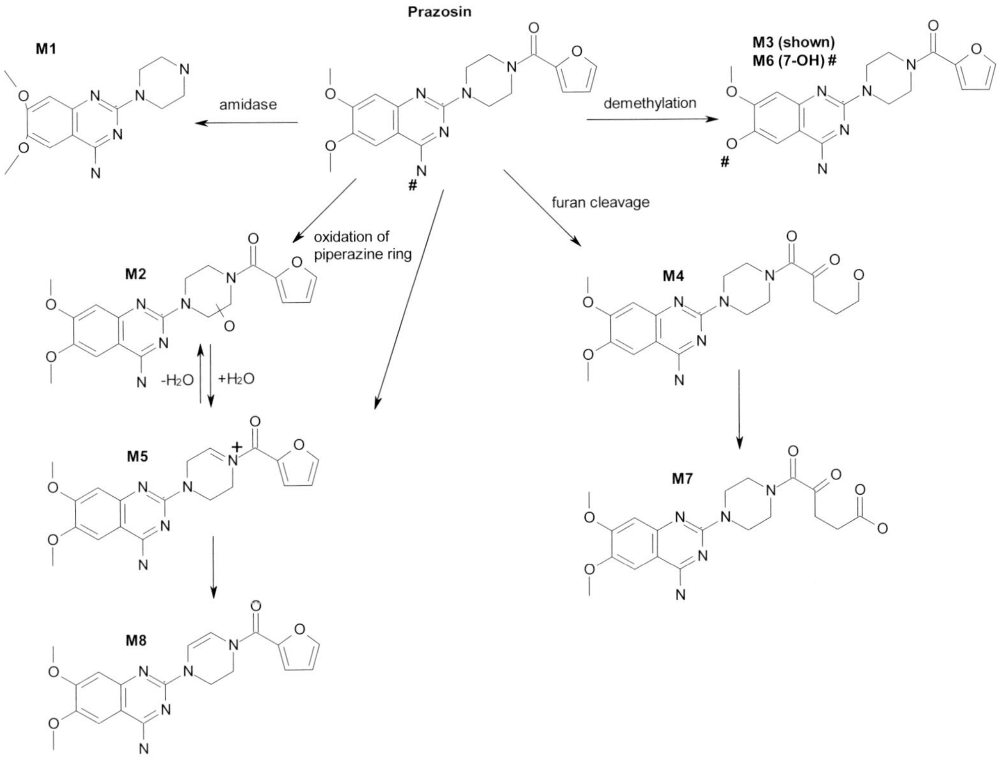

Figure 12.5 Metabolism of prazosin and conversions involved in the metabolism. Sites for *O*-glucuronidation are marked by the hash symbols (#).

Table 12.6 Pharmacokinetics, metabolism, and transport of the α_2-selective adrenergic receptor antagonist yohimbine [1, 9, 10, 41].

	Yohimbine
	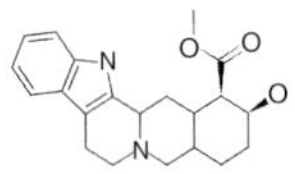
Bioavailability	7–87%
Half-life	30 min
Absorption	rapid
Excretion	extensive metabolism in liver and kidney
	mainly 11-OH-yohimbine; some 10-OH-yohimbine; 1000-fold variable; nonmetabolizers
Metabolizing enzymes	CYP2D6; (CYP3A4/5)
Transporters	inhibitor of P-gp (trimethoxybenzoylyohimbine)

nerve endings. This leads to the activation of α_1- and α_2-receptors in the heart and peripheral vasculature, and in this way increases the blood pressure. These actions are the opposite to those of clonidine–an α_2-agonist (Section 12.3.2). Yohimbine is mainly used to treat male sexual dysfunction.

12.4.3
β-Selective Adrenergic Receptor Antagonists

These drugs, also called β-blockers, are highly effective in the treatment of hypertension, ischemic heart disease, congestive heart failure, and certain arrhythmias, and are therefore widely used in clinical practice (Table 12.7). As catecholamines act in a chronotropic and ionotropic positive manner, β-adrenergic antagonists lower the heart rate and contractility. When the sympathetic nervous system is unstimulated, this effect is low. During exercise or stress (i.e., when β-receptors are stimulated), β-adrenergic antagonists attenuate the expected rise in heart rate. Additionally, these drugs cause a reduction in blood pressure in patients with hypertension, but not in patients with normal blood pressure. Nonselective β-adrenergic antagonists may lead to life-threatening bronchoconstriction in asthma and chronic obstructive pulmonary disease patients via blocking β_2-adrenergic receptors in bronchial smooth muscles.

Propranolol is a β-adrenergic receptor antagonist with equal affinity to β_1- and β_2-adrenergic receptors. Its absorption is high, but due to extensive first-pass metabolism only around 25% reaches the systemic circulation. The (–)- or *S*-enantiomer is the active form of the drug.

The major metabolites detected after incubations with human liver microsomes were 4- and 5-OH-propranolol and *N*-desisopropyl-propranolol (Figure 12.6). Correlation analyses and inhibitor studies identified CYP2D6 and CYP1A2 as responsible enzymes of hydroxylation and *N*-desisopropylation, respectively [45]. Metabolism is highly variable and affected by CYP genotypes [46]. Seventeen percent of the drug is glucuronidated by the enzymes UGT1A9, UGT2B4, and UGT2B7 at positions marked by the hash symbols (#). The highest activity in the glucuronidation of the pharmacologically active *S*-enantiomer was found for UGT1A9, which accounts, as UGT2B7, for around 5% of all expressed UGTs in liver, whereas UGT2B4 accounts for 35% [47].

Propranolol is transported by OCT2 [48] and P-gp [49].

12.5
Diuretics

By definition, drugs of this group increase the rate of urine flow. In addition, the rate of Na^+ excretion (natiuresis) is increased as NaCl is the major determinant of the body's extracellular fluid volume, which in most clinical applications of diuretics has to be reduced. Additionally, diuretics may alter the renal handling of other cations, anions, and uric acid. Treatment with different types of diuretics is

Table 12.7 Pharmacokinetics, metabolism, and transport of β-adrenergic receptor antagonists [1, 9, 10, 42–44].

	Propranolol (nonselective; first [t] generation)	Metoprolol (β_1-selective; second generation)	Carvedilol (nonselective; additional actions; third generation)	Nebivolol (β_1-selective; additional actions; third generation)
	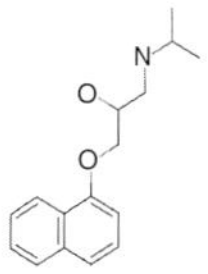	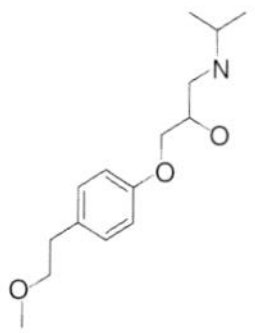	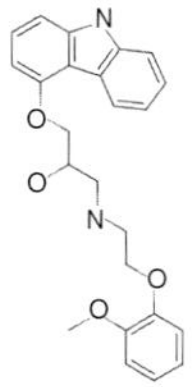	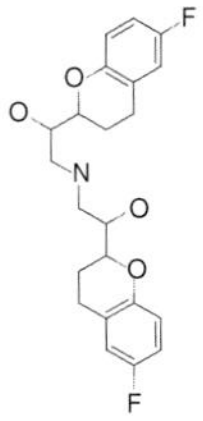
Bioavailability	30%	40–50%	30%	
Half-life	3–5 h	3–7 h	7–10 h	11–30 h
Absorption	>90%	100%	>90%	
Excretion	extensive first pass effect metabolites mainly renally excreted glucuronidation (UGT1A9, UGT2B4/7)	extensively metabolized in liver only 10% excreted unchanged renally	stereoselective first-pass metabolism; (rapid clearance of *S*-enantiomer) primarily hydroxylation followed by glucuronidation (UGT1A1, UGT2B4/7) and sulfation; demethylation	mono-, di-, and tri-hydroxylation *N*-dealkylation; glucuronidation
Metabolizing enzymes	CYP2D6, CYP1A2	CYP2D6	CYP2D6, CYP2C9	CYP2D6
Transporters	OCT2, P-gp inhibitor of OCT1 ($IC_{50} = 1.3\,\mu M$), OCT3 ($IC_{50} = 78\,\mu M$)	P-gp inhibitor of OCT1 ($IC_{50} = 53\,\mu M$)	P-gp inhibitor of OCT1 ($IC_{50} = 1.4\,\mu M$), OCT3 ($IC_{50} = 74\,\mu M$), OCTN1 ($IC_{50} = 73\,\mu M$)	

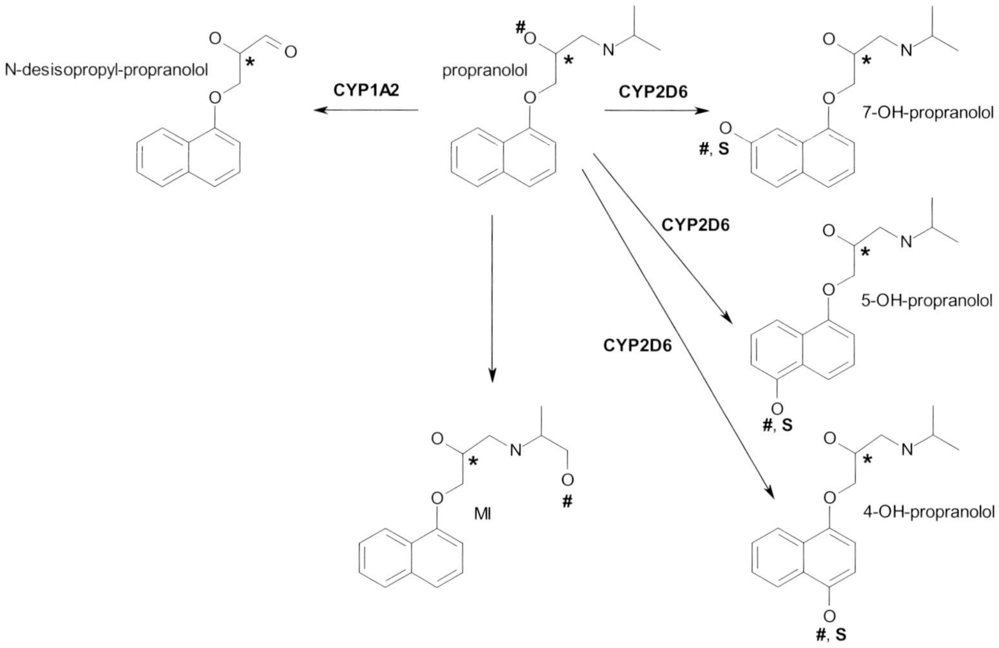

Figure 12.6 Metabolism of propranolol and responsible CYPs enzymes. Prazosin and its metabolites are enantiomers, and chirality centers are marked by asterisks. Sites for *O*-glucuronidation are marked by the hash symbols (#).

handled according to "Brater's algorithm" in chronic renal failure, nephritic syndrome, congestive heart failure, and cirrhosis [1].

Based on the mechanism of action, diuretics can be classified into six groups as detailed below.

12.5.1
Carbonic Anhydrase Inhibitors

These drugs act on a key enzyme of $NaHCO_3$ reabsorption and H^+ secretion in proximal tubuli. The Na^+ gradient of this section is created by the luminal Na^+–H^+ exchanger leading to Na^+ uptake. Carbonic anhydrase accelerates this action several thousand-fold by facilitating the transition $H_2O + CO_2 \rightarrow H_2CO_3$. Members of this group are acetazolamide and methazolamide (Table 12.8), but their clinical relevance is low.

12.5.2
Osmotic Diuretics

Glycerin, mannitol, and urea belong to this group of drugs, and act mainly in the loop of Henle and also in proximal tubuli by extracting water from intracellular

Table 12.8 Pharmacokinetics, metabolism, and transport of carbonic anhydrase inhibitors [1, 9, 10, 50].

	Acetazolamide	Methazolamide
	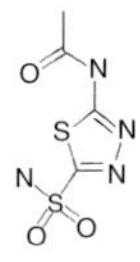	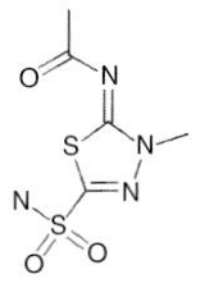
Bioavailability	100%	100%
Half-life	6–9 h	14 h
Absorption		
Excretion	renal	25% renal; 75% hepatic
Metabolizing enzymes	not metabolized	
Transporters	rOAT1	

compartments, leading to expanded extracellular fluid volume, decreased blood viscosity, and inhibited renin release. This reduces urinary excretion of Na^+, K^+, Ca^{2+}, Mg^{2+}, Cl^-, HCO_3^-, and phosphate.

12.5.3 Na^+–K^+–$2Cl^-$ Symport Inhibitors

Members of this class act on this transporter either in the ascending limb of the loop of Henle (high-ceiling diuretics) or in the distal convoluted tubule (thiazide or thiazide-like diuretics). The electrochemical Na^+ gradient established by the basolateral Na^+ pump is used by this symporter for "uphill" transport of K^+ and Cl^- into the cell. K^+ leaves the cell via an apical channel and Cl^- via a basolateral Cl^- channel.

The area of major reabsorptive capacity is the ascending limb of the loop of Henle (25% of filtered Na^+ is normally reabsorbed here) and high-ceiling diuretics acting mainly here are therefore highly efficacious. Hence, diuretics of this class like furosemide, ethacrynic acid, or torsemide (Table 12.9) allow a profound increase in urinary Na^+ and Cl^- excretion, and by abolition of the transepithelial potential difference also of Ca^{2+} and Mg^{2+}.

12.5.4 Thiazide or Thiazide-Like Diuretics

Unlike the above-mentioned diureticts, chlorothiazide, indapamide, or metolazone act in the distal convoluted tubule. As this part of the tubule is located past the highly absorptive area, these drugs (Table 12.10) are only moderately effective.

Table 12.9 Pharmacokinetics, metabolism, and transport of Na^{+}–K^{+}–$2Cl^{-}$ symport inhibitors [1, 9, 10, 50–54].

	Furosemide	**Torsemide**
	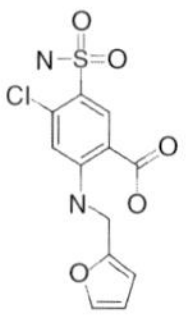	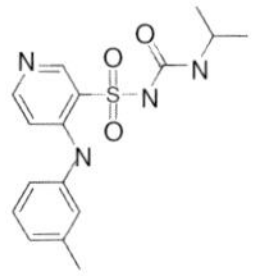
Bioavailability	60%	80%
Half-life	1.5 h	3.5 h
Absorption	60%	Rapid
Excretion	65% renal; 35% hepatic (only glucuronide metabolite)	20% renal; 80% hepatic (metabolites M1–M5; major: M5)
Metabolizing enzymes	?	CYP2C8
Transporters	rOAT1, OAT3, inhibitor of URAT1	Weak inhibitor of URAT1

Table 12.10 Pharmacokinetics, metabolism, and transport of thiazide or thiazide-like diuretics [1, 9, 10, 50, 53, 55].

	Chlorothiazide	**Indapamide**
	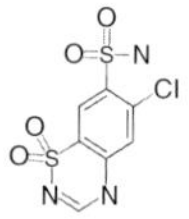	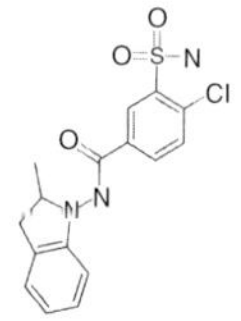
Bioavailability	9–56% (dose dependent)	93%
Half-life	1.5 h	14 h
Absorption	rapid	rapid
Excretion	renal	hepatic dehydrogenation hydroxylation and epoxidation
Metabolizing enzymes	not metabolized	CYP3A4
Transporters	inhibitor of OAT1 and rOAT1	

12.5.5 Nonspecific Cation Channel Inhibitors

These drugs are also called atrial natriuretic peptides (ANPs) and act mainly in the inner medullary collecting duct – the final absorptive site along the nephron. Five natriuretic peptides are produced in the human body and recombinant ANP or brain natriuretic peptide (BNP) are available as therapeutic agents. These peptides bind to the natriuretic peptide receptor, which increases intracellular cGMP resulting in the inhibition of a nonspecific cation channel. These peptide hormones are eliminated quickly by three ways: binding to natriuretic peptide receptor C, degradation by a neutral endopeptidase, and renal excretion. BNP (nesiritide), for example, has a half-life of 18 min.

12.5.6 Inhibitors of Renal Epithelial Na^+ Channels

These K^+-sparing diuretics act on Na^+ channels in the luminal membrane of cells in the late distal tubule and collecting duct, which allow Na^+ to follow the electrochemical gradient produced by Na^+ pumps in the basolateral membrane. This transepithelial potential difference is also important for the luminal secretion of K^+. The two drugs in this group – triamterene and amiloride (Table 12.11) – increase Na^+ excretion only minimally, whereas K^+, H^+, Ca^{2+}, and Mg^{2+} excretion rates are reduced.

Table 12.11 Pharmacokinetics, metabolism, and transport of inhibitors of renal epithelial Na^+ channels (K^+-sparing diuretics) [1, 9, 10, 56, 57].

	Triamterene	Amiloride
	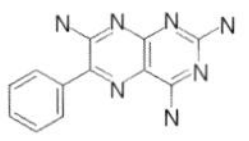	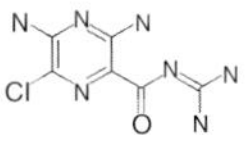
Bioavailability	around 50%	15–25%
Half-life	4 h (i.v.); OH-ester 3 h (i.v.)	21 h
Absorption	rapid, 50% of oral dose reaches urine	rapid
Excretion	renal, via sulfate conjugate	renal
Metabolizing enzymes	CYP1A2	not metabolized
Transporters	P-gp, BCRP	amiloride or metabolites are inhibitors of OCT1/2/3 and OCTN1/2

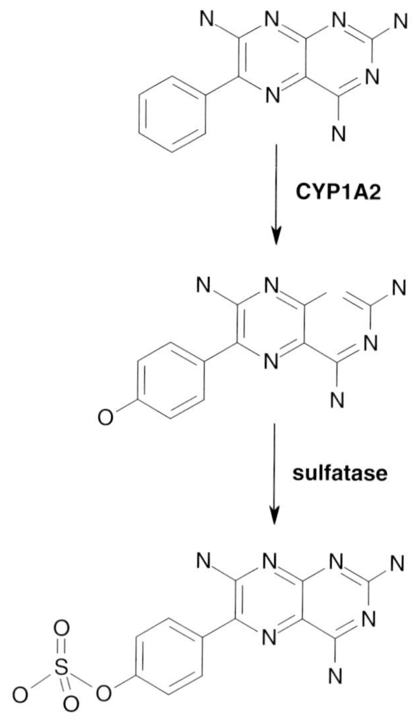

Figure 12.7 Metabolism of triamterene. The benzolic side-chain is hydroxylated by CYP1A2 and subsequently a substrate of sulfatases.

Triamterene is exclusively hydroxylated by CYP1A2, which converts it to the pharmacologically active *p*-OH-triamterene (Figure 12.7). The primary metabolite is the sulfate conjugate of OH-triamterene, of which the plasma levels greatly exceed the parent drug plasma levels [57]. The variability in CYP1A2 activity is changed by genetics, and highly affected by enzyme induction and inhibition. Important inducers are coffee or cigarette smoking. Triamterene is transported by P-gp and BCRP [58].

12.5.7 Mineralcorticoid Receptor Antagonists

Drugs of this class are also K^+-sparing diuretics and act on receptors, causing salt and water retention and increased K^+ and H^+ excretion after stimulation by mineralcorticoids like aldosterone. Therefore, receptor inhibition by spironolactone, canrenone, or eplerenone (Table 12.12) reduces the expression of aldosterone-induced proteins of cells in the late distal tubule and collecting duct, leading to similar effects as Na^+ channel inhibitors.

Table 12.12 Pharmacokinetics, metabolism, and transport of mineralocorticoid receptor antagonists (K^+-sparing diuretics) [1, 8–10, 59–62].

	Spironolactone	Eplerenone
	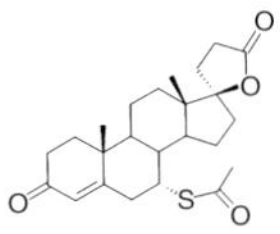	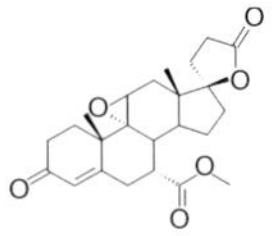
Bioavailability	65–100%	?
Half-life	10 min–1.6 h; metabolites 10–35 h	4–6 h
Absorption	rapid	
Excretion	hepatic; main metabolites are 7 α-thiomethylspirolactone, 6 β-OH-7-α-thiomethylspirolactone, and canrenone	5% unchanged; 66% via kidney as 6-β- and 21-OH-eplerenone
Metabolizing enzymes	by CYP enzymes lactone hydrolysis by PON3	CYP3A4
Transporters	Inhibitor of P-gp, rOatp1a1, rOatp1a3 OCT1 (IC_{50} = 1.2 μM), OCT3 (IC_{50} = 73 μM), OCTN1 (IC_{50} = 125 μM), OCTN2 (IC50 = 36 μM)	

12.6 Antiarrhythmics

12.6.1 Calcium Channel Blockers

Three different groups of calcium channel blockers are currently in clinical use (Table 12.13): hydropyridines (e.g., nifedipine, amlodipine), benzothiazepines (e.g., diltiazem), and phenylalkylamines (e.g., verapamil). All three are able to block the L-type calcium channels, but bind to different sites of the channel. Whereas the diltiazem and verapamil binding sites (D and V) overlap, the hydropyridine binding site (N) is located at a different part of the channel. Additionally, these groups show different affinities for different conformational stages of the calcium channel. Concerning the main site of drug action, hydropyridines have a higher potency for arterial vasodilation, whereas diltiazem and verapamil have stronger cardiac effects [63].

Verapamil is a synthetic papaverine derivate used for the treatment of angina, hypertension, and arrhythmia [64]. This calcium ion influx inhibitor (L-type

Table 12.13 Pharmacokinetics, metabolism, and transport of calcium channel blockers [1, 9, 10, 64, 66–75].

	Verapamil	**Amlodipine**	**Diltiazem**
	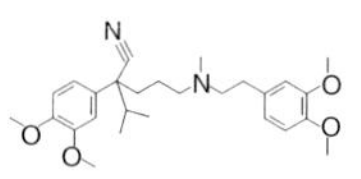	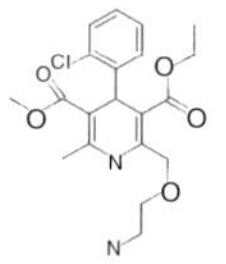	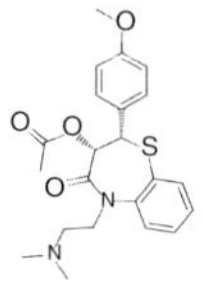
Bioavailability	22%	64–90%	
Half-life	2.8–7.4 h	30–50 h	3–4.5 h
Absorption	90%	around 100%	high
Excretion	70% renal as metabolites 3–4% unchanged 16% biliary	extensively metabolized renal: 10% of parent drug and 60% of metabolites	extensive first-pass effect; *N*-demethylation
Metabolizing enzymes	CYP3A4, CYP2C9	CYP3A4/5, stereoselective	CYP3A4
Transporters	OCTN1, OCTN2, P-gp (V + Nor-V + D-620 + D-617) inhibitor of OCT1 (IC_{50} = 1.2 μM), OCT3 (IC_{50} = 57 μM), OCTN1 (IC_{50} = 11 μM), OCTN2 (IC_{50} = 51 μM)	P-gp inhibitor of P-gp (IC_{50} = 22 μM) OCTN2 (inhibitor, K_i = 96 μM)	Inhibitor of P-gp (IC_{50} = 78 μM) OCT1 (IC_{50} = 1.7 μM), OCTN1 (IC_{50} = 126 μM)

calcium channel blocker) blocks depolarization of the atrioventricular (AV) node leading to decreased ventricular response by prolonged refractoriness and delayed AV node conduction. It is orally administered as a racemic mixture of (+)-*R*-verapamil and (−)-*S*-verapamil. Although having a similar spectrum of pharmacological effects, *S*-verapamil is 20 times more potent with regard to negative dromotropic effects on AV node conduction and only *R*-verapamil is able to reduce the mean arterial pressure [65].

Initial phase I metabolism of verapamil comprises *N*-dealkylation (formation of D-617), *N*-demethylation (formation of norverapamil), and *O*-demethylation (formation of D-703 and D-702) (Figure 12.8).

Data from cryopreserved hepatocytes showed that mainly norverapamil (around 30%), D-703, and D-617 (both around 20%) are produced in the liver [71]. *N*-dealkylation and *N*-demethylation are mainly catalyzed by CYP3A4/5 and CYP1A2. *O*-demethylation, however, is mainly catalyzed by CYP2C enzymes. Kinetic data from recombinant enzymes and expression data from human livers show

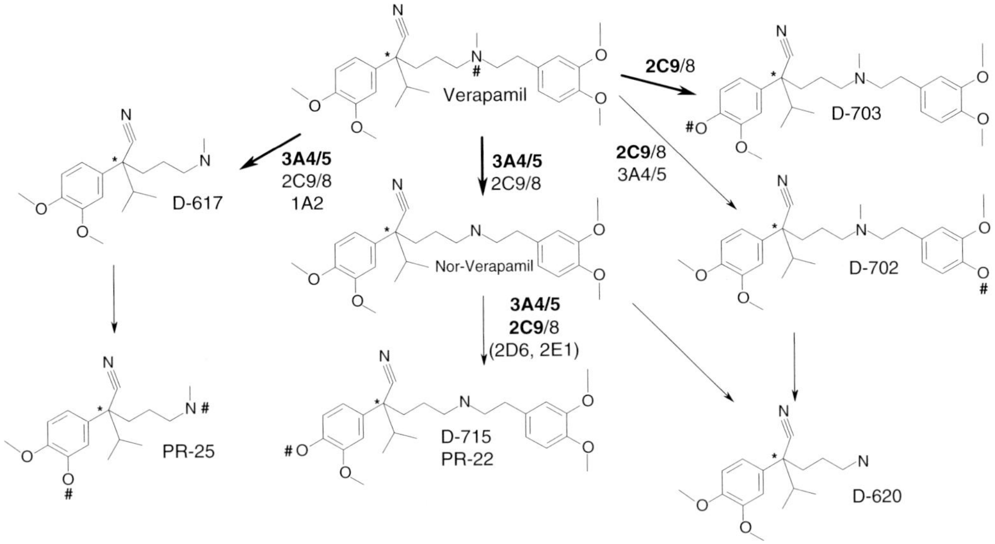

Figure 12.8 Metabolism of verapamil and responsible CYPs enzymes. Enzymes with major contribution are given in bold. Verapamil and its metabolites are an enantiomers and chirality centers are marked by asterisks. Possible sites for *N*- or *O*-glucuronidation [73] are marked by the hash symbols (#).

that CYP2C9 is the most important isozyme responsible for this reaction [66, 72, 76]. CYP2D6 and CYP2E1 play minor roles in the metabolism of norverapamil [76].

Phase II conjugation products have been described. Borlak *et al.* [73] were able to identify many glucuronides of verapamil and its metabolites in culture media of primary human hepatocytes and extracts of human urine. The responsible UGT enzymes have not yet been identified.

Transport of verapamil and its metabolites also shows high complexity. Whereas the *N*-dealkylated metabolites (D-617 and D-620) are good substrates of P-gp, the compounds with more functional units (verapamil, norverapamil, and D-703) are potent inhibitors of P-gp. Gut wall and liver express high levels of CYP and P-gp, making them the major sites of the complex interaction between verapamil metabolism and transport [74].

12.7 Anticoagulants

Drugs of this class have very different mechanisms of action, but are all aimed at altering the balance between procoagulant and anticoagulant reactions.

12.7.1 Heparin

This glycosaminoglycan serves as a catalytic template and increases thrombin–antithrombin binding 1000-fold, and in that way inhibits activated coagulation factors. It is clinically used to treat venous thrombosis and pulmonary embolism.

12.7.2 Vitamin K Antagonists

Drugs of this group, like warfarin, are oral anticoagulants. Several coagulation factors (II, VII, IX, X) require N-terminal glutamic acid carboxylation for their catalytic activity and the carboxylating enzyme requires reduced vitamin K for this reaction. Warfarin inhibits the vitamin K epoxide reductase (VKORC1). The drug is metabolized by CYP2C9 and carriers of the variant alleles *CYP2C9*2* or **3* (around 10–20% of the Caucasian population) with decreased enzymatic activity require a decreased drug dosage. Dose adjustment is also required according to *VKORC1* haplotype, with a 25% reduced dose in haplotype A heterozygotes and a 50% reduced dose in haplotype A homozygotes (with a frequency of around 40% in Caucasians, around 12% in African-Americans, and around 80% in Asians) [77–79].

12.7.3 Antiplatelet Drugs

These drugs inhibit the formation of the initial hemostatic plug at the site of vascular injury, and are therefore clinically highly relevant in the prevention of myocardial infarction, stroke, and peripheral vascular thromboses, and are used after angioplastic and vascular stent surgery. G-protein-coupled purinergic receptors in platelets (P2Y) are activated by ADP.

Clopidogrel – a thienopyridine prodrug – is an ADP P2Y12 receptor antagonist. It requires enzymatic conversion to the active thiol metabolite (Figure 12.9). Recently, it was shown that this activation is a two-step process involving an oxidation to 2-oxo-clopidogrel by the enzymes CYP2C19, CYP1A2, and CYP2B6 [80], and a hydrolysis reaction of the γ-thiobutyrolactone to the active drug by PON1 and PON3 [81] – a step that has also been described to be catalyzed by CYP3A4, CYP2B6, CYP2C19, and CYP2C9 [80]. Pharmacokinetic parameters of clopidogrel and warfarin are summarized in Table 12.14.

Additionally, CES1 and CES2, and to a minor amount butyrylcholinesterase, were described to be involved in the conversion to inactive carboxylic metabolites of clopidogrel, 2-oxo-clopidogrel, and the active thiol metabolite [81]. Furthermore, clopidogrel is a substrate of P-glycoprotein [82].

Interindividual variability in the antiplatelet response to this drug is high and most probably attributable to genetic effects. Genetic variability in the *CYP2C19* gene predicts variable clinical response to clopidogrel to considerable extent. A

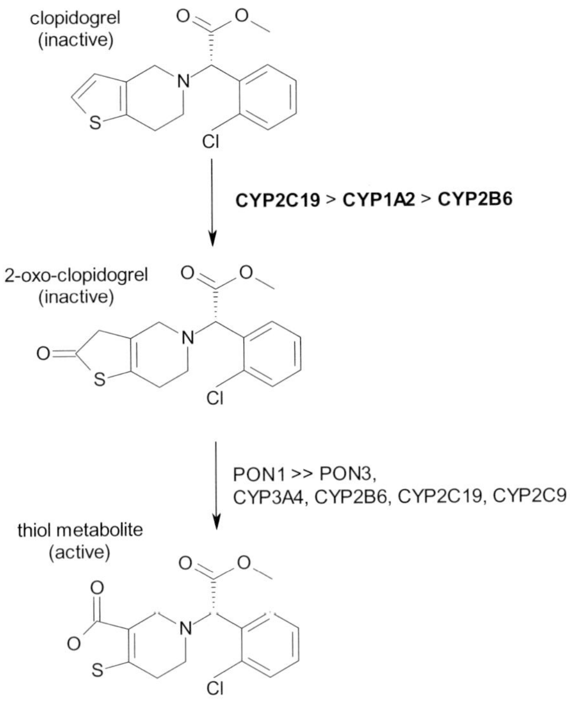

Figure 12.9 Metabolism of clopidogrel. Relative catalytic efficiencies of enzymes are shown and most important enzymes are printed in bold.

recent meta-analysis showed that carriers of a *CYP2C19* loss of function allele (specifically the most common **2* variant), compared to non-carriers, had a 1.5 to 2 times higher risk of cardiovascular events, and a 3 to 4 times higher risk of stent thrombosis after percutaneous coronary intervention.

The common *PON1 Q192R* variation considerably increased the risk for stent thrombosis in *Q192* homozygotes in one study [81], but this finding could not be reproduced in other studies [83, 84]. PON1 enzyme expression is mainly affected by various PON1 promoter polymorphisms including *–108C>T* and might therefore also be important [85].

12.8 Cholesterol-Lowering Drugs

High levels of low-density lipoproteins (LDLs) are a major cause of atherosclerosis, and associated with coronary heart disease, ischemic cerebrovascular disease, and peripheral vascular disease. Several types of drugs are used to treat hyperlipidemias.

Table 12.14 Pharmacokinetics, metabolism, and transport of anticoagulants [1, 9, 10, 77, 78, 80, 81].

	Clopidogrel	Warfarin
	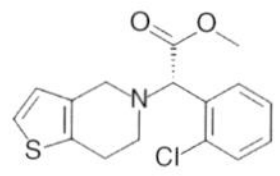	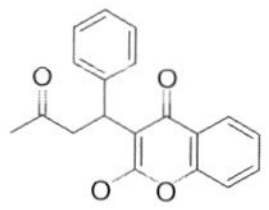
Bioavailability		around 100%
Half-life	8 h (carboxylic acid metabolites)	S-warfarin: 21–43 h R-warfarin: 37–89 h
Absorption	>50%	rapid
Excretion	50% renal, 46% biliary	
Metabolizing enzymes	CYP2C19, CYP1A2, CYP2B6, CYP3A4, PON1, PON3	S-warfarin by CYP2C9 (6-/7-OH) R-warfarin by CYP1A1, 1A2, and 3A4 glucuronidation at 6-/7-/8-OH UGT1A1 (UGT1A10)
Transporters	P-gp	OATPs (not clinically important)

12.8.1 Bile Acid Sequestrants

These resins are the oldest drugs of this group. They are not absorbed from the intestine and are able to lower LDL-cholesterol up to 25%, but may lead to gastrointestinal side-effects lowering compliance.

12.8.2 Cholesterol Uptake Inhibitors

Ezetimibe inhibits the transport protein NPC1L1 in jejunal enterocytes, reducing the uptake of cholesterol in the intestine and in that way reducing blood LDL-cholesterol levels by 15–20%. Ezetimibe is excreted in the form of glucuronides, 70% via feces and around 10% via urine. UGT1A1, 1A3, and 2B15 were found to produce the phenolic glucuronide, whereas UGT2B7 formed the benzylic glucuronide [86]. Ezetimibe and ezetimibe-glucuronide are substrates of MRP2 and P-gp [87].

12.8.3 Fibrates

This group of drugs also lowers LDL-cholesterol and, in addition, can increase the beneficial high-density lipoprotein (HDL)-cholesterol. The mechanism of action is still poorly understood, but involves fibrate binding to peroxisome proliferator-activated receptor-α, resulting in increased fatty acid oxidation, LPL synthesis, a reduced expression of apolipoprotein C III as well as increased expression of apolipoprotein AI and II, thereby stimulating an increase of HDL levels. The fibrate gemfibrozil is subject to oxidative metabolism and extensive glucuronidation [88] with UGT2B7 as the main UGT involved [89].

12.8.4 **Statins**

The most effective and most widely used drugs to lower LDL-cholesterol are 3-hydroxy-3-methyl-glutaryl (HMG)-CoA reductase inhibitors (statins, Table 12.15). They inhibit the rate-limiting enzyme in the biosynthesis of cholesterol. Resulting low levels of cholesterol in hepatocytes lead to an increased expression of LDL-cholesterol receptors on the hepatocyte membrane. In this way, more LDL-cholesterol is taken up from the plasma into the hepatocytes and plasma LDL levels are effectively reduced up to 55%. The statins are all structurally similar to HMG-CoA and are therefore reversible competitive inhibitors of the enzyme. In addition, statins were described to have positive effects independent of their effect on LDL-cholesterol. These pleiotropic effects influence endothelial function, plaque stability, coagulation, an anti-inflammatory function, and a decreased lipoprotein oxidation.

Atorvastatin – the entirely synthetic member of this group – is administered as an active drug in the statin acid conformation, but like many statins it is also found in its inactive lactone conformation with nearly equal AUCs. Both the acid and the lactone conformation are substrates of CYP3A4 and CYP3A5, resulting in *p*- and *o*-OH-metabolites (Figure 12.10). A comparison of the metabolism of acid and lactone revealed that the lactone had a 20-fold lower K_m, possibly due to higher lipophilicity resulting in better access to the hydrophobic substrate channel of the CYP enzyme near the membrane surface [93]. These results clearly indicated that the major elimination pathway of atorvastatin was via hydroxylation of atorvastatin lactone and not via hydroxylation of the parent compound. Inhibition or induction of CYP3A4 are reported to be associated with drug–drug interactions involving atorvastatin and other statins.

Recently, it was shown that UGT1A3 is responsible for the lactonization of atorvastatin in human liver. The parent compound is glucuronidated by this enzyme, leading to an unstable acyl-glucuronide which rapidly disintegrates to the pharmacologically inactive atorvastatin-lactone. The common *UGT1A3*2* haplotype was shown to increase this conversion around 2-fold *in vitro* and the lactone to acid AUC around 1.4-fold *in vivo* by an increased expression of the enzyme [94]. However, the atorvastatin-lactone is converted spontaneously and enzyme-dependently back to the parent compound at physiological pH. For this conversion, PON1 and PON3 were identified to be responsible. Although this conversion is not affected by common PON1 amino acid changes (L55M, Q192R), homozygous carriers of the common *PON1* promoter polymorphism *−108T>C* had a 1.7-fold higher lactone hydrolysis *in vitro* [85].

Table 12.15 Pharmacokinetics, metabolism, and transport of HMG-CoA reductase inhibitors [1, 9, 10, 90–92].

	Atorvastatin	Cerivastatin	Fluvastatin	Lovastatin	Pravastatin	Simvastatin	Rosuvastatin	Pitavastatin
	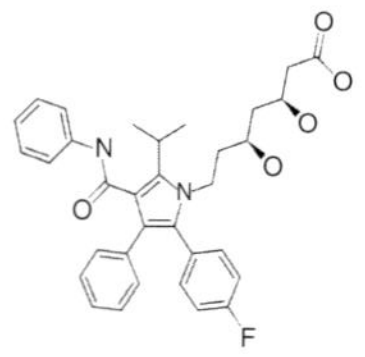	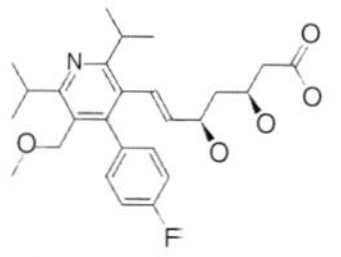	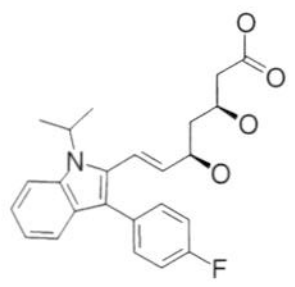	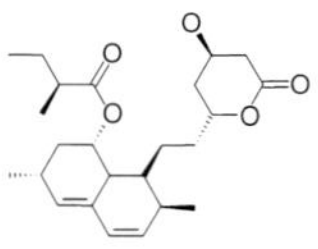	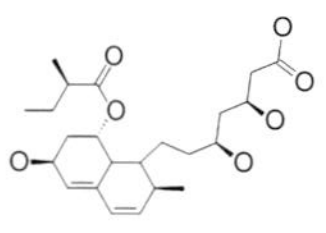	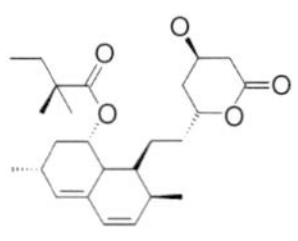	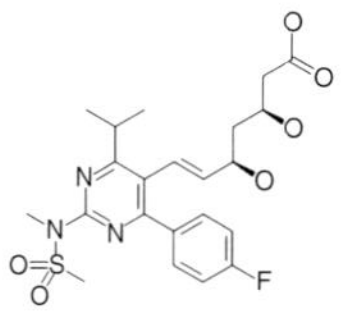	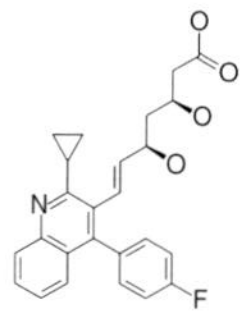
Bioavailability	12%	60%	24%	5%	18%	5%	20%	80%
Half-life	14 h OH-acids 20–30 h	2.5 h	1.2 h	3 h	1.8 h	2 h	19 h	11 h
Absorption	30%	>98%	98%	30%	35%	60–85%	50%	80%
Excretion	mainly biliary, <5% renal	30% renal	6% renal	10% renal	20% renal	13% renal	10% renal	NA
Metabolizing enzymes	CYP3A4, UGT1A3, PON1, PON3	CYP2C8, CYP3A4	CYP2C9	CYP3A4, CYP2C8?	low	CYP3A4, CYP2C8	low, CYP2C9 (CYP2C19)	low, (CYP2C9)
Transporters	OATP1B1, P-gp, MRP2, BCRP	OATP1B1, P-gp, MRP2, BCRP, BSEP	BSEP	P-gp	OATP1B1, OATP2B1, P-gp, OAT3, MRP2, BCRP, BSEP	OATP1B1, P-gp (lactone + acid)	OATP1B1	OATP1B1, OATP1B3, BSEP

BSEP, bile salt export pump (ABCB11).

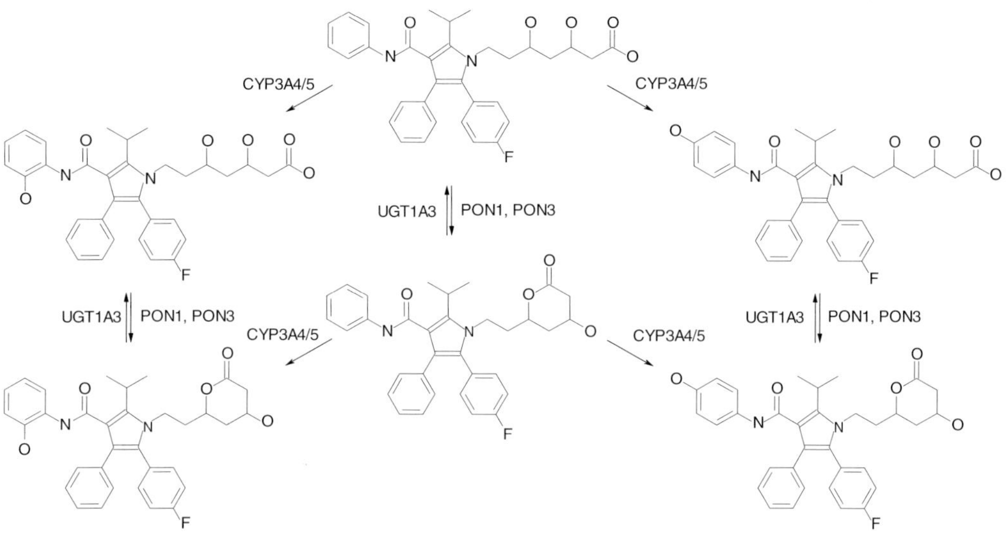

Figure 12.10 Metabolism of atorvastatin. *p*- and *o*-Hydroxyatorvastatin are pharmacologically active metabolites, whereas atorvastatin-lactone and its hydroxy metabolites are pharmacologically inactive. Due the fact that the lactone is a better substrate of CYP3A enzymes than the parent drug, the major metabolic pathway consists of UGT1A3-dependent lactonization followed by CYP3A-catalyzed hydroxylation. PON1 and PON3 are important for the hydrolysis of atorvastatin-lactones.

The uptake of atorvastatin into hepatocytes is mediated by the mostly liver expressed OATP1B1, OATP1B3, and the ubiquitously expressed OATP2B1 [95–97]. Plasma concentrations of many statins are 1.4-fold increased by the common amino acid variant V174A of OATP1B1. Additionally, drug–drug interactions via inhibition of OATP1B1 have been reported for several statins [98]. Focusing on the drug efflux, P-gp is known to export atorvastatin and its hydroxy metabolites [99]. Additionally, MRP1, 2, 3, and 6 were reported to be involved in atorvastatin transport [100]. Atorvastatin plasma concentrations were found to be affected by amino acid changes of P-gp (ABCB1) A893S/T or BCRP (ABCG2) Q141K, which had 1.6- or 1.7-fold higher plasma AUC of atorvastatin, respectively [101, 102].

References

1 Brunton, L.L., Chabner, B.A., and Knollmann, B.C. (eds) (2011) *Goodman and Gilman's The Pharmacological Basis of Therapeutics*, McGraw-Hill, New York.

2 Toutain, P.L. and Lefèbvre, H.P. (2004) Pharmacokinetics and pharmacokinetic/pharmacodynamic relationships for angiotensin-converting enzyme inhibitors. *J. Vet. Pharmacol. Ther.*, **27**, 515–525.

3 Verho, M., Luck, C., Stelter, W.J., Rangoonwala, B., and Bender, N. (1995) Pharmacokinetics, metabolism and biliary and urinary excretion of oral ramipril in man. *Curr. Med. Res. Opin.*, **13**, 264–273.

4 Shu, C., Shen, H., Hopfer, U., and Smith, D.E. (2001) Mechanism of intestinal absorption and renal reabsorption of an orally active ACE inhibitor: uptake and transport of fosinopril in cell cultures. *Drug Metab. Dispos.*, **29**, 1307–1315.

5 Vree, T.B., Dammers, E., Ulc, I., Horkovics-Kovats, S., Ryska, M., and Merkx, I. (2003) Lack of male–female differences in disposition and esterase hydrolysis of ramipril to ramiprilat in healthy volunteers after a single oral dose. *ScientificWorldJournal*, **3**, 1332–1343.

6 Li, B., Sedlacek, M., Manoharan, I., Boopathy, R., Duysen, E.G., Masson, P., *et al.* (2005) Butyrylcholinesterase, paraoxonase, and albumin esterase, but not carboxylesterase, are present in human plasma. *Biochem. Pharmacol.*, **70**, 1673–1684.

7 Yamada, S., Richardson, K., Tang, M., Halaschek-Wiener, J., Cook, V.J., Fitzgerald, J.M., *et al.* (2010) Genetic variation in carboxylesterase genes and susceptibility to isoniazid-induced hepatotoxicity. *Pharmacogenomics J.*, **10**, 524–536.

8 Draganov, D.I., Teiber, J.F., Speelman, A., Osawa, Y., Sunahara, R., and La Du, B.N. (2005) Human paraoxonases (PON1, PON2, and PON3) are lactonases with overlapping and distinct substrate specificities. *J. Lipid Res.*, **46**, 1239–1247.

9 Wishart, D.S., Knox, C., Guo, A.C., Shrivastava, S., Hassanali, M., Stothard, P., *et al.* (2006) DrugBank: a comprehensive resource for in silico drug discovery and exploration. *Nucleic Acids Res.*, **34**, D668–D672.

10 Ozawa, N., Shimizu, T., Morita, R., Yokono, Y., Ochiai, T., Munesada, K., Ohashi, A., Aida, Y., Hama, Y., Taki, K., Maeda, K., Kusuhara, H., and Sugiyama, Y. (2004) Transporter database, TPSearch: a web-accessible comprehensive database for research in pharmacokinetics of drugs. *Pharm. Res.*, **21**, 2133–2134.

11 Stearns, R.A., Chakravarty, P.K., Chen, R., and Chiu, S.H. (1995) Biotransformation of losartan to its active carboxylic acid metabolite in human liver microsomes. Role of cytochrome P4502C and 3A subfamily members. *Drug Metab. Dispos.*, **23**, 207–215.

12 Stearns, R.A., Miller, R.R., Doss, G.A., Chakravarty, P.K., Rosegay, A., Gatto, G.J., *et al.* (1992) The metabolism of DuP 753, a nonpeptide angiotensin II receptor antagonist, by rat, monkey, and human liver slices. *Drug Metab. Dispos.*, **20**, 281–287.

13 Iwanaga, T., Sato, M., Maeda, T., Ogihara, T. and Tamai, I. (2007) Concentration-dependent mode of interaction of angiotensin II receptor blockers with uric acid transporter. *J. Pharmacol. Exp. Ther.*, **320**, 211–217.

14 Alonen, A., Finel, M., and Kostiainen, R. (2008) The human UDP-glucuronosyltransferase UGT1A3 is highly selective towards N2 in the tetrazole ring of losartan, candesartan, and zolarsartan. *Biochem. Pharmacol.*, **76**, 763–772.

15 Yun, C.H., Lee, H.S., Lee, H., Rho, J.K., Jeong, H.G., and Guengerich, F.P. (1995) Oxidation of the angiotensin II receptor antagonist losartan (DuP 753) in human liver microsomes. Role of cytochrome P4503A(4) in formation of the active metabolite EXP3174. *Drug Metab. Dispos.*, **23**, 285–289.

16 Yasar, U., Tybring, G., Hidestrand, M., Oscarson, M., Ingelman-Sundberg, M., Dahl, M.L., *et al.* (2001) Role of CYP2C9 polymorphism in losartan oxidation. *Drug Metab. Dispos.*, **29**, 1051–1056.

17 Williamson, K.M., Patterson, J.H., McQueen, R.H., Adams, K.F., and Pieper, J.A. (1998) Effects of erythromycin or rifampin on losartan pharmacokinetics in healthy volunteers. *Clin. Pharmacol. Ther.*, **63**, 316–323.

18 Kaukonen, K.M., Olkkola, K.T., and Neuvonen, P.J. (1998) Fluconazole but not itraconazole decreases the metabolism of losartan to E-3174. *Eur. J. Clin. Pharmacol.*, **53**, 445–449.

19 Meadowcroft, A.M., Williamson, K.M., Patterson, J.H., Hinderliter, A.L., and Pieper, J.A. (1999) The effects of fluvastatin, a CYP2C9 inhibitor, on

losartan pharmacokinetics in healthy volunteers. *J. Clin. Pharmacol.*, **39**, 418–424.

20 Sandwall, P., Lo, M.W., Jonzon, B., Dalén, P., Furtek, C., Ritter, M., *et al.* (1999) Lack of polymorphism of the conversion of losartan to its active metabolite E-3174 in extensive and poor metabolizers of debrisoquine (cytochrome P450 2D6) and mephenytoin (cytochrome P450 2C19). *Eur. J. Clin. Pharmacol.*, **55**, 279–283.

21 Soldner, A., Benet, L.Z., Mutschler, E., and Christians, U. (2000) Active transport of the angiotensin-II antagonist losartan and its main metabolite EXP 3174 across MDCK-MDR1 and caco-2 cell monolayers. *Br. J. Pharmacol.*, **129**, 1235–1243.

22 Knütter, I., Kottra, G., Fischer, W., Daniel, H., and Brandsch, M. (2009) High-affinity interaction of sartans with H^+/peptide transporters. *Drug Metab. Dispos.*, **37**, 143–149.

23 Edwards, R.M., Stack, E.J., and Trizna, W. (1999) Transport of [^{3}H]losartan across isolated perfused rabbit proximal tubule. *J. Pharmacol. Exp. Ther.*, **290**, 38–42.

24 Yamashiro, W., Maeda, K., Hirouchi, M., Adachi, Y., Hu, Z., and Sugiyama, Y. (2006) Involvement of transporters in the hepatic uptake and biliary excretion of valsartan, a selective antagonist of the angiotensin II AT1-receptor, in humans. *Drug Metab. Dispos.*, **34**, 1247–1254.

25 Yamada, A., Maeda, K., Kamiyama, E., Sugiyama, D., Kondo, T., Shiroyanagi, Y., *et al.* (2007) Multiple human isoforms of drug transporters contribute to the hepatic and renal transport of olmesartan, a selective antagonist of the angiotensin II AT1-receptor. *Drug Metab. Dispos.*, **35**, 2166–2176.

26 Ibrahim, K.E., Midgley, J.M., Crowley, J.R., and Williams, C.M. (1983) The mammalian metabolism of *R*-(–)-*m*-synephrine. *J. Pharm. Pharmacol.*, **35**, 144–147.

27 Gumbhir, K. and Mason, W.D. (1996) High-performance liquid chromatographic determination of phenylephrine and its conjugates in human plasma using solid-phase extraction and electrochemical detection. *J. Pharm. Biomed. Anal.*, **14**, 623–630.

28 McInnes, G.T. (2008) *Clinical Pharmacology and Therapeutics of Hypertension*, Elsevier, Oxford.

29 van Zwieten, P.A. (1999) Centrally acting antihypertensive drugs. Present and future. *Clin. Exp. Hypertens.*, **21**, 859–873.

30 Claessens, A.J., Risler, L.J., Eyal, S., Shen, D.D., Easterling, T., and Hebert, M.F. (2010) CYP2D6 mediates 4-hydroxylation of clonidine *in vitro*: implication for pregnancy-induced changes in clonidine clearance. *Drug Metab Dispos.*, **38**, 1393–1396.

31 Faassen, F., Vogel, G., Spanings, H., and Vromans, H. (2003) Caco-2 permeability, P-glycoprotein transport ratios and brain penetration of heterocyclic drugs. *Int. J. Pharm.*, **263**, 113–122.

32 Bednarczyk, D., Ekins, S., Wikel, J.H., and Wright, S.H. (2003) Influence of molecular structure on substrate binding to the human organic cation transporter, hOCT1. *Mol. Pharmacol.*, **63**, 489–498.

33 Wu, X., Huang, W., Ganapathy, M.E., Wang, H., Kekuda, R., Conway, S.J., *et al.* (2000) Structure, function, and regional distribution of the organic cation transporter OCT3 in the kidney. *Am. J. Physiol. Renal Physiol.*, **279**, F449–F458.

34 Ohashi, R., Tamai, I., Yabuuchi, H., Nezu, J.I., Oku, A., Sai, Y., *et al.* (1999) Na^+-dependent carnitine transport by organic cation transporter (OCTN2): its pharmacological and toxicological relevance. *J. Pharmacol. Exp. Ther.*, **291**, 778–784.

35 Yabuuchi, H., Tamai, I., Nezu, J., Sakamoto, K., Oku, A., Shimane, M., *et al.* (1999) Novel membrane transporter OCTN1 mediates multispecific, bidirectional, and pH-dependent transport of organic cations. *J. Pharmacol. Exp. Ther.*, **289**, 768–773.

36 Sonders, R.C. (1986) Pharmacokinetics of terazosin. *Am. J. Med.*, **80**, 20–24.

37 Elliott, H.L., Meredith, P.A., and Reid, J.L. (1987) Pharmacokinetic overview of doxazosin. *Am. J. Cardiol.*, **59**, 78G–81G.

38 Pan, G., Winter, T.N., Roberts, J.C., Fairbanks, C.A., and Elmquist, W.F. (2010) Organic cation uptake is enhanced in bcrp1-transfected MDCKII cells. *Mol. Pharm.*, **7**, 138–145.

39 Dey, S., Ramachandra, M., Pastan, I., Gottesman, M.M., and Ambudkar, S.V. (1997) Evidence for two nonidentical drug-interaction sites in the human P-glycoprotein. *Proc. Natl. Acad. Sci. USA*, **94**, 10594–10599.

40 Hayer-Zillgen, M., Brüss, M., and Bönisch, H. (2002) Expression and pharmacological profile of the human organic cation transporters hOCT1, hOCT2 and hOCT3. *Br. J. Pharmacol.*, **136**, 829–836.

41 Le Corre, P., Parmer, R.J., Kailasam, M.T., Kennedy, B.P., Skaar, T.P., Ho, H., *et al.* (2004) Human sympathetic activation by alpha2-adrenergic blockade with yohimbine: bimodal, epistatic influence of cytochrome P450-mediated drug metabolism. *Clin. Pharmacol. Ther.*, **76**, 139–153.

42 Rau, T., Heide, R., Bergmann, K., Wuttke, H., Werner, U., Feifel, N., *et al.* (2002) Effect of the CYP2D6 genotype on metoprolol metabolism persists during long-term treatment. *Pharmacogenetics*, **12**, 465–472.

43 Bart, J., Dijkers, E.C.F., Wegman, T.D., de Vries, E.G.E., van der Graaf, W.T.A., Groen, H.J.M., *et al.* (2005) New positron emission tomography tracer [(11)C]carvedilol reveals P-glycoprotein modulation kinetics. *Br. J. Pharmacol.*, **145**, 1045–1051.

44 Gu, Z., *et al.* (2003) Metabolism study of ^{14}C nebivolol in humans with different CYP2D6 genotypes, AAPS Annual Meeting, Salt Lake City, UT, abstract (http://www.aapsj.org/abstracts/AM_2003/AAPS2003-002800.pdf).

45 Masubuchi, Y., Hosokawa, S., Horie, T., Suzuki, T., Ohmori, S., Kitada, M., *et al.* (1994) Cytochrome P450 isozymes involved in propranolol metabolism in human liver microsomes. The role of CYP2D6 as ring-hydroxylase and CYP1A2 as *N*-desisopropylase. *Drug Metab. Dispos.*, **22**, 909–915.

46 Ward, S.A., Walle, T., Walle, U.K., Wilkinson, G.R., and Branch, R.A. (1989) Propranolol's metabolism is determined by both mephenytoin and debrisoquin hydroxylase activities. *Clin. Pharmacol. Ther.*, **45**, 72–79.

47 Izukawa, T., Nakajima, M., Fujiwara, R., Yamanaka, H., Fukami, T., Takamiya, M., *et al.* (2009) Quantitative analysis of UGT1A and UGT2B expression levels in human livers. *Drug Metab. Dispos.*, **37**, 1759–1768.

48 Dudley, A.J., Bleasby, K., and Brown, C.D. (2000) The organic cation transporter OCT2 mediates the uptake of beta-adrenoceptor antagonists across the apical membrane of renal LLC-PK(1) cell monolayers. *Br. J. Pharmacol.*, **131**, 71–79.

49 D'Emanuele, A., Jevprasesphant, R., Penny, J., and Attwood, D. (2004) The use of a dendrimer-propranolol prodrug to bypass efflux transporters and enhance oral bioavailability. *J. Control Release*, **95**, 447–453.

50 Uwai, Y., Saito, H., Hashimoto, Y., and Inui, K.I. (2000) Interaction and transport of thiazide diuretics, loop diuretics, and acetazolamide via rat renal organic anion transporter rOAT1. *J. Pharmacol. Exp. Ther.*, **295**, 261–265.

51 Smith, D.E., Lin, E.T., and Benet, L.Z. (1980) Absorption and disposition of furosemide in healthy volunteers, measured with a metabolite-specific assay. *Drug Metab. Dispos.*, **8**, 337–342.

52 Yang, K.H., Choi, Y.H., Lee, U., Lee, J.H., and Lee, M.G. (2009) Effects of cytochrome P450 inducers and inhibitors on the pharmacokinetics of intravenous furosemide in rats: involvement of CYP2C11, 2E1, 3A1 and 3A2 in furosemide metabolism. *J. Pharm. Pharmacol.*, **61**, 47–54.

53 Race, J.E., Grassl, S.M., Williams, W.J., and Holtzman, E.J. (1999) Molecular cloning and characterization of two novel human renal organic anion transporters (hOAT1 and hOAT3). *Biochem. Biophys. Res. Commun.*, **255**, 508–514.

54 Hasannejad, H., Takeda, M., Taki, K., Shin, H.J., Babu, E., Jutabha, P., *et al.* (2004) Interactions of human organic anion transporters with diuretics. *J. Pharmacol. Exp. Ther.*, **308**, 1021–1029.

55 Sun, H., Moore, C., Dansette, P.M., Kumar, S., Halpert, J.R., and Yost, G.S. (2009) Dehydrogenation of the indoline-containing drug 4-chloro-*N*-(2-methyl-1-indolinyl)-3-sulfamoylbenzamide (indapamide) by CYP3A4: correlation with *in silico* predictions. *Drug Metab. Dispos.*, **37**, 672–684.

56 Brodie, R.R., Chasseaud, L.F., Darragh, A., Taylor, T., and Walmsley, L.M. (1982) Bioavailability of bemetizide and triamterene from a combination formulation. *Biopharm. Drug Dispos.*, **3**, 361–370.

57 Fuhr, U., Kober, S., Zaigler, M., Mutschler, E., and Spahn-Langguth, H. (2005) Rate-limiting biotransformation of triamterene is mediated by CYP1A2. *Int. J. Clin. Pharmacol. Ther.*, **43**, 327–334.

58 Enokizono, J., Kusuhara, H., Ose, A., Schinkel, A.H., and Sugiyama, Y. (2008) Quantitative investigation of the role of breast cancer resistance protein (Bcrp/Abcg2) in limiting brain and testis penetration of xenobiotic compounds. *Drug Metab. Dispos.*, **36**, 995–1002.

59 Kanai, N., Lu, R., Bao, Y., Wolkoff, A.W., and Schuster, V.L. (1996) Transient expression of oatp organic anion transporter in mammalian cells: identification of candidate substrates. *Am. J. Physiol.*, **270**, F319–F325.

60 Masuda, S., Ibaramoto, K., Takeuchi, A., Saito, H., Hashimoto, Y., and Inui, K.I. (1999) Cloning and functional characterization of a new multispecific organic anion transporter, OAT-K2, in rat kidney. *Mol. Pharmacol.*, **55**, 743–752.

61 Gardiner, P., Schrode, K., Quinlan, D., Martin, B.K., Boreham, D.R., Rogers, M.S., *et al.* (1989) Spironolactone metabolism: steady-state serum levels of the sulfur-containing metabolites. *J. Clin. Pharmacol.*, **29**, 342–347.

62 Cook, C.S., Berry, L.M., Kim, D.H., Burton, E.G., Hribar, J.D., and Zhang, L. (2002) Involvement of CYP3A in the metabolism of eplerenone in humans and dogs: differential metabolism by CYP3A4 and CYP3A5. *Drug Metab. Dispos.*, **30**, 1344–1351.

63 Golan, D.E. (2008) *Principles of Pharmacology*, Lippincott Williams & Wilkins, Baltimore, MD.

64 Eichelbaum, M., Ende, M., Remberg, G., Schomerus, M., and Dengler, H.J. (1979) The metabolism of DL-[^{14}C] verapamil in man. *Drug Metab. Dispos.*, **7**, 145–148.

65 Busse, D., Templin, S., Mikus, G., Schwab, M., Hofmann, U., Eichelbaum, M., *et al.* (2006) Cardiovascular effects of (*R*)- and (*S*)-verapamil and racemic verapamil in humans: a placebo-controlled study. *Eur. J. Clin. Pharmacol.*, **62**, 613–619.

66 Busse, D., Cosme, J., Beaune, P., Kroemer, H.K., and Eichelbaum, M. (1995) Cytochromes of the P450 2C subfamily are the major enzymes involved in the *O*-demethylation of verapamil in humans. *Naunyn Schmiedebergs Arch. Pharmacol.*, **353**, 116–121.

67 Grube, M., Ameling, S., Noutsias, M., Köck, K., Triebel, I., Bonitz, K., *et al.* (2011) Selective regulation of cardiac organic cation transporter novel type 2 (OCTN2) in dilated cardiomyopathy. *Am. J. Pathol.*, **178**, 2547–2559.

68 Diao, L., Ekins, S., and Polli, J.E. (2009) Novel inhibitors of human organic cation/carnitine transporter (hOCTN2) via computational modeling and *in vitro* testing. *Pharm. Res.*, **26**, 1890–1900.

69 Kim, K.-A., Park, P.-W., and Park, J.-Y. (2007) Effect of ABCB1 (MDR1) haplotypes derived from G2677T/C3435T on the pharmacokinetics of amlodipine in healthy subjects. *Br. J. Clin. Pharmacol.*, **63**, 53–58.

70 Takara, K., Sakaeda, T., Tanigawara, Y., Nishiguchi, K., Ohmoto, N., Horinouchi, M., *et al.* (2002) Effects of 12 Ca^{2+} antagonists on multidrug resistance, MDR1-mediated transport and MDR1 mRNA expression. *Eur. J. Pharm. Sci.*, **16**, 159–165.

71 Reder-Hilz, B., Ullrich, M., Ringel, M., Hewitt, N., Utesch, D., Oesch, F., *et al.* (2004) Metabolism of propafenone and

verapamil by cryopreserved human, rat, mouse and dog hepatocytes: comparison with metabolism *in vivo*. *Naunyn Schmiedebergs Arch. Pharmacol.*, **369**, 408–417.

72 Kroemer, H.K., Gautier, J.C., Beaune, P., Henderson, C., Wolf, C.R., and Eichelbaum, M. (1993) Identification of P450 enzymes involved in metabolism of verapamil in humans. *Naunyn Schmiedebergs Arch. Pharmacol.*, **348**, 332–337.

73 Borlak, J., Walles, M., Elend, M., Thum, T., Preiss, A., and Levsen, K. (2003) Verapamil: identification of novel metabolites in cultures of primary human hepatocytes and human urine by LC-MS^n and LC-NMR. *Xenobiotica*, **33**, 655–676.

74 Pauli-Magnus, C., von Richter, O., Burk, O., Ziegler, A., Mettang, T., Eichelbaum, M., *et al.* (2000) Characterization of the major metabolites of verapamil as substrates and inhibitors of P-glycoprotein. *J. Pharmacol. Exp. Ther.*, **293**, 376–382.

75 Klotz, U. (2007) Antiarrhythmics: elimination and dosage considerations in hepatic impairment. *Clin. Pharmacokinet.*, **46**, 985–996.

76 Tracy, T.S., Korzekwa, K.R., Gonzalez, F.J., and Wainer, I.W. (1999) Cytochrome P450 isoforms involved in metabolism of the enantiomers of verapamil and norverapamil. *Br. J. Clin. Pharmacol.*, **47**, 545–552.

77 Zielinska, A., Lichti, C.F., Bratton, S., Mitchell, N.C., Gallus-Zawada, A., Le, V.-H., *et al.* (2008) Glucuronidation of monohydroxylated warfarin metabolites by human liver microsomes and human recombinant UDP-glucuronosyltransferases. *J. Pharmacol. Exp. Ther.*, **324**, 139–148.

78 Frymoyer, A., Shugarts, S., Browne, M., Wu, A.H.B., Frassetto, L., and Benet, L.Z. (2010) Effect of single-dose rifampin on the pharmacokinetics of warfarin in healthy volunteers. *Clin. Pharmacol. Ther.*, **88**, 540–547.

79 Limdi, N.A. and Veenstra, D.L. (2008) Warfarin pharmacogenetics. *Pharmacotherapy*, **28**, 1084–1097.

80 Kazui, M., Nishiya, Y., Ishizuka, T., Hagihara, K., Farid, N.A., Okazaki, O., *et al.* (2010) Identification of the human cytochrome P450 enzymes involved in the two oxidative steps in the bioactivation of clopidogrel to its pharmacologically active metabolite. *Drug Metab. Dispos.*, **38**, 92–99.

81 Bouman, H.J., Schömig, E., van Werkum, J.W., Velder, J., Hackeng, C.M., Hirschhäuser, C., *et al.* (2011) Paraoxonase-1 is a major determinant of clopidogrel efficacy. *Nat. Med.*, **17**, 110–116.

82 Taubert, D., von Beckerath, N., Grimberg, G., Lazar, A., Jung, N., Goeser, T., *et al.* (2006) Impact of P-glycoprotein on clopidogrel absorption. *Clin. Pharmacol. Ther.*, **80**, 486–501.

83 Cuisset, T., Morange, P.-E., Quilici, J., Bonnet, J.L., Gachet, C., and Alessi, M.-C. (2011) Paraoxonase-1 and clopidogrel efficacy. *Nat. Med.*, **17**, 1039.

84 Sibbing, D., Koch, W., Massberg, S., Byrne, R.A., Mehilli, J., Schulz, S. *et al.* (2011) No association of paraoxonase-1 Q192R genotypes with platelet response to clopidogrel and risk of stent thrombosis after coronary stenting. *Eur. Heart J.*, **32**, 1605–1613.

85 Riedmaier, S., Klein, K., Winter, S., Hofmann, U., Schwab, M., and Zanger, U.M. (2011) Paraoxonase (PON1 and PON3) polymorphisms: impact on liver expression and atorvastatin-lactone hydrolysis. *Front. Pharmacol.*, **2**, 41.

86 Ghosal, A., Hapangama, N., Yuan, Y., Achanfuo-Yeboah, J., Iannucci, R., Chowdhury, S., Alton, K., Patrick, J.E., and Zbaida, S. (2004) Identification of human UDP-glucuronosyltransferase enzyme(s) responsible for the glucuronidation of ezetimibe (Zetia). *Drug Metab. Dispos.*, **32**, 314–320.

87 Oswald, S., Haenisch, S., Fricke, C., Sudhop, T., Remmler, C., Giessmann, T., Jedlitschky, G., Adam, U., Dazert, E., Warzok, R., Wacke, W., Cascorbi, I., Kroemer, H.K., Weitschies, W., von Bergmann, K., and Siegmund, W. (2006) Intestinal expression of P-glycoprotein (ABCB1), multidrug resistance associated protein 2 (ABCC2), and

uridine diphosphate-glucuronosyltransferase 1A1 predicts the disposition and modulates the effects of the cholesterol absorption inhibitor ezetimibe in humans. *Clin. Pharmacol. Ther.*, **79**, 206–217.

88 Nakagawa, A., Shigeta, A., Iwabuchi, H., Horiguchi, M., Nakamura, K., and Takahagi, H. (1991) Simultaneous determination of gemfibrozil and its metabolites in plasma and urine by a fully automated high performance liquid chromatographic system. *Biomed. Chromatogr.*, **5**, 68–73.

89 Mano, Y., Usui, T., and Kamimura, H. (2007) The UDP-glucuronosyltransferase 2B7 isozyme is responsible for gemfibrozil glucuronidation in the human liver. *Drug Metab. Dispos.*, **35**, 2040–2044.

90 Shitara, Y. and Sugiyama, Y. (2006) Pharmacokinetic and pharmacodynamic alterations of 3-hydroxy-3-methylglutaryl coenzyme A (HMG-CoA) reductase inhibitors: drug–drug interactions and interindividual differences in transporter and metabolic enzyme functions. *Pharmacol. Ther.*, **112**, 71–105.

91 Schachter, M. (2005) Chemical, pharmacokinetic and pharmacodynamic properties of statins: an update. *Fundam. Clin. Pharmacol.*, **19**, 117–125.

92 Neuvonen, P.J., Niemi, M., and Backman, J.T. (2006) Drug interactions with lipid-lowering drugs: mechanisms and clinical relevance. *Clin. Pharmacol. Ther.*, **80**, 565–581.

93 Jacobsen, W., Kuhn, B., Soldner, A., Kirchner, G., Sewing, K.F., Kollman, P.A., *et al.* (2000) Lactonization is the critical first step in the disposition of the 3-hydroxy-3-methylglutaryl-CoA reductase inhibitor atorvastatin. *Drug Metab. Dispos.*, **28**, 1369–1378.

94 Riedmaier, S., Klein, K., Hofmann, U., Keskitalo, J.E., Neuvonen, P.J., Schwab, M., *et al.* (2010) UDP-glucuronosyltransferase (UGT) polymorphisms affect atorvastatin lactonization *in vitro* and *in vivo*. *Clin. Pharmacol. Ther.*, **87**, 65–73.

95 Grube, M., Kock, K., Oswald, S., Draber, K., Meissner, K., Eckel, L., *et al.* (2006) Organic anion transporting polypeptide 2B1 is a high-affinity transporter for atorvastatin and is expressed in the human heart. *Clin. Pharmacol. Ther.*, **80**, 607–620.

96 Lau, Y.Y., Huang, Y., Frassetto, L., and Benet, L.Z. (2007) effect of OATP1B transporter inhibition on the pharmacokinetics of atorvastatin in healthy volunteers. *Clin. Pharmacol. Ther.*, **81**, 194–204.

97 Nishimura, M. and Naito, S. (2005) Tissue-specific mRNA expression profiles of human ATP-binding cassette and solute carrier transporter superfamilies. *Drug Metab. Pharmacokinet.*, **20**, 452–477.

98 Niemi, M., Pasanen, M.K., and Neuvonen, P.J. (2011) Organic anion transporting polypeptide 1B1: a genetically polymorphic transporter of major importance for hepatic drug uptake. *Pharmacol. Rev.*, **63**, 157–181.

99 Bogman, K., Peyer, A.K., Török, M., Küsters, E., and Drewe, J. (2001) HMG-CoA reductase inhibitors and P-glycoprotein modulation. *Br. J. Pharmacol.*, **132**, 1183–1192.

100 Chandra, P. and Brouwer, K.L.R. (2004) The complexities of hepatic drug transport: current knowledge and emerging concepts. *Pharm. Res.*, **21**, 719–735.

101 Keskitalo, J.E., Zolk, O., Fromm, M.F., Kurkinen, K.J., Neuvonen, P.J., and Niemi, M. (2009) ABCG2 polymorphism markedly affects the pharmacokinetics of atorvastatin and rosuvastatin. *Clin. Pharmacol. Ther.*, **86**, 197–203.

102 Keskitalo, J., Kurkinen, K., Neuvonen, P., and Niemi, M. (2008) ABCB1 haplotypes differentially affect the pharmacokinetics of the acid and lactone forms of simvastatin and atorvastatin. *Clin. Pharmacol. Ther.*, **84**, 457–461.

13
Anticancer Drugs

Matthias Schwab, Elke Schaeffeler, and Hiltrud Brauch

13.1
Introduction

Metabolism is a major determinant for the majority of anticancer drugs used in clinical practice. Since the variability in drug response to cancer agents still represents an important clinical problem, knowledge of drug metabolism is pertinent to clinicians and academic professionals. Within this chapter we describe the frequently used cancer agents listed by compound groups with a major focus on drug metabolism.

13.2
Alkylating Drugs

13.2.1
Oxazaphosphorine (Cyclophosphamide, Ifosphamide)

Cyclophosphamide (CP) is widely used in the treatment of a variety of tumor entities. Complex metabolic activation and inactivation reactions have been identified, and about 70–80% of a CP dose is metabolized to 4-OH-CP. Several cytochrome P450 (CYP) enzymes are involved in the 4-hydroxylation, including CYP2B6, 2C9, 2C19, 3A4,and 3A5, with a major contribution of CYP2B6 to the 4-hydroxylase activity [1]. The equilibrium between 4-OH-CP and the ring-opened aldehyde tautomer aldophosphamide is spontaneously converted to the phosphoramide mustard and acrolein. Phosphoramide mustard is believed to be the active alkylating metabolite. While 4-OH-CP and phosphoramide mustard are mainly catalyzed by glutathione *S*-transferase (GST) isoforms GSTA1 and GSTP1 to 4-glutathionyl-CP and di-glutathionyl-phosphoramide mustard, respectively [2], the metabolite aldophosphamide is converted to carboxyphosphamide via the aldehyde dehydrogenase (ALD) enzymes ALDH1A1 and ALDH3A1 [3]. Finally, CP side-chain oxidation by CYP3A4 and CYP3A5 results in the formation of 2-dechloroethyl-CP and chloroacetaldehyde, contributing to less than 5% of the total elimination of CP [4].

Metabolism of Drugs and Other Xenobiotics, First Edition. Edited by Pavel Anzenbacher, Ulrich M. Zanger.

CP metabolism is subject to profound autoinduction, resulting in an increased clearance of the parent drug and increased formation of CP metabolites.

13.2.2 Melphalan

High-dose melphalan is still an important agent in the consolidation of an initial therapy of multiple myeloma with biological agents such as lenalidomide and bortezomib as front-line therapy. About 10–15% of an administered melphalan dose is eliminated unchanged by renal excretion [5]. *In vitro* studies showed that melphalan is conjugated to glutathione by α-GST isozymes to form either a monoglutathione or diglutathione conjugate. Moreover, hydroxylated metabolites have been identified [6]. However, melphalan–GSH conjugates could not be detected in human bile during isolated *in situ* liver perfusion [7].

13.2.3 Ethyleneimines (Thiotepa)

Thiotepa is included in diverse regimens and used for the treatment of several cancers, including advanced or metastatic breast and ovarian cancer as well as tumors of the testis and various leukemias. In some instances it is considered as a high-dose regimen. Thiotepa and its desulfurated primary metabolite triethylenephosphoramide (TEPA) cause DNA strand breaks via cross-linking. Hepatic CYP3A4 followed by CYP2B6 is the major enzyme involved in the rapid formation of TEPA by oxidative desulfuration [8]. Thiotepa and TEPA are subject to further extensive metabolism, and are conjugated to glutathione via GSTA1-1 and P1-1 [9],with thiothepa and TEPA representing less than 10% of the excreted urinary compounds.

13.2.4 Busulfan

Busulfan is currently used for high-dose myeloablative regimens in patients with autologous or allogeneic stem cell transplantation. In individual cases, busulfan is used as a third-line therapy for various hematological disorders. Severe side-effects of busulfan are unpredictable pulmonary fibrosis, gastrointestinal mucosal damage, and hepatic veno-occlusive disease (VOD). In the first step of elimination, busulfan is conjugated to glutathione catalyzed mainly by GSTA1-1 with minor contributions of GSTM1-1 and GSTP1-1 to form γ-glutamyl-β-(*S*-tetrahydrothiophenium)-alanyl-glycine (THT^+) [10]. Further, metabolism via CYP enzymes towards inactive compounds has been considered. In addition to the liver, the small intestine contributes in part to the formation of THT^+ [11]. Since busulfan clearance is subject to considerable interindividual variability, therapeutic drug monitoring has been recommended to reduce severe side-effects such as VOD. Drug interactions between busulfan and anticonvulsants (e.g., phenytoin) given to protect against busulfan-related central nervous system toxicity are well known. Therefore, non-enzyme-inducing antiseizure agents like lorazepam should be used.

13.2.5
Methylhydrazines (Procarbazine)

Procarbazine is primarily used as a component of various chemotherapy regimens for Hodgkin's lymphoma (e.g., BEACOPP), primary central nervous system lymphoma, and high-grade gliomas [12]. Procarbazine is subject to multistep reactions involving CYP, monoamine oxidase (MAO), and cytosolic enzymes. After oxidation into azo-procarbazine and hydrogen peroxide, the subsequent conversion of azo-procarbazine to the isomer azoxy derivatives (methyl, benzylazoxy) is catalyzed exclusively by CYP [13]. Procarbazine metabolites are mainly excreted in the urine. It has been suggested that free radical intermediates produced during procarbazine metabolism may result in hepatic injury [14].

13.3
Platinum-Containing Agents

Platinum-containing agents are efficient anticancer drugs for a broad spectrum of tumors. This group of drugs is frequently used in the treatment of ovarian, bladder, head and neck, small-cell lung cancer, and colon cancer as well as testicular germ cell tumors, primarily in combination with other drugs. Three major platinum agents are currently in use: cisplatin, carboplatin, and oxaliplatin. Whereas metabolizing enzymes are of minor relevance, drug transport proteins substantially contribute to drug disposition and the observed drug resistance. Myeloperoxidase (MPO), NAD(P)H dehydrogenase quinone 1 (NQO1), GSTM1, GSTP1, and superoxide dismutase 1 (SOD1), albeit with different consequences on the alteration of intracellular concentrations, play a role in the clinical outcome such as drug resistance or sensitivity to ototoxicity and other side-effects of platinum-containing agents [15, 16]. By day 5, up to 45 % of the administered dose is excreted via the kidney, mostly covalently bound to protein and peptides.

13.4
Antimetabolites

13.4.1
Folic Acid Antagonist (Methotrexate)

Methotrexate (MTX) is used in the therapy of acute lymphoblastic childhood leukemia as high-dose treatment in remission induction and consolidation, and in maintenance of remission. Intravenous, intrathecal, and oral application are well-established routes of administration. In addition, MTX is used for the treatment of choriocarcinoma and related trophoblastic tumors, and as a component of several regimens for breast, ovarian, head and neck cancer, as well as non-Hodgkin's lymphoma. MTX is rapidly converted intracellular to the more active MTX polyglutamate (methotrexate polyglutamate MTXPGs) by folylpolyglutamate synthetase. Long-chain polyglutamates (MTXPG4–7) are more potent inhibitors of folate-dependent enzymes [17]. Lysosomal γ-glutamyl hydrolase (also termed folylpolyglutamate hydrolase) catalyzes the removal of γ-linked polyglutamates, converting long-chain MTXPG into shorter-chain MTXPG and ultimately to MTX [18]. About 90% of an oral dose of the parent drug MTX is excreted via the urine within the first 8–12 h. Hepatic metabolism of MTX is negligible. However, following intravenous high-dose application, 7-hydroxy-MTX can be detected – a metabolite that has been associated with a nephrotoxic potential.

13.4.2 Pyrimidine Analogs (5-Fluorouracil/Capecitabine/Tegafur)

5-Fluorouracl (5-FU) is frequently used in the treatment of solid tumors such as colorectal, breast as well as head and neck cancer, mainly in combination with other agents (e.g., oxaliplatin, irinotecan). Both catabolic and anabolic pathways play a role in 5-FU metabolism [19]. Dihydropyrimidine dehydrogenase (DPD) is the initial rate-limiting enzyme in the catabolism and accounts for approximately 85% of 5-FU metabolism. The inactive metabolite dihydro-FU is sequentially degraded via several enzymes (e.g., dihydropyrimidinase) to α-fluoro-β-alanine (FBAL) and carboxy-fluoro-β-alanine (CFBAL). In the anabolic pathway 5-FU is converted into nucleotides essential for its action. 5-Fluorouridine-5′-monophosphate (FUMP) is formed via the orotate phosphoribosyltransferase (OPRT). Via an alternative route and by sequential conversion, 5-FU is bioactivated into 5-fluoro-desoxy-uridine-5′-monophosphate (FdUMP) – the major active metabolite for the inhibition of thymidylate synthase (TS). Accordingly, only a small fraction of about 10–15% of the 5-FU dose is responsible for its antitumor activity. Capecitabine and tegafur are oral prodrugs of 5-FU. Capecitabine is converted into 5′-desoxy-5-fluorocytidine by hepatic carboxylesterase, subsequently metabolized into 5-desoxy-5-fluorouridine via cytidine deaminase, and finally converted into 5-FU by thymidine phosphorylase [20]. In the case of tegafur, CYP2A6, and, to a minor extent, CYP1A2 and CYP2C8 are involved in its bioactivation to 5-FU. The combination of tegafur with uracil results in a competitive inhibition of DPD via uracil, thereby increasing the anabolic pathway of 5-FU.

13.4.3 Cytidine Analogs

13.4.3.1 Cytarabine and Gemcitabine

The major application of cytarabine (cytosine arabinoside, ara-C) is the therapy of acute leukemia. Gemcitabine (dFdC) is used particularly in the treatment of solid tumors such as metastatic pancreatic cancer, non-small-cell lung cancer, but also bladder, ovarian, and head and neck tumors. The metabolism of ara-C and dFdC are quite similar, and both ara-C and dFdC are intracellularly phosphorylated into cytarabine monophosphate (dFdCMP or ara-CMP) via deoxycytidine kinase, which is the rate-limiting enzyme in the bioactivation process [21, 22]. Dephosphorylation of dFdCMP and ara-CMP via 5′-nucleotidase results in monophosphates that are sequentially converted into diphosphates (via dCMP kinase) and triphosphates (nucleoside diphosphate kinase). More than 90% of dFdCMP and ara-CMP dose is inactivated via cytidine deaminase into difluorodeoxyuridine (dFdU) and uracil arabinoside (ara-U), thus only a small proportion of the dFdCMP and ara-CMP dose executes the cytotoxic effects. Deoxycytidylate deaminase (DCTD) also inactivates gemcitabine to difluorodeoxyuridine monophosphate and dFdU [23].

13.4.3.2 **Azacitidine and Decitabine**

5-Azacitidine (azacitidine) and the deoxyribose derivative of azacitidine – 5-aza-2′-deoxycytidine (decitabine) – are inhibitors of DNA methylation, and are used for the treatment of myelodysplastic syndromes and acute leukemias, in particular acute myeloid leukemia. Decitabine is converted to 5-aza-2′-deoxycytidine-5′-monophosphate by deoxycytidine kinase. Following phosphorylation, decitabine triphosphate is formed that is efficiently incorporated into DNA. Decitabine is rapidly converted to 1-β-D-2′-deoxyribofuranosyl-3-guanylurea and several other products [24]. The exact route of elimination and metabolism is currently unknown. A high total body clearance and a total excretion in urine of the administered dose below 1% indicate elimination via extrahepatic enzymes such as cytidine deaminases in the intestine [25].

13.4.4
Purine Analogs

13.4.4.1 **6-Thiopurine Analogs**

6-Mercaptopurine (6-MP) and 6-thioguanine (6-TG) are predominantly used for treatment of acute leukemia, particularly in children. More than 50% of the 6-MP is detected in the urine 24 h after administration, and 48-h stool specimens contain about 12 and 22% of presumably unabsorbed 6-MP [26]. 6-MP is subject to extensive hepatic metabolism with anabolic and catabolic pathways being involved. The enzyme hypoxanthine guanine phosphoribosyltransferase (HPGRT) – responsible for the bioactivation of thiopurines – converts 6-MP into 6-thioinosine monophosphate, which is stepwise metabolized by several other intracellular enzymes (inosine monophosphate dehydrogenase, guanosine monophosphate synthetase) into 6-thioguanine nucleotide (TGN). Thiopurine *S*-methyltransferase (TPMT) and xanthine oxidase (XO) are the predominant catabolic enzymes in the metabolism of thiopurines. TPMT catalyzes the *S*-adenosyl-L-methionine dependent *S*-methylation of 6-MP and its metabolites. Oxidation by XO to the inactive 6-thiouric acid is an important catabolic step since a clinically relevant drug–drug interaction with allopurinol – a XO inhibitor – needs to be considered [27].

13.4.4.2 Fludarabine Phosphate

Fludarabine phosphate is used for the treatment of chronic lymphatic leukemia and low-grade lymphoma. In the circulation, fludarabine phosphate is immediately dephosphorylated to the nucleoside fludarabine. About 30–40% of nucleoside fludarabine is excreted into the urine. In addition, fludarabine is metabolized into a hypoxanthine metabolite also excreted in the urine [28]. Intracellularly, fludarabine is stepwise rephosphorylated to the active triphosphate. Deoxycytidine kinase is the dominant, if not the exclusive, enzyme for the formation of the monophosphate. Adenylate kinase and nucleoside diphosphate kinase are believed to be involved in the formation of the diphosphate and triphosphate, respectively [29].

13.5 Natural Products

13.5.1 Vinca Alkaloids (Vincristine)

Vincristine is given for the treatment of childhood leukemia for the induction of remission, but also in cases of non-Hodgkin's/Hodgkin's lymphoma, soft-tissue sarcomas, and other tumors (e.g., Wilms tumor). Since vincristine is given intravenously, subcutaneous extravasation is a major complication leading to severe ulceration. Vincristine is preferentially metabolized to a primary metabolite M1 – a secondary amine formed by CYP3A5 with a 9- to 14-fold higher intrinsic clearance than CYP3A4. Other CYPs, such as CYP2C19 and CYP2D6, play only a minor role in metabolism of vincristine and other vinca alkaloids [30]. Only 10–20% of the vincristine dose is excreted in the urine and approximately 80% is detected in the stool. Since CYP3A4 and CYP3A5 are involved in the metabolism, vincristine-related neurotoxicity has been linked with the interindividual variability of these enzymes.

13.5.2 Taxanes (Paclitaxel, Docetaxel)

Taxanes are frequently used in several cancer therapies, particularly metastatic ovarian, breast, head and neck, and lung tumors. Both paclitaxel and docetaxel are metabolized via CYP isozymes into inactive metabolites that are further eliminated via the bile route. Although both drugs have a similar chemical structure, they are oxidized by two different enzymes. CYP2C8 catalyzes the 6-hydroxylation on the taxane ring of paclitaxel, whereas CYP3A4 oxidizes docetaxel on the *tert*-butyl group of the lateral chain in C13 [31, 32]. CYP3A5 appears to be involved in docetaxel metabolism [33]. Drug interaction by inhibition or induction of CYP enzymes is important with significant consequences on pharmacokinetics (e.g., clearance).

13.5.3 Camptothecin Analogs

13.5.3.1 Topotecan

Topotecan is used in the treatment of ovarian and small-cell lung cancers following failure of a first-line treatment. The reversible conversion from the active closed-ring lactone form to an inactive open-ring hydroxyl acid strongly depends on the pH [34]. Following short-term intravenous infusion of topotecan, about 20–30% of the total dose is excreted in the urine within 24 h, predominantly as the open-ring inactive form [35]. Neither topotecan nor the hydroxyl acid are metabolized to any significant extent. Valid data on the metabolism of topotecan are limited. Hepatic *N*-demethylation forming *N*-desmethyl topotecan via CYP3A4 has been suggested [36], but represents only a minor metabolic pathway in the elimination of topotecan.

13.5.3.2 Irinotecan

Irinotecan is commonly used for the treatment of colorectal and lung cancers. Irinotecan is extensively metabolized in human liver. In a first step, the bipiperidinocarbonyl group of irinotecan is removed via hydrolysis by the carboxyesterases CES1 and CES2 resulting in the corresponding carboxylic acid and the active metabolite, 7-ethyl-10-hydroxy-camptothecin (SN-38) [37]. SN-38 is converted into the inactive SN-38 glucuronide (SN-38G) by UGT1A1 [38]. Moreover, irinotecan is sequentially oxidized via CYP3A4/5 to the inactive 7-ethyl-10-(4-*N*-(5-aminopentanoic acid)-1-piperidino)-carbonyloxy-camptothecin (APC) and 7-ethyl-10-(4-amino-1-piperidino)-carbonyloxy-camptothecin (NPC), which are not further metabolized to SN-38 [39]. Finally, several other metabolization steps occur in human plasma, including the formation of primary amines, decarboxylation of the irinotecan carboxylate form, and others [40]. Since only the lactone forms of the camptothecins are active, the interconversion of the carboxylate and lactone forms of both irinotecan and SN-38 is important.

13.5.4 Antibiotics

13.5.4.1 Dactinomycin

Dactonomycin (actinomycin D) is indicated in the treatment of solid tumors such as chorioncarcinoma, soft-tissue sarcoma, and specific tumors in children (e.g., Wilms tumor). Drug metabolism is of minor importance and about 70% of the parent drug is eliminated via renal excretion [41].

13.5.4.2 Anthracyclines

Doxorubicin (DOX) and daunorubicin are natural anthracyclines, whereas idarubicin and epirubicin are analogs. Daunorubicin and idarubicin are primarily effective in the treatment of acute myeloid leukemias mostly in combination with ara-C. Doxorubicin is active in a broader tumor spectrum and is used in malignant lymphoma, but also other solid tumors such as Ewing and soft-tissue sarcoma. Like epirubicin, DOX is a component of regimens for the treatment of breast cancer. Approximately 50% of DOX is removed unchanged from the body, whereas the other 50% undergoes metabolism, mainly by reduction to the C13-alcohol metabolite doxorubicinol (DOX-OL). Additional metabolites, mainly aglycones of DOX and DOX-OL, are detected at much lower concentrations than DOX-OL [42]. Reduction of DOX to DOX-OL is predominantly catalyzed by human carbonyl reductase 1 (CBR1) in the cytosol. In contrast, DOX reduction in the heart is mediated by aldo-keto reductase (AKR) 1A1 [43].

13.5.4.3 Epipodophyllotoxins

Etoposide as well as teniposide are given mostly intravenously with significant therapeutic efficiency during the treatment of testicular tumors, pediatric leukemia, lymphomas, and lung cancer. Following intravenous application, approximately 50% of the etoposide dose is recovered as unchanged etoposide and etoposide glucuronide in the urine [44]. Metabolism of etoposide includes different hydroxyacid derivatives, the *cis*-picrolactone, aglycone glucuronides, and sulfate conjugates of etoposide. CYP3A4 and CYP3A5 are involved in the 3-*O*-demethylation and the formation of active metabolites (semiquinone free radical, *o*-quinone, catechol) for the inhibition of topoisomerase II [45]. GST1/GSTP1 and UGT1A1 are the major inactivating enzymes, leading to glutathione conjugates and etoposide glucuronides, respectively.

13.6 Endocrine Therapy

13.6.1 Selective Estrogen Receptor Modulator (Tamoxifen)

Tamoxifen has for decades been a mainstay in the endocrine treatment of pre- and postmenopausal as well as male estrogen receptor-positive breast cancer [46]. Tamoxifen requires bioactivation via CYP enzymes to form the active 4-hydroxytamoxifen and endoxifen. Genetic polymorphisms in the key enzyme CYP2D6 explain the major interindividual variability of endoxifen plasma levels. CYP2D6 "poor metabolizer" patients have higher recurrence rates under tamoxifen compared to "extensive metabolizers" [47]. CYP2D6 inhibitors, such as selective serotonin reuptake inhibitors used as comedication to ameliorate postmenopausal symptoms, negatively impact serum endoxifen levels. Other enzymes involved in the metabolism of tamoxifen are CYP3A4/5, CYP2C9, CYP2B6, CYP2C19, and

CYP2C9, and as well as UGT1A4, UGT1A8, UGT1A10, UGT2B7, and UGT2B15, which lead in part to the formation of active metabolites [48].

13.6.2 Aromatase Inhibitors

Aromatase inhibitors are a major class of drugs of which the third-generation nonsteroidal anastrozole and letrozol as well as the steroidal exemestane represent novel approaches to the endocrine treatment of breast cancer patients [49]. Anastrozole is metabolized to pharmacologically inactive metabolites including triazole, hydroxyl-anastrozole (free and glucuronide conjugated) as well as anastrozole *N*-glucuronide [50]. Hydroxy-anastrozole is predominantly formed by CYP3A4, undergoing extensive glucuronidation predominantly by UGT1A4, and to a lesser extent by UGT2B7 and UGT1A3. Novel data indicate that anastrozole and not triazole hydroxylation represents the main oxidative metabolic pathway. Anastrozole *N*-glucuronidation represents the main conjugation pathway of the drug [51]. Approximately 60% of the administered dose is excreted in the urine as metabolites and less than 10% remains unchanged. Letrozole is metabolized to a pharmacologically inactive carbinol metabolite (4,4′-methanol-bisbenzonitrile) by CYP3A4 and CYP2A6 [52]. CYP2A6 forms both the carbinol metabolite and its ketone analog. Urinary fractions include 75% glucuronide conjugate of the alcoholic metabolite, 9% of two unidentified metabolites, and 6% unchanged letrozole.

13.7 Histone Deacetylase Inhibitor (Vorinostat)

Vorinostat (suberoylanilide hydroxamic acid (SAHA)) is an oral histone deacetylase inhibitor for the treatment of cutaneous T-cell lymphoma, but also for other types of lymphoma (e.g., B- and T cell lymphomas, myeloid leukemia) [53]. Vorinostat is subject to an extensive hepatic metabolism and is primarily glucuronidated via several UGTs (UGT1A9, UGT2B7, UGT2B17) into the inactive vorinostat glucuronide (SAHA-*O*-glucuronide) [54]. A second inactive metabolite – 4-anilino-4-oxobutanoic acid – is formed via hydrolysis followed by β-oxidation, but the specific enzymes responsible so far have not been investigated. In addition, the extrahepatic UGT1A8 and 1A1 enzymes showed high levels of activity against SAHA *in vitro*, suggesting that they may contribute to SAHA glucuronidation *in vivo* [55].

13.8 Tyrosine Kinase Inhibitors

Over the past 10 years, several tyrosine kinase inhibitors (TKIs) have been approved for use in cancer therapy. Multitargeted TKIs are pyrimidine (imatinib, dasatinib, nilotinib and pazopanib), pyridine (sorafenib), and pyrrole (sunitinib) derivates with activity towards several families of receptor (e.g., Bcr-Abl, c-kit, platelet-derived growth factor, vascular endothelial growth factor, fibroblast growth factor, B-RAF), and nonreceptor tyrosine kinases (e.g., Scr) [56]. All TKIs are primarily metabolized via CYP3A4; however, in the case of sorafenib, glucuronidation via UGT1A9 and *N*-oxidation via CYP3A4 are the main steps.

Active metabolites of imatinib and sunitinib contribute to the antitumor activity. As exemplarily shown by imatinib, TKI metabolism is complex and several pathways are involved, such as *N*-demethylation, piperazine ring oxidation with lactam formation, piperazine-*N*-4-oxidation, pyridine *N*-oxidation, benzylic hydroxylation, and oxidative desamination, with further oxidation to a carboxylic acid [57]. With respect to hepatic CYP enzymes, CYP3A4, CYP3A5, and CYP2C8 are of major importance, whereas CYP2D6, CYP1A2, CYP2C9, and CYP2C19 only contribute to a minor extent [58]. The *in vivo* relevance of extrahepatic CYP1A1 and CYP1B1 as well as the flavin-containing monooxygenase FMO3 involved in imatinib metabolism is currently unclear. Unchanged imatinib and its *N*-desmethyl metabolite are predominately identified in the plasma, urine and feces.

13.9
Proteasome Inhibitor (Bortezomib)

Bortezomib (PS-341, Velcade®) is a first-in-class proteasome inhibitor with antitumor activity against several hematologic and nonhematologic malignancies. Bortezomib received US Food and Drug Administration approval for the treatment of multiple myeloma patients. Bortezomib is metabolized by several CYP isozymes, leading to the formation of two carbinolamides. The primary enzyme involved is CYP3A4, followed by CYP2C19 and CYP1A2, while CYP2D6 and CYP2C9 contribute to a much less extent [59]. Secondary metabolism of the carbinolamides accounts for a large number of additional metabolites observed in human plasma, resulting in the formation of hydroxylcarbinolamides. Desaturation of the Leu moiety represents the second route of metabolism for bortezomib [60]. Drug–drug interaction with agents that inhibit particularly CYP3A may alter the pharmacokinetic and pharmacodynamic effects of bortezomib.

References

1 Roy, P., Yu, L.J., Crespi, C.L., and Waxman, D.J. (1999) Development of a substrate-activity based approach to identify the major human liver P-450 catalysts of cyclophosphamide and ifosfamide activation based on cDNA-expressed activities and liver microsomal P-450 profiles. *Drug Metab. Dispos.*, **27**, 655–666.

2 Dirven, H.A., van Ommen, B., and van Bladeren, P.J. (1994) Involvement of human glutathione *S*-transferase isoenzymes in the conjugation of cyclophosphamide metabolites

with glutathione. *Cancer Res.*, **54**, 6215–6220.
3 Sladek, N.E. (1999) Aldehyde dehydrogenase-mediated cellular relative insensitivity to the oxazaphosphorines. *Curr. Pharm. Des.*, **5**, 607–625.
4 de Jonge, M.E., Huitema, A.D., Rodenhuis, S., and Beijnen, J.H. (2005) Clinical pharmacokinetics of cyclophosphamide. *Clin. Pharmacokinet.*, **44**, 1135–1164.
5 Gera, S., Musch, E., Osterheld, H.K., and Loos, U. (1989) Relevance of the hydrolysis and protein binding of melphalan to the treatment of multiple myeloma. *Cancer Chemother. Pharmacol.*, **23**, 76–80.
6 Hall, A.G., Matheson, E., Hickson, I.D., Foster, S.A., and Hogarth, L. (1994) Purification of an alpha class glutathione *S*-transferase from melphalan-resistant Chinese hamster ovary cells and demonstration of its ability to catalyze melphalan–glutathione adduct formation. *Cancer Res.*, **54**, 3369–3372.
7 Vahrmeijer, A.L., Snel, C.A., Steenvoorden, D.P., Beijnen, J.H., Pang, K.S., Schutrups, J., Tirona, R., Keizer, H.J., van Dierendonck, J.H., van Dierendonck, V., and Mulder, G.J. (1996) Lack of glutathione conjugation of melphalan in the isolated *in situ* liver perfusion in humans. *Cancer Res.*, **56**, 4709–4714.
8 Jacobson, P.A., Green, K., Birnbaum, A., and Remmel, R.P. (2002) Cytochrome P450 isozymes 3A4 and 2B6 are involved in the *in vitro* human metabolism of thiotepa to TEPA. *Cancer Chemother. Pharmacol.*, **49**, 461–467.
9 Dirven, H.A., Dictus, E.L., Broeders, N.L., van Ommen, B., and van Bladeren, P.J. (1995) The role of human glutathione *S*-transferase isoenzymes in the formation of glutathione conjugates of the alkylating cytostatic drug thiotepa. *Cancer Res.*, **55**, 1701–1706.
10 Bredschneider, M., Klein, K., Murdter, T.E., Marx, C., Eichelbaum, M., Nussler, A.K., Neuhaus, P., Zanger, U.M., and Schwab, M. (2002) Genetic polymorphisms of glutathione *S*-transferase A1, the major glutathione *S*-transferase in human liver: consequences for enzyme expression and busulfan conjugation. *Clin. Pharmacol. Ther.*, **71**, 479–487.
11 Gibbs, J.P., Yang, J.S., and Slattery, J.T. (1998) Comparison of human liver and small intestinal glutathione *S*-transferase-catalyzed busulfan conjugation *in vitro*. *Drug Metab. Dispos.*, **26**, 52–55.
12 Diehl, V., Franklin, J., Pfreundschuh, M., Lathan, B., Paulus, U., Hasenclever, D., Tesch, H., Herrmann, R., Dorken, B., Muller-Hermelink, H.K., Duhmke, E., and Loeffler, M. (2003) Standard and increased-dose BEACOPP chemotherapy compared with COPP-ABVD for advanced Hodgkin's disease. *N. Engl. J. Med.*, **348**, 2386–2395.
13 Prough, R.A., Brown, M.I., Dannan, G.A., and Guengerich, F.P. (1984) Major isozymes of rat liver microsomal cytochrome P-450 involved in the *N*-oxidation of *N*-isopropyl-alpha-(2-methylazo)-*p*-toluamide, the azo derivative of procarbazine. *Cancer Res.*, **44**, 543–548.
14 Albano, E., Goria-Gatti, L., Clot, P., Jannone, A., and Tomasi, A. (1993) Possible role of free radical intermediates in hepatotoxicity of hydrazine derivatives. *Toxicol. Ind. Health*, **9**, 529–538.
15 Peters, U., Preisler-Adams, S., Hebeisen, A., Hahn, M., Seifert, E., Lanvers, C., Heinecke, A., Horst, J., Jurgens, H., and Lamprecht-Dinnesen, A. (2000) Glutathione *S*-transferase genetic polymorphisms and individual sensitivity to the ototoxic effect of cisplatin. *Anticancer Drugs*, **11**, 639–643.
16 Stoehlmacher, J., Park, D.J., Zhang, W., Groshen, S., Tsao-Wei, D.D., Yu, M.C., and Lenz, H.J. (2002) Association between glutathione *S*-transferase P1, T1, and M1 genetic polymorphism and survival of patients with metastatic colorectal cancer. *J. Natl. Cancer Inst.*, **94**, 936–942.
17 Barredo, J.C., Synold, T.W., Laver, J., Relling, M.V., Pui, C.H., Priest, D.G., and Evans, W.E. (1994) Differences in constitutive and post-methotrexate folylpolyglutamate synthetase activity in

B-lineage and T-lineage leukemia. *Blood*, **84**, 564–569.

18 Galivan, J., Ryan, T., Rhee, M., Yao, R., and Chave, K. (1999) Glutamyl hydrolase: properties and pharmacologic impact. *Semin. Oncol.*, **26** (Suppl. 6), 33–37.

19 Pinedo, H.M. and Peters, G.F. (1988) Fluorouracil: biochemistry and pharmacology. *J. Clin. Oncol.*, **6**, 1653–1664.

20 Kuhn, J.G. (2001) Fluorouracil and the new oral fluorinated pyrimidines. *Ann. Pharmacother*, **35**, 217–227.

21 Kufe, D.W. and Spriggs, D.R. (1985) Biochemical and cellular pharmacology of cytosine arabinoside. *Semin. Oncol.*, **12** (Suppl. 3), 34–48.

22 Wong, A., Soo, R.A., Yong, W.P., and Innocenti, F. (2009) Clinical pharmacology and pharmacogenetics of gemcitabine. *Drug Metab. Rev.*, **41**, 77–88.

23 Mini, E., Nobili, S., Caciagli, B., Landini, I., and Mazzei, T. (2006) Cellular pharmacology of gemcitabine. *Ann. Oncol.*, **17** (Suppl. 5), v7–12.

24 Liu, Z., Marcucci, G., Byrd, J.C., Grever, M., Xiao, J., and Chan, K.K. (2006) Characterization of decomposition products and preclinical and low dose clinical pharmacokinetics of decitabine (5-aza-2′-deoxycytidine) by a new liquid chromatography/tandem mass spectrometry quantification method. *Rapid Commun. Mass Spectrom.*, **20**, 1117–1126.

25 Bryan, J., Kantarjian, H., Garcia-Manero, G., and Jabbour, E. (2011) Pharmacokinetic evaluation of decitabine for the treatment of leukemia. *Expert Opin. Drug Metab. Toxicol.*, **7**, 661–672.

26 Elion, G.B. (1972) Significance of azathioprine metabolites. *Proc. R. Soc. Med.*, **65**, 257–260.

27 Teml, A., Schaeffeler, E., Herrlinger, K.R., Klotz, U., and Schwab, M. (2007) Thiopurine treatment in inflammatory bowel disease: clinical pharmacology and implication of pharmacogenetically guided dosing. *Clin. Pharmacokinet.*, **46**, 187–208.

28 Gandhi, V. and Plunkett, W. (2002) Cellular and clinical pharmacology of fludarabine. *Clin. Pharmacokinet.*, **41**, 93–103.

29 Avramis, V.I. and Plunkett, W. (1982) Metabolism and therapeutic efficacy of 9-beta-D-arabinofuranosyl-2-fluoroadenine against murine leukemia P388. *Cancer Res.*, **42**, 2587–2591.

30 Dennison, J.B., Jones, D.R., Renbarger, J.L., and Hall, S.D. (2007) Effect of CYP3A5 expression on vincristine metabolism with human liver microsomes. *J. Pharmacol. Exp. Ther.*, **321**, 553–563.

31 Cresteil, T., Monsarrat, B., Alvinerie, P., Treluyer, J.M., Vieira, I., and Wright, M. (1994) Taxol metabolism by human liver microsomes: identification of cytochrome P450 isozymes involved in its biotransformation. *Cancer Res.*, **54**, 386–392.

32 Cresteil, T., Monsarrat, B., Dubois, J., Sonnier, M., Alvinerie, P., and Gueritte, F. (2002) Regioselective metabolism of taxoids by human CYP3A4 and 2C8: structure–activity relationship. *Drug Metab. Dispos.*, **30**, 438–445.

33 Shou, M., Martinet, M., Korzekwa, K.R., Krausz, K.W., Gonzalez, F.J., and Gelboin, H.V. (1998) Role of human cytochrome P450 3A4 and 3A5 in the metabolism of taxotere and its derivatives: enzyme specificity, interindividual distribution and metabolic contribution in human liver. *Pharmacogenetics*, **8**, 391–401.

34 Underberg, W.J., Goossen, R.M., Smith, B.R., and Beijnen, J.H. (1990) Equilibrium kinetics of the new experimental anti-tumour compound SK&F 104864-A in aqueous solution. *J. Pharm. Biomed. Anal.*, **8**, 681–683.

35 Dennis, M.J., Beijnen, J.H., Grochow, L.B., and van Warmerdam, L.J. (1997) An overview of the clinical pharmacology of topotecan. *Semin. Oncol.*, **24** (Suppl. 5), S5.

36 Bai, F., Kirstein, M.N., Hanna, S.K., Iacono, L.C., Johnston, B., and Stewart, C.F. (2003) Determination of plasma topotecan and its metabolite *N*-desmethyl topotecan as both lactone and total form by reversed-phase liquid chromatography with fluorescence detection. *J. Chromatogr. B*, **784**, 225–232.

37 Satoh, T., Hosokawa, M., Atsumi, R., Suzuki, W., Hakusui, H., and Nagai, E.

(1994) Metabolic activation of CPT-11, 7-ethyl-10-[4-(1-piperidino)-1-piperidino] carbonyloxycamptothecin, a novel antitumor agent, by carboxylesterase. *Biol. Pharm. Bull.*, **17**, 662–664.

38 Iyer, L., King, C.D., Whitington, P.F., Green, M.D., Roy, S.K., Tephly, T.R., Coffman, B.L., and Ratain, M.J. (1998) Genetic predisposition to the metabolism of irinotecan (CPT-11). Role of uridine diphosphate glucuronosyltransferase isoform 1A1 in the glucuronidation of its active metabolite (SN-38) in human liver microsomes. *J. Clin. Invest.*, **101**, 847–854.

39 Santos, A., Zanetta, S., Cresteil, T., Deroussent, A., Pein, F., Raymond, E., Vernillet, L., Risse, M.L., Boige, V., Gouyette, A., and Vassal, G. (2000) Metabolism of irinotecan (CPT-11) by CYP3A4 and CYP3A5 in humans. *Clin. Cancer Res.*, **6**, 2012–2020.

40 Lokiec, F., du Sorbier, B.M., and Sanderink, G.J. (1996) Irinotecan (CPT-11) metabolites in human bile and urine. *Clin. Cancer Res.*, **2**, 1943–1949.

41 Estlin, E.J. and Veal, G.J. (2003) Clinical and cellular pharmacology in relation to solid tumours of childhood. *Cancer Treat. Rev.*, **29**, 253–273.

42 2005) Pharmacokinetics of low-dose doxorubicin and metabolites in patients with AIDS-related Kaposi sarcoma. *Cancer Chemother. Pharmacol.*, **55**, 488–496.

43 Kassner, N., Huse, K., Martin, H.J., Godtel-Armbrust, U., Metzger, A., Meineke, I., Brockmoller, J., Klein, K., Zanger, U.M., Maser, E., and Wojnowski, L. (2008) Carbonyl reductase 1 is a predominant doxorubicin reductase in the human liver. *Drug Metab. Dispos.*, **36**, 2113–2120.

44 D'Incalci, M., Rossi, C., Zucchetti, M., Urso, R., Cavalli, F., Mangioni, C., Willems, Y., and Sessa, C. (1986) Pharmacokinetics of etoposide in patients with abnormal renal and hepatic function. *Cancer Res.*, **46**, 2566–2571.

45 Relling, M.V., Nemec, J., Schuetz, E.G., Schuetz, J.D., Gonzalez, F.J., and Korzekwa, K.R. (1994) *O*-demethylation of epipodophyllotoxins is catalyzed by human cytochrome P450 3A4. *Mol. Pharmacol.*, **45**, 352–358.

46 Brauch, H., Murdter, T.E., Eichelbaum, M., and Schwab, M. (2009) Pharmacogenomics of tamoxifen therapy. *Clin. Chem.*, **55**, 1770–1782.

47 Schroth, W., Goetz, M.P., Hamann, U., Fasching, P.A., Schmidt, M., Winter, S., Fritz, P., Simon, W., Suman, V.J., Ames, M.M., Safgren, S.L., Kuffel, M.J., Ulmer, H.U., Bolander, J., Strick, R., *et al.* (2009) Association between CYP2D6 polymorphisms and outcomes among women with early stage breast cancer treated with tamoxifen. *JAMA*, **302**, 1429–1436.

48 Murdter, T.E., Schroth, W., Bacchus-Gerybadze, L., Winter, S., Heinkele, G., Simon, W., Fasching, P.A., Fehm, T., Eichelbaum, M., Schwab, M., and Brauch, H. (2011) Activity levels of tamoxifen metabolites at the estrogen receptor and the impact of genetic polymorphisms of phase I and II enzymes on their concentration levels in plasma. *Clin. Pharmacol. Ther.*, **89**, 708–717.

49 Smith, I.E. and Dowsett, M. (2003) Aromatase inhibitors in breast cancer. *N. Engl. J. Med.*, **348**, 2431–2442.

50 Lazarus, P. and Sun, D. (2010) Potential role of UGT pharmacogenetics in cancer treatment and prevention: focus on tamoxifen and aromatase inhibitors. *Drug Metab. Rev.*, **42**, 182–194.

51 Kamdem, L.K., Liu, Y., Stearns, V., Kadlubar, S.A., Ramirez, J., Jeter, S., Shahverdi, K., Ward, B.A., Ogburn, E., Ratain, M.J., Flockhart, D.A., and Desta, Z. (2010) *In vitro* and *in vivo* oxidative metabolism and glucuronidation of anastrozole. *Br. J. Clin. Pharmacol.*, **70**, 854–869.

52 Murai, K., Yamazaki, H., Nakagawa, K., Kawai, R., and Kamataki, T. (2009) Deactivation of anti-cancer drug letrozole to a carbinol metabolite by polymorphic cytochrome P450 2A6 in human liver microsomes. *Xenobiotica*, **39**, 795–802.

53 Richon, V.M., Garcia-Vargas, J., and Hardwick, J.S. (2009) Development of vorinostat: current applications and future perspectives for cancer therapy. *Cancer Lett.*, **280**, 201–210.

54 Kang, S.P., Ramirez, J., House, L., Zhang, W., Mirkov, S., Liu, W., Haverfield, E., and Ratain, M.J. (2010) A pharmacogenetic study of vorinostat glucuronidation. *Pharmacogenet. Genomics*, **20**, 638–641.

55 Balliet, R.M., Chen, G., Gallagher, C.J., Dellinger, R.W., Sun, D., and Lazarus, P. (2009) Characterization of UGTs active against SAHA and association between SAHA glucuronidation activity phenotype with UGT genotype. *Cancer Res.*, **69**, 2981–2989.

56 Agrawal, M., Garg, R.J., Cortes, J., and Quintas-Cardama, A. (2010) Tyrosine kinase inhibitors: the first decade. *Curr. Hematol. Malig. Rep.*, **5**, 70–80.

57 Di, G.P., Kanefendt, F., Lindauer, A., Scheffler, M., Doroshyenko, O., Fuhr, U., Wolf, J., and Jaehde, U. (2011) Clinical pharmacokinetics of tyrosine kinase inhibitors: focus on pyrimidines, pyridines and pyrroles. *Clin. Pharmacokinet.*, **50**, 551–603.

58 Nebot, N., Crettol, S., Esposito, F., Tattam, B., Hibbs, D.E., and Murray, M. (2010) Participation of CYP2C8 and CYP3A4 in the *N*-demethylation of imatinib in human hepatic microsomes. *Br. J. Pharmacol.*, **161**, 1059–1069.

59 Uttamsingh, V., Lu, C., Miwa, G., and Gan, L.S. (2005) Relative contributions of the five major human cytochromes P450, 1A2, 2C9, 2C19, 2D6, and 3A4, to the hepatic metabolism of the proteasome inhibitor bortezomib. *Drug Metab. Dispos.*, **33**, 1723–1728.

60 Pekol, T., Daniels, J.S., Labutti, J., Parsons, I., Nix, D., Baronas, E., Hsieh, F., Gan, L.S., and Miwa, G. (2005) Human metabolism of the proteasome inhibitor bortezomib: identification of circulating metabolites. *Drug Metab. Dispos.*, **33**, 771–777.

14
Antimicrobial Agents

Chantal Csajka, Oscar Marchetti, Oriol Manuel, Laurent Decosterd, and Amalio Telenti

14.1
Introduction

Infectious diseases are a major cause of morbidity and mortality worldwide. In 2008, the World Health Organization estimated that close to 9 million people died from infectious and parasitic diseases, representing over 15% of all causes of deaths. Correspondingly, the anti-infective market generated sales of US$91 billion in 2009 globally, representing close to 10% of the global pharmaceutical market [1].

The importance of infectious diseases worldwide and the widespread use of antimicrobials in human and veterinary medicine support the need for critical attention to the pharmacokinetics and pharmacodynamics of the various compounds. Antimicrobial agents provide good examples of improved clinical response as a consequence of individualization of treatment therapy based on therapeutic drug monitoring (TDM), which is especially true for those with narrow therapeutic intervals or highly subject to microbial resistance. The emerging field of pharmacogenetics also counts various success stories among these classes of compounds.

However, current knowledge and efforts are dwarfed by the size of the market, the incomplete understanding of diversity in metabolism across human populations, and the use of many of the drugs in unique settings (intensive care unit (ICU), immunosuppressed individuals, coinfection, pregnancy, and pediatric settings) that are subject to specific pharmacokinetics/pharmacodynamics circumstances and to drug interactions due to extensive comedication. In that respect, extension of drug individualization by incorporating both pharmacokinetics/pharmacodynamics indices would be of potential relevance to achieve optimal results for new and existing anti-infective drugs.

This chapter reviews pharmacokinetics/pharmacodynamics knowledge across various drug families – antibacterial, antiviral, and antifungal compounds. The text also provides a brief introduction to pharmacogenetics in the field.

Metabolism of Drugs and Other Xenobiotics, First Edition. Edited by Pavel Anzenbacher, Ulrich M. Zanger.

14.2
Pharmacokinetics/Pharmacodynamics of the Main Families of Antimicrobial Agents

14.2.1
Aminoglycosides

The aminoglycoside antibiotics represent a family of 13 molecules. Amikacin, gentamicin, and tobramycin are the most widely used drugs. Aminoglycosides are mainly combined with other antibacterial agents in the treatment of severe infections, in particular β-lactams, in order to broaden the antimicrobial spectrum in potentially multiresistant infections (e.g., severe sepsis or septic shock caused by Gram-negative bacteria) or to obtain an antibacterial synergism (e.g., in endocarditis or other endovascular infections caused by Gram-positive bacteria). All aminoglycosides have similar physical, chemical, and pharmacologic properties. They are bactericidal by inhibiting protein synthesis [2]. These drugs exhibit concentration-dependent bacterial killing and a postantibiotic effect allowing once-daily dosing (ODD) or extended-interval dosing (EID) regimens as alternatives to the traditional multiple-daily dosing (MDD) [3]. The advantages of the EID or ODD reside in optimal concentration-dependent activity while minimizing the risk of toxicity, in addition to decreased need for monitoring therapy [3, 4].

Aminoglycosides are highly polar cations with poor oral bioavailability that are administered as a short intravenous infusion or intramuscular injection. These drugs are highly soluble in water and their distribution is limited to the extracellular fluid compartment. Except for cells of the inner ear and the renal proximal tubule, which have active transport systems for aminoglycosides, these agents have a poor ability to cross lipid-containing cellular membranes and thus do not penetrate the majority of cells. They diffuse in most body fluids, such as synovial, peritoneal, and pleural fluids. Aminoglycosides are eliminated almost completely unchanged by the kidneys, primarily by glomerular filtration, and are actively reabsorbed by the proximal tubule. Mean half-life is approximately 2.5 h in patients with normal renal function, although there is a slow terminal elimination phase of 100 ± 150 h, related to distribution into extracellular compartments [4] and a volume of distribution of 0.15–0.25 l/kg.

Several conditions influence aminoglycoside pharmacokinetics, serum concentrations, and dosage requirements. Renal function is the most important determinant of drug levels as indicated by a proportional relationship between clearance of creatinine and aminoglycosides. Fluid balance determines the volume of distribution of aminoglycosides, which is increased by pathological conditions associated with fluid retention (e.g., ascites, overhydration). Burns and cystic fibrosis have also been reported to alter aminoglycoside pharmacokinetics. Obesity is associated with increased volume of distribution because of the extracellular fluid contained in adipose tissue. Newborn infants and, in particular, those born prematurely have a larger volume of distribution compared to adults, in addition to a lower aminoglycoside clearance, resulting in a decreased elimination.

Aminoglycosides exhibit a large interpatient variability of pharmacokinetics [5]. Differences in distribution and elimination have been mostly explained by variation in renal function, and in extracellular body fluid composition, body weight, and comorbidities. Interpatient differences in tissue uptake and release might also account for this variability, in particular for patients with rapid modification of renal function and/or fluid balance during the course of antibiotic therapy.

Ototoxicity and nephrotoxicity are the two most frequent adverse effects of aminoglycosides, associated with drug accumulation in the renal cortex and the inner ear [6, 7]. Both toxicities are reversible after early treatment discontinuation or decrease in drug exposure, but may become irreversible. Risk factors associated with aminoglycoside toxicity include age, impaired renal function, volume depletion, elevated drug concentrations, prior exposure to aminoglycosides, concurrent nephrotoxic or ototoxic drugs, total aminoglycoside dose, and duration of treatment [8]. Whether the incidence of toxicity differs among aminoglycosides remains matter of debate.

Numerous studies have been performed to evaluate the concentration–efficacy and concentration–toxicity relationships for these drugs. Since the reports of Moore *et al.* [9], other studies have demonstrated that a high ratio between peak plasma concentration (C_{max}) of the antibiotic and the minimum inhibitory concentration (MIC) of the infecting microorganism is a determinant for therapeutic response. A ratio of C_{max}/MIC that exceeds 8–10 : 1 has been associated with concentration-dependent bacterial killing predicting clinical response [10–12]. Increased peak levels might also lengthen the postantibiotic effect of this class of drugs. Therapeutic steady-state peak concentrations are 6–10 μg/ml for gentamicin and tobramycin, and 20–40 μg/ml for amikacin with the standard MDD regimen [4]. The ODD regimen in the adult population is better suited to fulfill this criterion, since a ratio C_{max}/MIC of 10 is easily achieved. However, no demonstration of a better microbiological killing has been shown when comparing the different dosing schedules with the same total daily dose [13]. In contrast, the synergistic effect of low-dose aminoglycosides with β-lactams (e.g., in the treatment of endocarditis) is not dependent on the C_{max}.

A higher risk of ototoxicity and nephrotoxicity has been associated with trough concentrations above 2 μg/ml for gentamicin or tobramycin and 10 μg/ml for amikacin [4]. Although early studies have suggested that nephrotoxicity and ototoxicity were related to peak concentrations as well (above 12 μg/ml for gentamicin and tobramycin, and above 35 μg/ml for amikacin) with conventional MDD, newer evidence suggest that the ODD, which produces higher peak concentrations, might be less toxic [3].

In the view of narrow therapeutic range, large interpatient variability in pharmacokinetics parameters, and well-defined concentration–efficacy/toxicity relationships, TDM of aminoglycosides has been largely used to optimize the benefit/risk balance. The recent move to the less-toxic ODD might, however, need a reassessment of the role of TDM.

14.2.2 Vancomycin

Vancomycin belongs with teicoplanin to the glycopeptide family, which acts by inhibition of the cell wall synthesis and by inhibition of RNA synthesis in Gram-positive bacteria. This antibacterial class is primarily used to treat Gram-positive infections due to organisms that are resistant to other antibiotics (e.g., methicillin-resistant *Staphylococcus aureus* (MRSA) or coagulase-negative staphylococci and ampicillin-resistant enterococci) or in patients allergic to β-lactams. Its use has increased dramatically since the mid-1980s as a result of the marked increase in the prevalence of MRSA. As opposed to aminoglycosides, vancomycin exhibits a time-dependent rather that concentration-dependent killing.

Owing to poor oral bioavailability (below 10%), vancomycin is administered by infusion to reach adequate systemic concentrations. Vancomycin can also be used orally for the local treatment of antibiotic-induced *Clostridium difficile* colitis. Vancomycin exhibits multiexponential kinetics, yielding first and terminal half-lives of 30 min to 1 h and 6–10 h, respectively. Its volume of distribution at steady-state is 0.5–0.9 l/kg in nonobese patients with normal renal function. Vancomycin is 50–55% bound to plasma proteins, and its penetration into tissues is variable and can be affected by inflammation [14]. It is eliminated mainly by glomerular filtration and undergoes tubular reabsorption. Approximately 80–90% of a dose is recovered unchanged in the urine. The liver is involved to a minor extent in its elimination.

Renal dysfunction is the most important condition that influences its disposition. Burn patients exhibit an increase in vancomycin elimination because of the increase in glomerular filtration rate. Its clearance is also increased in obese patients with normal renal function, but there is no or minor change in the volume of distribution. Vancomycin clearance is reduced in premature infants due to the immaturity of the kidneys, while in children aged from 3 months to 8 years clearance is higher than in adults [15]. A very large interpatient variability has been reported for the volume of distribution of vancomycin [16]. Several factors explain this variability, such as age, sex, and body weight. Fluid balance does not significantly affect the volume of distribution.

As for aminoglycosides, vancomycin is nephrotoxic and ototoxic; however, with a reduced toxic potential. This toxicity is dose-dependent and reversible if the antibiotic is withdrawn or doses appropriately adjusted. Other side-effects unrelated to drug levels include fever, chills, and phlebitis. The "red man syndrome," which manifests with flushing of the face, neck, and upper torso, has been associated with rapid drug infusion [14].

Although studies support a concentration-independent bactericidal action of vancomycin, some reports suggest that the achievement of a given level of exposure is required for efficacy. Optimal bactericidal effects are found at concentrations 3–5 times the organism's MIC [17]. Several monitoring parameters have been evaluated, including time over the MIC and the ratio of drug exposure on the MIC (area under the concentration–time curve (AUC)/MIC and C_{max}/MIC).

Current guidelines suggests that AUC/MIC > 350–400 is the best predictive parameter for vancomycin efficacy [14, 18]. Monitoring trough serum concentration is used as a surrogate marker for AUC since it represents the most accurate and practical method to guide vancomycin dosing. Target trough concentrations of 5–10 μg/ml have been proposed for the treatment of *S. aureus* and *Staphylococcus epidermidis* infections with MICs up to 1–2 μg/ml. For severe infections due to MRSA (e.g., endovascular or bone infections), trough concentrations of 15–20 μg/ml are recommended [19, 20]. Studies of the relationship between high-dose vancomycin and nephrotoxicity have indicated that trough concentrations exceeding 15 μg/ml increase the risk of renal damage [21], whereas ototoxicity is rare when vancomycin is administered without other ototoxic drugs. Associations of ototoxicity with serum vancomycin concentrations above 40 μg/ml have been suggested in the past, but these data are possibly biased by confounding factors [21].

Given the pharmacokinetics/pharmacodynamics relationships of vancomycin and its high interpatient variability, serial monitoring of vancomycin concentrations has been recommended. Data do not support monitoring peak vancomycin concentrations for predicting nephrotoxicity, whereas monitoring trough concentration is recommended for patients receiving high doses, in the case of coadministered nephrotoxic drugs, and in those with prolonged courses of therapy or altered renal function [21].

The emergence of vancomycin-resistant *S. aureus* and vancomycin-resistant *Enterococcus* spp. constitutes an additional challenge for the use of this drug. The efficacy of vancomycin for the treatment of MRSA bacteremia appears compromised when MICs approach 2 μg/ml. Daptomycin is the first-in-class cyclic lipopeptide antibiotic licensed for the treatment of complicated skin and soft-tissue infections, and for the treatment of infective endocarditis due to *S aureus*. This agent is an alternative for the treatment of MRSA bacteremia due to organisms with vancomycin MICs at or above 2 mg/l. However, the use of daptomycin in patients who have not responded to vancomycin may select for higher daptomycin MICs with impaired clinical response to this drug [22, 23]. The new lipoglycopeptides dalbavancin, oritavancin, and telavancin have a good activity against multidrug-resistant Gram-positive pathogens [24]. Whether such drugs will represent future therapeutic alternatives for pathogens with reduced vancomycin susceptibility or resistance or for vancomycin-related adverse events needs to be investigated.

14.2.3
β-Lactams

β-Lactam antibiotics are a major family of antibacterial agents. After the discovery of penicillin in the 1950s, multiples molecules of different classes with a common β-lactam ring have been developed during recent decades. β-Lactams are subdivided in three main classes: (i) penicillins, some combined with β-lactamase inhibitors, (ii) carbapenems, and (iii) cephalosporins. All share the same mode of action by binding to bacterial penicillin-binding proteins that inhibit the synthesis of bacterial cell wall peptidoglycans, resulting in cell lysis.

Broad-spectrum β-lactams are indicated for the treatment of severe infections due to Gram-negative and/or Gram-positive bacteria in hospitalized patients. The principal broad-spectrum β-lactams of the current antibacterial armamentarium include: the combination of penicillins with β-lactamase inhibitors (i.e., amoxicillin with clavulanic acid and piperacillin with tazobactam); the carbapenems imipenem (administered with the renal dehydropeptidase I inhibitor cilastatin), meropenem, and ertapenem; and the third- and fourth-generation cephalosporins ceftriaxone and cefepime, respectively. This section will focus on the four broad-spectrum anti-Gram-positive and anti-Gram-negative β-lactams most frequently used in the hospital: piperacillin/tazobactam, imipenem, meropenem, and cefepime. These antibiotics are administered intravenously, their percentage of plasma protein binding is low (2% meropenem; 20% cefepime and imipenem; 15–50% piperacillin), and they are eliminated at 70–80% by the kidney via glomerular filtration and tubular secretion. Their elimination half-lifes in healthy volunteers lie between 1 (imipenem, meropenem, and piperacillin) and 2 h (cefepime), and are highly dependent on the renal function. In adults, β-lactams dosage regimens are therefore selected according to patients' renal clearance and the severity of infection [25]. In hemodialysis and continuous veno-venous hemodiafiltration, reduced dosage regimens are proposed [25–28]. Algorithms (www.crrt.ch) have been developed for dose adjustment in critically ill patients under continuous renal replacement therapy. In neonatology, β-lactam dosages are given on a milligram per kilogram body weight basis and adjusted according to the renal function.

About 50% of ICU patients acquire an infection requiring treatment with antibiotics [29, 30]. Emergence of multiresistant Gram-positives and Gram-negatives is a major concern in this setting. As during the last decade the development of new antibacterial compounds did not keep pace with this evolution of the epidemiology, the appropriate use of the available agents has been recognized as a priority by clinicians. Actions have been focused on appropriate education, on indications and duration of antibacterial therapy, as well as appropriate dosing. β-Lactams are characterized by a so-called "time-dependent" antibacterial activity – the time interval during which the antibiotic concentration in plasma remains over the pathogen's *in vitro* MIC ($T >$ MIC) is critical for efficacy. TDM has traditionally been applied for the prevention of toxicity of antibiotics with a narrow therapeutic index (i.e., aminoglycosides, glycopeptides). This strategy has, however, not been widely applied for β-lactams because of the common perception that these antibiotics have favorable efficacy–safety profiles. However, extreme and unpredictable drug pharmacokinetics is common in ICU patients, putting them at risk of not achieving optimal antibiotic coverage for clinical response and prevention of the emergence of bacterial resistance. Several studies have revealed wide interindividual variability in plasma levels of β-lactams: imipenem in critically ill children [31] and adults [32], indicating that patients with severe infections may be exposed to insufficient antibiotic levels. Unpredictable exposure to cefepime has been also described in ICU patients [33]. Similarly, piperacillin serum concentrations were within the therapeutic target range in only 50% of critically ill patients [34].

Conversely, neurological toxicity (encephalopathy, convulsions) has been reported with patients treated with high-dose β-lactams (penicillins, carbapenems, and third- and fourth-generation cephalosporins), particularly in the presence of impaired renal function [33]. A recent study has reported a 50% probability of neurological toxicity at cefepime concentrations above 22 μg/ml in febrile neutropenic patients with mild impairment of renal function [35]. Other toxicities include nausea and vomiting (imipenem, meropenem, cefepime), and altered hepatic function tests (piperacillin/tazobactam).

The above issues suggest a potential role for TDM of high-dose β-lactam therapy in critically ill patients with severe infections and altered/fluctuating renal function or renal replacement techniques, making *a priori* β-lactam dose adjustment particularly complex and difficult. Since the therapeutic ranges for some β-lactam drugs are probably less large than expected, TDM-guided individualized adjustment of dosing regimens may be helpful for optimizing antibacterial efficacy, while avoiding severe toxic effects and insufficient β-lactam exposure associated with the risk of emergence of bacterial resistance. The objective in the treatment of life-threatening infections is the achievement of plasma levels above the MIC during the whole dosing interval. Target trough levels must therefore be above the MIC (when the sensitivity of strains isolated from patient has been determined) or above 1 μg/ml (imipenem, meropenem, and piperacillin) and 2 μg/ml (cefepime) for the treatment of sepsis, and are 2 times higher (2 μg/ml for imipenem, meropenem, and piperacillin; 4 μg/ml for cefepime) in the case of severe sepsis and septic shock. These minimal values are based on MIC_{90} values from most frequent strains according to the European Committee on Antimicrobial Susceptibility Testing (http.//www.srga.org/eucastwt/WTEUCAST.htm). Since β-lactams are only weakly bound to plasma proteins, the trough plasma can be considered accurate enough for the determination of the minimal threshold.

At the present time, TDM for β-lactams is being considered in the following clinical scenarios: (i) suspicion of insufficient dosage (lack of clinical response to β-lactam therapy), (ii) suspicion of overdosing in the presence of encephalopathy, seizures, nausea, and vomiting, (iii) alteration of renal function or during renal replacement therapy (hemodialysis and continuous veno-venous hemodiafiltration), (iv) severe sepsis, septic shock, or extended burns, which are associated with important alterations of pharmacokinetics parameters (distribution volume and elimination kinetics), (v) infections with decreased *in vitro* sensitivity, (vi) dosing regimens outside the recommended schedules, and (vii) drug interactions, in particular with uricosuric agents (i.e., probenecid), which are likely to increase β-lactam plasma levels via the inhibition of renal organic anion transporters (OATs). If TDM is considered for the efficient use of β-lactams, information on plasma levels must be available to clinicians for dose adjustment within 24–48 h.

Clinical laboratories equipped with mass spectrometry facilities are developing analytical methodologies with rapid turnaround times for simultaneous quantification of the blood levels of the most frequently used antibacterial drugs on a daily basis (Figure 14.1).

The antibacterial activity of β-lactam antibiotics depends on the duration of exposure to drug levels above the MIC and these molecules have short half-lives. This constitutes a pharmacokinetics/pharmacodynamics rationale for their administration by continuous infusion aimed at better achieving stable plasma levels above the MIC than with intermittent bolus injections [29, 36–39], while using lower total doses of antibiotics. However, this approach that has been investigated during decades [38] is not frequently used in clinical practice [34, 40–42]. Physicians have argued against its implementation based on concerns on the stability of β-lactams in reconstituted infusion solutions, the achievement of insufficient antibiotics concentration in tissues, and the required healthcare logistics, while benefits are insufficiently demonstrated.

Finally, β-lactams are a common cause of drug-induced immunoglobulin E-mediated anaphylaxis and allergies of the delayed type [43]. These adverse drug reactions are not concentration-dependent. An allergic cross-reactivity between penicillins and other β-lactams such as carbapenems and cephalosporins is described in up to 5–20% of cases [44].

14.2.4
Antifungal Agents

Invasive fungal infections, mainly due to *Candida* and *Aspergillus*, are increasingly frequent life-threatening complications occurring in hematological patients, hematopoietic or solid organ transplant recipients, and other immunocompromised and/or critically ill patients [45–49]. This section aims at describing the pharmacology of the systemic antifungal agents most frequently used for prevention and therapy in humans. Three drug classes are discussed (in parentheses the compounds licensed for clinical indications): the polyenes that disrupt the fungal cell permeability by binding to ergosterol in the cell membrane (amphotericin B deoxycholate, amphotericin B lipid complex, amphotericin B colloidal dispersion, liposomal amphotericin B), the azoles that inhibit the biosynthesis of ergosterol as an essential structural component of the cell membrane (fluconazole, itraconazole, posaconazole, voriconazole), and the echinocandins that inhibit β-glucan synthesis in the fungal cell wall (anidulafungin, caspofungin, micafungin). A fourth class of antifungals – the pyrimidine analogs (flucytosine) – is not included in the present section because of their limited clinical use [49].

Therapy for invasive fungal infections is often extended over weeks to months, and the availability of parenteral and oral agents is a determinant for the management during the acute phase requiring a rapid achievement of effective drug concentrations at the site of infection and for the consolidation of response until complete resolution of infection, respectively. In addition to efficacy, tolerability and substantially higher costs of the parenteral agents are major issues in

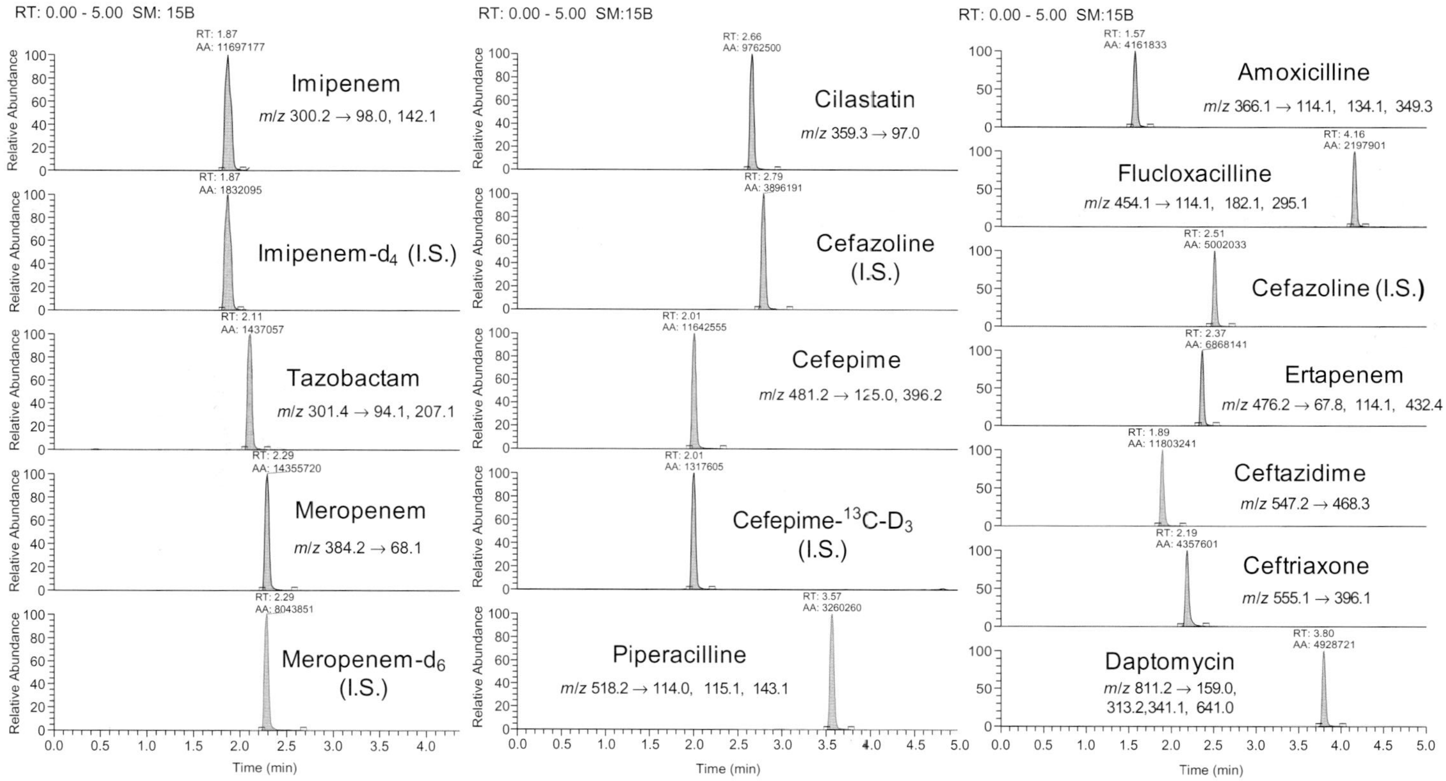

Figure 14.1 Multiplex analysis by ultra-high-performance liquid chromatography tandem mass spectroscopy of major currently-in-use β-lactams and daptomycin. Chromatographic profile of plasma quality control sample at 7.5 μg/ml for Pool 1 (left and center panels) and Pool 2 (right panel). Antibiotics are integrated in Pool 1 and Pool 2 according to the frequency of TDM drug measurement requests. Calibrations are established over the clinically relevant range of concentration of 0.1–100 μg/ml.

long-lasting antifungal therapy. Gastroinstestinal tract dysfunction, renal and hepatic failure as well as complex comedications are common characteristics in patients suffering of these severe infections. The choice of the appropriate antifungal therapy has thus to be based on multiple criteria, including the type of infection and the expected antifungal susceptibility of the involved pathogen, the patient's immune status, the management of the site of infection, the risk of toxicity, and the most cost-effective route of administration [49].

Amphotericin B and echinocandins have a very low oral bioavailability and are exclusively used as parenteral agents. In contrast, fluconazole, itraconazole, and voriconazole are used both as parenteral and oral forms. Only an oral form is available for the most recent agent, posaconazole, while a parenteral form is under development. Oral bioavailability is highest for fluconazole (above 90%), between 60 and 95% for voriconazole, and highly variable, in particular dependent on food and/or fat intake as well as gastric acidity, for itraconazole and posaconazole. With the exception of fluconazole, whose binding to plasma proteins is below 10%, the protein-bound fraction of all the other compounds is high, ranging from 60% for voriconazole to more than 80–95% for itraconazole, posaconazole, amphotericin B, and the echinocandins. All antifungal agents are widely distributed in the majority of tissues and body fluids. However, penetration in vitreous and cerebrospinal fluid as well as in the central nervous system is low to very low for amphotericin B and echinocandins, and ranges between 20 and 60% for azoles. Fluconazole is minimally metabolized in the liver and largely excreted as unchanged drug in the urine with renal function-dependent elimination kinetics. In contrast, liver function plays a central role in the elimination of the other agents. Itraconazole, posaconazole, and voriconazole are extensively transformed in the liver by the oxidative cytochrome P450 (CYP) system to antifungal active (OH-itraconazole) or inactive metabolites (e.g., NO-voriconazole) and by glucuronidation pathways (posaconazole). Genetic polymorphism of a CYP component strongly influences the elimination of voriconazole. The liver metabolism of azoles, however, is characterized by multiple interactions with concomitant medications, such as with cyclosporine and other calcineurin inhibitors, antiepileptic drugs, or rifampicin, which induce or inhibit the elimination of the antifungal compound or whose elimination is vice versa increased or decreased by the antifungal compound. Comedication needs thus to be carefully checked when azoles are prescribed. Among echinocandins, caspofungin and micafungin are metabolized by different hepatic pathways (hydrolysis, *N*-acetylation, CYP), whereas anidulafungin undergoes extrahepatic nonenzymatic degradation. Finally, the different forms of amphotericin B accumulate to variable degrees in the different tissues, and are excreted over weeks by the liver and kidneys; however, the specific pathways involved in their metabolism and elimination are unknown [49].

A concentration-dependent antifungal activity for the three drug classes has been demonstrated in experimental models of candidiasis, while data for other fungi are scarce or lacking. The ratio of peak blood concentration or AUC to the *in vitro* MIC of the drug for the fungal pathogen is the pharmacodynamic parameter best describing this dose–effect relationship. In tissues, similar quantitative relationships between drug exposure and antifungal action have been reported. In contrast, experimental data on the pharmacodynamics of toxicity are lacking [49, 50].

An important intra- and interindividual variability of drug blood concentrations is observed in patients treated with these three classes of antifungal agents. Lack of response of fungal infection to therapy and occurrence of breakthrough invasive infections during prophylaxis have been reported in patients with low blood concentrations of fluconazole, itraconazole, posaconazole, and voriconazole. High blood concentrations of voriconazole have been associated with the occurrence of a toxic encephalopathy and hepatopathy. Increasing clinical evidence thus supports the utility of TDM for guiding dosing of azole antifungal agents in order to optimize drug exposure on an individual basis. The lower threshold for trough blood concentrations – the most easily measurable pharmacokinetic parameter in clinical practice – has been set at the *in vitro* minimal inhibitory antifungal concentration required to inhibit growth of over 90% of the potentially implicated fungi (i.e., 1–2 μg/ml for itraconazole, posaconazole, and voriconazole, and 5–10 μg/ml for fluconazole). An upper concentration threshold of 4–6 μg/ml has been proposed for voriconazole based on clinical observations of a severe neurotoxicity occurring at higher trough concentrations. Itraconazole mean blood concentrations above 5–10 μg/ml have been associated with fluid retention and heart failure. For echinocandins and polyenes, a similar variability of blood concentrations has been described, but clinical data on its impact on efficacy and safety of therapy are lacking [51–54].

The antifungal armamentarium has been recently expanded with new agents of different classes, which have contributed to a substantial improvement of management and outcome in patients with invasive mycoses. Advances in the clinical application of the pharmacological principles have created the basis for optimizing individual antifungal dosing. Future investigations will focus on expanding our knowledge in this area, in particular by defining *a priori* the most appropriate individual dosing regimens by population pharmacokinetics studies associated with analyses of efficacy and toxicity outcomes, as well as the therapeutic drug concentration ranges needed for maximizing response while minimizing toxicity. The development of interdisciplinary platforms allowing the real-time measurement of antifungal blood concentrations with validated analytical techniques [55], and the joint interpretation of the results by infectious diseases specialists, pharmacologists, and microbiologists, will play a key role for the routine implementation of a clinically efficient TDM [49, 51, 56].

14.2.5
Antiviral Agents (Non-HIV)

This section presents the pharmacological characteristics of three main groups of antiviral drugs according to the type of viral infection targeted: herpes virus infection, viral hepatitis, and infection by respiratory viruses.

14.2.5.1 **Drugs for Herpes Virus Infection**

Acyclovir (and its prodrug valacyclovir) is mainly used for prophylaxis and treatment of herpes simplex virus (HSV) and varicella zoster virus (VZV) infections [57]. Oral acyclovir is used for treatment of mild infections, while intravenous acyclovir is the drug of choice for the treatment of HSV-1 encephalitis and disseminated zoster. Given the improved bioavailability of valacyclovir compared to acyclovir, this drug can be safely used in most moderate-to-severe HSV and VZV infections. Gancyclovir (and its prodrug valgancyclovir) is the drug of choice for prophylaxis and treatment of cytomegalovirus (CMV) infection [58]. Gancyclovir is also highly active against HSV and VZV, but the activity against other herpes viruses (Epstein–Barr virus, and human herpesvirus-6, -7, and -8) is less predictable. Other antiviral drugs that are less commonly used for the therapy of herpes virus infections include intravenous foscarnet and cidofovir (either intravenous or oral in a liposomal formulation). These drugs are used in the case of infection with gancyclovir-resistant virus or hematological toxicity due to gancyclovir.

The poor bioavailability of oral acyclovir and gancyclovir has been overcome with the introduction of valacyclovir and valgancyclovir, respectively [59]. Both are valylester prodrugs with a 10-fold higher bioavailability than the original drugs. In the intestine, both drugs are hydrolyzed to acyclovir/gancyclovir and released into the bloodstream. Acyclovir/gancyclovir clearance is significantly correlated to kidney function, so the dosage of these drugs should be adapted according to the glomerular filtration rate. In population pharmacokinetics studies, interpatient and intrapatient variability of gancyclovir plasma levels appears to be limited [60]. The pharmacokinetics/pharmacodynamics relationship of valgancyclovir and gancyclovir has been mainly assessed in solid-organ transplant recipients. Gancyclovir exposure correlates with the development of CMV viremia while the patient is on the drug, but not with subsequent CMV disease after the discontinuation of prophylaxis. Hematological toxicity is only marginally associated with gancyclovir exposure. Given the predictability of gancyclovir exposure using clinical variables (i.e., kidney function, weight), and the unclear relationship between gancyclovir exposure and efficacy and toxicity, TDM of gancyclovir is generally not recommended [59].

14.2.5.2 **Drugs for Viral Hepatitis**

Ribavirin is used for the treatment of chronic hepatitis C virus (HCV) infection in combination with α-(PEG)-interferon [61]. In addition, ribavirin has broad antiviral activity and is effective to treat paramyxovirus infections (respiratory syncytial virus, parainfluenza virus). The novel protease inhibitors telaprevir and boceprevir are promising molecules to additionally treat chronic HCV infection [62]. The arsenal of anti-hepatitis B virus (HBV) drugs includes lamivudine, emtricitabine, telbivudine, adefovir, tenofovir, and entecavir. These drugs are nucleoside or nucleotide analogs with a similar mechanism of action, but with different antiviral activity and resistance barrier. The precise indication for each drug in the treatment of HBV infection is beyond the scope of this chapter.

Ribavirin has a bioavailability of 30–40%, and it is mainly eliminated by hepatic metabolism and renal clearance. The anti-HBV nucleoside/nucleotide inhibitors have generally a good bioavailability, are not metabolized by the CYP system, and are eliminated by renal clearance. TDM of ribavirin has been proposed for the monitoring of efficacy/toxicity of the treatment of HCV infection. Some studies have correlated high plasma levels of ribavirin with improved response, but also with toxicity [63]. However, the optimal therapeutic range for ribavirin plasma levels has not yet been defined. Pharmacogenetics may also be of interest in patients receiving ribavirin; it has been recently shown that genetic variants leading to inosine triphosphatase deficiency protect against hemolytic anemia–a common adverse event of ribavirin therapy [64]. Regarding nucleoside/nucleotide inhibitors, most pharmacokinetics studies have been performed in the context of HIV infection. Currently, there are no recommendations for the routine use of TDM of anti-HBV drugs.

14.2.5.3 Drugs against Respiratory Viruses

Neuraminidase inhibitors are active against all types of influenza virus, and have replaced the M2 inhibitors amantadine and rimantadine as the drugs of choice to treat influenza [65]. Neuraminidase inhibitors include oral oseltamivir, inhaled and intravenous zanamivir and intravenous peramivir. As mentioned above, the only approved drug for the treatment of infections by other respiratory viruses is ribavirin, either orally, intravenously, or in aerosol.

In contrast to zanamivir and peramivir, oseltamivir has excellent bioavailability (80%) and it is the only neuraminidase inhibitor than can be administered in an oral formulation [66]. Zanamivir is administered by inhalation, which produces high drugs levels in sputum. Oseltamivir and zanamivir clearance is correlated with kidney function, although adjustment to kidney function is only recommended for oseltamivir. Experience with the intravenous neuraminidase inhibitors is limited to case series; there is scare data on pharmacokinetics of these drugs [67]. There is little intersubject variability of oseltamivir. In addition, there is no clear correlation between systemic oseltamivir exposure and antiviral activity or toxicity [66]. Therefore, it is not known whether TDM may be useful to improve the efficacy/safety profile of the drug. The short duration of therapy to treat influenza (5 days) would argue against the clinical use of TDM of neuraminidase inhibitors.

Overall, the improvement in the management of non-HIV viral infections thanks to the introduction of more efficacious and convenient antiviral drugs has not been accompanied by greater understanding of pharmacokinetics/pharmacodynamics relationships. Population pharmacokinetics analysis studies of some drugs have been performed in special populations, such as transplant recipients (e.g., valgancyclovir); for other drugs, data essentially come from studies in healthy volunteers. Finally, there are no current recommendations for TDM for any of these antiviral drugs.

14.2.6 Anti-HIV Agents

There are today over 20 different antiretroviral agents approved for clinical use. They belong to five families of compounds (protease inhibitors, nucleoside/nucleotide analog and non-nucleoside reverse transcriptase inhibitors, entry inhibitors, and integrase inhibitors). They are commonly used in triple-combination therapy to prevent viral resistance. The preferential choices for first-line therapy are generally well typified in international and national guidelines [68] – effectively reducing the number of potential drug combinations used in the clinics. The variety of compounds implicate various metabolic pathways, and are subject to drug–drug interaction – within the combination therapy and in association with other drugs used in the treatment of AIDS-associated complications. The pharmacology and interactions are well summarized in public domain resources such as www.hiv-druginteractions.org, www.clinicaloptions.com/hiv, and hivinsite.ucsf.edu.

Details on specific drugs and ADME (absorption, distribution, metabolism, and excretion) features are beyond the scope of this chapter. The family of antiretroviral agents is diverse; specific details on metabolism, pharmacokinetics, and approval histories can be accessed through the US Food and Drug Administration (Drugs@FDA), and in recent specialty reviews [69–71]. Non-nucleoside reverse transcriptase inhibitors and protease inhibitors are generally metabolized through CYP, the new integrase inhibitor raltegravir through glucuronidation, while the nucleoside analog reverse transcriptase inhibitors require intracellular anabolic phosphorylation to be converted into their triphosphorylated active metabolites. Various transporters have been implicated in uptake and elimination, access to selected biological compartments, and as determinants of intracellular concentrations.

It is important to emphasize the strategic use of some of pharmacokinetics interactions in benefit of treatment. Most notably is the use of the protease inhibitor ritonavir – a potent inhibitor of CYP3A – as agent to boost drug concentration of other protease inhibitors. However, given the fact that ritonavir can be poorly tolerated and that it retains antiviral activity – the dose used for pharmacoenhancing results in subtherapeutic antiviral levels – other molecules have been developed to achieve similar pharmacoenhancing goals. Cobicistat (GS-9350) is used in combination with the integrase inhibitor elvitegravir or protease inhibitor atazanavir [72]. A second compound – Sequoia Pharmaceuticals SPI-452 – is an inhibitor of CYP3A that has been used for boosting of various protease inhibitors.

Of relevance in antiretroviral therapy is the relative importance of so-called "special populations." This refers to the large numbers of pregnant women infected with HIV worldwide, to a substantial pediatric population, and to the importance of the simultaneous (or sequential) treatment of tuberculosis, hepatitis C, and other opportunistic infections [68]. Another important issue is the concept of viral reservoirs or compartments. These include organs, tissues, or cells proven or proposed to exhibit differences in pharmacokinetics, thus creating a setting where subtherapeutic drug levels may lead to viral escape. A third critical issue is the prevalence of short- and long-term adverse events of current therapies [73], some of which can be related to the pharmacokinetics profiles of the compounds (see below).

Another important features of these drugs is that they exhibit significant inter-individual variability, as observed in population pharmacokinetics analyses. Some demographic, physiopathological, and environmental factors have explained a small part of their variability. A number of drugs have been investigated by a novel approach using population pharmacokinetics/pharmacogenetics analyses: nevirapine [74, 75], atazanavir [76], lopinavir [77], efavirenz [78], and, recently, etravirine and raltegravir (unpublished). This approach can offer the possibility to capture the influence of genetic polymorphisms by generating accurate study phenotypes for extensive genetic and genomic discovery efforts [79] or for the integration of selected variables in a comprehensive population pharmacokinetics/pharmacogenetics model.

There is a level of complexity in establishing clear associations between pharmacokinetics profiles of antiretroviral drugs and antiviral action. (i) The antiretroviral agents are used in triple (or greater number of drugs)-combination therapy. (ii) There is likely a large therapeutic margin, at least when referring to the achievable plasma drug levels to the levels of viral susceptibility (described by the IC_{50} – the concentration that inhibits replication by 50%). (iii) Virological treatment failure is mostly driven by adherence or by pre-existing drug resistance. (iv) There is a limited understanding of the relationship between plasma drug levels and drug concentration at the sites of drug action – intracellular and compartments [80]. There is also limited understanding of the association of pharmacokinetics and toxicity [69]. There is a general agreement that the association is true for efavirenz neuropsychological adverse events and atazanavir hyperbilirubinemia; otherwise, the optimal therapeutic range has not been fully defined for a majority of the compounds.

Based on the considerations presented above, the use of TDM remains subject of discussion and research [81]. The last guidelines of the International Antiviral Society-USA indicate that [68]:

> . . . when assays are performed by a quality-assured laboratory, monitoring of [protease inhibitor] and [non-nucleoside reverse transcriptase inhibitor] levels may be useful in pregnant women, children, and patients with renal or liver impairment to minimize overexposure and adverse effects, manage potential drug–drug interactions, or evaluate virologic failure in the absence of resistance.

In general, the field of antiretroviral treatment remains an interesting field for clinical pharmacology because of the complexity of interactions, and the prevalence of treatment failure and toxicity. It is also a dynamic field because of the frequent use of TDM, and because of active research integrating pharmacogenetics in population pharmacokinetics models and advancing genetic prediction in clinical care.

14.3 Pharmacogenetics

There is increasing interest in identifying genetic and genomic markers of disease susceptibility, variants of drug ADME pathways, as well as of treatment response and toxicity. The approaches to this goal are multiple: from the detailed analysis of gene candidates, to the new generation of genome-wide association studies that explore up to 1 million common variants in the human genome. Those approaches have shared the importance of definition of the study phenotype or endpoint [82]. As indicated above, pharmacokinetics can be excellent to study traits. Severe toxicity is generally considered a priority target of genome-wide analyses, but may require large numbers of, generally, a rare event.

A number of studies in the field of antiretroviral therapy have investigated the association of variants in ADME genes and pharmacokinetics profiles. Efavirenz is a particularly interesting model because functional genetic variations in both principal and accessory metabolic pathways demonstrate a joint impact on efavirenz disposition [78]. The interindividual variability (65%) in average clearance is largely explained by CYP2B6 genetic variation (31%). CYP2A6 and CYP3A4 had a prominent influence on clearance when CYP2B6 was impaired. Dosage adjustment in accordance with the type of polymorphism is required in order to maintain efavirenz within the therapeutic target levels [83]. A similar approach to lopinavir/ritonavir pharmacokinetics results in a different message (Figure 14.2). Variants in two transporter genes – *SLCO1B1* and *ABCC2* – as well as in the *CYP3A* locus only explain 5% of lopinavir clearance variability. However, the limited variability explained at the population level does not negate the clinically relevant effects of variants for the rare individuals that are homozygous for the *SLCO1B1*4* alleles. This allele codes for a gain-of-function/change-of-substrate specificity variant of OATP1B1 – an uptake transporter of the OAT polypeptide superfamily. *SLCO1B1*4* homozygous individuals have a clearance of 12.6 l/h, compared to 5.4 l/h in the reference group [77].

Figure 14.2 Steps in the construction of a population pharmacokinetics/pharmacogenetics model. A number of studies have investigated the association of variants in ADME genes and pharmacokinetics profiles. The study of the antiretroviral fixed-dose combination agent lopinavir/ritonavir progressed through various steps. (a) Distribution of the lopinavir clearance ($LPV_{\eta CL}$) values: frequency histogram of interpatient variability on $LPV_{\eta CL}$ and the corresponding probits in a discovery population ($n = 638$). This representation allowed the identification of extremes: 121 individuals with a clear departure from the expected normal distribution (gray line) were selected as cases and the 92 individuals with values above percentile 85 were selected as controls. (b) Manhattan plot of results from the association study of cases and controls for 1330 single nucleotide polymorphisms (SNPs) analyzed in 20 chromosomes. The top line indicates the study-wide cut-off for significance, corresponding to Bonferroni correction of $P = 3.8 \times 10^{-5}$. The bottom line corresponds to the value at which the observed P values diverge from the null expectation. The y-axis presents the negative log of the association P value. Only one SNP, in a solute carrier transporter, reached study-wide significance; other candidate loci were re-evaluated in a independent validation population. (c) The resulting model for the discovery and validation steps that identified variants in two transporter genes *SLCO1B1* and *ABCC2*, as well as in the *CYP3A* locus that explain 5% of lopinavir clearance variability. (Adapted from Lubomirov *et al.* [77].)

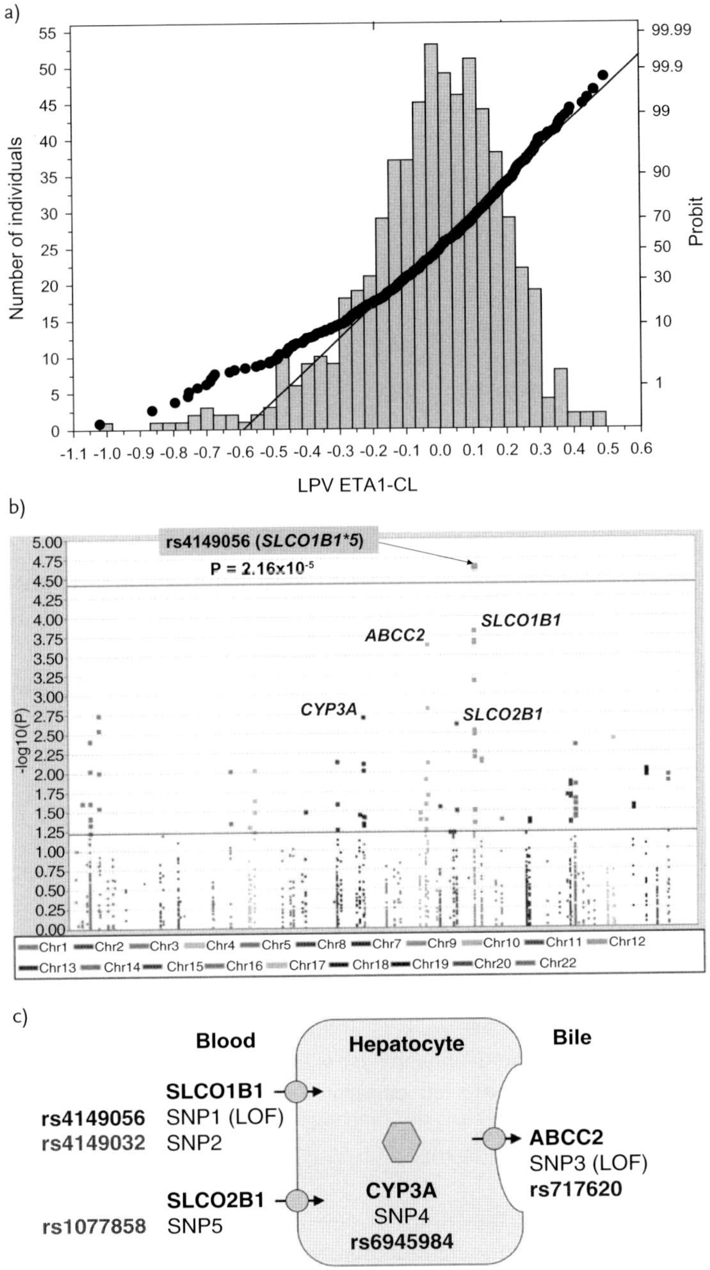

a)
Number of individuals
Probit
LPV ETA1-CL
b)
rs4149056 (SLCO1B1*5)
P = 2.16x10-5
-log10(P)
ABCC2
SLCO1B1
CYP3A
SLCO2B1
Chr1 Chr2 Chr3 Chr4 Chr5 Chr8 Chr7 Chr9 Chr10 Chr11 Chr12
Chr13 Chr14 Chr15 Chr16 Chr17 Chr18 Chr19 Chr20 Chr22
c)
Blood
Hepatocyte
Bile
SLCO1B1
rs4149056 SNP1 (LOF)
rs4149032 SNP2
SLCO2B1
rs1077858 SNP5
ABCC2
SNP3 (LOF)
rs717620
CYP3A
SNP4
rs6945984

For many drugs, toxicity is not dose-dependent. Thus, a number of valuable pharmacogenetic markers are not associated with a variation in ADME genes. A prominent example is hypersensitivity to abacavir–an antiretroviral agent. Individuals carriers of *HLA-B57:01* in the major histocompatibility complex locus are highly susceptible to developing severe systemic manifestations of hypersensitivity [84, 85]. This finding led to the first randomized pharmacogenetics-based clinical trial [86] and a formal reference to the molecular test in the drug label. *HLA-B57:01* also determines liver toxicity from the antibiotic flucloxacillin [87].

N-acetylation is important in the biotransformation of drugs such as isoniazid, sulfonamides, and dapsone. The human acetylation polymorphism is one of the first hereditary traits affecting drug response to be discovered [88]. This trait was first found in patients who developed numbness and tingling in the fingers and toes after responding to isoniazid treatment. Slow acetylators excreted less acetylisoniazid and were more prone to develop the neurologic toxicity. In humans, three *N*-acetyltransferase (NAT) genes are found, but only *NAT1* and *NAT2* are expressed [89], and over 25 *NAT2* allelic variants have been identified that account for 95% or more of alleles across populations. *NAT2**5A*, *NAT2**6A*, and *NAT2**7A* are associated with the slow acetylator phenotype.

Deficiency in the hereditary enzyme glucose 6-phosphate dehydrogenase (G6PD) causes hemolytic anemia after exposure to certain dietary substances, numerous drugs such as the 8-aminoquinolones, as well as other oxidant chemicals. G6PD is responsible for the oxidation of glucose-6-phosphate to 6-phosphogluconic acid. This reaction is necessary to produce NADPH, which functions as a proton donor in the glutathione reductase reaction. Reduced glutathione protects sulfhydryl-dependent enzymes and other cellular proteins against oxidation. The antimalarial drug primaquine induces hemolysis by causing a further reduction of the level of reduced glutathione in red cells that already have an impaired mechanism for the regeneration of NADPH. Over 400 variant alleles of *G6PD* have been reported, with a large number of coding variants identified as responsible for the defect.

Treatment of hepatitis C uses the combination of interferon-α and ribavirin. Two polymorphic genes have been recently identified through genome-wide association analyses that are important for treatment outcome and toxicity. Variants in *IL28B*–encoding interferon-λ–are markers of spontaneous and interferon-α-induced response [90, 91]. Inosine triphosphatase (ITPA) variants protect against hemolytic anemia in hepatitis-C-infected patients receiving ribavirin [64]. The importance of *IL28B* is such that it is currently recommended that hepatitis C trials that combine investigational agents with pegylated interferon should be stratified by *IL28B* genotypes [92].

There is intense debate about the future of personalized medicine based on pharmacogenetics. Experience in the field demonstrates that rather than a rapid revolution, there is progressive implementation of tests of genetic nature. The US Food and Drug Administration is adding information on genomic biomarkers to drug labels to describe drug exposure and clinical response variability, risk of adverse events, genotype-specific dosing, mechanisms of drug action, and polymorphic drug target and disposition genes (http://www.fda.gov/drugs/

scienceresearch/researchareas/pharmacogenetics/ucm083378.htm). The main limitations to the wider use of genetic tests are no longer costs, as genetic testing is becoming very cheap, but evaluation, validation, implementation, and assessment of cost-effectiveness.

A separate, but emerging issue is the inclusion of genetic consent, testing, and discovery in clinical trials of new medications. The standard was set by a clinical trial on pegylated interferon and ribavirin treatment of hepatitis C [61]. Re-analysis of the trial data through genome-wide association studies led to the rapid identification of the role of *IL28B* and *ITPA* variation described above. This is a good example of what should be aimed at in a state-of-the-art evaluation of treatment response and toxicity in the frame of clinical trials.

14.4 Conclusions

Despite the size of the world market of anti-infective drugs, and the widespread use of these agents across populations and in complex medical settings, there are important gaps in our understanding of principles of pharmacokinetics/pharmacodynamics/toxicity and dose adjustment through TDM. The field would benefit from more concerted action to systematically explore those aspects, if possible in the early postmarketing phase.

Among specific actions that would help advance the field (Table 14.1), we emphasize issues such as drug penetration into specific cells and compartments, and a better understanding of the determinants of intracellular drug concentration, comprehensive mapping of patterns of distribution of functional alleles of metabolizing enzymes across world populations, and a decisive move to integrate pharmacokinetics and pharmacogenetics/genomics in clinical trials. In addition,

Table 14.1 Key issues in pharmacokinetics, pharmacodynamics, and pharmacogenetics of anti-infective agents.

- The size of the anti-infective drug market justifies investment in a better understanding of the pharmacokinetics/pharmacodynamics/pharmacogenetics profiles under the guiding principles of evidence-based medicine.
- Treatment individualization of antibiotic, antiviral, and antifungal agents would have a significant impact on the efficacy, safety, and efficiency of prescription.
- There is a need for a better understanding of free circulating and intracellular drug concentration, and the determinants of drug penetration into specific cells and cellular compartments.
- Progress in genomics allows the comprehensive mapping of patterns of distribution of functional alleles of metabolizing enzymes and other ADME genes across world populations.
- Clinical trials and postmarketing studies should enhance the acquisition of pharmacokinetic and pharmacodynamic data as well as include provision for pharmacogenomics.

a better link between pharmacokinetics and pharmacodynamics models for treatment individualization of antibiotic, antiviral, and antifungal agents would have an enormous impact of the efficacy and efficiency of treatment. Progress in these areas would support the best use of the principles of evidenced-based medicine.

Acknowledgments

Supported by the Swiss National Science Foundation (grant 324730-124943).

References

1 Hamad, B. (2010) The antibiotics market. *Nat. Rev. Drug Discov.*, **9**, 675–676.

2 Kadurugamuwa, J.L., *et al.* (1993) Surface action of gentamicin on *Pseudomonas aeruginosa*. *J. Bacteriol.*, **175**, 5798–5805.

3 Nicolau, D.P., *et al.* (1995) Experience with a once-daily aminoglycoside program administered to 2184 adult patients. *Antimicrob. Agents Chemother.*, **39**, 650–655.

4 Begg, E.J. and Barclay, M.L. (1995) Aminoglycosides – 50 years on. *Br. J. Clin. Pharmacol.*, **39**, 597–603.

5 Zaske, D.E., *et al.* (1982) Gentamicin pharmacokinetics in 1640 patients: method for control of serum concentrations. *Antimicrob. Agents Chemother.*, **21**, 407–411.

6 Lopez-Novoa, J.M., *et al.* (2011) New insights into the mechanism of aminoglycoside nephrotoxicity: an integrative point of view. *Kidney Int.*, **79**, 33–45.

7 Guthrie, O.W. (2008) Aminoglycoside induced ototoxicity. *Toxicology*, **249**, 91–96.

8 Bertino, J.S., Jr, *et al.* (1993) Incidence of and significant risk factors for aminoglycoside-associated nephrotoxicity in patients dosed by using individualized pharmacokinetic monitoring. *J. Infect. Dis.*, **167**, 173–179.

9 Moore, R.D., Lietman, P.S., and Smith, C.R. (1987) Clinical response to aminoglycoside therapy: importance of the ratio of peak concentration to minimal inhibitory concentration. *J. Infect. Dis.*, **155**, 93–99.

10 Moore, R.D., Smith, C.R., and Lietman, P.S. (1984) Association of aminoglycoside plasma levels with therapeutic outcome in gram-negative pneumonia. *Am. J. Med.*, **77**, 657–662.

11 Moore, R.D., Smith, C.R., and Lietman, P.S. (1984) The association of aminoglycoside plasma levels with mortality in patients with Gram-negative bacteremia. *J. Infect. Dis.*, **149**, 443–448.

12 Zelenitsky, S.A., *et al.* (2003) Treatment and outcome of *Pseudomonas aeruginosa* bacteraemia: an antibiotic pharmacodynamic analysis. *J. Antimicrob. Chemother.*, **52**, 668–674.

13 Ali, M.Z. and Goetz, M.B. (1997) A meta-analysis of the relative efficacy and toxicity of single daily dosing versus multiple daily dosing of aminoglycosides. *Clin. Infect. Dis.*, **24**, 796–809.

14 Rybak, M.J., *et al.* (2009) Therapeutic monitoring of vancomycin in adults summary of consensus recommendations from the American Society of Health-System Pharmacists, the Infectious Diseases Society of America, and the Society of Infectious Diseases Pharmacists. *Pharmacotherapy*, **29**, 1275–1279.

15 Schaad, U.B., McCracken, G.H., Jr, and Nelson, J.D. (1980) Clinical pharmacology and efficacy of vancomycin in pediatric patients. *J. Pediatr.*, **96**, 119–126.

16 Thomson, A.H., *et al.* (2009) Development and evaluation of vancomycin dosage guidelines designed to achieve new target concentrations. *J. Antimicrob. Chemother.*, **63**, 1050–1057.

17 Ackerman, B.H., Vannier, A.M., and Eudy, E.B. (1992) Analysis of vancomycin time-kill studies with *Staphylococcus* species by using a curve stripping program to describe the relationship between concentration and pharmacodynamic response. *Antimicrob. Agents Chemother.*, **36**, 1766–1769.

18 Moise-Broder, P.A., *et al.* (2004) Pharmacodynamics of vancomycin and other antimicrobials in patients with *Staphylococcus aureus* lower respiratory tract infections. *Clin. Pharmacokinet.*, **43**, 925–942.

19 Liu, C., *et al.* (2011) Clinical practice guidelines by the Infectious Diseases Society of America for the treatment of methicillin-resistant *Staphylococcus aureus* infections in adults and children. *Clin. Infect. Dis.*, **52**, e18–e55.

20 Hidayat, L.K., *et al.* (2006) High-dose vancomycin therapy for methicillin-resistant *Staphylococcus aureus* infections: efficacy and toxicity. *Arch. Intern. Med.*, **166**, 2138–2144.

21 Rybak, M.J., *et al.* (1990) Nephrotoxicity of vancomycin, alone and with an aminoglycoside. *J. Antimicrob. Chemother.*, **25**, 679–687.

22 Pillai, S.K., *et al.* (2007) Daptomycin nonsusceptibility in *Staphylococcus aureus* with reduced vancomycin susceptibility is independent of alterations in MprF. *Antimicrob. Agents Chemother.*, **51**, 2223–2225.

23 Cui, L., *et al.* (2006) Correlation between reduced daptomycin susceptibility and vancomycin resistance in vancomycin-intermediate *Staphylococcus aureus*. *Antimicrob. Agents Chemother.*, **50**, 1079–1082.

24 Zhanel, G.G., *et al.* (2010) New lipoglycopeptides: a comparative review of dalbavancin, oritavancin and telavancin. *Drugs*, **70**, 859–886.

25 Sanford Guides (2008) The Sanford Guide to Antimicrobial Therapy, 38th edn, Antimicrobial Therapy, Sperryville, VA.

26 Trotman, R.L., *et al.* (2005) Antibiotic dosing in critically ill adult patients receiving continuous renal replacement therapy. *Clin. Infect. Dis.*, **41**, 1159–1166.

27 Pea, F., *et al.* (2007) Pharmacokinetic considerations for antimicrobial therapy in patients receiving renal replacement therapy. *Clin. Pharmacokinet.*, **46**, 997–1038.

28 Robatel, C., *et al.* (2003) Pharmacokinetics and dosage adaptation of meropenem during continuous venovenous hemodiafiltration in critically ill patients. *J. Clin. Pharmacol.*, **43**, 1329–1340.

29 Roberts, J.A., Hope, W.W., and Lipman, J. (2010) Therapeutic drug monitoring of beta-lactams for critically ill patients: unwarranted or essential? *Int. J. Antimicrob. Agents*, **35**, 419–420.

30 Vincent, J.L., *et al.* (2009) International study of the prevalence and outcomes of infection in intensive care units. *JAMA*, **302**, 2323–2329.

31 Giannoni, E., *et al.* (2006) Prospective determination of plasma imipenem concentrations in critically ill children. *Antimicrob. Agents Chemother.*, **50**, 2563–2568.

32 Lamoth, F., *et al.* (2009) Reassessment of recommended imipenem doses in febrile neutropenic patients with hematological malignancies. *Antimicrob. Agents Chemother.*, **53**, 785–787.

33 Chapuis, T.M., *et al.* (2010) Prospective monitoring of cefepime in intensive care unit adult patients. *Crit. Care*, **14**, R51.

34 Blondiaux, N., *et al.* (2010) Daily serum piperacillin monitoring is advisable in critically ill patients. *Int. J. Antimicrob. Agents*, **35**, 500–503.

35 Lamoth, F., *et al.* (2010) High cefepime plasma concentrations and neurological toxicity in febrile neutropenic patients with mild impairment of renal function. *Antimicrob. Agents Chemother.*, **54**, 4360–4367.

36 Roberts, J.A., *et al.* (2009) Meropenem dosing in critically ill patients with sepsis and without renal dysfunction: intermittent bolus versus continuous administration? Monte Carlo dosing simulations and subcutaneous tissue distribution. *J. Antimicrob. Chemother.*, **64**, 142–150.

37 Roberts, J.A., *et al.* (2007) Continuous infusion of beta-lactam antibiotics in severe infections: a review of its role. *Int. J. Antimicrob. Agents*, **30**, 11–18.

38 MacGowen, A.P. (2001) Role of pharmacokinetics and pharmacodynamics: does the dose matter? *Clin. Infect. Dis.*, **33** (Suppl. 3), S238–S239.

39 Roos, J.F., *et al.* (2006) Pharmacokinetic–pharmacodynamic rationale for cefepime dosing regimens in intensive care units. *J. Antimicrob. Chemother.*, **58**, 987–993.

40 Rappaz, I., *et al.* (2000) Continuous infusion of ceftazidime with a portable pump is as effective as thrice-a-day bolus in cystic fibrosis children. *Eur. J. Pediatr.*, **159**, 919–925.

41 Bodey, G.P., Ketchel, S.J., and Rodriguez, V. (1979) A randomized study of carbenicillin plus cefamandole or tobramycin in the treatment of febrile episodes in cancer patients. *Am. J. Med.*, **67**, 608–616.

42 Zeisler, J.A., *et al.* (1992) Cefuroxime by continuous infusion: a new standard of care? *Infect. Med.*, **9**, 54–60.

43 Joint Task Force on Practice Parameters, American Academy of Allergy, Asthma and Immunology, American College of Allergy, Asthma and Immunology, and The Joint Council of Allergy, Asthma and Immunology (2005) The diagnosis and management of anaphylaxis. *J. Allergy Clin. Immunol.*, **115**, S483–S523.

44 Frumin, J. and Gallagher, J.C. (2009) Allergic cross-sensitivity between penicillin, carbapenem, and monobactam antibiotics: what are the chances? *Ann. Pharmacother.*, **43**, 304–315.

45 Maertens, J., *et al.* (2011) European guidelines for antifungal management in leukemia and hematopoietic stem cell transplant recipients: summary of the ECIL 3-2009 Update. *Bone Marrow Transplant.*, **46**, 709–718.

46 Pappas, P.G., *et al.* (2009) Clinical practice guidelines for the management of candidiasis: 2009 update by the Infectious Diseases Society of America. *Clin. Infect. Dis.*, **48**, 503–535.

47 Walsh, T.J., *et al.* (2008) Treatment of aspergillosis: clinical practice guidelines of the Infectious Diseases Society of America. *Clin. Infect. Dis.*, **46**, 327–360.

48 Freifeld, A.G., *et al.* (2011) Clinical practice guideline for the use of antimicrobial agents in neutropenic patients with cancer: 2010 update by the Infectious Diseases Society of America. *Clin. Infect. Dis.*, **52**, e56–e93.

49 Dodds Ashley, E., *et al.* (2006) Pharmacology of systemic antifungal agents. *Clin. Infect. Dis.*, **43**, S28–S39.

50 Denning, D.W. (2003) Echinocandin antifungal drugs. *Lancet*, **362**, 1142–1151.

51 Andes, D., Pascual, A., and Marchetti, O. (2009) Antifungal therapeutic drug monitoring: established and emerging indications. *Antimicrob. Agents Chemother.*, **53**, 24–34.

52 Pascual, A., *et al.* (2008) Voriconazole therapeutic drug monitoring in patients with invasive mycoses improves efficacy and safety outcomes. *Clin. Infect. Dis.*, **46**, 201–211.

53 Walsh, T.J., *et al.* (2007) Treatment of invasive aspergillosis with posaconazole in patients who are refractory to or intolerant of conventional therapy: an externally controlled trial. *Clin. Infect. Dis.*, **44**, 2–12.

54 Lestner, J.M., *et al.* (2009) Toxicodynamics of itraconazole: implications for therapeutic drug monitoring. *Clin. Infect. Dis.*, **49**, 928–930.

55 Decosterd, L.A., *et al.* (2010) Multiplex ultra-performance liquid chromatography-tandem mass spectrometry method for simultaneous quantification in human plasma of fluconazole, itraconazole, hydroxyitraconazole, posaconazole, voriconazole, voriconazole-*N*-oxide, anidulafungin, and caspofungin. *Antimicrob. Agents Chemother.*, **54**, 5303–5315.

56 Bruggemann, R.J., *et al.* (2009) International interlaboratory proficiency testing program for measurement of azole antifungal plasma concentrations. *Antimicrob. Agents Chemother.*, **53**, 303–305.

57 Kempf, W., *et al.* (2007) Swiss recommendations for the management of varicella zoster virus infections. *Swiss Med. Wkly.*, **137**, 239–251.

58 Pescovitz, M.D. (2010) Valganciclovir: recent progress. *Am. J. Transplant.*, **10**, 1359–1364.

59 Perrottet, N., *et al.* (2009) Valganciclovir in adult solid organ transplant recipients: pharmacokinetic and pharmacodynamic characteristics and clinical interpretation of plasma concentration measurements. *Clin. Pharmacokinet.*, **48**, 399–418.

60 Perrottet, N., *et al.* (2009) Population pharmacokinetics of ganciclovir in solid-organ transplant recipients receiving oral valganciclovir. *Antimicrob. Agents Chemother.*, **53**, 3017–3023.

61 McHutchison, J.G., *et al.* (1998) Interferon alfa-2b alone or in combination with ribavirin as initial treatment for chronic hepatitis C. Hepatitis Interventional Therapy Group. *N. Engl. J. Med.*, **339**, 1485–1492.

62 McHutchison, J.G., *et al.* (2010) Telaprevir for previously treated chronic HCV infection. *N. Engl. J. Med.*, **362**, 1292–1303.

63 Chan, A.H., Partovi, N., and Ensom, M.H. (2009) The utility of therapeutic drug monitoring for ribavirin in patients with chronic hepatitis C – a critical review. *Ann. Pharmacother.*, **43**, 2044–2063.

64 Fellay, J., *et al.* (2010) ITPA gene variants protect against anaemia in patients treated for chronic hepatitis C. *Nature*, **464**, 405–408.

65 Moscona, A. (2005) Neuraminidase inhibitors for influenza. *N. Engl. J. Med.*, **353**, 1363–1373.

66 Widmer, N., *et al.* (2010) Oseltamivir in seasonal, avian H5N1 and pandemic 2009 A/H1N1 influenza: pharmacokinetic and pharmacodynamic characteristics. *Clin. Pharmacokinet.*, **49**, 741–765.

67 Gaur, A.H., *et al.* (2010) Intravenous zanamivir for oseltamivir-resistant 2009 H1N1 influenza. *N. Engl. J. Med.*, **362**, 88–89.

68 Thompson, M.A., *et al.* (2010) Antiretroviral treatment of adult HIV infection: 2010 recommendations of the International AIDS Society-USA panel. *JAMA*, **304**, 321–333.

69 Arab-Alameddine, M., *et al.* (2011) Antiretroviral drug toxicity in relation to pharmacokinetics, metabolic profile and pharmacogenetics. *Expert Opin. Drug Metab. Toxicol.*, Epub ahead of print. PubMed PMID: 21500966.

70 Dickinson, L., Khoo, S., and Back, D. (2010) Pharmacokinetics and drug–drug interactions of antiretrovirals: an update. *Antiviral Res.*, **85**, 176–189.

71 Brown, K.C., Paul, S., and Kashuba, A.D. (2009) Drug interactions with new and investigational antiretrovirals. *Clin. Pharmacokinet.*, **48**, 211–241.

72 Mathias, A.A., *et al.* (2010) Pharmacokinetics and pharmacodynamics of GS-9350: a novel pharmacokinetic enhancer without anti-HIV activity. *Clin. Pharmacol. Ther.*, **87**, 322–329.

73 Keiser, O., *et al.* (2007) Adverse events to antiretrovirals in the Swiss HIV Cohort Study: impact on mortality and treatment modification. *Antivir. Ther.*, **12**, 1157–1164.

74 Schipani, A., *et al.* (2011) Integration of population pharmacokinetics and pharmacogenetics: an aid to optimal nevirapine dose selection in HIV-infected individuals. *J. Antimicrob. Chemother.*, **66**, 1332–1339.

75 Chou, M., *et al.* (2010) Population pharmacokinetic–pharmacogenetic study of nevirapine in HIV-infected Cambodian patients. *Antimicrob. Agents Chemother.*, **54**, 4432–4439.

76 Schipani, A., *et al.* (2010) Population pharmacokinetic modeling of the association between 63396C→T pregnane X receptor polymorphism and unboosted atazanavir clearance. *Antimicrob. Agents Chemother.*, **54**, 5242–5250.

77 Lubomirov, R., *et al.* (2010) ADME pharmacogenetics: investigation of the pharmacokinetics of the antiretroviral agent lopinavir coformulated with ritonavir. *Pharmacogenet. Genomics*, **20**, 217–230.

78 Arab-Alameddine, M., *et al.* (2009) Pharmacogenetic-based population pharmacokinetic analysis of efavirenz in HIV-1 infected individuals. *Clin. Pharmacol. Ther.*, **85**, 485–494.

79 Lubomirov, R., Csajka, C., and Telenti, A. (2007) ADME pathway approach for pharmacogenetic studies of anti-HIV therapy. *Pharmacogenomics*, **8**, 623–633.

80 Bazzoli, C., *et al.* (2010) Intracellular pharmacokinetics of antiretroviral drugs in HIV-infected patients, and their

correlation with drug action. *Clin. Pharmacokinet.*, **49**, 17–45.

81 Kredo, T., *et al.* (2009) Therapeutic drug monitoring of antiretrovirals for people with HIV. *Cochrane Database Syst. Rev.*, **3**, CD007268.

82 Evangelou, E., *et al.* (2011) Impact of phenotype definition on genome-wide association signals: empirical evaluation in HIV-1 infection. *Am. J. Epidemiol.*, **173**, 1336–1342.

83 Mello, A.F., *et al.* (2011) Successful efavirenz dose reduction guided by therapeutic drug monitoring. *Antivir. Ther.*, **16**, 189–197.

84 Mallal, S., *et al.* (2002) Association between presence of HLA-B*5701, HLA-DR7, and HLA-DQ3 and hypersensitivity to HIV-1 reverse-transcriptase inhibitor abacavir. *Lancet*, **359**, 727–732.

85 Hetherington, S., *et al.* (2002) Genetic variations in HLA-B region and hypersensitivity reactions to abacavir. *Lancet*, **359**, 1121–1122.

86 Mallal, S., *et al.* (2008) HLA-B*5701 screening for hypersensitivity to abacavir. *N. Engl. J. Med.*, **358**, 568–579.

87 Daly, A.K., *et al.* (2009) HLA-B*5701 genotype is a major determinant of drug-induced liver injury due to flucloxacillin. *Nat. Genet.*, **41**, 816–819.

88 Bonicke, R. and Reif, W. (1953) Enzymatic inactivation of isonicotinic acid hydrazide in humans and animals. *Arch. Exp. Pathol. Pharmacol*, **220**, 321–333.

89 Grant, D.M. (1993) Molecular genetics of the *N*-acetyltransferases. *Pharmacogenetics*, **3**, 45–50.

90 Ge, D., *et al.* (2009) Genetic variation in IL28B predicts hepatitis C treatment-induced viral clearance. *Nature*, **461**, 399–401.

91 Rauch, A., *et al.* (2010) Genetic variation in IL28B is associated with chronic hepatitis C and treatment failure: a genome-wide association study. *Gastroenterology*, **138**, 1338–1345.

92 Thompson, A.J., *et al.* (2010) Hepatitis C trials that combine investigational agents with pegylated interferon should be stratified by interleukin-28B genotype. *Hepatology*, **52**, 2243–2244.

15
Drugs against Acute and Chronic Pain

Andrew A. Somogyi and Janet K. Coller

15.1
Introduction

A large number of drugs are used for acute or chronic pain, with many of the drugs often used in both settings. Here, we review how each drug is metabolized in humans, the identification of the principal cytochromes P450 (CYPs), UDP-glucuronosyltransferases (UGTs), and sulfotransferases (SULTs) mainly derived from human liver microsomal and expressed enzyme studies, and their relative contribution to overall metabolism where the information is available. We have divided the chapter in two sections – acute pain and chronic pain – noting a large section on opioids. It should be recognized that many drugs for acute pain are also used for chronic pain and *vice versa*. Table 15.1 summarizes, where possible, the principal CYP, UGT, and SULT enzymes involved in the metabolism of all the drugs used for acute and/or chronic pain cited in this chapter.

15.2
Acute Pain

15.2.1
Dexmedotomidine

This is an α_2-adrenoreceptor agonist used as an intravenous analgesic. It undergoes glucuronidation at positions *N*1 and *N*3 of the imidazole ring. In human liver microsomes, the *N*3-glucuronide is formed at a more than 3-fold greater extent than the *N*1-glucuronide. UGT1A4 forms the *N*3-glucuronide at a 6 times higher rate than the *N*1, while UGT2B10 equally forms both glucuronides, but at lower rates than UGT1A4. Two-enzyme kinetics describes the formation of the *N*3 (CL_{int} (V_{max}/K_m) values of 17 and 1 μl/min/mg) and *N*1 (7 and 0.2 μl/min/mg) metabolites. It would appear that the *N*3-glucuronide is the major metabolite and that UGT1A4 is the main enzyme [1].

Metabolism of Drugs and Other Xenobiotics, First Edition. Edited by Pavel Anzenbacher, Ulrich M. Zanger.

Table 15.1 Enzymes involved in metabolism of drugs and their metabolites used for acute and chronic pain.

Drug class	*Drug* Metabolite	Major enzymes
α_2-Adrenoreceptor agonist	*Dexmedotomidine*	
	*N*1-glucuronide	UGTs 1A4, 2B10
	*N*3-glucuronide	UGTs 1A4, 2B10
Analgesic/antipyretic	*Paracetamol/acetaminophen*	
	glucuronide	UGTs 1A6, 1A9
	sulfate	SULT1A1
	NAPQI	CYPs 3A4, 2E1, 2A6, 1A2, 2D6, 2C19, 2C9
	3-hydroxyparacetamol	CYPs 2E1, 2A6
NSAIDs	*S-(+)-ibuprofen*	
	2-hydroxy	CYPs 2C9, 2C8, 3A4, 2C19
	3-hydroxy	CYPs 2C9, 2C8, 3A4, 2C19
	acyl-glucuronide	UGTs 2B7, 1A9, 1A3, 2B4
	R-(−)-ibuprofen	
	2-hydroxy	CYPs 2C9, 2C8, 3A4, 2C19
	3-hydroxy	CYPs 2C9, 2C8, 3A4, 2C19
	acyl-glucuronide	UGTs 2B7, 1A9, 1A3, 2B4
	Diclofenac	
	4-hydroxydiclofenac	CYPs 2C9
	5-hydroxydiclofenac	CYPs 2C8, 3A4, 2C19
	acyl-glucuronide	UGTs 2B7, 2B4, 1A3, 1A9
	Naproxen	
	desmethylnaproxen	CYPs 2C9, 1A2
	glucuronide	UGT2B7
	Ketorolac	
	glucuronide	UGT2B7
	Ketoprofen	
	acyl-glucuronide	UGT2B7
	Flurbiprofen	
	4-hydroxyflurbiprofen	CYP2C9
	acyl-glucuronide	UGTs 2B7, 1A3, 1A9, 2B4
	4-hydroxy conjugate	
	3′,4′-dihydroxy conjugate	
	3′-hydroxy,4′-methoxy conjugate	
	Meloxicam	
	5-hydroxymethyl meloxicam	CYPs 2C9, 3A4
	5′-carboxy meloxicam	
Cyclooxygenase-2 selective inhibitors	*Celecoxib*	
	methyl hydroxy	CYPs 2C9, 3A4
	carboxylic acid	alcohol dehydrogenase

Table 15.1 (*Continued*)

Drug class	***Drug*** **Metabolite**	**Major enzymes**
	Etoricoxib	
	methyl hydroxy	CYPs 3A4, 2C9, 2D6, 1A2, 2C19
	N-oxide	
	Parecoxib	
	valdecoxib	
	valdecoxib methyl hydroxy	CYPs 2C9, 3A4
	valdecoxib *N*-glucuronide	
TCAs	*Amitriptyline*	
	nortriptyline	CYPs 2C19, 2C8, 2C9, 1A2, 2D6, 2B6, 3A4
	10-hydroxyamitriptyline	CYPs 2D6, 3A4
	amitriptyline *N*-oxide	
	amitriptyline *N*-glucuronide	UGT1A3, 1A4
	Nortriptyline	
	10-hydroxynortriptyline	CYPs 2D6, 3A4
	Imipramine	
	2-hydroxyimipramine	CYPs 2D6, 2C19, 1A2
	desmethylimipramine	CYPs 2C19, 1A2
	Desipramine	
	2-hydroxydesipramine	CYP2D6
SNRIs	*Duloxetine*	
	4-hydroxy	CYPs 2D6, 1A2
	5-hydroxy	CYPs 2D6, 1A2
	6-hydroxy	CYPs 2D6, 1A2
	Venlafaxine	
	O-desmethylvenlafaxine	CYPs 2D6, 2C19, 2C9
	N-desmethylvenlafaxine	CYPs 3A4, 2C19, 2C9
SSRIs	*Fluoxetine*	
	norfluoxetine	CYPs 2C9, 3A4, 2D6, 2C19, 1A2
	TFMP	CYPs 2C19, 3A4
	Paroxetine	
	M1 (BRL 36610)	CYP2D6
	M2 (BRL 36583)	CYP3A4
	Citalopram	
	desmethylcitalopram	CYPs 3A4, 2C19, 2D6
	didesmethylcitalopram	CYP2D6
NMDA antagonist	*Ketamine*	
	norketamine	CYPs 3A4, 2B6, 2C9
Antiepileptics	*Carbamazepine*	
	10,11-epoxide	CYPs 3A4, 2C8
	N-glucuronide	UGT2B7

(*Continued*)

Table 15.1 (*Continued*)

Drug class	*Drug* / Metabolite	Major enzymes
	Valproate	
	glucuronide	UGTs 2B7, 1A6, 1A9
Opioid	*Buprenorphine*	
	norbuprenorphine	CYPs 3A4, 2C8
	buprenorphine 3-glucuronide	UGTs 1A1, 2B7
	norbuprenorphine 3-glucuronide	UGTs 1A1, 1A3, 2B7
	Codeine	
	morphine	CYP2D6
	M3G	UGT2B7
	M6G	UGT2B7
	codeine-6-glucuronide	UGT2B7, UGT2B4
	norcodeine	CYP3A4
	normorphine	CYP3A4
	Dextropropoxyphene	
	nordextropropoxyphene	CYP3A4
	Dihydrocodeine	
	dihydromorphine	CYP2D6
	dihydromorphine-6-glucuronide	UGT2B7
	dihydromorphine-3-glucuronide	UGT2B7
	dihydrocodeine-6-glucuronide	
	nordihydrocodeine	CYP3A4
	Heroin (diamorphine)	
	6-monoacetylmorphine	
	morphine	esterases
	Hydrocodone	
	norhydrocodone	CYP3A4
	hydromorphone	CYP2D6
	Hydromorphone	
	dihydromorphine	ketone reductase
	norhydromorphone	
	hydromorphone-3-glucuronide	UGTs 1A3, 2B7
	Ketobemidone	
	norketobemidone	CYPs 2C9, 3A4
	ketobemidone glucuronide	
	LAAM	
	norLAAM	CYPs 3A4, 2B6, 2C19, 2C8, 2C9
	dinorLAAM	CYPs 3A4, 2B6, 2C19, 2C8, 2C9
	Levorphanol	
	3-glucuronide	UGT2B7

Table 15.1 (*Continued*)

Drug class	*Drug* Metabolite	Major enzymes
	Loperamide	
	desmethylloperamide	CYPs 3A4, 2C8, 2B6, 2D6
	Rac-methadone	
	EDDP	CYPs 3A4, 2B6, 2C19
	Morphine	
	M6G	UGTs 2B7, 1A8, 1A1
	M3G	UGTs 2B7, 1A8, 1A3, 1A10, 1A6, 1A1, 1A9
	normorphine	CYPs 3A4, 2C8
	Oxycodone	
	oxymorphone	CYP2D6
	noroxycodone	CYP3A4
	noroxymorphone	CYP3A4
	oxymorphone-3-glucuronide	UGT2B7
	oxymorphone 7,8-ketoreduction	unnamed reductase
	Pethidine	
	norpethidine	CYPs 2B6, 3A4, 2C19
	Tilidine	
	nortilidine	CYP3A
	Tramadol	
	O-desmethyltramadol, M1	CYP2D6
	N-desmethyltramadol, M2	CYPs 3A4, 2B6

15.2.2 Paracetamol/Acetaminophen

This weak analgesic is primarily conjugated to a glucuronide (around 50% dose) by UGTs 1A6 and 1A9, and a sulfate (around 30% dose) by SULT1A1 and possibly 2A1 to form paracetamol glucuronide and paracetamol sulfate, respectively [2]. A small percentage of the dose (below 10%) undergoes oxidative metabolism to form two metabolites–a hepatotoxic *N*-acetyl-*p*-benzoquinone imine (NAPQI) and 3-hydroxyparacetamol (nontoxic). The CYPs that contribute to this are traditionally acknowledged as CYP2E1 and CYP2A6. The intrinsic clearance values to these two metabolites are for NAPQI: CYP2E1, 5.2, CYP2A6, 1.7, and for 3-hydroxy paracetamol: CYP2E1, 0.6, CYP2A6, 6.5, all ml/min/nmol P450 [3]. However, more recent evidence has suggested a large role for CYP3A4 in NAPQI formation such that the CL_{int} was much greater than for CYP2E1 [4]. These investigators also found that the relative formation by CYP1A2 was 68% that of CYP3A4, 2D6 34%, 2C19 20%, and 2C9 below 5%.

15.2.3 Nonsteroidal Anti-Inflammatory Drugs

The major nonsteroidal anti-inflammatory drugs (NSAIDs) are ibuprofen, diclofenac, aspirin, ketoprofen, flurbiprofen, ketorolac, naproxen, and meloxicam. Less used in this context are indomethacin, mefenamic acid, piroxicam, tenoxicam, sulindac, and tiaprofenic acid. The NSAIDs are metabolized to various extents by glucuronidation and oxidation. UGT2B7 is the major UGT and CYP2C9 the major CYP.

15.2.3.1 Diclofenac

About 70% of the dose of diclofenac is recovered in urine and the remainder in bile. In urine, the major oxidative metabolite is 4-hydroxydiclofenac and this is mainly catalyzed by CYP2C9; CYPs 2C8, 3A4, and 2C19 catalyze the formation of the minor metabolite 5-hydroxydiclofenac. Both of these hydroxyl metabolites appear in urine as glucuronide conjugates (42% 4-hydroxyglucuronide; 12% 5-hydroxyglucuronide). In bile, of the almost 30% of the dose, 40% is the 4-hydroxy metabolite, 11% is the 5-hydroxy metabolite, and 5% is diclofenac, mostly as glucuronide conjugates [5]. There remains some controversy regarding the metabolic schema as it has been argued that most of the 4-hydroxydiclofenac glucuronide is derived from initial glucuronidation followed by oxidative metabolism of the glucuronide [6, 7].

A small proportion undergoes acyl glucuronidation (15% of the dose in urine and about 5% in bile), and using human liver microsomes and expressed enzymes and inhibitors, it appears that the rank order of intrinsic clearance values for this pathway is UGT2B7 and UGT2B4 > UGT1A3 = UGT1A9. The role of UGT2B17 appears unclear [8, 9].

15.2.3.2 Flurbiprofen

About 75% of an oral dose can be recovered in urine as unchanged flurbiprofen (less than 1%), an acyl glucuronide (24%), 4-hydroxy as a conjugate (45%), a 3′,4′ dihydroxy metabolite in conjugate form (around 2%), and 3′-hydroxy,4′-methoxy flurbiprofen as conjugate (around 7%) [10]. Details of any sequential metabolism are not apparent. It appears that CYP2C9 is the major CYP involved in the 4′-hydroxylation [11]. The glucuronidation of flurbiprofen is mainly via UGT2B7, with minor contributions from UGTs 1A3, 1A9, and 2B4 [8].

15.2.3.3 Ibuprofen

Metabolism of this NSAID is complicated by enantioselectivity, chiral inversion, and oxidative and conjugative reactions. For the much less active *R*-(−)-ibuprofen, about 60% of metabolism involves unidirectional chiral inversion to the active *S*-(+)-ibuprofen [12], acyl glucuronidation (about 9%), oxidative 2-hydroxylation (10%), and 3-hydroxylation (20%) [13].

For the active *S*-(+)-enantiomer, acyl glucuronidation represents 14% of metabolism, 2-hydroxylation 28%, and 3-hydroxylation 45% [14].

For the oxidative metabolism of both enantiomers, Chang *et al.* [15] summarized the relative CYP contribution using human liver microsomes as follows:

S-(+)-ibuprofen:

2-hydroxy: CYP2C9 (35%), CYP2C8 (8%), CYP3A4 (43%), CYP2C19 (7%).
3-hydroxy: CYP2C9 (92%), CYP2C8 (<1%), CYP3A4 (4%), CYP2C19 (2%).

R-(−)-ibuprofen:

2-hydroxy: CYP2C9 (32%), CYP2C8 (11%), CYP3A4 (42%), CYP2C19 (6%).
3-hydroxy: CYP2C9 (89%), CYP2C8 (2%), CYP3A4 (3%), CYP2C19 (3%).

These data indicate a major role for CYP2C9 in the oxidative metabolism of *S*- and *R*-ibuprofen, with relatively less or minor contributions from CYP2C8, 3A4, and 2C19. When Chang *et al.* [15] considered the other pathways of elimination (acyl glucuronidation, chiral inversion), they concluded that CYP2C9 and CYP2C8 contribute 50–70 and 13%, respectively, of the total clearance of *S*-(+)-ibuprofen, and 20–30 and 6%, for *R*-(−)-ibuprofen.

The chiral inversion of *R*-(−)- to *S*-(+)-ibuprofen involves aryl-CoA synthetase, epimerase, and acyl-CoA thioesterase [16]. For the acyl glucuronidation of racemic ibuprofen, using human liver microsomes and expressed enzymes and inhibitors, the rank order of intrinsic clearance values was UGT2B7 > UGT1A9 > UGT1A3 = UGT2B4 [8, 9].

15.2.3.4 Ketoprofen

About 80% of an oral dose is recovered in urine as the acyl glucuronide [17] and this is mainly by UGT2B7 [8].

15.2.3.5 Ketorolac

More than 90% of the dose of ketorolac is recovered in urine as a glucuronide and this is mainly via UGT2B7.

15.2.3.6 Meloxicam

The major pathway for metabolism is the initial formation of 5-hydroxymethyl meloxicam and then further oxidation to 5′-carboxy meloxicam. This pathway represents about 70% of the dose [18]. In human liver microsomes, the formation of the 5-hydroxymethyl metabolite is via CYPs 2C9 (high-affinity K_m of 15 μM) and 3A4 (low-affinity K_m 400 μM). The intrinsic clearance (V_{max}/K_m) value for the high-affinity component was about 10-fold higher than the low-affinity component [19]. Rodrigues [14] has estimated that the contribution of CYP2C9 is 60–80% and 3A4 20–40%, depending on the level of expression of the latter.

15.2.3.7 Naproxen

About 60% of an oral dose is recovered in urine as a glucuronide metabolite [20] and UGT2B7 appears to be the major UGT involved [21]. The remaining oral dose is mainly oxidatively metabolized to desmethylnaproxen, and CYPs 2C9 and 1A2 appear to be almost equally involved [22].

The metabolism of indomethacin, mefenamic acid, piroxicam, tenoxicam, sulindac, and tiaprofenic acid will not be covered due to limited data and very low use in pain therapy.

15.2.4 Cyclooxygenase-2 Selective Inhibitors

The three such inhibitors that will be reviewed are celecoxib, etoricoxib, and parecoxib. Lumaricoxib and rofecoxib were withdrawn from the market, and so will not be reviewed. For the three former coxibs, CYP3A4 and CYP2C9 in different proportions are the major enzymes involved [14].

15.2.4.1 Celecoxib

The major pathway (more than 85%) involves methyl hydroxylation and this is then converted to a carboxylic acid metabolite via alcohol dehydrogenase [23]. The initial methyl hydroxylation is via CYP2C9 (about 80%) and CYP3A4 (about 20%) [24, 25].

15.2.4.2 Etoricoxib

This coxib undergoes methyl hydroxylation (around 75% dose) and *N*-oxidation (below 10% dose) [26]. The former is via CYP3A4 around 60%, CYP2C9 by about 10%, with CYP2D6, CYP1A2, and CYP2C19 each contributing about 10% [27].

15.2.4.3 Parecoxib

This is a prodrug that undergoes rapid amide hydrolysis to the active moiety valdecoxib. This then undergoes minor *N*-glucuronidation (around 20% dose), but the majority undergoes methyl hydroxylation by CYP2C9 and CYP3A4 [14]. However, to date, it is difficult to find the proportion that each contributes [28, 29].

15.3 Chronic Pain

15.3.1 Tricyclic Antidepressants

15.3.1.1 Amitriptyline

This tricyclic is the most commonly used of this group of drugs that includes the tricyclic antidepressants (TCAs), serotonin–norepinephrine reuptake inhibitors (SNRIs), and selective serotonin reuptake inhibitors (SSRIs) (see below), as many studies have consistently shown a significant benefit in neuropathic pain [30]. Amitriptyline undergoes four different metabolic processes: *N*-demethylation to nortriptyline (around 65% dose, see below), aliphatic hydroxylation to 10-OH-amitriptyline (around 18%), *N*-oxidation to amitriptyline *N*-oxide (less than 1%), and glucuronidation to amitriptyline *N*-glucuronide (around 2%) [31]. At low substrate concentrations, *N*-demethylation occurs at a 2.5-fold higher rate than aliphatic hydroxylation, and *N*-oxidation and glucuronidation occur at even lower rates.

N-Demethylation At low substrate concentrations likely to be achieved in hepatocytes, this reaction is predominantly mediated by CYP2C19 with lesser contributions from CYP2C8/9 and 1A2, and even lesser contributions from CYP2D6, 2B6, and 3A4 [32]. However, at higher concentrations, there are similar contributions from CYP3A4 and 2C19/8/9.

Aliphatic Hydroxylation This represents a complicated metabolite profile as the process shows regio-, stereo-, and enantio-selectivity. Thus, the metabolites formed are (*E*)-10-hydroxy-(+)-amitriptyline, (*E*)-10-hydroxy-(–)-amitriptyline, (*Z*)-10-hydroxy-(+)-amitriptyline, and (*Z*)-10-hydroxy-(–)-amitriptyline. The (*E*)-geometric isomers are formed preferentially over the (*Z*)-geometric isomers by a factor of 3–14 and in urine the predominant isomer is the (–)-enantiomer (i.e., (*E*)-10-hydroxy-(–)-amitriptyline). In human liver microsomes, the predominant CYPs identified as catalyzing this aliphatic hydroxylation are CYP2D6 (35–88%) and CYP3A4 (12–65%). Thus, CYP2D6 is the major enzyme for aliphatic hydroxylation, but at only one of the four positions at the ethylene bridge. The CYPs involved in the other three positions are not known, but it is generally accepted that the (+)-(*Z*)-, and (–)-(*Z*)-10-OH and (+)-(*E*)-10-OH metabolites are formed in only small extents.

N-Glucuronidation The major enzymes involved are UGTs 1A3 and 1A4.

15.3.1.2 **Nortriptyline**
Similar to amitriptyline, the major metabolic pathway involves aliphatic hydroxylation to form (*E*)-10-hydroxy-(+)-nortriptyline, (*E*)-10-hydroxy-(–)-nortriptyline, (*Z*)-10-hydroxy-(+)-nortriptyline, and (*Z*)-10-hydroxy-(–)-nortriptyline.

Approximately 87% of aliphatic hydroxylation is to the (*E*)-geometric isomer and only 13% to the (*Z*)-geometric isomer. In addition, the (–)-isomer predominates over the (+)-isomer in a ratio of about 80 : 20. Human liver microsomal studies have shown two binding sites – a high-affinity site catalyzed by CYP2D6 and a low-affinity site catalyzed by CYP3A4. Venkatakrishnan *et al.* [33] have shown that CYP3A4 accounts for about 20% of the metabolism and CYP2D6 about 80%. For the formation of the minor (*E*)-10-OH-(+)-isomer, CYP2D6 plays a minor role. For the (*Z*)-geometric isomer, the enantiomeric selectivity is towards the (+)-enantiomer over the (–)-enantiomer by a factor of 4.

15.3.1.3 **Imipramine**
Similar to amitriptyline, imipramine undergoes oxidative metabolism to 2-hydroxyimipramine and to desmethylimipramine, which is then further hydroxylated to a 2-hydroxy metabolite. Using human liver microsomes, high- and

low-affinity components were identified for both *N*-demethylation and 2-hydroxylation reactions. Following the use of yeast-expressed enzymes and chemical inhibitors, it appears that for 2-hydroxylation, the high-affinity component (about 85%) is via CYP2D6 and the low-affinity component is mainly via CYP2C19 with minor contributions from CYP1A2 [34]. For the *N*-demethylation, the high-affinity component (70%) is via CYP2C19 and the low-affinity component (about 30%) via CYP1A2.

15.3.1.4 Desipramine

The major pathway is via 2-hydroxylation to 2-hydroxydesipramine, with minor pathways of 10-hydroxylation, desmethylation (to didesipramine), and dealkylation to an iminobenzyl metabolite [35]. Both the 2- and 10-hydroxyl metabolites undergo conjugation to glucuronide metabolites. In urine, about 45% of the dose is recovered as the total 2-hydroxy metabolite and less than 1% as the 10-hydroxy metabolite, and 30–40% was as unidentified metabolites. In CYP2D6 poor metabolizer (PM) subjects, the clearance of desipramine is decreased 7-fold and the clearance via 2-hydroxylation is decreased 40-fold, indicating that 2-hydroxylation is the major pathway and that it is almost entirely via CYP2D6.

15.3.2 SNRIs

15.3.2.1 Duloxetine

This drug undergoes primarily oxidative metabolism with the major plasma and urinary metabolite being the glucuronide conjugate of 4-hydroxyduloxetine. Other metabolites include conjugates of 5- and 6-hydroxy-, 4,6-dihydroxy-, and 6-hydroxy,5-methoxy-duloxetine (sulfate conjugate). We were unable to find any *in vitro* human metabolism studies, but Lantz *et al.* [36] cite in their paper unpublished results that ". . . CYP2D6 and CYP1A2 are the primary enzymes responsible for the oxidative metabolism at the 4-, 5-, or 6-position of the naphthyl ring."

15.3.2.2 Venlafaxine

This exists in *R*- and *S*-enantiomeric forms. Overall, urinary recovery data indicate almost exclusive oxidative metabolism to the active *O*-desmethylvenlafaxine (56% dose), *N*-desmethylvenlafaxine (around 1% of dose), and *N,O*-didesmethylvenlafaxine (16% of dose) [37]. These values are consistent to some extent with human liver microsomal studies indicating that *O*-demethylation accounts for about 90% and *N*-demethylation about 10% of oxidative metabolism [38]. These authors also showed that in CYP-transfected cells, the rank order of *O*-demethylation was CYP2D6 (90%), CYP2C19 (10%), and CYP2C9 (1%). Whereas for *N*-demethylation, it was CYP3A4 (36%), CYP2C19 (33%), and CYP2C9 (31%). Stereoselectivity has not been investigated comprehensively, but the ratio of plasma concentrations of *S*- to *R*-venlafaxine indicates that it is not significant [39]. Thus, CYP2D6 is the principal enzyme catalyzing the *O*-demethylation and

CYP3A4 the *N*-demethylation reactions [40]. However, although CYP2D6 is the major enzyme catalyzing the *O*-demethylation for both *R*- and *S*-venlafaxine, in CYP2D6 PM subjects the clearance of *R*-venlafaxine exceeds that of *S*-venlafaxine and there is a 12-fold reduction in *S*-venlafaxine clearance and only 2-fold for *R*-venlafaxine, indicating an additional CYP catalyzing *R*-venlafaxine.

15.3.3 SSRIs

15.3.3.1 Citalopram

This antidepressant consists of both *S*- and *R*-enantiomeric forms with the *S*-enantiomer being almost 110-fold more potent than the *R*-enantiomer, and is now marketed as escitalopram. The main metabolic pathways are *N*-demethylation to desmethylcitalopram, further demethylation at the secondary amine site to *N*-didesmethylcitalopram, *N*-oxidation to citalopram *N*-oxide, and there is a citalopram propionic acid derivative. In urine, 40% is recovered as unchanged citalopram (26%) and its *N*-glucuronide (14%), 19% as the desmethyl metabolite, 15% as the didesmethyl metabolite (unchanged 9%, *N*-glucuronide 6%), about 7% as the *N*-oxide, and 12% as an *O*-glucuronide of the propionic acid metabolite [41]. In the initial *N*-demethylation to desmethylcitalopram, CYP3A4, CYP2C19, and CYP2D6 contribute almost equally. However, the further *N*-demethylation to didesmethylcitalopram is catalyzed almost exclusively by CYP2D6 [42].

15.3.3.2 Fluoxetine

This SSRI also exits as two enantiomers – *S*-fluoxentine and *R*-fluoxetine. After oral dosing, 80% of the dose appears in urine and 15% in feces. In urine, 11% appears as fluoxetine plus 7% as an *N*-glucuronide, 7% as norfluoxetine, and an additional 8% as an *N*-glucuronide. About 20% appears as hippuric acid – a glycine conjugate of benzoic acid [43]. Thus, *N*-demethylation appears to be a major metabolic pathway. In human liver microsomes, Margolis *et al.* [44] found the following rank order of intrinsic clearance values (V_{max}/K_m) for *R*-fluoxetine, CYP2D6 > CY P2C9 > CYP3A4 > CYP2C19; and for *S*-fluoxetine, CYP2D6 > CYP3A4 > CYP2C 9 > CYP2C19. When upscaled to a human liver, for *R*-fluoxetine *N*-demethylation the relative contributions were, CYP2C9 (63%), CYP3A4 (18%), CYP2D6 (15%), CYP2C19 (3%), and CYP1A2 (2%); and for *S*-fluoxetine, CYP3A4 (39%), CYP2C9 (28%), CYP2D6 (25%), CYP2C19 (4%) and CYP1A2 (4%). It was also found that the intrinsic clearance of *R*-fluoxetine was greater than for *S*-fluoxetine by about 5-fold, but variability was extensive.

However, an *O*-dealkylation reaction to *p*-trifluoxetineoromethylphenol (TFMP) appears to be a major metabolic pathway. Liu *et al.* [45] examined the metabolism of racemic fluoxetine to this metabolite using human liver microsomes. A high-affinity component (about 86%) was via CYP2C19 and the lower-affinity component (14%) via CYP3A4. Enantioselectivity was not investigated and the contribution of this pathway to overall clearance remains to be firmly established.

15.3.3.3 Paroxetine

Paroxetine undergoes oxidative metabolism at the methylene-dioxyphenyl position to an unstable catechol, which then undergoes separate methylation at the two aliphatic alcohol positions *meta* and *para* to form Metabolite 1 (M1: BRL 36610) and M2 (BRL36583), respectively. M1 also then undergoes glucuronide and sulfate conjugation and M2 glucuronide conjugation. The catechol also undergoes metabolism to a M3 metabolite (BRL 35961). In healthy subjects, about 2% of an oral dose is excreted in urine as unchanged paroxetine, and 25–30% as conjugates of M1 and M2. In CYP2D6 PM subjects, the area under the concentration–time curve (AUC) of paroxetine increases about 7-fold and the metabolic clearance to the catechol is reduced about 15-fold following a single dose, but only about 2-fold after chronic dosing to the steady-state. However, even in CYP2D6 extensive metabolizers (EMs) after chronic dosing there is a substantial 10-fold decrease in clearance. In urine, in CYP2D6 PM subjects, the sulfate conjugate of M1 (the major metabolite) is reduced about 8-fold and by the same fold for M1 glucuronide, but no change in M2 glucuronide. After chronic dosing, M1 sulfate and M1 glucuronide are reduced 1.7-fold in CYP2D6 PM subjects, but M2 glucuronide is increased 1.8-fold. It has been deduced that M1 is formed by CYP2D6, and M2 by CYP3A4 and possibly other metabolites [46–48].

15.3.4 Ketamine

This old drug is mainly used for adjuvant analgesia in chronic pain management and it is the only *N*-methyl-D-aspartate (NMDA) antagonist that has successfully been used for such therapy. It exists as two enantiomers. *S*-(+)-ketamine is more potent and has less psychogenic effects than *R*-(−)-ketamine, and while the former is marketed in some countries, the racemate is used in most countries. As is the case with many old drugs, its metabolism is incompletely understood. Nevertheless, the major pathway is oxidative metabolism to norketamine [49]. Other pathways of oxidative metabolism are dehydronorketamine [50], and 4-hydroxy-, 5-hydroxy-, (*Z*)-6-hydroxy-, and norketamine, although the latter three are in very small amounts [51]. Kharash *et al.* [52], using human liver microsomes, showed that the intrinsic clearance (V_{max}/K_m) for the *S*-enantiomer was about 24% higher than for the *R*-enantiomer, that there was evidence of each enantiomer inhibiting each others metabolism, and that two enzymes contributed to norketamine formation – a high-affinity/low-capacity component (80–90%) and low-affinity/high-capacity component (10–20%). The CYPs involved in norketamine formation were identified as CYP3A4 (low-affinity/high-capacity), CYP2B6 (high-affinity/low-capacity), and CYP2C9 (low-affinity/high-capacity) [53]. Subsequently, Hijazi and Boulieu [54], based on a therapeutic plasma concentration of 5 μM, estimated that CYP3A4 would contribute about 62%, CYP2B6 31%, and CYP2C9 7%. However, ketamine as an adjuvant analgesic would achieve lower concentrations than 5 μM and therefore the relative contribution of CYP2B6 would increase.

15.3.5
Antiepileptics

15.3.5.1 Carbamazepine

This antiepileptic drug undergoes extensive metabolism as less than 5% is recovered unchanged in urine and over 70% of the dose as ^{14}C is recovered in urine [55]. Although many metabolites have been identified, three metabolic pathways predominate in humans. The main pathway involves formation of the 10,11-epoxide, which is then hydrolyzed to *trans*-10,11-dihydroxy-10,11-dihydrocarbamazepine (*trans*-CBZ-diol). In epileptic patients, the 10,11-epoxide accounts for less than 2% of the dose in urine, whereas the *trans*-CBZ-diol accounts for about 27% of the dose [56]. Kerr *et al.* [57] identified through a series of studies that CYP3A4 was the major CYP involved in the formation of the 10,11-epoxide, with a minor contribution from CYP2C8. Other metabolites of carbamazepine were 9-hydroxycarbamazepine (8% of dose), 2- and 3-hydroxycarbamazepine (less than 3% of dose, unconjugated), and an *N*-glucuronide formed by the enzyme UGT2B7 [58] and it is not readily apparent how much is recovered in urine.

15.3.5.2 Valproate

Valproate undergoes two major and one minor metabolic reaction. As it is a short-chain fatty acid, the pathways are glucuronidation (major), mitochondrial B-oxidation (major), and a CYP-mediated reaction via terminal desaturation (minor). The glucuronidation is catalyzed by UGTs 2B7, 1A6, and 1A9. Ethell *et al.* [59], using expressed isoforms and human liver microsomes, determined the kinetics of formation via the three UGTs with V_{max}/K_m values of 0.31, 0.22, and 0.19, respectively. The minor CYP pathway is considered likely to be due to CYP2C9 [60].

15.3.6
Miscellaneous

15.3.6.1 Gabapentin

This drug is almost completely renally excreted (more than 90% of the oral dose) [61] and will not be considered any further.

15.3.6.2 Pregabalin

This drug is almost completely renally excreted (more than 90% of the oral dose) [62] and will not be considered any further.

15.3.6.3 Tapentadol

This recently introduced drug has both μ-opioid agonist and blockade of norepinephrine uptake transport properties. It is almost exclusively metabolized, and the main metabolite (around 70% of dose) is the *O*-glucuronide formed by UGT1A9 and UGT2B7. About 27% of the dose is metabolized by the phase I system to a hydroxyl metabolite (less than 5% dose via CYP2D6) and a demethylated metabolite (less than 15% dose via CYP2C9 and CYP2C19) [63].

15.3.7
Opioids

Opioids are used to treat both acute and chronic malignant and nonmalignant pain. The metabolism of most opioids has been well described and, of clinical importance, can produce active metabolites with individual variability controlled by genetic polymorphisms (for a complete review, refer to [64]). In general, opioids undergo the following phase I metabolic reactions: *O*-dealkylation (alkyl ethers at the 3-phenolic hydroxyl group such as codeine, hydrocodone, and oxycodone, and opioids containing nitrogen atoms) mediated predominantly by CYP2D6; *N*-demethylation to their norderivatives (codeine, dihydrocodeine, morphine, oxycodone, tilidine, and tramadol) mediated predominantly by CYP3A4; and 6-ketoreduction (at C7-8 saturated molecules of the 4,5-epoxymorphinans, e.g., hydromorphone, hydrocodone, and oxycodone). With regard to phase II metabolism, glucuronidation reactions mainly mediated by UGT2B7 take place on free, aromatic, and alicyclic hydroxyl groups on opioids (e.g., morphine, oxymorphone, and nalbuphine).

15.3.7.1 Buprenorphine

As a 4,5-epoxymorphinan, buprenorphine is almost entirely hepatically cleared and its major metabolite is norbuprenorphine via *N*-dealkylation with a V_{max} in human liver microsomes of 2.3 nmol/(min · mg of protein) and an intrinsic clearance of 0.027 ml/(min · mg protein) [65]. This reaction is mediated predominantly by CYP3A4, with a minor role of CYP2C8 [65, 66]. Buprenorphine and norbuprenorphine both are glucuronidated to buprenorphine-3-glucuronide (UGT1A1 10% and 2B7 41%) and norbuprenorphine-3-glucuronide (UGT1A3 63%, 1A1 34%, and 2B7 minor role) [67]. Following sublingual administration (16 mg in combination with 4 mg naloxone) the percentage dose recovery in urine as buprenorphine, norbuprenorphine, buprenorphine-3-glucuronide, and norbuprenorphine-3-glucuronide was 0.014, 1.89, 1.01, and 7.76, respectively [68].

15.3.7.2 Butorphanol

Butorphanol is predominately hepatically cleared by hydroxylation to hydroxybutorphanol (60–80% at the cyclobutylmethyl group), by *N*-dealkylation to norbutorphanol (5–10% at the cyclobutylmethyl group), and by glucuronidation (less than 10% at the 3-hydroxy group), with further 3-glucuronidation of norbutorphanol and hydroxybutorphanol [69]. There are no published reports characterizing the CYP or UGT isoforms mediating butorphanol's metabolism.

15.3.7.3 Codeine

Codeine undergoes extensive phase I and phase II metabolism to codeine-6-glucuronide, norcodeine, norcodeine-6-glucuronide, morphine, normorphine,

morphine-6-glucuronide (M6G), and morphine-3-glucuronide (M3G) [70–72]. Codeine-6-glucuronide accounts for around 80% of the dose formed by UGTs 2B7 and 2B4 [73], such that the plasma AUC of codeine-6-glucuronide is 10–15 times higher than that of codeine [70–72]. Codeine also undergoes phase I metabolism with *O*-demethylation to morphine catalyzed almost exclusively by CYP2D6 [74] and *N*-demethylation to norcodeine mediated by CYP3A4 [75]. Up to 10% dose is converted to morphine in EMs, which is subsequently further metabolized (see morphine below; Section 15.3.7.16) [72]. However, in CYP2D6 PMs, the percentage of a 50-mg oral codeine dose recovered as morphine, M3G, and M6G, and normorphine is significantly reduced by 180-, 22-, 6-, and 52-fold, respectively [71]. Between 2.3 (CYP2D6 EMs) to 5.7% (CYP2D6 PMs) is recovered as norcodeine, with further glucuronidation to norcodeine-glucuronide representing 4.4 (CYP2D6 EMs) to 5.5% (CYP2D6 PMs) of the dose [71].

15.3.7.4 Dextromoramide

In contrast to the majority of opioids, little is known about its metabolism, with 2-hydroxydextromoramide possibly its major metabolite.

15.3.7.5 Dextropropoxyphene

Is a phenylheptylamine opioid. It undergoes *N*-demethylation by CYP3A4 to form its major metabolite nordextropropoxyphene [76], with plasma concentrations 3.3- and 5.8-fold higher following single and multiple dosing, respectively [77].

15.3.7.6 Dihydrocodeine

Not surprisingly, this 7,8-dihydro analog of codeine undergoes similar phase I and II metabolism as codeine [78]: *O*-demethylation to dihydromorphine (0.5%); *N*-demethylation to nordihydrocodeine (16%); and glucuronidation to 3-*O*- and 6-*O*-glucuronides of dihydromorphine (8.4%), dihydrocodeine-6-*O*-glucuronide (28%), and nordihydrocodeine glucuronide (6%) [79]. Formation of dihydromorphine is mediated by CYP2D6, with the urinary recovery and plasma concentrations reduced by 6.8-, and 7.3-fold, respectively, in CYP2D6 PMs [79]. In contrast to codeine, its glucuronidation is mediated by UGT2B7, but not 2B4 [80].

15.3.7.7 Alfentanil, Fentanyl, Sufentanil, and Remifentanil

These opioids have similar chemical structures centered on the phenylpiperidine chemical structure. Alfentanil, fentanyl, and sufentanil all undergo *N*-dealkylation by CYP3A4, and alfentanil also by 3A5 to produce norderivatives [81]. In contrast remifentanil – a derivative of fentanyl containing an ester linkage to propanoic acid – is metabolized by nonspecific esterases widespread throughout blood and tissues [82] to remifentanil acid, which is then predominantly (around 88%) renally cleared [83].

15.3.7.8 Heroin (Diamorphine (3,6-Diacetylmorphine))

A prodrug of morphine, it is very rapidly hydrolyzed to the active 6-acetylmorphine, which is subsequently hydrolyzed to morphine by esterases present in blood and liver [84, 85]. Indeed, following oral administration only the metabolites of heroin were detected in plasma [86]. The esterases mediating the initial hydrolysis were previously thought to be nonspecific, but recently a role for intestinal carboxylesterases has been shown [87]. 6-Acetylmorphine undergoes a small amount of glucuronidation to a 3-glucuronide [88], while morphine is further metabolized (see morphine below; Section 15.3.7.16) [86, 89].

15.3.7.9 Hydrocodone

Once again, the metabolic pathways for hydrocodone are similar to codeine: *N*-demethylation to norhydrocodone (mediated by CYP3A4 [90]), *O*-demethylation to hydromorphone (5–6% together with conjugated form, mediated by CYP2D6 [90, 91]), and 6-keto-reduction to dihydrocodeine and isodihydrocodeine (around 4%) [92]. A small percentage of the dose (0.2%) has also been recovered as dihydromorphine and isodihydromorphine [92].

15.3.7.10 Hydromorphone

The major metabolite is hydromorphone-3-glucuronide [93, 94] mediated by UGTs 1A3 and 2B7, while ketone reductase mediates the formation of dihydromorphine and isodihydromorphine [95]. Other minor detected metabolites include conjugated dihydromorphine and isodihydromorphine, hydromorphone-3-sulfate, norhydromorphone, and norisodihydromorphine [93, 94].

15.3.7.11 Ketobemidone

This opioid is *N*-demethylated to norketobemidone mediated by CYP2C9 and 3A4 [96], with no role for CYP2D6 or 2C19 [97]. The glucuronide conjugates of ketobemidone, norketobemidone, and hydroxymethoxyketobemidone have also been identified in human urine postintravenous administration of ketobemidone [98]; however, the role of specific UGT isoforms has not been reported.

15.3.7.12 L-α-Acetylmethadol

The major phase I metabolic pathway of L-α-acetylmethadol (LAAM) is N-demethylation to norLAAM and then subsequently to dinorLAAM [99], reaching 2-fold higher plasma concentrations [100]. *In vivo* relative contributions of the CYP isoforms mediating these demethylation reactions are as follows for LAAM and norLAAM, respectively: CYP3A4 (70 and 84%) > 2B6 (26 and 15%) > 2C19 (1.6 and 0.4%) > 2C8 (1.3 and 0.4%) = 2C9 (1.2 and 0.4%) [101].

15.3.7.13 Levorphanol

This morphinan undergoes phase II glucuronidation to a 3-glucuronide metabolite, mediated by UGT2B7 [102], reaching between 5- and 10-fold higher plasma concentrations than levorphanol [103].

15.3.7.14 Loperamide

A phenylpiperidine class opioid similar to fentanyl and pethidine, it undergoes *N*-demethylation to desmethylloperamide, that can undergo further *N*-demethylation to didesmethylloperamide. The *N*-demethylation in human liver microsomes is characterized by a high- and low-affinity component, and the rank order of formation by individual expressed CYP isoforms is 2C8 > 2B6 > 2D6 > 3A4 > 2C9, which is predicted to translate *in vivo* to major roles for CYPs 3A4 and 2C8, followed by 2B6 and 2D6 [104]. These metabolites then undergo glucuronidation (around 50%), although specific UGT isoforms have not been reported, and 40% is excreted as unchanged drug and metabolites in feces and urine.

15.3.7.15 Methadone

A diphenylheptylamine class of opioid, methadone is administered as a racemate and its major human metabolite is 2-ethylidene-1,5-dimethyl-3,3-diphenylpyrrolidine (EDDP); however, it has many more metabolites, of which some are active (e.g., α-(3*S*, 6*S*)-methadol, α-(3*S*, 6*S*)-*N*-desmethylmethadol) [105], both derived from the *S*-enantiomer. There has been some controversy regarding the stereoselective metabolism of methadone and the role of specific CYPs in the formation of EDDP. However, a recent report by Chang *et al.* [106] has shown, using a combined *in vitro* approach involving human liver microsomes, expressed CYP isoforms, and specific inhibitors, the following rank order of involvement scaled to relative *in vivo* expression levels: CYP3A4 (63–74%) > 2B6 (12–32%) > 2C19 (1.4–14%). Further, the *S*-EDDP was selectively formed by CYPs 2B6, 2D6, and 2C18, while *R*-EDDP was selectively formed by CYPs 2C19, 3A7, and 2C8, while CYP3A4 showed no stereoselectively.

15.3.7.16 Morphine

The major metabolic pathway is phase II glucuronidation to M3G (50%) and M6G (10%) [107, 108]. The formation of both M6G and M3G is mediated by multiple UGT isoforms, with the following rank order of *in vitro* K_m: M6G, UGT2B7 (both high and low-affinity binding sites) > 1A8 > 1A1; and M3G, UGT2B7 (both high- and low-affinity binding sites) > 1A8 > 1A3 > 1A10 > 1A6 = 1A1 > 1A9 [109, 110]. Other minor metabolites include morphine-3,6-diglucuronide, morphine-3-ethereal sulfate, normorphine, normorphine-6-glucuronide, and normorphine-3-glucuronide [88]. Several CYPs mediate the formation of normorphine, with a rank order of *in vitro* intrinsic clearance values by expressed enzymes of CYP3A4 > 2C8 = 2C19 > 2D6 > 2C9 [111]. This is predicted to equate to CYP3A4 and 2C8 forming around 90%, and 2C19, 2C9, and 2D6 forming the remaining 10% *in vivo*.

15.3.7.17 Nalbuphine

There is limited data on metabolism; however, nornalbuphine (likely formed by CYP3A) and 6-ketonalbuphine (likely formed by ketone reductases), with additional glucuronide conjugation, have been detected in urine [112].

15.3.7.18 Nicomorphine (3,6-Dinicotionylmorphine)

Another ester prodrug of morphine, intravenous nicomorphine is extremely rapidly hydrolyzed into the metabolites 6-nicotinoylmorphine and morphine, and morphine is then further metabolized (see morphine above; Section 15.3.7.16)

[113]. The specific CYP and UGT isoforms mediating the metabolism have not been reported.

15.3.7.19 Oxycodone

Similar to codeine and hydrocodone, oxycodone undergoes *N*-demethylation to noroxycodone, *O*-demethylation to oxymorphone predominantly via CYP3A4 and CYP2D6, respectively [114, 115], and 7-8 ketoreduction to 6-α- and 6-β-oxycodol [116]. Oxymorphone is further metabolized (see oxymorphone below; Section 15.3.7.20).

15.3.7.20 Oxymorphone

Similar to hydromorphone, the main metabolite is oxymorphone-3-glucuronide (40%), mediated predominantly by UGT2B7 [95]). However, 7-8 ketoreduction to 6-α- and 6-β-hydroxyoxymorphone and *N*-demethylation to noroxymorphone also occurs (less than 10%) [117, 118]. Noroxymorphone is further glucuronidated to form noroxymorphone-3-glucuronide [119].

15.3.7.21 Pentazocine

Pentazocine undergoes phase I hydroxylation to produce *cis*-hydroxy and *trans*-carboxylic acid metabolites, and also undergoes glucuronidation [120]. Although there is no report identifying specific CYP isoforms mediating the metabolism, smoking has been shown to induce metabolism, which suggests a role for CYPs 2E1 and/or 1A2.

15.3.7.22 Pethidine

A phenylpiperidine opioid, it undergoes *N*-demethylation to norpethidine and hydrolysis to pethidinic acid and its conjugate. The *in vitro* rank order of specific CYPs in the intrinsic clearance to norpethidine is CYP2B6 >> 3A4 > 2C19 [121].

15.3.7.23 Piritramide

Another phenylpiperidine opioid, little is known regarding the metabolism of this opioid; however, one study on the pharmacokinetics in five patients reported renal clearance to account for 1.7% of total clearance [122], leading the authors to comment "From the fact that renal elimination is negligible, it may be inferred that the elimination of the drug depends almost exclusively on hepatic metabolism." More recently, a Doctoral dissertation in German by Kahlich reported the formation of monohydroxy, dihydroxy, and dehydro metabolites [123]; however, no characterization of the individual enzymes involved was discussed.

15.3.7.24 Tilidine

Tilidine undergoes *N*-demethylation to nortilidine (less than 3%) that is further demethylated to bisnortilidine (less than 3%) and renally excreted by the kidney [124, 125]. The role of individual CYP isoforms in this metabolic pathway has not been characterized, but is thought to be largely mediated by the CYP3A family.

15.3.7.25 **Tramadol**

The metabolism of tramadol is highly complex with up to 33 metabolites reportedly formed in humans, dogs, and rats [126]. However, of these, only four were detected in human urine following a 100-mg dose at more than 5% and included: *O*-desmethyltramadol, M1, greater than 10%; *N*-desmethyltramadol, M2, more than 10%, *N,N*-didesmethyltramadol, M3, 5–10%; and *O,N*-didesmethyltramadol, M5, 5–10% [126]. *O*-Desmethyltramadol (M1) formation from tramadol and *O,N*-didesmethyltramadol (M5) formation from *N*-desmethyltramadol (M2) are mediated by CYP2D6 [127]; comparison studies between CYP2D6 PM and EM subjects revealed up to 4-fold lower plasma C_{max} and AUC of M1 in PM subjects [128–132]. *N*-desmethyltramadol (M2) formation from tramadol, *O,N*-didesmethyltramadol (M5) formation from *O*-desmethyltramadol (M1), and *N,N*-didesmethyltramadol (M3) formation from *N*-desmethyltramadol (M2) are likely mediated by CYP2B6 and CYP3A4 [127, 133]. In addition, *O*-desmethyltramadol (M1) and O,*N*-didesmethyltramadol (M5) also undergo glucuronidation [134]; however, the UGT isoforms mediating this reaction have not been reported.

References

1 Kaivosaari, S., Toivonen, P., Aitio, O., Sipilä, J., Koskinen, M., Salonen, J.S., and Finel, M. (2008) Regio- and stereospecific *N*-glucuronidation of medetomidine: the differences between UDP glucuronosyltransferase (UGT) 1A4 and UGT2B10 account for the complex kinetics of human liver microsomes. *Drug Metab. Dispos.*, **36**, 1529–1537.

2 Leeder, J.S. (2009) Developmental pharmacogenetics: a general paradigm for application to neonatal pharmacology and toxicology. *Clin. Pharmacol. Ther.*, **86**, 678–682.

3 Chen, W., Koenigs, L.L., Thompson, S.J., Peter, R.M., Rettie, A.E., Trager, W.F., and Nelson, S.D. (1998) Oxidation of acetaminophen to its toxic quinone imine and nontoxic catechol metabolites by baculovirus-expressed and purified human cytochromes P450 2E1 and 2A6. *Chem. Res. Toxicol.*, **11**, 295–301.

4 Laine, J.E., Auriola, S., Pasanen, M., and Juvonen, R.O. (2009) Acetaminophen bioactivation by human cytochrome P450 enzymes and animal microsomes. *Xenobiotica*, **39**, 11–21.

5 Stierlin, H. and Faigle, J.W. (1979) Biotransformation of diclofenac sodium (Voltaren) in animals and in man. II. Quantitative determination of the unchanged drug and principal phenolic metabolites, in urine and bile. *Xenobiotica*, **9**, 611–621.

6 Kumar, S., Samuel, K., Subramanian, R., Braun, M.P., Stearns, R.A., Chiu, S.H., Evans, D.C., and Baillie, T.A. (2002) Extrapolation of diclofenac clearance from *in vitro* microsomal metabolism data: role of acyl glucuronidation and sequential oxidative metabolism of the acyl glucuronide. *J. Pharmacol. Exp. Ther.*, **303**, 969–978.

7 Tang, W. (2003) The metabolism of diclofenac–enzymology and toxicology perspectives. *Curr. Drug Metab.*, **4**, 319–329.

8 Kuehl, G.E., Lampe, J.W., Potter, J.D., and Bigler, J. (2005) Glucuronidation of nonsteroidal anti-inflammatory drugs: identifying the enzymes responsible in human liver microsomes. *Drug Metab. Dispos.*, **33**, 1027–1035.

9 Sakaguchi, K., Green, M., Stock, N., Reger, T.S., Zunic, J., and King, C. (2004) Glucuronidation of carboxylic acid containing compounds by UDP-glucuronosyltransferase isoforms. *Arch. Biochem. Biophys.*, **424**, 219–225.

10 Szpunar, G.J., Albert, K.S., Bole, G.G., Dreyfus, J.N., Lockwood, G.F., and Wagner, J.G. (1987) Pharmacokinetics of flurbiprofen in man. I. Area/dose relationships. *Biopharm. Drug Dispos.*, **8**, 273–283.

11 Tracy, T.S., Marra, C., Wrighton, S.A., Gonzalez, F.J., and Korzekwa, K.R. (1996) Studies of flurbiprofen 4′-hydroxylation. Additional evidence suggesting the sole involvement of cytochrome P450 2C9. *Biochem. Pharmacol.*, **52**, 1305–1309.

12 Davies, N.M. (1998) Clinical pharmacokinetics of ibuprofen. The first 30 years. *Clin. Pharmacokinet.*, **34**, 101–154.

13 Rudy, A.C., Knight, P.M., Brater, D.C., and Hall, S.D. (1991) Stereoselective metabolism of ibuprofen in humans: administration of *R*-, *S*- and racemic ibuprofen. *J. Pharmacol. Exp. Ther.*, **259**, 1133–1139.

14 Rodrigues, A.D. (2005) Impact of CYP2C9 genotype on pharmacokinetics: are all cyclooxygenase inhibitors the same? *Drug Metab. Dispos.*, **33**, 1567–1575.

15 Chang, S.Y., Li, W., Traeger, S.C., Wang, B., Cui, D., Zhang, H., Wen, B., and Rodrigues, A.D. (2008) Confirmation that cytochrome P450 2C8 (CYP2C8) plays a minor role in (*S*)-(+)- and (*R*)-(–)-ibuprofen hydroxylation *in vitro*. *Drug Metab. Dispos.*, **36**, 2513–2522.

16 Hao, H., Wang, G., and Sun, J. (2005) Enantioselective pharmacokinetics of ibuprofen and involved mechanisms. *Drug Metab. Rev.*, **37**, 215–234.

17 Jamali, F. and Brocks, D.R. (1990) Clinical pharmacokinetics of ketoprofen and its enantiomers. *Clin. Pharmacokinet.*, **19**, 197–217.

18 Schmid, J., Busch, U., Heinzel, G., Bozler, G., Kaschke, S., and Kummer, M. (1995) Pharmacokinetics and metabolic pattern after intravenous infusion and oral administration to healthy subjects. *Drug Metab. Dispos.*, **23**, 1206–1213.

19 Chesné, C., Guyomard, C., Guillouzo, A., Schmid, J., Ludwig, E., and Sauter, T. (1998) Metabolism of Meloxicam in human liver involves cytochromes P4502C9 and 3A4. *Xenobiotica*, **28**, 1–13.

20 Vree, T.B., Van Den Biggelaar-Martea, M., Verwey-Van Wissen, C.P., Vree, M.L., and Guelen, P.J. (1993) The pharmacokinetics of naproxen, its metabolite *O*-desmethylnaproxen, and their acyl glucuronides in humans. Effect of cimetidine. *Br. J. Clin. Pharmacol.*, **35**, 467–472.

21 Bowalgaha, K., Elliot, D.J., Mackenzie, P.I., Knights, K.M., Swedmark, S., and Miners, J.O. (2005) *S*-Naproxen and desmethylnaproxen glucuronidation by human liver microsomes and recombinant human UDP-glucuronosyltransferases (UGT): role of UGT2B7 in the elimination of naproxen. *Br. J. Clin. Pharmacol.*, **60**, 423–433.

22 Miners, J.O., Coulter, S., Tukey, R.H., Veronese, M.E., and Birkett, D.J. (1996) Cytochromes P450, 1A2, and 2C9 are responsible for the human hepatic *O*-demethylation of *R*- and *S*-naproxen. *Biochem. Pharmacol.*, **51**, 1003–1008.

23 Paulson, S.K., Hribar, J.D., Liu, N.W., Hajdu, E., Bible R.H., Jr, Piergies, A., and Karim, A. (2000) Metabolism and excretion of [^{14}C]celecoxib in healthy male volunteers. *Drug Metab. Dispos.*, **28**, 308–314.

24 Tang, C., Shou, M., Mei, Q., Rushmore, T.H., and Rodrigues, A.D. (2000) Major role of human liver microsomal cytochrome P450 2C9 (CYP2C9) in the oxidative metabolism of celecoxib, a novel cyclooxygenase-II inhibitor. *J. Pharmacol. Exp. Ther.*, **293**, 453–459.

25 Sandberg, M., Yasar, U., Strömberg, P., Höög, J.O., and Eliasson, E. (2002) Oxidation of celecoxib by polymorphic cytochrome P450 2C9 and alcohol dehydrogenase. *Br. J. Clin. Pharmacol.*, **54**, 423–429.

26 Rodrigues, A.D., Halpin, R.A., Geer, L.A., Cui, D., Woolf, E.J., Matthews, C.Z., Gottesdiener, K.M., Larson, P.J., Lasseter, K.C., and Agrawal, N.G. (2003) Absorption, metabolism, and excretion of etoricoxib, a potent and selective cyclooxygenase-2 inhibitor, in healthy male volunteers. *Drug Metab. Dispos.*, **31**, 224–232.

27 Kassahun, K., McIntosh, I.S., Shou, M., Walsh, D.J., Rodeheffer, C., Slaughter, D.E., Geer, L.A., Halpin, R.A., Agrawal, N., and Rodrigues, A.D. (2001) Role of human liver cytochrome P4503A in the metabolism of etoricoxib, a novel cyclooxygenase-2 selective inhibitor. *Drug Metab. Dispos.*, **29**, 813–820.

28 Chavez, M.L. and DeKorte, C.J. (2003) Valdecoxib: a review. *Clin. Ther.*, **25**, 817–851.

29 Alsalameh, S., Burian, M., Mahr, G., Woodcock, B.G., and Geisslinger, G. (2003) Review article: the pharmacological properties and clinical use of valdecoxib, a new cyclo-oxygenase-2-selective inhibitor. *Aliment. Pharmacol. Ther.*, **17**, 489–501.

30 Finnerup, N.B., Sindrup, S.H., and Jensen, T.S. (2010) The evidence for pharmacological treatment of neuropathic pain. *Pain*, **150**, 573–581.

31 Breyer-Pfaff, U. (2004) The metabolic fate of amitriptyline, nortriptyline and amitriptylinoxide in man. *Drug Metab. Rev.*, **36**, 723–746.

32 Venkatakrishnan, K., von Moltke, L.L., and Greenblatt, D.J. (2001) Application of the relative activity factor approach in scaling from heterologously expressed cytochromes p450 to human liver microsomes: studies on amitriptyline as a model substrate. *J. Pharmacol. Exp. Ther.*, **297**, 326–337.

33 Venkatakrishnan, K., von Moltke, L.L., and Greenblatt, D.J. (1999) Nortriptyline *E*-10-hydroxylation *in vitro* is mediated by human CYP2D6 (high affinity) and CYP3A4 (low affinity): implications for interactions with enzyme-inducing drugs. *J. Clin. Pharmacol.*, **39**, 567–577.

34 Koyama, E., Chiba, K., Tani, M., and Ishizaki, T. (1997) Reappraisal of human CYP isoforms involved in imipramine *N*-demethylation and 2-hydroxylation: a study using microsomes obtained from putative extensive and poor metabolizers of *S*-mephenytoin and eleven recombinant human CYPs. *J. Pharmacol. Exp. Ther.*, **281**, 1199–1210.

35 Brøsen, K., Hansen, J.G., Nielsen, K.K., Sindrup, S.H., and Gram, L.F. (1993) Inhibition by paroxetine of desipramine metabolism in extensive but not in poor metabolizers of sparteine. *Eur. J. Clin. Pharmacol.*, **44**, 349–355.

36 Lantz, R.J., Gillespie, T.A., Rash, T.J., Kuo, F., Skinner, M., Kuan, H.Y., and Knadler, M.P. (2003) Metabolism, excretion, and pharmacokinetics of duloxetine in healthy human subjects. *Drug Metab. Dispos.*, **31**, 1142–1150.

37 Howell, S.R., Husbands, G.E., Scatina, J.A., and Sisenwine, S.F. (1993) Metabolic disposition of ^{14}C-venlafaxine in mouse, rat, dog, rhesus monkey and man. *Xenobiotica*, **23**, 349–359.

38 Fogelman, S.M., Schmider, J., Venkatakrishnan, K., von Moltke, L.L., Harmatz, J.S., Shader, R.I., and Greenblatt, D.J. (1999) *O*- and *N*-demethylation of venlafaxine *in vitro* by human liver microsomes and by microsomes from cDNA-transfected cells: effect of metabolic inhibitors and SSRI antidepressants. *Neuropsychopharmacology*, **20**, 480–490.

39 Gex-Fabry, M., Rudaz, S., Balant-Gorgia, A.E., Brachet, A., Veuthey, J.L., Balant, L.P., and Bertschy, G. (2002) Steady-state concentration of venlafaxine enantiomers: model-based analysis of between-patient variability. *Eur. J. Clin. Pharmacol.*, **58**, 323–331.

40 Otton, S.V., Ball, S.E., Cheung, S.W., Inaba, T., Rudolph, R.L., and Sellers, E.M. (1996) Venlafaxine oxidation *in vitro* is catalysed by CYP2D6. *Br. J. Clin. Pharmacol.*, **41**, 149–156.

41 Dalgaard, L. and Larsen, C. (1999) Metabolism and excretion of citalopram in man: identification of *O*-acyl- and *N*-glucuronides. *Xenobiotica*, **29**, 1033–1041.

42 Olesen, O.V. and Linnet, K. (1999) Studies on the stereoselective metabolism of citalopram by human liver microsomes and cDNA-expressed cytochrome P450 enzymes. *Pharmacology*, **59**, 298–309.

43 Altamura, A.C., Moro, A.R., and Percudani, M. (1994) Clinical pharmacokinetics of fluoxetine. *Clin. Pharmacokinet.*, **26**, 201–214.

44 Margolis, J.M., O'Donnell, J.P., Mankowski, D.C., Ekins, S., and Obach, R.S. (2000) (*R*)-, (*S*)-, and racemic fluoxetine *N*-demethylation by human

cytochrome P450 enzymes. *Drug Metab. Dispos.*, **28**, 1187–1191.
45 Liu, Z.Q., Zhu, B., Tan, Y.F., Tan, Z.R., Wang, L.S., Huang, S.L., Shu, Y., and Zhou, H.H. (2002) *O*-Dealkylation of fluoxetine in relation to CYP2C19 gene dose and involvement of CYP3A4 in human liver microsomes. *J. Pharmacol. Exp. Ther.*, **300**, 105–111.
46 Sindrup, S.H., Brøsen, K., Gram, L.F., Hallas, J., Skjelbo, E., Allen, A., Allen, G.D., Cooper, S.M., Mellows, G., Tasker, T.C., *et al.* (1992) The relationship between paroxetine and the sparteine oxidation polymorphism. *Clin. Pharmacol. Ther.*, **51**, 278–287.
47 Kaye, C.M., Haddock, R.E., Langley, P.F., Mellows, G., Tasker, T.C., Zussman, B.D., and Greb, W.H. (1989) A review of the metabolism and pharmacokinetics of paroxetine in man. *Acta Psychiatr. Scand. Suppl.*, **350**, 60–75.
48 Sawamura, K., Suzuki, Y., and Someya, T. (2004) Effects of dosage and CYP2D6-mutated allele on plasma concentration of paroxetine. *Eur. J. Clin. Pharmacol.*, **60**, 553–557.
49 White, P.F. (1989) Clinical uses of intravenous anesthetic and analgesic infusions. *Anesth. Analg.*, **68**, 161–171.
50 Köppel, C., Arndt, I., and Ibe, K. (1990) Effects of enzyme induction, renal and cardiac function on ketamine plasma kinetics in patients with ketamine long-term analgosedation. *Eur. J. Drug Metab. Pharmacokinet.*, **15**, 259–263.
51 Woolf, T.F. and Adams, J.D. (1987) Biotransformation of ketamine, (*Z*)-6-hydroxyketamine, and (*E*)-6-hydroxyketamine by rat, rabbit, and human liver microsomal preparations. *Xenobiotica*, **17**, 839–847.
52 Kharasch, E.D. and Labroo, R. (1992) Metabolism of ketamine stereoisomers by human liver microsomes. *Anesthesiology*, **77**, 1201–1207.
53 Yanagihara, Y., Kariya, S., Ohtani, M., Uchino, K., Aoyama, T., Yamamura, Y., and Iga, T. (2001) Involvement of CYP2B6 in *N*-demethylation of ketamine in human liver microsomes. *Drug Metab. Dispos.*, **29**, 887–890.
54 Hijazi, Y. and Boulieu, R. (2002) Contribution of CYP3A4, CYP2B6, and CYP2C9 isoforms to *N*-demethylation of ketamine in human liver microsomes. *Drug Metab. Dispos.*, **30**, 853–858.
55 Faigle, J.W. and Feldman, K.F. (1982) Carbamazepine biotransformation, in *Antiepileptic Drugs*, 2nd edn (eds D.M. Woodbury, J.K. Penry, and C.E. Pippenger), Raven Press, New York, pp. 483–495.
56 Eichelbaum, M., Tomson, T., Tybring, G., and Bertilsson, L. (1985) Carbamazepine metabolism in man. Induction and pharmacogenetic aspects. *Clin. Pharmacokinet.*, **10**, 80–90.
57 Kerr, B.M., Thummel, K.E., Wurden, C.J., Klein, S.M., Kroetz, D.L., Gonzalez, F.J., and Levy, R.H. (1994) Human liver carbamazepine metabolism. Role of CYP3A4 and CYP2C8 in 10,11-epoxide formation. *Biochem. Pharmacol.*, **47**, 1969–1979.
58 Staines, A.G., Coughtrie, M.W., and Burchell, B. (2004) *N*-glucuronidation of carbamazepine in human tissues is mediated by UGT2B7. *J. Pharmacol. Exp. Ther.*, **311**, 1131–1137.
59 Ethell, B.T., Anderson, G.D., and Burchell, B. (2003) The effect of valproic acid on drug and steroid glucuronidation by expressed human UDP-glucuronosyltransferases. *Biochem. Pharmacol.*, **65**, 1441–1449.
60 Anderson, G.D. (1998) A mechanistic approach to antiepileptic drug interactions. *Ann. Pharmacother.*, **32**, 554–563.
61 McLean, M.J. (1994) Clinical pharmacokinetics of gabapentin. *Neurology*, **44** (**6** Suppl. 5), S17–S22.
62 Bockbrader, H.N., Radulovic, L.L., Posvar, E.L., Strand, J.C., Alvey, C.W., Busch, J.A., Randinitis, E.J., Corrigan, B.W., Haig, G.M., Boyd, R.A., and Wesche, D.L. (2010) Clinical pharmacokinetics of pregabalin in healthy volunteers. *J. Clin. Pharmacol.*, **50**, 941–950.
63 Kneip, C., Terlinden, R., Beier, H., and Chen, G. (2008) Investigations into the drug–drug interaction potential of tapentadol in human liver microsomes and fresh human hepatocytes. *Drug Metab. Lett.*, **2**, 67–75.

64 Coller, J.K., Christrup, L.L., and Somogyi, A.A. (2009) Role of active metabolites in the use of opioids. *Eur. J. Clin. Pharmacol.*, **65**, 121–139.

65 Iribarne, C., Picart, D., Dréano, Y., Bail, J.-P., and Berthou, F. (1997) Involvement of cytochrome P450 3A4 in *N*-dealkylation of buprenorphine in human liver microsomes. *Life Sci.*, **60**, 1953–1964.

66 Moody, D.E., Slawson, M.H., Strain, E.C., Laycock, J.D., Spanbauer, A.C., and Foltz, R.L. (2002) A liquid chromatographic-electrospray ionization-tandem mass spectrometric method for determination of buprenorphine, its metabolite, norbuprenorphine, and a coformulant, naloxone, that is suitable for *in vivo* and *in vitro* metabolism studies. *Anal. Biochem.*, **306**, 31–39.

67 Rouguieg, K., Picard, N., Sauvage, F.L., Gaulier, J.M., and Marquet, P. (2010) Contribution of the different UDP-glucuronosyltransferase (UGT) isoforms to buprenorphine and norbuprenorphine metabolism and relationship with the main UGT polymorphisms in a bank of human liver microsomes. *Drug Metab. Dispos.*, **38**, 40–45.

68 Huang, W., Moody, D.E., and McCance-Katz, E.F. (2006) The *in vivo* glucuronidation of buprenorphine and norbuprenorphine determined by liquid chromatography-electrospray ionization-tandem mass spectrometry. *Ther. Drug Monit.*, **28**, 245–251.

69 Vachharajani, N.N., Shyu, W.C., Greene, D.S., and Barbhaiya, R.H. (1997) The pharmacokinetics of butorphanol and its metabolites at steady state following nasal administration in humans. *Biopharm. Drug Dispos.*, **18**, 191–202.

70 Chen, Z.R., Somogyi, A.A., Reynolds, G., and Bochner, F. (1991) Disposition and metabolism of codeine after single and chronic doses in one poor and seven extensive metabolisers. *Br. J. Clin. Pharmacol.*, **31**, 381–390.

71 Yue, Q.Y., Hasselstrom, J., Svensson, J.O., and Sawe, J. (1991) Pharmacokinetics of codeine and its metabolites in Caucasian healthy volunteers: comparisons between extensive and poor hydroxylators of debrisoquine. *Br. J. Clin. Pharmacol.*, **31**, 635–642.

72 Vree, T.B. and Verwey-Van Wissen, C.P. (1992) Pharmacokinetics and metabolism of codeine in humans. *Biopharm. Drug Dispos.*, **13**, 445–460.

73 Raungrut, P., Uchaipichat, V., Elliot, D.J., Janchawee, B., Somogyi, A.A., and Miners, J.O. (2010) *In vitro–in vivo* extrapolation predicts drug–drug interactions arising from inhibition of codeine glucuronidation by dextropropoxyphene, fluconazole, ketoconazole, and methadone in humans. *J. Pharmacol. Exp. Ther.*, **334**, 609–618.

74 Chen, Z.R., Somogyi, A.A., and Bochner, F. (1988) Polymorphic *O*-demethylation of codeine. *Lancet*, **2**, 914–915.

75 Caraco, Y., Tateishi, T., Guengerich, F.P., and Wood, A.J. (1996) Microsomal codeine *N*-demethylation: cosegregation with cytochrome P4503A4 activity. *Drug Metab. Dispos.*, **24**, 761–764.

76 Somogyi, A.A., Menelaou, A., and Fullston, S.V. (2004) CYP3A4 mediates dextropropoxyphene *N*-demethylation to nordextropropoxyphene: human *in vitro* and *in vivo* studies and lack of CYP2D6 involvement. *Xenobiotica*, **34**, 875–887.

77 Flanagan, R.J., Johnston, A., White, A.S., and Crome, P. (1989) Pharmacokinetics of dextropropoxyphene and nordextropropoxyphene in young and elderly volunteers after single and multiple dextropropoxyphene dosage. *Br. J. Clin. Pharmacol.*, **28**, 463–469.

78 Schmidt, H., Vormfelde, S.V., Klinder, K., Gundert-Remy, U., Gleiter, C.H., Skopp, G., Aderjan, R., and Fuhr, U. (2002) Affinities of dihydrocodeine and its metabolites to opioid receptors. *Pharmacol. Toxicol.*, **91**, 57–63.

79 Fromm, M.F., Hofmann, U., Griese, E.-U., and Mikus, G. (1995) Dihydrocodeine: a new opioid substrate for the polymorphic CYP2D6 in humans. *Clin. Pharmacol. Ther.*, **58**, 374–382.

80 Kirkwood, L.C., Nation, R.L., and Somogyi, A.A. (1997) Characterization of

the human cytochrome P450 enzymes involved in the metabolism of dihydrocodeine. *Br. J. Clin. Pharmacol.*, **44**, 549–555.

81 Guitton, J., Buronfosse, T., Desage, M., Lepape, A., Brazier, J.L., and Beaune, P. (1997) Possible involvement of multiple cytochrome P450S in fentanyl and sufentanil metabolism as opposed to alfentanil. *Biochem. Pharmacol.*, **53**, 1613–1619.

82 Beers, R. and Camporesi, E. (2004) Remifentanil update: clinical science and utility. *CNS Drugs*, **18**, 1085–1104.

83 Battershill, A.J. and Keating, G.M. (2006) Remifentanil: a review of its analgesic and sedative use in the intensive care unit. *Drugs*, **66**, 365–385.

84 Williams, F.M. (1985) Clinical significance of esterases in man. *Clin. Pharmacokinet.*, **10**, 392–403.

85 Lockridge, O., Mottershaw-Jackson, N., Eckerson, H.W., and La Du, B.N. (1980) Hydrolysis of diacetylmorphine (heroin) by human serum cholinesterase. *J. Pharmacol. Exp. Ther.*, **215**, 1–8.

86 Girardin, F., Rentsch, K.M., Schwab, M.A., Maggiorini, M., Pauli-Magnus, C., Kullak-Ublick, G.A., Meier, P.J., and Fattinger, K. (2003) Pharmacokinetics of high doses of intramuscular and oral heroin in narcotic addicts. *Clin. Pharmacol. Ther.*, **74**, 341–352.

87 Hatfield, M.J., Tsurkan, L., Hyatt, J.L., Yu, X., Edwards, C.C., Hicks, L.D., Wadkins, R.M., and Potter, P.M. (2010) Biochemical and molecular analysis of carboxylesterase-mediated hydrolysis of cocaine and heroin. *Br. J. Pharmacol.*, **160**, 1916–1928.

88 Yeh, S.Y., McQuinn, R.L., and Gorodetzky, C.W. (1977) Identification of diacetylmorphine metabolites in humans. *J. Pharm. Sci.*, **66**, 201–204.

89 Rentsch, K.M., Kullak-Ublick, G.A., Reichel, C., Meier, P.J., and Fattinger, K. (2001) Arterial and venous pharmacokinetics of intravenous heroin in subjects who are addicted to narcotics. *Clin. Pharmacol. Ther.*, **70**, 237–246.

90 Hutchinson, M.R., Menelaou, A., Foster, D.J.R., Coller, J.K., and Somogyi, A.A. (2003) CYP2D6 and CYP3A4 involvement in the primary oxidative metabolism of hydrocodone by human liver microsomes. *Br. J. Clin. Pharmacol.*, **57**, 287–297.

91 Otton, S.V., Schadel, M., Cheung, S.W., Kaplan, H.L., Busto, U.E., and Sellers, E.M. (1993) CYP2D6 phenotype determines the metabolic conversion of hydrocodone to hydromorphone. *Clin. Pharmacol. Ther.*, **54**, 463–472.

92 Cone, E.J., Darwin, W.D., Gorodetzky, C.W., and Tan, T. (1978) Comparative metabolism of hydrocodone in man, rat, guinea pig, rabbit, and dog. *Drug Metab. Dispos.*, **6**, 488–493.

93 Zheng, M., McErlane, K.M., and Ong, M.C. (2002) Hydromorphone metabolites: isolation and identification from pooled urine samples of a cancer patient. *Xenobiotica*, **32**, 427–439.

94 Baldacci, A. and Thormann, W. (2006) Capillary electrophoresis contributions to the hydromorphone metabolism in man. *Electrophoresis*, **27**, 2444–2457.

95 Armstrong, S.C. and Cozza, K.L. (2003) Pharmacokinetic drug interactions of morphine, codeine, and their derivatives: theory and clinical reality, part I. *Psychosomatics*, **44**, 167–171.

96 Yasar, U., Annas, A., Svensson, J.O., Lazorova, L., Artursson, P., and Al-Shurbaji, A. (2005) Ketobemidone is a substrate for cytochrome P4502C9 and 3A4, but not for P-glycoprotein. *Xenobiotica*, **35**, 785–796.

97 Al-Shurbaji, A. and Sawe, J. (2002) The pharmacokinetics of ketobemidone are not affected by CYP2D6 or CYP2C19 phenotype. *Eur. J. Clin. Pharmacol.*, **57**, 877–881.

98 Sundstrom, I., Hedeland, M., Bondesson, U., and Andren, P.E. (2002) Identification of glucuronide conjugates of ketobemidone and its phase I metabolites in human urine utilizing accurate mass and tandem time-of-flight mass spectrometry. *J. Mass. Spectrom.*, **37**, 414–420.

99 Kharasch, E.D., Whittington, D., Hoffer, C., Krudys, K., Craig, K., Vicini, P., Sheffels, P., and Lalovic, B. (2005) Paradoxical role of cytochrome P450 3A in the bioactivation and clinical effects of levo-alpha-acetylmethadol: importance

of clinical investigations to validate *in vitro* drug metabolism studies. *Clin. Pharmacokinet.*, **44**, 731–751.

100 Newcombe, D.A., Bochner, F., White, J.M., and Somogyi, A.A. (2004) Evaluation of levo-alpha-acetylmethdol (LAAM) as an alternative treatment for methadone maintenance patients who regularly experience withdrawal: a pharmacokinetic and pharmacodynamic analysis. *Drug Alcohol Depend.*, **76**, 63–72.

101 Neff, J.A. and Moody, D.E. (2001) Differential *N*-demethylation of l-alpha-acetylmethadol (LAAM) and norLAAM by cytochrome P450s 2B6, 2C18, and 3A4. *Biochem. Biophys. Res. Commun.*, **284**, 751–756.

102 Coffman, B.L., Rios, G.R., King, C.D., and Tephly, T.R. (1997) Human UGT2B7 catalyzes morphine glucuronidation. *Drug Metab. Dispos.*, **25**, 1–4.

103 Dixon, R., Crews, T., Inturrisi, C., and Foley, K. (1983) Levorphanol: pharmacokinetics and steady-state plasma concentrations in patients with pain. *Res. Commun. Chem. Pathol. Pharmacol.*, **41**, 3–17.

104 Kim, K.A., Chung, J., Jung, D.H., and Park, J.Y. (2004) Identification of cytochrome P450 isoforms involved in the metabolism of loperamide in human liver microsomes. *Eur. J. Clin. Pharmacol.*, **60**, 575–581.

105 Foster, D.J.R. (2001) An examination of the metabolism and pharmacokinetics of methadone with respect to stereoselectivity. Thesis, University of Adelaide.

106 Chang, Y., Fang, W.B., Lin, S.N., and Moody, D.E. (2011) Stereo-selective metabolism of methadone by human liver microsomes and cDNA-expressed cytochrome P450s: a reconciliation. *Basic Clin. Pharmacol. Toxicol.*, **108**, 55–62.

107 Lötsch, J., Stockmann, A., Kobal, G., Brune, K., Waibel, R., Schmidt, N., and Geisslinger, G. (1996) Pharmacokinetics of morphine and its glucuronides after intravenous infusion of morphine and morphine-6-glucuronide in healthy volunteers. *Clin. Pharmacol. Ther.*, **60**, 316–325.

108 Osborne, R., Joel, S., Trew, D., and Slevin, M. (1990) Morphine and metabolite behavior after different routes of morphine administration: demonstration of the importance of the active metabolite morphine-6-glucuronide. *Clin. Pharmacol. Ther.*, **47**, 12–19.

109 Stone, A.N., Mackenzie, P.I., Galetin, A., Houston, J.B., and Miners, J.O. (2003) Isoform selectivity and kinetics of morphine 3- and 6-glucuronidation by human UDP-glucuronosyltransferases: evidence for atypical glucuronidation kinetics by UGT2B7. *Drug Metab. Dispos.*, **31**, 1086–1089.

110 Ohno, S., Kawana, K., and Nakajin, S. (2008) Contribution of UDP-glucuronosyltransferase 1A1 and 1A8 to morphine-6-glucuronidation and its kinetic properties. *Drug Metab. Dispos.*, **36**, 688–694.

111 Projean, D., Morin, P.E., Tu, T.M., and Ducharme, J. (2003) Identification of CYP3A4 and CYP2C8 as the major cytochrome P450 s responsible for morphine *N*-demethylation in human liver microsomes. *Xenobiotica*, **33**, 841–854.

112 Yoo, Y.C., Chung, H.S., Kim, I.S., Jin, W.T., and Kim, M.K. (1995) Determination of nalbuphine in drug abusers' urine. *J. Anal. Toxicol.*, **19**, 120–123.

113 Koopman-Kimenai, P.M., Vree, T.B., Booij, L.H., Dirksen, R., and Nijhuis, G.M. (1993) Pharmacokinetics of intravenously administered nicomorphine and its metabolites in man. *Eur. J. Anaesthesiol.*, **10**, 125–132.

114 Rasmussen, I. (2000) Identification of cytochrome P450 isoforms involved in the metabolism of oxycodone. Thesis, University of Adelaide.

115 Lalovic, B., Phillips, B., Risler, L., Howald, W., and Shen, D.D. (2004) Quantitative contribution of CYP2D6 and CYP3A to oxycodone metabolism in human liver and intestinal microsomes. *Drug Metab. Dispos.*, **32**, 447–454.

116 Lalovic, B., Kharasch, E., Hoffer, C., Risler, L., Lui-Chen, L.-Y., and Shen,

D.D. (2006) Pharmacokinetics and pharmacodynamics of oral oxycodone in healthy human subjects: role of circulating active metabolites. *Clin. Pharmacol. Ther.*, **79**, 461–479.

117 Ishida, T., Oguri, K., and Yoshimura, H. (1979) Isolation and identification of urinary metabolites of oxycodone in rabbits. *Drug Metab. Dispos.*, **7**, 162–165.

118 Prommer, E. (2006) Oxymorphone: a review. *Support. Care Cancer*, **14**, 109–115.

119 Poyhia, R., Olkkola, K.T., Seppala, T., and Kalso, E. (1991) The pharmacokinetics of oxycodone after intravenous injection in adults. *Br. J. Clin. Pharmacol.*, **32**, 516–518.

120 Goldstein, G. (1985) Pentazocine. *Drug Alcohol Depend.*, **14**, 313–324.

121 Ramirez, J., Innocenti, F., Schuetz, E.G., Flockhart, D.A., Relling, M.V., Santucci, R., and Ratain, M.J. (2004) CYP2B6, CYP3A4, and CYP2C19 are responsible for the *in vitro N*-demethylation of meperidine in human liver microsomes. *Drug Metab. Dispos.*, **32**, 930–936.

122 Kietzmann, D., Briede, I., Bouillon, T., Gundert-Remy, U., and Kettler, D. (1996) Pharmacokinetics of piritramide after an intravenous bolus in surgical patients. *Acta Anaesthesiol. Scand.*, **40**, 898–903.

123 Kahlich, R. (2005) Studies on stereospecific pharmacokinetics and metabolism of phenprocoumon in adults and on pharmacokinetics and metabolism of piritramide in children by LC–MS-coupling. Thesis, Eberhard Karls Universitat Tubingen.

124 Vollmer, K.O., Thomann, P., and Hengy, H. (1989) Pharmacokinetics of tilidine and metabolites in man. *Arzneimittelforschung*, **39**, 1283–1288.

125 Thierry, C., Boeynaems, J.-M., and Paolo, M. (2005) Actions of tilidine and nortilidine on cloned opioid receptors. *Eur. J. Pharmacol.*, **506**, 205–208.

126 Grond, S. and Sablotzki, A. (2004) Clinical pharmacology of tramadol. *Clin. Pharmacokinet.*, **43**, 879–923.

127 Subrahmanyam, V., Renwick, A.B., Walters, D.G., Young, P.J., Price, R.J., Tonelli, A.P., and Lake, B.G. (2001) Identification of cytochrome P-450 isoforms responsible for *cis*-tramadol metabolism in human liver microsomes. *Drug Metab. Dispos.*, **29**, 1146–1155.

128 Poulsen, L., Arendt-Nielsen, L., Brøsen, K., and Sindrup, S. (1996) The hypoalgesic effect of tramadol in relation to CYP2D6. *Clin. Pharmacol. Ther.*, **60**, 636–644.

129 Borlak, J., Hermann, R., Erb, K., and Thum, T. (2003) A rapid and simple CYP2D6 genotyping assay–case study with analgetic tramadol. *Metabolism*, **52**, 1439–1443.

130 Fliegert, F., Kurth, B., and Gohler, K. (2005) The effects of tramadol on static and dynamic pupillometry in healthy subjects–the relationship between pharmacodynamics, pharmacokinetics and CYP2D6 metaboliser status. *Eur. J. Pharmacol.*, **61**, 257–266.

131 Slanar, O., Nobilis, M., Kvetina, J., Idle, J., and Perlik, F. (2006) *CYP2D6* polymorphism, tramadol pharmacokinetics and pupillary response. *Eur. J. Clin. Pharmacol.*, **62**, 75–76.

132 Slanar, O., Nobilis, M., Kvetina, J., Mikoviny, R., Zima, T., Idle, J., and Perlik, F. (2007) Miotic action of tramadol is determined by CYP2D6 genotype. *Physiol. Res.*, **56**, 129–136.

133 Gillen, C., Haurand, M., Kobelt, D.J., and Wnendt, S. (2000) Affinity, potency and efficacy of tramadol and its metabolites at the cloned human mu-opioid receptor. *Naunyn Schmiedebergs Arch. Pharmacol.*, **362**, 116–121.

134 Overbeck, P. and Blaschke, G. (1999) Direct determination of tramadol glucuronides in human urine by high-performance liquid chromatography with fluorescence detection. *J. Chromatogr. B*, **732**, 185–192.

16
Drugs of Abuse (Including Designer Drugs)

Markus R. Meyer and Hans H. Maurer

16.1
Introduction

Besides classic drugs of abuse such as morphine/heroin, cocaine, Δ^9-tetrahydrocannabinol (THC; marijuana), amphetamine/methamphetamine, lysergide (LSD), and phencyclidine (PCP), a series of new drug classes has appeared on the illicit drugs market in recent years. These drugs were derived from amphetamine [1–6], phenethylamine (so-called 2Cs) [7–12], cathinone [13, 14], phencyclidine [15–18], piperazine [19–27], pyrrolidinophenone [19, 28–35], or tryptamine [36–41]. In contrast to new medicaments, which are extensively studied in controlled clinical trials concerning metabolism, including cytochrome P450 (CYP) and UDP-glucuronosyltransferase (UGT) isozyme differentiation, and further pharmacokinetics, designer drugs are consumed without any safety testing. The corresponding data on the metabolism is mostly incomplete or even not available at all. However, data on the metabolism is strongly required. It is a prerequisite for toxicological risk assessment as well as for developing toxicological screening procedures, especially in urine.

Knowledge of the metabolism of drugs of abuse is of importance for the question of which drug can be detected in which body sample (urine, blood, saliva, sweat, hair, nails), via which target analyte (parent drug or metabolite), and for how long [42–44]. In addition, this knowledge is needed for the differentiation of whether a detected compound is formed by a licit (e.g., codeine) or illicit drug (e.g., heroin). For pharmacological and/or toxicological interpretation of the analytical results, pharmacokinetic calculations are often used as a basis [45]. Furthermore, knowledge on the isozymes involved in the particular metabolic steps of all used drugs is of great importance regarding drug–drug interactions and the impact of pharmacogenetic variability on, for example, drug transport and metabolism resulting in different pharmacokinetic behavior or toxic risks [46–55]. The main metabolic steps and the isozymes involved therein will be described for the above-mentioned drug classes if known. The metabolic data described in the text are summarized in Table 16.1, including main references.

Metabolism of Drugs and Other Xenobiotics, First Edition. Edited by Pavel Anzenbacher, Ulrich M. Zanger.

Table 16.1 Studied compounds, main metabolic reactions, and enzymes involved in the main metabolic reactions.

Compound	Main metabolic reactions	Enzyme	References
Classic drugs of abuse			
Morphine	conjugation	UGT2B7	[56–58]
Heroin	ester cleavage	hCE-1	[57, 59–61]
Cocaine	ester cleavage	hCE-1or hiCE	[57, 59, 60, 62–64]
THC	hydroxylation	CYP2C9	[65–68]
Amphetamine	hydroxylation	CYP2D6	[69, 70]
Methamphetamine	*N*-dealkylation, hydroxylation	CYP2D6	[69, 70]
LSD	hydroxylation	no data available	[71–75]
PCP	hydroxylation	CYP3A	[76]
Methylenedioxyamphetamines			
MDMA	demethylenation	CYP2D6	[77]
MDEA	demethylenation	CYP2D6	[78]
MBDB	demethylenation	CYP2D6	[79]
MDA	demethylenation	CYP2D6	[80]
BDB	demethylenation	CYP2D6	[80]
p-Substituted amphetamines			
PMA	*O*-demethylation	CYP2D6	[81–83]
PMMA	*O*-demethylation	CYP2D6	[84]
4-MTA	deamination/hydroxylation	no data available	[85–87]
2,5-Dimethoxyamphetamines			
DOB	*O*-demethylation	CYP2D6	[88]
DOC	*O*-demethylation	CYP2D6	[88]
DOI	*O*-demethylation	CYP2D6	[88]
MDOB	*O*-demethylation	CYP2D6	[88]
TMA-2	*O*-demethylation	CYP2D6	[88]
DOM	hydroxylation	CYP2D6	[88]
Phenethylamines (2Cs)			
2C-B	deamination	MAO-A, MAO-B	[89–92]
2C-I	deamination	MAO-A, MAO-B	[11, 92]
2C-D	deamination	MAO-A, MAO-B	[9, 92]
2C-E	deamination	MAO-A, MAO-B	[10, 92]
2C-T-2	deamination	MAO-A, MAO-B	[12, 92, 93]
2C-T-7	deamination	MAO-A, MAO-B	[7, 92, 94]

Table 16.1 (*Continued*)

Compound	Main metabolic reactions	Enzyme	References
Cathinones			
Methylone	initial reactions not given	no data available	[13]
Butylone	initial reactions not given	no data available	[14]
Ethylone	initial reactions not given	no data available	[14]
Mephedrone	initial reactions not given	no data available	[95]
Phencyclidine-derived designer drugs			
PCEPA	*O*-dealkylation	CYP2B6, CYP2C19, CYP2D6, CYP3A4	[96]
PCPr	*N*-dealkylation, ω-1 hydroxylation, 4-hydroxylation	CYP2B6	[16, 97]
PCEEA	*O*-dealkylation	CYP2B6, CYP2C9, CYP2C19, CYP3A4	[18, 97]
PCMEA	*O*-dealkylation	CYP2B6, CYP2C19	[18, 97]
PCMPA	*O*-dealkylation	CYP2B6, CYP2C19, CYP2D6	[17, 96]
Piperazines			
BZP	hydroxylation	no data available	[20, 26]
MDBP	demethylenation	no data available	[24]
TFMPP	hydroxylation	CYP2D6	[98]
mCPP	hydroxylation	CYP2D6	[99]
MeOPP	*O*-demethylation	CYP2D6	[100]
Pyrrolidinophenones			
PPP	2″-oxidation	no data available	[32]
MOPPP	*O*-demethylation	CYP2D6	[101]
MDPPP	demethylenation	CYP2D6	[102]
MPPP	4′-hydroxylation	CYP2D6	[103]
MPHP	4′-hydroxylation	CYP2D6, CYP2C19	[101]
MPBP	4′-hydroxylation	CYP1A2, CYP2C19, CYP2D6	[28, 104]
PVP	2″-oxidation	CYP2B6, CYP2C19, CYP2D6, CYP1A2	[29]
MDPV	demethylenation	CYP2D6/CYP2C19	[105]
Tryptamine-derived designer drugs			
5-MeO-DIPT	*O*-demethylation/*N*-deisopropylation glucuronidation and/or sulfation		[106, 107]

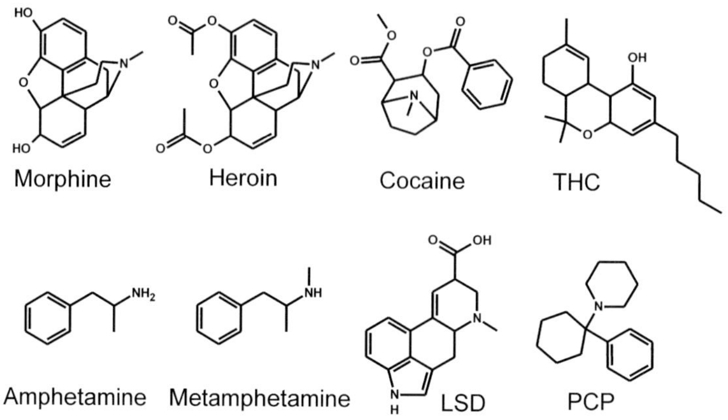

Figure 16.1 Chemical structure of classic drugs of abuse.

16.2
Classic Drugs of Abuse

Classic drugs of abuse such as morphine/heroin, cocaine, THC, amphetamine/ methamphetamine, LSD, and PCP have been abused for decades and are still in focus. Their chemical structures are shown in Figure 16.1.

16.2.1
Morphine and Heroin

Morphine is an alkaloid of the plant *Papaver somniferum* and is used as a potent analgesic, whereas its 3,6-diacetyl derivative heroin is a drug of abuse. The oral bioavailability of heroin is poor due to complete first-pass metabolism by hepatic and extrahepatic factors [57]. The metabolism of heroin to 6-monoacetylmorphine and morphine is catalyzed in the liver mainly by human cholinesterase (hCE)-1 and in part by hCE-2 [57, 59–61].

Morphine itself is directly conjugated mainly by UGT2B7 (besides many other isoforms) to the inactive metabolite morphine-3-glucuronide (M3G) and, to a less extent, to the pharmacologically active compound morphine-6-glucuronide (M6G) [56–58]. Finally, morphine is *N*-demethylated mainly by hepatic CYP3A4 [108].

16.2.2
Cocaine

Cocaine is a potent stimulant that is assumed to be primarily metabolized by pseudo-CE, and hCE-1 and -2) [57, 59, 60, 62, 64]. It is hydrolyzed by hCE-1 to benzoylecgonine or by pseudo-CE and hCE-2 to ecgonine methyl ester. In the presence of ethanol, hCE-1 catalyzes transesterification of cocaine to cocaethylene – a toxic metabolite that can be further hydrolyzed by hCE-1 to benzoylecgonine or by hCE-2 to ecgonine ethyl ester [60, 62, 64]. In contrast, a recent study showed that cocaine was not hydrolyzed by the human liver hCE-1, neither as highly active recombinant protein nor as enzyme isolated from human liver or intestinal extracts [63]. These results correlated well with computer-assisted molecular modeling studies that suggested that hydrolysis of cocaine by hCE-1 would be unlikely to occur. In that study, cocaine was a substrate of the intestinal CE (hiCE), as determined using both the recombinant protein and the tissue fractions. Again, these data were in agreement with the modeling results.

Apart from these steps, cocaine is *N*-demethylated to pharmacologically active norcocaine catalyzed by two pathways – one involving only CYP3A4 [109], and one involving other CYPs and flavin-containing monooxygenase (FMO) [110]. Norcocaine is further metabolized by *N*-hydroxylation at least partly catalyzed by several CYP subfamilies including 1A, 2A, 3A, and possibly 2B [111]. In addition, aromatic *m*- and *p*-hydroxylation of cocaine partly followed by hydrolysis to the corresponding hydroxy benzoylecgonine isomers was described [112, 113]. Unfortunately, the isozymes involved have not yet been identified.

16.2.3 THC

THC – a psychoactive ingredient of the plant *Cannabis sativa* – is substrate of CYP oxidation and subsequent UGT-dependent glucuronidation. The primary metabolite 11-hydroxy-THC (HO-THC) is formed by CYP2C9 [65–68] and further oxidized, probably by alcohol dehydrogenase (ADH) or microsomal alcohol oxygenase (MALCO), to the intermediate aldehyde 11-oxo-THC. Subsequently, it is oxidized to 11-nor-9-carboxy-THC (THC-COOH) by a microsomal aldehyde oxygenase (MALDO) followed by glucuronidation [68, 114–116]. Recent studies showed that HO-THC is mainly conjugated by UGT1A9 and UGT1A10, and THC-COOH mainly by UGT1A1 and UGT1A3 [117].

Further minor metabolic steps yield several hydroxy metabolites at C1′ to C5′ followed by β-oxidation to the corresponding carboxylic acids [67], two diastereomeric 8-hydroxy metabolites followed by dehydration [66, 67], an epoxide at C9–10 followed by hydrolysis or glutathione conjugation [66]. Formation of 8-hydroxy-THC and the epoxide are catalyzed by CYP3A4 [66]. Finally, several combinations of the metabolic steps have been described [67].

Given the high affinity of CYP2C9 for the hydroxylation of THC, the impact of the CYP2C9 polymorphism on the pharmacokinetics of orally administered THC was studied in 43 healthy volunteers. THC pharmacokinetics did not differ by CYP2C9*2 allele status. However, the median area under the concentration–time curve (AUC) of THC was 3- to 6-fold higher and that of 11-nor-9-carboxy-9-tetrahydrocannabinol was 70% lower in CYP2C9*3/*3 homozygotes than in CYP2C9*1/*1 homozygotes [118].

16.2.4
Amphetamine/Methamphetamine

Amphetamine and methamphetamine are stimulants acting as indirect sympathomimetic drugs. They are substrates of the monoamine transporter in the cell membrane of dopaminergic, noradrenergic, and adrenergic neurons, and in the membrane of the storage vesicles. They have no affinity to the adrenoceptors or dopamine receptors. Their effects result from a nonexocytotic, carrier-mediated release of neurotransmitters.

These two stimulants are not that extensively metabolized and are also excreted as unchanged parent compounds in urine [69, 70]. Nevertheless, the metabolic pathways of amphetamine and methamphetamine have been well known for several years: aromatic hydroxylation, aliphatic hydroxylation, *N*-demethylation, oxidative deamination, *N*-oxidation, and conjugation of the nitrogen. In addition, the phenolic metabolites are partly excreted as conjugates.

Using different *in vivo* and *in vitro* assays, it was shown that the ring hydroxylation of amphetamine and methamphetamine and the *N*-dealkylation of methamphetamine are mainly catalyzed by CYP2D6 isozymes [119, 120]. Interestingly, amphetamine and methamphetamine are substrates as well as competitive inhibitors of CYP2D6 [83]. Furthermore, amphetamine is oxidatively deaminated by monoamine oxidase (MAO). However, the deamination to phenylacetone seems to be also catalyzed by CYP2C [121].

16.2.5
LSD

LSD is a semisynthetic derivative of ergot alkaloids from the fungus *Claviceps purpurea*. LSD is supposed to act as a 5-HT_2 receptor agonist producing sensory alteration and euphoria [122]. It is metabolized to the following five metabolites: *N*-demethyl-LSD (nor-LSD), 2-oxo-LSD, 2-oxo-3-hydroxy-LSD, 13-hydroxy-LSD, and 14-hydroxy-LSD [72–74]. The 13- and 14-hydroxy metabolites are additionally excreted as glucuronides [74]. 2-Oxo-3-hydroxy-LSD was shown to be the main human urinary metabolite with concentrations 4–40 times higher than that of LSD [73–75]. In incubations of LSD with human liver microsomes and hepatocytes, 2,3-dihydroxy-LSD could be identified [71]. So far, the contribution and importance of specific enzymes in the formation of the LSD main metabolites such as 2-oxo-3-hydroxy-LSD still remains unclear.

16.2.6
PCP

PCP is a synthetic dissociative drug originally developed as a general anesthetic. Since clinical studies revealed that patients experienced delusions, severe anxiety, and agitation when emerging from the drug's effects, the use was stopped in 1965.

PCP is metabolized extensively in the body via a variety of metabolic routes. Primary metabolism involves hydroxylation of the alicyclic rings by CYPs. Hydroxylation of PCP at C2 of the piperidine ring (forming an unstable carbinolamine) leads to formation of polar, open-ring compounds. Hydroxylated metabolites are conjugated with glucuronic or sulfuric acid, or are further hydroxylated to dihydroxy derivatives that can also be conjugated. Studies suggest that several CYP isoforms contribute to PCP metabolism and that CYP3A isoforms play a major role in PCP biotransformation in human liver microsomes [76]. Furthermore, formation of highly reactive electrophilic metabolites of PCP has been demonstrated in microsomal preparations [123].

PCP is able to inactivate the activity of CYP2B6 in a concentration-, time-, and NADPH-dependent manner. Extensive dialysis of the PCP-inactivated CYP2B6 did not cause a return in catalytic activity, demonstrating PCP inactivation was irreversible [124]. The mechanism behind the observed inactivation of human CYP2B6 by PCP has been evaluated, suggesting that a reactive intermediate generated during the hydroxylation of the cyclohexane ring may be linked to CYP2B6 inactivation [124]. Following incubations with human and rat liver microsomes and recombinant CYP2B enzymes, a unique PCP bioactivation pathway involving initial *o*- or *p*-hydroxylation of the phenyl ring in PCP followed by spontaneous decomposition to piperidine and an electrophilic quinone methide intermediate was shown. If formed enzymatically *in vivo*, *p*-hydroxy-PCP may not require further metabolism to liberate the quinone methide, which can then react with macromolecules [125].

16.3 Designer Drugs of Abuse

In recent years, many new drug classes have appeared on the illicit drugs market (e.g., for use as rave drugs). Many derivatives have been "designed" to modify the effects and to avoid legal consequences as long as they are not yet scheduled. Although designer drugs have the reputation of being safe, several experimental studies in rats and humans and epidemiological studies indicated risks to humans; some of them should be caused by metabolites [35, 126].

16.3.1 Amphetamine Derivatives

The following section provides a comprehensive overview of the different kinds of amphetamine derivatives and their metabolism. Their chemical structures are shown in Figures 16.2 and 16.3.

16.3.1.1 Methylenedioxyamphetamines

One class of amphetamine-derived designer drug is made up of the methylenedioxy derivatives 3,4-methylenedioxymethamphetamine (MDMA, Ecstasy, Adam),

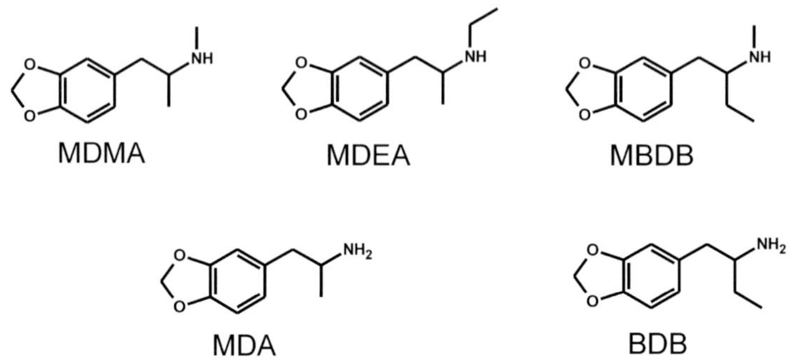

Figure 16.2 Chemical structure of methylenedioxyamphetamines.

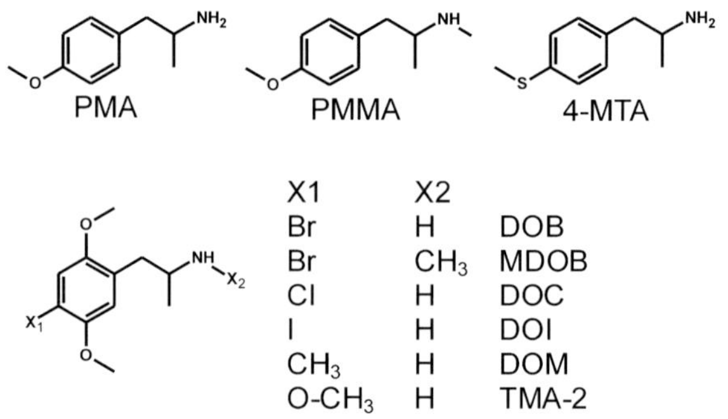

Figure 16.3 Chemical structure of *p*-substituted and 2,5-dimethoxyamphetamines.

3,4-methylenedioxyethylamphetamine (MDEA, Eve), *N*-methylbenzodioxolyl butanamine (MBDB, Eden), 4-methylenedioxyamphetamine (MDA), and benzodioxolylbutanamine (BDB). *In vivo* studies of MDMA, MDEA, and MBDB revealed two main metabolic steps: *N*-demethylation and demethylenation. The first pathway, predominant in humans, involves CYP-catalyzed *O*-demethylenation to the corresponding 3,4-dihydroxy compounds followed by catechol-*O*-methyltransferase (COMT)-catalyzed *O*-methylation to the 4-hydroxy-3-methoxy metabolites and *O*-conjugation with sulfate or glucuronic acid. The second entails initial *N*-dealkylation to MDA or BDB followed by deamination and oxidation to the corresponding benzoic acid derivatives conjugated with glycine [127–129]. Urinary recovery of MDMA represents about 15% of the MDMA dose, which indicates that the drug is mainly eliminated by metabolism [127]. MDA and BDB can also undergo *O*-demethylenation to the 3,4-dihydroxy compounds following *O*-methylation and *O*-conjugation with glucuronic acid or sulfate. The catechols, formed via metabolic demethylenation of the aforementioned drugs, can easily be oxidized to their corresponding *o*-quinones, which in turn can form adducts with glutathione and other thiol-containing compounds [130, 131].

It was shown that MDMA, MDEA, and MBDB are *N*-dealkylated mainly by CYP2B6, and demethylenated mainly by CYP2D6, CYP3A4, and CYP2C19, with a preference for the *S*-enantiomer [77–79]. Differences in the enantioselectivity of the involved isoforms where observed, indicating CYP2C19 to be the most selective in all cases. Furthermore, their *N*-dealkyl metabolites MDA and BDB are also demethylenated by CYP2D6 and CYP2C19 with a preference for their *S*-enantiomers, but these primary amines are not metabolized as enantioselectively as the secondary amines [80]. The catecholic phase I metabolites of the aforementioned designer drugs were investigated for enantioselective methylation and their *S*-enantiomers were also shown to be preferably formed [132]. Inhibition studies performed with DHMA, DHEA, and DHMBB clearly indicated an uncompetitive inhibition of the COMT catalyzed *O*-methylation of dopamine [132].

UGT1A1, UGT1A3, UGT1A8, UGT1A9, UGT2B4, UGT2B7, UGT2B15, and UGT2B17 were involved in the glucuronidation of 3-methoxymethamphetamine (HMMA). UGT2B15 showed the highest affinity and activity. UGT2B15, UGT2B17, and human liver microsomes were not considerably enantioselective, but showed slight preferences for *S*-HMMA. Marked enantioselectivity could only be observed for UGT1A9 with respect to the *S*-enantiomer and for UGT2B7 with respect to the *R*-enantiomer [133].

16.3.1.2 *p*-Substituted Amphetamines

_p_-Methoxyamphetamine (PMA) The *in vivo* metabolism of PMA in human was investigated in three subjects [82]. Two of them, showing the extensive metabolizer phenotype, excreted mainly 4-hydroxyamphetamine, free and conjugated, together with small amounts of the oxime metabolite and 4-hydroxynorephedrine. The third subject, showing the poor metabolizer phenotype, however, was defective in *O*-dealkylation. Only very small amounts of 4-hydroxyamphetamine were detected. The main excretion products were the unchanged PMA together with side-chain oxidized metabolites, 1-(*p*-methoxyphenyl)-propan-2-one oxime, 1-(*p*-methoxyphenyl)-propan-2-one, and, in contrast to the extensive metabolizers, side-chain degraded metabolites 4-methoxybenzoic acid and 4-hydroxybenzoic acid. Several studies were conducted on the metabolism of PMA in animals and deamination to the corresponding ketone 1-(*p*-methoxyphenyl)-propan-2-one and further reduction of the ketone to the corresponding alcohol were found besides *N*-hydroxylation and the formation of 1-(*p*-methoxyphenyl)-propan-2-one oxime metabolites were found [82, 134–136].

Furthermore, *O*-demethylation was reported as the main metabolic pathway in various animals mainly excreted as conjugate [82, 136]. In rat urine, 1-(*p*-methoxyphenyl)-propan-2-one oxime was detected as well as its glucuronide conjugate as minor metabolites, besides 4-hydroxyamphetamine, again mainly conjugated.

Further animal *in vivo* metabolites were described to be 4-hydroxy-3-methoxyamphetamine and the corresponding deaminated metabolites 1-(*p*-hydroxyphenyl)-propan-2-one and 1-(4-hydroxy-3-methoxyphenyl)-propan-2-one.

Further hydroxylation of the benzyl carbon of 1-(*p*-hydroxyphenyl)-propan-2-one was postulated.

Several studies indicated that CYP2D6 is the isoform mainly responsible for *O*-demethylation of PMA, and rates of *O*-demethylation of PMA and dextromethorphan were highly correlated in the panel of human microsomes, and that the CYP2D6 inhibitors quinine and quinidine showed significant inhibition of the monitored reaction [81–83].

p-Methoxymethamphetamine (PMMA) PMMA was extensively metabolized via *O*-demethylation of the methoxy moiety to 4-hydroxy methamphetamine and aromatic hydroxylation to dihydroxymethamphetamine followed by methylation to 4′-hydroxy-3′-methoxymethamphetamine in male Wistar rats [137]. The isomer 3′-hydroxy-4′-methoxymethamphetamine was only formed to a very small extent and *N*-demethylation of PMMA to PMA was only observed to a minor extent. The metabolite 4-hydroxyamphetamine was formed via PMMA *N*-demethylation to PMA followed by *O*-demethylation [82, 136]. 1-Hydroxylation of hydroxymethamphetamine led to the formation of oxilofrine. The phenolic metabolites were partially excreted as conjugates. Glucuronide and sulfate conjugation was postulated, and sulfation was already described for 4-hydroxymethamphetamine [138–141].

CYP2D6 was identified as the only isozyme capable of demethylating PMMA, which was further supported by significant inhibition of the metabolite formation by the CYP2D6 inhibitor quinidine and by a significantly lower metabolite formation rate in poor metabolizer human liver microsomes [84].

p-Methylthioamphetamine (4-MTA) The metabolism of 4-MTA was studied in CD1 mice [85]. β-Hydroxylation to 4-methylthiophenylpropanolamine and 4-methylthiocathine, and degradation of the side-chain to 4-methylthiobenzoic acid, were observed. Furthermore, hydroxylation at the aromatic ring or at the methylthio group were discussed. 4-MTA was only poorly metabolized using several *in vitro* methods [86]. 4-Methylthiobenzoic acid was identified as the major metabolite in human, monkey, dog, rabbit, and mouse hepatocytes, but no metabolite was identified in rat hepatocytes, indicating qualitative interspecies differences. 4-Methylthiophenylpropanolamin and 4-methylthiocathine were identified as metabolites in the *in vivo* study in mice [85]. Two metabolites – a hydroxylated metabolite and a sulfoxide – were reported in a case report on a fatality after 4-MTA consumption [87].

16.3.1.3 **2,5-Dimethoxyamphetamines**

Typical drugs of this class are 4-bromo-2,5-dimethoxyamphetamine (DOB), 4-chloro-2,5-dimethoxyamphetamine (DOC), 4-iodo-2,5-dimethoxyamphetamine (DOI), 2,5-dimethoxy-4-methyl-amphetamine (DOM), 4-bromo-2,5-dimethoxy methamphetamine (MDOB), and 2,4,5-trimethoxyamphetamine (TMA-2).

The metabolism of these drugs has been studied in detail using male Wistar rats [2–6, 88, 142, 143]. These studies show that the 2,5-dimethoxyamphetamine designer drugs DOB, DOC, DOI, MDOB, and TMA-2 were mainly metabolized by *O*-demethylation, and in the case of DOM by hydroxylation. Further steps were side-chain hydroxylation and the oxidative deamination. As metabolic phase II reactions, partial glucuronidation and/or sulfation were observed. Furthermore, combinations of these steps as well as minor metabolites were also detected [3–6, 88].

In vitro studies showed that CYP2D6 was the only isoform catalyzing the demethylation of the DOB, DOC, DOI, MDOB, and TMA-2, and the hydroxylation of DOM.

Although for all of these drugs, demethylation of one of the 2,5-methoxy groups by CYP2D6 was observed, these drugs were found to be more or less potent CYP2D6 inhibitors [88].

16.3.2 Phenethylamines (2Cs)

The abuse of phenethylamine itself is not common due to its rapid metabolism [144]. However, its derivatives such as 2C-B, 2C-I, 2C-D, 2C-E, 2C-T-2, and 2C-T-7 are known drugs of abuse [145]. Their chemical structures are shown in Figure 16.4.

16.3.2.1 2C-B

Metabolism of 2C-B was investigated in rat urine, rat hepatocytes, and whole rats [89–91, 146]. The major metabolites in rat hepatocytes were 2-*O*-desmethyl-2C-B and its carboxylic acid derivative. Further metabolites were the alcohol derivative 2-*O*-demethyl-*N*-acetyl-2C-B and 5-*O*-demethyl-*N*-acetyl-2C-B. Further metabolites identified were a deaminohydroxy side-chain hydroxy, an *O*-demethyl deaminohydroxy side-chain hydroxy, and an *O*-demethyldeaminohydroxy side-chain oxo metabolite.

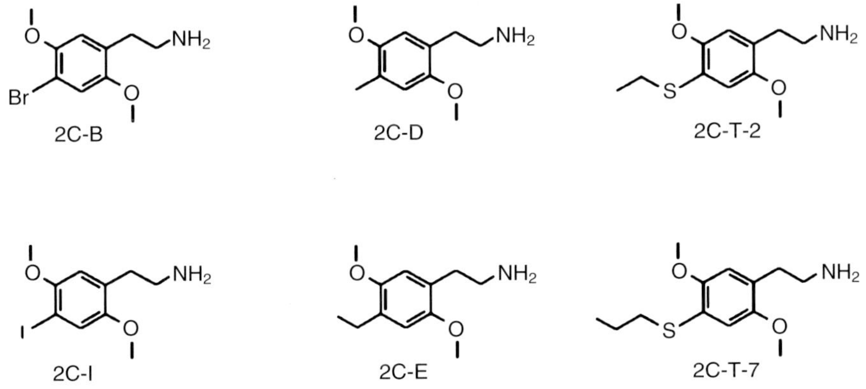

Figure 16.4 Chemical structure of 2Cs.

After incubation of 2C-B with human hepatocytes, six metabolites could be identified, described to be 4-bromo-2,5-dimethoxyphenylacetic acid, 4-bromo-2-hydroxy-5-methoxy-phenylacetic acid, 4-bromo-2,5-dimethoxybenzoic acid, 2-(4-bromo-2,5-dimethoxyphenyl)-ethanol, 2-(4-bromo-2-hydroxy-5-methoxyphenyl)-ethanol, and 4-bromo-2,5-dimethoxy-phenol [147, 148].

16.3.2.2 **2C-I**

The following metabolic steps were postulated for 2C-I [11]. *O*-demethylation of the parent compound in position 2 and 5 of the aromatic ring, respectively, followed either by partial glucuronidation/sulfation or by *N*-acetylation with subsequent partial glucuronidation/sulfation or by deamination to the corresponding aldehyde, followed by oxidation to the corresponding acid or reduction to the corresponding alcohol, followed by partial glucuronidation/sulfation. The latter alcohol was further hydroxylated in the β-position and further oxidized to the corresponding oxo metabolite. Another metabolic pathway was the deamination of the parent compound to the corresponding aldehyde, followed by oxidation to the corresponding acid or reduction to the corresponding alcohol with subsequent partial glucuronidation/sulfation.

16.3.2.3 **2C-D**

The following metabolic steps were postulated after application of 2C-D to male Wistar rats. *O*-demethylation of the parent compound in position 2 or 5, followed by *N*-acetylation or by deamination with oxidation to the corresponding acid or reduction to the corresponding alcohol [9]. Furthermore, 2C-D was hydroxylated at the methyl moiety in position 4 and deaminated followed by oxidation to the corresponding acid or by reduction to the corresponding alcohol.

16.3.2.4 **2C-E**

After application of 2C-E to male Wistar rats, the following metabolic steps could be postulated: *O*-demethylation of the parent compound in position 2 or 5, followed by *N*-acetylation and hydroxylation at C2′, or by deamination with oxidation to the corresponding acid or reduction to the corresponding alcohol [10]. *N*-acetylation of the parent compound followed by hydroxylation at position C1′ of the ethyl side-chain with subsequent dealkylation and oxidation to the corresponding ketone or followed by β-hydroxylation were described. Apart from these steps, hydroxylation of the parent compound at position C2′ of the ethyl side-chain followed by *N*-acetylation and oxidation of the hydroxy group to the corresponding acid was observed. A further pathway was the deamination of the parent compound followed by reduction to the corresponding alcohol or by oxidation to the corresponding acid. The latter was hydroxylated at position C2′ or C1′ followed by oxidation to the corresponding ketone or aldehyde.

16.3.2.5 **2C-T-2**

In rats, 2C-T-2 forms an aldehyde metabolite by deamination and subsequent oxidation and/or reduction [93]. The amino group is acetylated to form the metabolites 1-acetoamino-2-(2-hydroxy-4-ethylthio-5-methoxyphenyl)-ethane and 1-

acetoamino-2- (2-methoxy-4-ethylsulfanyl-5-hydroxyphenyl)-ethane. Other studies proposed the following metabolic steps: sulfoxidation of the parent compound to the corresponding sulfone, followed by *N*-acetylation and either *O*-demethylation of one methoxy group or hydroxylation of the *S*-alkyl side-chain. A second pathway was the *O*-demethylation of the parent compound, followed by *N*-acetylation and sulfoxidation to the corresponding sulfone. A third pathway was the *N*-acetylation of the parent compound, followed either by *O*-demethylation and sulfoxidation or by *S*-deethylation to the corresponding thiol with subsequent methylation of the thiol moiety [12].

16.3.2.6 2C-T-7

2C-T-7 is metabolized by hydroxylation of the propyl side-chain followed by *N*-acetylation and sulfoxidation, and by deamination followed by oxidation to the corresponding acid. Apart from these steps, it is transformed to the corresponding alcohol and *S*-dealkylated followed by *N*-acetylation, *S*-methylation, and sulfoxidation [7]. The following pathways could be postulated. Hydroxylation of the propyl side-chain to 2,5-dimethoxy-4-hydroxypropylthio-β-phenethylamine followed by *N*-acetylation and sulfoxidation. The second pathway led to the corresponding acid or (reduced) to the corresponding alcohol, followed by partial glucuronidation and/or sulfation. The third pathway led via *N*-acetylation and *S*-depropylation to the corresponding thiol, followed by methylation of the thiol moiety. Further metabolic steps were the sulfoxidation of the methylated thiol to the corresponding sulfoxide and the corresponding sulfone [94].

16.3.2.7 Enzymes Involved in the Metabolism of 2,5-Dimethoxyamphetamines

The deamination and rapid reduction or oxidation to the respective alcohols or carboxylic acids are major metabolic steps of the phenethylamines [7–12, 86, 89–91]. For 2C-D, 2C-E, 2C-T-2, and 2C-T-7, CYP2D6 was involved in deamination, but with low formation rates [92]. Kinetic data for MAO isoforms A and B showed that the 2Cs have a slightly higher affinity for MAO-A than for MAO-B. As MAO-A and MAO-B are involved in one of the major metabolic steps of the 2Cs, the 2Cs might be susceptible to drug–drug interactions with MAO inhibitors.

16.3.3 Cathinones

The so-called cathinones have appeared as a new class of designer drugs on the black market in many countries [13, 149, 150]. Due to their chemical similarity to amphetamines or methcathinone and the use as alternatives for these drugs, a similar stimulant effect of the cathinones could be postulated. Their chemical structures are shown in Figure 16.5.

16.3.3.1 Methylone

Metabolism of methylone was investigated using rat and human urine samples [13, 95]. The human and rat urine samples were collected 36 or over 24 h after administration, respectively. In rat urine, 4-hydroxy-3-methoxymethcathinone

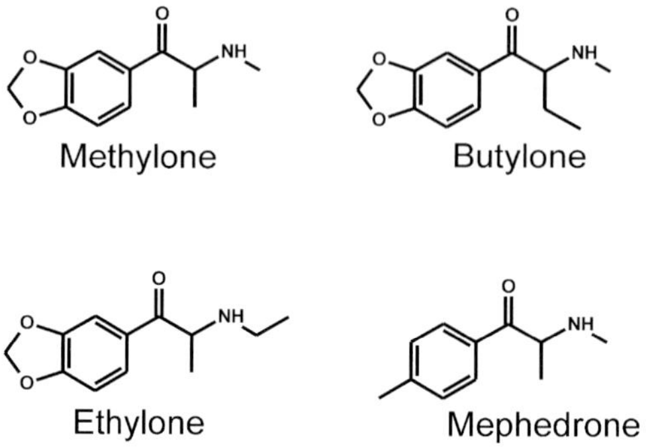

Figure 16.5 Chemical structure of cathinones.

(HMMC) and 3-hydroxy-4-methoxymethcathinone (3-OH-4-MeO-MC) were detected, which is in line with other findings concerning similar β-keto compounds [28–34, 151]. Over 80% of the excreted urinary HMMC and 3-OH-4-MeO-MC were found to be conjugated. In human urine, methylone, 3,4-methylenedioxycathinone (MDC), HMMC, and 3-OH-4-MeO-MC were detected. Among them, HMMC was the most abundant and characteristic metabolite of methylone.

16.3.3.2 **Butylone**

Similar to methylone, the metabolites of butylone were also identified in human urine [14]. The following metabolic steps could be postulated. *N*-demethylation, demethylenation followed by methylation, and reduction of the keto group. In conclusion, *N*-demethylation was the minor step and demethylenation followed by methylation the predominant one.

16.3.3.3 **Ethylone**

Metabolites of ethylone in human urine were identified to be 2-amino-1-(3,4-methylenedioxyphenyl)propan-1-one (bk-MDA), 2-ethylamino-1-(4-hydroxy-3-methoxyphenyl)propan-1-one (bk-4,3-HMEA), 2-ethylamino-1-(3-hydroxy-4-methoxyphenyl)propan-1-one (bk-3,4-HMEA), and 2-ethylamino-1-(3,4-methylenedioxyphenyl)propan-1-ol (β-hydroxy-MDEA) [14]. bk-4,3-HMEA was the most abundant among the identified metabolites and the same pathways as described for bk-MBDB were true also for bk-MDEA.

16.3.3.4 **Mephedrone**

The metabolism of mephedrone was studied in rat and human urine [95]. The following metabolites were deduced: nor-mephedrone, nor-dihydro mephedrone, hydroxytolyl mephedrone, and nor-hydroxytolyl mephedrone. Apart from these metabolites, the parent drug mephedrone was also detected. Hydroxytolyl mephedrone and nor-hydroxytolyl mephedrone were partly excreted as glucuronides and/or sulfates. In human urine samples a further metabolite – 4-carboxy-dihydro mephedrone – could be identified by the authors of the study.

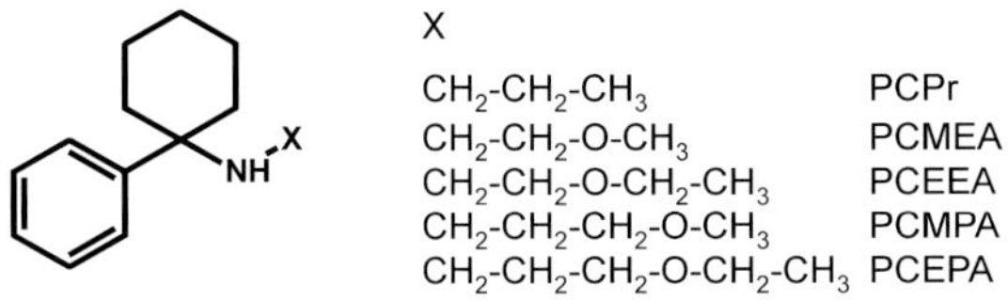

Figure 16.6 Chemical structure of phencyclidine derivatives.

16.3.4 Phencyclidine Derivatives

Only little information on the pharmacological properties of these compounds is available [152]. Due to structural similarities, they might be assumed to be similar to those of PCP or ketamine, which both act as antagonists at *N*-methyl-D-aspartate (NMDA) receptors and have psychotomimetic as well as anesthetic properties [153]. Furthermore, it has been reported that (1-phenylcyclohexyl)-amine – a known metabolite of PCP and of the above-mentioned PCP-derived compounds [15–18] – produced a long-lasting dose-dependent effect on the efflux of dopamine in the rat [154]. The chemical structures of the phencyclidine derivatives are shown in Figure 16.6.

16.3.4.1 *N*-(1-Phenylcyclohexyl)-3-ethoxypropylamine (PCEPA) and *N*-(1-Phenylcyclohexyl)-3-methoxypropanamine (PCMPA)

Postulated metabolic pathways of PCEPA are the following: *N*-dealkylation; *O*-de-ethylation partially followed by oxidation to the corresponding acids; hydroxylation of the cyclohexyl ring at different positions; *O*-deethylation followed by *N*-dealkylation; *O*-deethylation followed by hydroxylation of the cyclohexyl ring and *N*-dealkylation; *O*-deethylation followed by hydroxylation of the cyclohexyl ring and aromatic hydroxylation and oxidation to the corresponding acid; and *O*-deethylation followed by oxidation to the corresponding acid and aromatic hydroxylation followed by hydroxylation of the cyclohexyl ring [15].

PCMPA was mainly metabolized to the same metabolites as PCEPA [17]. Therefore, common metabolic pathways of PCMPA and PCEPA were concluded with the exception of monohydroxylation of the parent drug, which was observed for PCEPA, but not for PCMPA.

16.3.4.2 *N*-(1-Phenylcyclohexyl)propanamine (PCPr)

Combinations of the different possibilities of hydroxylation of the cyclohexyl ring, the aromatic system, and the side-chain were shown for PCPr [16]. Furthermore, *N*-dealkylation, hydroxylation of the cyclohexyl ring at different positions and of the aromatic system as well as of the side-chain were observed. Metabolites hydroxylated at the side-chain were postulated to be hydroxylated in omega-1 position. Almost all non-*N*-dealkylated metabolites were excreted in conjugated form.

16.3.4.3 *N*-(1-Phenylcyclohexyl)-2-ethoxyethanamine (PCEEA) and *N*-(1-Phenylcyclohexyl)-2-methoxyethanamine (PCMEA)

For PCEEA and PCMEA, the following steps were deduced: *N*-dealkylation; *O*-dealkylation partially followed by oxidation to the corresponding acid; hydroxylation of the cyclohexyl ring at different positions of *N*-dealkyl metabolites; *O*-dealkyl metabolites and of the corresponding acids; and finally aromatic hydroxylation of the *O*-dealkyl metabolites [18].

16.3.4.4 Enzymes Involved in the Metabolism of Phencyclidine Derivatives

In vitro initial screening studies were performed on the influence of CYP isozymes on the metabolism of phencyclidine-derived designer drugs [96, 97].

According to the results of the relative activity factor (RAF approach), CYP2B6 should be the most relevant CYP for *O*-dealkylation of PCEEA and PCMEA, accounting for 53% (PCEEA) and 91% (PCMEA) of the net clearance. Concerning PCEPA and PCMPA, CYP2D6 was the most important enzyme, and accounted for 30% (PCEPA) and 40% (PCMPA) of the net clearance. Furthermore, the decreasing side-chain length of the compounds was associated with a higher contribution of CYP2B6. In accordance with the decreasing involvement of CYP2B6, the number of CYPs involved and their contributions increased with increasing side-chain length [97].

Considering this major involvement of CYP2B6, simultaneous intake of potent CYP2B6 inhibitors such as triethylenethiophosphoramide (thiotepa), ticlopedine, clopidogrel [155, 156], or several antidepressants [157] might lead to a decreased clearance of PCMEA or PCPr and, consequently, to elevated plasma concentrations. However, the clinical relevance of such interactions remains to be established [96, 97].

16.3.5 Piperazines

The piperazines (containing a piperazine heterocycle) can be divided into two subclasses, the benzylpiperazines (BZPs; MDBP) and the phenylpiperazines (TFMPP, mCPP, and MeOPP).

Studies revealed amphetamine-like effects of BZP and central serotoninomimetic action, which involves serotonin (5-HT) uptake inhibition and 5-HT_1 receptor agonistic effects [158]. Furthermore, weak inhibition of serotonin transporters, norepinephrine release, and interactions with the dopaminergic system were described [159–162]. Studies with healthy volunteers corroborated the amphetamine-like effects also *in vivo* [163]. TFMPP shows central activity and serotonergic properties [164–170]. Owing to its serotonergic properties, TFMPP has been widely used as a pharmacological probe drug for drug discrimination procedures in animals [171–174]. Detailed information on its pharmacological effects can be found in [175].

Interestingly, mCPP is an active metabolite of therapeutics such as trazodone [176–179], nefazodone [176, 180], etoperidone [178, 181–183], and mepiprazol

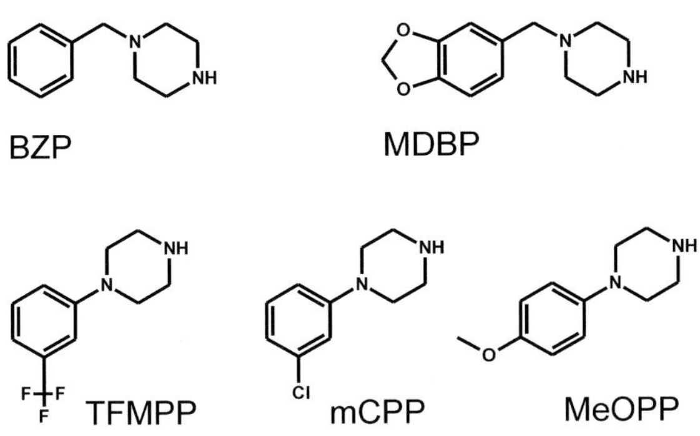

Figure 16.7 Chemical structure of piperazines.

[178]. Serotonin release by acting as a substrate for serotonin transporter proteins [170, 184–187] has been found. Inhibition of serotonin reuptake [186], slight dopamine release [185], as well as interactions with adrenergic and dopaminergic receptors [188] have also been reported. The chemical structures of the piperazines are shown in Figure 16.7.

16.3.5.1 **N-BZP**

BZP was not that extensively metabolized and also excreted as unchanged parent compound [20, 26]. The aromatic ring was metabolically altered by single or double hydroxylation followed by methylation to *N*-(4-hydroxy-3-methoxy-benzyl)piperazine and formation of the corresponding glucuronides and/or sulfates was postulated. The piperazine heterocycle was degraded by *N*-dealkylation, leading either to the formation of benzylamine or to *N*-benzylethylenediamine, depending on the positions of these metabolic reactions.

16.3.5.2 **1-(3,4-Methylenedioxybenzyl)piperazine (MDBP)**

The metabolism of MDBP was also studied in male Wistar rats [24]. Similar to BZP, MDBP was mainly excreted as unchanged parent compound. Demethylenation of the 3,4-methylenedioxy moiety to the corresponding catechol and further methylation to *N*-(4-hydroxy-3-methoxybenzyl)piperazine followed by partial glucuronidation or sulfation led to formation of metabolites common with BZP. Furthermore, *N*-dealkylation at the benzyl carbon, leading to piperazine, was described. Degradation of the piperazine heterocycle by double *N*-dealkylation led to the corresponding *N*-benzylethylenediamine, and benzylamine derivatives *N*-(3,4-methylenedioxybenzyl)ethylenediamine and 3,4-methylenedioxybenzylamine.

16.3.5.3 **1-(3-Trifluoromethylphenyl)piperazine (TFMPP)**

In contrast to the two afore-mentioned benzylpiperazines, TFMPP was extensively metabolized and almost exclusively excreted as metabolites [21]. Aromatic hydroxylation to hydroxy TFMPP followed by partial glucuronidation or sulfation was described. Degradation of the piperazine heterocycle by double *N*-dealkylation could be observed for the parent compound TFMPP, leading to the formation of *N*-(3-trifluoromethylphenyl)ethylenediamine or to 3-trifluoromethylaniline, as well as for its hydroxylated metabolite hydroxy TFMPP, leading to the formation of *N*-(hydroxy-3-trifluoromethylphenyl)ethylenediamine or to hydroxy-3-trifluoromethylaniline. Partial *N*-acetylation was observed of the aniline derivatives.

The hydroxylation of TFMPP to hydroxy TFMPP was studied *in vitro* [98]. CYP2D6 was the most important isozyme, accounting for 80% of predicted total TFMPP hydroxylation clearance by all individual CYPs in pooled human liver microsomes. CYP1A2 and CYP3A4 were responsible for 12 and 8%, respectively.

16.3.5.4 1-(3-Chlorophenyl)piperazine (mCPP)

Extensive metabolism of mCPP was reported and *p*-hydroxy mCPP was identified as the major metabolite [22, 189]. In addition to the aromatic hydroxylation, degradation of the piperazine heterocycle by *N*-dealkylation of mCPP to *N*-(3-chlorophenyl)ethylenediamine or to 3-chloroaniline was observed. Hydroxy-3-chloroaniline was the only metabolite resulting from degradation of the piperazine moiety of hydroxy mCPP. The aniline metabolites were partially *N*-acetylated. In studies on the mCPP precursor drug trazodone, the formation of mCPP *N*-glucuronides was reported [179, 190].

CYPs involved in the hydroxylation of mCPP – the major metabolic reaction – were also investigated *in vitro* [191, 192]. These studies concluded, in accordance with clinical studies, increased steady-state plasma mCPP concentrations in CYP2D6 poor metabolizers receiving treatment with the mCPP precursor drug nefazodone that CYP2D6 is mainly responsible for the described reaction [99].

16.3.5.5 1-(4-Methoxyphenyl)piperazine (MeOPP)

As with the two other phenylpiperazines, MeOPP was extensively metabolized [100]. *O*-demethylation of the methoxy moiety was the major metabolic step. The formed metabolite hydroxyphenylpiperazine was subsequently conjugated by partial glucuronidation or sulfation as concluded from studies with a mixture of β-glucuronidase and arylsulfatase. *N*-(4-Methoxyphenyl)ethylenediamine and 4-methoxyaniline were formed by degradation of the piperazine moiety of MeOPP and 4-hydroxyaniline could be detected as the piperazine-degraded metabolite of hydroxyphenylpiperazine. 4-Hydroxyaniline was found to be partially glucuronidated, sulfated, or *N*-acetylated.

The influence of human CYP isozymes on the major metabolic reaction – the *O*-demethylation of MeOPP – was studied *in vitro*, showing CYP2D6 to be the only isozyme capable of demethylating MeOPP [100].

16.3.6 Pyrrolidinophenones

Information about the dosage as well as the pharmacological and toxicological effects of the pyrrolidinophenones is rare. However, they may be expected to be

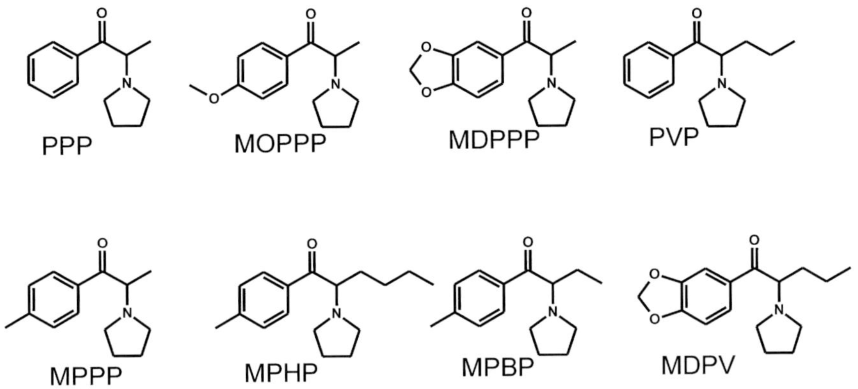

Figure 16.8 Chemical structure of pyrrolidinophenones.

very similar to those of pyrovalerone (4-methyl-pyrrolidinovalerophenone) due to their close structural relation to this drug. Pyrovalerone is a psychostimulant that acts by releasing dopamine and norepinephrine from the respective nerve terminals [193–195]. The chemical structures of the discussed pyrrolidinophenones are shown in Figure 16.8.

16.3.6.1 **α-Pyrrolidinopropiophenone (PPP)**

PPP was extensively metabolized in male Wistar rats and almost exclusively excreted as metabolites [32]. The pyrrolidine ring of PPP was either hydroxylated at the 2″-position followed by dehydrogenation to the corresponding lactam or metabolically degraded by double dealkylation to the corresponding primary amine cathinone. Partial subsequent reduction of the keto group to the corresponding secondary alcohol leads to norephedrine diastereomers. Hydroxylation of PPP in position 4′ led to the formation of an acidic metabolite. This metabolite as well as the norephedrine metabolites were shown to be partially conjugated.

16.3.6.2 **4′-Methoxy-α-pyrrolidinopropiophenone (MOPPP)**

The metabolism of MOPPP was also described in male Wistar rats [31]. *O*-demethylation of the methoxy group led to the formation of 4′-hydroxy-pyrrolidinopropiophenone, followed by aromatic hydroxylation at position 3′ to the corresponding catechol and 3′-methylation to 4′-hydroxy-3′-methoxy-pyrrolidinopropiophenone. Deamination resulted in the formation of 4′-methoxy-2-oxo-propiophenone, 4′-hydroxy-2-oxo-propiophenone, and 4′-hydroxy-3′-methoxy-2-oxo-propiophenone. Hydroxylation of the 2″-position of the pyrrolidine ring followed by dehydrogenation to the corresponding lactam was also observed. The phenolic metabolites were partially excreted as glucuronides and/or sulfates.

16.3.6.3 **Methylenedioxy-α-pyrrolidinopropiophenone (MDPPP)**

Demethylenation of the methylenedioxy followed by COMT-catalyzed methylation to 4′-hydroxy-3′-methoxy-pyrrolidinopropiophenone was the major metabolic pathway for MDPPP [30]. Furthermore, MDPPP and its altered metabolites at the methylenedioxy moiety were either oxidative deaminated to the corresponding 2-oxo compounds (3′,4′-methylenedioxy-2-oxo-propiophenone, 3′,4′-dihydroxy-2-oxo-propiophenone, or 4′-hydroxy-3′-methoxy-2-oxo-propiophenone) or its pyrrolidine ring was oxidized to the corresponding lactams (2″-oxo-MDPPP, 3′,4′-dihydroxy-2″-oxo-pyrrolidinopropiophenone, and 3′-hydroxy-4′-methoxy-2″-oxo-pyrrolidinopropiophenone). Oxidative deamination of these lactams would also yield the 2-oxo compound. The phenolic metabolites were partially excreted as glucuronides and/or sulfates, again as concluded from studies with a mixture of β-glucuronidase and arylsulfatase.

CYP2C19 and CYP2D6 were identified to be able to catalyze the MOPPP *O*-demethylation and MDPPP demethylenation. Calculations using a RAF approach [103, 196–200] to correct recombinant CYP formation rates for native human liver enzyme activity showed that CYP2D6 accounted for about 80–95% of the net intrinsic clearance of MOPPP and for about 55% of the net intrinsic clearance of MDPPP [101, 102].

16.3.6.4 4′-Methyl-α-pyrrolidinopropiophenone (MPPP)

Apart from oxidation of the tolyl methyl group to the corresponding carboxylic acid and/or hydroxylation of the 2″-position of the pyrrolidine ring followed by dehydrogenation to the corresponding lactam, the side-chain of MPPP is mainly metabolically altered [33]. Oxidative deamination of the carboxylic acid metabolite 2″-oxo-4′-carboxy-pyrrolidinopropiophenone and/or of the further at the pyrrolidine ring oxidized metabolite 2″-oxo-4′-carboxy-pyrrolidinopropiophenone to 2-oxo-4′-carboxy-propiophenone, which was further metabolized by side-chain degradation to the 4′-carboxybenzoic acid was observed. The carboxy acid metabolites were partially excreted as conjugates.

The influence of human CYP isozymes on hydroxylation of the tolyl methyl group of MPPP – the initial oxidation step – showed that CYP2D6 accounted for about 80% of the net intrinsic clearance of MPPP besides CYP2C19 [103].

16.3.6.5 4′-Methyl-α-pyrrolidinohexanophenone (MPHP)

MPHP was extensively metabolized in male Wistar rats [34]. Hydroxylation of the tolyl methyl group mostly followed by dehydrogenation to the corresponding carboxy compounds and hydroxylation of the 2″-position of the pyrrolidine ring followed by dehydrogenation to the corresponding lactam was observed. Reduction of the keto group to the corresponding secondary alcohol diastereomers could also be detected. It is further hydroxylated of the side-chain, leading to diastereomers and possibly to positional isomers. The hydroxylated metabolites and the carboxy metabolites were excreted as glucuronides and/or sulfates.

As for its α-pyrrolidinopropiophenone analog MPPP, the influence of CYP isozymes on the hydroxylation of the tolyl methyl group was investigated for MPHP [101]. CYP1A2, CYP2B6, CYP2C9, and CYP2D6 were capable of catalyzing this reaction, with CYP2D6 and CYP2C19 having the highest affinity towards MPHP. In addition, CYP2C19 exhibited the highest turnover rate and CYP2D6

– the enzyme with the highest affinity – showed the lowest capacity. Furthermore, CYP2B6, CYP2C9, and CYP2C19 were identified to be capable of hydroxylating the side-chain. However, side-chain hydroxylation was only a minor metabolic pathway.

16.3.6.6 4′-Methyl-α-pyrrolidinobutyrophenone (MPBP)

The following metabolic pathway could be deduced from the rat model [28]. Hydroxylation of the 4′-methyl group to the corresponding alcohol followed by oxidation to the corresponding carboxylic acid; hydroxylation of the 2″-position of the pyrrolidine ring followed by dehydrogenation to the corresponding lactams; reduction of the keto group of 4′-carboxy metabolites to the corresponding secondary alcohols; and oxidative deamination of 4′-carboxy-PBP to the corresponding 2-oxo compound. The 4′-carboxy-2-oxo-, 4′-hydroxy-, and 1-dihydro-4′-carboxy-2″-oxo metabolites were partly excreted as glucuronides and/or sulfates.

CYP2C19, CYP2D6, and CYP1A2 were markedly capable of catalyzing the hydroxylation of the 4′-methyl moiety of MPBP [104]. According to the results of the RAF approach, CYP2D6 (54%) and CYP2C19 (30%) accounted for more than 80% of the net clearance.

16.3.6.7 4′-Methyl-α-pyrrolidinovalerophenone (PVP)

The urinary metabolites of PVP were also identified using male Wistar rats leading to the following partly overlapping metabolic pathways [29]. Hydroxylation of the side-chain followed by dehydrogenation to the corresponding ketone; hydroxylation of the 2″-position of the pyrrolidine ring followed by dehydrogenation to the corresponding lactams or followed by ring opening to the respective aliphatic aldehyde and further oxidation to the respective carboxylic acid; degradation of the pyrrolidine ring to the corresponding primary amines; hydroxylation of the phenyl ring, most probably in the 4′-position resulting in a phenylogous carboxylic acid. HO-phenyl-PVP, hydroxyphenyl- 2″-oxo-PVP, di-HO-PVP, HO-phenyl-amino-PVP, and HO-alkyl-PVP were partly excreted as glucuronides and/or sulfates. Concerning PVP, solely an initial screening study with nine human hepatic CYPs was performed [29].

16.3.6.8 3′,4′-Methylenedioxypyrovalerone (MDPV)

MDPV is the latest of the pyrrolidinophenones to have appeared on the drug market. Its metabolism was investigated in rat and human urine [105]. The studies revealed the following phase I main metabolic steps: demethylenation followed by methylation, aromatic and side-chain hydroxylation and oxidation of the pyrrolidine ring to the corresponding lactam as well as ring opening to the corresponding carboxylic acid. Furthermore, phase II metabolites of the respective compounds were identified.

As for all pyrrolidino-oxo metabolites of all pyrrolidinophenones, the exact position of the oxo group could not be determined. However, the 2″-position seems to be the most likely as lactam formation is common in the metabolism of pyrrolidino compounds such as prolintane and nicotine [201].

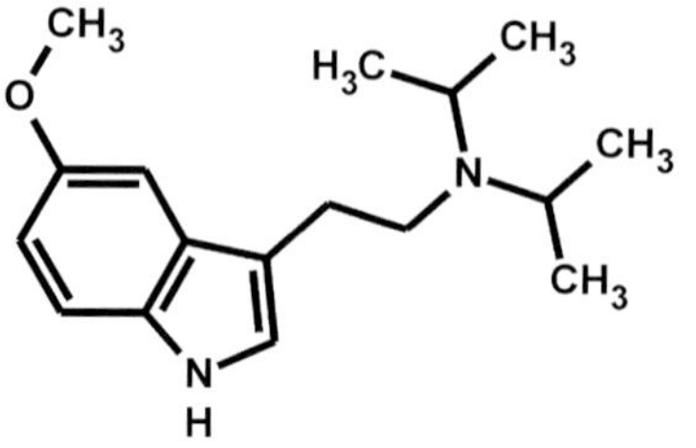

Figure 16.9 Chemical structure of tryptamines.

The formation of the initial MDPV metabolite–demethylenyl-MDPV–was detected in incubations of human liver microsomes, and CYP2C19, CYP2D6, and CYP1A2 [105].

16.3.7 Tryptamines

In general, tryptamines have high affinity for the serotonin 5-HT_2 receptors; hallucinogenic potencies are well correlated with the relative affinity of these compounds for the 5-HT_2 receptor [202]. Tryptamine derivatives that have been identified as synthetic hallucinogenic designer drugs include 5-MeO-DIPT (Foxy, Foxy Methoxy). The chemical structure is shown in Figure 16.9.

16.3.7.1 5-Methoxy-diisopropyl-tryptamine (5-MeO-DIPT)

The following metabolic steps of 5-MeO-DIPT were deduced from identified metabolites [106, 107, 203, 204]: *O*-demethylation to 5-hydroxy-DIPT and hydroxylation at position 6 to 6-hydroxy-5-MeO-DIPT, – both steps followed by conjugation to sulfates and glucuronides. *N*-Dealkylation of the side-chain led to the corresponding secondary amine. 5-Hydroxy-DIPT and 6-hydroxy-5-MeO-DIPT were found to be the major metabolites. Another study reported 5-methoxyindoleacetic acid in addition to the *O*-demethyl and *N*-dealkyl metabolites to be formed in the rat model [205]. In poor metabolizer human liver microsomes, *O*-demethylation was the major step and *N*-dealkylation the minor one. In rat liver microsomes, *O*-demethylation was predominant in a low substrate concentration range, while *N*-dealkylation became important in a high substrate concentration range [107, 204].

CYP2D6 is the major and preferred human CYP enzyme for the *O*-demethylation of 5-MeO-DIPT [107, 204].

References

1 Balikova, M. (2005) Nonfatal and fatal DOB (2,5-dimethoxy-4-bromoamphetamine) overdose. *Forensic Sci. Int.*, **153**, 85–91.

2 Ewald, A.H., Ehlers, D., and Maurer, H.H. (2008) Metabolism and toxicological detection of the designer drug 4-chloro-2,5-dimethoxyamphetamine in rat urine using gas chromatography-mass spectrometry. *Anal. Bioanal. Chem.*, **390**, 1837–1842.

3 Ewald, A.H., Fritschi, G., Bork, W.R., and Maurer, H.H. (2006) Designer drugs 2,5-dimethoxy-4-bromoamphetamine (DOB) and 2,5-dimethoxy-4-bromomethamphetamine (MDOB): studies on their metabolism and toxicological detection in rat urine using gas chromatographic/mass spectrometric techniques. *J. Mass Spectrom.*, **41**, 487–498.

4 Ewald, A.H., Fritschi, G., and Maurer, H.H. (2006) Designer drug 2,4,5-trimethoxyamphetamine (TMA-2): studies on its metabolism and toxicological detection in rat urine using gas chromatographic/mass spectrometric techniques. *J. Mass Spectrom.*, **41**, 1140–1148.

5 Ewald, A.H., Fritschi, G., and Maurer, H.H. (2007) Metabolism and toxicological detection of the designer drug 4-iodo-2,5-dimethoxy-amphetamine (DOI) in rat urine using gas chromatography-mass spectrometry. *J. Chromatogr. B*, **857**, 170–174.

6 Ewald, A.H., Puetz, M., and Maurer, H.H. (2008) Designer drug 2,5-dimethoxy-4-methyl-amphetamine (DOM, STP): involvement of the cytochrome P450 isoenzymes in formation of its main metabolite and detection of the latter in rat urine as proof of a drug intake using gas chromatography-mass spectrometry. *J. Chromatogr. B*, **862**, 252–256.

7 Theobald, D.S., Fehn, S., and Maurer, H.H. (2005) New designer drug 2,5-dimethoxy-4-propylthiophenethylamine (2C-T-7): studies on its metabolism and toxicological detection in rat urine using gas chromatography/mass spectrometry. *J. Mass Spectrom.*, **40**, 105–116.

8 Theobald, D.S., Fritschi, G., and Maurer, H.H. (2007) Studies on the toxicological detection of the designer drug 4-bromo-2,5-dimethoxy-beta-phenethylamine (2C-B) in rat urine using gas chromatography-mass spectrometry. *J. Chromatogr. B*, **846**, 374–377.

9 Theobald, D.S. and Maurer, H.H. (2006) Studies on the metabolism and toxicological detection of the designer drug 2,5-dimethoxy-4-methyl-beta-phenethylamine (2C-D) in rat urine using gas chromatographic-mass spectrometric techniques. *J. Mass Spectrom.*, **41**, 1509–1519.

10 Theobald, D.S. and Maurer, H.H. (2006) Studies on the metabolism and toxicological detection of the designer drug 4-ethyl-2,5-dimethoxy-beta-phenethylamine (2C-E) in rat urine using gas chromatographic-mass spectrometric techniques. *J. Chromatogr. B*, **842**, 76–90.

11 Theobald, D.S., Putz, M., Schneider, E., and Maurer, H.H. (2006) New designer drug 4-iodo-2,5-dimethoxy-beta-phenethylamine (2C-I): studies on its metabolism and toxicological detection in rat urine using gas chromatographic/mass spectrometric and capillary electrophoretic/mass spectrometric techniques. *J. Mass Spectrom.*, **41**, 872–886.

12 Theobald, D.S., Staack, R.F., Puetz, M., and Maurer, H.H. (2005) New designer drug 2,5-dimethoxy-4-ethylthio-beta-phenethylamine (2C-T-2): studies on its metabolism and toxicological detection in rat urine using gas chromatography/mass spectrometry. *J. Mass Spectrom.*, **40**, 1157–1172.

13 Kamata, H.T., Shima, N., Zaitsu, K., Kamata, T., Miki, A., Nishikawa, M., Katagi, M., and Tsuchihashi, H. (2006) Metabolism of the recently encountered designer drug, methylone, in humans and rats. *Xenobiotica*, **36**, 709–723.

14 Zaitsu, K., Katagi, M., Kamata, H.T., Kamata, T., Shima, N., Miki, A., Tsuchihashi, H., and Mori, Y. (2009) Determination of the metabolites of the new designer drugs bk-MBDB and bk-MDEA in human urine. *Forensic Sci. Int.*, **188**, 131–139.

15 Sauer, C., Peters, F.T., Staack, R.F., Fritschi, G., and Maurer, H.H. (2006)

New designer drug (1-(1-phenylcyclohexyl)-3-ethoxypropylamine (PCEPA)): studies on its metabolism and toxicological detection in rat urine using gas chromatography/mass spectrometry. *J. Mass Spectrom.*, **41**, 1014–1029.

16 Sauer, C., Peters, F.T., Staack, R.F., Fritschi, G., and Maurer, H.H. (2008) Metabolism and toxicological detection of a new designer drug, *N*-(1-phenylcyclohexyl)propanamine, in rat urine using gas chromatography-mass spectrometry. *J. Chromatogr. A*, **1186**, 380–390.

17 Sauer, C., Peters, F.T., Staack, R.F., Fritschi, G., and Maurer, H.H. (2008) Metabolism and toxicological detection of the designer drug *N*-(1-phenylcyclohexyl)-3-methoxypropanamine (PCMPA) in rat urine using gas chromatography-mass spectrometry. *Forensic Sci. Int.*, **181**, 47–51.

18 Sauer, C., Peters, F.T., Staack, R.F., Fritschi, G., and Maurer, H.H. (2008) New designer drugs *N*-(1-phenylcyclohexyl)-2-ethoxyethanamine (PCEEA) and *N*-(1-phenylcyclohexyl)-2-methoxyethanamine (PCMEA): studies on their metabolism and toxicological detection in rat urine using gas chromatographic/mass spectrometric techniques. *J. Mass Spectrom.*, **43**, 305–316.

19 Maurer, H.H., Kraemer, T., Springer, D., and Staack, R.F. (2004) Chemistry, pharmacology, toxicology, and hepatic metabolism of designer drugs of the amphetamine (ecstasy), piperazine, and pyrrolidinophenone types, a synopsis. *Ther. Drug Monit.*, **26**, 127–131.

20 Staack, R.F., Fritschi, G., and Maurer, H.H. (2002) Studies on the metabolism and the toxicological analysis of the new piperazine-like designer drug *N*-benzylpiperazine in urine using gas chromatography-mass spectrometry. *J. Chromatogr. B*, **773**, 35–46.

21 Staack, R.F., Fritschi, G., and Maurer, H.H. (2003) New designer drug 1-(3-trifluoromethylphenyl)piperazine (TFMPP): gas chromatography/mass spectrometry and liquid chromatography/mass spectrometry studies on its phase I and II metabolism and on its toxicological detection in rat urine. *J. Mass Spectrom.*, **38**, 971–981.

22 Staack, R.F. and Maurer, H.H. (2003) Piperazine-derived designer drug 1-(3-chlorophenyl)piperazine (mCPP): GC-MS studies on its metabolism and its toxicological detection in urine including analytical differentiation from its precursor drugs trazodone and nefazodone. *J. Anal. Toxicol.*, **27**, 560–568.

23 Staack, R.F. and Maurer, H.H. (2003) Toxicological detection of the new designer drug 1-(4-methoxyphenyl) piperazine and its metabolites in urine and differentiation from an intake of structurally related medicaments using gas chromatography-mass spectrometry. *J. Chromatogr. B*, **798**, 333–342.

24 Staack, R.F. and Maurer, H.H. (2004) New designer drug 1-(3,4-methylene dioxybenzyl) piperazine (MDBP): studies on its metabolism and toxicological detection in rat urine using gas chromatography/mass spectrometry. *J. Mass Spectrom.*, **39**, 255–261.

25 Tsutsumi, H., Katagi, M., Miki, A., Shima, N., Kamata, T., Nakajima, K., Inoue, H., Kishi, T., and Tsuchihashi, H. (2005) Isolation, identification and excretion profile of the principal urinary metabolite of the recently banned designer drug 1-(3-trifluoromethylphenyl)piperazine (TFMPP) in rats. *Xenobiotica*, **35**, 107–116.

26 Tsutsumi, H., Katagi, M., Miki, A., Shima, N., Kamata, T., Nakajima, K., Inoue, H., Kishi, T., and Tsuchihashi, H. (2006) Metabolism and the urinary excretion profile of the recently scheduled designer drug *N*-benzylpiperazine (BZP) in the rat. *J. Anal. Toxicol.*, **30**, 38–43.

27 Tsutsumi, H., Katagi, M., Miki, A., Shima, N., Kamata, T., Nishikawa, M., Nakajima, K., and Tsuchihashi, H. (2005) Development of simultaneous gas chromatography-mass spectrometric and liquid chromatography-electrospray ionization mass spectrometric determination method for the new

designer drugs, N-benzylpiperazine (BZP), 1-(3-trifluoromethylphenyl) piperazine (TFMPP) and their main metabolites in urine. *J. Chromatogr. B*, **819**, 315–322.

28 Peters, F.T., Meyer, M.R., Fritschi, G., and Maurer, H.H. (2005) Studies on the metabolism and toxicological detection of the new designer drug 4′-methyl-alpha-pyrrolidinobutyrophenone (MPBP) in urine using gas chromatography-mass spectrometry. *J. Chromatogr. B*, **824**, 81–91.

29 Sauer, C., Peters, F.T., Haas, C., Meyer, M.R., Fritschi, G., and Maurer, H.H. (2009) New designer drug alpha-pyrrolidinovalerophenone (PVP): studies on its metabolism and toxicological detection in rat urine using gas chromatographic/mass spectrometric techniques. *J. Mass Spectrom.*, **44**, 952–964.

30 Springer, D., Fritschi, G., and Maurer, H.H. (2003) Metabolism and toxicological detection of the new designer drug 3′,4′-methylenedioxy-alpha-pyrrolidinopropiophenone studied in urine using gas chromatography-mass spectrometry. *J. Chromatogr. B*, **793**, 377–388.

31 Springer, D., Fritschi, G., and Maurer, H.H. (2003) Metabolism and toxicological detection of the new designer drug 4′-methoxy-α-pyrrolidinopropiophenone studied in rat urine using gas chromatography-mass spectrometry. *J. Chromatogr. B*, **793**, 331–342.

32 Springer, D., Fritschi, G., and Maurer, H.H. (2003) Metabolism of the new designer drug alpha-pyrrolidinopropiophenone (PPP) and the toxicological detection of PPP and 4′methyl-alpha-pyrrolidinopropiophenone (MPPP) studied in urine using gas chromatography-mass spectrometry. *J. Chromatogr. B*, **796**, 253–266.

33 Springer, D., Peters, F.T., Fritschi, G., and Maurer, H.H. (2002) Studies on the metabolism and toxicological detection of the new designer drug 4′-methyl-alpha-pyrrolidinopropiophenone in urine using gas chromatography-mass spectrometry. *J. Chromatogr. B*, **773**, 25–33.

34 Springer, D., Peters, F.T., Fritschi, G., and Maurer, H.H. (2003) New designer drug 4′-methyl-alpha-pyrrolidinohexanophenone: studies on its metabolism and toxicological detection in urine using gas chromatography-mass spectrometry. *J. Chromatogr. B*, **789**, 79–91.

35 Staack, R.F. and Maurer, H.H. (2005) Metabolism of designer drugs of abuse. *Curr. Drug Metab.*, **6**, 259–274.

36 Meatherall, R. and Sharma, P. (2003) Foxy, a designer tryptamine hallucinogen. *J. Anal. Toxicol.*, **27**, 313–317.

37 Muller, A.A. (2004) New drugs of abuse update: Foxy Methoxy. *J. Emerg. Nurs.*, **30**, 507–508.

38 Sanders, B., Lankenau, S.E., Bloom, J.J., and Hathazi, D. (2008) "Research chemicals": tryptamine and phenethylamine use among high-risk youth. *Subst. Use Misuse*, **43**, 389–402.

39 Shulgin, A.T. and Carter, M.F. (1980) *N,N*-Diisopropyltryptamine (DIPT) and 5-methoxy-*N,N*-diisopropyltryptamine (5-MeO-DIPT). Two orally active tryptamine analogs with CNS activity. *Commun. Psychopharmacol.*, **4**, 363–369.

40 Tanaka, E., Kamata, T., Katagi, M., Tsuchihashi, H., and Honda, K. (2006) A fatal poisoning with 5-methoxy-*N,N*-diisopropyltryptamine, Foxy. *Forensic Sci. Int.*, **163**, 152–154.

41 Wilson, J.M., McGeorge, F., Smolinske, S., and Meatherall, R. (2005) A foxy intoxication. *Forensic Sci. Int.*, **148**, 31–36.

42 Maurer, H.H. (2004) Position of chromatographic techniques in screening for detection of drugs or poisons in clinical and forensic toxicology and/or doping control. *Clin. Chem. Lab. Med.*, **42**, 1310–1324.

43 Vandevenne, M., Vandenbussche, H., and Verstraete, A. (2000) Detection time of drugs of abuse in urine. *Acta Clin. Belg.*, **55**, 323–333.

44 Verstraete, A.G. (2004) Detection times of drugs of abuse in blood, urine, and oral fluid. *Ther. Drug Monit.*, **26**, 200–205.

45 Toennes, S.W.H. and Maurer, H.H. (1997) Microsoft Excel in pharmacokinetics – an easy way to solve kinetic problems in clinical toxicology, legal medicine or doping control, in *Proceedings of the 34th International TIAFT Meeting* (eds H. Sachs, W. Bernhard, and A. Jaeger), Molina Press, Leipzig, pp. 201–204.
46 Antoniou, T. and Tseng, A.L. (2002) Interactions between recreational drugs and antiretroviral agents. *Ann. Pharmacother.*, **36**, 1598–1613.
47 Eichelbaum, M., Ingelman-Sundberg, M., and Evans, W.E. (2006) Pharmacogenomics and individualized drug therapy. *Annu. Rev. Med.*, **57**, 119–137.
48 Evans, W.E. and McLeod, H.L. (2003) Pharmacogenomics – drug disposition, drug targets, and side effects. *N. Engl. J. Med.*, **348**, 538–549.
49 Howard, L.A., Sellers, E.M., and Tyndale, R.F. (2002) The role of pharmacogenetically-variable cytochrome P450 enzymes in drug abuse and dependence. *Pharmacogenomics*, **3**, 185–199.
50 Lotsch, J., Skarke, C., Liefhold, J., and Geisslinger, G. (2004) Genetic predictors of the clinical response to opioid analgesics: clinical utility and future perspectives. *Clin. Pharmacokinet.*, **43**, 983–1013.
51 Pritzker, D., Kanungo, A., Kilicarslan, T., Tyndale, R.F., and Sellers, E.M. (2002) Designer drugs that are potent inhibitors of CYP2D6. *J. Clin. Psychopharmacol.*, **22**, 330–332.
52 Rendic, S. (2002) Summary of information on human CYP enzymes: human P450 metabolism data. *Drug Metab. Rev.*, **34**, 83–448.
53 Tang, C., Lin, J.H., and Lu, A.Y. (2005) Metabolism-based drug–drug interactions: what determines individual variability in cytochrome P450 induction? *Drug Metab. Dispos.*, **33**, 603–613.
54 Zanger, U.M., Raimundo, S., and Eichelbaum, M. (2004) Cytochrome P450 2D6: overview and update on pharmacology, genetics, biochemistry. *Naunyn Schmiedebergs Arch. Pharmacol.*, **369**, 23–37.
55 Zhang, Z.Y. and Wong, Y.N. (2005) Enzyme kinetics for clinically relevant CYP inhibition. *Curr. Drug Metab.*, **6**, 241–257.
56 Kilpatrick, G.J. and Smith, T.W. (2005) Morphine-6-glucuronide: actions and mechanisms. *Med. Res. Rev.*, **25**, 521–544.
57 Kreek, M.J., Bart, G., Lilly, C., LaForge, K.S., and Nielsen, D.A. (2005) Pharmacogenetics and human molecular genetics of opiate and cocaine addictions and their treatments. *Pharmacol. Rev.*, **57**, 1–26.
58 Stone, A.N., Mackenzie, P.I., Galetin, A., Houston, J.B., and Miners, J.O. (2003) Isoform selectivity and kinetics of morphine 3- and 6-glucuronidation by human UDP-glucuronosyltransferases: evidence for atypical glucuronidation kinetics by UGT2B7. *Drug Metab. Dispos.*, **31**, 1086–1089.
59 Bencharit, S., Morton, C.L., Xue, Y., Potter, P.M., and Redinbo, M.R. (2003) Structural basis of heroin and cocaine metabolism by a promiscuous human drug-processing enzyme. *Nat. Struct. Biol.*, **10**, 349–356.
60 Brzezinski, M.R., Spink, B.J., Dean, R.A., Berkman, C.E., Cashman, J.R., and Bosron, W.F. (1997) Human liver carboxylesterase hCE-1: binding specificity for cocaine, heroin, and their metabolites and analogs. *Drug Metab. Dispos.*, **25**, 1089–1096.
61 Kamendulis, L.M., Brzezinski, M.R., Pindel, E.V., Bosron, W.F., and Dean, R.A. (1996) Metabolism of cocaine and heroin is catalyzed by the same human liver carboxylesterases. *J. Pharmacol. Exp. Ther.*, **279**, 713–717.
62 Dean, R.A., Christian, C.D., Sample, R.H., and Bosron, W.F. (1991) Human liver cocaine esterases: ethanol-mediated formation of ethylcocaine. *FASEB J.*, **5**, 2735–2739.
63 Hatfield, M.J., Tsurkan, L., Hyatt, J.L., Yu, X., Edwards, C.C., Hicks, L.D., Wadkins, R.M., and Potter, P.M. (2010) Biochemical and molecular analysis of carboxylesterase-mediated hydrolysis of

cocaine and heroin. *Br. J. Pharmacol.*, **160**, 1916–1928.

64 Laizure, S.C., Mandrell, T., Gades, N.M., and Parker, R.B. (2003) Cocaethylene metabolism and interaction with cocaine and ethanol: role of carboxylesterases. *Drug Metab. Dispos.*, **31**, 16–20.

65 Bland, T.M., Haining, R.L., Tracy, T.S., and Callery, P.S. (2005) CYP2C-catalyzed delta9-tetrahydrocannabinol metabolism: kinetics, pharmacogenetics and interaction with phenytoin. *Biochem. Pharmacol.*, **70**, 1096–1103.

66 Bornheim, L.M., Lasker, J.M., and Raucy, J.L. (1992) Human hepatic microsomal metabolism of delta 1-tetrahydrocannabinol. *Drug Metab. Dispos.*, **20**, 241–246.

67 Halldin, M.M., Widman, M., Bahr, V., Lindgren, J.E., and Martin, B.R. (1982) Identification of *in vitro* metabolites of delta 1-tetrahydrocannabinol formed by human livers. *Drug Metab. Dispos.*, **10**, 297–301.

68 Watanabe, K., Matsunaga, T., Yamamoto, I., Funae, Y., and Yoshimura, H. (1995) Involvement of CYP2C in the metabolism of cannabinoids by human hepatic microsomes from an old woman. *Biol. Pharm. Bull.*, **18**, 1138–1141.

69 Kraemer, T. and Maurer, H.H. (2002) Toxicokinetics of amphetamines: metabolism and toxicokinetic data of designer drugs, of amphetamine, methamphetamine and their *N*-alkyl derivatives. *Ther. Drug Monit.*, **24**, 277–289.

70 Musshoff, F. (2000) Illegal or legitimate use? Precursor compounds to amphetamine and methamphetamine. *Drug Metab. Rev.*, **32**, 15–44.

71 Klette, K.L., Anderson, C.J., Poch, G.K., Nimrod, A.C., and ElSohly, M.A. (2000) Metabolism of lysergic acid diethylamide (LSD) to 2-oxo-3-hydroxy LSD (O-H-LSD) in human liver microsomes and cryopreserved human hepatocytes. *J. Anal. Toxicol.*, **24**, 550–556.

72 Nelson, C.C. and Foltz, R.L. (1992) Chromatographic and mass spectrometric methods for determination of lysergic acid diethylamide (LSD) and metabolites in body fluids. *J. Chromatogr.*, **580**, 97–109.

73 Poch, G.K., Klette, K.L., Hallare, D.A., Manglicmot, M.G., Czarny, R.J., McWhorter, L.K., and Anderson, C.J. (1999) Detection of metabolites of lysergic acid diethylamide (LSD) in human urine specimens: 2-oxo-3-hydroxy-LSD, a prevalent metabolite of LSD. *J. Chromatogr. B*, **724**, 23–33.

74 Reuschel, S.A., Eades, D., and Foltz, R.L. (1999) Recent advances in chromatographic and mass spectrometric methods for determination of LSD and its metabolites in physiological specimens. *J Chromatogr. B*, **733**, 145–159.

75 Verstraete, A.G. and Van de Velde, E.J. (1999) 2-Oxo-3-hydroxy-LSD: an important LSD metabolite? *Acta Clin. Belg. Suppl.*, **1**, 94–96.

76 Laurenzana, E.M. and Owens, S.M. (1997) Metabolism of phencyclidine by human liver microsomes. *Drug Metab. Dispos.*, **25**, 557–563.

77 Meyer, M.R., Peters, F.T., and Maurer, H.H. (2008) The role of human hepatic cytochrome P450 isozymes in the metabolism of racemic 3,4-methylenedioxy-methamphetamine and its enantiomers. *Drug Metab. Dispos.*, **36**, 2345–2354.

78 Meyer, M.R., Peters, F.T., and Maurer, H.H. (2009) The role of human hepatic cytochrome P450 isozymes in the metabolism of racemic 3,4-meth ylenedioxyethylamphetamine and its single enantiomers. *Drug Metab. Dispos.*, **37**, 1152–1156.

79 Meyer, M.R., Peters, F.T., and Maurer, H.H. (2009) Stereoselective differences in the cytochrome P450-dependent dealkylation and demethylenation of *N*-methyl-benzodioxolyl-butanamine (MBDB, Eden) enantiomers. *Biochem. Pharmacol.*, **77**, 1725–1734.

80 Meyer, M.R., Peters, F.T., and Maurer, H.H. (2009) Investigations on the human hepatic cytochrome P450 isozymes involved in the metabolism of 3,4-methylenedioxy-amphetamine (MDA) and benzodioxolyl-butanamine

(BDB) enantiomers. *Toxicol. Lett.*, **190**, 54–60.

81 Bach, M.V., Coutts, R.T., and Baker, G.B. (1999) Involvement of CYP2D6 in the *in vitro* metabolism of amphetamine, two *N*- alkylamphetamines and their 4-methoxylated derivatives. *Xenobiotica*, **29**, 719–732.

82 Kitchen, I., Tremblay, J., Andre, J., Dring, L.G., Idle, J.R., Smith, R.L., and Williams, R.T. (1979) Interindividual and interspecies variation in the metabolism of the hallucinogen 4-methoxyamphetamine. *Xenobiotica*, **9**, 397–404.

83 Wu, D., Otton, S.V., Inaba, T., Kalow, W., and Sellers, E.M. (1997) Interactions of amphetamine analogs with human liver CYP2D6. *Biochem. Pharmacol.*, **53**, 1605–1612.

84 Staack, R.F., Theobald, D.S., Paul, L.D., Springer, D., Kraemer, T., and Maurer, H.H. (2004) Identification of human cytochrome p450 2D6 as major enzyme involved in the *O*-demethylation of the designer drug *p*-methoxymethamphetamine. *Drug Metab. Dispos.*, **32**, 379–381.

85 Carmo, H., de Boer, D., Remiao, F., Carvalho, F., dos Reys, L.A., and Bastos, M.L. (2002) Identification of 4-methylthioamphetamine and some of its metabolites in mouse urine by GC-MS after acute administration. *J. Anal. Toxicol.*, **26**, 228–232.

86 Carmo, H., Hengstler, J.G., de Boer, D., Ringel, M., Carvalho, F., Fernandes, E., Remiao, F., dos Reys, L.A., Oesch, F., and De Lourdes, B.M. (2004) Comparative metabolism of the designer drug 4-methylthioamphetamine by hepatocytes from man, monkey, dog, rabbit, rat and mouse. *Naunyn Schmiedebergs Arch. Pharmacol.*, **369**, 198–205.

87 Elliott, S.P. (2000) Fatal poisoning with a new phenylethylamine: 4-methylthioamphetamine (4-MTA). *J. Anal. Toxicol.*, **24**, 85–89.

88 Ewald, A.H. and Maurer, H.H. (2008) 2,5-Dimethoxyamphetamine-derived designer drugs: studies on the identification of cytochrome P450 (CYP) isoenzymes involved in formation of their main metabolites and on their capability to inhibit CYP2D6. *Toxicol. Lett.*, **183**, 52–57.

89 Kanamori, T., Inoue, H., Iwata, Y., Ohmae, Y., and Kishi, T. (2002) *In vivo* metabolism of 4-bromo-2,5-dimethoxyphenethylamine (2C-B) in the rat: identification of urinary metabolites. *J. Anal. Toxicol.*, **26**, 61–66.

90 Kanamori, T., Tsujikawa, K., Ohmae, Y., Iwata, Y., Inoue, H., Inouye, Y., and Kishi, T. (2003) Excretory profile of 4-bromo-2,5-dimethoxy-phenethylamine (2C-B) in rat. *J. Health Sci.*, **49**, 166–169.

91 Kanamori, T., Tsujikawa, K., Ohmae, Y., Iwata, Y.T., Inoue, H., Kishi, T., Nakahama, T., and Inouye, Y. (2005) A study of the metabolism of methamphetamine and 4-bromo-2,5-dimethoxyphenethylamine (2C-B) in isolated rat hepatocytes. *Forensic Sci. Int.*, **148**, 131–137.

92 Theobald, D.S. and Maurer, H.H. (2007) Identification of monoamine oxidase and cytochrome P450 isoenzymes involved in the deamination of phenethylamine-derived designer drugs (2C-series). *Biochem. Pharmacol.*, **73**, 287–297.

93 Lin, L.C., Liu, J.T., Chou, S.H., and Lin, C.H. (2003) Identification of 2,5-dimethoxy-4-ethylthiophenethylamine and its metabolites in the urine of rats by gas chromatography-mass spectrometry. *J. Chromatogr. B*, **798**, 241–247.

94 Kanamori, T., Kuwayama, K., Tsujikawa, K., Miyaguchi, H., Iwata, Y.T., Inoue, H., and Kishi, T. (2007) *In vivo* metabolism of 2,5-dimethoxy-4-propylthiophenethylamine in rat. *Xenobiotica*, **37**, 679–692.

95 Meyer, M.R., Wilhelm, J., Peters, F.T., and Maurer, H.H. (2010) Beta-keto amphetamines: studies on the metabolism of the designer drug mephedrone and toxicological detection of mephedrone, butylone, and methylone in urine using gas chromatography-mass spectrometry. *Anal. Bioanal. Chem.*, **397**, 1225–1233.

96 Sauer, C., Peters, F.T., Schwaninger, A.E., Meyer, M.R., and Maurer, H.H. (2008) Identification of cytochrome P450

enzymes involved in the metabolism of the designer drugs *N*-(1-phenylcyclohexyl)-3-ethoxypropanamine (PCEPA) and *N*-(1-phenylcyclohexyl)-3-methoxypropanamine (PCMPA). *Chem. Res. Toxicol.*, **21**, 1949–1955.

97 Sauer, C., Peters, F.T., Schwaninger, A.E., Meyer, M.R., and Maurer, H.H. (2009) Investigations on the cytochrome P450 (CYP) isoenzymes involved in the metabolism of the designer drugs *N*-(1-phenylcyclohexyl)-2-ethoxyethanamine and *N*-(1-phenylcyclohexyl)-2-methoxyethanamine. *Biochem. Pharmacol.*, **77**, 444–450.

98 Staack, R.F., Paul, L.D., Springer, D., Kraemer, T., and Maurer, H.H. (2004) Cytochrome P450 dependent metabolism of the new designer drug 1-(3-trifluoromethylphenyl)piperazine (TFMPP). *In vivo* studies in Wistar and Dark Agouti rats as well as *in vitro* studies in human liver microsomes. *Biochem. Pharmacol.*, **67**, 235–244.

99 Barbhaiya, R.H., Shukla, U.A., and Greene, D.S. (1995) Single-dose pharmacokinetics of nefazodone in healthy young and elderly subjects and in subjects with renal or hepatic impairment. *Eur. J. Clin. Pharmacol.*, **49**, 221–228.

100 Staack, R.F., Theobald, D.S., Paul, L.D., Springer, D., Kraemer, T., and Maurer, H.H. (2004) *In vivo* metabolism of the new designer drug 1-(4-methoxyphenyl) piperazine (MeOPP) in rat and identification of the human cytochrome P450 enzymes responsible for the major metabolic step. *Xenobiotica*, **34**, 179–192.

101 Springer, D., Paul, L.D., Staack, R.F., Kraemer, T., and Maurer, H.H. (2003) Involvement of human hepatic cytochrome P450 isoenzymes in the metabolism of the new pyrrolidinophenone designer drugs MPPP, MOPPP, MDPPP and MPHP, in *Proceedings of the GTFCh Symposium* (eds F. Pragst and R. Aderjan), Helm, Heppenheim, pp. 204–211.

102 Springer, D., Paul, L.D., Staack, R.F., Kraemer, T., and Maurer, H.H. (2005) Identification of cytochrome P450 enzymes involved in the metabolism of 3′,4′-methylenedioxy-α-pyrrolidinopropiophenone (MDPPP), a designer drug, in human liver microsomes. *Xenobiotica*, **35**, 227–237.

103 Springer, D., Paul, L.D., Staack, R.F., Kraemer, T., and Maurer, H.H. (2003) Identification of the cytochrome P450 enzymes involved in the metabolism of 4′-methyl-(alpha)-pyrrolidinopropiophenone, a novel scheduled designer drug, in human liver microsomes. *Drug Metab. Dispos.*, **31**, 979–982.

104 Peters, F.T., Meyer, M.R., Theobald, D.S., and Maurer, H.H. (2008) Identification of cytochrome P450 enzymes involved in the metabolism of 4′-methyl-pyrrolidino-butyrophenone (MPBP), a new designer drug, in human liver microsomes. *Drug Metab. Dispos.*, **36**, 163–168.

105 Meyer, M.R., Du, P., Schuster, F., and Maurer, H.H. (2010) Studies on the metabolism of the alpha-pyrrolidinophenone designer drug methylenedioxy-pyrovalerone (MDPV) in rat urine and human liver microsomes using GC-MS and LC-high-resolution-MS and its detectability in urine by GC-MS. *J. Mass Spectrom.*, **45**, 1426–1442.

106 Kamata, T., Katagi, M., Kamata, H.T., Miki, A., Shima, N., Zaitsu, K., Nishikawa, M., Tanaka, E., Honda, K., and Tsuchihashi, H. (2006) Metabolism of the psychotomimetic tryptamine derivative 5-methoxy-*N*,*N*-diisopropyltryptamine in humans: identification and quantification of its urinary metabolites. *Drug Metab. Dispos.*, **34**, 281–287.

107 Narimatsu, S., Yonemoto, R., Saito, K., Takaya, K., Kumamoto, T., Ishikawa, T., Asanuma, M., Funada, M., Kiryu, K., Naito, S., Yoshida, Y., Yamamoto, S., and Hanioka, N. (2006) Oxidative metabolism of 5-methoxy-*N*,*N*-diisopropyltryptamine (Foxy) by human liver microsomes and recombinant cytochrome P450 enzymes. *Biochem. Pharmacol.*, **71**, 1377–1385.

108 Projean, D., Morin, P.E., Tu, T.M., and Ducharme, J. (2003) Identification of CYP3A4 and CYP2C8 as the major cytochrome P450 s responsible for

morphine *N*-demethylation in human liver microsomes. *Xenobiotica*, **33**, 841–854.

109 LeDuc, B.W., Sinclair, P.R., Shuster, L., Sinclair, J.F., Evans, J.E., and Greenblatt, D.J. (1993) Norcocaine and *N*-hydroxynorcocaine formation in human liver microsomes: role of cytochrome P-450 3A4. *Pharmacology*, **46**, 294–300.

110 Kloss, M.W., Rosen, G.M., and Rauckman, E.J. (1983) *N*-demethylation of cocaine to norcocaine. Evidence for participation by cytochrome P-450 and FAD-containing monooxygenase. *Mol. Pharmacol.*, **23**, 482–485.

111 Pellinen, P., Kulmala, L., Konttila, J., Auriola, S., Pasanen, M., and Juvonen, R. (2000) Kinetic characteristics of norcocaine *N*-hydroxylation in mouse and human liver microsomes: involvement of CYP enzymes. *Arch. Toxicol.*, **74**, 511–520.

112 Cone, E.J., Tsadik, A., Oyler, J., and Darwin, W.D. (1998) Cocaine metabolism and urinary excretion after different routes of administration. *Ther. Drug Monit.*, **20**, 556–560.

113 Zhang, J.Y. and Foltz, R.L. (1990) Cocaine metabolism in man: identification of four previously unreported cocaine metabolites in human urine. *J. Anal. Toxicol.*, **14**, 201–205.

114 Nadulski, T., Pragst, F., Weinberg, G., Roser, P., Schnelle, M., Fronk, E.M., and Stadelmann, A.M. (2005) Randomized, double blind, placebo-controlled study about the effects of cannabidiol (CBD) on the pharmacokinetics of delta9-tetrahydrocannabinol (THC) after oral application of THC verses standardized cannabis extract. *Ther. Drug Monit.*, **27**, 799–810.

115 Wall, M.E., Sadler, B.M., Brine, D., Taylor, H., and Perez-Reyes, M. (1983) Metabolism, disposition, and kinetics of delta-9-tetrahydrocannabinol in men and women. *Clin. Pharmacol. Ther.*, **34**, 352–363.

116 Williams, P.L. and Moffat, A.C. (1980) Identification in human urine of delta 9-tetrahydrocannabinol-11-oic acid glucuronide: a tetrahydrocannabinol metabolite. *J. Pharm. Pharmacol.*, **32**, 445–448.

117 Mazur, A., Lichti, C.F., Prather, P.L., Zielinska, A.K., Bratton, S.M., Gallus-Zawada, A., Finel, M., Miller, G.P., Radominska-Pandya, A., and Moran, J.H. (2009) Characterization of human hepatic and extrahepatic UDP-glucuronosyltransferase enzymes involved in the metabolism of classic cannabinoids. *Drug Metab. Dispos.*, **37**, 1496–1504.

118 Sachse-Seeboth, C., Pfeil, J., Sehrt, D., Meineke, I., Tzvetkov, M., Bruns, E., Poser, W., Vormfelde, S.V., and Brockmoller, J. (2009) Interindividual variation in the pharmacokinetics of Delta9-tetrahydrocannabinol as related to genetic polymorphisms in CYP2C9. *Clin. Pharmacol. Ther.*, **85**, 273–276.

119 Law, M.Y., Slawson, M.H., and Moody, D.E. (2000) Selective involvement of cytochrome P450 2D subfamily in *in vivo* 4-hydroxylation of amphetamine in rat. *Drug Metab. Dispos.*, **28**, 348–353.

120 Lin, L.Y., Di Stefano, E.W., Schmitz, D.A., Hsu, L., Ellis, S.W., Lennard, M.S., Tucker, G.T., and Cho, A.K. (1997) Oxidation of methamphetamine and methylenedioxymethamphetamine by CYP2D6. *Drug Metab. Dispos.*, **25**, 1059–1064.

121 Shiiyama, S., Soejima, O.T., Honda, S., Kumagai, Y., Cho, A.K., Yamada, H., Oguri, K., and Yoshimura, H. (1997) Major role of the CYP2C isozymes in deamination of amphetamine and benzphetamine: evidence for the quinidine-specific inhibition of the reactions catalysed by rabbit enzyme. *Xenobiotica*, **27**, 379–387.

122 Passie, T., Halpern, J.H., Stichtenoth, D.O., Emrich, H.M., and Hintzen, A. (2008) The pharmacology of lysergic acid diethylamide: a review. *CNS Neurosci. Ther.*, **14**, 295–314.

123 Holsztynska, E.J. and Domino, E.F. (1985) Biotransformation of phencyclidine. *Drug Metab. Rev.*, **16**, 285–320.

124 Jushchyshyn, M.I., Kent, U.M., and Hollenberg, P.F. (2003) The mechanism-based inactivation of human cytochrome

P450 2B6 by phencyclidine. *Drug Metab. Dispos.*, **31**, 46–52.

125 Driscoll, J.P., Kornecki, K., Wolkowski, J.P., Chupak, L., Kalgutkar, A.S., and O'Donnell, J.P. (2007) Bioactivation of phencyclidine in rat and human liver microsomes and recombinant P450 2B enzymes: evidence for the formation of a novel quinone methide intermediate. *Chem. Res. Toxicol.*, **20**, 1488–1497.

126 Meyer, M.R. and Maurer, H.H. (2010) Metabolism of designer drugs of abuse: an updated review. *Curr. Drug Metab.*, **11**, 468–482.

127 de la Torre, R., Farre, M., Roset, P.N., Pizarro, N., Abanades, S., Segura, M., Segura, J., and Cami, J. (2004) Human pharmacology of MDMA: pharmacokinetics, metabolism, and disposition. *Ther. Drug Monit.*, **26**, 137–144.

128 Maurer, H.H. (1996) On the metabolism and the toxicological analysis of methylenedioxyphenylalkylamine designer drugs by gas chromatography-mass spectrometry. *Ther. Drug Monit.*, **18**, 465–470.

129 Maurer, H.H., Bickeboeller-Friedrich, J., Kraemer, T., and Peters, F.T. (2000) Toxicokinetics and analytical toxicology of amphetamine-derived designer drugs ("Ecstasy"). *Toxicol. Lett.*, **112**, 133–142.

130 Hiramatsu, M., Kumagai, Y., Unger, S.E., and Cho, A.K. (1990) Metabolism of methylenedioxymethamphetamine: formation of dihydroxymethamphetamine and a quinone identified as its glutathione adduct. *J. Pharmacol. Exp. Ther.*, **254**, 521–527.

131 Miller, R.T., Lau, S.S., and Monks, T.J. (1995) Metabolism of 5-(glutathion-*S*-yl)-alpha-methyldopamine following intracerebroventricular administration to male Sprague-Dawley rats. *Chem. Res. Toxicol.*, **8**, 634–641.

132 Meyer, M.R. and Maurer, H.H. (2009) Enantioselectivity in the methylation of the catecholic phase-I metabolites of methylenedioxy designer drugs and their capability to inhibit COMT catalyzed dopamine 3-methylation. *Chem. Res. Toxicol.*, **22**, 1205–1211.

133 Schwaninger, A.E., Meyer, M.R., Zapp, J., and Maurer, H.H. (2009) The role of human UDP-glucuronyltransferases on the formation of the methylenedioxymethamphetamine (Ecstasy) phase II metabolites *R*- and *S*-3-methoxymethamphetamine 4-*O*-glucuronides. *Drug Metab. Dispos.*, **37**, 2212–2220.

134 Beckett, A.H. and Midha, K.K. (1974) The indentification of four metabolic products after incubation of *p*-methoxyamphetamine with liver preparations of various species. *Xenobiotica*, **4**, 297–311.

135 Hubbard, J.W., Bailey, K., Midha, K.K., and Cooper, J.K. (1981) 3-*O*-methyl-alpha-methyldopamine, a urinary metabolite of *p*-methoxyamphetamine in dog and monkey. *Drug Metab. Dispos.*, **9**, 250–254.

136 Hubbard, J.W., Midha, K.K., and Cooper, J.K. (1977) The metabolism of *p*-methoxyamphetamine in dog and monkey. *O*-demethylation as a major route. *Drug Metab. Dispos.*, **5**, 329–334.

137 Staack, R.F., Fehn, J., and Maurer, H.H. (2003) New designer drug *para*-methoxymethamphetamine: studies on its metabolism and toxicological detection in urine using gas chromatography-mass spectrometry. *J. Chromatogr. B*, **789**, 27–41.

138 Petzsche, M. and Furst, W. (1988) [Preparation, detection and pharmacokinetic behavior of pholedrine sulfuric acid ester. 5. Methods for determining pholedrine and pholedrine sulfuric acid esters in plasma]. *Pharmazie*, **43**, 867–868.

139 Petzsche, M. and Furst, W. (1988) [Preparation, detection and pharmacokinetic behavior of pholedrine sulfuric acid esters. 4. Detection and determination of pholedrine sulfuric acid esters in urine]. *Pharmazie*, **43**, 291–292.

140 Petzsche, M., Furst, W., Fahr, A., and Sziegoleit, W. (1988) [Preparation, detection and pharmacokinetic behavior of pholedrine sulfuric acid ester. 6. Determination of pholedrine and pholedrine sulfuric acid esters in plasma

after oral administration of pholedrine]. *Pharmazie*, **43**, 875.

141 Petzsche, M., Neubert, R., and Furst, W. (1988) [Production, analysis and pharmacokinetic behavior of pholedrin sulfuric acid esters. 1. Production and analysis of pholedrin sulfuric acid esters]. *Pharmazie*, **43**, 46–47.

142 Ho, B.T., Estevez, V., and Fritchie, G.E. (1971) The fate of 2,5-dimethoxy-4-methylamphetamine (STP, DOM) in monkey and rat brains. *Brain Res.*, **29**, 166–169.

143 Ho, B.T., Estevez, V., Tansey, L.W., Englert, L.F., Creaven, P.J., and McIsaac, W.M. (1971) Analogs of amphetamine. 5. Studies of excretory metabolites of 1-(2,5-dimethoxy-4-methylphenyl)-2-aminopropane (DOM) in rats. *J. Med. Chem.*, **14**, 158–160.

144 Shulgin, A. (1991) *Pihkal: A Chemical Love Story*, Transform Press, Berkley, CA.

145 de Boer, D. and Bosman, I. (2004) A new trend in drugs-of-abuse; the 2C-series of phenethylamine designer drugs. *Pharm. World Sci.*, **26**, 110–113.

146 Maurer, H.H., Pfleger, K., and Weber, A.A. (2007) *Mass Spectral and GC Data of Drugs, Poisons, Pesticides, Pollutants and Their Metabolites*, Wiley-VCH Verlag GmbH, Weinheim.

147 Carmo, H., Boer, D., Remiao, F., Carvalho, F., Reys, L.A., and Bastos, M.L. (2004) Metabolism of the designer drug 4-bromo-2,5-dimethoxyphenethylamine (2C-B) in mice, after acute administration. *J. Chromatogr. B*, **811**, 143–152.

148 Carmo, H., Hengstler, J.G., de Boer, D., Ringel, M., Remiao, F., Carvalho, F., Fernandes, E., dos Reys, L.A., Oesch, F., and De Lourdes, B.M. (2005) Metabolic pathways of 4-bromo-2,5-dimethoxyphenethylamine (2C-B): analysis of phase I metabolism with hepatocytes of six species including human. *Toxicology*, **206**, 75–89.

149 Bossong, M.G., Van Dijk, J.P., and Niesink, R.J. (2005) Methylone and mCPP, two new drugs of abuse? *Addict. Biol.*, **10**, 321–323.

150 Shimizu, E., Watanabe, H., Kojima, T., Hagiwara, H., Fujisaki, M., Miyatake, R., Hashimoto, K., and Iyo, M. (2007) Combined intoxication with methylone and 5-MeO-MIPT. *Prog. Neuropsychopharmacol. Biol. Psychiatry*, **31**, 288–291.

151 Springer, D., Peters, F.T., Fritschi, G., and Maurer, H.H. (2002) GC-MS studies on the metabolism and toxicological analysis of the new pyrrolidino-hexanophenone designer drug 4′-methyl-alpha-pyrrolidinohexanophenone (MPHP). *Ann. Toxicol. Anal.*, **14**, 212.

152 Maddox, V.H., Godefroi, E.F., and Parcell, R.F. (1965) Synthesis of phencyclidine and other 1-arylcyclohexylamines. *J. Med. Chem.*, **8**, 230–235.

153 Rang, H.P., Dale, M.M., and Ritter, J.M. (1999) *Pharmacology*, Churchill Livingston, London.

154 Takeda, H., Gazzara, R.A., and Howard, S.G. (1986) Phenylcyclohexylamine: effect of a metabolite of phencyclidine on the efflux of dopamine in the rat. *Neuropharmacology*, **25**, 1341–1345.

155 Rae, J.M., Soukhova, N.V., Flockhart, D.A., and Desta, Z. (2002) Triethylenethiophosphoramide is a specific inhibitor of cytochrome P450 2B6: implications for cyclophosphamide metabolism. *Drug Metab. Dispos.*, **30**, 525–530.

156 Turpeinen, M., Raunio, H., and Pelkonen, O. (2006) The functional role of CYP2B6 in human drug metabolism: substrates and inhibitors *in vitro, in vivo* and *in silico*. *Curr. Drug Metab.*, **7**, 705–714.

157 Hesse, L.M., Venkatakrishnan, K., Court, M.H., von Moltke, L.L., Duan, S.X., Shader, R.I., and Greenblatt, D.J. (2000) CYP2B6 mediates the *in vitro* hydroxylation of bupropion: potential drug interactions with other antidepressants. *Drug Metab. Dispos.*, **28**, 1176–1183.

158 Tekes, K., Tothfalusi, L., Malomvolgyi, B., Herman, F., and Magyar, K. (1987) Studies on the biochemical mode of action of EGYT-475, a new antidepressant. *Pol. J. Pharmacol. Pharm.*, **39**, 203–211.

159 Hashimoto, K., Maeda, H., and Goromaru, T. (1992) Effects of benzylpiperazine derivatives on the neurotoxicity of 3,4-meth ylenedioxymethamphetamine in rat brain. *Brain Res.*, **590**, 341–344.

160 Magyar, K., Fekete, M.I., Tekes, K., and Torok, T.L. (1986) The action of trelibet, a new antidepressive agent on [^{3}H] noradrenaline release from rabbit pulmonary artery. *Eur. J. Pharmacol.*, **130**, 219–227.

161 Oberlander, C., Euvrard, C., Dumont, C., and Boissier, J.R. (1979) Circling behaviour induced by dopamine releasers and/or uptake inhibitors during degeneration of the nigrostriatal pathway. *Eur. J. Pharmacol.*, **60**, 163–170.

162 Szucks, Z., Szentendrei, T., and Fekete, M.I. (1987) The effect of EGYT-475 (Trelibet) and its metabolites on the potassium-stimulated ^{3}H-noradrenaline release from cortical slices of rat brain. *Pol. J. Pharmacol. Pharm.*, **39**, 185–193.

163 Bye, C., Munro, F.A., Peck, A.W., and Young, P.A. (1973) A comparison of the effects of 1-benzylpiperazine and dexamphetamine on human performance tests. *Eur. J. Clin. Pharmacol.*, **6**, 163–169.

164 Caccia, S., Fong, M.H., and Urso, R. (1985) Ionization constants and partition coefficients of 1-arylpiperazine derivatives. *J. Pharm. Pharmacol.*, **37**, 567–570.

165 Cunningham, K.A. and Appel, J.B. (1986) Possible 5-hydroxytryptamine1 (5-HT$_1$) receptor involvement in the stimulus properties of 1-(*m*-trifluoromethylphenyl)piperazine (TFMPP). *J. Pharmacol. Exp. Ther.*, **237**, 369–377.

166 Fuller, R.W., Snoddy, H.D., Mason, N.R., and Molloy, B.R. (1978) Effect of 1-(*m*-trifluoromethylphenyl)-piperazine on ^{3}H-serotonin binding to membranes from rat brain *in vitro* and on serotonin turnover in rat brain *in vivo*. *Eur. J. Pharmacol.*, **52**, 11–16.

167 Glennon, R.A. (1987) Central serotonin receptors as targets for drug research. *J. Med. Chem.*, **30**, 1–12.

168 Hoyer, D., Clarke, D.E., Fozard, J.R., Hartig, P.R., Martin, G.R., Mylecharane, E.J., Saxena, P.R., and Humphrey, P.P. (1994) International Union of Pharmacology classification of receptors for 5-hydroxytryptamine (Serotonin). *Pharmacol. Rev.*, **46**, 157–203.

169 Middlemiss, D.N. and Tricklebank, M.D. (1992) Centrally active 5-HT receptor agonists and antagonists. *Neurosci. Biobehav. Rev.*, **16**, 75–82.

170 Pettibone, D.J. and Williams, M. (1984) Serotonin-releasing effects of substituted piperazines *in vitro*. *Biochem. Pharmacol.*, **33**, 1531–1535.

171 Hernandez, E.J., Williams, P.A., and Dudek, F.E. (2002) Effects of fluoxetine and TFMPP on spontaneous seizures in rats with pilocarpine-induced epilepsy. *Epilepsia*, **43**, 1337–1345.

172 Herndon, J.L., Pierson, M.E., and Glennon, R.A. (1992) Mechanistic investigation of the stimulus properties of 1-(3-trifluoromethylphenyl)piperazine. *Pharmacol. Biochem. Behav.*, **43**, 739–748.

173 Schechter, M.D. (1988) Serotonergic-dopaminergic mediation of 3,4-meth ylenedioxymethamphetamine (MDMA, "ecstasy"). *Pharmacol. Biochem. Behav.*, **31**, 817–824.

174 Schechter, M.D. (1988) Use of TFMPP stimulus properties as a model of 5-HT$_{1B}$ receptor activation. *Pharmacol. Biochem. Behav.*, **31**, 53–57.

175 Murphy, D.L., Lesch, K.P., Aulakh, C.S., and Pigott, T.A. (1991) Serotonin-selective arylpiperazines with neuroendocrine, behavioral, temperature, and cardiovascular effects in humans. *Pharmacol. Rev.*, **43**, 527–552.

176 Caccia, S. (1990) In-vivo metabolism of 4-substituted arylpiperazines to pharmacologically active 1-arylpiperazines. *Boll. Chim. Farm.*, **129**, 183–189.

177 Caccia, S., Ballabio, M., Samanin, R., Zanini, M.G., and Garattini, S. (1981) (–)-*m*-Chlorophenyl-piperazine, a central 5-hydroxytryptamine agonist, is a metabolite of trazodone. *J. Pharm. Pharmacol.*, **33**, 477–478.

178 Fong, M.H., Garattini, S., and Caccia, S. (1982) 1-*m*-Chlorophenylpiperazine is an active metabolite common to the psychotropic drugs trazodone, etoperidone and mepiprazole. *J. Pharm. Pharmacol.*, **34**, 674–675.

179 Melzacka, M., Boksa, J., and Maj, J. (1979) 1-(*m*-Chlorophenyl)piperazine: a metabolite of trazodone isolated from rat urine. *J. Pharm. Pharmacol.*, **31**, 855–856.

180 Mayol, R.F., Cole, C.A., Luke, G.M., Colson, K.L., and Kerns, E.H. (1994) Characterization of the metabolites of the antidepressant drug nefazodone in human urine and plasma. *Drug Metab. Dispos.*, **22**, 304–311.

181 Caldwell, G.W., Wu, W.N., and Masucci, J.A. (2001) Evaluation of the absorption, excretion and metabolism of [^{14}C] etoperidone in man. *Xenobiotica*, **31**, 823–839.

182 Holland, M.L. and Heebner, E.T. (1991) High-performance liquid chromatographic assay with ultraviolet detection for the determination of etoperidone and two active metabolites, 5-(1-hydroxyethyl) etoperidone and 1-(3-chlorophenyl)piperazine, in plasma. *J. Chromatogr.*, **567**, 433–440.

183 Yan, Z., Caldwell, G.W., Wu, W.N., McKown, L.A., Rafferty, B., Jones, W., and Masucci, J.A. (2002) *In vitro* identification of metabolic pathways and cytochrome P450 enzymes involved in the metabolism of etoperidone. *Xenobiotica*, **32**, 949–962.

184 Baumann, M.H., Mash, D.C., and Staley, J.K. (1995) The serotonin agonist *m*-chlorophenylpiperazine (mCPP) binds to serotonin transporter sites in human brain. *Neuroreport.*, **6**, 2150–2152.

185 Eriksson, E., Engberg, G., Bing, O., and Nissbrandt, H. (1999) Effects of mCPP on the extracellular concentrations of serotonin and dopamine in rat brain. *Neuropsychopharmacology*, **20**, 287–296.

186 Gobbi, M., Moia, M., Pirona, L., Ceglia, I., Reyes-Parada, M., Scorza, C., and Mennini, T. (2002) *p*-Methylthioamphetamine and 1-(*m*-chlorophenyl)piperazine, two non-neurotoxic 5-HT releasers *in vivo*, differ from neurotoxic amphetamine derivatives in their mode of action at 5-HT nerve endings *in vitro*. *J. Neurochem.*, **82**, 1435–1443.

187 Rothman, R.B. and Baumann, M.H. (2002) Therapeutic and adverse actions of serotonin transporter substrates. *Pharmacol. Ther.*, **95**, 73–88.

188 Hamik, A. and Peroutka, S.J. (1989) 1-(*m*-chlorophenyl)piperazine (mCPP) interactions with neurotransmitter receptors in the human brain. *Biol. Psychiatry*, **25**, 569–575.

189 Mayol, R.F., Cole, C.A., Colson, K.E., and Kerns, E.H. (1994) Isolation and identification of the major urinary metabolite of *m*-chlorophenylpiperazine in the rat. *Drug Metab. Dispos.*, **22**, 171–174.

190 Caccia, S., Fong, M.H., Garattini, S., and Zanini, M.G. (1982) Plasma concentrations of trazodone and 1-(3-chlorophenyl)piperazine in man after a single oral dose of trazodone. *J. Pharm. Pharmacol.*, **34**, 605–606.

191 Rotzinger, S., Fang, J., Coutts, R.T., and Baker, G.B. (1998) Human CYP2D6 and metabolism of *m*-chlorophenylpiperazine. *Biol. Psychiatry*, **44**, 1185–1191.

192 von-Moltke, L.L., Greenblatt, D.J., Granda, B.W., Grassi, J.M., Schmider, J., Harmatz, J.S., and Shader, R.I. (1999) Nefazodone, meta-chlorophenylpiperazine, and their metabolites *in vitro*: cytochromes mediating transformation, and P450-3A4 inhibitory actions. *Psychopharmacology*, **145**, 113–122.

193 Fauquet, J.P., Morel, E., Demarty, C., and Rapin, J.R. (1976) [Role of central catecholamines in the psychostimulant activity of pyrovalerone]. *Arch. Int. Pharmacodyn. Ther.*, **224**, 325–337.

194 Goldberg, J., Gardos, G., and Cole, J.O. (1973) A controlled evaluation of pyrovalerone in chronically fatigued volunteers. *Int. Pharmacopsychiatry*, **8**, 60–69.

195 Servin, A., Fauquet, J.P., Jacquot, C., and Rapin, J.R. (1978) Effects of pyrovalerone on peripheral noradrenergic mechanisms. *Biochem. Pharmacol.*, **27**, 1693–1694.

196 Crespi, C.L. (1995) Xenobiotic-metabolizing human cells as tools for pharmacological and toxicological research, in *Advances in Drug Research* (eds B. Testa and U.A. Meyer), Academic Press, London, pp. 179–235.

197 Crespi, C.L. and Miller, V.P. (1999) The use of heterologously expressed drug metabolizing enzymes – state of the art and prospects for the future. *Pharmacol. Ther.*, **84**, 121–131.

198 Crespi, C.L. and Penman, B.W. (1997) Use of cDNA-expressed human cytochrome P450 enzymes to study potential drug–drug interactions. *Adv. Pharmacol.*, **43**, 171–188.

199 Springer, D., Staack, R.F., Paul, L.D., Kraemer, T., and Maurer, H.H. (2003) Identification of cytochrome P450 enzymes involved in the metabolism of 4′-methoxy-pyrrolidinopropiophenone (MOPPP), a designer drug, in human liver microsomes. *Xenobiotica*, **33**, 989–998.

200 Venkatakrishnan, K., von Moltke, L.L., Court, M.H., Harmatz, J.S., Crespi, C.L., and Greenblatt, D.J. (2000) Comparison between cytochrome P450 (CYP) content and relative activity approaches to scaling from cDNA-expressed CYPs to human liver microsomes: ratios of accessory proteins as sources of discrepancies between the approaches. *Drug Metab. Dispos.*, **28**, 1493–1504.

201 Vickers, S. and Polsky, S.L. (2000) The biotransformation of nitrogen containing xenobiotics to lactams. *Curr. Drug Metab.*, **1**, 357–389.

202 O'Brien, C.P. (1996) Drug addiction and abuse, in *Goodman and Gilman's The Pharmacological Basis of Therapeutics* (eds J.G. Hardman, L.E. Limbird, P.M. Molinoff, R.W. Ruddon, and A. Gilman), McGraw-Hill, New York, p. 573.

203 Fantegrossi, W.E., Harrington, A.W., Kiessel, C.L., Eckler, J.R., Rabin, R.A., Winter, J.C., Coop, A., Rice, K.C., and Woods, J.H. (2006) Hallucinogen-like actions of 5-methoxy-*N*,*N*-diisopropyltryptamine in mice and rats. *Pharmacol. Biochem. Behav.*, **83**, 122–129.

204 Narimatsu, S., Yonemoto, R., Masuda, K., Katsu, T., Asanuma, M., Kamata, T., Katagi, M., Tsuchihashi, H., Kumamoto, T., Ishikawa, T., Naito, S., Yamano, S., and Hanioka, N. (2008) Oxidation of 5-methoxy-*N*,*N*-diisopropyltryptamine in rat liver microsomes and recombinant cytochrome P450 enzymes. *Biochem. Pharmacol.*, **75**, 752–760.

205 Kanamori, T., Kuwayama, K., Tsujikawa, K., Miyaguchi, H., Iwata, Y., Inoue, H., and Kishi, T. (2006) *In vivo* metabolism of 5-methoxy-*N*,*N*-diisopropyltryptamine in rat. *J. Health Sci.*, **52**, 425–430.

17
Nicotine Metabolism and its Implications

Andy Z.X. Zhu and Rachel F. Tyndale

17.1
Introduction

This chapter will focus on the absorption of nicotine from tobacco smoking, the distribution of nicotine in the body, the hepatic metabolism and renal excretion of nicotine, as well as the sources of variation in the rates of nicotine metabolism and the implications of this variability.

Currently, there are approximately 1.3 billion smokers worldwide [1] and tobacco smoking is the largest cause of preventable death globally. Although not a direct cause of tobacco-related diseases, nicotine is the main psychoactive ingredient of tobacco [2]; it is highly addictive and is responsible for the reinforcing properties of tobacco [3, 4]. Moreover, nicotine is also used medically as nicotine replacement therapy, and experimentally to treat Parkinson's disease, attention-deficit hyperactivity disorder, Tourette's syndrome, ulcerative colitis, and Alzheimer's disease [5–7]. A thorough understanding of the metabolism and disposition of nicotine is required to provide the fundamental knowledge necessary for more effective, personalized therapeutic interventions for smoking cessation as well as other diseases.

17.2
Absorption and Distribution of Nicotine

17.2.1
Absorption

A typical cigarette contains about 10–14 mg of nicotine [8], but only 1–1.5 mg is absorbed into the body during smoking [9]. Nicotine's absorption kinetics during smoking are important to its pharmacology and addictive properties. When tobacco is burned and the smoke is inhaled, nicotine is carried by the tar droplets (also known as particulate matter) into the lungs. Since nicotine is a tertiary amine with a weakly basic pK_a of 8.0, the absorption of nicotine across the biological

Metabolism of Drugs and Other Xenobiotics, First Edition. Edited by Pavel Anzenbacher, Ulrich M. Zanger.

membranes is highly pH-dependent. It was initially thought that the smoke from most flue-cured cigarettes was acidic (pH ~ 5.3) [10], which would minimize the buccal absorption of nicotine. However, more recent evidence suggests that the pH of the cigarette smoke is between 6.0 and 7.8 [11]. At this pH range, between 1 and 36% of nicotine is in the unionized form, and can be absorbed by the buccal membrane and the respiratory tract [11]. In contrast to flue-cured cigarette products, the smoke from air-cured tobacco products, such as cigars and pipes, is more basic. Hence, a large amount of nicotine is unionized and is mostly absorbed buccally [12]. Likewise, chewing tobacco generally has a basic pH, which allows the maximum absorption of nicotine across the buccal mucosa [13].

Following inhalation of cigarette smoke, the tar droplets containing nicotine reach the small airways and alveoli of the lung, and nicotine is rapidly absorbed into the bloodstream. After a puff, it takes only 10–20 s for high levels of nicotine to reach the brain and activate the dopaminergic rewarding system [14]. This rapid absorption/distribution of nicotine makes smoking the most reinforcing route of nicotine administration [14]. Moreover, the short time needed for nicotine to enter the brain allows smokers to manipulate the inhalation depth and puff volume to reach a desirable nicotine level [15]. This is supported by the fact that when smokers are provided with lower nicotine yield cigarettes or when their nicotine renal clearance is enhanced, they will smoke more cigarettes to obtain more nicotine [16–18].

17.2.2 Distribution

After being absorbed, nicotine is extensively distributed into different body tissues. This is reflected by the large volume of distribution (2.6 l/kg) of nicotine [19, 20] (Table 17.1). Nicotine is not extensively protein bound in the plasma (less than 5%) and the distribution half-life is around 8 min [19] (Table 17.1). The arterial concentration of nicotine after smoking a cigarette is usually in the range of 20–60 ng/ml [14, 21–23] (Table 17.1). The mean increase in venous nicotine concentration after smoking a cigarette is around 11 ng/ml [36], but this number can be as high as 30 ng/ml depending on how a cigarette is smoked [23, 37]. The venous nicotine concentration in smokers generally ranges from 10 to 50 ng/ml [37, 38].

17.3 Excretion of Nicotine

The renal clearance of unchanged nicotine is a minor route of total clearance (Figure 17.1); only 8–10% of the absorbed nicotine is excreted unchanged, whereas the majority of nicotine is metabolized before excretion [39, 50]. Nicotine is excreted from the body by glomerular filtration and tubular secretion. The normal renal clearance rate of nicotine is in the range of 35–123 ml/min [24, 25, 51] (Table 17.1), but it is highly dependent on urinary pH. For example, in acidic urine, where nicotine is highly ionized, there is little tubular reabsorption and renal clearance

Table 17.1 Pharmacokinetic parameters for nicotine.

	Route of Administration	Absorption Pharmacokinetics			Distribution and eliminatior pharmacokinetics						Reference
		C_{max} (ng/ml)	T_{max} (min)	Bioavailability (%)	$t_{1/2}$ distribution (min)	$t_{1/2}$ elimination (min)	Clearance (ml/min)	Renal clearance (ml/min)	Nonrenal clearance (ml/min)	V_d (l/kg)	
Nicotine	smoking (one cigarette)	10–30 (venous) 20–60 (arterial)	5–8 (venous) 3–5 (arterial)	80–90 of inhaled nicotine							[14, 19–34]
	intravenous (2 μg/kg/min)	30 (venous) 50 (arterial)	30 (venous) 30 (arterial)	100	8	100–150	1110–1500	35–123	1050–1460	2.6	
	oral solution (2 mg)	4.7	51	20–44							
Cotinine	intravenous infusion (2 μg/kg/min)	90 (venous)	30 (venous)	100		770–1130	42–55	3–9	36–52	0.69–0.93	[20, 27, 35]
Trans-3′ -hydroxycotinine	intravenous infusion (4 μg/kg/min)					396	82	50	32	0.67	[30]

C_{max}, maximum concentration; T_{max}, time to maximum concentration; $T_{1/2}$ distribution, distribution half-life; $t_{1/2}$, elimination, elimination half-life; V_d, volume of distribution.

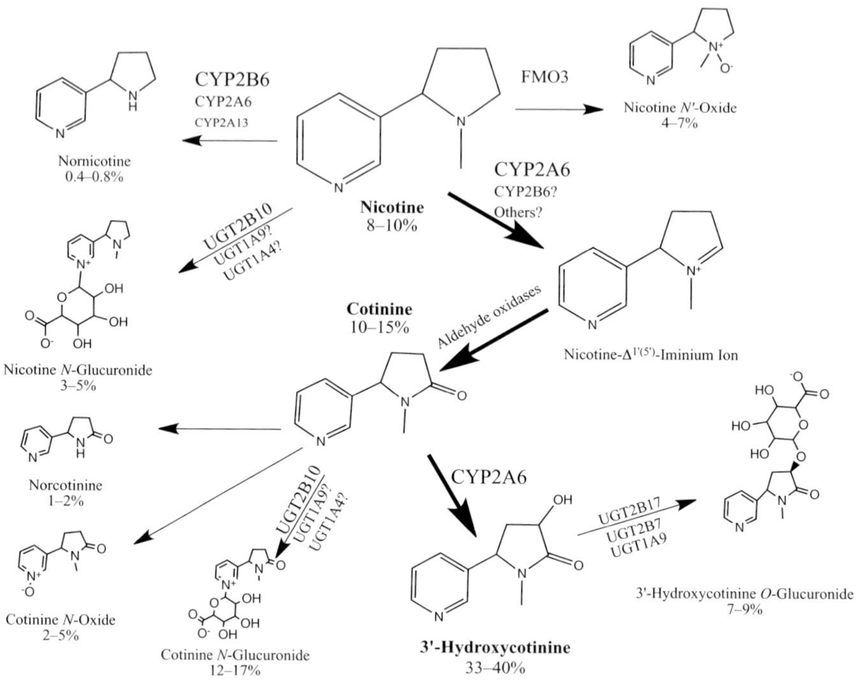

Figure 17.1 Quantitative scheme of nicotine metabolism pathways. The percentage below each metabolite is an estimate of the average excretion of this metabolite as a percentage of total urinary nicotine equivalent or the nicotine dose. This figure represents broad estimates as the data were gathered by different studies using various methods [27, 35, 39–49].

rates can be as high as 600 ml/min [18]. In contrast, in basic urine the renal clearance of nicotine can be as low as 17 ml/min [18]. Twin studies suggest a significant genetic contribution to nicotine renal clearance [52]. However, the molecular mechanism(s) explaining the variation in nicotine renal clearance is largely unknown. Genetic variation in the renal cation transporter systems may contribute to the variation in nicotine renal clearance [52].

17.4 Metabolism of Nicotine

17.4.1 Primary Metabolites of Nicotine

Nicotine is metabolized by the liver to a number of primary metabolites such as cotinine, nicotine *N*′-oxide, nornicotine, and nicotine *N*′-glucuronide (Figure 17.1), and minor metabolites such as nicotine isomethonium ion and 2′-hydroxynicotine. Cotinine is the major metabolite of nicotine. In humans, approximately 70–80% of intravenously infused nicotine is metabolized to cotinine [20]. The metabolism of nicotine to cotinine is a two-step process. The first step is a cytochrome P450 (CYP)-mediated oxidation of nicotine to the nicotine-$\Delta^{1'(5')}$-iminium ion [53–55] and the second step involves the conversion of the nicotine-$\Delta^{1'(5')}$-iminium ion to cotinine by aldehyde oxidases [40, 56]. This second step is generally not considered as the rate-limiting step in cotinine formation [40, 55]. The final urinary concentration of cotinine is only 10–15% of the nicotine dose given due to the extensive metabolism of cotinine [20].

In humans, 90% of the oxidation step is mediated by CYP2A6 [41, 42, 57], with possibly a minor contribution from CYP2B6 and other CYPs [57]. A number of *in vitro* studies support the dominant role of CYP2A6 in nicotine *C*-oxidation. For example, in human liver microsomes the rate of nicotine *C*-oxidation correlates highly with immunochemically determined hepatic CYP2A6 levels and coumarin 7-hydroxylase activities – a phenotypic marker for CYP2A6 activity [41, 58]. cDNA-expressed CYP2A6 demonstrates the highest rate of cotinine formation among all CYPs [41]. CYP2A6 inhibitors and inhibitory antibodies against CYP2A6 prevent cotinine formation from nicotine [41, 42]. *In vivo* studies further confirm the essential role of CYP2A6 in nicotine *C*-oxidation. Notably, individuals homozygous for the *CYP2A6* deletion allele have very low plasma cotinine levels after nicotine administration [26, 59–62] and excrete very small amounts of cotinine in urine compared to individuals with the functional *CYP2A6* gene [63–65]. Methoxsalen – a chemical inhibitor of CYP2A6 – significantly reduces the first-pass metabolism of oral nicotine [66]. In addition to CYP2A6, other CYPs may play a minor role in nicotine *C*-oxidation. For example, cDNA-expressed CYP2B6 can catalyze nicotine *C*-oxidation, but the affinity is 10 times lower compared to CYP2A6 [57]. More recent data from a human liver bank suggest that CYP2B6 plays little role in nicotine metabolism [67]. Likewise, CYP2A13 was also able to mediate nicotine *C*-oxidation [68, 69]. However, due to the limited hepatic expression of this enzyme, CYP2A13 is unlikely to contribute substantially to systemic nicotine *C*-oxidation [70, 71].

In humans, only 4–7% of the nicotine dose is found in urine as nicotine *N'*-oxide [27] and the formation of nicotine *N'*-oxide is generally thought to be mediated by the flavin-containing monooxygenase FMO3 (Figure 17.1) [43, 72]. Nicotine *N'*-oxide is directly excreted in urine without further metabolism.

In humans, less than 1% of nicotine is excreted as nornicotine in urine [27, 44]. In pooled human liver microsomes, the rate of nicotine *N*-demethylation is biphasic, suggesting possible contributions from two different enzymes [45]. Subsequent cDNA expression experiments suggest that CYP2B6 has the highest nicotine *N*-demethylase activity, followed by CYP2A6 and CYP2A13 [45].

In addition to the oxidative pathways, nicotine can also undergo glucuronidation to nicotine *N'*-β-glucuronide [20, 44] (Figure 17.1). In humans, about 3–5% of nicotine is excreted as nicotine *N'*-β-glucuronide [20]. However, this percentage may increase in individuals with reduced nicotine *C*-oxidation [73]. Consistent evidence suggests that the same UDP-glucuronosyltransferase (UGT) isoform mediates the conjugation of both nicotine and cotinine [27, 74]. UGT1A4 was initially thought to be the main enzyme catalyzing nicotine glucuronidation with a minor contribution from UGT1A9 [74, 75]. However, recent evidence suggests that nicotine and cotinine glucuronidation may be largely mediated by UGT2B10 [46–48].

Another minor nicotine metabolic pathway is the 2′-hydroxylation of nicotine to produce 4-(methylamino)-1-(3-pyridyl)-1-butanone with 2′-hydroxynicotine as an intermediate [76]. This pathway is interesting as 4-(methylamino)-1-(3-pyridyl)-1-butanone can potentially be converted to carcinogenic nitrosamines [76]. However, the formation of nitrosamines is either extremely low or not detected in long-term nicotine transdermal patch users [77], suggesting this may not be a pathway of particular clinical relevance.

17.4.2 Secondary Metabolites of Nicotine

Although the majority of nicotine is metabolized to cotinine, only a small percentage of cotinine is excreted unchanged [9, 20]. Six metabolites of cotinine have been reported in humans; the two major ones are 3′-hydroxycotinine and cotinine *N*′-glucuronide.

Most of the cotinine is metabolized to 3′-hydroxycotinine in humans with approximately 40–50% of absorbed nicotine excreted as 3′-hydroxycotinine and its glucuronide in urine [20, 50, 78]. Interestingly, the formation of 3′-hydroxycotinine in humans is highly selective toward the *trans* isomer with less than 5% excreted as the *cis* isomer in urine [79, 80]. The formation of 3′-hydroxycotinine from cotinine is exclusively catalyzed by CYP2A6 in humans. This is supported by multiple lines of evidence: cDNA-expressed CYP2A6 has very high cotinine 3′-hydroxylase activity [49]; in human liver microsomes cotinine 3′-hydroxylase activity is highly correlated with immunoreactive CYP2A6 protein levels and coumarin 7′-hydroxylase activities [49]; chemical CYP2A6 inhibitors and inhibitory antibodies against CYP2A6 inhibit 3′-hydroxycotinine formation from cotinine in human liver microsomes [49]; and no 3′-hydroxycotinine is detected in individuals homozygous for the *CYP2A6* deletion allele [26, 81].

In addition to the oxidative pathways, about 16–17% of the absorbed nicotine is excreted in urine as cotinine *N*-glucuronide in humans [27]. Recent evidence suggests that UGT2B10 is the most efficient enzyme mediating cotinine glucuronidation [46, 47] and individuals with a loss-of-function *UGT2B10* allele excrete significantly less cotinine glucuronides compared to individuals with wild-type alleles [46].

17.4.3 Tertiary Metabolite of Nicotine

Like nicotine and cotinine, 3′-hydroxycotinine can also undergo glucuronidation; however, in contrast to the *N*-glucuronide conjugates of nicotine and cotinine, only 3′-hydroxycotinine *O*-glucuronide can be detected in urine [44]. In humans, about 8% of the absorbed nicotine is secreted as 3′-hydroxycotinine *O*-glucuronide with possibly contributions from UGT2B17, UGT2B7, and UGT1A9 [27, 39].

17.5 Sources of Variation in Nicotine Metabolism

17.5.1 Genetic

Twin studies have suggested that there is a significant heritable (around 60%) contribution to nicotine clearance and metabolism [82]. While genetic variation in the main nicotine-metabolizing enzyme, CYP2A6, has been studied extensively, the influence of genetic variation in other nicotine-metabolizing enzymes is less well characterized.

17.5.1.1 CYP2A6 and Nicotine *C*-Oxidation

A substantial amount of interindividual variation is observed in nicotine *C*-oxidation *in vivo* as well as in hepatic CYP2A6 mRNA, protein levels, and *in vitro* catalytic activity [26, 83, 84]. The human *CYP2A6* gene consists of nine exons and spans 6700 bp on the long arm of chromosome 19 [85]. Studies over the past decade have revealed the complexity of the genetic variation in *CYP2A6*. Currently, 35 numbered and two duplication alleles have been identified (http://www.cypalleles.ki.se/cyp2a6.htm).

Based on both *in vitro* and *in vivo* data, *CYP2A6* variant alleles with lower activity are generally grouped into loss-of-function alleles or reduction-of-function alleles (Table 17.2). *CYP2A6* slow metabolizers are defined as individuals with one or more copies of loss-of-function alleles or two copies of reduction-of-function alleles. Individuals with one copy of a reduction-of-function allele are generally considered as intermediate metabolizers [96, 117, 118]. The most profound effects on nicotine metabolism are observed in individuals with two loss-of-function *CYP2A6* alleles. For example, individuals with two copies of the *CYP2A6*4* allele, which is the *CYP2A6* whole gene deletion allele [86, 99–101, 129], have higher nicotine plasma levels, higher peak nicotine levels, and lower oral nicotine clearance compared to those without **4* alleles [26, 62]. Furthermore, *CYP2A6*4/*4* individuals excrete only 11–15% of the cotinine levels that wild-type individuals excrete after a similar amount of smoking [63, 64]; they also excrete no 3′-hydroxycotinine [26, 81].

Currently, while many of the variant alleles identified to date have a substantial impact on nicotine metabolism, only a small percentage of the interindividual variation in nicotine metabolism can be explained by characterized *CYP2A6* variants and there is a wide variability in nicotine clearance among people without known variants [26]. Thus, a phenotypic marker may be useful, as it can account for the known and unknown genetic variation, as well as the environmental influences on CYP2A6 activity *in vivo*. However, like all phenotype markers, it may be susceptible to the transitory effects of inducers and inhibitors.

17.5.1.2 Using the 3′-Hydroxycotinine : Cotinine Ratio as an *In Vivo* Probe for CYP2A6 Activity

The 3′-hydroxycotinine : cotinine ratio (also known as the nicotine metabolite ratio) can be used as a noninvasive probe for CYP2A6 activity and nicotine clearance

Table 17.2 Common genetic variants in nicotine-metabolizing enzymes.

Alleles	Allele frequencies					Allele description	*In vivo* activity	*In vitro* activity	*In vivo* grouping	Reference
	Caucasians	African-American	Korean	Japanese	Chinese					
*CYP2A6*1A*						reference allele				
*CYP2A6*1B*	29–35	13–20	57	48–55	43–51	higher transcription by mRNA stabilization; associated with faster nicotine clearance *in vivo*	↑	↑		[86–93]
*CYP2A6*1D*	30–39	48		18	9	50% lower transcription *in vitro*; unclear impact *in vivo*				[87, 94, 95]
*CYP2A6*2*	1–5	0.3–1	0	0	0	unstable, fails to incorporate heme and inactive protein *in vivo*; inactive *in vivo*	none	none	loss	[86, 88, 96–98]
*CYP2A6*4*[a)]	0–4	2	11	17–24	5–15	deletion of CYP2A6 gene caused by unequal crossover; inactive *in vivo*	none	none	loss	[87, 92, 93, 96, 99–104]
*CYP2A6*5*	0–0.3	0	0.5	2	0.5–1	unstable and inactive enzyme *in vitro*; unclear impact *in vivo*		none		[86, 87, 91, 93, 96, 102]
*CYP2A6*7*	0	0	11	10–13	6–10	unstable enzyme *in vitro*; inactive towards nicotine *in vivo*	none	↓	loss	[62, 87, 91, 93, 96, 104–106]
*CYP2A6*8*	0	0	0–2	0–1	0–1	unclear *in vivo* impact		→	→	[62, 87, 91, 93, 106, 107]

*CYP2A6*9*	5–8	7–9	16	19–20	16	lower transcription *in vivo*; reduced activity *in vivo*	↓	↓	reduction	[87, 94, 96, 104, 106, 108, 109]
*CYP2A6*10*	0	0	1–4	2–3	2–4	inactive *in vivo*	none		loss	[62, 87, 91, 93, 106, 107]
*CYP2A6*11*	0	0	1	0.5		lower activity *in vitro*; unclear impact *in vivo*		↓		[87, 110]
*CYP2A6*12*	0–3	0–0.4	0	0–1	0	unstable enzyme *in vitro*; reduced activity *in vivo*	↓	↓	reduction	[87, 96, 109, 111, 112]
*CYP2A6*13*	0	0	0.2	1		likely to exhibit reduced activity as it has the same –48T>G SNP as CYP2A9*9	↓?			[87, 113, 114]
*CYP2A6*14*	4	1	0	0		unclear impact *in vivo*				[87, 113]
*CYP2A6*15*	0	0	1	2		likely to exhibit reduced activity as it has the same –48T>G SNP as CYP2A9*9	↓?			[87, 113, 114]
*CYP2A6*16*	0.3	0–2	0	0		unclear impact *in vivo*				[87, 113]
*CYP2A6*17*	0	7–11	0	0		lower activity *in vitro*; inactive *in vivo*	none	↓	loss	[87, 115]
*CYP2A6*18*	2	0	0	0.5		similar nicotine *C*-oxidation activity as the wild-type *in vitro*		→		[116]
*CYP2A6*19*	0	0	0.5	0		lower nicotine *C*-oxidation activity *in vitro*; likely to exhibit reduced activity as it has the same 6558T>C SNP as CYP2A6*7 and CYP2A6*10	↓?	↓		[116]

(*Continued*)

Table 17.2 (*Continued*)

Alleles	Allele frequencies					Allele description	*In vivo* activity	*In vitro* activity	*In vivo* grouping	Reference
	Caucasians	African-American	Korean	Japanese	Chinese					
*CYP2A6*20*	0	1–2	0	0		truncated protein; inactive *in vivo*	none	none	loss	[117–119]
*CYP2A6*21*	0.5–2	1	0	0		similar activity toward nicotine *in vivo*	→			[114, 120]
*CYP2A6*22*	0.3	0	0	0		likely to exhibit reduced activity *in vivo* as it alters the same amino acid as CYP2A9*2				[114]
*CYP2A6*23*	0	2		0	0	lower activity *in vitro*; inactive *in vivo*	none	↓	loss	[117, 118, 121]
*CYP2A6*24*		1				similar nicotine *C*-oxidation activity as the wild-type *in vitro*	→	→		[117, 118]
*CYP2A6*25*		0.5–1				similar nicotine *C*-oxidation activity as the wild-type *in vitro*; associated with reduced activity *in vivo*	↓	→	loss	[117, 118]
*CYP2A6*26*		0.7				no detectable amount of protein *in vitro*; associated with greatly reduced activity *in vivo*	↓	↓	loss	[117, 118]

*CYP2A6*27*		0.7				no detectable amount of protein *in vitro*; associated with greatly reduced activity *in vivo*	↓	↓	loss	[117, 118]
*CYP2A6*28*		1–2				similar nicotine *C*-oxidation activity as the wild-type *in vitro*; inconsistent *in vivo* impact		→		[117, 118]
*CYP2A6*31*		1				associated with reduced activity (unpublished data)	↓		loss	Unpublished observation
*CYP2A6*34*										
*CYP2A6*35*		2–3		0.8	0.5	decreased thermal stability and activity *in vitro*; associated with reduced activity *in vivo*	↓	↓	loss	[117, 122]
*CYP2A6*1X2A*	0–1	2	0	0.4		unclear impact *in vivo*	↑			[123]
*CYP2A6*1X2B*	0	2	0	0		unclear impact *in vivo*	↑			[123, 124]
*CYP2B6*4*	4	0	4.5	6		mixed *in vivo* impact on nicotine metabolism	?			[125–127]
*CYP2B6*6*	25.6	32.8	15.9	18		mixed *in vivo* impact on nicotine metabolism	?			[125–128]
*UGT2B10*2 (D67Y)*	11	8.3				associated with reduced nicotine and cotinine glucuronidation *in vivo*	↓			[46, 48]

a) Different studies looked at different version of *4s (i.e., *4A versus *4B).

in vivo. The 3′-hydroxycotinine : cotinine ratio is used since cotinine has a long half-life (Table 17.1), resulting in cotinine plasma levels in regular smokers that show little fluctuation [130]. Additionally, 3′-hydroxycotinine is completely formation-dependent, which makes the 3′-hydroxycotinine : cotinine ratio very stable over time. Furthermore, the 3′-hydroxycotinine : cotinine ratio has several advantages as a phenotypic marker. (i) Unlike most of the phenotypic probes, the 3′-hydroxycotinine : cotinine ratio can be assessed from a single smokers' plasma or saliva sample with no need for a period of abstinence followed by administration of the probe drug and subsequent assessment of metabolites at a specified time [131]. (ii) Since the 3′-hydroxycotinine : cotinine ratio is stable over time, samples can be taken at any time of the day [130, 131]. (iii) The 3′-hydroxycotinine : cotinine ratio is highly specific toward CYP2A6 activity; individuals with two *CYP2A6* deletion alleles have no detectable amount of 3′-hydroxycotinine after oral nicotine administration, making it a good CYP2A6 phenotype [26]. (iv) The 3′-hydroxycotinine : cotinine ratio correlates highly with total nicotine clearance *in vivo*, making it useful as a surrogate measure of total nicotine clearance [26].

17.5.1.3 **Interethnic Variability in Nicotine *C*-Oxidation**

There is substantial interethnic variation in nicotine *C*-oxidation (Table 17.2). Although nongenetic factors such as dietary differences may contribute to this variation, important genetic differences in nicotine-metabolizing enzymes are also observed between ethnicities. For example, the frequencies of *CYP2A6* alleles vary substantially between ethnicities; loss/reduction-of-function *CYP2A6* alleles are more prevalent in Asians followed by African-Americans then Caucasians [84, 132], and the combined frequencies of individuals with at least one copy of loss/reduction-of-function *CYP2A6* alleles are 55, 47, and 23% for Japanese, African-Americans, and Caucasians, respectively [87, 117, 133, 134] (Table 17.2). The higher frequency of loss/reduction-of-function *CYP2A6* alleles results in lower CYP2A6 protein levels and activity in Asians compared to Caucasians [135]. This *in vitro* finding is supported by the interethnic variation observed in nicotine pharmacokinetics. Asian-Americans and African-Americans metabolize nicotine and cotinine more slowly than Caucasian Americans [25, 35].

17.5.1.4 **Genetic Influences on Other Nicotine-Metabolizing Enzymes**

CYP2B6 Like *CYP2A6*, the human *CYP2B6* gene is also highly polymorphic with 29 numbered alleles identified (http://www.cypalleles.ki.se/cyp2b6.htm). *In vitro* experiments suggest that cDNA-expressed CYP2B6 can convert nicotine to cotinine, albeit with relatively low affinity compared CYP2A6. *In vivo* association studies have yielded mixed and inconclusive results; while some studies observed associations between *CYP2B6*4* or **6* and increased nicotine metabolism as well as clearance [125, 128], other studies did not [67, 126]. A study in a human liver bank found that *CYP2B6*6* is associated with reduced protein levels, but once levels of CYP2A6 were controlled for, there was no evidence of slower nicotine *C*-oxidation with a *CYP2B6*6* allele [67].

UGT2B10 and Other Enzymes Genetic variation in *UGT2B10* can also alter nicotine metabolism. Human livers with an *UGT2B10*2 (D67Y)* allele exhibit significant reduction in nicotine and cotinine glucuronidation activities, and individuals with one copy of a *UGT2B10*2 (D67Y)* allele have lower nicotine and cotinine glucuronide conjugation *in vivo* [48]. There is also considerable interethnic variation in nicotine and cotinine glucuronidation. The formation of nicotine and cotinine glucuronides is bimodal in African-Americans, with evidence of both fast and slow formers, whereas the formation of nicotine and cotinine glucuronides is unimodal in Caucasians [25]. This interethnic variation cannot be explained by the *UGT2B10*2* allele alone [25, 48], suggesting additional genetic or environmental factors may also modulate nicotine glucuronidation. Genetic variation has also been identified in other nicotine-metabolizing enzymes, such as FMOs and aldehyde oxidases, but their impact *in vivo* has not been explicitly demonstrated.

17.5.2 Gender and Pregnancy

Female gender is associated with faster nicotine and cotinine metabolism compared to males [136]. Furthermore, estrogen-containing oral contraceptive usage can further enhance the metabolism of nicotine and cotinine [136]. Since cotinine is a low extraction drug, its metabolism is highly dependent on drug-metabolizing enzyme activities and less dependent on the hepatic blood flow (Figure 17.2). Therefore, the fact that females have higher cotinine as well as nicotine clearance suggests that this increase is, at least in part, due to an increase in CYP2A6 activity. This is further supported by the fact that females have a higher 3′-hydroxycotinine : cotinine ratio (suggesting faster CYP2A6-mediated 3′-hydroxycotinine formation)

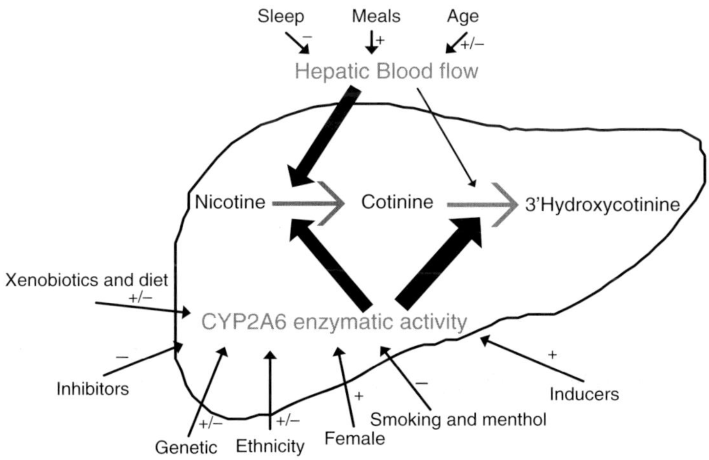

Figure 17.2 Factors influencing nicotine metabolism *in vivo*. A number of factors, including genetics, gender, pregnancy, age, meals, diet, smoking, and xenobiotics, can influence nicotine metabolism. These factors generally affect nicotine metabolism by either influencing hepatic blood flow or nicotine-metabolizing enzyme activity.

compared to males [117, 125], and that female livers have significantly higher CYP2A6 mRNA, protein, and activity comparing to male livers [83].

This gender difference in CYP2A6 activity is likely caused by hormones. For example, *in vitro* data indicates that estrogen induces CYP2A6 via an estrogen receptor-dependent transcriptional upregulation [137]. Moreover, estrogen-containing oral contraceptives usage can increase CYP2A6 activity (as measured by caffeine phenotyping), and nicotine and cotinine clearance [136, 138], while progesterone-containing contraceptives do not alter nicotine clearance [136]. Menopausal or postmenopausal women, who have low estrogen levels, have similar nicotine and cotinine clearance compared to men [136]. Hence, these data support the hypothesis that the increase in nicotine and cotinine metabolism in females and female oral contraceptive users is due to the induction of CYP2A6 by female sex hormones, likely estrogen.

Supporting this is the finding that the clearance of nicotine and cotinine is also significantly higher during pregnancy, when female sex hormone levels are elevated [139]. In fact, the clearance of nicotine increases by 60% during pregnancy, whereas the clearance of cotinine increases by 140% [139]. That pregnancy increases cotinine clearance more than it does nicotine likely indicates an impact on increasing CYP2A6 activity. Therefore, it is possible that the elevated levels of female sex hormone during pregnancy induce CYP2A6 activity, resulting in increased nicotine and cotinine clearance. However, the menstrual cycle has no detectable effect on nicotine and cotinine pharmacokinetics in nonsmoking females [140], which suggests that the temporary alterations in sex hormone levels may not be sufficient to alter the rate of nicotine metabolism or that there is not sufficient change in estrogen levels during menstrual cycle to alter nicotine metabolism.

17.5.3 Age

Generally, there are no age-related differences in nicotine metabolism, except in neonates and the elderly where nicotine metabolism is slower. Neonates have a longer nicotine half-life compared to adults; however, the cotinine half-life is similar [141, 142] and the CYP2A6 protein level is only slightly lower in neonates [143]. Since cotinine clearance is less dependent on hepatic blood flow compared to nicotine and unaltered in neonates, the reduction of nicotine metabolism in neonates is more likely explained by a reduction in hepatic blood flow [144]. In adolescents and adults, there is no correlation between age and CYP2A6 protein levels or activity [83, 145], suggesting a limited impact of age on nicotine metabolism. Furthermore, no differences in steady-state nicotine plasma concentrations are observed between adult age groups when given the same dose of nicotine [146, 147]. In agreement with this, the rate of coumarin metabolism (a specific CYP2A6 probe) is similar across wide age ranges [148, 149], suggesting CYP2A6 activity does not change with age. Notably, the clearance of nicotine is slower in the elderly [150]. This is likely explained by decreases in hepatic blood flow, since no age-associated reductions in CYP2A6 protein or *in vitro* nicotine metabolism have been observed [42, 83].

17.5.4
Meals and the Chronopharmacokinetics of Nicotine

Nicotine clearance exhibits a circadian variation [151]. It generally increases after a meal as hepatic blood flow increases [151, 152], but decreases during sleep, likely as hepatic blood flow decreases [39]. Consequently, nicotine clearance decreases by as much as 17% between 6:00 p.m. (i.e., high at dinner time) and 3:00 a.m. (i.e., low during sleep) [151].

17.5.5
Xenobiotics

Xenobiotics can also influence nicotine metabolism. For example, nicotine metabolism can be induced by a number of prototypical CYP inducers, such as rifampicin, dexamethasone, and phenobarbital [83, 153–158]. Rifampicin treatment increases both CYP2A6 mRNA and activity in human primary hepatocytes [153, 156]. However, the magnitude of induction varies between individuals [153, 156, 159]. Interestingly, rifampicin can also act as an inhibitor of CYP2A6 [160], thus some of the variability observed in CYP2A6 activity upon rifampicin treatment may be explained by the fact that this drug can both inhibit and induce CYP2A6 activity.

Phenobarbital can also induce CYP2A6 [83, 153]. Liver microsomes from phenobarbital-treated patients exhibit higher amounts of CYP2A6 protein than those of untreated patients [43]. As little as 2 days of phenobarbital treatment results in increased *ex vivo* nicotine *C*-oxidation activity [155].

The inducers of nicotine metabolism are generally nuclear receptor ligands or activators that regulate nicotine-metabolizing enzymes via transcriptional activation [156, 161, 162]. Specifically, upon activation by their respective ligand or activator, rifampicin and phenobarbital, the pregnane X receptor (PXR) and the constitutive active androstane receptor (CAR) translocate to the nucleus. There, they dimerize with the retinoid X receptor (RXR)-α and bind to the DR-4 sites upstream of the *CYP2A6* gene to increase its transcription [163].

A number of compounds are known to inhibit nicotine *C*-oxidation *in vitro*, including methoxsalen, menthol, tryptamine, coumarin, tranylcypromine, and selegiline [41, 42, 164–168]. These compounds generally have reasonable selectivity toward CYP2A6 [164, 165]. Clinically, oral methoxsalen administration inhibits the first-pass metabolism of oral nicotine *in vivo* [66] and also decreases the clearance of nicotine following subcutaneous nicotine injections [169]. It can also reduce the number of cigarettes smoked, suggesting titration of consumption to compensate for prolonged nicotine levels [169]. In addition to the compounds known to inhibit nicotine *C*-oxidation, compounds that inhibit CYP2A6-mediated coumarin 7-hydroxylation are predicted to inhibit nicotine *C*-oxidation as both of these processes are mediated by CYP2A6. Examples of coumarin 7-hydroxylation inhibitors include pilocarpine, metyrapone, ketoconazole, and rifampicin [170, 171].

17.5.6
Smoking

The clearance of nicotine is significantly slower in smokers compared to nonsmokers [28] and a 7-day smoking abstinence period increases nicotine nonrenal clearance within the same subjects [51]. This reduction in nicotine clearance among smokers may be caused by reduced CYP2A6 activity, which is supported by the fact that smoking also decreases the metabolism of coumarin – another CYP2A6 substrate [172, 173]. The tobacco component that inhibits CYP2A6 activity or reduces CYP2A6 protein expression has not yet been identified. However, *in vivo* studies demonstrate that cotinine and carbon monoxide are not responsible for the reduction of nicotine clearance in smokers [29, 51]. Some animal and *in vitro* expression evidence suggests that nicotine might be inhibiting its own metabolism and/or downregulating CYP2A6 [174, 175], although a more recent human *in vivo* study does not support this [176]. Thus, there is a possibility that some other substance in tobacco may be inhibiting nicotine metabolism. One of the potential candidates is β-nicotyrine – a nicotine-related alkaloid in tobacco [174]. Interestingly, although smoking significantly reduces nicotine clearance, it does not affect cotinine clearance [51]. This observation complicates the interpretation of the data; however, it remains clear that smoking reduces nicotine metabolism and CYP2A6-mediated coumarin metabolism to an extent that may be clinically relevant.

17.5.7
Menthol

Menthol is an additive in food, personal care products, and cigarettes. In human liver microsomes, menthol weakly inhibits nicotine *C*-oxidation and coumarin 7-hydroxylation [167], suggesting a possible inhibitory effect on CYP2A6. Similarly, *in vivo* studies also demonstrate that smoking mentholated cigarettes is associated with a lower 3′-hydroxycotinine : cotinine ratio compared to smoking nonmentholated cigarettes [117], suggesting that menthol can inhibit CYP2A6 activity *in vivo*. In agreement, menthol decreases nicotine clearance and increases nicotine systemic exposure in human laboratory studies [177]. Together, this evidence suggests that menthol increases nicotine systemic exposure *in vivo*, at least in part, by weakly inhibiting CYP2A6 activity.

17.5.8
Other Factors

A number of other factors can also alter nicotine metabolism; for example, kidney failure can decrease the renal clearance of nicotine and cotinine [178]. Dietary components, such as grapefruit juice and broccoli, can also potentially influence the rate of nicotine metabolism. Grapefruit can inhibit coumarin 7-hydroxylation and nicotine *C*-oxidation *in vivo*, suggesting a possible inhibitory effect on CYP2A6 [24, 179, 180]. In contrast to the inhibitory effect of grapefruit juice, broccoli is a possible dietary inducer of nicotine metabolism [181].

17.6 Implications of Variation in Nicotine Metabolism and CYP2A6 Activity

17.6.1 Variation in Nicotine Metabolism is Associated with Altered Smoking Behaviors

A number of studies have provided evidence that variation in *CYP2A6* may alter smoking acquisition among adolescents [102, 111, 182]. The current hypothesis is that *CYP2A6* slow metabolizers acquire dependence sooner than normal metabolizers, but plateau at a lower level of nicotine dependence and at lower levels of cigarette consumption. In adult dependent smokers, *CYP2A6* slow metabolizers smoke fewer cigarettes per day, are less likely to smoke within 5 min after waking, and have reduced inhalation depth compared with those that are normal metabolizers [96, 108, 183, 184], which suggests that they are also less nicotine-dependent [108]. Moreover, CYP2A6 slow metabolizers quit smoking more easily than CYP2A6 normal metabolizers without any active drug treatment [117, 185], consistent with their increased likelihood of being former smokers versus current smokers [96, 186]. Together, these data suggest that the rate of nicotine metabolism could have a profound influence on smoking behaviors. However, some reports did not find any associations between *CYP2A6* genotype and smoking behavior [187, 188]. This may be explained, in part, by the differences in genotyping methods, the number of alleles tested for, as well as the phenotypes used (i.e., the tobacco dependence scales used).

17.6.2 Variation in Nicotine Metabolism May Alter the Health Consequences of Smoking

Reduced CYP2A6 activity may be associated with reduced risk for the health consequences of smoking. Since smokers smoke to maintain satisfactory levels of nicotine in the body, reduced nicotine metabolism results in lower numbers of cigarettes smoked [96] and consequently lower exposure to the dangerous chemicals in cigarettes. Moreover, CYP2A6 can activate the carcinogenic nitrosamines in cigarettes. Therefore, individuals with reduced CYP2A6 activity may have less activation of nitrosamines [169] and potentially lower risk of cancer [189]. In fact, a recent genome-wide association study suggests an association between *CYP2A6* and smoking behaviors as well as lung cancer risk [190]. This protective effect of the reduction in CYP2A6 activity may be the result of lowered nitrosamine activation, in addition to lower smoke exposure, since after controlling for the amount of cigarettes smoked, *CYP2A6* slow metabolizers still have a decreased risk of smoking-related cancers [189]. Human laboratory studies demonstrate that CYP2A6 inhibitors can significantly increase the amount of nicotine-derived nitrosamine ketone (NNK) that is metabolically reduced to the inactive 4-(methylnitrosamino)-1-(3-pyridyl)-1-butanol glucuronide (NNAL-glucuronide), suggesting less NNK activation by CYP2A6 [169]. Together, these data suggest reduced CYP2A6 activity decreases the number of cigarettes smoked, and may directly and/or indirectly decrease lung cancer risk.

17.6.3 Variation in Nicotine Metabolism Alters Smoking Cessation Outcomes

The rate of nicotine metabolism can significantly alter an individual's ability to quit smoking and his/her response to pharmacotherapies, such as the nicotine replacement patch. For example, a number of studies demonstrate that slow nicotine metabolism (assessed by the 3′-hydroxycotinine : cotinine ratio or by *CYP2A6* genotype) is associated with higher smoking cessation rates in the placebo-treated arm of a clinical trial indicating higher frequencies of spontaneous quitting [96, 117, 191]. Furthermore, individuals with low 3′-hydroxycotinine : cotinine ratios, or *CYP2A6* slow metabolizers by genotype, have significantly better smoking cessation rates on nicotine patch compared to individuals with normal rates of nicotine metabolism [108, 134, 185]. This can be explained, in part, by the higher nicotine plasma concentrations, resulting from a slower nicotine metabolism, in combination with the higher quit rates found in the absence of any active treatment. Interestingly, no differences in quit rates were observed between *CYP2A6* slow metabolizers and normal metabolizers when using nicotine nasal spray treatment [108, 185]. This is likely due to the fact that when using nicotine nasal spray, the subjects altered the amount of nicotine usage, resulting in a titration of their nicotine plasma levels in response to their different rates of nicotine metabolism [108]. No associations were found between the 3′-hydroxycotinine : cotinine ratio and the clinical response to bupropion therapy [191]. This is consistent with the idea that bupropion is not a CYP2A6 substrate and may act downstream of nicotinic receptors; hence, the rate of nicotine metabolism does not appear to alter abstinence rates. Together, this evidence strongly suggests that the rate of nicotine metabolism can have significant effects on smoking cessation outcomes. This suggests that slow metabolizers should be treated with behavioral counseling and/or nicotine patches (perhaps for extended duration), while normal metabolizers benefit substantially more from bupropion than placebo/behavioral counseling. However, prospective testing is needed before genetically tailored treatments should be widely implemented.

Before the translation of genetic research into clinical practice, the results should be replicated in multiple independent studies and the cost-effectiveness of the genetically tailored treatments should be validated. To date, the association between CYP2A6 activity and smoking cessation rates has been replicated in a number of independent studies [117, 134, 185, 191] and the 3′-hydroxycotinine : cotinine ratio consistently predicts cessation outcomes. The cost-effectiveness of implementing genetically tailored therapy is dependent on the distribution of the relevant genetic polymorphism, costs involved in phenotyping or genotyping, and the subsequent effectiveness of the tailored versus untailored therapies [192]. Although no cost-effectiveness analyses have been carried out on tailored smoking cessation treatments based on the 3′-hydroxycotinine : cotinine ratio, pharmacoeconomic simulations suggests that genetically tailored cessation treatments based on the dopamine receptor genotypes can be more cost-effective (cost per quality adjusted life years saved) compared to standard nicotine replacement treatment [193].

17.7
Conclusions

Herein, we have discussed the different pathways of nicotine metabolism and the genetic, physiological as well as the environmental factors influencing them. Nicotine disposition kinetics are highly variable between individuals and ethnicities. Twin studies suggest that a large proportion of this variation is heritable, but environmental factors also play a role. Nicotine metabolism involves multiple genetically polymorphic enzymes. Among them, CYP2A6 plays a dominant role in nicotine *C*-oxidation and genetic variation in *CYP2A6* has profound influences on nicotine metabolism. However, a substantial amount of variability in the rate of nicotine metabolism is still observed within the CYP2A6 "wild-type" individuals. Moreover, it is unclear how genetic variation in other nicotine-metabolizing enzymes, such as *AOXI*, *UGTs*, *FMOs*, *CYP2A13*, and *CYP2B6*, influence nicotine metabolism, and subsequently affect smoking behavior and cessation outcomes.

In addition to genetic factors, gender, pregnancy, age, diet, circadian rhythm, smoking, and exposure to xenobiotics can also influence nicotine metabolism. These factors generally affect nicotine metabolism via two mechanisms. The first mechanism is by altering the nicotine-metabolizing enzyme activities; ethnicity, smoking status, gender, xenobiotic inducers, and inhibitors are thought to act via by this mechanism. The second mechanism is by altering hepatic blood flow; the effects of meals, circadian rhythm, and age are thought to act via this mechanism.

Although the neurobiology of smoking is not fully understood, the implications of the variation in nicotine metabolism are straightforward: to compensate for slower rates of nicotine metabolic inactivation, individuals self-administer less nicotine. Thus, the rate of nicotine metabolism is associated with the amount of cigarette consumption. Furthermore, since the same enzyme–CYP2A6–metabolizes both nicotine and the carcinogenic nitrosamines, CYP2A6 activity may directly (by activation of nitrosamines) and/or indirectly (by influencing smoking behavior) alter smoking-related cancer risks. With regard to smoking cessation treatments, individuals with a slower nicotine metabolism rate quit better on placebo and respond better to nicotine patch treatment. The better nicotine patch responses may be explained, in part, by the higher nicotine plasma concentrations resulting from a slower nicotine metabolism rate in combination with the higher quit rates found in the absence of any active treatment. Thus, significant advances have been made in understanding the sources of variation in nicotine metabolism, and its impact on smoking behaviors, cancer risk, and cessation outcomes.

Acknowledgments

We acknowledge the support of CRC (RFT), CIHR grant MOP86471 and NIH grant UO1 DA020830, CAMH, and the CAMH foundation.

Conflict of Interest

Dr. Tyndale owns shares and participates in Nicogen Research Inc. and has consulted for Novartis and McNeil.

References

1 Wipfli, H. and Samet, J.M. (2009) Global economic and health benefits of tobacco control: part 1. *Clin. Pharmacol. Ther.*, **86**, 263–271.

2 Benowitz, N.L. (2009) Pharmacology of nicotine: addiction, smoking-induced disease, and therapeutics. *Annu. Rev. Pharmacol. Toxicol.*, **49**, 57–71.

3 Le Foll, B. and Goldberg, S.R. (2006) Nicotine as a typical drug of abuse in experimental animals and humans. *Psychopharmacology*, **184**, 367–381.

4 Le Foll, B. and Goldberg, S.R. (2009) Effects of nicotine in experimental animals and humans: an update on addictive properties. *Handb. Exp. Pharmacol.*, **192**, 335–367.

5 Potter, A.S. and Newhouse, P.A. (2004) Effects of acute nicotine administration on behavioral inhibition in adolescents with attention-deficit/hyperactivity disorder. *Psychopharmacology*, **176**, 182–194.

6 McGrath, J., McDonald, J.W., and Macdonald, J.K. (2004) Transdermal nicotine for induction of remission in ulcerative colitis. *Cochrane Database Syst. Rev.*, **4**, CD004722.

7 Howson, A.L., *et al.* (2004) Clinical and attentional effects of acute nicotine treatment in Tourette's syndrome. *Eur. Psychiatry*, **19**, 102–112.

8 Kozlowski, L.T., *et al.* (1998) Filter ventilation and nicotine content of tobacco in cigarettes from Canada, the United Kingdom, and the United States. *Tob. Control*, **7**, 369–375.

9 Benowitz, N.L. and Jacob, P., 3rd (1984) Daily intake of nicotine during cigarette smoking. *Clin. Pharmacol. Ther.*, **35**, 499–504.

10 Brunnemann, K.D. and Hoffmann, D. (1974) The pH of tobacco smoke. *Food Cosmet. Toxicol.*, **12**, 115–124.

11 Pankow, J.F., *et al.* (2003) Percent free base nicotine in the tobacco smoke particulate matter of selected commercial and reference cigarettes. *Chem. Res. Toxicol.*, **16**, 1014–1018.

12 Armitage, A., *et al.* (1978) Absorption of nicotine from small cigars. *Clin. Pharmacol. Ther.*, **23**, 143–151.

13 Benowitz, N.L. (1988) Nicotine and smokeless tobacco. *CA Cancer J. Clin.*, **38**, 244–247.

14 Henningfield, J.E. and Keenan, R.M. (1993) Nicotine delivery kinetics and abuse liability. *J. Consult. Clin. Psychol.*, **61**, 743–750.

15 Herning, R.I., *et al.* (1983) How a cigarette is smoked determines blood nicotine levels. *Clin. Pharmacol. Ther.*, **33**, 84–90.

16 Benowitz, N.L., *et al.* (1983) Smokers of low-yield cigarettes do not consume less nicotine. *N. Engl. J. Med.*, **309**, 139–142.

17 National Cancer Institute (2001) *Risks Associated with Smoking Cigarettes with Low Machine-Measured Yields of Tar and Nicotine (Smoking and Tobacco Control Monograph)*, Department of Health and Human Services, Bethesda, MD.

18 Benowitz, N.L. and Jacob, P., 3rd (1985) Nicotine renal excretion rate influences nicotine intake during cigarette smoking. *J. Pharmacol. Exp. Ther.*, **234**, 153–155.

19 Benowitz, N.L., *et al.* (1991) Stable isotope studies of nicotine kinetics and bioavailability. *Clin. Pharmacol. Ther.*, **49**, 270–277.

20 Benowitz, N.L. and Jacob, P., 3rd (1994) Metabolism of nicotine to cotinine studied by a dual stable isotope method. *Clin. Pharmacol. Ther.*, **56**, 483–493.

21 Armitage, A.K., *et al.* (1975) Absorption and metabolism of nicotine from cigarettes. *BMJ*, **4**, 313–316.

22 Rose, J.E., *et al.* (1999) Arterial nicotine kinetics during cigarette smoking and intravenous nicotine administration: implications for addiction. *Drug Alcohol Depend.*, **56**, 99–107.

23 Lunell, E., *et al.* (2000) Site of nicotine absorption from a vapour inhaler–comparison with cigarette smoking. *Eur. J. Clin. Pharmacol.*, **55**, 737–741.

24 Hukkanen, J., Jacob, P., 3rd, and Benowitz, N.L. (2006) Effect of grapefruit juice on cytochrome P450 2A6 and nicotine renal clearance. *Clin. Pharmacol. Ther.*, **80**, 522–530.

25 Benowitz, N.L., *et al.* (1999) Ethnic differences in *N*-glucuronidation of nicotine and cotinine. *J. Pharmacol. Exp. Ther.*, **291**, 1196–1203.

26 Dempsey, D., *et al.* (2004) Nicotine metabolite ratio as an index of cytochrome P450 2A6 metabolic activity. *Clin. Pharmacol. Ther.*, **76**, 64–72.

27 Benowitz, N.L., *et al.* (1994) Nicotine metabolic profile in man: comparison of cigarette smoking and transdermal nicotine. *J. Pharmacol. Exp. Ther.*, **268**, 296–303.

28 Benowitz, N.L. and Jacob, P., 3rd (1993) Nicotine and cotinine elimination pharmacokinetics in smokers and nonsmokers. *Clin. Pharmacol. Ther.*, **53**, 316–323.

29 Zevin, S., Jacob, P., 3rd, and Benowitz, N. (1997) Cotinine effects on nicotine metabolism. *Clin. Pharmacol. Ther.*, **61**, 649–654.

30 Benowitz, N.L. and Jacob, P., 3rd (2001) *Trans*-3′-hydroxycotinine: disposition kinetics, effects and plasma levels during cigarette smoking. *Br. J. Clin. Pharmacol.*, **51**, 53–59.

31 Gourlay, S.G. and Benowitz, N.L. (1997) Arteriovenous differences in plasma concentration of nicotine and catecholamines and related cardiovascular effects after smoking, nicotine nasal spray, and intravenous nicotine. *Clin. Pharmacol. Ther.*, **62**, 453–463.

32 Russell, M.A. and Feyerabend, C. (1978) Cigarette smoking: a dependence on high-nicotine boli. *Drug Metab. Rev.*, **8**, 29–57.

33 Compton, R.F., *et al.* (1997) A dose-ranging pharmacokinetic study of nicotine tartrate following single-dose delayed-release oral and intravenous administration. *Aliment. Pharmacol. Ther.*, **11**, 865–874.

34 Zins, B.J., *et al.* (1997) Pharmacokinetics of nicotine tartrate after single-dose liquid enema, oral, and intravenous administration. *J. Clin. Pharmacol.*, **37**, 426–436.

35 Benowitz, N.L., *et al.* (2002) Slower metabolism and reduced intake of nicotine from cigarette smoking in Chinese-Americans. *J. Natl. Cancer Inst.*, **94**, 108–115.

36 Patterson, F., *et al.* (2003) Individual differences in nicotine intake per cigarette. *Cancer Epidemiol. Biomarkers Prev.*, **12**, 468–471.

37 Schneider, N.G., *et al.* (2001) The nicotine inhaler: clinical pharmacokinetics and comparison with other nicotine treatments. *Clin. Pharmacokinet.*, **40**, 661–684.

38 Benowitz, N.L. (1990) Clinical pharmacology of inhaled drugs of abuse: implications in understanding nicotine dependence. *NIDA Res. Monogr.*, **99**, 12–29.

39 Hukkanen, J., Jacob, P., 3rd, and Benowitz, N.L. (2005) Metabolism and disposition kinetics of nicotine. *Pharmacol. Rev.*, **57**, 79–115.

40 Brandange, S. and Lindblom, L. (1979) The enzyme "aldehyde oxidase" is an iminium oxidase. Reaction with nicotine delta 1′(5′) iminium ion. *Biochem. Biophys. Res. Commun.*, **91**, 991–996.

41 Nakajima, M., *et al.* (1996) Role of human cytochrome P4502A6 in *C*-oxidation of nicotine. *Drug Metab. Dispos.*, **24**, 1212–1217.

42 Messina, E.S., Tyndale, R.F., and Sellers, E.M. (1997) A major role for CYP2A6 in nicotine C-oxidation by human liver microsomes. *J. Pharmacol. Exp. Ther.*, **282**, 1608–1614.

43 Cashman, J.R., *et al.* (1992) Metabolism of nicotine by human liver microsomes: stereoselective formation of *trans*-nicotine *N*′-oxide. *Chem. Res. Toxicol.*, **5**, 639–646.

44 Byrd, G.D., *et al.* (1992) Evidence for urinary excretion of glucuronide conjugates of nicotine, cotinine, and

trans-3′-hydroxycotinine in smokers. *Drug Metab. Dispos.*, **20**, 192–197.

45 Yamanaka, H., *et al.* (2005) CYP2A6 AND CYP2B6 are involved in nornicotine formation from nicotine in humans: interindividual differences in these contributions. *Drug Metab. Dispos.*, **33**, 1811–1818.

46 Chen, G., *et al.* (2007) Glucuronidation of nicotine and cotinine by UGT2B10: loss-of-function by the UGT2B10 codon 67 (Asp>Tyr) polymorphism. *Cancer Res.*, **67**, 9024–9029.

47 Kaivosaari, S., *et al.* (2007) Nicotine glucuronidation and the human UDP-glucuronosyltransferase UGT2B10. *Mol. Pharmacol.*, **72**, 761–768.

48 Berg, J.Z., *et al.* (2010) Nicotine metabolism in African Americans and European Americans: variation in glucuronidation by ethnicity and UGT2B10 haplotype. *J. Pharmacol. Exp. Ther.*, **332**, 202–209.

49 Nakajima, M., *et al.* (1996) Characterization of CYP2A6 involved in 3′-hydroxylation of cotinine in human liver microsomes. *J. Pharmacol. Exp. Ther.*, **277**, 1010–1015.

50 Neurath, G.B. (1994) Aspects of the oxidative metabolism of nicotine. *Clin. Investig.*, **72**, 190–195.

51 Benowitz, N.L. and Jacob, P., 3rd (2000) Effects of cigarette smoking and carbon monoxide on nicotine and cotinine metabolism. *Clin. Pharmacol. Ther.*, **67**, 653–659.

52 Benowitz, N.L., Lessov-Schlaggar, C.N., and Swan, G.E. (2008) Genetic influences in the variation in renal clearance of nicotine and cotinine. *Clin. Pharmacol. Ther.*, **84**, 243–247.

53 Murphy, P.J. (1973) Enzymatic oxidation of nicotine to nicotine 1′(5′) iminium ion. A newly discovered intermediate in the metabolism of nicotine. *J. Biol. Chem.*, **248**, 2796–2800.

54 Peterson, L.A., Trevor, A., and Castagnoli, N., Jr (1987) Stereochemical studies on the cytochrome P-450 catalyzed oxidation of (*S*)-nicotine to the (*S*)-nicotine delta 1′(5′)-iminium species. *J. Med. Chem.*, **30**, 249–254.

55 Obach, R.S. and van Vunakis, H. (1990) Radioimmunoassay of nicotine-delta 1′(5′)-iminium ion, an intermediate formed during the metabolism of nicotine to cotinine. *Drug Metab. Dispos.*, **18**, 508–513.

56 Gorrod, J.W. and Hibberd, A.R. (1982) The metabolism of nicotine-delta 1′(5′)-iminium ion, *in vivo* and *in vitro*. *Eur. J. Drug Metab. Pharmacokinet.*, **7**, 293–298.

57 Yamazaki, H., *et al.* (1999) Roles of CYP2A6 and CYP2B6 in nicotine *C*-oxidation by human liver microsomes. *Arch. Toxicol.*, **73**, 65–70.

58 Berkman, C.E., *et al.* (1995) In vitro-*in vivo* correlations of human (*S*)-nicotine metabolism. *Biochem. Pharmacol.*, **50**, 565–570.

59 Nakajima, M., *et al.* (2000) Deficient cotinine formation from nicotine is attributed to the whole deletion of the CYP2A6 gene in humans. *Clin. Pharmacol. Ther.*, **67**, 57–69.

60 Nakajima, M., *et al.* (2001) Relationship between interindividual differences in nicotine metabolism and CYP2A6 genetic polymorphism in humans. *Clin. Pharmacol. Ther.*, **69**, 72–78.

61 Kwon, J.T., *et al.* (2001) Nicotine metabolism and CYP2A6 allele frequencies in Koreans. *Pharmacogenetics*, **11**, 317–323.

62 Xu, C., *et al.* (2002) An *in vivo* pilot study characterizing the new CYP2A6*7, *8, and *10 alleles. *Biochem. Biophys. Res. Commun.*, **290**, 318–324.

63 Kitagawa, K., *et al.* (1999) The significance of the homozygous CYP2A6 deletion on nicotine metabolism: a new genotyping method of CYP2A6 using a single PCR-RFLP. *Biochem. Biophys. Res. Commun.*, **262**, 146–151.

64 Yang, M., *et al.* (2001) Individual differences in urinary cotinine levels in Japanese smokers: relation to genetic polymorphism of drug-metabolizing enzymes. *Cancer Epidemiol. Biomarkers Prev.*, **10**, 589–593.

65 Zhang, X., *et al.* (2002) Effects of whole deletion of CYP2A6 on nicotine metabolism in humans. *Drug Chem. Toxicol.*, **25**, 203–213.

66 Sellers, E.M., Kaplan, H.L., and Tyndale, R.F. (2000) Inhibition of cytochrome P450 2A6 increases nicotine's oral

bioavailability and decreases smoking. *Clin. Pharmacol. Ther.*, **68**, 35–43.

67 Al Koudsi, N. and Tyndale, R.F. (2010) Hepatic CYP2B6 is altered by genetic, physiologic, and environmental factors but plays little role in nicotine metabolism. *Xenobiotica*, **40**, 381–392.

68 Murphy, S.E., Raulinaitis, V. and Brown, K.M. (2005) Nicotine 5′-oxidation and methyl oxidation by P450 2A enzymes. *Drug Metab. Dispos.*, **33**, 1166–1173.

69 Bao, Z., *et al.* (2005) Metabolism of nicotine and cotinine by human cytochrome P450 2A13. *Drug Metab. Dispos.*, **33**, 258–261.

70 Su, T., *et al.* (2000) Human cytochrome P450 CYP2A13: predominant expression in the respiratory tract and its high efficiency metabolic activation of a tobacco-specific carcinogen, 4-(methylnitrosamino)-1-(3-pyridyl)-1-butanone. *Cancer Res.*, **60**, 5074–5079.

71 Koskela, S., *et al.* (1999) Expression of CYP2A genes in human liver and extrahepatic tissues. *Biochem. Pharmacol.*, **57**, 1407–1413.

72 Park, S.B., *et al.* (1993) Stereoselective metabolism of (*S*)-(–)-nicotine in humans: formation of *trans*-(*S*)-(–)-nicotine *N*-1′-oxide. *Chem. Res. Toxicol.*, **6**, 880–888.

73 Yamanaka, H., *et al.* (2004) Metabolic profile of nicotine in subjects whose CYP2A6 gene is deleted. *Eur. J. Pharm. Sci.*, **22**, 419–425.

74 Nakajima, M., *et al.* (2002) Characterization of nicotine and cotinine *N*-glucuronidations in human liver microsomes. *Drug Metab. Dispos.*, **30**, 1484–1490.

75 Kuehl, G.E. and Murphy, S.E. (2003) *N*-glucuronidation of nicotine and cotinine by human liver microsomes and heterologously expressed UDP-glucuronosyltransferases. *Drug Metab. Dispos.*, **31**, 1361–1368.

76 Hecht, S.S., *et al.* (2000) 2′-Hydroxylation of nicotine by cytochrome P450 2A6 and human liver microsomes: formation of a lung carcinogen precursor. *Proc. Natl. Acad. Sci. USA*, **97**, 12493–12497.

77 Stepanov, I., *et al.* (2009) Evidence for endogenous formation of *N*′-nitrosonornicotine in some long-term nicotine patch users. *Nicotine Tob. Res.*, **11**, 99–105.

78 McKennis, H., Jr, Schwartz, S.L., and Bowman, E.R. (1964) Alternate routes in the metabolic degradation of the pyrrolidine ring of nicotine. *J. Biol. Chem.*, **239**, 3990–3996.

79 Jacob, P., 3rd, Shulgin, A.T., and Benowitz, N.L. (1990) Synthesis of (3′*R*,5′*S*)-*trans*-3′-hydroxycotinine, a major metabolite of nicotine. Metabolic formation of 3′-hydroxycotinine in humans is highly stereoselective. *J. Med. Chem.*, **33**, 1888–1891.

80 Voncken, P., Rustemeier, K., and Schepers, G. (1990) Identification of *cis*-3′-hydroxycotinine as a urinary nicotine metabolite. *Xenobiotica*, **20**, 1353 1356.

81 Mwenifumbo, J.C., *et al.* (2010) New CYP2A6 gene deletion and conversion variants in a population of Black African descent. *Pharmacogenomics*, **11**, 189–198.

82 Swan, G.E., *et al.* (2005) Nicotine metabolism: the impact of CYP2A6 on estimates of additive genetic influence. *Pharmacogenet. Genomics*, **15**, 115–125.

83 Al Koudsi, N., *et al.* (2010) Hepatic CYP2A6 levels and nicotine metabolism: impact of genetic, physiological, environmental, and epigenetic factors. *Eur. J. Clin. Pharmacol.*, **66**, 239–251.

84 Mwenifumbo, J.C. and Tyndale, R.F. (2007) Genetic variability in CYP2A6 and the pharmacokinetics of nicotine. *Pharmacogenomics*, **8**, 1385–1402.

85 Hoffman, S.M., *et al.* (1995) Organization and evolution of the cytochrome P450 CYP2A-2B-2F subfamily gene cluster on human chromosome 19. *J. Mol. Evol.*, **41**, 894–900.

86 Oscarson, M., *et al.* (1999) Identification and characterisation of novel polymorphisms in the CYP2A locus: implications for nicotine metabolism. *FEBS Lett.*, **460**, 321–327.

87 Nakajima, M., *et al.* (2006) Comprehensive evaluation of variability in nicotine metabolism and CYP2A6 polymorphic alleles in four ethnic

populations. *Clin. Pharmacol. Ther.*, **80**, 282–297.
88 Yamano, S., Tatsuno, J., and Gonzalez, F.J. (1990) The CYP2A3 gene product catalyzes coumarin 7-hydroxylation in human liver microsomes. *Biochemistry*, **29**, 1322–1329.
89 Wang, J., Pitarque, M., and Ingelman-Sundberg, M. (2006) 3′-UTR polymorphism in the human CYP2A6 gene affects mRNA stability and enzyme expression. *Biochem. Biophys. Res. Commun.*, **340**, 491–497.
90 Mwenifumbo, J.C., *et al.* (2008) Identification of novel CYP2A6*1B variants: the CYP2A6*1B allele is associated with faster *in vivo* nicotine metabolism. *Clin. Pharmacol. Ther.*, **83**, 115–121.
91 Nurfadhlina, M., *et al.* (2006) CYP2A6 polymorphisms in Malays, Chinese and Indians. *Xenobiotica*, **36**, 684–692.
92 Gambier, N., *et al.* (2005) Association of CYP2A6*1B genetic variant with the amount of smoking in French adults from the Stanislas cohort. *Pharmacogenomics J.*, **5**, 271–275.
93 Gyamfi, M.A., *et al.* (2005) High prevalence of cytochrome P450 2A6*1A alleles in a black African population of Ghana. *Eur. J. Clin. Pharmacol.*, **60**, 855–857.
94 Pitarque, M., *et al.* (2004) A nicotine *C*-oxidase gene (CYP2A6) polymorphism important for promoter activity. *Hum. Mutat.*, **23**, 258–266.
95 von Richter, O., *et al.* (2004) Polymorphic NF-Y dependent regulation of human nicotine *C*-oxidase (CYP2A6). *Pharmacogenetics*, **14**, 369–379.
96 Schoedel, K.A., *et al.* (2004) Ethnic variation in CYP2A6 and association of genetically slow nicotine metabolism and smoking in adult Caucasians. *Pharmacogenetics*, **14**, 615–626.
97 Benowitz, N.L., Griffin, C., and Tyndale, R. (2001) Deficient C-oxidation of nicotine continued. *Clin. Pharmacol. Ther.*, **70**, 567.
98 Benowitz, N.L., Jacob, P., 3rd, and Sachs, D.P. (1995) Deficient *C*-oxidation of nicotine. *Clin. Pharmacol. Ther.*, **57**, 590–594.
99 Nunoya, K., *et al.* (1998) A new deleted allele in the human cytochrome P450 2A6 (CYP2A6) gene found in individuals showing poor metabolic capacity to coumarin and (+)-*cis*-3,5-dimethyl-2-(3-pyridyl)thiazolidin-4-one hydrochloride (SM-12502). *Pharmacogenetics*, **8**, 239–249.
100 Nunoya, K.I., *et al.* (1999) A new CYP2A6 gene deletion responsible for the *in vivo* polymorphic metabolism of (+)-*cis*-3,5-dimethyl-2-(3-pyridyl) thiazolidin-4-one hydrochloride in humans. *J. Pharmacol. Exp. Ther.*, **289**, 437–442.
101 Oscarson, M., *et al.* (1999) Characterisation and PCR-based detection of a CYP2A6 gene deletion found at a high frequency in a Chinese population. *FEBS Lett.*, **448**, 105–110.
102 Huang, S., *et al.* (2005) CYP2A6, MAOA, DBH, DRD4, and 5HT2A genotypes, smoking behaviour and cotinine levels in 1518 UK adolescents. *Pharmacogenet. Genomics*, **15**, 839–850.
103 Ariyoshi, N., *et al.* (2000) Structural characterization of a new variant of the CYP2A6 gene (CYP2A6*1B) apparently diagnosed as heterozygotes of CYP2A6*1A and CYP2A6*4C. *Pharmacogenetics*, **10**, 687–693.
104 Minematsu, N., *et al.* (2006) Limitation of cigarette consumption by CYP2A6*4, *7 and *9 polymorphisms. *Eur. Respir. J.*, **27**, 289–292.
105 Ariyoshi, N., *et al.* (2001) A single nucleotide polymorphism of CYP2b6 found in Japanese enhances catalytic activity by autoactivation. *Biochem. Biophys. Res. Commun.*, **281**, 1256–1260.
106 Yoshida, R., *et al.* (2002) Genetic polymorphisms in human CYP2A6 gene causing impaired nicotine metabolism. *Br. J. Clin. Pharmacol.*, **54**, 511–517.
107 Mwenifumbo, J.C., *et al.* (2005) Ethnic variation in CYP2A6*7, CYP2A6*8 and CYP2A6*10 as assessed with a novel haplotyping method. *Pharmacogenet. Genomics*, **15**, 189–192.
108 Malaiyandi, V., *et al.* (2006) Impact of CYP2A6 genotype on pretreatment smoking behaviour and nicotine levels from and usage of nicotine replacement therapy. *Mol. Psychiatry*, **11**, 400–409.

109 Benowitz, N.L., *et al.* (2006) CYP2A6 genotype and the metabolism and disposition kinetics of nicotine. *Clin. Pharmacol. Ther.*, **80**, 457–467.

110 Daigo, S., *et al.* (2002) A novel mutant allele of the CYP2A6 gene (CYP2A6*11) found in a cancer patient who showed poor metabolic phenotype towards tegafur. *Pharmacogenetics*, **12**, 299–306.

111 Audrain-McGovern, J., *et al.* (2007) The role of CYP2A6 in the emergence of nicotine dependence in adolescents. *Pediatrics*, **119**, e264–e274.

112 Oscarson, M., *et al.* (2002) Characterization of a novel CYP2A7/CYP2A6 hybrid allele (CYP2A6*12) that causes reduced CYP2A6 activity. *Hum. Mutat.*, **20**, 275–283.

113 Kiyotani, K., *et al.* (2002) Twenty one novel single nucleotide polymorphisms (SNPs) of the CYP2A6 gene in Japanese and Caucasians. *Drug Metab. Pharmacokinet.*, **17**, 482–487.

114 Haberl, M., *et al.* (2005) Three haplotypes associated with CYP2A6 phenotypes in Caucasians. *Pharmacogenet. Genomics*, **15**, 609–624.

115 Fukami, T., *et al.* (2004) A novel polymorphism of human CYP2A6 gene CYP2A6*17 has an amino acid substitution (V365M) that decreases enzymatic activity *in vitro* and *in vivo*. *Clin. Pharmacol. Ther.*, **76**, 519–527.

116 Fukami, T., *et al.* (2005) Characterization of novel CYP2A6 polymorphic alleles (CYP2A6*18 and CYP2A6*19) that affect enzymatic activity. *Drug Metab. Dispos.*, **33**, 1202–1210.

117 Ho, M.K., *et al.* (2009) Association of nicotine metabolite ratio and CYP2A6 genotype with smoking cessation treatment in African-American light smokers. *Clin. Pharmacol. Ther.*, **85**, 635–643.

118 Mwenifumbo, J.C., *et al.* (2008) Novel and established CYP2A6 alleles impair *in vivo* nicotine metabolism in a population of Black African descent. *Hum. Mutat.*, **29**, 679–688.

119 Fukami, T., *et al.* (2005) A novel CYP2A6*20 allele found in African-American population produces a truncated protein lacking enzymatic activity. *Biochem. Pharmacol.*, **70**, 801–808.

120 Al Koudsi, N., *et al.* (2006) Characterization of the novel CYP2A6*21 allele using *in vivo* nicotine kinetics. *Eur. J. Clin. Pharmacol.*, **62**, 481–484.

121 Ho, M.K., *et al.* (2008) A novel CYP2A6 allele, CYP2A6*23, impairs enzyme function *in vitro* and *in vivo* and decreases smoking in a population of Black-African descent. *Pharmacogenet. Genomics*, **18**, 67–75.

122 Al Koudsi, N., *et al.* (2009) A novel CYP2A6 allele (CYP2A6*35) resulting in an amino-acid substitution (Asn438Tyr) is associated with lower CYP2A6 activity *in vivo*. *Pharmacogenomics J.*, **9**, 274–282.

123 Rao, Y., *et al.* (2000) Duplications and defects in the CYP2A6 gene: identification, genotyping, and *in vivo* effects on smoking. *Mol. Pharmacol.*, **58**, 747–755.

124 Fukami, T., *et al.* (2007) A novel duplication type of CYP2A6 gene in African-American population. *Drug Metab. Dispos.*, **35**, 515–520.

125 Johnstone, E., *et al.* (2006) Determinants of the rate of nicotine metabolism and effects on smoking behavior. *Clin. Pharmacol. Ther.*, **80**, 319–330.

126 Lee, A.M., *et al.* (2007) CYP2B6 genotype does not alter nicotine metabolism, plasma levels, or abstinence with nicotine replacement therapy. *Cancer Epidemiol. Biomarkers Prev.*, **16**, 1312–1314.

127 Klein, K., *et al.* (2005) Genetic variability of CYP2B6 in populations of African and Asian origin: allele frequencies, novel functional variants, and possible implications for anti-HIV therapy with efavirenz. *Pharmacogenet. Genomics*, **15**, 861–873.

128 Ring, H.Z., *et al.* (2007) Gene–gene interactions between CYP2B6 and CYP2A6 in nicotine metabolism. *Pharmacogenet. Genomics*, **17**, 1007–1015.

129 Nunoya, K., *et al.* (1999) Homologous unequal cross-over within the human CYP2A gene cluster as a mechanism for the deletion of the entire CYP2A6 gene associated with the poor metabolizer phenotype. *J. Biochem.*, **126**, 402–407.

130 Lea, R.A., Dickson, S., and Benowitz, N.L. (2006) Within-subject variation of

the salivary 3HC/COT ratio in regular daily smokers: prospects for estimating CYP2A6 enzyme activity in large-scale surveys of nicotine metabolic rate. *J. Anal. Toxicol.*, **30**, 386–389.

131 Levi, M., *et al.* (2007) Prediction methods for nicotine clearance using cotinine and 3-hydroxy-cotinine spot saliva samples II. Model application. *J. Pharmacokinet. Pharmacodyn.*, **34**, 23–34.

132 Malaiyandi, V., Sellers, E.M., and Tyndale, R.F. (2005) Implications of CYP2A6 genetic variation for smoking behaviors and nicotine dependence. *Clin. Pharmacol. Ther.*, **77**, 145–158.

133 Mwenifumbo, J.C. and Tyndale, R.F. (2009) Molecular genetics of nicotine metabolism. *Handb. Exp. Pharmacol.*, **192**, 235–259.

134 Lerman, C., *et al.* (2010) Genetic variation in nicotine metabolism predicts the efficacy of extended-duration transdermal nicotine therapy. *Clin. Pharmacol. Ther.*, **87**, 553–557.

135 Shimada, T., Yamazaki, H., and Guengerich, F.P. (1996) Ethnic-related differences in coumarin 7-hydroxylation activities catalyzed by cytochrome P4502A6 in liver microsomes of Japanese and Caucasian populations. *Xenobiotica*, **26**, 395–403.

136 Benowitz, N.L., *et al.* (2006) Female sex and oral contraceptive use accelerate nicotine metabolism. *Clin. Pharmacol. Ther.*, **79**, 480–488.

137 Higashi, E., *et al.* (2007) Human CYP2A6 is induced by estrogen via estrogen receptor. *Drug Metab. Dispos.*, **35**, 1935–1941.

138 Krul, C. and Hageman, G. (1998) Analysis of urinary caffeine metabolites to assess biotransformation enzyme activities by reversed-phase high-performance liquid chromatography. *J. Chromatogr. B*, **709**, 27–34.

139 Dempsey, D., Jacob, P., 3rd, and Benowitz, N.L. (2002) Accelerated metabolism of nicotine and cotinine in pregnant smokers. *J. Pharmacol. Exp. Ther.*, **301**, 594–598.

140 Hukkanen, J., *et al.* (2005) Influence of menstrual cycle on cytochrome P450 2A6 activity and cardiovascular effects of nicotine. *Clin. Pharmacol. Ther.*, **77**, 159–169.

141 Leong, J.W., *et al.* (1998) The elimination half-life of urinary cotinine in children of tobacco-smoking mothers. *Pulm. Pharmacol. Ther.*, **11**, 287–290.

142 Dempsey, D., Jacob, P., 3rd, and Benowitz, N.L. (2000) Nicotine metabolism and elimination kinetics in newborns. *Clin. Pharmacol. Ther.*, **67**, 458–465.

143 Tateishi, T., *et al.* (1997) A comparison of hepatic cytochrome P450 protein expression between infancy and postinfancy. *Life Sci.*, **61**, 2567–2574.

144 Gow, P.J., *et al.* (2001) Neonatal hepatic drug elimination. *Pharmacol. Toxicol.*, **88**, 3–15.

145 Parkinson, A., *et al.* (2004) The effects of gender, age, ethnicity, and liver cirrhosis on cytochrome P450 enzyme activity in human liver microsomes and inducibility in cultured human hepatocytes. *Toxicol. Appl. Pharmacol.*, **199**, 193–209.

146 Gourlay, S.G. and Benowitz, N.L. (1996) The benefits of stopping smoking and the role of nicotine replacement therapy in older patients. *Drugs Aging*, **9**, 8–23.

147 Mwenifumbo, J.C., Sellers, E.M., and Tyndale, R.F. (2007) Nicotine metabolism and CYP2A6 activity in a population of black African descent: impact of gender and light smoking. *Drug Alcohol Depend.*, **89**, 24–33.

148 Shimada, T., *et al.* (1994) Interindividual variations in human liver cytochrome P-450 enzymes involved in the oxidation of drugs, carcinogens and toxic chemicals: studies with liver microsomes of 30 Japanese and 30 Caucasians. *J. Pharmacol. Exp. Ther.*, **270**, 414–423.

149 Pasanen, M., *et al.* (1997) Hepatitis A impairs the function of human hepatic CYP2A6 *in vivo*. *Toxicology*, **123**, 177–184.

150 Molander, L., Hansson, A., and Lunell, E. (2001) Pharmacokinetics of nicotine in healthy elderly people. *Clin. Pharmacol. Ther.*, **69**, 57–65.

151 Gries, J.M., Benowitz, N., and Verotta, D. (1996) Chronopharmacokinetics of nicotine. *Clin. Pharmacol. Ther.*, **60**, 385–395.

152 Lee, B.L., *et al.* (1989) Food and nicotine metabolism. *Pharmacol. Biochem. Behav.*, **33**, 621–625.
153 Madan, A., *et al.* (2003) Effects of prototypical microsomal enzyme inducers on cytochrome P450 expression in cultured human hepatocytes. *Drug Metab. Dispos.*, **31**, 421–431.
154 Sotaniemi, E.A., *et al.* (1995) CYP3A4 and CYP2A6 activities marked by the metabolism of lignocaine and coumarin in patients with liver and kidney diseases and epileptic patients. *Br. J. Clin. Pharmacol.*, **39**, 71–76.
155 Kyerematen, G.A., *et al.* (1990) Metabolism of nicotine by hepatocytes. *Biochem. Pharmacol.*, **40**, 1747–1756.
156 Rae, J.M., *et al.* (2001) Rifampin is a selective, pleiotropic inducer of drug metabolism genes in human hepatocytes: studies with cDNA and oligonucleotide expression arrays. *J. Pharmacol. Exp. Ther.*, **299**, 849–857.
157 Mattes, W.B. and Li, A.P. (1997) Quantitative reverse transcriptase/PCR assay for the measurement of induction in cultured hepatocytes. *Chem. Biol. Interact.*, **107**, 47–61.
158 Maurice, M., *et al.* (1991) Isolation and characterization of a cytochrome P450 of the IIA subfamily from human liver microsomes. *Eur. J. Biochem.*, **200**, 511–517.
159 Meunier, V., *et al.* (2000) Expression and induction of CYP1A1/1A2, CYP2A6 and CYP3A4 in primary cultures of human hepatocytes: a 10-year follow-up. *Xenobiotica*, **30**, 589–607.
160 Xia, X.Y., *et al.* (2002) *In vitro* metabolic characteristics of cytochrome P-450 2A6 in Chinese liver microsomes. *Acta Pharmacol. Sin.*, **23**, 471–476.
161 Donato, M.T., *et al.* (2000) CYP2A5/CYP2A6 expression in mouse and human hepatocytes treated with various *in vivo* inducers. *Drug Metab. Dispos.*, **28**, 1321–1326.
162 Maglich, J.M., *et al.* (2002) Nuclear pregnane X receptor and constitutive androstane receptor regulate overlapping but distinct sets of genes involved in xenobiotic detoxification. *Mol. Pharmacol.*, **62**, 638–646.
163 Itoh, M., *et al.* (2006) Induction of human CYP2A6 is mediated by the pregnane X receptor with peroxisome proliferator-activated receptor-gamma coactivator 1alpha. *J. Pharmacol. Exp. Ther.*, **319**, 693–702.
164 Zhang, W., *et al.* (2001) Evaluation of methoxsalen, tranylcypromine, and tryptamine as specific and selective CYP2A6 inhibitors *in vitro*. *Drug Metab. Dispos.*, **29**, 897–902.
165 Taavitsainen, P., Juvonen, R., and Pelkonen, O. (2001) *In vitro* inhibition of cytochrome P450 enzymes in human liver microsomes by a potent CYP2A6 inhibitor, *trans*-2-phenylcyclopropylamine (tranylcypromine), and its nonamine analog, cyclopropylbenzene. *Drug Metab. Dispos.*, **29**, 217–222.
166 Siu, E.C. and Tyndale, R.F. (2008) Selegiline is a mechanism-based inactivator of CYP2A6 inhibiting nicotine metabolism in humans and mice. *J. Pharmacol. Exp. Ther.*, **324**, 992–999.
167 MacDougall, J.M., *et al.* (2003) Inhibition of human liver microsomal (*S*)-nicotine oxidation by (–)-menthol and analogues. *Chem. Res. Toxicol.*, **16**, 988–993.
168 Le Gal, A., *et al.* (2001) Human cytochrome P450 2A6 is the major enzyme involved in the metabolism of three alkoxyethers used as oxyfuels. *Toxicol. Lett.*, **124**, 47–58.
169 Sellers, E.M., *et al.* (2003) The effect of methoxsalen on nicotine and 4-(methylnitrosamino)-1-(3-pyridyl)-1-butanone (NNK) metabolism *in vivo*. *Nicotine Tob. Res.*, **5**, 891–899.
170 Draper, A.J., Madan, A., and Parkinson, A. (1997) Inhibition of coumarin 7-hydroxylase activity in human liver microsomes. *Arch. Biochem. Biophys.*, **341**, 47–61.
171 Pelkonen, O., *et al.* (2000) CYP2A6: a human coumarin 7-hydroxylase. *Toxicology*, **144**, 139–147.
172 Poland, R.E., *et al.* (2000) Effect of cigarette smoking on coumarin metabolism in humans. *Nicotine Tob. Res.*, **2**, 351–354.
173 Iscan, M., *et al.* (1994) Interindividual variability of coumarin 7-hydroxylation

in a Turkish population. *Eur. J. Clin. Pharmacol.*, **47**, 315–318.

174 Denton, T.T., Zhang, X., and Cashman, J.R. (2004) Nicotine-related alkaloids and metabolites as inhibitors of human cytochrome P-450 2A6. *Biochem. Pharmacol.*, **67**, 751–756.

175 Schoedel, K.A., *et al.* (2003) Down-regulation of hepatic nicotine metabolism and a CYP2A6-like enzyme in African green monkeys after long-term nicotine administration. *Mol. Pharmacol.*, **63**, 96–104.

176 Hukkanen, J., *et al.* (2010) Effects of nicotine on cytochrome P450 2A6 and 2E1 activities. *Br. J. Clin. Pharmacol.*, **69**, 152–159.

177 Benowitz, N.L., Herrera, B., and Jacob, P., 3rd (2004) Mentholated cigarette smoking inhibits nicotine metabolism. *J. Pharmacol. Exp. Ther.*, **310**, 1208–1215.

178 Molander, L., *et al.* (2000) Pharmacokinetics of nicotine in kidney failure. *Clin. Pharmacol. Ther.*, **68**, 250–260.

179 Merkel, U., Sigusch, H., and Hoffmann, A. (1994) Grapefruit juice inhibits 7-hydroxylation of coumarin in healthy volunteers. *Eur. J. Clin. Pharmacol.*, **46**, 175–177.

180 Runkel, M., *et al.* (1997) The character of inhibition of the metabolism of 1,2-benzopyrone (coumarin) by grapefruit juice in human. *Eur. J. Clin. Pharmacol.*, **53**, 265–269.

181 Hakooz, N. and Hamdan, I. (2007) Effects of dietary broccoli on human *in vivo* caffeine metabolism: a pilot study on a group of Jordanian volunteers. *Curr. Drug Metab.*, **8**, 9–15.

182 O'Loughlin, J., *et al.* (2004) Genetically decreased CYP2A6 and the risk of tobacco dependence: a prospective study of novice smokers. *Tob. Control*, **13**, 422–428.

183 Strasser, A.A., *et al.* (2007) An association of CYP2A6 genotype and smoking topography. *Nicotine Tob. Res.*, **9**, 511–518.

184 Gu, D.F., *et al.* (2000) The use of long PCR to confirm three common alleles at the CYP2A6 locus and the relationship between genotype and smoking habit. *Ann. Hum. Genet.*, **64**, 383–390.

185 Lerman, C., *et al.* (2006) Nicotine metabolite ratio predicts efficacy of transdermal nicotine for smoking cessation. *Clin. Pharmacol. Ther.*, **79**, 600–608.

186 Iwahashi, K., Waga, C., and Takimoto, T. (2004) Whole deletion of CYP2A6 gene (CYP2A6AST;4C) and smoking behavior. *Neuropsychobiology*, **49**, 101–104.

187 Munafo, M., *et al.* (2004) The genetic basis for smoking behavior: a systematic review and meta-analysis. *Nicotine Tob. Res.*, **6**, 583–597.

188 Carter, B., Long, T., and Cinciripini, P. (2004) A meta-analytic review of the CYP2A6 genotype and smoking behavior. *Nicotine Tob. Res.*, **6**, 221–227.

189 Fujieda, M., *et al.* (2004) Evaluation of CYP2A6 genetic polymorphisms as determinants of smoking behavior and tobacco-related lung cancer risk in male Japanese smokers. *Carcinogenesis*, **25**, 2451–2458.

190 Thorgeirsson, T.E., *et al.* (2010) Sequence variants at CHRNB3–CHRNA6 and CYP2A6 affect smoking behavior. *Nat. Genet.*, **42**, 448–453.

191 Patterson, F., *et al.* (2008) Toward personalized therapy for smoking cessation: a randomized placebo-controlled trial of bupropion. *Clin. Pharmacol. Ther.*, **84**, 320–325.

192 Roden, D.M., *et al.* (2006) Pharmacogenomics: challenges and opportunities. *Ann. Intern. Med.*, **145**, 749–757.

193 Heitjan, D.F., *et al.* (2008) Cost-effectiveness of pharmacogenetic testing to tailor smoking-cessation treatment. *Pharmacogenomics J.*, **8**, 391–399.

18
Metabolism of Alcohol and its Consequences

Helmut K. Seitz and Sebastian Mueller

18.1
Introduction

Ethanol – a simple two-carbon molecule – is metabolized in every tissue and every cell of the human body, and also by gastrointestinal bacteria. Ethanol is metabolized via alcohol dehydrogenase (ADH), cytochrome P450 (CYP) 2E1, and by catalase, resulting primarily in the generation of acetaldehyde, which is further metabolized via acetaldehyde dehydrogenase (ALDH) to acetate. Acetate is then channeled as acetyl-CoA into the citric acid cycle. Since seven isoenzymes of ADH exist and two of the ADHs are polymorphic, ethanol metabolism varies considerably interindividually, resulting in the generation of different acetaldehyde concentrations. As acetaldehyde is toxic and carcinogenic, the rate of its generation and of its degradation predicts the individual risk for organ toxicity and cancer development. In addition to acetaldehyde, reducing equivalents in the form of NADH are also generated via the ADH reaction, resulting in a severe change of the intracellular redox state and leading to severe alterations of the intermediary metabolism, which may explain various pathologies.

Ethanol metabolism via CYP2E1 is quantitatively lower. However, CYP2E1 is inducible by chronic alcohol consumption and, therefore, the rate of ethanol metabolism via CYP2E1 increases in the chronic alcohol abuser. Ethanol metabolism via CYP2E1 also generates reactive oxygen species (ROS), resulting in tissue toxicity and DNA damage. Since CYP2E1 is not only responsible for ethanol metabolism, but also for the metabolism of various drugs, xenobiotics, and procarcinogens, an interaction between these substances and alcohol metabolism occurs. As a result, changes of drug blood concentrations are observed and an increased toxicity of certain drugs is seen. These interactions are of clinical importance. Thus, ethanol metabolism is not only an important prerequisite to explain ethanol toxicity in various organs such as the liver, but also plays an important role to explain the interaction with drugs, xenobiotics, procarcinogens, and retinoids.

The present chapter not only focuses on various aspects of ethanol metabolism, including genetics, but also emphasizes the consequences of ethanol metabolism

Metabolism of Drugs and Other Xenobiotics, First Edition. Edited by Pavel Anzenbacher, Ulrich M. Zanger.

with respect to ethanol-associated pathologies and diseases as well as alterations of the metabolism of drugs, xenobiotics, procarcinogens, and retinoids, which is of major clinical relevance. The knowledge of these complex interactions is a major prerequisite for pharmacologists to understand ethanol effects, and for clinicians to diagnose and treat alcohol-induced, -mediated, or -associated disorders.

18.2 Properties and Sources of Ethanol

18.2.1 Chemical Properties of Ethanol

Molecular weight 46.07, C_2H_6O (52.14% C,13.13% H, 34.74% O), density 0.789 at 15.56 °C (60 °F), boiling point 78.5 °C, refraction index *n*20/*D* 1.361 for 20 °C and sodium light, solid if below −130 °C, water soluble, LD_{50} orally in rats 13.7 g/kg.

18.2.2 Ethanol Content of Alcoholic Beverages

Ethanol concentrations of various alcoholic beverages are given in Table 18.1.

18.2.3 Ethanol Generation in the Human Body

Endogenous ethanol production may occur through bacterial fermentation of carbohydrates in the gastrointestinal tract, especially in the stomach. Gastric bacte-

Table 18.1 Alcoholic content of various alcoholic beverages.

Beverage	Ethanol content (vol%)	Ethanol content (g/100 ml; approximate values)
Alcohol-free beer	max. 0.5	0.4
Low-strength beer	2	1.6
Standard beer (e.g., lager)	3–4	2.4–3
Pilsner, weiss beer	4–5.7	3.1–4.5
Bock beer	7–8	5.5–6.4
Fruit wine	8–14	6–11.5
White wine, red wine, sparkling wine	8–15	6.3–12
Liqueur	25–45	2.0–3.5
Spirits (brandy, cognac)	30–40	2.3–3.2
Whiskey, gin	35–45	2.7–3.6
Fruit brandy, slivovitz, vodka	40–50	3.1–4.0
Spirit of Melissa	60–70	4.7–5.5
Rum	40–70	3.1–5.5

rial overgrowth observed in atrophic gastritis may lead to the generation of ethanol intragastrically. In addition, *Candida* species may also generate ethanol, resulting in relatively high concentrations of blood alcohol up to 25 mmol/l [1–3].

18.3 Ethanol Absorption and Elimination

18.3.1 Ethanol Absorption and Ethanol Blood Levels

Blood alcohol concentrations (BACs) reflect gastrointestinal absorption, diffusion, metabolism, and unchanged excretion of ethanol. Thus, absorption of ethanol associated with increasing BAC has to be distinguished from elimination with decreasing BAC. At the end of alcohol absorption a peak is detectable, which may change to a plateau if alcohol is further consumed continuously.

Alcohol is absorbed from the upper gastrointestinal tract by simple diffusion. This is a fast process due to the small molecule of alcohol and its excellent solubility in water, but not in fat. Delayed gastric emptying and food in the upper gastrointestinal tract may lead to lower BAC, while a higher BAC is observed after gastrointestinal bypass surgery and after consumption of highly concentrated alcoholic beverages such as liquors compared to low concentrated beverages like beer and wine [4, 5]. Gastrointestinal absorption of ethanol depends on various factors, including the ethanol concentration of the beverage, blood perfusion of the stomach and duodenum, simultaneous food intake, rate of gastric emptying, body temperature, and menstrual cycle [4, 5].

Twenty percent of alcohol is absorbed from the stomach and 80% from the upper small intestine. In the gastric mucosa, alcohol can be metabolized by various ADHs. This is called gastric first-pass metabolism (FPM) of alcohol [6]. No such metabolism has been observed in the small intestine. The rest of the ethanol enters the liver via the portal vein. There is a partial metabolism of alcohol in the liver, but also a release of alcohol without metabolism. Ethanol is metabolized to more than 90% in the liver after multiple passages through the liver, to 5–10% in the gastric mucosa, and approximately 3–5% of the orally absorbed ethanol is excreted unchanged through the lungs, skin, and kidneys [4, 5].

Ethanol is primarily metabolized through ADHs. Their kinetic parameters, localization, and substrate specificity are given in Table 18.2 [7]. In addition, ethanol can also be oxidized by a CYP2E1-dependent microsomal ethanol oxidizing system (MEOS) in various cells, but predominantly in hepatocytes [8–10].

The ethanol distribution space (body water) is smaller in women than in men and smaller in the elderly than in younger individuals. As a consequence, the same ethanol consumption per kilogram body weight results in higher ethanol blood concentrations [11, 12]. This is also true for overweight or obese persons since ethanol is almost insoluble in fat. The ethanol elimination rate is also higher in men compared to women. A maximal amount of 150 mg ethanol/kg body weight/h

Table 18.2 Characteristics of human ADHs.

Gene/locus	Allele	Protein subunit	K_m ethanol (mM)	V_{max} (min^{-1})	Ethnic/nutritional distribution	Location
ADH1A	ADH1A	α	4.0	30	Europe, Africa	liver
ADH1B	ADH1B*1	β1	0.05	4	Europe, Africa	liver, lung
	ADH1B*2	β2	0.9	350	Asia	
	ADH1B*3	β3	40	300	Africa, Native American	
ADH1C	ADH1C*1	γ1	1.0	87	all	liver, stomach, blood vessels (intima and media mainly ADH1B)
	ADH1C*2	γ2	0.63	40	Europe	
	ADH1C*3	–	–	–	Native American	
ADH4	ADH4	π	30	20	all Sweden	Liver
ADH5	ADH5	X	>1000	100	all	all tissues
ADH6	ADH6		?	?	all	
ADH7	ADH-IV	σ, μ	30	1800	all	stomach, upper aerodigestive tract, and other tissues

can be metabolized by a healthy man. This represents approximately 10 g ethanol in a 70-kg person per 1 h or 240 g ethanol in a 70-kg person per 24 h. The ethanol elimination rate is about 13 mg/100 ml/h. Chronic ethanol consumption increases the ethanol elimination rate significantly due to the induction of CYP2E1 [13]. It is noteworthy that no feedback mechanisms exist for ethanol metabolism. Organs with a high blood supply, such as the liver, kidney and brain, have an increased uptake of ethanol in the resting condition compared to skeletal muscles.

18.3.2
Calculation of Ethanol Elimination Using the Widmark Equation

Widmark was the first to describe quantitatively the slope of the blood alcohol elimination curve. The postabsorption phase of the elimination kinetic can be expressed by a simple equation:

$$C_t = C_o - (\beta \times t)$$

This equation resembles an open one-compartment model with zero-order elimination kinetics. C_o is the relationship between ethanol dose and body weight, whereas body weight is reduced by r – a dimensionless factor. This reduction factor was installed to equalize ethanol concentration in the blood to that of the total body. The Widmark factor r represents the water distribution space of ethanol, which is approximately the total water content of the body. When C_o is eliminated the following equation results:

$$\text{ethanol uptake (g)} = \text{body weight (kg)} \times r \times (C_t + \beta_t)$$

to calculate the amount of ethanol ingested by knowing BAC in the postabsorption phase or:

$$C_t = \text{ethanol uptake (g)}/(\text{body weight (kg)} \times r) - (\beta_t)$$

to calculate BAC following a defined amount of ingested alcohol at certain time points.

Prerequisite is a stable distribution space r, complete absorption, distribution, and a negligible FPM. If these prerequisites are not fulfilled, a so-called absorption deficit needs to be defined.

The Widmark factor r is approximately 0.7 in man and 0.6 in women, and the loss of resorption β_t is approximately 10%. For more information, the reader is referred to more detailed calculations [14–16]. In principle, ethanol elimination is an enzymatic process that follows a Michaelis–Menten kinetic. One equation can reflect linear elimination at higher BACs with an exponential phase at low BAC:

$$-\mathrm{d}C/\mathrm{d}T = (V_{\max} \times C)/(K_{\mathrm{m}} + C)$$

where $-\mathrm{d}C/\mathrm{d}T$ is the change in concentration per unit of time, $V_{\max}$ is the maximal reaction velocity, K_{m} is the Michaelis–Menten constant, and C is the ethanol concentration.

Despite the fact that a single pharmacokinetic model does not describe completely the fate of ethanol in the body, the Widmark equation has been found to be a useful tool, especially in forensic medicine.

18.4 Ethanol Metabolism

Ethanol is metabolized by oxidation to acetaldehyde by the enzyme ADH, by the CYP2E1-dependent MEOS, or by catalase and further to acetate by ALDH (Figure 18.1).

18.4.1 Ethanol Metabolism via ADH

ADH is localized in the cytoplasm of all cells, but predominantly in hepatocytes. ADH requires as cofactor NAD^+, which is reduced to $NADH + H^+$ during the metabolism of ethanol to acetaldehyde. ADH is a zinc-containing enzyme with a molecular weight of 80 000 and a predominant location around the central vein within the hepatic lobule. It is a dimer consisting of three polypeptide chains (α, β, and γ) [7].

$$CH_3CH_2OH + NAD^+ \xrightarrow{\text{ADH}} CH_3CHO + NADH^+ + H^+$$

$$CH_3CH_2OH + NADPH + H^+ + O_2 \xrightarrow{\text{MEOS}} CH_3CHO + NADP^+ + 2H_2O$$

$$NADPH + H^+ + O_2 \xrightarrow{\text{NADPH O xidase}} NADP^+ + H_2O_2$$

+

$$H_2O_2 + CH_3CH_2OH \xrightarrow{\text{Catalase}} 2H_2O + CH_3CHO$$

$$HYPOXANTHINE + H_2O + O_2 \xrightarrow{\text{Xanthine Oxidase}} XANTHINE + H_2O_2$$

+

$$H_2O_2 + CH_3CH_2OH \xrightarrow{\text{Catalase}} 2H_2O + CH_3CHO$$

Figure 18.1 Ethanol metabolism via ADH, MEOS, and catalase. The catalase reaction needs either NADH oxidase or xanthine oxidase to produce H_2O_2, which reacts with alcohol to produce acetaldehyde.

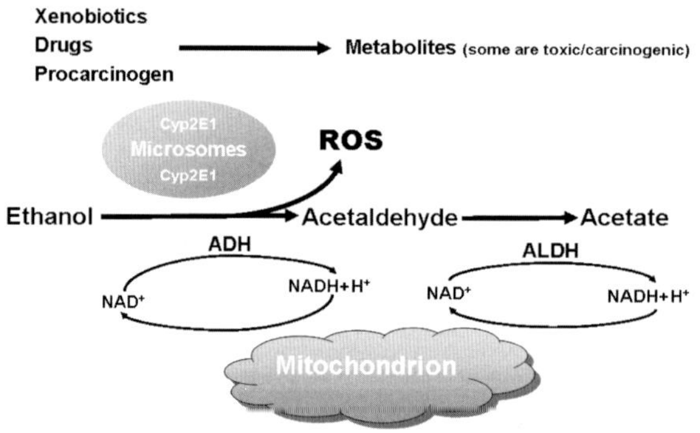

Figure 18.2 Ethanol metabolism through microsomal CYP2E1. Ethanol is metabolized to a lower extent by microsomal ethanol oxidation to acetaldehyde. ROS are generated in this process, which may have toxic effects on the cell. In addition, various xenobiotics, drugs, and procarcinogens use the same CYP2E1 that is induced by chronic alcohol consumption for their metabolism, resulting in an increased metabolism of these compounds and sometimes leading to the generation of toxic metabolites.

ADH oxidizes ethanol first to acetaldehyde, which is then further oxidized to acetate (Figure 18.2). The reactions involve an intermediate carrier of electrons, NAD^+, which is reduced to NADH. The electrons that originated in ethanol to produce NADH are ultimately transferred to oxygen via a number of other intermediate carriers in the mitochondrial electron transport chain and oxygen is reduced to water at the terminal enzyme (cytochrome oxidase). The final oxidation creates energy as ATP (1 g of ethanol equivalents 7.1 kcal). This intramitochondrial electron transport may generate ROS if not controlled adequately. A small portion of oxygen that is reduced in the mitochondria is released as the one-electron-reduced form – superoxide. Increased mitochondrial activity and NADH use generate more superoxide. As a protection against intramitochondrially generated ROS, the mitochondria possess manganese superoxide dismutase, which destroys superoxide.

Multiple ADH and ALDH enzymes exist that are encoded by different genes. They are characterized in Table 18.2 [17]. Some of these genes have several alleles and the enzyme encoded by these alleles can differ in the rate of ethanol metabolism. These alleles influence drinking behavior, and the risk of developing alcohol dependency and alcohol-associated organ damage. The mechanisms by which these alleles influence alcoholism risk are elevated acetaldehyde concentrations either through more rapid ethanol oxidation via ADH or slower acetaldehyde oxidation via ALDH.

Acetaldehyde is toxic and carcinogenic [18], and its accumulation results in a so-called flush syndrome (see below) similar to after the administration of disulfiram, which results in discouragement of further drinking. Most of the alleles of ADH and ALDH are single nucleotide polymorphisms. The *ADH* genes are located along a small region of chromosome 4.

Class I ADH – the major ADH in the liver – has a Michaelis–Menten constant for ethanol of 0.5–1.0 mM. This equals 0.02–0.05 mg/ml ethanol. Thus, class I ADH (ADH1A, ADH1B, and ADH1C) encode the α, β, and γ subunits, which can form homodimers or heterodimers and react at a relatively low ethanol concentration. Ethanol metabolism via ADH can neither be increased with increasing ethanol concentrations nor after chronic alcohol consumption.

ADH4 encodes π-ADH, which contributes to ethanol oxidation at higher concentrations and which is present only in the liver. ADH5 encodes χ-ADH – a formaldehyde dehydrogenase with low affinity for ethanol. ADH6 mRNA is present in the liver, but the enzyme has not been isolated so far. ADH7 encodes σ-ADH present primarily in the stomach and in the retina, and responsible for gastric FPM of ethanol and retinol oxidation [19].

ADH1B and ADH1C show polymorphisms, resulting in the production of enzymes with different kinetic properties and different ethanol-oxidizing capacities. There are three different ADH1B alleles that alter the amino sequence of the encoded β subunit. In both the β2 and β3 subunit, the amino acid substitution occurs at an amino acid that contacts with NAD. This substitution results in enzymes that have a 70- to 80-fold higher turnover rate than the β_1 subunit since the coenzyme is released more rapid at the end of the reaction [7]. ADH1B1 contributes approximately 20% to ethanol metabolism in the liver.

ADH1C has also three alleles. The ADH1C*1 allele encodes the γ_1 subunit and the ADH1C*2 allele encodes the γ_2 subunit. ADH consisting of two γ_1 subunits has a 70% higher turnover rate as compared to the γ_2 enzyme. While the ADH1B2 allele encodes for an enzyme that is approximately 40 times more active in producing acetaldehyde as compared to the enzyme encoded by the ADH1B1 allele, the ADH1C1 allele encodes for an enzyme with 2.5 times more acetaldehyde production as compared to the ADH1C2 allele. This has severe consequences with respect to ethanol drinking behavior and ethanol-associated cancer development. With respect to alcoholism and liver disease, the presence of the ADH1B2 allele seems to be strongly protective, since individuals with this gene produce enormous amounts of acetaldehyde following alcohol ingestion [17, 20–22]. Under these circumstances severe side-effects of acetaldehyde such as tachycardia, sweating, flushing, nausea, and vomiting occur (flush syndrome), and therefore these individuals avoid alcohol.

With respect to ADH1C polymorphism, individuals homozygous for the ADH1C1 allele with a small but significant greater production of acetaldehyde do not show such side-effects. However, they seem to be at increased risk for the development of cancer of the upper aerodigestive tract, breast, and colorectum [19, 23–25]. ADH1C1 contributes approximately 40% to ethanol metabolism in the liver.

Metabolic consequences of the ADH reaction are either due to an increase in NADH or acetaldehyde. Production of NADH leads to a change in the cellular redox potential and has a severe influence on the intermediary cell metabolism. This is especially pronounced in the liver and includes [5, 13, 26]:

i) An increase in NADPH which results in the presence of induced CYP2E1 in an increase of ROS [26].

ii) A change in transcription regulation by affecting C-terminal binding protein and the silent information regulator, resulting in enhanced histone acetylation and reduced deacetylation associated with epigenetic changes and activation of certain inflammatory genes [26].

iii) An effect on signaling proteins such as NF-κB, c-Jun N-terminal kinase (JNK), and p38 mitogen-activated protein kinase [26].

Clinical consequences of a change in the redox state are [5, 13, 26]:

- Activation of the nuclear transcription factor SREBP-1c and inhibition of peroxisome proliferator-activated receptor-α, resulting in a stimulation of fatty acids and triglyceride synthesis, and inhibition of β-oxidation of fatty acids. As a result, fatty liver and also hyperlipoproteinemia type IV and V according to Fredricksen may occur.

- Decreased pyruvate and increased lactate concentrations in the liver. As a consequence, an inhibition of gluconeogenesis due to a lack of pyruvate with hypoglycemia may occur especially in individuals with liver disease in the fasted state. Also, lactacidosis occurs followed by low urinary pH and increased tubular reabsorption of uric acid leading to hyperuricemia. The increase in lactate also stimulates hepatic stellate cells (HSCs) to produce collagen.

- Disturbed porphyrin metabolism with the occurrence of secondary porphyria [27]

- Decreased production of testosterone in the Leydig cells of the gonads resulting in feminization (body fat, gynekomastia, body hair) [28].
- Reduced generation of UDP-glucuronic acid from UDP-glucose, and thus inhibition of hepatic glucuronidation of phenolphtaleien, trichlorethane, and diethyldithiocarbamate [29].

The generation of acetaldehyde leads to [5, 13, 26]:

- Mitochondrial damage with alteration of the respiratory chain and decreased ATP production. As a morphological consequence hepatic megamitochondria may occur.
- Damage of the microtubular system with an altered secretion of proteins, such as albumin, transferrin, and very-low-density lipoproteins. As a morphological equivalent, ballooning of the hepatocyte may occur.
- A decrease in glutathione, and thus an alteration of the detoxification of xenobiotics and ROS.
- An inhibition of the nuclear repair systems with an enhancement of carcinogenesis [30].
- A disturbed methyl transfer with decreased levels of the active methyl donor *S*-adenosylmethionine and an increase of homocysteine, which produces endoplasmic reticulum stress resulting in fatty liver, as well as a decrease in mitochondrial glutathione and increased apoptosis. As a consequence, membrane damage and hypomethylation of DNA may occur. Aberrant methylation causes an inflammatory response and tissue injury, and DNA hypomethylation may cause liver cancer [31].
- Binding of acetaldehyde to proteins with generation of neoantigens, activation of the immune system, and production of antibodies [32].
- Binding of acetaldehyde to DNA and generation of mutagenic DNA lesions [33].
- Stimulation of fibrogenesis by activation of stellate cells [5, 13].

The increased formation of acetate leads to:

- An increased acetylation of histones associated with epigenetic changes (see above).
- An increased acetylation of certain compounds such as sulfanilamide [34].

Since ethanol metabolism primarily via ADH effects hepatic intermediary metabolism, the occurrence of various metabolic diseases is favored by chronic ethanol consumption, including hypoglycemia, hyperlactacedemia (lactacidosis), hyperuricemia, hyperhomocysteinemia, porphyria, and an altered testosterone : estrogen ratio.

Ethanol competes with some substrates at the ADH binding site. Most importantly, the conversion of retinol to retinal and retinoic acid is inhibited in the

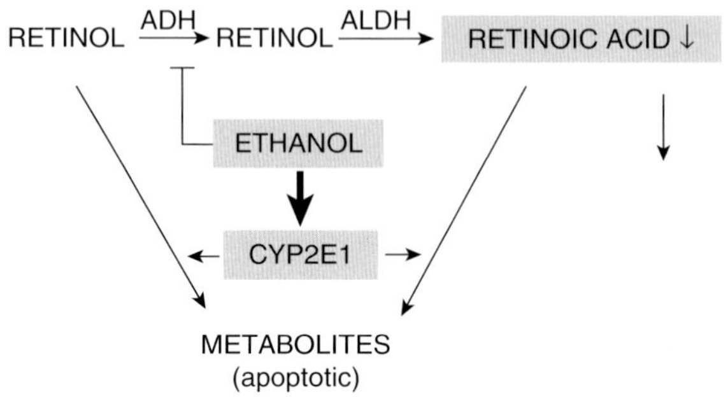

Figure 18.3 Metabolism of retinol to retinal and retinoic acid is inhibited by alcohol due to competitive inhibition of ADH and ALDH. As a result, levels of retinoic acid are low. In addition, chronic alcohol consumption induces CYP2E1, which is involved in the metabolism of retinol and retinoic acid. An induced CYP2E1 state results in an increased metabolism of these two compounds, generating apoptotic metabolites. As a result, retinol and retinoic acids levels decrease and apoptotic/toxic metabolites increase.

Table 18.3 Factors influencing gastric FPM.

Concentration of alcohol consumed
Polymorphism of ADH1C
Ethnicity (a lack of σ-ADH expression has been observed in Asians)
Gender
Age
Drugs (cimetidine, ranitidine, aspirin)
Gastric mucosal injury (atrophic gastritis, *H. pylori*-associated gastritis)
Rate of gastric emptying

presence of ethanol. This is one mechanism to explain low levels of retinoic acid in the liver after chronic ethanol consumption (Figure 18.3) [35].

Ethanol metabolism through class I ADH is inhibited by chlorpromazine and chloralhydrate [36]. The later inhibits ethanol metabolism through trichlorethane, a competitive inhibitor of ADH, whereas cimetidine inhibits ethanol metabolism via ADH7 in the stomach, resulting in elevated serum ethanol concentrations (see Section 18.4.2) [37].

18.4.2
Gastric FPM of Ethanol

As mentioned above, ethanol is metabolized in the stomach by various ADHs (Table 18.2). This so-called gastric FPM of alcohol is primarily due to σ-ADH encoded by ADH7 with a K_m of 41 mM. However, γ-ADH encoded by ADH1C and χ-ADH encoded by ADH5 also contribute to gastric alcohol metabolism. Various factors affecting gastric ADH activity and thus gastric ethanol metabolism are summarized in Table 18.3 [4, 5].

Women have a lower gastric σ-ADH activity than men [38]. However, with age, the ADH activity of men decreases and reaches the level of female activities at the age of 65 years or older [39]. Furthermore, some drugs bind to gastric σ-ADH and inhibit its activity (e.g., cimetidine) [40]. Other drugs such as aspirin may injure the gastric mucosa, leading to a decrease in gastric ADH activity and thus to a decrease in gastric FPM of ethanol [4, 41]. Finally, ranitidine also decreases gastric FPM. However, this decrease is due to an enhanced gastric emptying with a decreased contact time of ethanol to gastric ADH [42]. In all these situations gastric FPM is decreased, which results in increased ethanol blood concentration following alcohol consumption. Gastric emptying is a modulator of gastric FPM [43]. Delayed gastric emptying increases gastric FPM and enhanced gastric emptying decreases gastric FPM. This may be of relevance when alcohol is taken together with food such as fat, which delays gastric emptying, or in diabetic patients with gastroparesis.

Gastric morphology also has an influence on gastric ethanol metabolism. Atrophic gastritis or gastric atrophy decreases gastric parietal cell mass and therefore the amount of ADH in the stomach, leading to a decreased gastric FPM [4, 44]. The presence of bacteria in the stomach has also an effect; for example, *Helicobacter pylori* possesses ADH activity and produces acetaldehyde from ethanol as may do other microbes [45]. Although *H. pylori* metabolizes ethanol, the *H. pylori*-associated gastric mucosal damage counteracts this metabolism and therefore the FPM of alcohol is decreased in the presence of *H. pylori* [46]. Gastric bacteria do not contribute much to overall alcohol metabolism; however, they are capable of producing acetaldehyde from alcohol, and acetaldehyde is a powerful toxin and carcinogen. This may be relevant with respect to gastric mucosal damage and the pathogenesis of upper aerodigestive tract cancer [1]. In summary, gastric FPM of ethanol is modified by various factors (Table 18.4). Its overall contribution to alcohol metabolism is, however, not more than 5–10% *in vivo* [43, 47].

σ-ADH is also able to detoxify the dietary carcinogen nitrobenzaldehyde [48]. It has been shown that Japanese who lack this enzyme exhibit an increased risk for stomach cancer. In the colon, ADH isozymes may also activate dimethylhydrazine – a well-known colon carcinogen.

Table 18.4 CYP species involved in ethanol metabolism.

CYP isoenzyme	MEOS activity (nmol acetaldehyde/min/nmol CYP)
1A2	10.90
2A6	3.75
2B6	2.89
2D6	0.70
2E1	11.51
3A4	3.38

18.4.3 Ethanol Metabolism via the MEOS

The hepatic MEOS is located in the endoplasmic reticulum of the hepatocytes. The MEOS requires molecular oxygen and NADPH as a cofactor (Figures 18.1 and 18.2). It has an activity optimum of pH 6.9–7.5 and a K_m of 7–11 mM for ethanol. The MEOS metabolizes not only ethanol, but also other primary aliphatic alcohols such as methanol, propanol, butanol, and pentanol, as well secondary alcohols such as isopropanol and tertiary alcohols such as *t*-butanol [5, 9, 10, 13]. The activity of the MEOS is gender-dependent with higher activities in the male gender. Castration, ovariectomy, and substitution with sex hormones affect the MEOS activity. The MEOS activity decreases with age, and may depend on diets with higher activities following hypocaloric carbohydrate-deficient diets and lower activities following protein malnutrition [5]. The MEOS activity can also be induced by certain drugs. Major components of the MEOS are CYP2E1 and NADPH, cytochrome *c* reductase as well as phospholipids. The reaction occurs within the smooth endoplasmic reticulum and involves P450 reductase [8–10]. This protein transfers electrons to the CYP2E1 heme iron after first accepting them from the reduced NADPH (Figure 18.4). CYP2E1 catalyzes the oxidation of small organic compounds such as the production of glucose from ketones such as acetone and acetol during starvation [49].

The ethanol metabolism via CYP2E1 produces first *gem*-diol – an unstable product that disintegrates to acetaldehyde (Figure 18.5) [49]. Since oxygen is used in this CYP2E1-dependent reaction, ROS can occur. CYP2E1 also catalyzes the formation of hydroxyethyl radicals directly from ethanol. Importantly, when oxygen is used in the reaction, sometimes the reaction does not continue and ROS may be generated [50–52].

The MEOS is localized in the smooth endoplasmic reticulum of the hepatocyte, which proliferates following chronic alcohol consumption associated with an increase in MEOS activity and an increase in CYP2E1 [13, 53, 54]. As a result, ethanol metabolism is increased, associated with an increased generation of acetaldehyde and with an increase of ROS. This increased oxidative stress is of special importance as a pathogenetic mechanism of alcoholic liver disease and will be discussed separately. Various CYP species are involved in MEOS activity (Table 18.4). The isoenzyme form of CYP2E1 has the highest metabolic activity for ethanol. The genetic polymorphism for CYP2E1 is well known; however, it may not play an important role with respect to alcoholic liver disease or alcohol-mediated cancer [55]. It has, however, been reported that the highly active CYP2E1 is associated with an increased toxicity of isoniacid [56]. CYP2E1 is not only localized in the endoplasmic reticulum, but also in the nucleus and in the plasma membranes. CYP2E1 and CYP3A4 are also found in the epithelium of the intra- and extrahepatic bile ducts. CYP2E1 is also present in Kupffer cells, but not in HSCs, where CYP3A4 has been described [5]. CYP2E1 is unique since it is one out of 57 different CYPs in humans that accepts electrons to generate ROS even in the absence of a substrate.

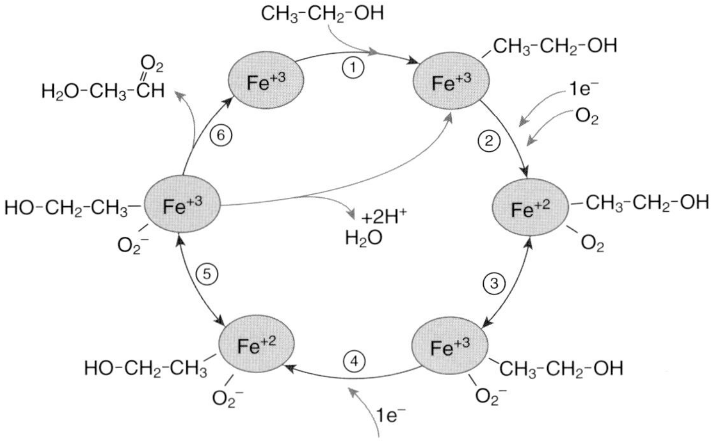

Figure 18.4 Generation of reactive oxygen by CYP2E1. CYP2E1 is represented by the heme iron in the shaded ovals. When CYP2E1 uses oxygen to metabolize alcohol, ROS can be generated by the following chain of events. Ethanol first binds to the enzyme (step 1). As the first electron is passed to the heme of CYP2E1 and oxygen is bound (step 2), the electron can move and exist on the oxygen, essentially generating superoxide bound to the heme of CYP2E1 (step 3). Occasionally, the superoxide will break down, releasing free superoxide and generating the starting enzyme. If the second electron is added to the enzyme (step 4), then a second form of reduced oxygen is produced that is identical to a heme-bound form of the two-electron-reduced oxygen (i.e., peroxide) (step 5). When this product breaks down, it picks up to hydrogens to generate hydrogen peroxide. The production of these ROS by CYP2E1 is referred to as an "uncoupled reaction" because the oxygen does not end up in the substrate. If the reduced oxygen species remains bound, the enzyme will transfer one oxygen atom to the substrate and the other atom becomes water, producing an unstable intermediate (i.e., a *gem*-diol) product that decomposes to acetaldehyde (step 6). (Reproduced from [49] with permission from Dr Koop.)

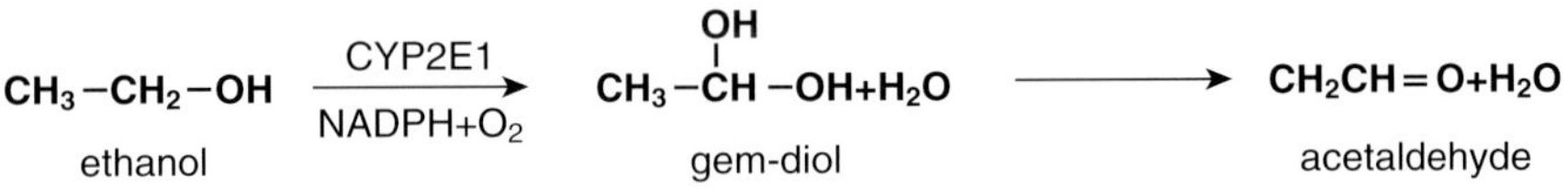

Figure 18.5 CYP2E1-catalyzed metabolism of alcohol produces an unstable intermediate (i.e., a *gem*-diol) that will decompose to produce acetaldehyde.

The amount of CYP2E1 in the liver and in other tissue is variable, and may vary up to 8-fold. Induction of CYP2E1 by chronic ethanol ingestion occurs not only in the liver, but has also been reported in the mucosa cells of the small and large intestine, in the pancreas, in the lung, and in the brain [57–59]. CYP2E1 is also induced by 4-methylpyrazole–an ADH inhibitor–and by acetone and free fatty acids, which may possibly be of importance in the pathogenesis of nonalcoholic fatty liver disease [53].

Chronic ethanol ingestion even at relatively low doses such as 40 g ethanol/day and even after a short period of time such as 1 week results in a significant induction of CYP2E1 [60]. However, this induction varies interindividually. Some individuals have a strong induction and some have no induction at all [60]. The enhanced metabolism of ethanol after chronic alcohol consumption is due the induction of CYP2E1, and it is important to note that CYP2E1 activity needs NADPH and reutilizes reducing equivalents from the ADH reaction as NADPH from NADH.

An enhanced ethanol metabolism in the CYP2E1-induced state with increased ethanol clearance from the blood explains the fact that chronic alcohol abusers are rarely drunk and still are able to function even at a blood alcohol concentration over 150 mg/100 ml.

The mechanisms for regulating the enzyme concentration are complex. CYP2E1 is lower in the fed sate and higher during starvation or in obesity. In addition to control mechanisms for translation and transcription, an inhibition of CYP2E1 degradation by the ubiquitin–proteasome pathway may additionally contribute to the increase of CYP2E1 following ethanol consumption [61]. Thus, various factors contribute to the large variation of CYP2E1 after alcohol ingestion.

The metabolic and clinical consequences of ethanol metabolism via MEOS are multiple.

Major consequences are:

- Production of ROS including hydroxyl-ethyl radicals, superoxide anions, and hydrogen peroxide, which contribute to liver damage and cancer [18]. ROS results in lipid peroxidation with lipid peroxidation products such as 4-hydroxynonenal or malondialdehyde. 4-Hydroxynonenal binds to DNA, forming highly carcinogenic exocyclic etheno–DNA adducts [62].
- Interaction of the microsomal ethanol metabolism with the metabolism of various drugs, leading to decreased drug blood levels and increased drug toxicity (Table 18.5) [5, 13].
- Interaction of CYP2E1 ethanol metabolism with the metabolism of various xenobiotics and carcinogens, leading to increased toxicity and carcinogenesis (Table 18.6) [63].
- Interaction of CYP2E1 ethanol metabolism with the metabolism of retinol and retinoic acid, leading to vitamin deficiency and increased toxicity, including enhanced carcinogenesis (Figures 18.3 and 18.6) [18, 64].

The interaction with drugs needs closer inspection due to its importance in clinical pharmacology.

Since a variety of xenobiotics are also metabolized via CYP2E1, competition at the binding site of CYP2E1 occurs. In the presence of certain drugs, ethanol metabolism is preferred. In such a situation the metabolism of many drugs is inhibited, resulting in an enhanced drug effect at the target site. This is predominantly relevant for psychoactive drugs such as meprobamate, pentobarbital [65],

Table 18.5 Drugs that are metabolized via CYP and ADH, and therefore interact with ethanol metabolism, as well as drugs that can initiate an antabus reaction due to their interaction with ALDH.

CYP2E1	CYP1A2	ADH	ALDH
paracetamol	theophylline	cimetidine	sulfonylureas
barbiturates	caffeine	aspirin	sulfonamide
isoniazid	tamoxifen	chlorpromazine	metronidazole
cyclophosphamide	phenytoin	chloral hydrate	griseofulvin
halothane	barbiturates		tolazoline
methadone	clozapine/olanzapine		procarbazine
phenylbutazone	imipramine		quinacrine
propranolol	ciprofloxacin		disulfiram
rifampicin	norafloxacin		calcium carbimide
warfarin	methadone		cephalosporins
tolbutamide	estradiol		mepacrine
tranquilizers			furazolidone
retinol/retinoic acid			chloramphenicol

Table 18.6 Xenobiotics and procarcinogens that are activated by CYP2E1, resulting in toxic or carcinogenic metabolites.

Chemicals	Carcinogens
Acetone	acetylaminofluorene
Butanol	2-aminofluorene
Pentanol	4-aminobiphenyl
Aniline	aflatoxin
Benzene	amino acid
Bromobenzene	pyrrolysates
CCl_4	benzo[*a*]pyrene
Solvents	dimethylhydrazine
Vinyl chloride	nitrosamine

diazepam [66], lorazepam [67], chlomethiazole [68], or phenytoin, but also for warfarin [69], tolbutamide [70], phenothiazine [71], acetaminophen [72], and caffeine [73]. Amitryptiline – a tricyclic antidepressant – reveals additive pharmacodynamic as well as pharmacokinetic interactions with ethanol, resulting in increased blood concentrations and severe side-effects with alcohol [74].

More recently, it has been shown that the administration of 50 mg hydroxyzine – an antihistaminic drug (H_1 receptor antagonist) – produced a significant impairment of central nervous system function when given together with alcohol already 1 h after drug intake. This was not the case with fexofenadine – a third-generation drug [75].

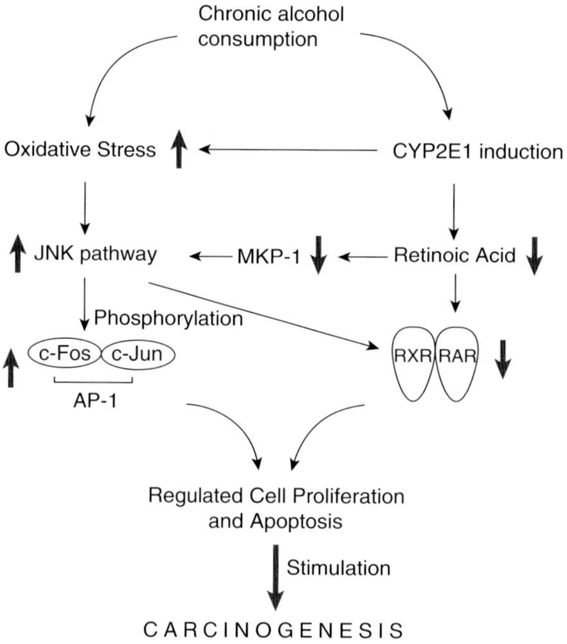

Figure 18.6 Effect of chronic alcohol consumption and CYP2E1 induction with its consequences. CYP2E1 induction results in an increase of oxidative stress and in a decrease of retinoic acid (see Figure 18.3). As a consequence, mitogen-activated protein kinase phosphatase-1 (MPK-1) decreases and the JNK pathway increases, leading to activation of the AP-1 gene and to a decrease in retinoic acid receptors. As a final, result cell proliferation increases and carcinogenesis is stimulated.

Six days of daily moderate alcohol consumption (20 g) resulted in a significant increase in the area under the curve for the 3-hydroxy-3-methyl-glutaryl (HMG)-CoA reductase inhibitor fluvastatin and in a greater time to maximum concentration as compared to fluvastatin alone. However, the lipid-lowering efficacy was not affected by concomitant ethanol administration. The longer T_{max} of fluvastatin in patients with alcohol reflects prolonged absorption and may be explained by delayed gastric emptying during alcohol consumption [76].

A prerequisite for an increased drug metabolism is the absence of blood alcohol at the time of drug intake. For example, chronic ethanol consumption in the evening already at a level of 40 g/day results in CYP2E1 induction, which is associated with an increased degradation of drugs taken in the morning when no alcohol can compete for the CYP2E1 binding site. This can lead to a decrease of therapeutic blood concentrations of drugs, which requires doses adaptation (Table 18.5).

Drugs with a hepatic FPM also show an interaction with ethanol. There is an increased bioavailability of mephenytoin [77] and propoxyphene [78] in the presence of alcohol.

Some drugs are metabolized via CYP2E1 to toxic metabolites, resulting in liver injury. The best-known drug in this respect is acetaminophen, which exerts its toxicity already at lower doses when chronic ethanol consumption has induced CYP2E1 and may then lead to severe liver, injury including acute hepatic failure [79, 80] due to an ethanol-associated deficiency of glutathione.

Another drug is of clinical importance is isoniazid, since alcoholics have an increased risk for tuberculosis. The metabolism of isoniazid–a tuberculostatic drug–is severely affected by ethanol. It has clearly been shown that slow acetylators of isoniazid as well as rapid metabolizers of the intermediate acetylhydrazine have an increased risk for hepatotoxicity. Thus, patients with the homozygous wild genotype CYP2E1 *c1/c1* have a higher risk for liver damage as compared to those with mutant allele *c2*. If CYP2E1 *c1/c2* or *c2/c2* genotype combined with a rapid acetylator status was regarded as the reference group, the risk for hepatotoxicity increased from 3.9 for CYP2E1 *c1/c1* with rapid acetylator status to 7.4 for CYP2E1 *c1/c1* with slow acetylator status. Thus, CYP2E1 genetic polymorphism may be associated with a change in susceptibility to the tuberculostatic drug isoniacid [56].

Also, a severe interaction between methadone, cocaine, and ethanol exists [81–83]. It has been known for decades that the microsomal demethylation of methadone is inhibited by ethanol, resulting in elevated levels of methadone in the brain and the liver [81]. More recently, it has been shown that the concomitant intake of ethanol and cocaine produced a greater increase in heart rate and euphoria as compared with the effects of cocaine alone [82]. Cardiovascular changes induced by the combination caused an increase in myocardial oxygen consumption and increased cardiovascular toxicity. Ethanol increased cocaine and norcocaine plasma concentrations, and induced the synthesis of cocaethylene and norcocaethylene [82]. This is of considerable importance since many individuals consume cocaine and alcohol together.

Finally, it is noteworthy that CYP2E1 can be inhibited by chlormethiazol (CMZ)–a muscle relaxant [84]. CMZ is therefore used experimentally to assess the role of CYP2E1 in alcohol-mediated metabolic disturbances and organ damage. Since CMZ inhibits alcoholic liver disease in animals it was concluded that CYP2E1 plays an important role in the pathogenesis of alcoholic liver disease [85].

In addition to increased drug metabolism, various procarcinogens can also be activated by CYP2E1 and this enhanced activation may be important in ethanol-associated carcinogenesis. This has been intensively investigated with nitrosamines [86], but also with other carcinogens including polycyclic hydrocarbons [62]. In addition, chemicals used at the working place such as various solvents in the car industry or chemicals in the dry cleaning industry are also activated by CYP2E1 to toxins and may produce liver injury [87].

Finally, retinol and retinoic acid are also metabolized by CYP2E1 to polar metabolites with toxic and apoptotic properties [88, 89]. As a result, both retinol and retinoic acid concentrations are low in the livers of alcoholics, resulting in the activation of activator protein-1 (AP-1) with severe effects on cell cycle and hyperproliferation, and increased carcinogenesis [35, 64]. These low levels of retinoids are also responsible for night blindness and sexual dysfunction. The substitution of retinoids may be toxic due to its increased CYP2E1-mediated metabolism to toxic intermediates [89]. Therefore, a small therapeutic window exists for the application of retinoids [35, 64, 88, 89].

18.4.4
Ethanol Metabolism via Catalase

Catalase is localized in the peroxisomes of the hepatocyte and is able to oxidize ethanol to acetaldehyde by using H_2O_2 (Figure 18.2). However, due to the low generation of H_2O_2 in the liver, catalase does not contribute significantly to ethanol metabolism.

18.4.5
Nonoxidative Metabolism of Ethanol

Nonoxidative metabolism of ethanol includes the generation of fatty acid ethyl ester (FAEE) [90, 91], phosphatidylethanol (Peth) [92, 93] as well as ethylglucuronide (EtG) and ethylsulfate (EtS) [94, 95]. While FAEEs have been implicated in the pathogenesis of organ injury, especially in the pancreas, the later compounds have been used in forensic medicine as markers for chronic or acute alcohol ingestion.

Peth is generated from phosphatidylcholine with phospholipase D. Peth has a high specificity for ethanol since it has a low rate of degradation. The median half-life is approximately 14 days and, therefore, it can be found even 2 weeks after abstinence. However, Peth is only detectable at an alcohol ingestion of more than 40–60 g/day for a longer period of time.

EtG can be found in the urine up to 5 days after alcohol ingestion. EtG can also be determined in hairs (if more than 20 g ethanol/day is consumed). The detection of EtG and FAEE in hairs of more than 1 ng/mg demonstrates excessive ethanol consumption. Since EtG can be degraded by bacteria (urinary tract infection), the measurement of EtS seems superior. Other ethanol metabolites are ethylphosphate and ethylnitrite in very low concentrations.

18.4.6
Acetaldehyde Metabolism via ALDH

Among the 19 known human ALDHs, mitochondrial ALDH2 and, to a lesser extent, cytosolic ALDH1 have been shown to play a major role in acetaldehyde oxidation and elimination (Figure 18.2) [96]. Both enzymes–homotetramers with a 55-kDa subunit–exhibit low K_m constants for acetaldehyde (i.e., 3.2 and 180 μM for human ALDH2 and ALDH1A1, respectively) [97]. Since acetaldehyde injures mitochondria, mitochondrial function also decreases as described above including the activity of ALDH2. As a result acetaldehyde further increases and a vicious cycle is induced.

The best-known variation of alcohol-metabolizing enzymes is associated with the *ALDH2* gene. A coding variant known as ALDH2*2 allele leads to the substitution of Lys for Glu at position 504. This substitution results in the production of a nearly inactive ALDH2 enzyme [7].

Fifty percent of Asians have this mutation at the ALDH2 gene, resulting in low activity of the ALDH2 enzyme. In 10% of the Japanese this mutation is homozygous and associated with zero ALDH activity. These individuals cannot drink ethanol at all since they develop severe side-effects such as flushing, tachycardia, nausea, and vomiting. They are completely protected from alcohol drinking. Forty percent of Japanese, however, are heterozygotes. They may consume alcohol with an ALDH2 activity of approximately 10–15% compared to those of normal Caucasians. They also develop a flushing syndrome. However, this can be tolerated, so that they continue to drink. As a result, acetaldehyde levels increase in the blood, in the liver, and in the saliva [1]. Since acetaldehyde is a carcinogen, these individuals have a high risk for alcohol-associated cancer development, such as cancer of the upper alimentary tract and the colon [98]. The presence of even a single ALDH2*2 allele is strongly protective against alcohol dependence. Compared with an individual carrying two active ALDH2*1 alleles and two copies of the normal ADH1B*1 allele, the odd ratios for risk for alcoholism for a man carrying one inactive ALDH2*2 allele and two ADH1B*1 alleles is 0.33. If, in addition to the ALDH2*2 allele, the man also carries at least one overactive ADH1B*2 allele, the odds ratio declines further to 0.05 [7].

The protective effect of the ALDH2*2 allele can, however, be modulated by the environment. In Japan, the percentage of alcoholics with the ALDH2*2 allele has increased over the years from less than 3% to over 12% due to a sociological change of increased alcohol consumption in Japan [7].

ALDH2 can also be inhibited by various drugs leading to a flush reaction (Table 18.5). Disulfiram has been used in alcoholics to obtain abstinence.

Most recently, another human low-K_m ALDH has been characterized as ALDH1B1, being actively involved in ethanol metabolism, especially in the intestinal mucosa [99]. Similar to the ADH genes, many noncoding variations in the ALDH2 gene exist and several promoter polymorphisms in the ALDH1A1 gene affect gene expression *in vitro*.

Acknowledgments

Original studies were supported by grants of the Dietmar Hopp and Manfred Lautenschläger Foundations.

References

1 Salaspuro, M. (2009) Acetaldehyde as a common denominator and cumulative carcinogen indigestive tract cancers. *Scand. J. Gastroenterol.*, **44**, 912–925.

2 Spinucci, G., Guidetti, M., Lanzoni, E., and Pironi, L. (2006) Endogenous ethanol production in a patient with chronic intestinal pseudo-obstruction and small intestinal bacterial overgrowth. *Eur. J. Gastroenterol. Hepatol.*, **18**, 799–802.

3 Yajima, D., Motani, H., Kamei, K., Sato, Y., Hayakawa, M., and Iwase, H. (2006) Ethanol production by *Candida albicans* in postmortem human blood samples: effects of blood glucose level and dilution. *Forensic Sci. Int.*, **164**, 116–121.

4 Seitz, H.K. and Poschl, G. (1997) The role of gastrointestinal factors in alcohol metabolism. *Alcohol Alcohol.*, **32**, 543–549.

5 Seitz, H. and Mueller, S. (2010) Alcoholic liver disease, in *Principles and Practice of Hepatobiliary Disease* (ed. H. Dancygier), Springer, New York, pp. 1111–1152.

6 DiPadova, C., Worner, T.M., Julkunen, R.J., and Lieber, C.S. (1987) Effects of fasting and chronicalcohol consumption on the first-pass metabolism of ethanol. *Gastroenterology*, **92**, 1169–1173.

7 Edenberg, H.J. (2007) The genetics of alcohol metabolism: role of alcohol dehydrogenase and aldehyde dehydrogenase variants. *Alcohol Res. Health*, **30**, 5–13.

8 Lieber, C.S. and DeCarli, L.M. (1968) Ethanol oxidation by hepatic microsomes: adaptive increase after ethanol feeding. *Science*, **162**, 917–918.

9 Lieber, C.S. and DeCarli, L.M. (1970) Hepatic microsomal ethanol-oxidizing system. *In vitro* characteristics and adaptive properties *in vivo*. *J. Biol. Chem.*, **245**, 2505–2512.

10 Lieber, C.S. (1999) Microsomal ethanol-oxidizing system (MEOS): the first 30 years (1968–1998) – a review. *Alcohol. Clin. Exp. Res.*, **23**, 991–1007.

11 Gaertner, U., Schmier, M., Bogusz, M., and Seitz, H. (1996) [Blood alcohol concentrations after oral alcohol administration – effect of age and sex]. *Z. Gastroenterol.*, **34**, 675–679.

12 Vestal, R.E., McGuire, E.A., Tobin, J.D., Andres, R., Norris, A.H., and Mezey, E. (1977) Aging and ethanol metabolism. *Clin. Pharmacol. Ther.*, **21**, 343–354.

13 Lieber, C.S. (1994) Alcohol and the liver: 1994 update. *Gastroenterology*, **106**, 1085–1105.

14 Gullberg, R.G. (2007) Estimating the uncertainty associated with Widmark's equation as commonly applied in forensic toxicology. *Forensic Sci. Int.*, **172**, 33–39.

15 Gullberg, R.G. and Jones, A.W. (1994) Guidelines for estimating the amount of alcohol consumed from a single measurement of blood alcohol concentration: re-evaluation of Widmark's equation. *Forensic Sci. Int.*, **69**, 119–130.

16 Thieden, H.I. and Hunding, A. (1991) A new approach to the determination of ethanol elimination rate *in vivo*: an extension of Widmark's equation. *Pharmacol. Toxicol.*, **68**, 51–56.

17 Hurley, T., Edenberg, H., and Li, T. (2002) Pharmacogenomics of alcoholism, in *Pharmacogenomics – The Search for Individualized Therapies* (eds J. Licinio and M. Wong), Wiley-VCH Verlag GmbH, Weinheim, pp. 417–441.

18 Seitz, H.K. and Stickel, F. (2007) Molecular mechanisms of alcohol-mediated carcinogenesis. *Nat. Rev. Cancer*, **7**, 599–612.

19 Parés, X. and Farrés, J. (1996) Alcohol and aldehyde deydrogenases in the gastrointestinal tract, in *Alcohol and the Gastrointestinal Tract* (ed. V.E.W. Preedy and R.R. Watson), CRC Press, Boca Raton, FL, pp. 57–68.

20 Crabb, D.W., Matsumoto, M., Chang, D., and You, M. (2004) Overview of the role of alcohol dehydrogenase and aldehyde dehydrogenase and their variants in the genesis of alcohol related pathology. *Proc. Nutr. Soc.*, **63**, 49–63.

21 Luczak, S.E., Glatt, S.J., and Wall, T.L. (2006) Meta-analyses of ALDH2 and ADH1B with alcohol dependence in Asians. *Psychol. Bull.*, **132**, 607–621.

22 Whitfield, J.B. (2002) Alcohol dehydrogenase and alcohol dependence: variation in genotype-associated risk between populations. *Am. J. Hum. Genet.*, **71**, 1247–1250; author reply 1250–1.

23 Homann, N., Stickel, F., Konig, I.R., Jacobs, A., Junghanns, K., Benesova, M., Schuppan, D., Himsel, S., Zuber-Jerger, I., Hellerbrand, C., Ludwig, D., Caselmann, W.H., and Seitz, H.K. (2006) Alcohol dehydrogenase 1C*1 allele is a

genetic marker for alcohol-associated cancer in heavy drinkers. *Int. J. Cancer*, **118**, 1998–2002.

24 Homann, N., Konig, I.R., Marks, M., Benesova, M., Stickel, F., Millonig, G., Mueller, S., and Seitz, H.K. (2009) Alcohol and colorectal cancer: the role of alcohol dehydrogenase 1C polymorphism. *Alcohol. Clin. Exp. Res.*, **33**, 551–556.

25 Harty, L.C., Caporaso, N.E., Hayes, R.B., Winn, D.M., Bravo-Otero, E., Blot, W.J., Kleinman, D.V., Brown, L.M., Armenian, H.K., Fraumeni, J.F., Jr, and Shields, P.G. (1997) Alcohol dehydrogenase 3 genotype and risk of oral cavity and pharyngeal cancers. *J. Natl. Cancer Inst.*, **89**, 1698–1705.

26 Zakhari, S. (2006) Overview: how is alcohol metabolized by the body? *Alcohol Res. Health*, **29**, 245–254.

27 Doss, M., Baumann, H., and Sixel, F. (1982) Alcohol in acute porphyria. *Lancet*, **i**, 1307.

28 Noth, R.H. and Walter, R.M., Jr (1984) The effects of alcohol on the endocrine system. *Med. Clin. North Am.*, **68**, 133–146.

29 Moldeus, P., Andersson, B., and Norling, A. (1978) Interaction of ethanol oxidation with glucuronidation in isolated hepatocytes. *Biochem. Pharmacol.*, **27**, 2583–2588.

30 Garro, A.J., Espina, N., Farinati, F., and Salvagnini, M. (1986) The effects of chronic ethanol consumption on carcinogen metabolism and on O^6-methylguanine transferase-mediated repair of alkylated DNA. *Alcohol. Clin. Exp. Res.*, **10**, 73S–77S.

31 Stickel, F., and Seitz, H.K. (2004) Ethanol and Methyltransfer: 1st role in liver disease and hepatocarcinogenesis, in *Nutrition and Alcohol* (eds R. Watson and V. Preedy), CRC Press, Boca Raton, FL, pp. 57–72.

32 Niemela, O. (2007) Acetaldehyde adducts in circulation. *Novartis Found. Symp.*, **285**, 183–192; discussion 193–197.

33 Theruvathu, J.A., Jaruga, P., Nath, R.G., Dizdaroglu, M., and Brooks, P.J. (2005) Polyamines stimulate the formation of mutagenic 1,*N*2-propanodeoxyguanosine adducts from acetaldehyde. *Nucleic Acids Res.*, **33**, 3513–3520.

34 Olson, H. and Morland, J. (1978) Ethanol-induced increase in drug acetylation in man and isolated rat liver cells. *Br. Med. J.*, **2**, 1260–1262.

35 Wang, X.D., Liu, C., Chung, J., Stickel, F., Seitz, H.K., and Russell, R.M. (1998) Chronic alcohol intake reduces retinoic acid concentration and enhances AP-1 (c-Jun and c-Fos) expression in rat liver. *Hepatology*, **28**, 744–750.

36 Sellers, E.M., Carr, G., Bernstein, J.G., Sellers, S., and Koch-Weser, J. (1972) Interaction of chloral hydrate and ethanol in man. II. Hemodynamics and performance. *Clin. Pharmacol. Ther.*, **13**, 50–58.

37 Seitz, H.K., Veith, S., Czygan, P., Bosche, J., Simon, B., Gugler, R., and Kommerell, B. (1984) *In vivo* interactions between H2-receptor antagonists and ethanol metabolism in man and in rats. *Hepatology*, **4**, 1231–1234.

38 Frezza, M., di Padova, C., Pozzato, G., Terpin, M., Baraona, E., and Lieber, C.S. (1990) High blood alcohol levels in women. The role of decreased gastric alcohol dehydrogenase activity and first-pass metabolism. *N. Engl. J. Med.*, **322**, 95–99.

39 Seitz, H.K., Egerer, G., and Simanowski, U. (1990) High blood alcohol levels in women. *N. Engl. J. Med.*, **323**, 58–59.

40 Seitz, H.K., Simanowski, U.A., Egerer, G., Waldherr, R., and Oertl, U. (1992) Human gastric alcohol dehydrogenase: *in vitro* characteristics and effect of cimetidine. *Digestion*, **51**, 80–85.

41 Roine, R., Gentry, R.T., Hernandez-Munoz, R., Baraona, E., and Lieber, C.S. (1990) Aspirin increases blood alcohol concentrations in humans after ingestion of ethanol. *JAMA*, **264**, 2406–2408.

42 Amir, I., Anwar, N., Baraona, E., and Lieber, C.S. (1996) Ranitidine increases the bioavailability of imbibed alcohol by accelerating gastric emptying. *Life Sci.*, **58**, 511–518.

43 Oneta, C.M., Simanowski, U.A., Martinez, M., Allali-Hassani, A., Pares, X., Homann, N., Conradt, C., Waldherr, R., Fiehn, W., Coutelle, C., and Seitz, H.K. (1998) First pass metabolism of ethanol is strikingly influenced by the

speed of gastric emptying. *Gut*, **43**, 612–619.

44 Pedrosa, M.C., Russell, R.M., Saltzman, J.R., Golner, B.B., Dallal, G.E., Sepe, T.E., Oates, E., Egerer, G., and Seitz, H.K. (1996) Gastric emptying and first-pass metabolism of ethanol in elderly subjects with and without atrophic gastritis. *Scand. J. Gastroenterol.*, **31**, 671–677.

45 Salmela, K.S., Roine, R.P., Hook-Nikanne, J., Kosunen, T.U., and Salaspuro, M. (1994) Acetaldehyde and ethanol production by *Helicobacter pylori*. *Scand. J. Gastroenterol.*, **29**, 309–312.

46 Simanowski, U.A., Egerer, G., Oneta, C., Keil, T., Pares, X., Conradt, C., Arce, L., Waldherr, R., Stickel, F., Russell, R.M., Aderjan, R., Klee, F., and Seitz, H.K. (1998) *Helicobacter pylori* infection decreases gastric alcohol dehydrogenase activity and first-pass metabolism of ethanol in man. *Digestion*, **59**, 314–320.

47 Ammon, E., Schafer, C., Hofmann, U., and Klotz, U. (1996) Disposition and first-pass metabolism of ethanol in humans: is it gastric or hepatic and does it depend on gender? *Clin. Pharmacol. Ther.*, **59**, 503–513.

48 Baraona, E., Yokoyama, A., Ishii, H., Hernandez-Munoz, R., Takagi, T., Tsuchiya, M., and Lieber, C.S. (1991) Lack of alcohol dehydrogenase isoenzyme activities in the stomach of Japanese subjects. *Life Sci.*, **49**, 1929–1934.

49 Koop, D.R. (2006) Alcohol metabolism's damaging effects on the cell: a focus on reactive oxygen generation by the enzyme cytochrome P450 2E1. *Alcohol Res. Health*, **29**, 274–280.

50 Lieber, C.S. (2004) The discovery of the microsomal ethanol oxidizing system and its physiologic and pathologic role. *Drug Metab. Rev.*, **36**, 511–529.

51 Dey, A. and Cederbaum, A.I. (2007) Induction of cytochrome P450 2E1 (corrected) promotes liver injury in *ob/ob* mice. *Hepatology*, **45**, 1355–1365.

52 Gonzales, F.J. (2005) Role of cytochrome P450 in chemical toxicity and oxidative stress: studies with CYP2E1. *Mutat. Res.*, **569**, 101–110.

53 Lieber, C.S. (2004) CYP2E1: from ASH to NASH. *Hepatol. Res.*, **28**, 1–11.

54 Lieber, C.S. (1997) Cytochrome P-4502E1: its physiological and pathological role. *Physiol. Rev.*, **77**, 517–544.

55 Stickel, F. and Osterreicher, C.H. (2006) The role of genetic polymorphisms in alcoholic liver disease. *Alcohol Alcohol.*, **41**, 209–224.

56 Huang, Y.S., Chern, H.D., Su, W.J., Wu, J.C., Chang, S.C., Chiang, C.H., Chang, F.Y., and Lee, S.D. (2003) Cytochrome P450 2E1 genotype and the susceptibility to antituberculosis drug-induced hepatitis. *Hepatology*, **37**, 924–930.

57 Seitz, H.K., Korsten, M.A., and Lieber, C.S. (1979) Ethanol oxidation by intestinal microsomes: increased activity after chronic ethanol administration. *Life Sci.*, **25**, 1443–1448.

58 Seitz, H.K., Bosche, J., Czygan, P., Veith, S., and Kommerell, B. (1982) Microsomal ethanol oxidation in the colonic mucosa of the rat. Effect of chronic ethanol ingestion. *Naunyn Schmiedebergs Arch. Pharmacol.*, **320**, 81–84.

59 Pikkarainen, P.H., Baraona, E., Jauhonen, P., Seitz, H.K., and Lieber, C.S. (1981) Contribution of oropharynx microflora and of lung microsomes to acetaldehyde in expired air after alcohol ingestion. *J. Lab. Clin. Med.*, **97**, 631–636.

60 Oneta, C.M., Lieber, C.S., Li, J., Ruttimann, S., Schmid, B., Lattmann, J., Rosman, A.S., and Seitz, H.K. (2002) Dynamics of cytochrome P4502E1 activity in man: induction by ethanol and disappearance during withdrawal phase. *J. Hepatol.*, **36**, 47–52.

61 French, S.W. and Barderyg-Gorce, F. (2005) Ubiquitin–proteasome pathway in the pathogenesis of liver disease, in *Signaling Pathways in Liver Diseases* (eds J. Dafour and R. Clavier), Springer, Berlin, pp. 377–390.

62 Wang, Y., Millonig, G., Nair, J., Patsenker, E., Stickel, F., Mueller, S., Bartsch, H., and Seitz, H.K. (2009) Ethanol-induced cytochrome P4502E1 causes carcinogenic etheno-DNA lesions in alcoholic liver disease. *Hepatology*, **50**, 453–461.

63 Seitz, H.K. and Osswald, B. (1992) Effect of ethanol on procarcinogen activation, in *Alcohol and Cancer* (ed. R. Watson), CRC Press, Boca Raton, FL, pp. 55–72.

64 Wang, X.D. (2005) Alcohol, vitamin A, and cancer. *Alcohol*, **35**, 251–258.

65 Rubin, E., Gang, H., Misra, P.S., and Lieber, C.S. (1970) Inhibition of drug metabolism by acute ethanol intoxication. A hepatic microsomal mechanism. *Am. J. Med.*, **49**, 801–806.

66 Hoyumpa, A.M., Jr, Desmond, P.V., Roberts, R.K., Nichols, S., Johnson, R.F., and Schenker, S. (1980) Effect of ethanol on benzodiazepine disposition in dogs. *J. Lab. Clin. Med.*, **95**, 310–322.

67 Hoyumpa, A.M., Patwardhan, R., Maples, M., Desmond, P.V., Johnson, R.F., Sinclair, A.P., and Schenker, S. (1981) Effect of short-term ethanol administration on lorazepam clearance. *Hepatology*, **1**, 47–53.

68 Hoyumpa, A.M., Jr and Schenker, S. (1982) Major drug interactions: effect of liver disease, alcohol, and malnutrition. *Annu. Rev. Med.*, **33**, 113–149.

69 Kater, R.M., Roggin, G., Tobon, F., Zieve, P., and Iber, F.L. (1969) Increased rate of clearance of drugs from the circulation of alcoholics. *Am. J. Med. Sci.*, **258**, 35–39.

70 Carulli, N., Manenti, F., Gallo, M., and Salvioli, G.F. (1971) Alcohol–drugs interaction in man: alcohol and tolbutamide. *Eur. J. Clin. Invest.*, **1**, 421–424.

71 Milner, G. and Landauer, A.A. (1971) Alcohol, thioridazine and chlorpromazine effects on skills related to driving behaviour. *Br. J. Psychiatry*, **118**, 351–352.

72 Sato, C. and Lieber, C.S. (1981) Mechanism of the preventive effect of ethanol on acetaminophen-induced hepatoxicity. *J. Pharmacol. Exp. Ther.*, **218**, 811–815.

73 Mitchell, M.C., Hoyumpa, A.M., Schenker, S., Johnson, R.F., Nichols, S., and Patwardhan, R.V. (1983) Inhibition of caffeine elimination by short-term ethanol administration. *J. Lab. Clin. Med.*, **101**, 826–834.

74 Dorian, P., Sellers, E.M., Reed, K.L., Warsh, J.J., Hamilton, C., Kaplan, H.L., and Fan, T. (1983) Amitriptyline and ethanol: pharmacokinetic and pharmacodynamic interaction. *Eur. J. Clin. Pharmacol.*, **25**, 325–331.

75 Ridout, F., Shamsi, Z., Meadows, R., Johnson, S., and Hindmarch, I. (2003) A single-center, randomized, double-blind, placebo-controlled, crossover investigation of the effects of fexofenadine hydrochloride 180 mg alone and with alcohol, with hydroxyzine hydrochloride 50 mg as a positive internal control, on aspects of cognitive and psychomotor function related to driving a car. *Clin. Ther.*, **25**, 1518–1538.

76 Smit, J.W., Wijnne, H.J., Schobben, F., Sitsen, A., De Bruin, T.W., and Erkelens, D.W. (1995) Effects of alcohol and fluvastatin on lipid metabolism and hepatic function. *Ann. Intern. Med.*, **122**, 678–680.

77 Zysset, T., Preisig, R., and Bircher, J. (1980) Increased systemic availability of drugs during acute ethanol intoxication: studies with mephenytoin in the dog. *J. Pharmacol. Exp. Ther.*, **213**, 173–178.

78 Oguma, T. and Levy, G. (1981) Acute effect of ethanol on hepatic first-pass elimination of propoxyphene in rats. *J. Pharmacol. Exp. Ther.*, **219**, 7–13.

79 Zimmerman, H.J. and Maddrey, W.C. (1995) Acetaminophen (paracetamol) hepatotoxicity with regular intake of alcohol: analysis of instances of therapeutic misadventure. *Hepatology*, **22**, 767–773.

80 Lauterburg, B.H. and Velez, M.E. (1988) Glutathione deficiency in alcoholics: risk factor for paracetamol hepatotoxicity. *Gut*, **29**, 1153–1157.

81 Borowsky, S.A. and Lieber, C.S. (1978) Interaction of methadone and ethanol metabolism. *J. Pharmacol. Exp. Ther.*, **207**, 123–129.

82 Farre, M., de la Torre, R., Gonzalez, M.L., Teran, M.T., Roset, P.N., Menoyo, E., and Cami, J. (1997) Cocaine and alcohol interactions in humans: neuroendocrine effects and cocaethylene metabolism. *J. Pharmacol. Exp. Ther.*, **283**, 164–176.

83 Smith, A.C., Freeman, R.W., and Harbison, R.D. (1981) Ethanol enhancement of cocaine-induced hepatotoxicity. *Biochem. Pharmacol.*, **30**, 453–458.

84 Gebhardt, A.C., Lucas, D., Menez, J.F., and Seitz, H.K. (1997) Chlormethiazole inhibition of cytochrome P450 2E1 as assessed by chlorzoxazone hydroxylation in humans. *Hepatology*, **26**, 957–961.

85 Gouillon, Z., Lucas, D., Li, J., Hagbjork, A.L., French, B.A., Fu, P., Fang, C., Ingelman-Sundberg, M., Donohue, T.M., Jr, and French, S.W. (2000) Inhibition of ethanol-induced liver disease in the intragastric feeding rat model by chlormethiazole. *Proc. Soc. Exp. Biol. Med.*, **224**, 302–308.

86 Garro, A.J., Seitz, H.K., and Lieber, C.S. (1981) Enhancement of dimethylnitrosamine metabolism and activation to a mutagen following chronic ethanol consumption. *Cancer Res.*, **41**, 120–124.

87 Seitz, H., Lieber, S., and Simanowski, U. (2000) *Alkohol und Interaktionen mit Arzneimitteln, Xenobiotika, Arbeitsplatztoxinen und Prokarzinogenen Handbuch Alkohol, Alkoholismus, alkoholbedingte Organschäden*, J. A. Barth, Heidelberg.

88 Liu, C., Russell, R.M., Seitz, H.K., and Wang, X.D. (2001) Ethanol enhances retinoic acid metabolism into polar metabolites in rat liver via induction of cytochrome P4502E1. *Gastroenterology*, **120**, 179–189.

89 Dan, Z., Popov, Y., Patsenker, E., Preimel, D., Liu, C., Wang, X.D., Seitz, H.K., Schuppan, D., and Stickel, F. (2005) Hepatotoxicity of alcohol-induced polar retinol metabolites involves apoptosis via loss of mitochondrial membrane potential. *FASEB J.*, **19**, 845–847.

90 De Jersey, J. and Treloar, T. (1994) Biosynthesis and possible pathological significance of fatty acid ethyl esters. *Alcohol Alcohol. Suppl.*, **2**, 171–176.

91 Lange, L.G. (1991) Mechanism of fatty acid ethyl ester formation and biological significance. *Ann. NY Acad. Sci.*, **625**, 802–805.

92 Wurst, F.M., Thon, N., Aradottir, S., Hartmann, S., Wiesbeck, G.A., Lesch, O., Skala, K., Wolfersdorf, M., Weinmann, W., and Alling, C. (2010) Phosphatidylethanol: normalization during detoxification, gender aspects and correlation with other biomarkers and self-reports. *Addict. Biol.*, **15**, 88–95.

93 Varga, A. and Alling, C. (2002) Formation of phosphatidylethanol *in vitro* in red blood cells from healthy volunteers and chronic alcoholics. *J. Lab. Clin. Med.*, **140**, 79–83.

94 Kissack, J.C., Bishop, J., and Roper, A.L. (2008) Ethylglucuronide as a biomarker for ethanol detection. *Pharmacotherapy*, **28**, 769–781.

95 Halter, C.C., Dresen, S., Auwaerter, V., Wurst, F.M., and Weinmann, W. (2008) Kinetics in serum and urinary excretion of ethyl sulfate and ethyl glucuronide after medium dose ethanol intake. *Int. J. Legal Med.*, **122**, 123–128.

96 Vasiliou, V. and Pappa, A. (2000) Polymorphisms of human aldehyde dehydrogenases. Consequences for drug metabolism and disease. *Pharmacology*, **61**, 192–198.

97 Klyosov, A.A., Rashkovetsky, L.G., Tahir, M.K., and Keung, W.M. (1996) Possible role of liver cytosolic and mitochondrial aldehyde dehydrogenases in acetaldehyde metabolism. *Biochemistry*, **35**, 4445–4456.

98 Okoyama, A., Muramatsu, T., Ohmori, T., Yokoyama, T., Okuyama, K., Takahashi, H., Hasegawa, Y., Higuchi, S., Maruyama, K., Shirakura, K., and Ishii, H. (1998) Alcohol-related cancers and aldehyde dehydrogenase-2 in Japanese alcoholics. *Carcinogenesis*, **19**, 1383–1387.

99 Stagos, D., Chen, Y., Brocker, C., Donald, E., Jackson, B.C., Orlicky, D.J., Thompson, D.C., and Vasiliou, V. (2010) Aldehyde dehydrogenase 1B1: molecular cloning and characterization of a novel mitochondrial acetaldehyde-metabolizing enzyme. *Drug Metab. Dispos.*, **38**, 1679–1687.

Part Three
Metabolism of Natural Compounds

19
Introduction and Overview

Michael Murray

19.1
Introduction

19.1.1
Sources and Functional Importance of Natural Products

Natural product chemicals are present in many different species, including bacteria, fungi, and other microorganisms, and marine invertebrates and mammals, but most of the agents that have been widely studied to date are derived from plants. Although the functions of these agents in the host are not always completely clear, many appear to protect against predation or to assist in pollination. The unpleasant taste and aromatic nature of simple monoterpenoids and alkaloids, for example, deters ingestion of the host plants by herbivores. In contrast, the color and taste of certain natural products in ripe fruit and nectar attracts birds, insects, and foraging animals, which facilitates seed dispersal.

Humans and other mammals are exposed to natural products through their diets, the environment, and by contact with products that contain these agents, including herbal medicines, cosmetics, cleaning products, and even certain insecticides. Structurally, natural product chemicals are very complex and there is a mystique associated with their use as drugs. Certain plant products, such as the cardiac glycoside digoxin, are still in routine therapeutic use. Indeed, the mining of plant species has yielded numerous agents of value in the treatment of important human ailments. The identification of active agents from plant sources has also led to the development of semisynthetic molecules that have been designed to possess superior potency. Thus, natural products may be used as drugs in their own right or may be lead compounds for the rational synthesis of effective new agents.

Metabolism of Drugs and Other Xenobiotics, First Edition. Edited by Pavel Anzenbacher, Ulrich M. Zanger.

19.1.2
Plant Products as Drugs: A Historical Perspective

Information on the use of plants for therapeutic purposes arose from the civilizations of Mesopotamia and Egypt prior to 1500 BC [1]. The Greeks and Romans advanced these approaches further. In parallel, the ancient Chinese and Ayurvedic (Indian) literature detailed the use of plant-derived extracts in Eastern societies, and attempted to standardize their therapeutic applications. Subsequently, medicinal plants were developed further in the nineteenth and twentieth centuries with the isolation and identification of active molecules, such as the alkaloids morphine and quinine. Structural characterization and quantification of molecules from plant preparations using modern spectroscopic approaches became practical in the second half of the twentieth century. Thus, technology has underpinned the present development of a wide range of natural products and their semisynthetic derivatives as drugs.

19.1.3
Considerations with the Use of Natural Products as Drugs

Natural products are now used extensively in Western medicine, but this may have unforeseen consequences, including toxicity and the precipitation of pharmacokinetic interactions with conventional drugs. It is now accepted that interactions between natural product-containing therapies and conventional agents are due to competition for biotransformation enzymes and transporters for elimination [2]. Thus, phase I oxidation by cytochrome P450 (CYP) enzymes, phase II conjugations by UDP-glucuronosyltransferases (UGTs), sulfotransferases (SULTs), and glutathione *S*-transferases (GSTs), and cellular influx/efflux by the ATP-binding cassette (ABC) and solute carrier (SLC) transporters are all important in the biotransformation and disposition of natural products as well as conventional drugs.

Owing to the ready access that patients have to many natural products, they often self-medicate without informing their physicians [3]. One recent study reported that the combined use of natural products and conventional drugs led to pharmacokinetic interactions in around 40% of subjects [4]. Pharmacokinetic interactions may exaggerate or nullify the anticipated clinical benefits from drugs by altering the rate at which they are eliminated. Decreased elimination may enhance the therapeutic effect because plasma concentrations and systemic exposure, as reflected by the area under the concentration–time curve (AUC), are increased. However, induction of biotransformation enzymes and transporters may increase the elimination of therapeutic substances and lead to decreased exposure. Interactions are particularly significant when they involve natural products and drugs that have narrow therapeutic indexes (i.e., the ratio of the drug dose that produces an undesired effect to the dose that produces the desired effect). To appreciate the potential consequences of natural product–drug combinations it is essential to have information on the toxicity of the agents involved and their pathways of biotransformation.

19.1.4
Biotransformation of Natural Products

There are several reasons why understanding the biotransformation of natural products is important. (i) As is the case with conventional drugs and chemicals, the conversion of natural products to metabolites that are more readily eliminated usually decreases their duration of action. (i) Many natural products are toxic. If toxicity is due to the parent chemical this can be limited by biotransformation. However, a number of natural products, such as the monoterpenoid pulegone and the pyrrolizidine alkaloids, undergo biotransformation to reactive intermediates that bind covalently to cell macromolecules and initiate cell injury [5–8]. Similarly, the furanocoumarins are converted to reactive intermediates that irreversibly inactivate CYP enzymes that mediate their formation [9, 10].

Many natural products have been found to inhibit the biotransformation of coadministered drugs. The macrolide antibiotic erythromycin and the methylenedioxyphenyl-substituted alkaloids that are present in the herbal agent goldenseal elicit clinically significant pharmacokinetic interactions [11, 12]. Although studied less frequently, it is also possible that the inhibition of phase II biotransformation enzymes and transporters could mediate pharmacokinetic interactions. Importantly, some natural products activate receptors that regulate genes that mediate xenobiotic and endobiotic biotransformation. One of the best-described examples is that of St John's Wort, which contains hyperforin, which activates the pregnane X receptor (PXR) – a member of the nuclear receptor superfamily [13]. This leads to marked induction of CYP3A and enhances the elimination of numerous coadministered drugs that are also cleared by the enzyme [14].

19.1.5
Classes of Natural Products

There are essentially four major classes of natural products found in plants: terpenoids, polyketides, shikimic acid derivatives, and alkaloids. In some cases it is difficult to assign natural products unequivocally to a single class because they contain overlapping structural features. Moreover, the number and structural diversity of plant-derived natural product chemicals is extreme, and detailed information on their biotransformation is not always available. Some studies clearly define the roles of specific enzymes and transporters in biotransformation and disposition, while others focus on qualitative identification of metabolites. Whereas a number of studies have taken a biochemical approach, others have been clinically based and describe the pharmacokinetic behavior of natural products. In view of the diverse nature of this information, the present chapter discusses the principal mechanisms and consequences of natural product biotransformation using examples from one of the major classes of natural products – the terpenoids.

19.2
Terpenoids: A Structurally Complex Group of Natural Products

19.2.1
Terpenoid Biosynthesis

The biosynthesis of terpenoids begins with condensation of the five-carbon isoprenoid subunits dimethylallylpyrophosphate (DMP) and its isomer isopentenyl pyrophosphate (IPP) (Figure 19.1) [15]. The product is the 10-carbon geranyl pyrophosphate that gives rise to simple aliphatic monoterpenes, such as β-citronellol and linalool, and which may be converted enzymically to a wider range of aliphatic monoterpenoids. Geranyl pyrophosphate also undergoes cyclization to produce more complex monoterpenes, such as limonine, perillaldehyde, and pulegone. Further modification of terpenoids occurs by oxidation to hydroxylated, carboxylated, or carbonyl-containing derivatives. Many aliphatic and cyclic monoterpenoids derived from geranyl pyrophosphate are constituents of essential oils that are used in medicine, such as clove oil, or in fragrances and cleaning products, such as eucalyptol.

Higher terpenoids are synthesized from simple terpenoid precursors in further condensation reactions (Figure 19.1). Sesquiterpenoids are formed when the 10-carbon geranyl pyrophosphatase reacts with another molecule of IPP to produce the 15-carbon farnesyl pyrophosphate. Deterpenoids are produced when farnesyl pyrophosphate condenses with another molecule of IPP to produce the 20-carbon derivative geranylgeranyl pyrophosphate (GGPP) (Figure 19.1). Alternately, condensation of two molecules of farnesyl pyrophosphate produces hexaprenyl pyrophosphate that is converted to the triterpenoid squalene. Squalene is the precursor to cholesterol that undergoes further biotransformation in mammalian tissues to generate gonadal and adrenal steroids, bile acids, and the biologically active form of vitamin D_3 (Figure 19.2). Finally, condensation of two molecules of GGPP produces the 40-carbon tetraterpenoid phytoene that is converted to the carotenoids, such as β-carotene and lycopene (Figure 19.1). β-Carotene is an important molecule because it undergoes enzymic cleavage in mammalian cells to generate two equivalents of vitamin A (Figure 19.3), which is a critical regulator of embryonic development and cellular differentiation, and is also used therapeutically in dermatology and oncology [16–18].

Considered together, the terpenoids constitute a large and diverse group of natural products. The simplest terpenoids contain two isoprenoid units (C10 monoterpenoids) but, as outlined above, the condensation with additional subunits produces larger derivatives, such as the di- and triterpenoids. As the number of component isoprenoid subunits increases, so the potential for structural complexity increases. In this section aspects of terpenoid biotransformation will be

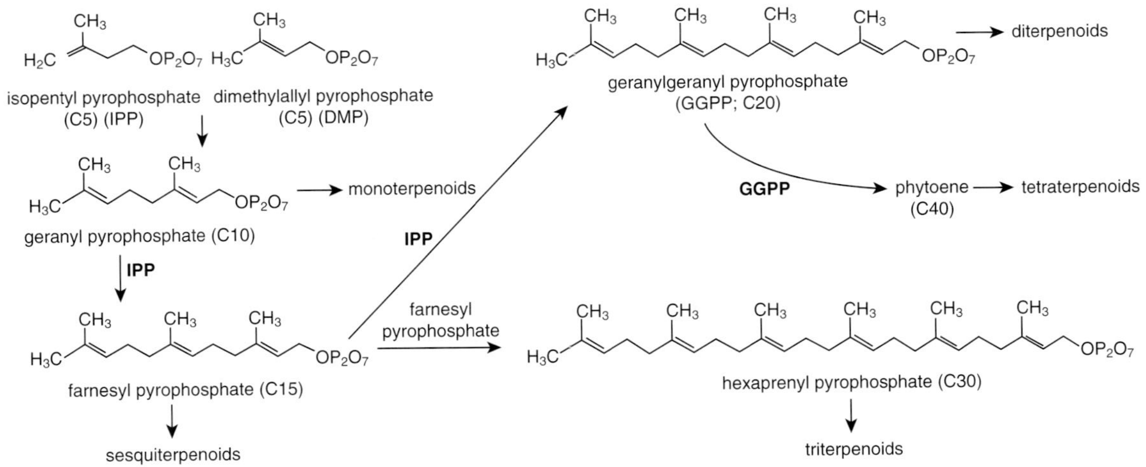

Figure 19.1 Biosynthesis of monoterpenoids and higher terpenoids from the isoprenoid subunits IPP and DMP, and the related intermediates farnesyl pyrophosphate and GGPP.

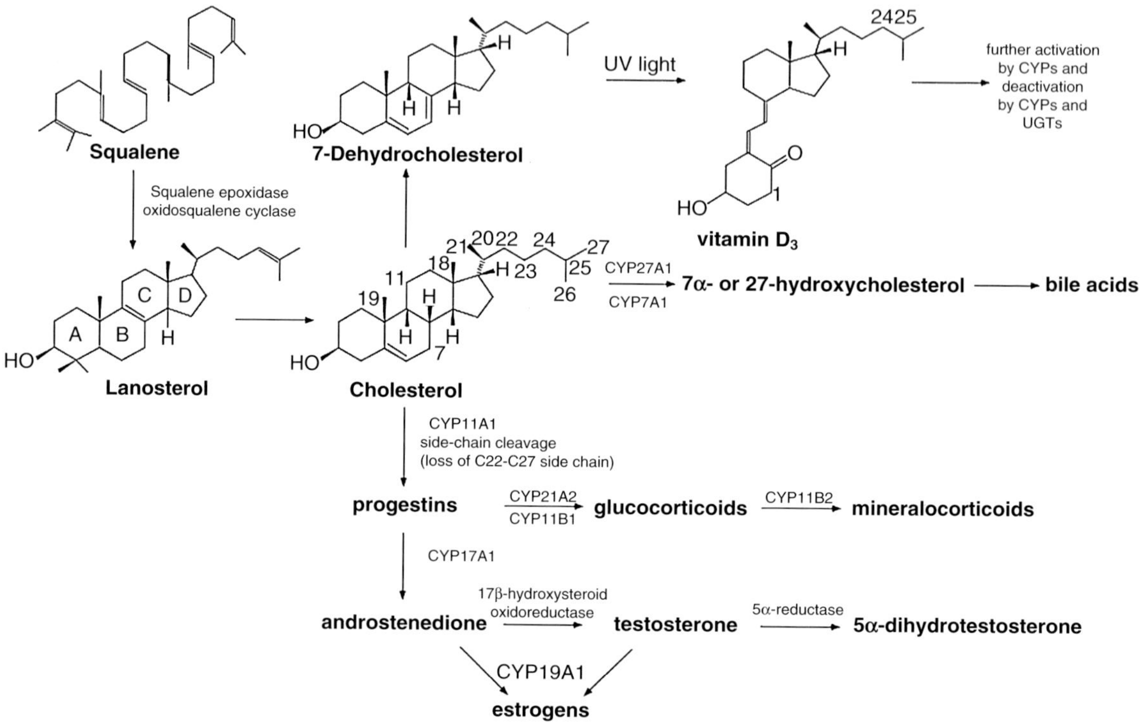

Figure 19.2 Synthesis of cholesterol from the triterpenoid squalene via lanosterol. Cholesterol then undergoes a series of biotransformation reactions mediated by specialized CYPs and other enzymes in multiple cell types to produce bile acids, adrenal, and gonadal steroids. Cholesterol is also activated to vitamin D_3. The A–D rings in lanosterol are shown as is the numbering of important carbon atoms in cholesterol and vitamin D_3.

used to illustrate processes that are representative of natural products in general. Where appropriate, how biotransformation of terpenoids generates molecules that regulate cellular homeostasis will be discussed.

19.2.2
Biotransformation of Terpenoids

19.2.2.1 Monoterpenoids

One of the simplest aliphatic monoterpenoids is citral–the major component of lemongrass oil present in citrus fruits, which is used extensively in the food, cosmetic, and detergent industries. Citral is a mixture of the alicyclic monoterpenoids geranial ((*E*)-3,7-dimethyl-2,6-octadienal) and neral ((*Z*)-3,7-dimethyl-2,6-octadienal). Biotransformation occurs by reduction and oxidation to the corresponding alcohols and acids, and is mediated by alcohol and aldehyde dehydrogenases, respectively, and by CYPs to produce the 8-hydroxy derivatives

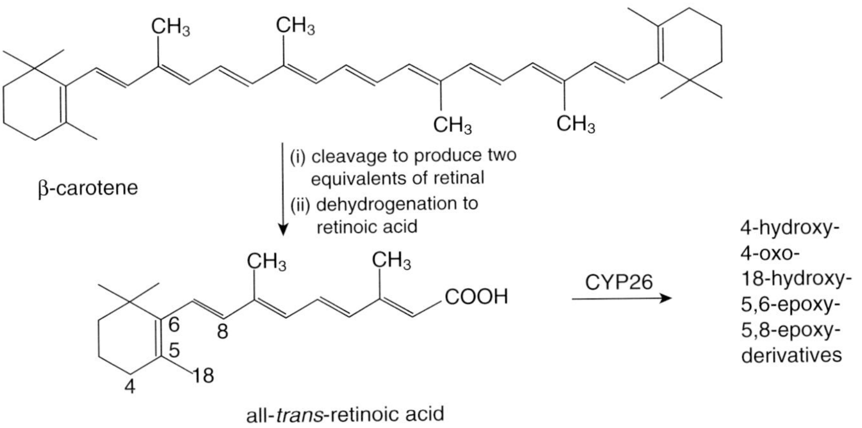

Figure 19.3 β-Carotene undergoes enzymic cleavage to generate two stoichiometric equivalents of all-*trans*-retinal that is dehydrogenated to the active all-*trans*-retinoic acid. CYP26 enzymes generate oxidized metabolites of all-*trans*-retinoic acid. Carbon atoms in all-*trans*-retinoic acid that undergo biotransformation by CYPs are indicated.

that may undergo further oxidation to the 8-carboxylate derivative (Figure 19.4a; [19, 20]). In rabbits, geraniol (the *trans*-alcohol derived from geranial) is metabolized to the 1,8-dicarboxylate, which is also formed in the rat, as well as to the 1,8-diol and the 8-carboxylate [20]. Glucuronides of these metabolites have been identified in bile, thus implicating UGT enzymes in the phase II biotransformation of simple monoterpenoids. Indeed, enterohepatic circulation is apparently important in the metabolism of citral because the amount excreted in bile is around 4-fold greater than that excreted in feces [21]. This likely reflects deconjugation of the glucuronide metabolites by gut flora, followed by reabsorption and re-excretion of the monoterpenoids and/or their phase I metabolites.

Pulegone is a cyclic monoterpenoid present in pennyroyal oil that undergoes extensive biotransformation in the rat to at least 14 urinary metabolites [22, 23]. Major metabolic pathways in rats include (i) hydroxylation at C-5 and C-9, (ii) reduction of the olefinic bond to yield menthone, followed by hydroxylation, (iii) glucuronidation of hydroxylated metabolites, and (iv) Michael addition of glutathione to pulegone and further processing to mercapturic acids (Figure 19.4b). In the rat, glutathione conjugates have been detected in bile, but not urine, which implicates transporter-facilitated excretion [24, 25]. In humans, pulegone is oxidized by CYP2E1, with minor contributions from CYP1A2 and CYP2C19 [6]. However, at present there is no information concerning possible roles of human UGTs, GSTs, and transporters in pulegone disposition.

(*R*)-(+)-Pulegone undergoes CYP-dependent biotransformation to a hepatotoxic metabolite, which appears to be an electrophilic α,β-unsaturated γ-ketoenal [26]. It has been proposed that the activated ketoenal could arise from allylic oxidation or epoxidation of menthofuran (Figure 19.4b) [5, 26–28]. Once formed, the ketoenal may react with nucleophilic groups on adjacent proteins to form covalent

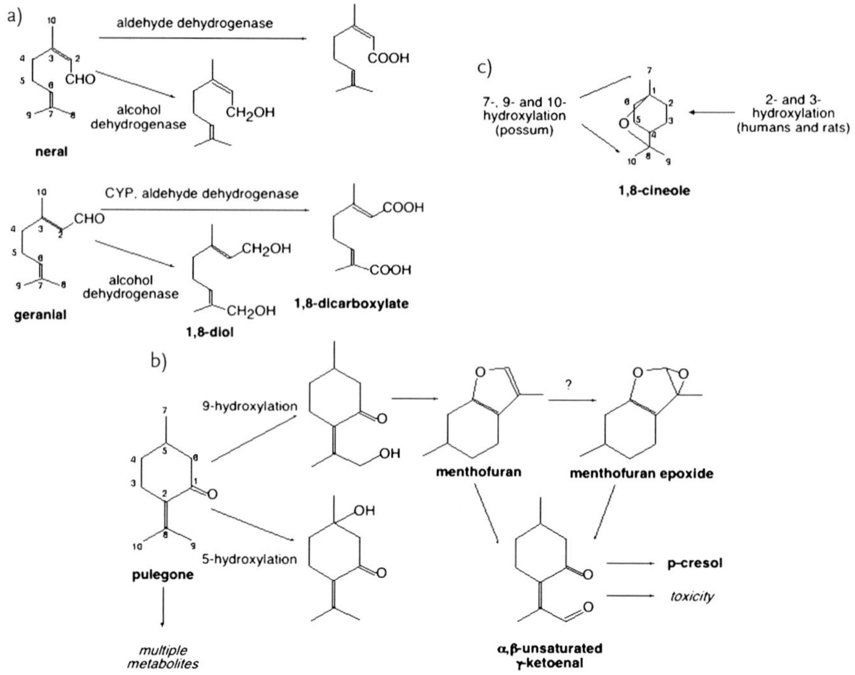

Figure 19.4 (a) Biotransformation of the aliphatic monoterpenoids neral and geranial, (b) conversion of pulegone to stable and reactive metabolites, including the putative toxic intermediates menthofuran epoxide and the α,β-unsaturated γ-ketoenal, and (c) species-dependent oxidation of the fused-ring monoterpenoid 1,8-cineole.

adducts. *p*-Cresol is also formed from pulegone and has been suggested as a potential alternate mediator of toxicity. However, this seems unlikely because *p*-cresol formation is disproportionately high compared to the observed toxicity. Instead, by depleting cellular glutathione [29], it is feasible that *p*-cresol could potentiate the toxicity of *R*-(+)-pulegone by decreasing the amount of glutathione available for conjugation with reactive pulegone metabolites, which might indirectly enhance covalent binding.

1,8-Cineole (eucalyptol) is a monoterpenoid cyclic ether present in eucalyptus oil that has been used principally in nasal sprays and disinfectants. Its unusual fused-ring system indicates the structural complexity that may occur within the monoterpenoids. In rat and human liver microsomes 1,8-cineole is oxidized preferentially at C-2 and C-3 in the ring system by CYP3A enzymes; this creates two pairs of stereoisomers at these carbons (Figure 19.4c [30]). However, arboreal marsupials, such as the possum and the koala bear, feed on eucalyptus foliage and ingest large quantities of 1,8-cineole that would prove toxic in other mammals. Recent findings indicate that possums may have a well-adapted biotransformation system that enables them to eliminate 1,8-cineole efficiently. Thus, Boyle *et al.* identified a large number of hydroxylated and acidic metabolites and their glucuronides in the urine and feces of 1,8-cineole-fed possums [31]. Apart from oxidation at C-2 and C-3 in the carbocyclic system, major alcoholic metabolites were also formed at the exocyclic C-7, C-9, and C-10 [31–34]. 9-Hydroxylation was inhibited by ketoconazole, thus implicating CYP3A enzymes in the pathway, although this remains to be established unequivocally [35]. The C-7 and C-9 hydroxylated metabolites were oxidized further to the carboxylic acids; conjugation of these metabolites was extensive. Considered together, findings with 1,8-cineole indicate that important species differences exist for the biotransformation of certain monoterpenoids in mammals. It would now be of particular interest to compare the structure and function of possum CYP3A with orthologous enzymes from other mammals in order to account for the unusual catalytic capacity of that enzyme toward 1,8-cineole.

1,4-Cineole is an isomer of 1,8-cineole in which the intramolecular ether linkage occurs between C-1 and C-4, which gives rise to five-membered oxygen-containing cyclic systems rather than the six-membered systems in 1,8-cineole. Like the 1,8-isomer, 1,4-cineole undergoes 2- and 3-oxidation in rat and human liver microsomes with CYP3A enzymes again implicated [36, 37]. 1,8-Cineole occupies a larger molecular volume than the 1,4-isomer; however, despite this, the former appears to be a better substrate for CYP oxidation. This conclusion was reached from kinetic experiments that found a lower K_m and greater V_{max} for oxidation of 1,8-cineole, and because 1,8-cineole inhibited the oxidation of 1,4-cineole, while the converse was not true. These findings suggest that relatively small structural differences in cyclic monoterpenoids may contribute significantly to differences in their capacity to undergo biotransformation.

19.2.2.2 **Sesquiterpenoids**

The tricyclic sesquiterpenoid lactone endoperoxide artemisinin is an effective agent against resistant strains of the malarial parasite *Plasmodium falciparum*. Structurally, artemisinin possesses a C-12 keto group in the lactone ring and undergoes reduction to the lactol dihydroartemisinin (DHA), which is the biologically active form of the drug. Hepatic metabolism appears to be the main route of artemisinin elimination. When administered to male rats biliary excretion was important, with the principal metabolite being α-DHA-β-glucuronide. Additional metabolites were formed by ring hydroxylation, rearrangement of the endoperoxide bridge to produce desoxy-DHA and a ring-contracted DHA derivative, as well as the corresponding glucuronides [38]. In human liver microsomes and in cDNA-expressed systems artemisinin oxidation was mediated by CYPs 2B6, and, to a lesser extent, 3A4 and 2A6 [39]. In addition, glucuronidation by UGT1A9, and possibly also UGT2B7, was the predominant pathway of DHA clearance in humans, but sulfation was nonsignificant [40].

The pharmacokinetics of artemisinin illustrates some important points relating to the therapeutic use of this terpenoid. Artemisinin elimination has a short half-life of 2–5 h with biotransformation to the active DHA occurring rapidly [41]. However, in a study of healthy, male Vietnamese adults, the AUC of artemisinin, which reflects systemic drug availability, was markedly decreased after 7 days of intake compared to the AUC at the commencement of treatment [42]. After a 2-week washout period the AUC had essentially normalized, consistent with a reversible autoinductive effect on metabolism. In accord with these observations, artemisinin was found to induce CYP2C19 and CYP2B6 after *in vivo* administration [42, 43]. Since CYP2B6 is involved in artemisinin elimination [39], induction of this enzyme would account for the observed effects during therapy [42]. It was found subsequently that artemisinin activates the PXR and constitutive androstane receptor (CAR) that mediate the induction of CYP2B6 [44]. Although receptor activation required relatively high artemisinin concentrations, these might be achievable in intestinal epithelium and liver during treatment with the drug. The potential significance of these findings is high because it is recommended that artemisinin should be used in combination with other drugs to prevent the development of parasite resistance. Thus, artemesinin-mediated CYP induction via PXR and CAR could compromise the effectiveness of coadministered agents by enhancing their clearance.

19.2.2.3 **Diterpenoids**

Possibly the most important diterpenoid derivatives in man are the cannabinoids. Cannabinoid formation starts with the condensation of geranyl pyrophosphate with olivetolic acid to produce cannabigerol, which then undergoes conversion to cannabidiol and cannabichromene along separate enzymic pathways that yield cannabinoids with side-chains of different length [45]. Cannabidiol undergoes cyclization to tetrahydrocannabinol (THC) – the principal psychoactive component of marijuana.

As the cannabinoids have high lipid solubility they are good substrates for CYP enzymes. Oxidation of THC to the 11- and 8-alcohols is mediated by human CYP2C9 and CYP3A4, respectively [46]; the alkyl side-chain is also subject to CYP oxidation [47]. Further oxidation of the hydroxylated metabolites to the corresponding carboxylates has been reported, which facilitates UGT-dependent glucuronidation. While the parent cannabinoids such as THC are poor substrates for human UGTs, 11-hydroxy-THC was glucuronidated efficiently by UGT1A9 and the extrahepatic enzyme UGT1A10, whereas 11-carboxy-THC was glucuronidated by UGT1A3 [48]. Cannabinol and cannabidiol also underwent glucuronidation by multiple UGTs [48]. Thus, it emerges that different UGTs contribute to the conjugation and elimination of cannabinoids and their metabolites.

In vivo evidence has suggested that cannabinoids are potent inhibitors of hepatic drug metabolism in mammals. In the mouse, CYPs 2C and 3A oxidize THC and cannabidiol to reactive metabolites, possibly the quinone derivatives, that inactivate the enzymes [49, 50]. Similar inactivation of human CYP3A4 by cannabidiol has also been demonstrated [50, 51]. Thus, during CYP-mediated biotransformation of cannabinoids both stable and highly reactive metabolites are produced.

19.2.2.4 **Triterpenoids**

Paclitaxel Paclitaxel may be the most important of the triterpenoids in current clinical use because it is an essential agent in the treatment of ovarian, breast, and non-small-cell lung cancer. In man, paclitaxel undergoes CYP2C8-dependent 6α-hydroxylation within the taxane ring system to produce pharmacologically inactive metabolites [52] that are eliminated in bile; biliary excretion may be mediated by the ABC transporters P-glycoprotein (ABCB1), multidrug-resistance protein-2 (ABCC2), and possibly also multidrug-resistance protein-5 (ABCC5) [53].

Steroid Synthesis from Triterpenoid Precursors In eukaryotes, squalene synthase catalyzes the condensation of two molecules of farnesyl pyrophosphate and generates the triterpenoid squalene ($C_{30}H_{50}$) [15]. The product undergoes epoxidation at the 2,3-olefinic bond, which is then cyclized by the enzyme squalene oxidocyclase to lanosterol (Figure 19.2). In this way, the long-chain aliphatic and highly conjugated squalene is converted to the carbocyclic molecule lanosterol. Lanosterol then undergoes conversion to cholesterol in a concerted series of enzymic reactions that removes three methyl groups, reduces two double bonds, and introduces another double bond between C-5 and C-6 of the B-ring [15]. Once formed, cholesterol is the precursor to a number of important molecules that regulate homeostasis in mammals, including the adrenal and gonadal steroids, bile acids, and vitamin D.

The initial step in the conversion of the 27-carbon cholesterol to adrenal and gonadal steroids is the cleavage of a six-carbon-containing fragment by the mitochondrial side-chain cleavage CYP11A1 to produce pregnenolone (Figure 19.2) [15]. Pregnenolone may be converted to progesterone by the enzyme hydroxysteroid dehydrogenase (HSD) 3B2. CYP enzymes then convert pregnenolone and progesterone to biologically important steroid derivatives in a cell-type-specific manner. In the adrenal cortex progesterone undergoes biotransformation to glucocorticoids, which regulate carbohydrate metabolism, and mineralocorticoids, which regulate sodium and potassium homeostasis. Thus, CYP21A2 hydroxylates progesterone at C-21 to produce the glucocorticoid deoxycorticosterone, while the mineralocorticoid aldosterone is produced from deoxycorticosterone by CYP11B2 (aldosterone synthase) [15].

Peptide hormones secreted by the pituitary gland regulate CYP11A1 expression in the ovary and testis. The increase in cholesterol side-chain cleavage activity is the first step in the biosynthesis of androgens and estrogens [15]. Thus, the formation of pregnenolone and progesterone occurs in an analogous fashion to that in the adrenal. The action of CYP17A1 then removes the three-carbon side-chain from C-17 and generates the weak androgen androstenedione, which is reduced to testosterone by the microsomal 17β-hydroxysteroid dehydrogenase (Figure 19.2). Testosterone undergoes A-ring 5α-reduction to the active androgen dihydrotestosterone or may be oxidized to estradiol by CYP19A1 aromatase.

Adrenal and gonadal steroids regulate the transcription of target genes by acting as specific ligands for highly specialized steroid hormone receptors [54]. In addition to playing a central role in the formation of these steroids in multiple cell types, biotransformation also terminates their biological actions. The hepatic drug-metabolizing CYPs, especially CYP3A4 in man, mediate the 6β-hydroxylation of many steroids prior to their conjugation and elimination as glucuronide and sulfate conjugates [55, 56].

The cholesterol 7α- and 27-hydroxylases (CYP7A1 and CYP27A1, respectively) catalyze alternate pathways of hepatic bile acid biosynthesis (Figure 19.2), with subsequent steps mediated by the microsomal 3β-hydroxy-C27-steroid dehydrogenase/isomerase and the oxysterol 7α-hydroxylase (CYP7B1) [57]. Expression of these enzymes is tightly regulated in rodent liver by substrates that include the triterpenoid-derived cholesterol, oxysterols, and bile acids [58]. The rat *CYP7A1* gene is regulated by liver X receptor (LXR), which is activated by oxysterols [59], and farnesoid X receptor (FXR), which is activated by bile acids [57]. The oxysterol–LXR complex activates CYP7A1 expression while the bile acid–FXR complex downregulates the gene in a negative feedback loop [60]. Thus, not only does the natural product triterpenoid squalene undergo biotransformation in mammalian cells to a range of steroidal molecules derived from cholesterol, but the products also act as ligands for a family of specialized steroid and nuclear receptors. These receptors mediate the biological actions of steroidal metabolites, including the regulation of genes that control their further biotransformation.

Precursors of vitamin D, such as cholecalciferol, are generated in the skin following the isomerization of 7-deoxycholesterol by exposure to UV light (Figure 19.2). Cholecalciferol then undergoes activation by hepatic CYP27A1 to generate 25-hydroxyvitamin D_3, which is further activated in the kidney by CYP27B1 to 1α,25-dihydroxyvitamin D_3 [61]. The nuclear vitamin D receptor mediates the actions of vitamin D_3 on gene expression. Termination of the action of vitamin D_3 by 24-hydroxylation to 1α,24,25-trihydroxyvitamin D_3 occurs in the renal tubule and other vitamin D target cells that express CYP24A1.

19.2.2.5 **Triterpenoids**

The tetraterpenoid β-carotene is the most abundant carotenoid in fruit and vegetables, and serves as an important dietary source of vitamin A, which is essential for normal vision and development. After absorption, the intestinal β-carotenoid 15,15′-dioxygenase cleaves β-carotene to generate two stoichiometric equivalents of all-*trans*-retinal (Figure 19.3). The retinal formed in this way is reduced to retinol, esterified, and transported as retinyl esters via the lymphatic system to the liver for storage [62]. When required at extrahepatic tissues, the stored retinyl esters are hydrolyzed and the retinol that is produced is transported in plasma in the form of a ternary complex with retinol binding protein and transthyretin. Once delivered to the cell retinol undergoes oxidative biotransformation by several short-chain dehydrogenase/reductase enzymes to retinal and then by cell-specific retinaldehyde dehydrogenases to all-*trans*-retinoic acid [63]. The latter is an important ligand for the retinoic acid nuclear receptors.

CYP26A1 mediates the oxidation of all-*trans*-retinoic acid to its 4-hydroxy, 4-oxo, 18-hydroxy, 5,6-epoxy, and 5,8-epoxy metabolites (Figure 19.3) [64]. The more recently identified CYP26B1 and CYP26C1 exhibit different developmental- and tissue-specific expression, and slightly different substrate specificities [65, 66]. Although members of the *CYP26* gene family mediate the initial step in the oxidative biotransformation of all-*trans*-retinoic acid, some hydroxylated metabolites retain biological activity by acting as ligands for retinoid receptors [67]. Apart from

CYP26, it has also been reported that hepatic drug-metabolizing CYPs have the capacity to oxidize all-*trans*-retinoic acid to the 4-hydroxy metabolite. Indeed, several studies have implicated CYP2C8, CYP3A4, and possibly other human CYPs in this pathway [68, 69]. Glucuronides may be formed from retinol, retinoic acids, and their biotransformation products; these are probably destined for excretion in bile and urine [70]. It remains to be established how the "specialized" CYP26 retinoic acid hydroxylases function in relation to the "nonspecialized" hepatic CYPs that also mediate retinoid oxidation. However, it seems feasible that CYPs 26 primarily generate oxidized metabolites of vitamin A in extrahepatic tissues; these might be used for local activation of retinoid receptors. In contrast, the hepatic drug-metabolizing CYPs appear to contribute to the oxidative biotransformation of excess retinoic acid and to enhance clearance.

It is evident from the foregoing discussion that several important points have emerged from considerations of terpenoid biotransformation: (i) terpenoids generate a large number of metabolites, (ii) biotransformation is a crucial determinant of the clearance of terpenoids and their potential toxicity, (iii) the higher terpenoids in particular are converted enzymically to important signaling molecules, and (iv) specialized receptors have evolved in mammals that accommodate these biotransformation products from higher terpenoids as ligands. Thus, terpenoid biotransformation products are important modulators of cellular homeostasis.

19.3 Other Classes of Natural Products

In this chapter important aspects relating to the biotransformation of natural products have been illustrated with reference to the terpenoids. However, as mentioned, there are three other major groups of natural products: polyketides, shikimates, and alkaloids. The following section briefly describes some of the most important agents in these classes for which human biotransformation pathways and their significance have been well defined.

19.3.1 Biosynthesis of Polyketides, Shikimates, and Alkaloids

The polyketides are composed of two carbon subunits that are activated by esterification with coenzyme A to form acetyl-CoA [71]. Condensation reactions with malonyl-CoA generates larger molecules containing additional carbon atoms that may adopt both extended chain and cyclic structures.

Shikimate is the precursor of the aromatic amino acids Tyr, Trp, and Phe, and is used in the biosynthesis of a range of polyphenolic aromatic compounds, including the phenylpropenes, coumarins, flavonoids, and stilbenes. In the first step of shikimate biosynthesis the biochemical intermediates phosphoenol pyruvate and erythrose 4-phosphate are condensed to produce 3-hydroquinate. Consecutive dehydration and reduction reactions yield shikimate, which is then converted to aromatic amino acids and to the range of polyphenolics mentioned above [72].

Phenylpropenes are the simplest shikimate-derived natural products and are formed from the deamination of phenylalanine [72]. More complex derivatives arise following intramolecular cyclization reactions in which substituted shikimates produce bicyclic systems that contain either lactone (coumarins) or pyrone rings (flavonoids). The flavonoids have been well studied for their antioxidant potency and their capacity to modulate the activity of intracellular signaling kinases, and are discussed in greater detail in Chapter 20.

The alkaloids are a large and diverse group of natural products that contain a range of nitrogen heterocyclic systems and are present in about 20% of plant species. Briefly, important alkaloids include the pyridine alkaloids nicotine and coniine from tobacco and hemlock, respectively, and the pyrrolizidine alkaloids, exemplified by senecionine and riddelliine, that are important in agriculture because of their hepatotoxic potential in grazing animals. Quinine and its isomer quinidine from *Cinchona* bark are quinoline alkaloids that have antimalarial and antiarrhythmic activity, respectively. Important benzylisoquinoline alkaloids include the morphinans morphine and codeine, which are also the basis for the semisynthetic narcotic analgesics.

19.3.2
Biotransformation of Important Polyketides, Shikimates, and Alkaloids in Man

Oxidation by CYP3A enzymes is important in the biotransformation of three widely used polyketide drugs in man: cyclosporine, erythromycin, and lovastatin (Table 19.1). Aoyama *et al.* reported that CYP3A converted the immunosuppressant cyclosporine to several metabolites, with the regioselectivity of substrate

Table 19.1 Well-defined biotransformation pathways for polyketides, shikimates, and alkaloids in man.

Natural product	Comments	References
Polyketides		
Cyclosporine	several metabolites by CYP3A	[73]
Erythromycin	*N*-desmethylation by CYP3A	[74]
Lovastatin	6′-hydroxylation by CYP3A	[75]
	6-*exo*-methylene by CYP3A	[75]
Shikimates		
Bergamottin	mechanism-based inactivation-reactive metabolite by CYP3A4	[10]
	mechanism-based inactivation-reactive metabolite by CYP2B6 and CYP3A5	[76]
Coumarin	7-hydroxylation by CYP2A6	[77]

Table 19.1 (*Continued*)

Natural product	Comments	References
Estragole	1′-hydroxylation by CYP1A2 and CYP2A6	[78]
Eugenol	1′-hydroxylation by CYP1A2, CYP2C9, CYP2C19, and CYP2D6	[79]
8-methoxypsoralen	4′,5′-epoxidation by CYP2A6	[9]
Myristicin	5-allyl-1-methoxy-2,3-catechol by CYP3A4 and CYP1A2	[80]
Resveratrol	3′-hydroxylation by CYP1A2	[81]
	3-*O*- and 4′-*O*-glucuronidation by UGT1A1 and UGT1A9	[82]
	3-*O*- and 4′-*O*-sulfation, and 3,4-*O*-disulfation by SULT1A1, SULT1A2, and SULT1A2/1A3	[83]
Safrole	1′-hydroxylation by CYP2C9, CYP2A6, CYP2D6, and CYP2E1	[84, 85]
Alkaloids		
Caffeine	3-demethylation by CYP1A2	[86]
Codeine	*O*-demethylation by CYP2D6	[87]
Colchicine	2- and 3-hydroxylation by CYP3A4	[88]
Emetine	9-*O*-demethylation by CYP3A4 and CYP2A6	[89]
	10-*O*-demethylation by CYP3A4	
Harmaline	*O*-demethylation by CYP1A2, CYP2C9, and CYP2D6	[90]
Harman	3- and 6-hydroxylation by CYP1A	[91]
	2-oxidation by CYP2E1	[91]
Harmine	*O*-demethylation by CYP1A2, CYP2C9, and CYP2D6	[90]
Morphine	3- and 6-glucuronidation by UGT2B7	[92, 93]
Nicotine	cotinine by CYP2A6	[94]
	N-glucuronidation by UGT2B10	[95]
Norharman	3- and 6-hydroxylation by CYP1A	[91]
	2-oxidation by CYP2E1	[91]
Pilocarpine	3-hydroxylation by CYP2A6	[96]
Quinine	3-hydroxylation and 2′-quininone formation by CYP3A4	[97]
Riddelliine	dehydrogenation and *N*-oxidation by CYP3A4	[8]
Senecionine	*N*-glucuronidation by UGT1A2	[98]
	dehydrogenation and *N*-oxidation by CYP3A4	[7]

Natural products are included if information was derived in part from *in vitro* studies that used multiple active systems, and where metabolites were identified and quantified. Pharmacokinetic studies that quantified metabolite formation but did not identify the enzymes that mediated metabolite formation have been excluded.

oxidation differing between CYPs 3A4 and 3A5 [73]. Similarly, the fungal-derived macrolide antibiotic erythromycin undergoes CYP3A-dependent *N*-demethylation [74]. Indeed, erythromycin may be used as a selective *in vivo* probe for the activity of CYP3A in human subjects. CYP3A enzymes also catalyze the oxidation of the hypocholesterolemic agent lovastatin at the 6′-carbon to generate the 6′-hydroxy and 6-*exo*-methylene metabolites [75].

CYPs 3A and 2B6 are important enzymes in the oxidation of the shikimate-derived furanocoumarin (psoralen) derivative bergamottin; in the process these enzymes are inactivated by a reactive metabolite [10, 76]. As a consequence bergamottin–a constituent of grapefruit juice–elicits clinically significant effects, including increased toxicity with a number of coadministered drugs [99]. Interestingly a different profile of CYP biotransformation has been reported for the structurally similar 8-methoxypsoralen. Rather than CYPs 3A, CYP2A6 appears most susceptible to inactivation during the biotransformation of 8-methoxypsoralen, which has been attributed to a reactive epoxide or γ-ketoenal intermediate (Figure 19.5) [10]. The factors that determine the relative CYP specificity for biotransformation of different furanocoumarins remains to be established, but it is noteworthy that coumarin itself is also a substrate for CYP2A6 [77]. It is feasible that the 5-substituent in bergamottin increases the susceptibility of CYPs 3A and 2B6 to inactivation.

The biotransformation of several phenylpropene derivatives that are found in essential oils has been described. CYP1A2 has been found to catalyze the 1′-hydroxylation of estragole and eugenol, with additional contributions from CYP2A6, and CYPs 2C9, 2C19, and 2D6, respectively [78, 79]. In contrast, safrole 1′-hydroxylation is mediated by several CYPs from family 2 [84, 85]. Again, it is not yet clear why a different profile of CYPs mediates the side-chain oxidation of

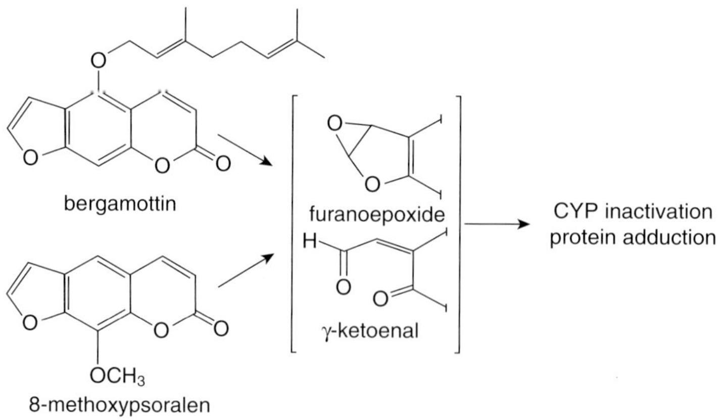

Figure 19.5 Putative reactive epoxide and γ-ketoenal metabolites formed from the furanocoumarins bergamottin and 8-methoxypsoralen that inactivate CYPs by covalent adduct formation.

safrole, but it could be related to the presence of the methylenedioxyphenyl moiety (Table 19.1). Indeed, in the case of myristicin, this system undergoes oxidation by CYPs 1A2 and 3A4 within the methylenedioxyphenyl system to produce 5-allyl-1-methoxy-2,3-catechol [80].

Stilbenes resemble the flavonoids, but possess a bis-benzilic structure rather than the fused-ring system present in the latter. There has been particular recent interest in the stilbene resveratrol because of its potential as an anticancer and anti-inflammatory agent. As it is produced by grapes, some of the reported heath benefits of red wine have been attributed to resveratrol. The 3′-hydroxylation of resveratrol is mediated by CYP1A2 [81], but, probably because this molecule is already polyhydroxylated, phase II conjugation by UGTs and SULTs appears to be more prominent than oxidation. Recent studies have defined the roles of several UGT and SULT enzymes in the conjugation of the hydroxyl groups of resveratrol (Table 19.1) [82, 83].

In terms of therapeutic significance, the role of CYP2D6 in the *O*-demethylation of the alkaloid codeine to its active metabolite morphine is of major importance [87]. Individuals who do not express active CYP2D6 (the poor metabolizers) experience minimal pain relief from codeine, whereas individuals who express multiple active copies of CYP2D6 genes (the so-called ultrarapid metabolizers) may experience toxicity due to morphine over-production [100]. Morphine is itself conjugated efficiently and eliminated by UGT2B7 [92, 93]. CYP3A enzymes are important in the biotransformation of several alkaloids, including colchicine [88], emetine [89], quinine [97], and the hepatotoxic pyrrolizidine alkaloids such as riddelliine [8] and senecionine [7]. Conjugation of the latter alkaloids is mediated by UGT1A2, which is likely to be important in minimizing toxicity [98].

Several human CYPs have been found to oxidize the psychotropic β-carboline alkaloids, which may limit their duration of action. Thus, CYP1A enzymes mediate the 3- and 6-hydroxylation of harman and norharman [91], and contribute along with CYPs 2C9 and 2D6 to the *O*-demethylation pathway [90]. In contrast, CYP2A6 mediates 3-hydroxylation of the imidazole alkaloid pilocarpine [96] and 2′- and 5′-hydroxylation of the pyridine alkaloid nicotine to cotinine [94]. Indeed, rapid clearance induces nicotine craving, so that inhibitors of CYP2A6 have been used in patients to decrease nicotine clearance and minimize cigarette smoking [101]. Glucuronidation is an important pathway of elimination for nicotine and its metabolites. Recent studies have implicated human UGT2B10 in this pathway [95]. Biotransformation of the xanthine-based alkaloid caffeine is extensive, yielding several metabolites, and involving the enzymes CYP1A2, xanthine oxidase and *N*-acetyltransferase [86]. Owing to the established role of CYP1A2 in paraxanthine formation (3-demethylation), caffeine has been used as a substrate for selective *in vivo* phenotyping of CYP1A2 activity in man [102].

In summary, the polyketides, shikimates, and alkaloids are classes of natural products that include a very large number of structurally diverse derivatives. Many of these agents have been used in pharmacognosy for centuries, but important aspects of their biotransformation have emerged only relatively recently. However, although our capacity to study biotransformation pathways of natural products is now well developed, there has been a focus on a limited number of agents that are molecules of therapeutic importance in man.

19.4 Summary and Conclusions

Like conventional drugs, natural products undergo biotransformation by hepatic phase I and phase II enzymes, and are substrates for transporter proteins. Thus, the propensity for drug interactions that lead to toxicity or decreased efficacy is high. It has also emerged that the biotransformation products of certain natural products serve as ligands for a number of closely related nuclear receptors that modulate target gene expression. Thus, natural product metabolites, including those derived from vitamins A and D and the higher terpenoids, regulate cellular homeostasis and modulate the expression and function of CYP genes. This aspect highlights the particular significance of the biotransformation of some natural products. It is likely that the number of natural products used in human therapeutics will continue to increase in the future, and that some of these will be derived from marine and other nonplant sources. How biotransformation influences the pharmacological and toxicological actions of these agents will be of interest, and may lead to the identification of important new biological paradigms.

Acknowledgments

Work in the author's laboratory has been funded by the Australian National Health and Medical Research Council and the State Cancer Council, NSW.

References

1 Ji, H.-F., Li, X.-J., and Zhang, H.-Y. (2009) Natural products and drug discovery. *EMBO Rep.*, **10**, 194–200.

2 Ioannides, C. (2002) Pharmacokinetic interactions between herbal remedies and medicinal drugs. *Xenobiotica*, **32**, 451–478.

3 Kennedy, J., Wang, C.C., and Wu, C.H. (2008) Patient disclosure about herb and supplement use among adults in the US. *Evid. Based Complement. Alternat. Med.*, **5**, 451–456.

4 Bush, T.M., Rayburn, K.S., Holloway, S.W., Sanchez-Yamamoto, D.S., Allen, B.L., Lam, T., So, B.K., Tran de, H., Greyber, E.R., Kantor, S., and Roth, L.W. (2007) Adverse interactions between herbal and dietary substances and prescription medications: a clinical survey. *Altern. Ther. Health Med.*, **13**, 30–35.

5 Madyastha, K.M. and Raj, C.P. (1990) Biotransformations of *R*-(+)-pulegone and menthofuran *in vitro*: chemical basis for toxicity. *Biochem. Biophys. Res. Commun.*, **173**, 1086–1092.

6 Khojasteh-Bakht, S.C., Chen, W., Koenigs, L.L., Peter, R.M., and Nelson, S.D. (1999) Metabolism of *(R)*-(+)-pulegone and *(R)*-(+)-menthofuran by

human liver cytochrome P-450s: evidence for formation of a furan epoxide. *Drug Metab. Dispos.*, **27**, 574–580.

7 Miranda, C.L., Reed, R.L., Guengerich, F.P., and Buhler, D.R. (1991) Role of cytochrome P450IIIA4 in the metabolism of the pyrrolizidine alkaloid senecionine in human liver. *Carcinogenesis*, **12**, 515–519.

8 Xia, Q., Chou, M.W., Kadlubar, F.F., Chan, P.C., and Fu, P.P. (2003) Human liver microsomal metabolism and DNA adduct formation of the tumorigenic pyrrolizidine alkaloid, riddelliine. *Chem. Res. Toxicol.*, **16**, 66–73.

9 Koenigs, L.L. and Trager, W.F. (1998) Mechanism-based inactivation of cytochrome P450 2B1 by 8-methoxypsoralen and several other furanocoumarins. *Biochemistry*, **37**, 13184–13193.

10 He, K., Iyer, K.R., Hayes, R.N., Sinz, M.W., Woolf, T.F., and Hollenberg, P.F. (1998) Inactivation of cytochrome P450 3A4 by bergamottin, a component of grapefruit juice. *Chem. Res. Toxicol.*, **11**, 252–259.

11 Larrey, D., Funck-Brentano, C., Breil, P., Vitaux, J., Theodore, C., Babany, G., and Pessayre, D. (1983) Effects of erythromycin on hepatic drug metabolizing enzymes in humans. *Biochem. Pharmacol.*, **32**, 1063–1068.

12 Gurley, B.J., Swain, A., Hubbard, M.A., Hartsfield, F., Thaden, J., Williams, D.K., Gentry, W.B., and Tong, Y. (2008) Supplementation with goldenseal (*Hydrastis canadensis*), but not kava kava (*Piper methysticum*), inhibits human CYP3A activity *in vivo*. *Clin. Pharmacol. Ther.*, **83**, 61–69.

13 Moore, L.B., Goodwin, B., Jones, S.A., Wisely, G.B., Serabjit-Singh, C.J., Willson, T.M., Collins, J.L., and Kliewer, S.A. (2000) St. John's wort induces hepatic drug metabolism through activation of the pregnane X receptor. *Proc. Natl. Acad. Sci. USA*, **97**, 7500–7502.

14 Roby, C.A., Anderson, G.D., Kantor, E., Dryer, D.A., and Burstein, A.H. (2000) St John's Wort: effect on CYP3A4 activity. *Clin. Pharmacol. Ther.*, **67**, 451–457.

15 McMurry, J.E. and Begley, T.P. (eds) (2005) *The Organic Chemistry of Biological Pathways*, Roberts, Greenwood Village, CO, pp. 93–160.

16 Zile, M.H. (2001) Function of vitamin A in vertebrate embryonic development. *J. Nutr.*, **131**, 705–708.

17 Zouboulis, C.C. (2001) Retinoids: which dermatological indications will benefit in the near future? *Skin Pharmacol. Appl. Skin Physiol.*, **14**, 303–315.

18 Tallman, M.S. (2004) Acute promyelocytic leukemia as a paradigm for targeted therapy. *Semin. Hematol.*, **41** (Suppl. 4), 27–32.

19 Ishida, T., Toyota, M., and Asakawa, Y. (1989) Terpenoid biotransformation in mammals. V. Metabolism of (+)-citronellal, (±)-7-hydroxycitronellal, citral, (−)-perillaldehyde, (−)-myrtenal, cuminaldehyde, thujone, and (±)-carvone in rabbits. *Xenobiotica*, **19**, 843–855.

20 Diliberto, J.J., Usha, G., and Birnbaum, L.S. (1988) Disposition of citral in male Fischer rats. *Drug Metab. Dispos.*, **16**, 721–727.

21 Diliberto, J.J., Srinivas, P., Overstreet, D., Usha, G., Burka, L.T., and Birnbaum, L.S. (1990) Metabolism of citral, an α,β-unsaturated aldehyde, in male F344 rats. *Drug Metab. Dispos.*, **18**, 866–875.

22 Chen, L.-J., Lebetkin, E.H., and Burka, L.T. (2001) Metabolism of (*R*)-(+)-pulegone in F344 rats. *Drug Metab. Dispos.*, **29**, 1567–1577.

23 Madyastha, K.M. and Gaikwad, N.W. (1998) Metabolic fate of *S*-(−)-pulegone in rat. *Xenobiotica*, **28**, 723–734.

24 Thomassen, D., Pearson, P.G., Slattery, J.T., and Nelson, S.D. (1991) Partial characterization of biliary metabolites of pulegone by tandem mass spectrometry. *Drug Metab. Dispos.*, **19**, 997–1003.

25 Chen, L.J., Lebetkin, E.H., and Burka, L.T. (2003) Comparative disposition of (*R*)-(+)-pulegone in B6C3F1 mice and F344 rats. *Drug Metab. Dispos.*, **31**, 892–899.

26 Nelson, S.D., McClanahan, R.H., Thomassen, D., Gordon, W.P., and

Knebel, N. (1992) Investigations of mechanisms of reactive metabolite formation from (*R*)-(+)-pulegone. *Xenobiotica*, **22**, 1157–1164.

27 Madyastha, K.M. and Raj, C.P. (1992) Metabolic fate of menthofuran in rats. Novel oxidative pathways. *Drug Metab. Dispos.*, **20**, 295–301.

28 Thomassen, D., Knebel, N., Slattery, J.T., McClanahan, R.H., and Nelson, S.D. (1992) Reactive intermediates in the oxidation of menthofuran by cytochromes P-450. *Chem. Res. Toxicol.*, **5**, 123–130.

29 Thompson, D.C., Perera, K., Fisher, R., and Brendel, K. (1994) Cresol isomers: comparison of toxic potency in rat liver slices. *Toxicol. Appl. Pharmacol.*, **125**, 51–58.

30 Miyazawa, M., Shindo, M., and Shimada, T. (2001) Oxidation of 1,8-cineole, the monoterpene cyclic ether originated from eucalyptus polybractea, by cytochrome P450 3A enzymes in rat and human liver microsomes. *Drug Metab. Dispos.*, **29**, 200–205.

31 Boyle, R., McLean, S., and Davies, N.W. (2000) Biotransformation of 1,8-cineole in the brushtail possum (*Trichosurus vulpecula*). *Xenobiotica*, **30**, 915–932.

32 Southwell, I.A., Flynn, T.M., and Degabriele, R. (1980) Metabolism of α- and β-pinene, *p*-cymene and 1,8-cineole in the brushtail possum, *Trichosurus vulpecula*. *Xenobiotica*, **10**, 17–23.

33 Carman, R.M. and Rayner, A.C. (1994) 2α,4-Dihydroxy 1,8 cineole. A new possum urinary metabolite. *Aust. J. Chem.*, **47**, 2087–2097.

34 Bull, S.D., Carman, R.M., Carrick, F.N., and Klika, K.D. (1993) 7-Hydroxy-1,8-cineole and 7-cineolic acid. Two new possum urinary metabolites. *Aust. J. Chem.*, **46**, 441–447.

35 Pass, G.J. and McLean, S. (2002) Inhibition of the microsomal metabolism of 1,8-cineole in the common brushtail possum (*Trichosurus vulpecula*) by terpenes and other chemicals. *Xenobiotica*, **32**, 1109–1126.

36 Miyazawa, M., Shindo, M., and Shimada, T. (2001) Roles of cytochrome P450 3A enzymes in the 2-hydroxylation of 1,4-cineole, a monoterpene cyclic ether, by rat and human liver microsomes. *Xenobiotica*, **31**, 713–723.

37 Duisken, M., Sandner, F., Blömeke, B., and Hollender, J. (2005) Metabolism of 1,8-cineole by human cytochrome P450 enzymes: identification of a new hydroxylated metabolite. *Biochim. Biophys. Acta*, **1722**, 304–311.

38 Maggs, J.L., Madden, S., Bishop, L.P., O'Neill, P.M., and Park, B.K. (1997) The rat biliary metabolites of dihydroartemisinin, an antimalarial endoperoxide. *Drug Metab. Dispos.*, **25**, 1200–1204.

39 Svensson, U.S. and Ashton, M. (1999) Identification of the human cytochrome P450 enzymes involved in the *in vitro* metabolism of artemisinin. *Br. J. Clin. Pharmacol.*, **48**, 528–535.

40 Ilett, K.F., Ethell, B.T., Maggs, J.L., Davis, T.M., Batty, K.T., Burchell, B., Binh, T.Q., Thu le, T.A., Hung, N.C., Pirmohamed, M., Park, B.K., and Edwards, G. (2002) Glucuronidation of dihydroartemisinin *in vivo* and by human liver microsomes and expressed UDP-glucuronosyltransferases. *Drug Metab. Dispos.*, **30**, 1005–1012.

41 Lee, I.S. and Hufford, C.D. (1990) Metabolism of antimalarial sesquiterpene lactones. *Pharmacol. Ther.*, **48**, 345–355.

42 Simonsson, U.S., Jansson, B., Trinh, N.H., Dinh, X.H., Tybring, G., and Ashton, M. (2003) Artemisinin autoinduction is caused by involvement of cytochrome P450 2B6 but not 2C9. *Clin. Pharmacol. Ther.*, **74**, 32–43.

43 Mihara, K., Svensson, U.S., Tybring, G., Trinh, N.H., Bertilsson, L., and Ashton, M. (1999) Stereospecific analysis of omeprazole supports artemisinin as a potent inducer of CYP2C19. *Fundam. Clin. Pharmacol.*, **13**, 671–675.

44 Burk, O., Arnold, K.A., Nussler, A.K., Schaeffeler, E., Efimova, E., Avery, B.A., Avery, M.A., Fromm, M.F., and Eichelbaum, M. (2005) Antimalarial artemisinin drugs induce cytochrome P450 and MDR1 expression by activation of xenosensors pregnane X receptor and constitutive androstane

receptor. *Mol. Pharmacol.*, **67**, 1954–1965.

45 Shoyama, Y., Hirano, H., and Nishioka, I. (1984) Biosynthesis of propyl cannabinoid acid and its biosynthetic relationship with pentyl and methyl cannabinoid acids. *Phytochemistry*, **23**, 1909–1912.

46 Watanabe, K., Yamaori, S., Funahashi, T., Kimura, T., and Yamamoto, I. (2007) Cytochrome P450 enzymes involved in the metabolism of tetrahydrocannabinols and cannabinol by human hepatic microsomes. *Life Sci.*, **80**, 1415–1419.

47 Bornheim, L.M., Lasker, J.M., and Raucy, J.L. (1992) Human hepatic microsomal metabolism of Δ^1-tetrahydrocannabinol. *Drug Metab. Dispos.*, **20**, 241–246.

48 Mazur, A., Lichti, C.F., Prather, P.L., Zielinska, A.K., Bratton, S.M., Gallus-Zawada, A., Finel, M., Miller, G.P., Radominska-Pandya, A., and Moran, J.H. (2009) Characterization of human hepatic and extrahepatic UDP-glucuronosyltransferase enzymes involved in the metabolism of classic cannabinoids. *Drug Metab. Dispos.*, **37**, 1496–1504.

49 Bornheim, L.M. and Correia, M.A. (1990) Selective inactivation of mouse liver cytochrome P-450IIIA by cannabidiol. *Mol. Pharmacol.*, **38**, 319–326.

50 Jaeger, W., Benet, L.Z., and Bornheim, L.M. (1996) Inhibition of cyclosporine and tetrahydrocannabinol metabolism by cannabidiol in mouse and human microsomes. *Xenobiotica*, **26**, 275–284.

51 Bornheim, L.M. and Grillo, M.P. (1998) Characterization of cytochrome P450 3A inactivation by cannabidiol: possible involvement of cannabidiol-hydroxyquinone as a P450 inactivator. *Chem. Res. Toxicol.*, **11**, 1209–1216.

52 Cresteil, T., Monsarrat, B., Dubois, J., Sonnier, M., Alvinerie, P., and Gueritte, F. (2002) Regioselective metabolism of taxoids by human CYP3A4 and 2C8: structure–activity relationship. *Drug Metab. Dispos.*, **30**, 438–445.

53 Václavíková, R., Boumendjel, A., Ehrlichová, M., Kovár, J., and Gut, I. (2006) Modulation of paclitaxel transport by flavonoid derivatives in human breast cancer cells. Is there a correlation between binding affinity to NBD of P-gp and modulation of transport? *Bioorg. Med. Chem.*, **14**, 4519–4525.

54 Beato, M. (1989) Gene regulation by steroid hormones. *Cell*, **56**, 335–344.

55 Niwa, T., Yabusaki, Y., Honma, K., Matsuo, N., Tatsuta, K., Ishibashi, F., and Katagiri, M. (1998) Contribution of human hepatic cytochrome P450 isoforms to regioselective hydroxylation of steroid hormones. *Xenobiotica*, **28**, 539–547.

56 Adlercreutz, H. (1974) Hepatic metabolism of estrogens in health and disease. *N. Engl. J. Med.*, **290**, 1081–1083.

57 Chiang, J.Y.L. (2002) Bile acid regulation of gene expression: roles of nuclear hormone receptors. *Endocr. Rev.*, **23**, 443–463.

58 Waxman, D.J. (1999) P450 gene induction by structurally diverse xenochemicals: central role of nuclear receptors CAR, PXR, and PPAR. *Arch. Biochem. Biophys.*, **369**, 11–23.

59 Janowski, B.A., Willy, P.J., Devi, T.R., Falck, J.R., and Mangelsdorf, D.J. (1996) An oxysterol signalling pathway mediated by the nuclear receptor LXRα. *Nature*, **383**, 728–731.

60 Chiang, J.Y.L. and Stroup, D. (1994) Identification and characterization of a putative bile acid-responsive element in cholesterol 7α-hydroxylase gene promoter. *J. Biol. Chem.*, **269**, 17502–17507.

61 Sakaki, T., Kagawa, N., Yamamoto, K., and Inouye, K. (2005) Metabolism of vitamin D_3 by cytochromes P450. *Front. Biosci.*, **10**, 119–134.

62 Goodman, D.S. (1969) Biosynthesis of vitamin A from beta-carotene. *Am. J. Clin. Nutr.*, **22**, 963–965.

63 Pares, X., Farres, J., Kedishvili, N., and Duester, G. (2008) Medium-chain and short-chain dehydrogenases/reductases in retinoid metabolism. *Cell. Mol. Life Sci.*, **65**, 3936–3949.

64 Abu-Abed, S., Dollé, P., Metzger, D., Beckett, B., Chambon, P., and Petkovich, M. (2001) The retinoic acid-metabolizing enzyme, CYP26A1, is essential for

normal hindbrain patterning, vertebral identity, and development of posterior structures. *Genes Dev.*, **15**, 226–240.
65 Xi, J. and Yang, Z. (2008) Expression of RALDHs (ALDH1As) and CYP26s in human tissues and during the neural differentiation of P19 embryonal carcinoma stem cell. *Gene Expr. Patterns*, **8**, 438–442.
66 Uehara, M., Yashiro, K., Mamiya, S., Nishino, J., Chambon, P., Dolle, P., and Sakai, Y. (2007) CYP26A1 and CYP26C1 cooperatively regulate anterior–posterior patterning of the developing brain and the production of migratory cranial neural crest cells in the mouse. *Dev. Biol.*, **302**, 399–411.
67 Idres, N., Marill, J., Flexor, M.A., and Chabot, G.G. (2002) Activation of retinoic acid receptor-dependent transcription by all-*trans*-retinoic acid metabolites and isomers. *J. Biol. Chem.*, **277**, 31491–31498.
68 Nadin, L. and Murray, M. (1999) Participation of CYP2C8 in retinoic acid 4-hydroxylation in human hepatic microsomes. *Biochem. Pharmacol.*, **58**, 1201–1208.
69 McSorley, L.C. and Daly, A.K. (2000) Identification of human cytochrome P450 isoforms that contribute to all-*trans*-retinoic acid 4-hydroxylation. *Biochem. Pharmacol.*, **60**, 517–526.
70 Genchi, G., Wang, W., Barua, A., Bidlack, W.R., and Olson, J.A. (1996) Formation of β-glucuronides and of β-galacturonides of various retinoids catalyzed by induced and noninduced microsomal UDP-glucuronosyltransferases of rat liver. *Biochim. Biophys. Acta*, **1289**, 284–290.
71 Staunton, J. and Weissman, K.J. (2001) Polyketide biosynthesis: a millennium review. *Nat. Prod. Rep.*, **18**, 380–416.
72 Knaggs, A.R. (2001) The biosynthesis of shikimate metabolites. *Nat. Prod. Rep.*, **18**, 334–355.
73 Aoyama, T., Yamano, S., Waxman, D.J., Lapenson, D.P., Meyer, U.A., Fischer, V., Tyndale, R., Inaba, T., Kalow, W., Gelboin, H.V., and Gonzalez, F.J. (1989) Cytochrome P-450 hPCN3, a novel cytochrome P-450 IIIA gene product that is differentially expressed in adult human liver. cDNA and deduced amino acid sequence and distinct specificities of cDNA-expressed hPCN1 and hPCN3 for the metabolism of steroid hormones and cyclosporine. *J. Biol. Chem.*, **264**, 10388–10395.
74 Hunt, C.M., Watkins, P.B., Saenger, P., Stave, G.M., Barlascini, N., Watlington, C.O., Wright, J.T., Jr, and Guzelian, P.S. (1992) Heterogeneity of CYP3A isoforms metabolizing erythromycin and cortisol. *Clin. Pharmacol. Ther.*, **51**, 18–23.
75 Wang, R.W., Kari, P.H., Lu, A.Y., Thomas, P.E., Guengerich, F.P., and Vyas, K.P. (1991) Biotransformation of lovastatin: IV. Identification of cytochrome P450 3A proteins as the major enzymes responsible for the oxidative metabolism of lovastatin in rat and human liver microsomes. *Arch. Biochem. Biophys.*, **290**, 355–361.
76 Lin, H.L., Kent, U.M., and Hollenberg, P.F. (2005) The grapefruit juice effect is not limited to cytochrome P450 (P450) 3A4: evidence for bergamottin-dependent inactivation, heme destruction, and covalent binding to protein in P450s 2B6 and 3A5. *J. Pharmacol. Exp. Ther.*, **313**, 154–164.
77 Yamano, S., Tatsuno, J., and Gonzalez, F.J. (1990) The CYP2A3 gene product catalyzes coumarin 7-hydroxylation in human liver microsomes. *Biochemistry*, **29**, 1322–1329.
78 Jeurissen, S.M., Punt, A., Boersma, M.G., Bogaards, J.J., Fiamegos, Y.C., Schilter, B., van Bladeren, P.J., Cnubben, N.H., and Rietjens, I.M. (2007) Human cytochrome P450 enzyme specificity for the bioactivation of estragole and related alkenylbenzenes. *Chem. Res. Toxicol.*, **20**, 798–806.
79 Jeurissen, S.M., Bogaards, J.J., Boersma, M.G., ter Horst, J.P., Awad, H.M., Fiamegos, Y.C., van Beek, T.A., Alink, G.M., Sudhölter, E.J., Cnubben, N.H., and Rietjens, I.M. (2006) Human cytochrome P450 enzymes of importance for the bioactivation of methyleugenol to the proximate carcinogen 1′-hydroxymethyleugenol. *Chem. Res. Toxicol.*, **19**, 111–116.
80 Yun, C.H., Lee, H.S., Lee, H.Y., Yim, S.K., Kim, K.H., Kim, E., Yea, S.S., and

Guengerich, F.P. (2003) Roles of human liver cytochrome P450 3A4 and 1A2 enzymes in the oxidation of myristicin. *Toxicol. Lett.*, **137**, 143–150.

81 Piver, B., Fer, M., Vitrac, X., Merillon, J.M., Dreano, Y., Berthou, F., and Lucas, D. (2004) Involvement of cytochrome P450 1A2 in the biotransformation of *trans*-resveratrol in human liver microsomes. *Biochem. Pharmacol.*, **68**, 773–782.

82 Brill, S.S., Furimsky, A.M., Ho, M.N., Furniss, M.J., Li, Y., Green, A.G., Bradford, W.W., Green, C.E., Kapetanovic, I.M., and Iyer, L.V. (2006) Glucuronidation of *trans*-resveratrol by human liver and intestinal microsomes and UGT isoforms. *J. Pharm. Pharmacol.*, **58**, 469–479.

83 Miksits, M., Maier-Salamon, A., Aust, S., Thalhammer, T., Reznicek, G., Kunert, O., Haslinger, E., Szekeres, T., and Jaeger, W. (2005) Sulfation of resveratrol in human liver: evidence of a major role for the sulfotransferases SULT1A1 and SULT1E1. *Xenobiotica*, **35**, 1101–1119.

84 Ueng, Y.F., Hsieh, C.H., Don, M.J., Chi, C.W., and Ho, L.K. (2004) Identification of the main human cytochrome P450 enzymes involved in safrole 1′-hydroxylation. *Chem. Res. Toxicol.*, **17**, 1151–1156.

85 Jeurissen, S.M., Bogaards, J.J., Awad, H.M., Boersma, M.G., Brand, W., Fiamegos, Y.C., van Beek, T.A., Alink, G.M., Sudhölter, E.J., Cnubben, N.H., and Rietjens, I.M. (2004) Human cytochrome P450 enzyme specificity for bioactivation of safrole to the proximate carcinogen 1′-hydroxysafrole. *Chem. Res. Toxicol.*, **17**, 1245–1250.

86 Rasmussen, B.B. and Brøsen, K. (1996) Determination of urinary metabolites of caffeine for the assessment of cytochrome P4501A2, xanthine oxidase, and *N*-acetyltransferase activity in humans. *Ther. Drug Monit.*, **18**, 254–262.

87 Dayer, P., Desmeules, J., Leemann, T., and Striberni, R. (1988) Bioactivation of the narcotic drug codeine in human liver is mediated by the polymorphic monooxygenase catalyzing debrisoquine 4-hydroxylation (cytochrome P-450 dbl/bufI). *Biochem. Biophys. Res. Commun.*, **152**, 411–416.

88 Tateishi, T., Soucek, P., Caraco, Y., Guengerich, F.P., and Wood, A.J. (1997) Colchicine biotransformation by human liver microsomes. Identification of CYP3A4 as the major isoform responsible for colchicine demethylation. *Biochem. Pharmacol.*, **53**, 111–116.

89 Asano, T., Kushida, H., Sadakane, C., Ishihara, K., Wakui, Y., Yanagisawa, T., Kimura, M., Kamei, H., and Yoshida, T. (2001) Metabolism of ipecac alkaloids cephaeline and emetine by human hepatic microsomal cytochrome P450s, and their inhibitory effects on P450 enzyme activities. *Biol. Pharm. Bull.*, **24**, 678–682.

90 Yu, A.M., Idle, J.R., Krausz, K.W., Küpfer, A., and Gonzalez, F.J. (2003) Contribution of individual cytochrome P450 isozymes to the *O*-demethylation of the psychotropic β-carboline alkaloids harmaline and harmine. *J. Pharmacol. Exp. Ther.*, **305**, 315–322.

91 Herraiz, T., Guillén, H., and Arán, V.J. (2008) Oxidative metabolism of the bioactive and naturally occurring β-carboline alkaloids, norharman and harman, by human cytochrome P450 enzymes. *Chem. Res. Toxicol.*, **21**, 2172–2180.

92 Miners, J.O., Lillywhite, K.J., and Birkett, D.J. (1998) *In vitro* evidence for the involvement of at least two forms of human liver UDP-glucuronosyltransferase in morphine 3-glucuronidation. *Biochem. Pharmacol.*, **37**, 2839–2845.

93 Stone, A.N., Mackenzie, P.I., Galetin, A., Houston, J.B., and Miners, J.O. (2003) Isoform selectivity and kinetics of morphine 3- and 6-glucuronidation by human UDP-glucuronosyltransferases: evidence for atypical glucuronidation kinetics by UGT2B7. *Drug Metab. Dispos.*, **31**, 1086–1089.

94 Hecht, S.S., Hochalter, J.B., Villalta, P.W., and Murphy, S.E. (2000) 2′-Hydroxylation of nicotine by cytochrome P450 2A6 and human liver microsomes: formation of a lung

carcinogen precursor. *Proc. Natl. Acad. Sci. USA*, **97**, 12493–12497.

95 Kaivosaari, S., Toivonen, P., Hesse, L.M., Koskinen, M., Court, M.H., and Finel, M. (2007) Nicotine glucuronidation and the human UDP-glucuronosyltransferase UGT2B10. *Mol. Pharmacol.*, **72**, 761–768.

96 Endo, T., Ban, M., Hirata, K., Yamamoto, A., Hara, Y., and Momose, Y. (2007) Involvement of CYP2A6 in the formation of a novel metabolite, 3-hydroxypilocarpine, from pilocarpine in human liver microsomes. *Drug Metab. Dispos.*, **35**, 476–483.

97 Mirghani, R.A., Yasar, U., Zheng, T., Cook, J.M., Gustafsson, L.L., Tybring, G., and Ericsson, O. (2002) Enzyme kinetics for the formation of 3-hydroxyquinine and three new metabolites of quinine *in vitro*; 3-hydroxylation by CYP3A4 is indeed the major metabolic pathway. *Drug Metab. Dispos.*, **30**, 1368–1371.

98 He, Y.Q., Liu, Y., Zhang, B.F., Liu, H.X., Lu, Y.L., Yang, L., Xiong, A.Z., Xu, L.L., Wang, C.H., Yang, L., and Wang, Z.T. (2010) Identification of the UDP-glucuronosyltransferase isozyme involved in senecionine glucuronidation in human liver microsomes. *Drug Metab. Dispos.*, **38**, 626–634.

99 Lown, K.S., Bailey, D.G., Fontana, R.J., Janardan, S.K., Adair, C.H., Fortlage, L.A., Brown, M.B., Guo, W., and Watkins, P.B. (1997) Grapefruit juice increases felodipine oral availability in humans by decreasing intestinal CYP3A protein expression. *J. Clin. Invest.*, **99**, 2545–2553.

100 Yue, Q.Y., Alm, C., Svensson, J.O., and Säwe, J. (1997) Quantification of the *O*- and *N*-demethylated and the glucuronidated metabolites of codeine relative to the debrisoquine metabolic ratio in urine in ultrarapid, rapid, and poor debrisoquine hydroxylators. *Ther. Drug Monit.*, **19**, 539–542.

101 Sellers, E.M., Kaplan, H.L., and Tyndale, R.F. (2000) Inhibition of cytochrome P450 2A6 increases nicotine's oral bioavailability and decreases smoking. *Clin. Pharmacol. Ther.*, **68**, 35–43.

102 Ghassabian, S., Chetty, M., Tattam, B.N., Glen, J., Rahme, J., Stankovic, Z., Ramzan, I., Murray, M., and McLachlan, A.J. (2009) A high-throughput assay using liquid chromatography-tandem mass spectrometry for simultaneous *in vivo* phenotyping of 5 major cytochrome P450 enzymes in patients. *Ther. Drug Monit.*, **31**, 239–246.

20
Flavonoids

Petr Hodek

20.1
Flavonoids – Plant Phytochemicals

The flavonoids are a large group of plant secondary metabolites categorized as phenolic compounds. Their wide distribution in plants makes them the most abundant phenolics in the human diet. Owing to a wide range of biological activities, flavonoids have been extensively studied for several decades. Although flavonoids provide numerous beneficial properties to human health, they are foreign compounds (xenobiotics), the administration of which into the human body should be considered with caution. The aim of this chapter is to summarize our knowledge about flavonoid metabolism and the interactions of flavonoids with important metabolic pathways in mammalian systems. Special attention will be paid to the human health aspects related to flavonoid consumption.

20.1.1
Classification of Flavonoids and Their Physicochemical Properties

Flavonoids share the common C6–C3–C6 carbon framework of their basic structure. These compounds (Figure 20.1) are derivatives of bicyclic chromene (benzopyran) having its heterocyclic ring C substituted with an aromatic ring (B). Depending on the position of the aromatic ring B linkage to chromene these flavans may be classified into three groups: position 2 – flavonoids (2-phenylbenzopyrans); position 3 – isoflavonoids (3-phenylbenzopyrans); and position 4 – neoflavonoids (4-phenylbenzopyrans). Further, the flavonoids are subdivided according to their oxidation status of ring C: the introduction of an oxo group in position 4 provides flavanones; a double bond between C2 and C3 is characteristic for flavones (compounds with quinone-like properties); the presence an additional double bond in ring C (instead of a C4-oxo group) results in a group of anthocyanidins. Formerly, chalcones (derivatives of diphenylpropane skeleton),

Metabolism of Drugs and Other Xenobiotics, First Edition. Edited by Pavel Anzenbacher, Ulrich M. Zanger.

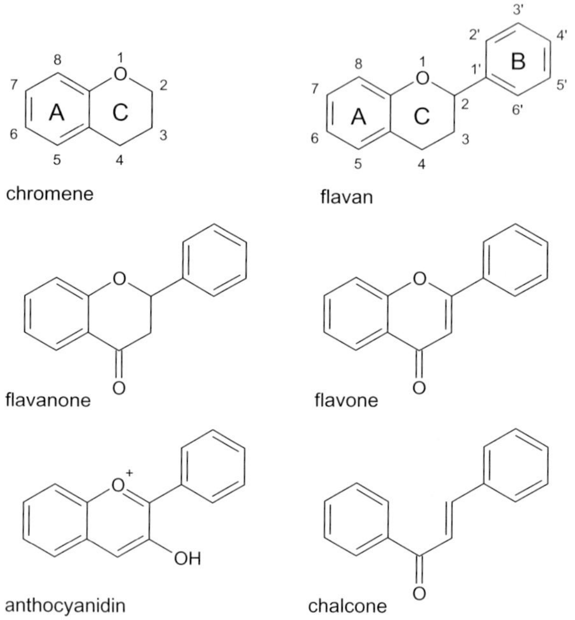

Figure 20.1 Structures of basic flavonoid skeletons and chalcone.

which are precursors of some flavonoids, were also counted among flavonoids. More than 8000 compounds with a flavonoid structure have been identified [1]. The large number of compounds arises from various combinations of multiple hydroxyl and methoxyl groups, substituting the basic flavonoid skeleton. Moreover, natural flavonoids usually occur as glycosides (e.g., glucosides, rhamnoglucosides, rutinosides) and even as more complex structures (e.g., oligomeric forms of procyanidins, flavonolignans, catechin esters, or prenylated chalcones) [2].

Physicochemical properties of flavonoids as well as their physiological activities are closely related to the oxidation level of the C ring (number of double bonds, presence of oxo groups), hydroxylation pattern of the whole flavonoid skeleton, and the extent of glycosylation or methylation of hydroxyl groups. According to their water solubility, flavonoids can be basically classified into two types: hydrophilic flavonoids (highly hydroxylated flavonoids, glycosides, and anthocyanins) and nonpolar flavonoids (aglycones, methylated, or alkylated flavonoids). All flavonoids are UV-light-absorbing chemicals and some of them are colorful compounds, such as the well-known anthocyanins, showing pH-sensitive color transitions. Flavonoids are frequently referred to as powerful antioxidants. The efficiency of their antioxidant activity depends on their flavonoid hydroxylation pattern, in particular on the 3′,4′-dihydroxy catechol structure in the B ring and the presence of 2,3-unsaturation in conjunction with the 4-oxo group in the C ring [3].

20.1.2
Biosynthesis of Flavonoids and Their Biological Function in Plants

Flavonoids in plants were disregarded by some as byproducts or unwanted compounds with no obvious purpose. Recently, we have been gradually discovering that their production is of great importance for plants, since these compounds play numerous roles in plant physiology, development, and ecology. One of the most obvious functions for flavonoids is to serve as UV-light shields (i.e., protecting against solar UV-B–the irradiation that is damaging to DNA) [4]. Flavonoids mentioned above as antioxidants can exert antioxidant properties for the benefit of the plant against potential oxidative stress. Flavonoids are also able to mediate specific interactions between plants and insect pollinators (e.g., sweet taste, color, smell), and/or symbiotic plants and microorganisms (e.g., attraction of nitrogen-fixing bacteria). Moreover, some flavonoids are required for germination of pollen grains and for successful pollen growth [4]. In addition to these positive functions for plants, flavonoids may serve as attractants for pathogenic fungi and bacteria [5].

The biosynthesis of flavonoids starts with the condensation of a cinnamic acid with three malonyl-CoA moieties. All flavonoids arise from this initial reaction, via the chalcone intermediate (for structure see Figure 20.1), which is usually converted into phenylbenzopyran (flavan), and further elaboration leads to the flavones, isoflavones, flavonols, or anthocyanins [6]. Next, the glycosylation (even multiple) of the flavonoid skeleton potentiates the huge variety of flavonoid phytochemicals present in plants [7].

20.2
Absorption and Metabolism of Flavonoids

Flavonoids of the vegetable diet are known to provide multiple pharmacological effects on mammalian systems. To achieve this, these phytochemicals need to be first absorbed from the gastrointestinal tract. The flavonoids from ingested food are usually not absorbed into blood circulation in their native form. They are frequently converted via endogenous and/or microbial enzymes into derivatives or forms allowing their absorption. Thus, bioavailability of flavonoids is closely related to their metabolism. It should be noted that flavonoid species exerting a detectable effect on the target organ, tissue, or protein most likely differ from those present in the original plant material. Hence, the assignment of some health-promoting effect to a particular flavonoid is definitely not simple and straightforward, and requires an extensive study of the metabolic fate of that flavonoid.

20.2.1
Flavonoid Bioavailability

Obtaining reliable data on average flavonoid amounts consumed daily throughout the world is quite difficult because of significant differences in the sources of flavonoids available, and dietary habits and preferences. The total flavonoid intake probably reaches up to 1 g/day in people who eat several servings of fruit and vegetables per day [8]. For the United States, it was calculated by Kuhnau [9] that dietary flavonoid intake consisted of the following: 16% flavonols, flavones, and flavanones; 17% anthocyanins; 20% catechins; and 45% "biflavones" (dimeric flavonoids). Current knowledge allowed revising the original data and gives us a better estimate of a typical mean intake that is in the range 450–600 mg as aglycones [10]. More precise data is available for the intake of individual classes of flavonoids. For instance, anthocyanin consumption (based on data from Finland) was found to be 82 mg/day on average, although some intakes exceeded 200 mg/day [11]. The consumption of flavonols has been estimated at 20–25 mg/day in the United States [12]. For isoflavones, an average dietary intake of 30–40 mg/day was determined in Asian countries, where soy products are frequently consumed [13]. Although flavonoids belong to xenobiotics, which daily intake in diet is rather high (10–100 mg of a single compound), their plasma concentrations hardly reach the micromolar range and thus the concentrations are typically in the range of tens to hundreds of nanomoles per liter.

The great majority of natural flavonoids occur as glycosylated forms that negatively influence their absorption. Although much remains unknown about the mechanisms of gastrointestinal flavonoid absorption, it is assumed that flavonoids (i.e., their glycosides) are too hydrophilic to penetrate the gut wall [8]. Thus, only flavan-3-ols – flavonoids naturally occurring as aglycones – may be absorbed intact. Moreover, it is speculated that the uptake of glucosides of cyanidin and quercetin proceeds specifically via the sodium-dependent glucose transporter [14]. At first glance the connection between bioavailability and metabolism of most flavonoids reminds us of the "chicken and egg" causality dilemma – to be absorbed into the circulation system and metabolized in the liver, flavonoids need to be bioavailable; however, their bioavailability depends on their metabolic conversion. It is generally believed that the removal of the glycosidic moiety is necessary prior to flavonoid absorption. The released aglycone is thought then to undergo passive diffusion across the intestine brush border. Cleavage of flavonoid glycosides is catalyzed by hydrolytic enzymes – glycosidases – either cytosolic or secreted into gastrointestinal tract as well as extensively provided by colonic microflora. The important role of glycosidases for flavonoid absorption is evident from the comparison of the time course of quercetin conjugate concentrations in plasma after quercetin aglycone and rutin. The time to reach the peak of quercetin concentration was markedly delayed after rutin administration, which is consistent with the necessity of rutin hydrolysis into quercetin in the more distal part of the small intestine [15].

The extent of absorption of dietary flavonoids in the small intestine is relatively low depending on the particular flavonoid. Baicalin (baicalein 7-*O*-β-glucopyranuronoside) is an example of a well-absorbed flavonoid, with bioavailability determined to be about 2.2 and 27.8%, based on baicalin and its conjugated metabolites, respectively [16]. However, for chrysin, after an oral dose of 400 mg, there were only trace amounts of this lipid-soluble flavonoid in plasma, corresponding to an estimated bioavailability of 0.003–0.02% [17]. Similarly, orally administered quercetin (8–50 mg) allows us to detect quercetin conjugates in plasma, although almost no aglycone [15]. Thus, a major part of the flavonoids ingested (75–99%) is not found in urine [18]. This finding implies low bioavailability of released aglycones and/or their rapid further metabolism, including, for example, conjugation reactions and even the breakdown of the flavonoid skeleton catalyzed by colonic microflora (see Section 20.2.2). In addition, the bioavailability of some flavonoids might be reduced by multidrug resistance-associated proteins (MRPs) serving as effective efflux transporters. For instance, epicatechin-3-gallate – a neutral tea flavonoid – was shown to be a substrate of MRPs [19].

To conclude, some polyphenols may be less efficiently absorbed than others, but nevertheless reach equivalent plasma concentrations because of lower secretion toward the intestinal lumen, and lower metabolism and elimination [8]. Apparently, the absorption of flavonoids from the gastrointestinal tract is a rather complex process, whose full understanding requires much more information on the fate of ingested flavonoids.

20.2.2 Metabolism of Flavonoids

In general, metabolism of flavonoids proceeds via phase I and phase II biotransformation similarly to other xenobiotics. The major task of this process is their fast detoxification and excretion from the body. However, metabolism of flavonoids is unusual in two aspects. (i) The majority of ingested flavonoids are already conjugated with polar compounds, saccharides (glycosides), which should be final products of phase II of biotransformation. (ii) Flavonoids, even though considered health-promoting compounds (see Section 20.4), are paradoxically eliminated from the body.

The first principal site of flavonoid metabolism is the small intestine. Flavonoid glycosides are at first subjected to enzymatic hydrolysis, resulting in the formation of free aglycone ready for flavonoid absorption as well as for the *C*-hydroxylation of the skeleton and/or *O*-demethylation [20]. In the next step, flavonoids undergo *O*-methylation and conjugation with glucuronate, sulfate, or glycine (and their combinations) via endogenous phase II enzymes. Moreover, flavonoids and their derivatives are exposed to a huge enzyme machinery of colonic microflora, which is even able to degrade flavonoids completely into carbon dioxide [21].

In addition to the intestinal tract, the second key site of flavonoid metabolism is the liver, where the absorbed flavonoids are metabolized further. Resulting derivatives, mostly flavonoid glucuronates and sulfates, are transported by the biliary route into the small intestine and/or to plasma, from where a substantial part of metabolites is excreted in urine. Interestingly, the flavonoid dose determines the primary site of metabolism. Large doses are metabolized mostly in the liver, while small doses may be metabolized in the small intestine with the liver playing a secondary role to further modify flavonoid conjugates from the small intestines. A much smaller portion of flavonoid metabolism, mainly deglycosylation, can be assigned to other tissues. Surprisingly, enzymes present in human saliva are also involved (e.g., in hydrolysis of rutin into quercetin).

20.2.2.1 **Intestinal Metabolism**

As mentioned in Section 20.2.1, only a few of the naturally occurring flavonoids are aglycones – the forms suitable for their absorption; others are present as the conjugated form, mainly with saccharide moieties. Thus, intestinal flavonoid metabolism begins with the hydrolytic cleavage of the *O*-glycosidic bond of glycosides, resulting in the liberation of free flavonoid aglycone. This reaction is catalyzed by glycosidases present in food (endogenous plant enzymes), produced by cells of the gastrointestinal mucosa, or secreted by colon microflora. Whereas human cells express various β-glucosidases, which are specific for the cleavage of the attached glucose (possibly arabinose and xylose) from flavonoids [18], plants and namely bacteria provide glycosidases with a much wider range of hydrolytic activities. These enzyme data can explain the delayed (more than 5 h) maximum of quercetin in plasma after *per os* administration of quercetin-3-*O*-rhamnoglucoside compared to that of quercetin-4′-*O*-glucoside [22]. *O*-glucoside is both rapidly deglycosylated and actively absorbed from the small intestine, whereas quercetin-3-*O*-rhamnoglucoside is absorbed only after a deglycosylation later in the colon by microflora. Apart from cytosolic β-glucosidases, another deglycosylation pathway involves the lactase phloridzine hydrolase – a glucosidase of the brush border membrane – that catalyzes extracellular hydrolysis of some glucosides [23]. Both enzymes are probably involved, but their relative contribution for the various glucosides remains to be clarified.

After deconjugation, flavonoids are conjugated again, but with other compounds than in plants. Most frequently, flavonoid glucoronates are formed in phase II of their biotransformation. The reaction is catalyzed by UDP-glucuronosyltransferase (UGT). In human intestinal mucosa, there are two isoforms – UGT1A8 and UGT1A10 – that are absent in the liver [24]. The extent of glucuronidation seems to be dependent on the flavonoid structure; it is obviously sensitive to the position(s) of hydroxyl group(s) on the B ring. When the flavonoids are hydroxylated in positions 3′,4, the glucuronidation of them (e.g., quercetin) occurred predominantly at the 5- and 7-positions on the A ring [14]. Flavan-3-ols are much more often subjected to *O*-methylation of hydroxyls via catechol-*O*-methyltransferase (COMT) than other flavonoids. *O*-methylated flavonoids may be glucuronidated, as is common with catechins. In addition to *O*-methylation and conjugation with glucuronate, flavonoid sulfates are formed in the small intestine, but probably to a much less extent than in the liver. It has been shown that some flavonoids can inhibit human cytosolic sulfotransferases (SULTs), while the others are readily transformed into sulfate conjugates.

Although the total mass of cytochromes P450 (cytochrome P450CYPs) in the entire small intestine has been estimated to be less than 1% of that in the liver, human studies have demonstrated that enteric CYPs (i.e., the major forms of the

CYP3A subfamily) can contribute significantly to the overall first-pass metabolism of foreign compounds [25]. Only limited information is available on the role of CYP-mediated *O*-demethylation and/or *C*-hydroxylation in flavonoid metabolism in the human small intestine. Similarly, the function of glutathione *S*-transferase (GST), *N*-acetyltransferase (NAT), and epoxide hydrolase remains unclear.

20.2.2.2 **Decisive Role of Colonic Microflora**

Flavonoids, their derivatives, oligomers, or other forms not suitable for absorption into the portal circulation, are faced with the enormous catalytic and hydrolytic potential of colonic microflora. Bacterial degradation of flavonoids includes, for example, hydrolysis, dehydroxylation, demethylation, decarboxylation, repeated deconjugation of glucuronates, and ring cleavage, resulting in breakdown products such as phenolic and carboxylic acids [8]. Thus, the processing of flavonoids by the colonic microflora generates a large variety of new metabolites and their conjugates. For example, as a breakdown product of quercetin-3-*O*-rhamnoglucoside, 3,4-dihydroxyphenylacetic acid and 4-hydroxybenzoic acid were found. A typical glycine conjugate of benzoic acid – hippuric acid – is attributed to the action of intestinal bacteria, too. Interestingly, colon microflora mediates reductive metabolic conversion of soy isoflavone diadzein into equol (isoflavan), exhibiting even stronger estrogenic activity than daidzein [26].

It is assumed that for flavonoids that are not easily absorbed from the small intestine the microbial metabolism can be higher than that in all human tissues involved. Many bacterial metabolites and conjugates are then absorbed, as is clear from their detection in the human urine. Hence, the precise determination of microbial metabolites is turning out to be an important direction of flavonoid research since microbial metabolites may have physiologic effects originally assigned to flavonoid aglycones.

As the flavonoids themselves can exert influence on the microflora, it is possible that flavonoid-induced changes in the composition of the colonic bacterial population may affect the metabolic capacity of the microflora and, consequently, the overall metabolism of xenobiotics as well as the health of the individual [14].

20.2.2.3 **Metabolism in Liver**

In the liver, flavonoids can be further metabolized via metabolic pathways generally similar to those in the small intestine. These reactions include hydrolytic deconjugation of flavonoid glucuronides by β-glucuronidases as well as a reverse aglycone conjugation with glucoronate by UGTs and/or with "active sulfate" by SULTs. *In vivo* studies demonstrate the liberation of aglycone, such as quercetin from glucuronides, which is catalyzed by liver β-glucuronidase [27]. Flavonoid hydroxyl groups may also undergo their methylation by COMT and hydroxymethyl group demethylation by CYPs. Flavonoids with monohydroxymethylated B rings, which can hardly form glucuronides in the small intestine, may be efficiently glucuronidated by liver enzymes. In addition to CYP *O*-demethylation of methoxylated flavonoids, the CYP monooxygenase system also catalyzes *C*-hydroxylation of the flavonoid skeleton. Data from *in vitro* experiments with liver microsomal samples suggest CYP-mediated *C*-hydroxylation of various flavonoids with no or one hydroxyl group on the B ring, such as chrysin or apigenin. The presence of two or more hydroxyl groups on this ring prevents the further hydroxylation by CYPs [28]. Similarly, the *O*-demethylation of hydroxymethyl groups is significantly affected by the hydroxylation pattern of the B-ring. While CYPs catalyze *O*-demethylation at the 4′-position (e.g., tamarixetin, tangeretin and hesperitin), no reaction is performed at the 3′-position (e.g., isorhamnetin) [28]. It has been shown that CYP1A2 plays a major role in hydroxylation and demethylation of flavonoids. The involvement of isoforms 3A4, 2C9, and probably 2E1 and 2B6 is suggested, too, but their relevance for the metabolism of flavonoids *in vivo* seems to be limited [29]. The most prevailing flavonoid metabolites formed in the liver are products of flavonoid conjugation reactions (i.e., glucuronidation and sulfation) and methylation in various mixed and multiple combinations. The CYP-mediated oxidation of flavonoids seems to be of a minor importance compared to the conjugation reactions. However, in *O*-demethylation of flavonoids containing multiple hydroxymethyl groups (e.g., five in tangeretin), CYPs are apparently involved since demethylated derivatives were found in the urine of tangeretin-treated rats [30]. The participation of other xenobiotic-metabolizing enzymes (e.g., NATs, GSTs, and epoxy hydrolases) is not considered to be important for flavonoid metabolism.

Large amounts of methylated, glucuronidated, and sulfated metabolites are transported via the bile to the small intestine and subjected to the next absorption cycle. This enterohepatic flavonoid cycling may cause significant retention of these compounds within the body. At this point it is worth emphasizing that the use of *in vivo* experimental models based on living animals missing the gall bladder (e.g., rats) and biliary route to predict the metabolic fate of flavonoids in the human body may easily be erroneous.

20.2.2.4 **Flavonoid Excretion**

Ingested flavonoids are excreted from the body via two main routes – in urine and in feces. When the flavonoid carbon backbone is degraded by colonic microflora, the final product is carbon dioxide, released by lungs, and carboxylic acids, occurring possibly in sweat secreted by skin. Recovery of total excreted radioactivity in human subjects was determined after an oral dose of [^{14}C]quercetin (100 mg). The average values for urine, feces, and expired air (carbon dioxide trapped) are 4.6, 1.9, and 52.1%, respectively [21]. As an inner excretory mechanism the transport of flavonoid metabolites from the liver into the bile should be considered. Furthermore, on a cellular level the excretion of flavonoid metabolites is performed through active efflux mediated by MRPs.

Flavonoids are predominantly excreted in the form of glucuronidated and sulfated (mixed or multiple) conjugates. The urinary route is preferred by small conjugates such as monosulfates, whereas extensively conjugated metabolites are more likely transported in the bile [8]. Biliary excretion of flavonoids in humans may differ greatly from that in rats because of the existence of the gall bladder in humans; however, this has never been examined [8]. From animal studies, biliary excretion seems to be a major pathway for the elimination of, for example, genistein [31] and epigallocatechin gallate [32]. As aglycones are present, if at all, in rather low concentrations in blood and are effectively conjugated in the liver, they should be generally absent in the urine. Nevertheless, free aglycons of isoflavones, daidzein, and genistein were detected in urine in quantities ranging from nondetectable concentrations (below 0.3%) up to 18% of the total daidzein content and below 0.3–22% for free genistein after acute dosing (up to 500 mg/day). The explanation for this may lie in the instability of the isoflavone glycosides against glycosidases present in plasma and/or extrahepatic tissues. The pattern of daidzein conjugates consists of 7-glucuronide (54%), 4′-glucuronide (25%), monosulfates (13%), sulfoglucuronides (0.9%), diglucuronide (0.4%), and disulfate (0.1%) [33]. The composition of hydrophilic flavonoid metabolites in urine is usually proportional to that determined in the plasma. The total amount of metabolites excreted in urine is roughly correlated with maximum plasma concentrations. Epigallocatechin gallate, however, constitutes an exception to this rule, because this compound is present at high concentrations in plasma, but no detectable amounts were found in urine [34]. The urinary excretion is quite high; for instance, for citrus flavanones, up to 30% of the intake for naringenin, and for soy isoflavones, up to 66% for daidzein. However, low urinary excretion was determined for anthocyanins, ranging from 0.005 to 0.1% of their intake [8]. Low recovery of anthocyanins in urine may be indicative of their high biliary excretion, extensive metabolism (bacterial or endogenous), and possibly complexing with plasma proteins. Thus, based on numerous human and animal studies, it is possible to estimate that, on average, the major part of the flavonoids ingested (75–99%) is not found in urine [18]. A similar conclusion has been drawn more recently based on reviewing a study of 97 flavonoids. The excretion in urine ranged from 0.3 to 43% of the dose recalculated to 50 mg aglycone [35]. This general statement cannot, however, entirely reflect all possible variables; specific properties of any particular flavonoid, microflora status (strain diversity), diet matrix components (content of fiber or fat), and other factors, such as a the diuretic effect of ethanol, consumed simultaneously.

While hydrophilic flavonoid metabolites of various kinds are excreted in bile and urine, only hardly bioavailable, large flavonoid molecules and derivatives are retained in feces. These residual compounds either escaped from absorption or bacterial degradation because of their insolubility or binding to undigested fiber and other food constituents. The limited absorption through the gut barrier is typical for proanthocyanidins (i.e., their oligomeric forms). Experiments with their dimers resulted in the detection of large amounts of unmetabolized/unconjugated epicatechin monomers that were retained [14].

20.2.3
Overall Flavonoid Fate in Organisms

This section summarizes the overall absorption, distribution, and metabolic fate of ingested flavonoids discussed in detail in the previous Sections 20.2.1 and

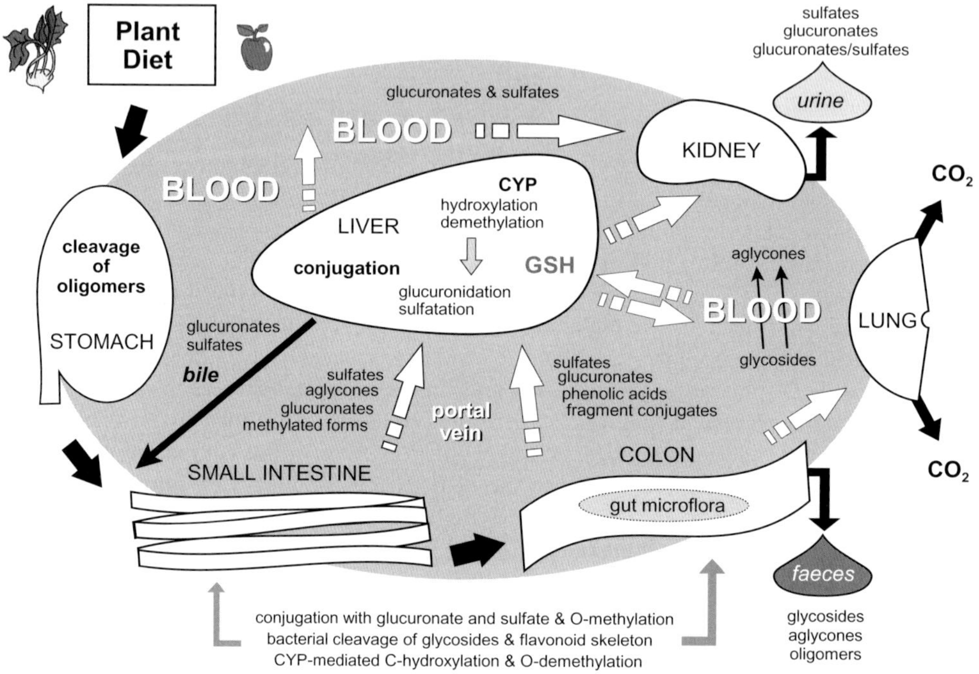

Figure 20.2 Overall flavonoid fate in an organism.

20.2.2. The general scheme showing the prevailing routes and pathways is presented in Figure 20.2. The key site of flavonoid metabolism/absorption is the small intestine. Ingested oligomeric flavonoids (proanthocyanidins) can be hydrolyzed in the acidic stomach juice prior to entering the small intestine. Flavonoid glycosides are then hydrolyzed by β-glucosidases to liberate free aglycones suitable for absorption. Most flavonoids that are taken up by enterocytes are metabolized before they reach the portal blood. They are partially resecreted into the intestinal lumen (e.g., MRP efflux). Flavonoids absorbed in the duodenum enter the circulation again as conjugates produced by a combination of methylation, sulfate conjugation, glucuronide conjugation plus glycine conjugation in the case of phenolic acids. Only a very small amount of flavonoids consumed (5 to 10%) enters the plasma as unchanged plant flavonoids (e.g., glucosides via transporter) [36]. Not yet absorbed flavonoids proceed to lower colonic parts and are metabolized by the gut microflora.

Further flavonoid metabolism takes place in the liver, where conjugates are possible cleaved (glycosidases), flavonoid hydroxyl groups may be methylated (COMT), and hydroxymethyl groups demethylated (CYPs) or the flavonoid skeleton *C*-hydroxylated. In the liver, an additional (mixed/multiple) conjugation with sulfate and glucuronate frequently occurs. However, deconjugation to free aglycone takes place rapidly, too. Thus, for example, the actual glucuronidation yield of flavonoids in the liver reflects the balance between the activity of UGT and β-glucuronidase, which is regularly shifted toward the conjugated forms. From the liver, the flavonoid metabolites are secreted into the bile (returning back to the small intestine) and transferred to plasma for the kidney-mediated excretion of flavonoid metabolites. In addition to enterohepatic cycling, liver uptake of circulating flavonoid metabolites is also possible. In the scheme, the cleavage of conjugates into aglycones by plasma glycosidases (e.g., β-glucuronidases) is also considered.

20.2.3.1 Plasma Levels and Pharmacokinetics of Flavonoids

It is rather difficult to carry out precise pharmacokinetic analyzes with flavonoids because neither ingested conjugates of these compounds nor their aglycones are detectable in plasma. Pharmacokinetic data are usually based on the concentrations of aglycones obtained after specific hydrolysis of conjugates in plasma or urine. However, not all the conjugates are equally sensitive to enzymic or chemical hydrolysis, which makes the results of analyses misleading to some extent. That is why this kind of methodology is referred to as "pseudo-pharmacokinetics."

Isoflavones are clearly the best-absorbed flavonoids – plasma concentrations of 1.4–4 μmol/l are reached in adults after intake of about 50 mg isoflavones [8]. Plasma concentrations up to 5 μmol/l are reported for citrus flavanones and soy isoflavones [8]. Proanthocyanidins may serve as an example of flavonoids that are hardly absorbed from the small intestine into circulation. However, hydroxylated flavan-3-ols with a galloyl moiety (e.g., epigallocatechin gallate and epigallocatechin) reach the blood mainly as the aglycon form (up to 80–90%) [29]. For an extensive overview of flavonoid plasma concentrations, please refer to review articles by Clifford [10] and Manach [35].

Although flavonoids may vary among their subclasses in their pharmacokinetics, it is possible to estimate T_{max} values for plasma concentrations of their metabolites. For flavonoids absorbed in the duodenum, T_{max} values range from 1 to 2.5 h, whereas for those that require metabolism by colonic microflora prior to absorption, T_{max} values increase up to 5–12 h. Consequently, elimination half-lives are highly variable (1–20 h) [10] and even up to 42 h has determined after an oral dose of [^{14}C]quercetin [21]. High values may be related to a biphasic elimination, including enterohepatic circulation of a significant portion of metabolites (e.g., glucuronides), followed by their deconjugation and further degradation by colonic microflora before they enter the circulation. The methylation appears to provide higher metabolic stability as well as higher membrane transport properties and thus may extend their half-lives. As methylated flavones are missing free hydroxyl groups, they cannot serve as acceptors for conjugating glucuronic and sulfate groups. They can be *O*-demethylated by CYPs and then conjugated [37]. It is generally accepted that most flavan-3-ols should be cleared from the body within 10–20 h. A few studies, however, reported appreciable plasma levels 24 h after flavonoid consumption [38].

20.3
Interactions of Flavonoids with Mammalian Proteins with Possible Implications for Drug Metabolism

Flavonoids belong to remarkable biologically active phytochemicals exerting various effects on living systems, including humans [39]. Although these compounds are well-known antioxidants *per se*, a much wider range of their activities is manifested through their interactions with proteins (i.e., receptors and enzymes) involved in cell regulation and metabolic pathways of endogenous and foreign compounds. For health concerns arising from these interactions, see Sections 20.4 and 20.5. Thus, flavonoids have to be viewed as foreign compounds (xenobiotics) with potential health beneficial as well as negative activities [40].

20.3.1
Plasma Proteins

Very little is known about the interactions of flavonoids with plasma proteins in general. Weak flavonoid binding has been reported, for example, for α_1-glycoprotein (quercetin); for fibronectin, fibrinogen, and histidine-rich glycoprotein (flavan-3-ols having a 3-*O*-galloyl moiety); and for apolipoprotein A1 of high-density lipoproteins (catechins) [41]. However, most of the data are available for the interaction of flavonoids with serum albumin – the principal carrier protein of many endogenous and exogenous compounds in blood plasma. This highly abundant protein (blood concentration of about 7.0×10^{-4} M) affects the pharmacokinetics of many drugs and, thus, for instance, flavonoid binding in a competitive manner increasing the concentration of free drug can be of a great significance. Fortunately, that is not the case when the common flavonoid quercetin is present in the binding cavity of human serum albumin (HSA). The binding site of HSA is large enough to accommodate additional ligands such as salicylate and warfarin [41]. In addition, the binding of endogenous compounds to HSA may affect the binding affinity of some flavonoids. This effect has been shown for oleate, which effectively binds HSA. In the presence of oleate, the affinity of daidzein, genistein, naringenin, and quercetin for the albumin decreased up to 2-fold (as judged from dissociation equilibrium constants) [42].

Since the binding of ligand with the serum albumin cavity is mainly driven by dispersion interactions (such as a hydrophobic effect), it is to be expected that lipophilic flavonoids (e.g., aglycones with low number of hydroxyl groups) circulate in blood as albumin complexes rather than in their free form. The influence of aglycone glycosylation, methylation, and sulfation on albumin binding has been assessed. Glucoside of quercetin (quercetin-3-*O*-β-D-glucoside) shows the binding affinity lowered by 3-fold compared to the parent compound. On the contrary, the glucuronyl moiety that is typical of most flavonoid conjugates does not change the binding to HSA, at least in the case of baicalin (5,6,7-trihydroxyflavone-7-*O*-β-D-glucuronide) when compared to baicalein (5,6,7-trihydroxyflavone). Similarly, methylation of 4′-OH of quercetin, resulting in tamarixetin, gave a high binding constant for HSA. In addition, a single sulfation of quercetin (quercetin-7-*O*-sulfate) does not affect HSA binding affinity, whereas an additional sulfation of 4′-OH markedly weakens the binding [41]. From these examples, it is clear that flavonoid–albumin complexation does not follow the simple logic of the lipophilicity rule, but a more complex mode of interactions is involved. Usually, site-specific conjugations of the flavonoid skeleton (e.g., with glucuronate) as well as the presence of free hydroxyl groups in certain positions are prerequisites for an effective HSA binding.

20.3.2 ATP-Binding Proteins

Flavonoids were shown to interfere with the function of several ATP-binding proteins, such as various ATPases, protein kinases, topoisomerase II, and MRPs. It is assumed that their inhibition is possibly caused by flavonoid binding to the ATP-binding site. Two major groups of ATP-binding proteins – MRPs and kinases – that are of the major interest from the viewpoint of pharmacology and drug metabolism are discussed in following sections.

20.3.2.1 MRPs

The phenomenon of so-called "multidrug resistance" is defined as the resistance of tumor cells against drugs used in cancer chemotherapy. One mechanism of multidrug resistance is via the active efflux of drugs through the cellular membrane, which is mediated by MRPs. This group of proteins contains the ATP-dependent xenobiotic transporters (ABC family), namely P-glycoprotein (P-gp/MDR1), MRPs (e.g., MRP1, MRP2), and breast cancer resistant protein (BCRP) [43].

The inhibitory mechanisms of flavonoids on P-gp function may involve ATPase activity inhibition and/or binding to the P-gp substrate site. For example, flavonoids such as morin inhibited P-gp substrate binding, while ATPase activity was inhibited by epigallocatechin-3-gallate [44]. Furthermore, some flavones and flavon-3-ols may act as dual inhibitors whose binding site overlaps both ATP- and xenobiotic-binding sites. Using multidrug-resistant human epidermal carcinoma cell line KB-C2 cells, which overexpress P-gp, and daunorubicin as P-gp substrate, the structure requirements for the inhibitory effects of flavonoids were suggested. For flavonoids missing large substituents, the planarity of the skeleton and the hydrophobicity are important for the interaction with P-gp. Nonplanar flavonoids, having large substituents like the galloyl group (e.g., tea catechins), require the presence of both a hydrophobic region and neighboring hydrophilic hydroxyl groups for the interaction with P-gp [45]. Contrary to the efflux inhibition, several flavonols, such as galangin, kaempferol, fisetin, and quercetin, were shown to be effective in increasing P-gp-mediated efflux of the drug doxorubicin from HCT-15 colon cells, while flavanols catechin and epicatechin did not exert any effect on the P-gp efflux [46]. Interestingly, catechins with a gallate moiety (epigallocatechin-3-gallate and epicatechin-3-gallate) are, in accordance with previous data, inhibitors of P-gp-mediated xenobiotic transport.

The MRP members (i.e., MRP1, MRP2, and MRP3) exhibit similar substrate specificity to P-gp and are also able to transport xenobiotic metabolites, including their glutathione, glucuronide, and sulfate conjugates. Thus, various flavonoids are substrates of MRPs. In the intestinal cell line Caco-2, quercetin, chrysin, epicatechin, epicatechin gallate, genistein as well as some of their glycosides and other conjugated metabolites are secreted via MRP2 [29]. Hence, efflux transporters limit the intestinal absorption of flavonoid glycosides and metabolites. However, flavon-3-ols substituted with a pyrogallol group in the B ring (e.g., myricetin, robinetin) were shown to inhibit MRP2 in MDCKII cells expressing this protein. In addition, the effect of quercetin conjugation after phase II metabolism on its capacity to inhibit MRP1 and MRP2 was investigated. While 4′-*O*-methylation of quercetin appeared to reduce the potential to inhibit both MRP1 and MRP2, glucuronidation, resulting in 7-*O*-glucuronosyl quercetin, significantly increased the potential of quercetin to affect MRPs – the inhibition of MRP1-mediated transport of the model drug, calcein, being more effective than that of MRP2 [47]. This particular finding for quercetin suggests that even flavonoid metabolites could enhance the inhibitory potential of the parent compound in order to overcome MRP-mediated multidrug resistance.

In addition to P-gp and MRPs, BCRP is responsible for multidrug resistance in some cancer cells. This transporter is also expressed in various normal human tissues and cells, where it transports physiologic substrates such as sulfated estrogens. Several flavonoids (e.g., genistein, naringenin) were demonstrated to diminish the function of BCRP as an efflux pump and thus reverse BCRP-mediated resistance to anticancer agents [48]. More recently, flavonoid compounds from various classes were screened for their BCRP-inhibitory activity [49]. Among 20 active compounds, 3′,4′,7-trimethoxyflavone showed the strongest anti-BCRP activity so far. In other studies with the tamoxifen-resistant MCF-7 cell line, cell treatment with epigallocatechin-3-gallate resulted in strong inhibition of BCRP efflux of the drug mitoxantrone and a significant downregulation of BCRP activity [50]. Thus, the green tea catechin – epigallocatechin-3-gallate – seemed to provide a double action on BCRP in this cell line. Although the accumulating evidence suggests flavonoids as promising multidrug resistance modulators, it is quite difficult to draw a more general picture of their role in this process as the majority of data was obtained with cancer cell lines overexpressing MRPs, which were exposed to unrealistically high flavonoid concentrations.

20.3.2.2 **Kinases**

Phosphotransferases (kinases) represent a large group of enzymes involved in phosphorylation of proteins (at Ser, Thr, and Tyr residues) or low-molecular-weight compounds such as lipids, carbohydrates, amino acids, and nucleotides. The phosphorylation of the target molecule usually triggers intracellular signal transduction important for various cellular functions as well as for metabolism regulation. Flavonoids are able to interact with various protein kinases, and thus interfere with cellular signaling pathways controlling, for example, the cell cycle, differentiation, apoptosis, angiogenesis, and metastasis. The majority of flavonoids share the same mechanism of action based on the competitive inhibition at the catalytic ATP-binding site of the kinase; however, some flavonoids have been found to bind to an allosteric site on protein kinases rather than the ATP pocket. For instance, the flavonoids luteolin, apigenin, and quercetin exhibited high affinity for the catalytic ATP domain of protein kinase C, or myricetin inhibited mitogen-activated protein kinase 4 directly by competing with ATP [51, 52]. Quercetin and, likely, delphinidin are examples of inhibitory flavonoids not binding the ATP site of the mitogen-activated protein kinase/extracellular signal-regulated kinase 1 (MEK1) and Fyn kinase, respectively [53, 54]. Actually, the most reviewed kinase inhibitor is epigallocatechin gallate. This versatile catechin was described as a specific inhibitor of numerous protein kinases, including MEK1/2, extracellular signal-regulated protein kinase 1/2, c-Jun N-terminal kinase, Akt kinase, dual-specificity tyrosine phosphorylation-regulated kinase 1A, and cyclin-dependent kinase 1 and 2 [55]. Via affecting kinase cascades, flavonoids can act as inhibitor of carcinogenesis, namely on the cell cycle and apoptosis levels (for review, see [55]). Contrary to inhibitory effects, several flavonoids, such as epigallocatechin gallate, quercetin, and resveratrol, have been shown to activate AMP-activated protein kinases – key regulators of the metabolic pathways [56]. By modulation of these kinases, flavonoids could help to prevent the development of numerous metabolic diseases (e.g., diabetes, obesity, cardiac hypertrophy, and even cancer).

20.3.3 Flavonoid-Binding Receptors

20.3.3.1 Estrogen Receptor

The estrogen receptor (ER) is a ligand-inducible nuclear transcription factor, which depending on ligand binding mediates activation or repression of the target genes. Two forms – ER-α and ER-β – were discovered to be expressed differently in various tissues. It was found that some flavonoids (i.e., present in soybeans and to a lesser extent in other legumes) bind this receptor like the endogenous steroidal ligand 17β-estradiol. These so-called phytoestrogens, belonging to the group of isoflanones, are structurally similar to 17β-estradiol and thus have estrogenic effects. The typical isoflavone phytoestrogens are daidzein and genistein, their naturally occurring glucosides, daidzin and genistin, and their methyl ether precursors, formononetin and biochanin A. These precursors are converted to daidzein and genistein by intestinal glucosidases. Intestinal bacteria further metabolize daidzein to isoflavan equol and nonflavonoid *O*-desmethylangolensin [57]. It is interesting to note that isoflavonoids, genistein, and daidzein preferentially bind ER-β, while endogenous estrogen ligand binds both ERs with similar affinities. The affinity of, for example, genistein for ER-α and ER-β is 0.7 and 13% of that for the endogenous ligand 17β-estradiol, respectively [58]. Equol has been found to be a much more potent ER-α agonist compared to either genistein or daidzein, while it acts similarly to daidzein on ER-β [59]. Although isoflavonoids exert only limited estrogenic potency (compared to steroids), their rather high levels in humans under certain dietary conditions could result in significant biological effects. Epidemiological studies suggest that the intake of isoflavone-rich soy foods is inversely correlated with the risk of prostate and breast cancers, and helps to overcome health problems associated with the menopause [57].

20.3.3.2 **GABA-A Receptor**

GABA-A receptors are transmembrane proteins regulating a chloride flux through their ion channel in response to binding γ-aminobutyric acid (GABA) – the major inhibitory neurotransmitter. In addition to the GABA-binding site, the receptor contains a number of different allosteric binding sites such as the benzodiazepine (BDZ)-binding site, where variety of neuroactive ligands, including flavones, bind and thus indirectly modulate the receptor activity [60]. Chrysin – 5,7-dihydroxyflavone from the folk medicine *Passiflora coerulea* – was the first flavonoid reported to be a competitive ligand for the BDZ site, with anxiolytic activities [61]. Similar activity was described also for apigenin – a component of *Matricicaria recutita* flowers [62]. A flavonoid purified from *Scutellaria baicalensis* Georgi – 5,7,2′-trihydroxy-6,8-dimethoxyflavone – manifested a high affinity for the BDZ site comparable to that of diazepam [63]. Studies using sets of neuroactive flavonoids revealed a number of structural moieties important for their binding to the BDZ site. For instance, 2′-hydroxyl substitution of the skeleton plays a critical role for BDZ site affinities for some flavonoids. Hydroxyl moieties at positions 5 and 7 had negligible effects on the affinity of flavone, whereas hydroxylation at positions 3, 3′, and 4′ resulted in reduced affinity [60]. In addition, the substitution at position 6 affects the BDZ site binding. Hispidulin (4′,5,7-trihydroxy-6-methoxyflavone) – the 6-methoxy derivative of apigenin – was 30 times more potent that apigenin in displacing flumazenil binding [64]. Accordingly, semisynthetic nitroflavones were prepared and their binding affinity compared. Two nitroderivatives – 6-methyl-3′-nitroflavone and 6-methyl-3′,5-dinitroflavone – were effective agonistics, binding the BDZ site with a potency comparable of flumazenil [65]. At anxiolytic doses, these compounds exert minimal sedative action.

20.3.3.3 **Aryl Hydrocarbon Receptor**

Flavonoids are well-known compounds that can upregulate gene expression and consequently levels of xenobiotic-metabolizing enzymes in the body. This is an adaptive mechanism enabling herbivores to metabolize xenobiotics administered in the diet in order to detoxicate and excrete them. Flavonoids induce xenobiotic-metabolizing enzymes via activation of a soluble ligand-dependent transcription factor – the aryl hydrocarbon receptor (AhR). After ligand (flavonoid) binding, the activated AhR in collaboration with associated proteins binds to a AhR-specific DNA recognition site – the xenobiotic-responsive element (XRE) – and finally activates the gene promoter. The most responsive genes are, for example, *CYP1A1*, *CYP1A2*, and *CYP1B1*, *GST*, *UGT*, and *NADPH quinone reductase* [66]. In numerous investigations, many flavonoids have been screened as agonists or antagonists of AhR. In fact, they may exhibit weak AhR agonist and/or partial antagonist activities.

Tests of AhR activation by flavonoids are mostly based on the use of aryl hydrocarbon-responsive cancer cells or cell lines containing a stably transfected *AhR-responsive luciferase reporter* gene. Results of these *in vitro* assays are significantly affected by the cell context and flavonoid concentrations used. In aryl hydrocarbon-responsive MCF-7 human breast cells, HepG2 human liver cancer cells, and mouse Hepa-1 cells, chrysin and baicalein (both at 10 μM) induced luciferase activity, while galangin, genistein, daidzein, apigenin, and diosmin were active only in stably transfected Hepa-1. However, kaempferol, quercetin, myricetin, and luteolin behaved as AhR antagonists depending on the cell lines used [67]. A more recent study confirmed these data; for example, apigenin (weak agonist) showed notable inhibitory effects on the *in vitro* activation of AhR induced by 2,3,7,8-tetrachlorodibenzo-*p*-dioxin (TCDD). Moreover, it has been suggested that glycosides, in general, show lower or no AhR responses than the corresponding aglycones [68].

Flavonoid–AhR interactions could be also examined indirectly in *in vivo* experiments by determination of the AhR-responsive gene products, such as transcribed mRNAs or expressed proteins. This approach, which provides more consistent results than *in vitro* assays with cells, is being used for the responsive gene products (e.g., the *CYP1 family*). In this respect, synthetic 5,6-benzoflavone, known as β-naphthoflavone (BNF), may serve as a prototype CYP1A1/2 inducer and, thus, AhR agonist [69]. In addition, several natural flavonoids have been proven to induce CYP1A1/2 [70]. In experiments where rats were treated with tested flavonoids by gavage, quercetin glycosides, rutin, isoquercitrin, and aglycone morin caused CYP1A1 induction in the small intestine, while flavone, rutin, and isoquercitrin, and partially quercetin, increased levels of CYP1A2 in the liver, but always to a less extent than BNF did [71, 72]. The possible drawback of this approach, which allows potential metabolic conversion of administered flavonoids, is the uncertainty as to what is the ultimate flavonoid form (derivative) that binds to AhR as its agonist.

Since AhR-responsive gene products are involved in the metabolism of drugs and in the processes of chemical carcinogenesis, interactions of flavonoids with AhR give rise to several important issues. By induction of xenobiotic-metabolizing enzymes, flavonoids might dramatically affect the plasma concentrations of pharmaceutical drugs, resulting in either overdose or loss of their therapeutic effect [70]. These potential drug–flavonoid interactions are discussed in Sections 20.4 and 20.5.

20.3.4
Redox Enzyme Activity Modulation

Flavonoid anticancer, antioxidant, and anti-inflammatory activities are at least in part associated with the direct inhibition of enzymes dealing with reactive oxygen species (ROS) in their catalytic cycle. The inhibition of CYPs, lipoxygenases (LOXs), cyclooxygenases (COXs), and xanthine oxidase (XO) are well documented examples of flavonoid interaction with redox enzymes. Inhibitory flavonoids may interfere with the formation of ROS and/or products of enzyme reactions, such as leukotrienes and prostaglandins (LOXs and COXs), and activated carcinogens (CYPs). However, redox enzymes can convert flavonoids into reactive pro-oxidant forms (e.g., the flavonoid semiquinone radical resulting from one-electron oxidation via peroxidase) [73].

20.3.4.1 **Xenobiotic-Metabolizing Enzymes**

Among enzymes involved in phase I metabolism of xenobiotics, CYPs play a key role, since they comprise 70–80% of all phase I enzymes. Although CYPs generally convert xenobiotics (e.g., drugs, carcinogens, food components, pollutants) to less-toxic products, the reactions frequently involve the formation of reactive intermediates or allow the leakage of free radicals capable of causing toxicity. Flavonoids interact with CYPs at least in three ways. (i) As mentioned in the Section 20.3.3, flavonoids are able to increase the xenobiotic-metabolizing capacity by inducing the expression of, for example, members of the CYP1 family via AhR activation. The induction of CYP2B1 in the liver and small intestine after administration of flavone (*per os* to rats) is an example of another induction mechanism than via AhR activation [71]. (ii) Flavonoids may undergo *O*-demethylation and/or *C*-hydroxylation catalyzed by CYPs to be conjugated by phase II enzymes (see Section 20.2.2). (iii) Flavonoids can modulate CYP activities as inhibitors by direct binding to CYP enzymes; for a comprehensive study on 33 flavonoids, see Shimada *et al.* [74].

Numerous mainly *in vitro* studies have been devoted to screening flavonoids for CYP inhibition ability in order to apply them as protective compounds against CYP-mediated carcinogen activation. Synthetic and naturally occurring flavonoids are effective inhibitors of five CYPs – xenobiotic-metabolizing CYP1A1, 1A2, 1B1, 2C9, and 3A4 – and one steroidogenic CYP19 (for reviews, see [40, 74–76]). Summarizing CYP1A1 and 1A2 inhibitory studies, the structure–function relationship of flavonoids can be explored. The CYP1A1 active site has a preference for binding 7-hydroxyl-substituted flavones. A prerequisite for binding to CYP1A2 is the presence of multiple hydroxyl groups (preferably two in positions 5 and 7) on the flavone skeleton and an additional hydroxyl substitution of C2 in the case of flavon-3-ols (e.g., morin). Planar molecules with a small volume : surface ratio turn out to possess high inhibitory activity of CYP1A2. That is why flavanones and flavanes (missing the C2–C3 double bond), having a phenyl group (B ring) nearly perpendicular to the rest of the molecule, showed a decreased inhibitory efficiency. Glycosylation as well as the presence of several hydroxyl groups and/or addition of methoxy groups results in a drastic decrease in their inhibitory activities. Based on the observation that catechins had no effect on CYP enzyme activity, the oxo group (position C4) in the C ring is also an essential factor for enzyme inhibition. The most potent CYP1A2 inhibitors are chrysin (5,7-dihydroxyflavone) and 3,5,7-trihydroxyflavone, followed by apigenin (5,7,4′-trihydroxyflavone) and morin (3,5,7,2′,4′-pentahydroxyflavone) [74, 77]. For CYP1B1, acacetin (5,7-dihydroxy-4′-methoxyflavone), in addition to galangin (3,5,7-trihydroxyflavone), seems to be the most selective and potent inhibitor with an IC_{50} that is more than 10 times lower than that of CYP1A1 and 1A2 [78]. Similarly, hesperetin (5,7,3′-trihydroxy-4′-methoxyflavone) is a selective inhibitor of expressed CYP1B1 in lymphoblastoid microsomes. Prenylated flavonoids from hops are highly effective inhibitors of CYP1 family enzymes. At 0.01 mM concentration, prenylated chalcone–xanthohumol–almost completely inhibited CYP1A1 and totally eliminated CYP1B1 activity [79]. The most effective inhibitors of CYP1A2 were 8-prenylnaringenin and isoxanthohumol. These findings are in agreement with the suggested similarities of the binding sites of CYP1A1 and 1B1 when compared to that of CYP1A2. CYP2C9 was more inhibited by 7-hydroxy-, 5,7-dihydroxy-, and 3,5,7-trihydroxyflavones than by flavone, but was weakly inhibited by 3- and 5-hydroxyflavone. Of 33 tested flavonoids, 3,5,7-trihydroxyflavone was the most potent inhibitor of CYP3A4 with an IC_{50} of 2.3 μM [74]. The described studies shed some light on our understanding of structural principles of flavonoid–CYP interactions [70, 74].

There is accumulating evidence that the metabolic activity of several CYPs (e.g., the CYP1A, CYP2C, and CYP3A families) is stimulated by inhibitors of other CYPs. While specific activities of CYP1A1 and CYP1B1 were inhibited by various flavonoids, certain metabolic activities of CYP1A2 and CYP3A4 were also stimulated by flavonoids–α-naphthoflavone and tangeretin, respectively [80, 81]. Several heterotropic cooperativity models are used to explain this stimulatory effect of flavonoids (i.e., in CYP3A4) [82]. Usually, the balance between the positive cooperativity and inhibition of these CYPs is a matter of a compound concentration. The effect of other quercetins on the mutagenicity of 2-amino-3,4-dimethylimidazo[4,5-*f*] quinoline (MeIQ) was tested in a system expressing human CYP1A2 and NADPH : CYP reductase. Mutagenicity of MeIQ was enhanced 50 and 42% by quercetin at 0.1 and 1 μM, respectively, but suppressed 82 and 96% at 50 and 100 μM, respectively [83]. Thus, the MeIQ-induced mutation is a concentration-dependent process showing both stimulation, at low concentrations, and inhibition of CYP1A2 activity, at high concentrations of the flavonoid used. This example of a dose-dependent manner of stimulation or inhibition of carcinogen activation emphasizes the need for chemopreventive compound testing even at low concentrations, which likely occur in the human body after compound (food) ingestion [40].

In addition to the phase I enzymes, flavonoids affect enzymes of phase II of xenobiotic biotransformation. For instance, flavanone and flavone, but not tangeretin and quercetin, induced UGT [84]. Moreover, tangeretin, chrysin, and flavanone were found to be the most potent inhibitors of UGT. Also the activities of other phase II enzymes, such as GSTs and SULTs, are induced and/or inhibited by flavonoids. For more detailed data, refer to the review by Moon *et al.* [75].

20.3.4.2 **LOXs, COXs, and XOs**

LOXs and COXs are involved in the biosynthesis of leukotrienes and prostaglandins from arachidonic acid. Mammalian LOX (15-LOX1) has been proposed as an enzyme oxidizing low-density lipoproteins at an early stage in atherosclerosis. The most potent inhibitors of LOX ($IC_{50} \sim 1$ mM) are luteolin, baicalein, and fisetin [41]. The mechanism of LOX inhibition is proposed to be a combination of direct inhibition (noncompetitively to fatty acid) and radical scavenging.

Flavonoids can interfere with COX-1 and COX-2 metabolic activities. For example, flavonoids such as apigenin, luteolin, kaempferol, and quercetin were shown to be inhibitors of COX-1, reducing the development of inflammatory responses [85]. Interestingly, apigenin and luteolin exert COX-2/5–LOX dual-inhibitory activity [86].

XO catalyzes simultaneous biosynthesis of uric acid from xanthine and the formation of superoxide/peroxide. Flavonoids can perform two roles – they act as enzyme inhibitors and/or as scavengers of ROS. The planarity of the C ring (flavones) is important for XO inhibition. Thus, catechins show significantly reduced interaction with XO. The presence of hydroxy groups in positions 5 and 7 on the flavone C ring (e.g., chrysin, galagin, apigenin, luteolin, kaempferol, quercetin, and myricetin) seems to be an important prerequisite for XO inhibition [87]. Morin (3,5,7,2′,4′-pentahydroxyflavone), having reduced inhibitory ability, suggests a role for the hydroxylation position on the flavone B ring. Moreover, flavonols with a hydroxylated B ring (e.g., quercetin, myricetin, fisetin) show in addition to XO inhibition also ROS-scavenging activity. Glycosylation of the flavonoids mostly abolishes XO inhibition (e.g., quercitrin (quercetin-3-*O*-rhamnoside) retained superoxide scavenging, but lost the inhibition of XO) [41].

20.4 Dietary Flavonoids – Health Issues

Flavonoids are generally accepted as health-promoting compounds present in a plant diet. Since these compounds are able to provide a wide variety of biological activities (i.e., as powerful antioxidants and anticancer agents), they are frequently called chemopreventive compounds. In addition to a regular intake from a plant diet, some flavonoids are used as food supplements and even drugs. These compounds, especially when administered in high doses (food supplements), are not necessarily beneficial for the organism. In Section 20.3, flavonoids were shown to target a large number of proteins involved in gene regulation or in metabolic pathways and cell signaling. Although the wide intake of flavonoids is psychologically acceptable due to their plant origin, potential threats resulting from, for example, drug interactions, effect on metabolism of endogenic compounds should be regarded. Unfortunately, much of the research in this area is focused on simplified *in vitro* systems, which cannot take into account the complexity of flavonoid interactions with living systems. Moreover, processes such as absorption and biotransformation are often ignored when "beneficial" flavonoid activities are declared.

20.4.1 Antioxidant and Pro-Oxidant Properties

Many of the beneficial activities of flavonoids have been attributed to their antioxidant properties. Flavonoids act as antioxidants *per se* or affect ROS status through more complex mechanisms (e.g., via modulation of redox enzymes and/or signaling pathways) (reviewed by Williams *et al.* [88]). Structurally features that define antioxidant activity are mainly the presence of 3′,4′-dihydroxy groups (catechol structure) in the B ring, and 2,3-unsaturation and a 4-oxo group in the C ring. In addition, some flavonoids are effective scavengers of reactive nitrogen species (peroxynitrite), chelators of transition metal ions (Fe-mediated ROS), and quenchers of singlet oxygen [89].

However, depending on the hydroxylation pattern, flavonoids can also act as pro-oxidants. Flavonoids promote the generation of hydroxyl radicals in the presence of metal ions (Fenton reaction). Moreover, the scavenging of ROS (antioxidant activity) leads to the oxidation of the flavonoid molecule and its conversion into a potential pro-oxidant. Flavones containing a 3′,4′-dihydroxy substituent in their B ring (e.g., quercetin) may undergo autoxidation and/or enzymatic oxidation (tyrosinase, peroxidase), resulting in the formation of semiquinone- and quinone-type metabolites. These quinones may covalently bind to cellular macromolecules (proteins, DNA) as well as provide the capability for efficient redox cycling, resulting in the production of ROS. The mutagenicity of quercetin is an example of a harmful effect ascribed to the formation of such alkylating quinone-type metabolites [73]. 3-Hydroxyflavone, apigenin (5,7,4′-trihydroxyflavone), and luteolin (5,7,3′,4′-tetrahydroxyflavone) were shown to be cytotoxic for human lung embryonic fibroblasts (TIG-1 cells) due to their intracellular ROS-generating ability [90]. Thus, it is obvious that even a single flavonoid can act as a pro-oxidant as well as antioxidant, depending on the experimental settings, especially flavonoid concentration, cell type, and/or culture conditions.

20.4.2 Antiviral, Antibacterial, and Antifungal Agents

Flavonoids have been found to be active against a wide range of animal (e.g., poliovirus, adenovirus, herpes simplex virus, HIV, rotavirus) and plant viruses (e.g., tobacco mosaic virus). Although the biological properties of the flavonoids are well studied, the mechanisms of action underlying their antiviral properties have not been fully elucidated. Current results suggest a combination of effects on both the virus and the host cell. For instance, isoflavones have been reported to affect virus binding, entry, replication, viral protein translation, and formation of certain virus envelope glycoprotein complexes. Isoflavones also affect a variety of host cell signaling processes, including induction of gene transcription factors and secretion of cytokines [91]. Furthermore, the flavonoid baicalein has been shown to be active against human cytomegalovirus. The flavonoid seems to interfere with virus infection through inhibiting its entry into cells and its replication [92]. Green tea constituents seem to be effective against HIV. Epigallocatechin-3-gallate caused the destruction of viral particles and inhibited viral attachment to cells, post-adsorption entry into cells, reverse transcription, and viral production [93]. In the most recent comparative study, the authors evaluated the *in vitro* antirotavirus activity of 60 flavonoids, of which 34 compounds showed at least moderate antiviral activity [94]. The analysis of structure–activity relationships indicates that the A ring substitution with a methoxyl group is important for flavonoid antirotavirus activity.

In line with the assumption that flavonoids are produced by plants as one of their defense mechanisms against microbial infections, flavonoids have been shown to exert potent antimicrobial activity in general, even to human pathogens. The efficacy of flavonoids against a variety of microorganisms can be attributed to their impact on the permeability of the cell wall, membrane integrity, and the porins in the outer membrane. Combinations of flavonoids were shown to act synergistically and more effectively against Gram-negative microorganisms [95]. Flavonoids having free hydroxyl groups in the A ring at C5 and C7 positions seem to be more active than others [96]. Thus, apigenin exhibited a potent activity (minimum inhibitory concentration (MIC) 3.9–15.6 μg/ml) against 20 strains of methicillin-resistant *Staphylococcus aureus*. Another common flavonoid containing a 5,7-dihydroxylated A ring – kaempferol – effectively inhibited strains of bacteria, such as *Salmonella typhi* and *Shigella dysenteriae* (Gram-negative) and *Bacillus subtilis* (Gram-positive), all with a MIC of 2.4–9.7 μg/ml, and moreover showed activity against *Candida glabrata* (MIC 2.4 μg/ml), but hardly any to *Candida albicans* [97]. Even flavone glycoside, 4′,5,7-trihydroxy-3′-*O*-β-D-glucuronic acid-6″-methylester – a compound named vitegnoside – was effective against other yeasts *Trichophyton mentagrophytes* and *Cryptococcus neoformans* (MICs both 6.25 μg/ml) in comparison to the standard antifungal drug fluconazole (MIC 2.0 μg/ml) [98]. Thus, flavonoids could be a promising and effective alternative to conventional antibiotics in the treatment of infections caused especially by antibiotic-resistant microorganisms.

20.4.3 Other Biological Activities of Flavonoids

Due to the frequent targeting of mammalian proteins (including enzymes), flavonoids are able to modulate various physiological and pathological processes in the body. As mentioned in Section 20.3.2, flavonoids through their interactions with ATP-binding proteins (e.g., kinases) can affect important processes proceeding in cells and tissues, such as cell differentiation, apoptosis, angiogenesis, and metastasis. In addition, because of binding to specific receptor macromolecules (e.g., ER and GABA receptors; see Section 20.3.3), flavonoids show estrogenic/antiestrogenic and anxiolytic activities, respectively.

In traditional herbal medicine, flavonoids are also known for their anti-inflammatory activity. Via inhibition of LOXs and COXs – enzymes that are involved in the biosynthesis of leukotrienes and prostaglandins (see Section 20.3.4) – flavonoids reduce the formation and release of proinflammatory cytokines and mediators. The mechanism of flavonoid anti-inflammatory activity is, however, much more complex. It includes, for example, blockage of histamine release, inhibition of phosphodiesterase and protein kinases, and activation of transcriptase. For a review dealing with several suggested mechanisms of flavonoid anti-inflammatory action, see [99]. At the cellular level flavonoids exert their anti-inflammatory property by inhibition of neutrophil degranulation, which is a direct way to diminish the release of arachidonic acid by neutrophils and other immune cells [99]. Citrus polymethoxy flavones were reported to suppress production of the cytokine–tumor necrosis factor-α–via inhibition of phosphodiesterase [100]. Moreover, epigallocatechin-3-gallate inhibits the expression of inducible nitric oxide synthase, producing another inflammatory agent–nitric oxide. Another target of flavonoid action is inhibition of kinases–the key regulatory enzymes in the initiation of inflammation and the immune response. For instance, myricetin has been shown to inhibit IκB kinase–the enzyme important for the activation of the nuclear transcription factor NF-κB, which elicit various biological responses through induction of target genes. Surprisingly, apigenin and kaempferol were almost devoid of any IκB kinase inhibitory effect [101].

A number of investigations have revealed that flavonoids exhibit antithrombotic activities and thus flavonoids are believed to provide protection against the development of cardiovascular disease [102]. The antithrombotic activity of flavonoids is likely elicited by their already-mentioned ability to inhibit the activity of COX and LOX pathways as well as to scavenge free radicals. Flavonoids present in red wine and purple grape juice were shown to exert antioxidant and antiplatelet properties. Both *in vitro* incubation platelets and human oral supplementation with purple grape juice decreased platelet aggregation and enhanced release of platelet-derived nitric oxide [103]. However, a recent overview evaluating the role of flavonoids in protection against cardiovascular disease (via antiplatelet effect) does not come up with as many promising conclusions as the results from early *in vitro* studies. Of 25 intervention studies, one consistent finding was that cocoa-related products containing flavonols have platelet-inhibiting effects when consumed in moderate amounts [104]. Owing to the inconsistency in the obtained results, it is not possible to conclude whether flavonoids from black tea, coffee, and alcoholic beverages have beneficial effects on platelet function when consumed in moderate amounts in the diet.

In addition, flavonoids make a major contribution to the flavor of fruits, in particular the bitterness of citrus fruits (grapefruit) [105]. For instance, citrus naringin (4′,5,7-trihydroxyflavanone-7-rhamnoglucoside), tangeretin, quercetin, and neohesperidin are very bitter. In red wine, catechins and epicatechins are responsible for its bitter taste. On the other side of the scale, hesperidin dihydrochalcone is intensely sweet. The most powerful sweetener was found to be 3′-carboxyhesperetin dihydrochalcone, which was shown to be about 3400 times sweeter than a 6% aqueous solution of sucrose [106].

20.4.4
Flavonoids as Nutraceuticals

In the previous sections, flavonoids were presented as remarkable biologically active compounds affecting directly or indirectly a large variety of processes in living systems. Many studies suggest positive correlations between the intake of flavonoid-containing food and the prevention of several human diseases. Epidemiological studies have shown that frequent consumption of, for example, a soy diet high in isoflavonoids (daidzein, genistein) is correlated with a low incidence for breast and prostate cancers as well as reduced menopausal symptoms, such as osteoporosis. Similarly, frequent drinking of green tea is suggested to be associated with a lowered risk of stomach cancer, most likely due to the protective effect of catechins [107]. As a result, plant-based food containing significant amounts of these versatile compounds is nowadays called "functional food." The term "nutraceuticals," which was coined from "nutrition" and "pharmaceuticals," is reserved for "functional food" used intentionally in order to provide medical or health benefits, including the prevention and/or treatment of a disease [108]. In addition, another closely related term – "dietary supplement" – is used as a term to describe a product (pill, capsule, tablet, or liquid form) that is intended to supplement the diet by increasing the total daily intake of one or a combination of dietary ingredients. Flavonoids definitely span all these categories. Moreover, some particular flavonoids are also used as constituents of drugs. For example, rutin (quercetin-3-rutinoside) strengthens the capillaries, decreases their permeability, and inhibits platelet aggregation. The semisynthetic flavonoid diosmin, frequently in combination with hesperidin, is a major component of a phlebotropic drug used in the treatment of venous disease (i.e., chronic venous insufficiency and hemorrhoidal disease) [109].

Based on *in vitro* and *ex vivo* experiments and epidemiological studies, flavonoids seem to be a "panacea;" however, data from clinical trials can hardly meet any of the described health-promoting activities of flavonoids [110]. There are at least two obvious reasons that may explain this discrepancy of *in vitro* and *in vivo* results. (i) *In vitro* studies are mostly carried out with unrealistic flavonoid concentrations, which cannot be reached under *in vivo* conditions because of the rather low bioavailability of flavonoids and metabolism that significantly reduce their plasma levels. In such experiments, concentrations of tested compounds are orders of magnitude greater than achievable in humans, which rarely exceed the nanomolar range. (ii) Intake of a single compound is rarely as effective as that compound in a complex dietary mixture in which multiple compounds and/or multiple interacting regulatory molecules underlie the biological effect. Apparently, additive and synergistic effects of flavonoids with each other and with other compounds are prerequisites of many of the observed beneficial effects assigned to "functional food." Hence, it is clear that reliable assessment of the alleged heath benefits resulting from human flavonoid intake has to be based on much more developed authentic models (i.e., considering realistic flavonoid dosage, long-term exposure, and flavonoid absorption and metabolism).

20.4.4.1 **Cytotoxic and Cytoprotective Effects**

Flavonoids are frequently referred to as chemopreventive (chemoprophylactic) compounds due to their ability to protect cells from damage caused by ROS and other reactive intermediates. As discussed in Section 20.4.1, flavonoids provide great antioxidant potential as both radical scavengers and metal cation chelators, or inhibitors of enzymes involved in ROS production. These mechanisms underlie the protective effect of flavonoids such as epicatechin and quercetin, which have been shown to reduce the neurotoxicity induced by oxidized low-density lipoprotein [111]. Moreover, flavonoids act as anticancer agents via blocking of enzymes (e.g., CYPs) at expression or activity levels, which activate carcinogens into DNA-modifying intermediates [112] (see Section 20.3.4). For instance, baicalein inhibits 7,12-dimethylbenz[*a*]anthracene–DNA adduct formation by modulating CYP1A1 activity at both expression and activity levels [113]. Flavonoids may also protect cells by other mechanisms; one of them is based on flavonoid interference with the process of apoptosis. These compounds can affect this process in mitochondria, which play pivotal roles in both the life and the death of the cell. Flavonoids specifically block mitochondria-dependent apoptotic pathways by reduction of cytochrome *c* directly or by preventing its oxidation and thus protect the cells [114].

However, it is necessary to note that flavonoids are also reported as cytotoxic compounds. In addition to their antioxidant properties, flavonoids at same time may act as pro-oxidants, especially at high doses. Flavonoids, such as quercetin, have been shown to be cytotoxic in many cell systems by mechanisms involving the production of oxygen radicals through an auto-oxidation process. Moreover, this quercetin paradox is even more pronounced when quercetin is scavenging free radicals that result in the formation of thiol-reactive quercetin quinones depleting, for example, GSH in the cells [115]. Similarly, cytotoxicity toward cultured normal human cells through increasing intracellular ROS levels was also reported for apigenin, luteolin, kaemphero, and 1- and 3-hydroxyflavone [90]. Although cytotoxic, flavonoids with this activity are invited to eradicate cancer cells. Flavonoids act in a similar way as known anticancer drugs do–binding and cleavage of DNA, and the generation of ROS in the presence of transition metal ions [116]. Thus, the pro-oxidant action of flavonoids rather than their antioxidant activity may be important for their anticancer and apoptosis-inducing properties. The ability of flavonoids to induce mitochondria-mediated apoptosis was: apigenin > quercetin > myricetin > kaempferol [114]. Flavonoids may also induce tumor cell apoptosis by inhibiting DNA topoisomerase II and p53 downregulation or by causing mitochondrial toxicity, which initiates mitochondrial apoptosis [117].

In conclusion, it is possible to summarize that the issue of chemoprevention versus cytotoxicity is rather complex, and the assessment of flavonoid activity is strongly dependent on the target cells under consideration. Thus, analogously to drugs, although the flavonoid cytotoxic effect is desired against cancer cells, it is adverse for normal cells and vice versa. This complexity can be illustrated by the example of genistein, which at high doses (50–100 μM) inhibits the growth of human breast cancer cells *in vitro*, whereas it induces proliferation at lower doses (0.01–10 μM), [118].

20.4.5
Flavonoid Interference with the Metabolism of Endo- and Xenobiotics

In addition to the already described flavonoid activities, these phytochemicals can modulate enzymes involved in the metabolism of endogenous and foreign compounds. Thus, administration of flavonoid-based dietary supplements and/or nutraceuticals has to be considered with caution since flavonoids have the potential to cause pathological or even life-threatening changes in an organism's physiology. Section 20.5 is devoted to the broad issue of flavonoid–drug interactions.

20.4.5.1 Flavonoid Impact on the Metabolism of Endogenous Compounds

Apparently, numerous beneficial/adverse effects of flavonoids are associated with their impact on the metabolism of physiological substrates. However, much more data are needed to ascribe the found effects to flavonoid intake.

In some particular cases, the role of flavonoids has been suggested. In addition to the already-mentioned inhibition of various enzymes (e.g., kinases, phosphodiesterases, LOXs, COXs, XOs, and DNA topoisomerase II) of physiological significance, flavonoids exert inhibitory activity on the biosynthesis of hormones. Some plant isoflavonoids – genistein and daidzein from soya – inhibit thyroperoxidase that catalyzes iodination and thyroid hormone biosynthesis. Moreover, in millet the hypothyroid effect is attributed to vitexin – a *C*-glycosyl flavone that inhibits *in vitro* thyroid peroxidase [119]. This flavonoid antithyroid effect seems to explain endemic goiter. It is also suggested that early maternal hypothyroxinemia may produce morphological brain changes leading to autism [120].

Another well-documented example of flavonoid interference with hormone synthesis is the antiestrogenic action of flavones and flavanones. The conversion of androgens (e.g., androstenedione, testosterone) to estrogens (e.g., estrone, estradiol) is catalyzed by CYP19 (aromatase) via aromatization of the A ring of androgens. The presence of a C4-oxo group in the flavonoid skeleton seems to be crucial for inhibition. Moreover, one to three hydroxyl groups in certain positions are a prerequisite for a high inhibitory potency. Hydroxylation at C7 or C8 of flavone increases significantly the aromatase inhibition activity, while the presence of a single hydroxyl group in positions C3, C5, or C6 drastically reduces the inhibitory effect. Thus, 7-hydroxyflavone, chrysin (5,7-dihydroxyflavone), and apigenin (5,7,4′-trihydroxyflavone) show IC_{50} values in the low micromolar range. Isoflavones, such as genistein and daidzein, which are known as ligands of ERs, are far less effective as aromatase inhibitors. The inhibition of aromatase causes complex changes, inducing a shift in the overall hormonal balance of the individual, resulting in various effects, such as infertility and retardation of cell proliferation [70]. However, these potential problems should be balanced against the chemopreventive (beneficial) roles of flavonoids.

20.4.5.2 Effect of Flavonoids on Carcinogen Activation

Increased consumption of flavonoids seems to be associated with decreased risk of various kinds of cancers. Beneficial effects of flavonoids in prevention and cancer therapy are often linked to their antioxidant activity, anti-inflammatory properties, activation of immune response against cancer cells, induction of apoptosis in premalignant or cancerous cells, suppression of growth and proliferation of various types of tumor cells via induction of cell cycle arrest, modulation of drug resistance, and antiangiogenic action [121]. Much less attention is paid to the role of flavonoids in the direct protection against carcinogen activation. The xenobiotic-metabolizing enzymes (e.g., CYPs) that are involved in carcinogen activation are discussed in detail in Section 20.3.4 in view of their interactions with flavonoids. Here, flavonoids are presented as compounds acting both beneficially and adversely in the process of carcinogen activation. The complexity and ambiguity of the effects of flavonoids on the carcinogenicity of chemicals will be shown first at the level of activity modulation of xenobiotic-metabolizing enzymes and then at the level of the induction of these enzyme.

Flavonoids and carcinogens are xenobiotics, whose metabolism proceeds usually via phase I and phase II of their biotransformation. Most carcinogens are initially metabolized by the CYP enzymes (phase I) to inactive metabolites as well as to chemically reactive metabolites that covalently bind to DNA and initiate a carcinogenic process. Considering the CYP monooxygenase system to be responsible for the activation of a particular carcinogen, the inhibition of these enzymes by flavonoids should block the initialization phase of carcinogenesis. Accordingly, flavones (apigenin) and flavonoles (myricetin, quercetin, and kaempferol) are shown to be potent inhibitors of CYP1A1-catalyzed epoxidation of 7,8-diol-benz[*a*]anthracene, forming the major benz[*a*]anthracene metabolite with carcinogenic properties [122]. This straightforward interpretation of the role of flavonoids in carcinogenesis inhibition, however, does not necessarily meet all the consequences of flavonoid interactions with the CYP monooxygenase system. Multiple CYPs are possibly involved in carcinogen metabolism, some of them responsible for carcinogen activation, others playing detoxification roles. Thus, the inhibition of the detoxification pathway allows the carcinogen to be preferentially metabolized via the activation pathway. Flavonoids, similarly to carcinogens, frequently undergo phase II metabolism mediated by conjugation enzymes (UGTs, SULTs). At this step of carcinogen metabolism, flavonoids may compete with chemically reactive metabolites for the conjugation reactions and cause the accumulation of mutagenic intermediates. Moreover, flavonoids such as α-naphthoflavone and tangeretin are able to stimulate CYP enzyme activity, and thus enhance carcinogen activation [80, 81]. A stimulatory effect of flavonoids was described also for the activity of NADPH : CYP reductase. α-Naphthoflavone increases the NADPH : CYP reductase-catalyzed activation of aristolochic acid I into intermediates covalently binding DNA [123]. On the contrary, hydroxylated flavonoids such as quercetin and morin exerted inhibitory effects, similar to α-lipoic acid that is a known NADPH : CYP reductase inhibitor [124].

In addition to the ability of flavonoids to modulate the activity of xenobiotic-metabolizing enzymes by their direct binding, these phytochemicals are inducers of phase I and phase II enzyme expression (see Section 20.3.3). Inducer effects on the carcinogenicity of a certain chemical will depend on the inducer impact on the ratio of carcinogen metabolism to inactive and active metabolites by these enzymes [125]. Paradoxically, the induction of CYP1A1/1A2 involved in the activation of the majority of carcinogens might be protective against the formation of DNA-modifying intermediates from other carcinogens. This protective mechanism was shown for activation of aflatoxin B1. Induction of rats with β-naphthoflavone, which stimulates the CYP1A1/1A2 hepatic metabolism of aflatoxin B1 to aflatoxin M1 (an inactivation pathway), inhibits the hepatocarcinogenic activity of aflatoxin B1 [126]. Enzymes of phase II biotransformation (conjugation enzymes) are generally considered to be protective because of the neutralization of reactive intermediates originating from phase I, but under specific conditions their induction is associated with carcinogen activation. That is the case for carcinogens that are present in amino acid pyrrolysates of high-temperature cooked meat. One of these carcinogenic heterocyclic amines – 2-amino-1-methyl-6-phenylimidazo[4,5-*b*]pyridine (PhIP) – is *N*-hydroxylated by CYP1A2 and consequently esterified by NAT or *N*-SULT, that results in the highly mutagenic nitrenium ion [127]. Since, for example, quercetin induces expression of NAT in human volunteers by 88.7%, this popular chemopreventive flavonoid may potentiate the formation of the ultimate carcinogen from PhIP [128].

When combining both concepts of flavonoid induction and inhibition of CYPs, the potential risk of carcinogenesis may evolve from sequential administration of a protective flavonoid and carcinogen. Ingestion of a protective flavonoid, such as rutin (quercetin-3-rutinoside) and isoquercitrin (quercetin-3-β-D-glucoside), causes *in vivo* induction of CYPs 1A1 and 1A2, and thus increases the carcinogen activation potential [72]. Then, within 48–76 h, the carcinogen is administered, but its activation is not inhibited by already excreted protective flavonoid; however, the activation is considerably enhanced.

Although there is a widely accepted assumption that flavonoids are solely active in anticancer actions, the above-mentioned examples show possible opposite activity leading to enhanced carcinogen activation.

20.5 Flavonoid–Drug Interactions

From 1989, when the first report of a grapefruit juice–drug interaction was published, there has been accumulating evidence documenting the significance of food–drug, herb–drug, and also flavonoid–drug interactions. The majority of studies are devoted to the evaluation of the inhibitory properties of various herbal medicines, but much less attention has been paid to certain chemicals that are behind the herb activities; for reviews, see, for example, papers by Ioannides [129] and Izzo and Ernst [130].

Drugs and flavonoids are handled in the organism as foreign compounds, thus similar or identical enzyme systems are involved in the metabolism of these compounds. This implies flavonoids are potential modulators of drug metabolism with all the anticipated impacts on drugs pharmacokinetics and consequent therapeutic effects. In fact, there are two basic possibilities for how the flavonoid may interfere with the drug therapeutic action. (i) The induction of drug-metabolizing enzymes and/or stimulation of their activity by flavonoids can result either in speeded up elimination from the body and loss of therapeutic action, or when the drug is administered as a prodrug, in raising the concentrations of therapeutically active drug. (ii) The flavonoid-mediated inhibition of drug-metabolizing enzymes may either obstruct drug excretion and cause drug accumulation in the body or prevent conversion of the prodrug into the active compound. In other words, flavonoid–drug interactions may result in loss of therapeutic action or drug overdosing, which both are possibly life threatening. Moreover, due to the interactions of flavonoids with proteins and enzymes involved in various signaling pathways, flavonoids may affect the fate of the drug in an organism in a very specific way, which is hardly predictable. In the special case of xenobiotic transporters (MRP, P-gp), by blocking the efflux of antitumor drug, flavonoids can increase the efficiency of chemotherapy. Quite surprisingly, the inhibition of these transporters by flavonoids (e.g., chrysin) did not lead to drug-mediated apoptosis of cancer cells. The tested flavonoid was suggested to increase cancer cell survival by enhanced expression of xenobiotic transporters in cancer cells [131]. Moreover, the flavonoid effect on the signaling pathway associated with the process of apoptosis is also considered.

Although it is virtually impossible to map and predict all food-based flavonoid–drug interactions, this phenomenon has received increasing attention and some of the most pronounced interactions have already been described. In Section 20.3.4, some flavonoids were shown as CYP inducers/inhibitors/stimulators and the basic structure–function relationships were defined. Since CYP3A4 is a predominant human CYP enzyme and is responsible for the metabolism of a large number of therapeutic agents, the interaction of flavonoids with this xenobiotic-metabolizing enzyme is of high importance with the respect to flavonoid–drug interactions. Selected examples will be presented in this section to illustrate the extent of possible flavonoid–drug (food–drug) interactions.

In herb extracts from medicinal herbs, such as milk thistle (*Silybum marianum*) and St John's Wort (*Hypericum perforatum*), in addition to other active compounds, CYP3A4 inhibitors silymarin (mixture of flavonolignans) and I3,II8-biapigenin, respectively, were found. The biflavonoid I3,II8-biapigenin was shown to be a potent, competitive inhibitor of CYP3A4, 2C9, and 1A2 activities with K_i values of 0.038, 0.32, and 0.95 μM, respectively [132]. Silymarin, in addition to efficient inhibition of CYP3A4, 2C19, and 2D6, proved to be a strong inhibitor of UGT in cell cultures [133, 134]. The citrus flavonoid naringenin (5,7,4′-trihydroxyflavanone), which is present in grapefruit juice, also exerts an inhibitory effect on CYP3A4 in some experimental models [135]. Interestingly, an *in vivo* study with a furanocoumarin-free and a regular grapefruit juice does not establish flavonoids, but furanocoumarins (e.g., bergamottin, dihydroxybergamottin), as the mediators of the grapefruit juice–drug interactions enhancing the systemic exposure of the drug felodipine [136]. Another citrus flavonoid – tangeretin – completely blocked the therapeutic inhibitory effect of tamoxifen on mammary cancer in mice [137]. However, simultaneous administration of tamoxifen and genistein showed a synergistic effect on the inhibition of the growth of ER-negative breast cancer cells [138].

Only a limited number of studies have been undertaken to examine the effect of common flavonoids, present in the human diet, on the expression of CYPs or conjugation enzymes and on the consequent flavonoid–drug interactions. For instance, ethinylestradiol (EE), which is one of the major components of oral contraceptives, is mainly metabolized by flavonoid-inducible hepatic CYP3A4 and intestinal CYP1A1 [139]. Therefore, increased EE elimination (even attenuated pharmacological effects of EE) similar to omeprazole users and smokers should be expected after ingestion of high flavonoid food or food supplements (for CYP induction, refer to Section 20.3.4). The opposite effect (i.e., EE retention) may occur after ingestion of quercetin, which is an efficient inhibitor of human cytosolic SULT1E1 – the enzyme that is involved in EE sulfation at clinically relevant concentrations [140]. Moreover, SULT1E1 does not seem to be inducible by flavonoids such as β-naphthoflavone, contrary to other SULTs (e.g., SULT1A3) [141]. In general, the inhibition of SULT1E1 by quercetin, resulting in elevated estrogen hormone levels in tissues, may be a potentially harmful effect in relation to cancer development. Flavonoid–drug interactions may result also in some cases in health-promoting outcomes. This is documented, for example, by interaction of baicalein and acetaminophen. Baicalein significantly decreased acetaminophen-induced hepatotoxicity associated with the formation of the acetaminophen metabolite, *N*-acetyl-*p*-benzoquinoneimine. This hepatoprotective effect of baicalein against acetaminophen overdose may be due to its ability to block the bioactivation of acetaminophen by inhibiting CYP2E1 expression [142].

Apart from the enzymes of drug biotransformation, transporters of xenobiotics are also potential targets of flavonoid–drug interactions. The stimulation of activity of xenobiotic transporters (MRP, P-gp), involved in the efflux of antitumor drugs, by flavonoids can significantly reduce the efficiency of the cancer chemotherapy. Conversely, quercetin, genistein, naringenin, and xanthohumol reduced the efflux of cimetidine – a P-gp substrate – in both Caco-2 and LLC-PK1 cells [143]. That is an example of a flavonoid–drug interaction resulting in a desired increase of cellular uptake of the drug that is caused by flavonoid inhibition of P-gp-mediated drug efflux. Likewise, flavone may increase the effectiveness of some other antineoplastic agents such as paclitaxel. Coadministration of paclitaxel with flavone in rats significantly increased the peak plasma level of paclitaxel and its half-life in comparison to control animals. It is suggested that the bioavailability of paclitaxel coadministered with flavone was enhanced by both the inhibition of the P-gp efflux pump and CYPs in the intestinal mucosa [144]. Lethal consequences of flavonoid–drug interactions have been reported for pigs coadministered with digoxin and quercetin, which both interact with P-gp as a substrate and modulator, respectively. The simultaneous administration of this cardiac drug (at nontoxic dose) and quercetin via gavage increased significantly the bioavailability of the drug and elevated (4-fold) its plasma peak compared to controls, which resulted in sudden death of two of three animals [145]. Similar severe interactions should be considered for other drugs with a very narrow therapeutic range.

The opposite view of flavonoid–drug interactions is represented by the study examining the effect of antibiotics on the absorption and metabolism of baicalin in the gastrointestinal tract [146]. Coadministration of aminoglycoside antibiotics with baicalin resulted in dramatically decreased levels of baicalin derivatives in plasma, most likely because of the antibiotic bactericidal effect on intestinal bacteria mediating baicalin hydrolysis, which is the rate-limiting step for its absorption.

These selected examples highlight the wide range of possible ways flavonoids impact on the pharmacokinetics of commonly used drugs, from the direct competition of flavonoid and drug for a certain protein (enzyme or receptor) to indirect flavonoid–drug interactions represented by, for example, flavonoid induction of the drug-metabolizing enzyme. Most of the effects shown, however, require flavonoid concentrations at micromolar concentrations, which are not regularly achieved with a common intake of a plant-based diet. Thus, extrapolating *in vitro* findings to conditions *in vivo* should be done with caution. Although flavonoids seem to be less active in drug interactions than other well-known phytochemicals interfering with drug bioavailability (e.g., furocoumarins, hyperforin), their simultaneous ingestion with prescribed drugs should be considered as potentially deleterious since knowledge of flavonoid–drug interactions altering drug pharmacokinetics is very incomplete at present. This is especially true for food supplements containing concentrated flavonoids.

20.6
Conclusion – Double-Edged Sword Properties of Flavonoids

Flavonoids are plant xenobiotics known mostly for their antioxidant properties. Moreover, they may exert a huge array of biological activities via binding to proteins (receptors, enzymes, transporters) of living systems. Epidemiologic studies show plant-based food containing flavonoids to be health promoting. As a result, a flavonoid-rich diet is advised as nutraceuticals to prevent and/or cure numerous "civilization diseases." Likewise, concentrated herb extracts and certain flavonoids are marketed as food supplements. However, the majority of data proving the beneficial activities of flavonoids are based on *in vitro* studies with unrealistically high doses, disregarding flavonoid absorption, distribution, and metabolism in the body. In *in vivo* systems exposed to a regular plant diet, the beneficial effects of flavonoids are hardly seen, mainly because of their rather low bioavailability. In addition, concentrations of ingested flavonoids are reduced by their metabolism mediated by xenobiotic-metabolizing enzymes and colon microflora, and followed by excretion of metabolites from the body. Similarly, clinical trials with flavonoids applied at physiological doses during short-term regimen do not meet the expectations extrapolated from *in vitro* investigations. Owing to the metabolism of flavonoids, it is entirely misleading to attribute the potential health-promoting effect(s) to certain compound(s) found in the plant diet. If any beneficial activities of flavonoids are implied from epidemiologic studies, one has to keep in mind that the desired effects are not most likely caused by a sole dietary flavonoid, but by the complex mixture of various phytochemicals acting additively and/or synergistically.

Although consumption of a plant-rich diet and flavonoid nutraceuticals seems to be, with a few exemptions (e.g., soya milk), safe, the administration of herb extracts and flavonoid-based food supplements may even cause life-threatening effects. It is worth noting that flavonoids, in addition to their popular health beneficial activities, are potentially detrimental. For instance, they are both cytoprotective and cytotoxic, antioxidant and pro-oxidant, anticarcinogenic and cocarcinogenic or mutagenic, and antiestrogenic and estrogenic. These equivocal properties strongly depend on the manner in which the flavonoid compound is applied (i.e., on the dose, route of administration, duration of exposure, subject medication, exposure to other xenobiotics or carcinogens) as well as on the particular compound used and cells or tissues effected. Moreover, genetic polymorphisms, especially of xenobiotic-metabolizing enzymes, may also play an important role in the final effect of flavonoids. The major issues to consider in this respect are flavonoid–drug interactions, which can cause unpredictable changes in drug pharmacokinetics, possibly resulting in a severe impact on human health. This concern is of a special importance regarding the risk–benefit assessment of flavonoids intended for prolonged prophylactic human use. Bearing in mind that flavonoids are clearly not a "panacea" given to mankind, but are regular xenobiotics, it is necessary to evaluate carefully the double-edged sword properties of these compounds.

References

1 Pietta, P.G. (2000) Flavonoids as antioxidants. *J. Nat. Prod.*, **63**, 1035–1042.

2 Andersen, Ø.M. and Markham, K.R. (2006) *Flavonoids: Chemistry, Biochemistry and Applications*, CRC Press, Boca Raton, FL.

3 Rice-Evans, C.A., Miller, N.J., and Paganga, G. (1996) Structure–antioxidant activity relationships of flavonoids and phenolic acids. *Free Radic. Biol. Med.*, **20**, 933–956.

4 Bohm, B.A. (1998) Flavonoid functions in nature, in *Introduction to Flavonoids* (ed. B.A. Bohm), Harwood, Amsterdam, pp. 339–365.

5 Treutter, D. (2006) Significance of flavonoids in plant resistance: a review. *Environ. Chem. Lett.*, **4**, 147–157.

6 Packer, L. and Sies, H., eds (2001) Flavonoids and other polyphenols, in *Methods in Enzymology 335*, Academic Press, New York.

7 Stafford, H.A. (1990) *Flavonoid Metabolism*, CRC Press, Boca Raton, FL.

8 Manach, C., Scalbert, A., Morand, C., Remesy, C., and Jimenez, L. (2004) Polyphenols: food sources and bioavailability. *Am. J. Clin. Nutr.*, **79**, 727–747.

9 Kuhnau, J. (1976) The flavonoids. A class of semi-essential food components: their role in human nutrition. *World Rev. Nutr. Diet.*, **24**, 117–191.

10 Clifford, M.N. (2004) Diet-derived phenols in plasma and tissues and their implications for health. *Planta Med.*, **70**, 1103–1114.

11 Heinonen, M. (2001) Anthocyanins as dietary antioxidants, *Proceedings of the Third International Conference on Natural Antioxidants and Anticarcinogens in Food, Health, and Disease, Helsinki.*

12 Sampson, L., Rimm, E., Hollman, P.C., de Vries, J.H., and Katan, M.B. (2002) Flavonol and flavone intakes in US health professionals. *J. Am. Diet. Assoc.*, **102**, 1414–1420.

13 Kimira, M., Arai, Y., Shimoi, K., and Watanabe, S. (1998) Japanese intake of flavonoids and isoflavonoids from foods. *J. Epidemiol.*, **8**, 168–175.

14 Spencer, J.P.E., Rice-Evans, C.A., and Singh Srai, S.K. (2003) Metabolism in the small intestine and gastrointestinal

tract, in *Flavonoids in Health and Disease* (eds L. Packer and C.A. Rice-Evans), Dekker, New York, pp. 363–391.

15 Erlund, I., Kosonen, T., Alfthan, G., Maaenpaa, J., Perttunen, K., Kenraali, J., Parantainen, J., and Aro, A. (2000) Pharmacokinetics of quercetin from quercetin aglycone and rutin in healthy volunteers. *Eur. J. Clin. Pharmacol.*, **56**, 545–553.

16 Xing, J., Chen, X., and Zhong, D. (2005) Absorption and enterohepatic circulation of baicalin in rats. *Life Sci.*, **78**, 140–146.

17 Walle, T., Otake, Y., Brubaker, J.A., Walle, U.K., and Halushka, P.V. (2001) Disposition and metabolism of the flavonoid chrysin in normal volunteers. *Br. J. Clin. Pharmacol.*, **51**, 143–146.

18 Scalbert, A. and Williamson, G. (2000) Dietary intake and bioavailability of polyphenols. *J. Nutr.*, **130**, 2073S–2085S.

19 Vaidyanathan, J.B. and Walle, T. (2003) Cellular uptake and efflux of the tea flavonoid (–)-epicatechin-3-gallate in the human intestinal cell line Caco-2. *J. Pharmacol. Exp. Ther.*, **307**, 745–752.

20 Walle, T. (2004) Absorption and metabolism of flavonoids. *Free Radic. Biol. Med.*, **36**, 829–837.

21 Walle, T., Walle, U.K., and Halushka, P.V. (2001) Carbon dioxide is the major metabolite of quercetin in humans. *J. Nutr.*, **131**, 2648–2652.

22 Hollman, P.C., Bijsman, M.N., van Gameren, Y., Cnossen, E.P., de Vries, J.H., and Katan, M.B. (1999) The sugar moiety is a major determinant of the absorption of dietary flavonoid glycosides in man. *Free Radic. Res.*, **31**, 569–573.

23 Day, A.J., Canada, F.J., Diaz, J.C., Kroon, P.A., Mclauchlan, R., Faulds, C.B., Plumb, G.W., Morgan, M.R., and Williamson, G. (2000) Dietary flavonoid and isoflavone glycosides are hydrolysed by the lactase site of lactase phlorizin hydrolase. *FEBS Lett.*, **468**, 166–170.

24 Cheng, Z., Radominska-Pandya, A., and Tephly, T.R. (1999) Studies on the substrate specificity of human intestinal UDP-lucuronosyltransferases 1A8 and 1A10. *Drug Metab. Dispos.*, **27**, 1165–1170.

25 Paine, M.F., Hart, H.L., Ludington, S.S., Haining, R.L., Rettie, A.E., and Zeldin, D.C. (2006) The human intestinal cytochrome P450 "pie". *Drug Metab. Dispos.*, **34**, 880–886.

26 Setchell, K.D. and Clerici, C. (2010) Equol: history, chemistry, and formation. *J. Nutr.*, **140**, 1355S–1362S.

27 Prior, R.L., Wu, X., and Gu, L. (2006) Flavonoid metabolism and challenges to understanding mechanisms of health effects. *J. Sci. Food Agric.*, **86**, 2487–2491.

28 Nielsen, S.E., Breinholt, V.M., Justesen, U., Cornett, C., and Dragsted, L.O. (1998) *In vitro* biotransformation of flavonoids by rat liver microsomes. *Xenobiotica*, **28**, 389–401.

29 Cermak, R. and Wolffram, S. (2006) The potential of flavonoids to influence drug metabolism and pharmacokinetics by local gastrointestinal mechanisms. *Curr. Drug Metab.*, **7**, 729–744.

30 Nielsen, S.E., Breinholt, V.M., Cornett, C., and Dragsted, L.O. (2000) Biotransformation of the citrus flavone tangeretin in rats. Identification of metabolites with intact flavane nucleus. *Food Chem. Toxicol*, **38**, 739–746.

31 Sfakianos, J., Coward, L., Kirk, M., and Barnes, S. (1997) Intestinal uptake and biliary excretion of the isoflavone genistein in rats. *J. Nutr.*, **127**, 1260–1268.

32 Kohri, T., Nanjo, F., Suzuki, M., Nanjo, F., Hara, Y., and Oku, N. (2001) Synthesis of (–)-[4-^{3}H]epigallocatechin gallate and its metabolic fate in rats after intravenous administration. *J. Agric. Food Chem.*, **49**, 1042–1048.

33 Clarke, D.B., Lloyd, A.S., Botting, N.P., Oldfield, M.F., Needs, P.W., and Wiseman, H. (2002) Measurement of intact sulfate and glucuronide phytoestrogen conjugates in human urine using isotope dilution liquid chromatography–tandem mass spectrometry with [^{13}C3]isoflavone internal standards. *Anal. Biochem.*, **309**, 158–172.

34 Chow, H.-H.S., Cai, Y., Albert, D.S., Hakim, I., Dorr, R., Shahi, F., Crowell, J., Yang, C., and Hara, Y. (2001) Phase I pharmacokinetic study of tea

polyphenols following single-dose administration of epigallocatechin gallate and polyphenon E. *Cancer Epidemiol. Biomark. Prev.*, **10**, 53–58.
35 Manach, C., Williamson, G., Morand, C., Scalbert, A., and Remesy, C. (2005) Bioavailability and bioefficacy of polyphenols in humans. I. Review of 97 bioavailability studies. *Am. J. Clin. Nutr.*, **81**, 230S–242S.
36 Clifford, M. and Brown, J.E. (2006) Dietary flavonoids and health – broadening the perspective, in *Flavonoids: Chemistry, Biochemistry and Applications* (eds Ø.M. Andersen and K.R. Markham), CRC Press, Boca Raton, FL, pp. 320–344.
37 Walle, T. (2009) Methylation of dietary flavones increases their metabolic stability and chemopreventive effects. *Int. J. Mol. Sci.*, **10**, 5002–5019.
38 Donovan, J.L. and Waterhouse, A.L. (2003) Bioavailability of flavanol monomers, in *Flavonoids in Health and Disease* (eds L. Packer and C.A. Rice-Evans), Dekker, New York, pp. 413–441.
39 Han, X., Shen, T., and Lou, H. (2007) Dietary polyphenols and their biological significance. *Int. J. Mol. Sci.*, **8**, 950–988.
40 Hodek, P., Krizkova, J., Burdova, K., Sulc, M., Kizek, R., Hudecek, J., and Stiborova, M. (2009) Chemopreventive compounds – view from the other side. *Chem. Biol. Interact.*, **180**, 1–9.
41 Dangles, O. and Dufour, C. (2006) Flavonoid–protein interactions, in *Flavonoids: Chemistry, Biochemistry and Applications* (eds Ø.M. Andersen and K.R. Markham), CRC Press, Boca Raton, FL, pp. 443–464.
42 Bolli, A., Marino, M., Rimbach, G., Fanali, G., Fasano, M., and Ascenzi, P. (2010) Flavonoid binding to human serum albumin. *Biochem. Biophys. Res. Commun.*, **398**, 444–449.
43 Perez-Tomas, R. (2006) Multidrug resistance: retrospect and prospects in anti-cancer drug treatment. *Curr. Med. Chem.*, **13**, 1859–1876.
44 Zhang, S. and Morris, M.E. (2003) Effects of the flavonoids biochanin A, morin, phloretin, and silymarin on P-glycoprotein-mediated transport. *J. Pharmacol. Exp. Ther.*, **304**, 1258–1267.
45 Kitagawa, S. (2006) Inhibitory effects of polyphenols on P-glycoprotein-mediated transport. *Biol. Pharm. Bull.*, **29**, 1–6.
46 Critchfield, J.W., Welsh, C.J., Phang, J.M., and Yeh, G.C. (1994) Modulation of adriamycin accumulation and efflux by flavonoids in HCT-15 colon cells. Activation of P-glycoprotein as a putative mechanism. *Biochem. Pharmacol.*, **48**, 1437–1445.
47 van Zanden, J.J., van der Woude, H., Vaessen, J., Usta, M., Wortelboer, H.M., Cnubben, N.H., and Rietjens, I.M. (2007) The effect of quercetin phase II metabolism on its MRP1 and MRP2 inhibiting potential. *Biochem. Pharmacol.*, **74**, 345–351.
48 Imai, Y., Tsukahara, S., Asada, S., and Sugimoto, Y. (2004) Phytoestrogen/flavonoids reverse breast cancer resistance protein/ABCG2-mediated multidrug resistance. *Cancer Res.*, **64**, 4346–4352.
49 Katayama, K., Masuyama, K., Yoshioka, S., Hasegawa, H., Mitsuhashi, J., and Sugimoto, Y. (2007) Flavonoids inhibit breast cancer resistance protein-mediated drug resistance: transporter specificity and structure–activity relationship. *Cancer Chemother. Pharmacol.*, **60**, 789–797.
50 Farabegoli, F., Papi, A., Bartolini, G., Ostan, R., and Orlandi, M. (2010) (–)-Epigallocatechin-3-gallate downregulates Pg-P and BCRP in a tamoxifen resistant MCF-7 cell line. *Phytomedicine*, **17**, 356–362.
51 Singh, S., Malik, B.K., and Sharma, D.K. (2007) Protein kinase C in prostate cancer and herbal products: a bioinformatics approach. *Int. J. Integrat. Biol.*, **1**, 72–87.
52 Kim, J.E., Kwon, J.Y., Lee, D.E., Kang, N.J., Heo, Y.S., Lee, K.W., and Lee, H.J. (2009) MKK4 is a novel target for the inhibition of tumor necrosis factor-α-induced vascular endothelial growth factor expression by myricetin. *Biochem. Pharmacol.*, **77**, 412–421.
53 Lee, K.W., Kang, N.J., Heo, Y.S., Rogozin, E.A., Pugiliese, A., Hwang, M.K., Bowden, G.T., Bode, A.M., Lee,

H.J., and Dong, Z. (2008) Raf and MEK protein kinases are direct molecular targets for the chemopreventive effect of quercetin, a major flavonol in red wine. *Cancer Res.*, **68**, 946–955.

54 Hwang, M.K., Kang, N.J., Heo, Y.S., Lee, K.W., and Lee, H.J. (2009) Fyn kinase is a direct molecular target of delphinidin for the inhibition of cyclooxygenase-2 expression induced by tumor necrosis factoralpha. *Biochem. Pharmacol.*, **77**, 1213–1222.

55 Lamoral-Theys, D., Pottier, L., Dufrasne, F., Neve, J., Dubois, J., Kornienko, A., Kiss, R., and Ingrassia, L. (2010) Natural polyphenols that display anticancer properties through inhibition of kinase activity. *Curr. Med. Chem.*, **17**, 812–825.

56 Hwang, J.T., Kwon, D.Y., and Yoon, S.H. (2009) AMP-activated protein kinase: a potential target for the diseases prevention by natural occurring polyphenols. *N. Biotechnol.*, **26**, 17–22.

57 Wiseman, H. (2006) Isoflavonoids and human, in *Flavonoids: Chemistry, Biochemistry and Applications* (eds Ø.M. Andersen and K.R. Markham), CRC Press, Boca Raton, FL, pp. 371–388.

58 Kuiper, G.G., Lemmen, J.G., Carlsson, B., Corton, J.C., Safe, S.H., van der Saag, P.T., van der Burg, B., and Gustafsson, J.A. (1998) Interaction of estrogenic chemicals and phytoestrogens with estrogen receptor β. *Endocrinology*, **139**, 4252–4263.

59 Ricketts, M.L., Moore, D.D., Banz, W.J., Mezei, O., and Shay, N.F. (2005) Molecular mechanisms of action of the soy isoflavones includes activation of promiscuous nuclear receptors. A review. *J. Nutr. Biochem.*, **16**, 321–330.

60 Wang, F., Shing, M., Huen, Y., Tsang, S.Y., and Xue, H. (2005) Neuroactive flavonoids interacting with GABAA receptor complex. *Curr. Drug Targets CNS Neurol. Disord.*, **4**, 575–585.

61 Wolfman, C., Viola, H., Paladini, A.C., Dajas, D., and Medina, J.H. (1994) Possible anxiolytic effects of chrysin, a central benzodiazepine receptor ligand isolated from *Passiflora coerulea*. *Pharmacol. Biochem. Behav.*, **47**, 1–4.

62 Viola, H., Wasowski, C., Levi de Stein, M., Wolfman, C., Silveira, R., Dajas, F., Medina, J.H., and Paladini, A.C. (1995) Apigenin, a component of *Matricaria recutita* flowers, is a central benzodiazepine receptors-ligand with anxiolytic effects. *Plant Med.*, **61**, 213–216.

63 Huen, M.S., Hui, K.M., Leung, J.W., Sigel, E., Baur, R., Wong, J.T., and Xue, H. (2003) Naturally occurring 2′-hydroxyl-substituted flavonoids as high-affinity benzodiazepine site ligands. *Biochem. Pharmacol.*, **66**, 2397–2407.

64 Johnston, G.A. (2005) GABA(A) receptor channel pharmacology. *Curr. Pharm. Des.*, **11**, 1867–1885.

65 Dekermendjian, K., Kahnberg, P., Witt, M.R., Sterner, O., Nielsen, M., and Liljefors, T. (1999) Structure–activity relationships and molecular modeling analysis of flavonoids binding to the benzodiazepine site of the rat brain GABA(A) receptor complex. *J. Med. Chem.*, **42**, 4343–4350.

66 Denison, M.S., Phelan, D., and Elferink, C.J. (1998) The Ah receptor signal transduction pathway, in *Toxicant–Receptor Interactions* (eds M.S. Denison and W.G. Helferich), Taylor & Francis, Philadelphia, PA, pp. 3–33.

67 Zhang, S., Qin, C., and Safe, S.H. (2003) Flavonoids as aryl hydrocarbon receptor agonists/antagonists: effects of structure and cell context. *Environ. Health Perspect.*, **111**, 1877–1882.

68 Amakura, Y., Tsutsumi, T., Sasaki, K., Nakamura, M., Yoshida, T., and Maitani, T. (2008) Influence of food polyphenols on aryl hydrocarbon receptor-signaling pathway estimated by *in vitro* bioassay. *Phytochemistry*, **69**, 3117–3130.

69 Ioannides, C. and Parke, D.V. (1993) Induction of cytochrome P4501 as an indicator of potential chemical carcinogenesis. *Drug Metab. Rev.*, **25**, 485–501.

70 Hodek, P., Trefil, P., and Stiborova, M. (2002) Flavonoids–potent and versatile biologically active compounds interacting with cytochromes P450. *Chem. Biol. Interact.*, **139**, 1–21.

71 Krizkova, J., Burdova, K., Hudecek, J., Stiborova, M., and Hodek, P. (2008) Induction of cytochromes P450 in small

intestine by chemopreventive compounds. *Neuro Endocrinol. Lett.*, **29**, 717–721.

72 Krizkova, J., Burdova, K., Stiborova, M., Kren, V., and Hodek, P. (2009) Effect of selected flavonoids on cytochromes P450 in rat liver and small intestine. *Interdisc. Toxicol.*, **2**, 201–204.

73 Awad, H.M., Boersma, M.G., Boeren, S., van Bladeren, P.J., Vervoort, J., and Rietjens, I.M. (2001) Structure–activity study on the quinone/quinone methide chemistry of flavonoids. *Chem. Res. Toxicol.*, **14**, 398–408.

74 Shimada, T., Tanaka, K., Takenaka, S., Murayama, N., Martin, M.V., Foroozesh, M.K., Yamazaki, H., Guengerich, F.P., and Komori, M. (2010) Structure–function relationships of inhibition of human cytochromes P450 1A1, 1A2, 1B1, 2C9, and 3A4 by 33 flavonoid derivatives. *Chem. Res. Toxicol.*, **23**, 1921–1935.

75 Moon, Y.J., Wang, X., and Morris, M.E. (2006) Dietary flavonoids: effects on xenobiotic and carcinogen metabolism. *Toxicol. In Vitro*, **20**, 187–210.

76 Androutsopoulos, V.P., Papakyriakou, A., Vourloumis, D., Tsatsakis, A.M., and Spandidos, D.A. (2010) Dietary flavonoids in cancer therapy and prevention: substrates and inhibitors of cytochrome P450 CYP1 enzymes. *Pharmacol. Ther.*, **126**, 9–20.

77 Lee, H., Yeom, H., Kim, Y.G., Yoon, C.N., Jin, C., Choi, J.S., Kim, B.R., and Kim, D.H. (1998) Structure-related inhibition of human hepatic caffeine *N*3-demethylation by naturally occurring flavonoids. *Biochem. Pharmacol.*, **55**, 1369–1375.

78 Doostdar, H., Burke, M.D., and Mayer, R.T. (2000) Bioflavonoids: selective substrates and inhibitors for cytochrome P450 CYP1A and CYP1B1. *Toxicology*, **144**, 31–38.

79 Henderson, M.C., Miranda, C.L., Stevens, J.F., Deinzer, M.L., and Buhler, D.R. (2000) *In vitro* inhibition of human P450 enzymes by prenylated flavonoids from hops, *Humulus lupulus*. *Xenobiotica*, **30**, 235–251.

80 Tsyrlov, I.B., Goldfarb, I.S., and Gelboin, H.V. (1993) Enzyme-kinetic and immunochemical characteristics of mouse cDNA-expressed, microsomal, and purified CYP1A1 and CYP1A2. *Arch. Biochem. Biophys.*, **307**, 259–266.

81 Borek-Dohalsk, L., Hodek, P., Sulc, M., and Stiborova, M. (2001) Alpha-naphthoflavone acts as activator and reversible or irreversible inhibitor of rabbit microsomal CYP3A6. *Chem. Biol. Interact.*, **138**, 85–106.

82 Ueng, Y.F., Kuwabara, T., Chun, Y.J., and Guengerich, F.P. (1997) Cooperativity in oxidations catalyzed by cytochrome P450 3A4. *Biochemistry*, **36**, 370–381.

83 Kang, I.H., Kim, H.J., Oh, H., Park, Y.I., and Dong, M.S. (2004) Biphasic effects of the flavonoids quercetin and naringenin on the metabolic activation of 2-amino-3,5-dimethylimidazo[4,5-*f*] quinoline by *Salmonella typhimurium* TA1538 co-expressing human cytochrome P450 1A2, NADPH-cytochrome P450 reductase, and cytochrome b_5. *Mutat. Res.*, **545**, 37–47.

84 Canivenc-Lavier, M.C., Vernevaut, M.F., Totis, M., Siess, M.H., Magdalou, J., and Suschetet, M. (1996) Comparative effects of flavonoids and model inducers on drug-metabolizing enzymes in rat liver. *Toxicology*, **114**, 19–27.

85 Kim, H.P., Son, K.H., Chang, H.W., and Kang, S.S. (2004) Anti-inflammatory plant flavonoids and cellular action mechanisms. *J. Pharm. Sci.*, **96**, 229–245.

86 Kim, J.S., Kim, J.C., Shim, S.H., Lee, E.J., Jin, W., Bae, K., Son, K.H., Kim, H.P., Kang, S.S., and Chang, H.W. (2006) Chemical constituents of the root of *Dystaenia takeshimana* and their anti-inflammatory activity. *Arch. Pharm. Res.*, **29**, 617–623.

87 Van Hoorn, D.E., Nijveldt, R.J., Van Leeuwen, P.A., Hofman, Z., M'Rabet, L., De Bont, D.B., and Van Norren, K. (2002) Accurate prediction of xanthine oxidase inhibition based on the structure of flavonoids. *Eur. J. Pharmacol.*, **451**, 111–118.

88 Williams, R.J., Spencer, J.P., and Rice-Evans, C. (2004) Flavonoids: antioxidants or signalling molecules? *Free Radic. Biol. Med.*, **36**, 838–849.

89 Spencer, J.P.E., Schroeter, H., and Rice-Evans, C.A. (2003) Cytoprotective and cytotoxic effects of flavonoids, in *Flavonoids in Health and Disease* (eds L. Packer and C.A. Rice-Evans), Dekker, New York, pp. 309–349.

90 Matsuo, M., Sasaki, N., Saga, K., and Kaneko, T. (2005) Cytotoxicity of flavonoids toward cultured normal human cells. *Biol. Pharm. Bull.*, **28**, 253–259.

91 Andres, A., Donovan, S.M., and Kuhlenschmidt, M.S. (2009) Soy isoflavones and virus infections. *J. Nutr. Biochem.*, **20**, 563–569.

92 Evers, D.L., Chao, C.F., Wang, X., Zhang, Z., Huong, S.M., and Huang, E.S. (2005) Human cytomegalovirus-inhibitory flavonoids: studies on antiviral activity and mechanism of action. *Antiviral Res.*, **68**, 124–134.

93 Yamaguchi, K., Honda, M., Ikigai, H., Hara, Y., and Shimamura, T. (2002) Inhibitory effects of (–)-epigallocatechin gallate on the life cycle of human immunodeficiency virus type 1 (HIV-1). *Antiviral Res.*, **53**, 19–34.

94 Savi, L.A., Caon, T., de Oliveira, A.P., Sobottka, A.M., Werner, W., Reginatto, F.H., Schenkel, E.P., Barardi, C.R., and Simões, C.M. (2010) Evaluation of antirotavirus activity of flavonoids. *Fitoterapia*, **81**, 1142–1146.

95 Alvarez, M.A., Debattista, N.B., and Pappano, N.B. (2008) Antimicrobial activity and synergism of some substituted flavonoids. *Fol. Microbiol.*, **53**, 23–28.

96 Saleem, M., Nazir, M., Ali, M.S., Hussain, H., Lee, Y.S., Riaz, N., and Jabbar, A. (2010) Antimicrobial natural products: an update on future antibiotic drug candidates. *Nat. Prod. Rep.*, **27**, 238–254.

97 Kuete, V., Nguemeving, J.R., Beng, V.P., Azebaze, A.G., Etoa, F.X., Meyer, M., Bodo, B., and Nkengfack, A.E. (2007) Antimicrobial activity of the methanolic extracts and compounds from *Vismia laurentii* De Wild (Guttiferae). *J. Ethnopharmacol.*, **109**, 372–379.

98 Sathiamoorthy, B., Gupta, P., Kumar, M., Chaturvedi, A.K., Shukla, P.K., and Maurya, R. (2007) New antifungal flavonoid glycoside from *Vitex negundo*. *Bioorg. Med. Chem. Lett.*, **17**, 239–242.

99 Rathee, P., Chaudhary, H., Rathee, S., Rathee, D., Kumar, V., and Kohli, K. (2009) Mechanism of action of flavonoids as anti-inflammatory agents: a review. *Inflamm. Allergy Drug Targets*, **8**, 229–235.

100 Manthey, J.A., Grohmann, K., Montanari, A., Ash, K., and Manthey, C.L. (1999) Polymethoxylated flavones derived from citrus suppress tumor necrosis factor-α expression by human monocytes. *J. Nat. Prod.*, **62**, 441–444.

101 Tsai, S.-H., Liang, Y.-C., Lin-Shiau, S.-Y., and Lin, J.-K. (1999) Suppression of TNFα-mediated NFκB activity by myricetin and other flavonoids through downregulating the activity of IKK in ECV304 cells. *J. Cell. Biochem.*, **74**, 606–615.

102 Vita, J.A. (2005) Polyphenols and cardiovascular disease: effects on endothelial and platelet function. *Am. J. Clin. Nutr.*, **81**, 292S–297S.

103 Freedman, J.E., Parker, C., 3rd, Li, L., Perlman, J.A., Frei, B., Ivanov, V., Deak, L.R., Iafrati, M.D., and Folts, J.D. (2001) Select flavonoids and whole juice from purple grapes inhibit platelet function and enhance nitric oxide release. *Circulation*, **103**, 2792–2798.

104 Ostertag, L.M., O'Kennedy, N., Kroon, P.A., Duthie, G.G., and de Roos, B. (2010) Impact of dietary polyphenols on human platelet function – a critical review of controlled dietary intervention studies. *Mol. Nutr. Food Res.*, **54**, 60–81.

105 Drewnowski, A. and Gomez-Carneros, C. (2000) Bitter taste, phytonutrients, and the consumer: a review. *Am. J. Clin. Nutr.*, **72**, 1424–1435.

106 Bohm, B.A. (1998) Human use of flavonoids, in *Introduction to Flavonoids* (ed. B.A. Bohm), Harwood, Amsterdam, pp. 365–395.

107 Le Marchand, L. (2002) Cancer preventive effects of flavonoids – a review. *Biomed. Pharmacother.*, **56**, 296–301.

108 Kalra, E.K. (2003) Nutraceutical – definition and introduction. *AAPS PharmSci.*, **5**, 27–28.

109 Ramelet, A.A. (2001) Clinical benefits of Daflon 500 mg in the most severe stages of chronic venous insufficiency. *Angiology*, **52**, S49–S56.

110 Meyskens, F.L., Jr and Szabo, E. (2005) Diet and cancer: the disconnect between epidemiology and randomized clinical trials. *Cancer Epidemiol. Biomarkers Prev.*, **14**, 1366–1369.

111 Schroeter, H., Spencer, J.P., Rice-Evans, C., and Williams, R.J. (2001) Flavonoids protect neurons from oxidized low-density-lipoprotein-induced apoptosis involving c-Jun N-terminal kinase (JNK), c-Jun and caspase-3. *Biochem. J.*, **358**, 547–557.

112 Kale, A., Gawande, S., and Kotwal, S. (2008) Cancer phytotherapeutics: role for flavonoids at the cellular level. *Phytother. Res.*, **22**, 567–577.

113 Chan, H.Y., Chen, Z.Y., Tsang, D.S., and Leung, L.K. (2002) Baicalein inhibits DMBA–DNA adduct formation by modulating CYP1A1 and CYP1B1 activities. *Biomed. Pharmacother.*, **56**, 269–275.

114 Boyd, C.S. and Cadenas, E. (2003) Mitochondrial actions of flavonoids and isoflavonoids, in *Flavonoids in Health and Disease* (eds L. Packer and C.A. Rice-Evans), Dekker., New York, pp. 273–301.

115 Boots, A.W., Li, H., Schins, R.P., Duffin, R., Heemskerk, J.W., Bast, A., and Haenen, G.R. (2007) The quercetin paradox. *Toxicol. Appl. Pharmacol.*, **222**, 89–96.

116 Rahman, A., Shahabuddin, A., Hadi, S.M., and Parish, J.H. (1990) Complexes involving quercetin, DNA and Cu(II). *Carcinogenesis*, **11**, 2001–2003.

117 Galati, G. and O'Brien, P.J. (2004) Potential toxicity of flavonoids and other dietary phenolics: significance for their chemopreventive and anticancer properties. *Free Radic. Biol. Med.*, **37**, 287–303.

118 Hsieh, C.Y., Santell, R.C., Haslam, S.Z., and Helferich, W.G. (1998) Estrogenic effects of genistein on the growth of estrogen receptor-positive human breast cancer (MCF-7) cells *in vitro* and *in vivo*. *Cancer Res.*, **58**, 3833–3838.

119 Gaitan, E., Cooksey, R.C., Legan, J., and Lindsay, R.H. (1995) Antithyroid effects *in vivo* and *in vitro* of vitexin: a *C*-glucosylflavone in millet. *J. Clin. Endocrinol. Metab.*, **80**, 1144–1147.

120 Román, G.C. (2007) Autism: transient *in utero* hypothyroxinemia related to maternal flavonoid ingestion during pregnancy and to other environmental antithyroid agents. *J. Neurol. Sci.*, **262**, 15–26.

121 Fresco, P., Borges, F., Diniz, C., and Marques, M.P. (2006) New insights on the anticancer properties of dietary polyphenols. *Med. Res. Rev.*, **26**, 747–766.

122 Schwarz, D. and Roots, I. (2003) *In vitro* assessment of inhibition by natural polyphenols of metabolic activation of procarcinogens by human CYP1A1. *Biochem. Biophys. Res. Commun.*, **303**, 902–907.

123 Stiborova, M., Frei, E., Hodek, P., Wiessler, M., and Schmeiser, H.H. (2005) Human hepatic and renal microsomes, cytochromes P450 1A1/2, NADPH : cytochrome P450 reductase and prostaglandin H synthase mediate the formation of aristolochic acid-DNA adducts found in patients with urothelial cancer. *Int. J. Cancer*, **113**, 189–197.

124 Hodek, P., Tepla, M., Krizkova, J., Sulc, M., and Stiborova, M. (2009) Modulation of cytochrome P450 enzyme system by selected flavonoids. *Neuro Endocrinol. Lett.*, **30**, S67–S71.

125 Conney, A.H. (2003) Enzyme induction and dietary chemicals as approaches to cancer chemoprevention: the Seventh DeWitt S. Goodman Lecture. *Cancer Res.*, **63**, 7005–7031.

126 Gurtoo, H.L., Koser, P.L., Bansal, S.K., Fox, H.W., Sharma, S.D., Mulhern, A.I., and Pavelic, Z.P. (1985) Inhibition of aflatoxin B1-hepatocarcinogenesis in rats by β-naphthoflavone. *Carcinogenesis*, **6**, 675–678.

127 Nakagama, H., Nakanishi, M., and Ochiai, M. (2005) Modeling human colon cancer in rodents using a food-borne carcinogen, PhIP. *Cancer Sci.*, **96**, 627–636.

128 Chen, Y., Xiao, P., Ou-Yang, D.S., Fan, L., Guo, D., Wang, Y.N., Han, Y., Tu,

J.H., Zhou, G., Huang, Y.F., and Zhou, H.H. (2009) Simultaneous action of the flavonoid quercetin on cytochrome P450 (CYP) 1A2, CYP2A6, *N*-acetyltransferase and xanthine oxidase activity in healthy volunteers. *Clin. Exp. Pharmacol. Physiol.*, **36**, 828–833.

129 Ioannides, C. (2002) Pharmacokinetic interactions between herbal remedies and medicinal drugs. *Xenobiotica*, **32**, 451–478.

130 Izzo, A.A. and Ernst, E. (2009) Interactions between herbal medicines and prescribed drugs: an updated systematic review. *Drugs*, **69**, 1777–1798.

131 Schumacher, M., Hautzinger, A., Rossmann, A., Holzhauser, S., Popovic, D., Hertrampf, A., Kuntz, S., Boll, M., and Wenzel, U. (2010) Chrysin blocks topotecan-induced apoptosis in Caco-2 cells in spite of inhibition of ABC-transporters. *Biochem. Pharmacol.*, **80**, 471–479.

132 Obach, R.S. (2000) Inhibition of human cytochrome P450 enzymes by constituents of St. John's Wort, an herbal preparation used in the treatment of depression. *J. Pharmacol. Exp. Ther.*, **294**, 88–95.

133 Venkataramanan, R., Ramachandran, V., Komoroski, B.J., Zhang, S., Schiff, P.L., and Strom, S.C. (2000) Milk thistle, a herbal supplement, decreases the activity of CYP3A4 and uridine diphosphoglucuronosyl transferase in human hepatocyte cultures. *Drug Metab. Dispos.*, **28**, 1270–1273.

134 Doehmer, J., Tewes, B., Klein, K.U., Gritzko, K., Muschick, H., and Mengs, U. (2008) Assessment of drug–drug interaction for silymarin. *Toxicol. In Vitro*, **22**, 610–617.

135 Bailey, D.G., Dresser, G.R., Kreeft, J.H., Munoz, C., Freeman, D.J., and Bend, J.R. (2000) Grapefruit–felodipine interaction: effect of unprocessed fruit and probable active ingredients. *Clin. Pharmacol. Ther.*, **68**, 468–477.

136 Paine, M.F., Widmer, W.W., Hart, H.L., Pusek, S.N., Beavers, K.L., Criss, A.B., Brown, S.S., Thomas, B.F., and Watkins, P.B. (2006) A furanocoumarin-free grapefruit juice establishes furanocoumarins as the mediators of the grapefruit juice–felodipine interaction. *Am. J. Clin. Nutr.*, **83**, 1097–1105.

137 Bracke, M.E., Depypere, H.T., Boterberg, T., Van Marck, V.L., Vennekens, K.M., Vanluchene, E., Nuytinck, M., Serreyn, R., and Mareel, M.M. (1999) Influence of tangeretin on tamoxifen's therapeutic benefit in mammary cancer. *J. Natl. Cancer Inst.*, **91**, 354–359.

138 Shen, F., Xue, X., and Weber, G. (1999) Tamoxifen and genistein synergistically down-regulate signal transduction and proliferation in estrogen receptor-negative human breast carcinoma MDA-MB-435 cells. *Anticancer Res.*, **19**, 1657–1662.

139 Wang, B., Sanchez, R.I., Franklin, R.B., Evans, D.C., and Huskey, S.E. (2004) The involvement of CYP3A4 and CYP2C9 in the metabolism of 17 alpha-ethinylestradiol. *Drug Metab. Dispos.*, **32**, 1209–1212.

140 Schrag, M.L., Cui, D., Rushmore, T.H., Shou, M., Ma, B., and Rodrigues, A.D. (2004) Sulfotransferase 1E1 is a low K_m isoform mediating the 3-O-sulfation of ethinyl estradiol. *Drug Metab. Dispos.*, **32**, 1299–1303.

141 Miyano, J., Yamamoto, S., Hanioka, N., Narimatsu, S., Ishikawa, T., Ogura, K., Watabe, T., Nishimura, M., Ueda, N., and Naito, S. (2005) Involvement of SULT1A3 in elevated sulfation of 4-hydroxypropranolol in Hep G2 cells pretreated with beta-naphthoflavone. *Biochem. Pharmacol.*, **69**, 941–950.

142 Jang, S.I., Kim, H.J., Hwang, K.M., Jekal, S.J., Pae, H.O., Choi, B.M., Yun, Y.G., Kwon, T.O., Chung, H.T., and Kim, Y.C. (2003) Hepatoprotective effect of baicalin, a major flavone from *Scutellaria radix*, on acetaminophen-induced liver injury in mice. *Immunopharmacol. Immunotoxicol.*, **25**, 585–594.

143 Taur, J.S. and Rodriguez-Proteau, R. (2008) Effects of dietary flavonoids on the transport of cimetidine via P-glycoprotein and cationic transporters in Caco-2 and LLC-PK1 cell models. *Xenobiotica*, **38**, 1536–1550.

144 Choi, J.S., Choi, H.K., and Shin, S.C. (2004) Enhanced bioavailability of paclitaxel after oral coadministration with flavone in rats. *Int. J. Pharm.*, **275**, 165–170.
145 Wang, Y.H., Chao, P.D.L., Hsiu, S.L., Wen, K.C., and Hou, Y.C. (2004) Lethal quercetin–digoxin interaction in pigs. *Life Sci.*, **74**, 1191–1197.
146 Xing, J., Chen, X., Sun, Y., Luan, Y., and Zhong, D. (2005) Interaction of baicalin and baicalein with antibiotics in the gastrointestinal tract. *J. Pharm. Pharmacol.*, **57**, 743–750.

Acknowledgment

The author wish to thank the Grant Agency of the Czech Republic (P303/12/G163) for financial support.

21
St John's Wort (*Hypericum perforatum* L.)

Miroslav Dostalek and Anna-Katarina Stark

21.1
The Name Hypericum

The generic name *Hypericum* derives from *hyper* (above) and *eikon* (a figure, possibly an unwanted apparition), which relates to the ancient use of the plant to exorcise evil spirits or influences. It may have been placed over religious icons as a symbol of protection. The second term, *perforatum*, is derived from Latin for perforated because the leaves, when held to the light, reveal translucent dots, giving the impression that the leaf is perforated. The popular name St John's Wort (old English "wort" means plant) is said to be in honor of the Knights of St John of Jerusalem who used this herb to treat battlefield wounds. Early Christian authors claimed the red spots symbolized the blood of St John and appeared on the leaves of *Hypericum* on 29 August – the anniversary of the saint's beheading by Herod. Others considered the best day to pick the plant was 24 June – the day of St John's feast.

21.2
Chemical Constituents of *Hypericum perforatum*

H. perforatum extracts are among the best-characterized herbal medicines [1]. More than 150 ingredients, or groups of ingredients, with a multiplicity of additive, synergistic, and partly antagonistic effects, have been identified so far [2–4]. Still, 30–50% of its compounds are, as yet, not structurally defined; some of these might well contribute to the clinical effects [2]. The analytical composition of this herbal drug is reported in Table 21.1 [2, 5, 6].

St John's Wort is currently available as standardized extracts, tea leaves, and oil infusions for topical use. The *H. perforatum* extracts are usually prepared by extracting the *hyperici herba* with mixtures of ethanol or methanol/water. Based on various factors, *H. perforatum* extract contains variable amounts of active compound (Table 21.2). These factors are growth environment, quantities of the

Metabolism of Drugs and Other Xenobiotics, First Edition. Edited by Pavel Anzenbacher, Ulrich M. Zanger.

Table 21.1 Constituents and percentage of St John's Wort herbal drug.

Component group (%)	Component	Percent of herbal drug	Plant parts	Action	Activity
Naphthodianthrone derivates (0.05–0.15)	hypericin	0.003–3.0	flowers, buds	inhibition of MAO, PKC, and dopamine-β-hydroxylase; inhibition of 5-HT and noradrenaline reuptake; inhibition of σ and M receptors	antidepressant, antiviral, photosensitizing
	pseudohypericin	0.2			
Phloroglucinol derivates (2–5)	hyperforin	2.0–4.0	flowers, buds	inhibition of 5-HT, dopamine, noradrenaline, L-glutamate reuptake	antidepressant, antibiotic
	adhyperforin	0.2–1.9			
Flavonol derivates (2–5)	hyperoside	0.5–2.0	leaves, stalk, buds	inhibition of MAO, COMT, inhibition of ion channels, bound to benzodiazepine receptors	antidepressant, antiphlogistic
	rutin	0.3–1.6			
	quercetrin	0.3–0.5			
	isoquercetrin	0.3			
	quercetin	2.0–4.0			
	kaempferol				
	myricetin				
	luteolin				
	mangiferin				
Biflavonol derivates	biapigenin	0.1–0.5	flowers	bound to benzodiazepine receptors	sedating, antiphlogistic
	amentoflavone	0.01–0.05			

Xanthone derivates (0.01)	kielcorin	0.01	roots, flowers	inhibition of MAO and COMT	antidepressant
	tetrahydroxanthon	0.0004			
Phenolic acids	caffeic acid	0.1	flowers, leaves	spasmolytic activity	
	chlorogenic acid	<1.0			
	ferulic acid				
Tannin and proanthrocyanidin derivates (6–15)	tannins	6.0–12	aerial parts, flowers, buds		antiphlogistic, antioxidant
	catechin	2.0–4.0			
	epicatechin				
	procyanidin B2				
Terpenes (0.1–1)			flowers, leaves		
n-Alkenes/ *n*-alkanols (0.1–1)			flowers, leaves		
Amino acids (0.01)	GABA	0.0007	flowers, leaves		antidepressant
	melatonin				sedating
Sterols	β-sitosterol				
Vitamins	vitamin A				
	vitamin C				

different plant parts used (leaf, stem, and/or flowers), harvest time (flowering or fruiting time), drying procedures, and storage conditions [1]. Thus, the *European Pharmacopoeia* requires not less than 0.08% naphthodianthrones of the hypericin group–calculated as hypericin using UV spectrophotometry analysis for herbal drug [7].

Table 21.2 Commercially available *H. perforatum* extracts evaluated for drug interactions [8].

Extract type/ brand name	Standardization	Pharmaceutical form	Distributor
Esbericum®	hyperforin 1.47%	capsules containing 60 mg of St John's Wort dried extract	Schaper & Bruemmer, Germany
Hypericum 2000 plus®	hypericin 0.055%, hyperforin 0.75%	capsules containing St John's Wort dried extract equivalent to 2 g dry herb and *Ginkgo biloba* equivalent to 100 mg dry leaf	Nutra-Life, New Zealand
Jarsin 300®	hypericin 0.28%	tablets containing 300 mg of St John's Wort dried extract (LI 160)	Lichtwer Pharma AG, Germany
Kira®	hypericin 0.28%	tablets containing 100 mg of St John's Wort dried extract (LI 160)	Lichtwer Pharma AG, Germany
LI 160®	hypericin 0.12–0.28%	Dried extract of St John's Wort flowers and leaves	Lichtwer Pharma AG, Germany
Neuroplant®	hypericin 0.12–0.28, hyperforin 3.0–6.0%	tablets containing 300 mg WS 5570 extract	Dr Willmar Schwabe Pharmaceuticals, Germany
Neuroplant® AKTIV	hypericin 0.12–0.28, hyperforin 3.0–6.0%	tablets containing 600 mg WS 5570 extract	Dr Willmar Schwabe Pharmaceuticals, Germany
Movina®	hyperforin 3.0–6.0%	capsules containing 300 mg of St John's Wort dried extract	Boehringer Ingelheim AB, Sweden
WS® 5570	hypericin 0.12–0.28%, hyperforin 3.0–6.0%	soft gel containing 300 mg of St John's Wort dried extract	Dr Willmar Schwabe Pharmaceuticals, Germany
ZE 117®	hypericin 0.12–0.28, hyperforin <0.5%	dried extract of St John's Wort flowers and leaves	Zeller AG, Switzerland

21.3
Clinical Pharmacology of *H. perforatum*

21.3.1
Antidepressive Activity

St John's Wort is the most common herbal supplement used for mild-to-moderate depression, although the underlying mechanisms have not been elucidated. Early *in vitro* work reported inhibition of monoamine oxidase (MAO)-A and -B [9, 10]; Thiede and Walper found MAO and catechol *O*-methyltransferase (COMT) inhibition [11]. Recent studies show that St John's Wort's antidepressant activity is mediated by serotonergic, noradrenergic, and dopaminergic systems [2, 12–15], as well as by means of γ-aminobutyric acid (GABA) and glutamate amino acid neurotransmitters [16–19]. The weak activity *in vitro* suggests a combination of multiple mechanisms [12]. Several systematic reviews report St John's Wort to be more effective than placebo [13–15, 18–29], and equally effective as systemic antidepressant drugs, in short-term treatment of depressive disorder, including major depression [14, 15, 23, 27, 30–40].

21.3.2
Photodynamic Therapy and Cancer

The pro-oxidant photodynamic properties of hypericin have been exploited for the photodynamic therapy of cancer. Hypericin, in combination with light, effectively induces apoptosis and/or necrosis of cancer cells [41]. It has also been shown that upon light activation hypericin inhibits protein kinase C (PKC) and other growth factor-stimulated protein kinases [42–45], induces peroxidation of membrane lipids [28, 29, 46], increases superoxide dismutase activity, decreases cellular glutathione levels [29, 47], and impairs mitochondrial functions [46–50].

21.3.3
Antiviral Activity

Hypericin, and to a lesser extent pseudohypericin, has been the topic of intense research concerning antiviral properties. It has been shown to exhibit virucidal activity by inhibiting viral infectivity in a hypericin-preincubation and light-dependent inactivation reaction, as well as antiviral activity by inhibiting viral replication in cell cultures. Additionally, hypericin has shown *in vitro* activity against a variety of viruses (i.e., influenza virus [35], vesiculostomatitis virus [51], and herpes viruses [35]). Moreover, interaction studies of hypericin with HIV-1 reverse transcriptase and HIV-1 protease have also been reported [36].

21.3.4
Other Pharmacological Activities

The traditional uses of St John's Wort include treatment for bacterial infections, respiratory conditions, skin wounds, peptic ulcers, and inflammation [52].

21.4
Pharmacokinetics and Pharmacokinetic Interactions of *H. perforatum*

H. perforatum contains a wide range of different natural product classes. Best known are the naphthodianthrones, with hypericin and pseudohypericin as main compounds, and the prenylated phloroglucinols group containing hyperforin. Moreover, typical natural product groups comprise xanthones, flavonoids, and biflavonoids.

21.4.1
Phloroglucinols: Hyperforin

Maximal plasma levels of hyperforin were observed 3–3.5 h after oral administration. Biotransformation is decreased after once-daily high-dose extract. A two-compartment model was described for hyperforin with an elimination time of distribution and elimination half-life of approximately 3 and 9 h, respectively. No significant difference in the mean clearance could be found between the 300- and 600-mg doses. By contrast, the difference in the mean clearance between the 300- and 1200-mg doses was statistically significant. Thus, the pharmacokinetics of hyperforin seems to be linear up to a 600-mg dose of an extract (Table 21.3).

21.4.2
Naphthodianthrones: Hypericin and Pseudohypericin

Hypericin and pseudohypericin are structurally similar compounds; however, their absorption rates after oral administration differ significantly. Plasma concen-

Table 21.3 Pharmacokinetic parameters of hyperforin after single- and repeated-dose oral administration.

Study	Dosage form	Extract	Dosage (mg)	Hyperforin (mg)	C_{max} (ng/ml)	t_{max} (min)	AUC (ng·min/ml)	$t_{1/2}$ (min)	CL (ml/min)
Biber [53]	tablet	WS 5572	300	14.8	153.15	211.8	1335.9	567.6	199.3
Biber [53]	tablet	WS 5572	600	29.6	301.8	210	2214.6	511.2	238.2
Biber [53]	tablet	WS 5572	900	4.5	20.7	180	254	960	283
Biber [53]	tablet	WS 5572	900	42.84	246	186	2336	672	266
Biber [53]	tablet	WS 5572	1200	59.2	437.3	169.8	3377.9	579	340.3
Agrosi [54]	soft gelatin capsule	–	300	15	168.35	150	1482.7	–	–
Agrosi [54]	hard gelatin capsule	–	300	15	84.25	184.8	583.65	–	–
Cui [37]	capsule	–	1800	8.55	27.6	264	–	210	561.6

Table 21.4 Pharmacokinetic parameters of hypericin after single- and repeated-dose oral administration.

Study	Extract	Dosage form	Dosage (mg)	Hypericin (mg)	C_{max} (ng/ml)	t_{max} (min)	AUC (ng·min/ml)	$t_{1/2}$ (min)	*CL* (ml/min)
Weiser [38]	LI 160	tablet	300, 600, 1200	–	4.3	2.5	–	6	–
Staffeldt [55]	LI 160	tablet	300	0.25	1.5	5.2	1920	24.8	–
Staffeldt [55]	LI 160	tablet	900	0.75	7.5	4.1	8820	26	–
Staffeldt [55]	LI 160	tablet	1800	1.5	14.2	5.9	23090	26.5	–
Brockmoller [56]	LI 160	tablet	900	1.1	18	7.1	7250	27.8	45
Brockmoller [56]	LI 160	tablet	3 × 300	2.18	36	6.0	59580	29.1	40
Brockmoller [56]	LI 160	tablet	3600	4.36	91	6.5	150180	27.5	36.6
Brockmoller [56]	LI 160	tablet	1800	2.18	29		16200	41.7	44.7
Kerb [57]	LI 160	tablet	300	0.25	1.3	5.5	2484	24.5	101
Kerb [57]	LI 160	tablet	900	0.75	7.2	6.0	11880	43.1	63.3
Kerb [57]	LI 160	tablet	3 × 300	1.5	16.6	5.7	29640	48.2	51
Kerb [57]	LI 160	tablet	900	0.75	8.8	–	3690	41.3	68.2

tration of hypericin is detected after a lag time of approximately 2 h, whereas almost no lag time has been observed for pseudohypericin. The low bioavailability of naphthodianthrones reflects their poor water solubility. However, the presence of additional flavanol glycosides in the extracts may enhance water solubility of naphthodianthrone derivates, thereby increasing the bioavailability (Tables 21.4 and 21.5).

21.4.3 Flavonoids: Rutin and Quercetin

The flavonoids are widespread compounds found in the plant kingdom. St John's Wort extract without the flavonoid rutin showed less therapeutic efficiency than extract containing generally present amounts of rutin [58]. However, the role of flavonoids in the treatment of depression remains unclear. Graefe *et al.* [39] demonstrated the presence of four or five quercetin glucuronides in human plasma, instead of free quercetin and rutin. A report by Day *et al.* [40] identified seven different quercetin conjugates in human plasma; major compounds were quercetin-3-glucuronide, 3-methylquercetin-glucuronide (approximately 20%), and quercetin 3-sulfate (approximately 35%) (Table 21.6).

Table 21.5 Pharmacokinetic parameters of pseudohypericin after single- and repeated-dose oral administration.

Study	Extract	Dosage form	Dosage (mg)	Pseudohypericin (mg)	C_{max} (ng/ml)	t_{max} (min)	AUC (ng·min/ml)	$t_{1/2}$ (min)	*CL* (ml/min)
Weiser [38]	LI 160	tablet	300, 600, 1200	–	–	–	–	–	–
Staffeldt [55]	LI 160	tablet	300	0.526	2.7	2.7	1900	16.3	–
Staffeldt [55]	LI 160	tablet	900	1.58	11.7	3.0	7130	36.0	–
Staffeldt [55]	LI 160	tablet	1800	3.16	30.6	3.2	19910	22.8	–
Brockmoller [56]	LI 160	tablet	900	1.72	10	3.3	8280	19.4	235
Brockmoller [56]	LI 160	tablet	1800	3.44	25	3.2	20040	16.1	205
Brockmoller [56]	LI 160	tablet	3600	6.89	68	3.5	50100	17.5	190
Brockmoller [56]	LI 160	tablet	3 × 600	3.44	29	–	9900	22.8	116
Kerb [57]	LI 160	tablet	300	0.526	3.4	3.0	2700	18.2	195
Kerb [57]	LI 160	tablet	900	1.578	12.1	3.0	8400	24.8	188
Kerb [57]	LI 160	tablet	3 × 300	3.156	29.7	3.0	17100	19.5	185
Kerb [57]	LI 160	tablet	900	1.578	8.5	–	3054	18.8	172

Table 21.6 Pharmacokinetics parameters or quercetin and rutin after single-dose oral administration.

Study	Source	Quercetin (mg)	C_{max} (ng/ml)	t_{max} (min)	AUC (ng·min/ml)	$t_{1/2}$ (min)	*CL* (ml/min)
Graefe [39]	onions	100	2.31	0.68	582	10.9	13.3
	quercetin -4-glucoside	100	2.12	0.70	504	11.9	17.4
	buckwheat tea	200	0.64	4.32	228	10.3	131
	pure rutin	200	0.32	6.98	150	11.8	159
Erlund [59]	pure quercetin	8	0.0414	1.90	37.8	17.1	–
	pure quercetin	20	0.0661	2.70	63.5	17.7	–
	pure quercetin	50	0.0861	4.90	79.4	15.1	–
	pure rutin	~8	0.0235	6.50	28.7	–	–
	pure rutin	~20	0.0476	7.40	47.6	–	–
	pure rutin	~50	0.0899	7.50	72.1	–	–
Erlund [60]	pure quercetin	25	0.02–0.044	–	–	–	–
Hollman [61]	onions	68	0.224	0.70	139.8	28 ± 92	–
	apple	98	92	2.51	62.8	23 ± 32	–
	pure rutin	100	90	9.30	59.0	–	–
Ishii [44]	pure rutin	500	0.063	5.00	–	2.5	–

21.5 *In Vitro* Studies

Numerous studies have reported the inductive and inhibitory effects of St John's Wort on cytochrome P450 (CYP) and P-glycoprotein (P-gp). These findings indicate that St John's Wort can both induce and inhibit CYPs and P-gp. Studies performed *in vitro* have demonstrated that St John's Wort extract (hyperforin) is a potent inducer of CYP2B6, 2C9, and 3A4 [45, 62–64]. Hyperforin has also been shown to be a potent ligand (K_i = 27 nmol) for the pregnane X receptor (PXR) [63], which is responsible for the regulation of CYP2B6 and 3A4 expression [62, 64, 65].

The flavonoid I3,II8-biapigenin has been shown to be an inhibitor of four of the most important drug-metabolizing CYPs: CYP3A4 ($K_i = 0.038 \pm 0.006\,\mu M$, competitive inhibition), 2C9 ($K_i = 0.32 \pm 0.14\,\mu M$, competitive inhibition), 2D6 ($K_i = 2.3 \pm 1.8\,\mu M$, competitive inhibition), and 1A2 ($K_i = 0.95 \pm 0.22\,\mu M$, competitive inhibition). Hyperforin was found to be an inhibitor of CYP2D6 ($K_i = 1.5 \pm 0.9\,\mu M$, noncompetitive inhibition), 2C9 ($K_i = 1.8 \pm 0.9\,\mu M$, competitive inhibition), and 3A4 ($K_i = 0.49 \pm 0.24\,\mu M$, competitive inhibition) [66]. Additionally, hypericin inhibited CYP2C9 ($K_i = 1.1 \pm 1.1\,\mu M$, competitive inhibition), 2D6 ($K_i = 2.6 \pm 0.9\,\mu M$, competitive inhibition), and 3A4 ($K_i = 4.6 \pm 2.2\,\mu M$, competitive inhibition). Similar results were observed with quercetin for CYP1A2 ($K_i = 3.3 \pm 0.6\,\mu M$, competitive inhibition) [66] (Table 21.7).

The occurrence of drug interactions *in vivo* is likely if the maximum unbound plasma concentration $K_i > 0.2$ [67]. The maximum plasma concentration of hyperforin is reported to be 0.17–0.50 μM in humans following a single administration (300 mg) of standardized *Hypericum* extracts containing 5% hyperforin [53, 54]. Thus, a maximum unbound plasma concentration K_i of 0.35–1.04 μM for CYP3A4, 0.11–0.33 μM for CYP2C9, and 0.09–0.28 μM for CYP2D6 would be expected, increasing the risk of possible drug interactions with a number of CYP substrates.

Several studies indicate that St John's Wort induces expression and activity of intestinal P-gp *in vitro* and *in vivo* [65, 68, 69]. Oral administration of St John's

Table 21.7 Inhibition of the most common drug-metabolizing CYPs by St John's Wort constituents [66].

Inhibitor	IC_{50} (μM)				
	CYP1A2 phenacetin	CYP2C9 diclofenac	CYP2C19 mephenytoin	CYP2D6 bufuralol	CYP3A4 Testosterone
Hyperforin	>100	4.4	31	1.6	2.3
I3,II8-biapigenin	3.7	4.0	28	5.7	0.082
Quercetin	7.5	47	>100	24	22
Chlorogenic acid	>100	>100	–	>100	>100
Hypericin	>100	3.4	37	8.5	8.7

Wort at 900 mg/day for 14 days in healthy volunteers resulted in a 1.4-fold increase in P-gp expression [65].

21.6
In Vivo Studies

St John's Wort has been reported to interact with medications that are substrates for CYP3As or P-gp [70–74]. However, the effect of St John's Wort is usually observed after more than 10 days of treatment [74–77]. Long-term St John's Wort administration (2 weeks) at 900 mg resulted in significant and selective induction in the CYP3A activity [78]. Oral clearance of midazolam (CYP3As substrate) was increased from 121.8 ± 70.7 to 254.5 ± 127.8 l/h with a corresponding decrease in oral bioavailability from 0.28 ± 0.15 to 0.17 ± 0.06 and area under the concentration–time curve (AUC) from 41.1 ± 34.5 to 19.6 ± 9.9 μg·h/l [78]. Thus, long-term St John's Wort administration did not alter the CYP1A2 (caffeine), 2C9 (tolbutamide), and 2D6 (dextromethorphan) activities [78]. Similar results have been observed by Ruschitzka *et al.* [49], Roby *et al.* [50], and Ereshefsky *et al.* [79] using the urinary 6β-hydroxy cortisol/cortisol ratio as a marker of CYP3As activity. However, short-term administration (3–4 days) of St John's Wort at the same dose had no effect on CYP3As (alprazolam, midazolam), 1A2 (caffeine), 2C9 (tolbutamide), and 2D6 (dextromethorphan) activity in human volunteers [78, 80].

A majority of the interactions of St John's Wort appear to be associated with the hyperforin content [81]. Clinical results suggest that the hyperforin content determines the magnitude of St John's Wort interactions. Extracts with low hyperforin content showed weak or no effect on both CYPs and P-gp probe drugs [51, 82–86]; for example, low hypericin content had no effect on CYP3A (alprazolam, midazolam) [83, 86], 2C9 (tolbutamide) [83], and P-gp (digoxin, cyclosporine) [83, 84]. High hyperforin concentrations activate the nuclear PXR, which results in induction of CYP3A and P-gp production [63, 65].

The market and interest for herbal medicines and supplements in the western world has markedly increased in recent years, and, not surprisingly, reports of interactions with conventional drugs have increased. The most well-known and documented example is the interaction of St John's Wort with a variety of concomitantly used drugs [87, 88]. Based on clinical and experimental data, coadministration of St John's Wort extract should be avoided in patients who are taking drugs with a narrow therapeutic range. Many case reports showing interactions between St John's Worth with anticonvulsants [89], anti-HIV drugs [52, 90, 91], antidepressants [53, 92, 93], immunosuppressant agents [49, 54, 59, 94–105], and oral contraceptives [63, 89] have been published (Table 21.8).

Acknowledgments

We acknowledge Professor F. Peter Guengerich, Vanderbilt University School of Medicine, Nashville, TN, in appreciation of his mentoring.

Table 21.8 Clinical trials reporting interaction between St John's Wort and concomitantly used drugs.

Compound	Male/female	Dose/day	Pharmacokinetic parameters without St John's Wort versus with St John's Wort	Reference
Alprazolam	4/3	900 mg/3 days	AUC = 179 ± 164 versus 106 ± 62 ng·h/ml $t_{1/2}$ = 7.6 ± 5.6 versus 5.8 ± 2.5 h C_{max} = 12.4 ± 8.4 versus 14.2 ± 11.2 ng/ml	[80]
	6/6	900 mg/14 days	AUC = 565 ± 121 versus 262 ± 71 ng·h/ml CL/F = 3.7 ± 0 9 versus 8.4 ± 3.2 l/h $t_{1/2}$ = 12.4 ± 3.9 versus 6.0 ± 2.4 h C_{max} = 34 ± 9 versus 31 ± 7 ng/ml	[106]
	18/10	120 mg/10 days	Single dose AUC = 149 (109–272) versus 177 (129–301) μg·h/l C_{max} = 14.1 (10.8–29.9) versus 16.4 (8.4–26.1) μg/l t_{max} = 1.0 (0.6–3.0) versus 1.0 (0.5–3.9) h $t_{1/2}$ = 11.8 (7.8–37.6) versus 12.2 (8.6–26.4) h Repeated dose (change, %) AUC = 1.2 (−40–54) versus 14.2 (−23–43) C_{max} = −0.6 (−7.9–15.5) versus 0.4 (−15.1–7.3) $t_{1/2}$ = 0.8 (−15.5–14.8) versus 1.5 (−3.6–16.4)	[64]
Amitriptyline	3/9	900 mg/14 days	AUC = 709 ± 118 versus 555 ± 76 μg·h/l C_{max} = 69.8 ± 11.8 versus 54.1 ± 7.4 μg/l	[65]
Atorvastatin	10/6	600 mg/4 weeks	ND	[107]
Carbamazepine	5/3	900 mg/2 weeks	AUC = 142.4 ± 12.9 versus 143.8 ± 27.2 mg·h/l CL/F = 2.8 ± 0.3 versus 2.9 ± 0.6 l/h C_{max} = 7.2 ± 1.0 versus 7.6 ± 1.3 mg/l	[108]
Caffeine	7	120 mg/10 days	AUC = 11.1 (4.4–23.4) versus 10.7 (5.9–20.9) mg·h/l C_{max} = 2.3 (0.9–3.1) versus 2.3 (1.4–3.3) mg/l $t_{1/2}$ = 3.5 (1.7–6.4) versus 3.8 (1.0–7.1) h AUC = −1.5 (−4.2–0.4) versus −0.3 (5.9–6.3) mg·h/l C_{max} = −0.3 (−1.9–0.5) versus 0.1 (−1.3–0.7) mg/l $t_{1/2}$ = −0.7 (−5.9–0.8) versus 0.3 (−5.1–4.2) h	[64]

(*Continued*)

Table 21.8 (*Continued*)

Compound	Male/female	Dose/day	Pharmacokinetic parameters without St John's Wort versus with St John's Wort	Reference
	7/5	900 mg/1 day	AUC = 39.1 ± 24.8 versus 42.5 ± 41.5 mg·h/l CL/F = 5.1 ± 2.0 versus 4.7 ± 2.3 l/h C_{max} = 4.3 ± 1.4 versus 4.2 ± 1.7 mg/l $t_{1/2}$ = 5.1 ± 4.0 versus 6.3 ± 3.8 h	[78]
	7/5	900 mg/14 days	AUC = 39.1 ± 24.8 versus 37.1 ± 23.6 mg·h/l CL/F = 5.1 ± 2.0 versus 5.4 ± 2.5 l/h C_{max} = 4.3 ± 1.4 versus 3.8 ± 1.1 mg/l $t_{1/2}$ = 5.1 ± 4.0 versus 6.1 ± 4.0 h	[78]
	8/8	900 mg/14 days	17 1-methylxanthine (MX)/137MX (saliva) 0.54 (0.24–0.63) versus 0.54 (0.26–0.91) (5-acetylamino-6-formylamino-3-methyl uracil (AFMU) + 1MX + 1 1-methyluric acid (MU))/17MU (urine) 3.5 (1.8–5.3) versus 3.8 (2.0–6.5)	[69]
	12/0	900/14 days	17X/137X *2C19*1/*1* = 0.49 ± 0.18 versus 0.43 ± 0.13 *2C19*2/*2 and *3* = 0.36 ± 0.08 versus 0.36 ± 0.09	[109]
	6/6	900 mg/28 days	ND	[71]
	6/6	900 mg/28 days	paraxanthine/caffeine 0.526 (0.315–0.736) versus 0.520 (0.364–0.676)	[72]
Chlorzoxazone	6/6	900 mg/28 days	ND	[71]
	6/6	900 mg/28 days	hydroxyl chlorzoxazone (OH-CZX)/chlorzoxazone (CZX) 0.393 (0.295–0.491) versus 0.496 (0.378–0.613)	[72]
Cyclosporine	10/10	900 mg/12 days	C_{max} = 1123 ± 162 versus 805 ± 185 ng/ml CL/F = 728 ± 195 versus 1155 ± 236 ml/min $t_{1/2}$ = 3.9 ± 0.6 versus 3.8 ± 1.0 h	[110]
	9/1 (renal transplants)	900 mg/14 days	high hyperforin AUC = 3473 ± 715 versus 1671 ± 313 ng·h/ml C_{max} = 979 ± 199 versus 562 ± 117 ng/ml low hyperforin AUC = 3333 ± 699 versus 3110 ± 527 ng·h/ml C_{max} = 1001 ± 286 versus 894 ± 187 ng/ml	[73]

Debrisoquine	6/6	900 mg/28 days	ND	[71]
	6/6	900 mg/28 days	4-hydroxydebrisoquine (HDEB)/(HDEB + DEB) 0.623 (0.499–0.746) versus 0.634 (0.520–0.748)	[72]
	8/8	900 mg/14 days	HDEB/(HDEB + debrisoquine (DEB)) 0.606 (0.522–0.691) versus 0.620 (0.537–0.703)	[74]
Dextromethorphan	8/5	900 mg/1 day	dextromethorphan (DEM)/dextrorphan (DOR) 0.42 ± 0.85 versus 0.62 ± 1.35	[78]
	8/5	900 mg/14 days	DEM/DOR 0.42 ± 0.85 versus 0.59 ± 0.59	[78]
	4/9	900 mg/14 days	ND	[76]
	6/6	900 mg/14 days	DEM/DOR 0.006 ± 0.010 versus 0.014 ± 0.025	[106]
	4/3	900 mg/3 days	$\log_{10}$ DMR −2.24 ± 0.82 versus −2.50 ± 0.69	[80]
	8/8	900 mg/14 days	DOR/DEM 485 (66–1226) versus 432 (157–1110)	[69]
Digoxin	13/12	900 mg/10 days	ND	[77]
	96	0.5–4.0 g/14 days	*Hypericum* powder 4 g/day AUC = 31.4 ± 5.6 versus 22.9 ± 4.0 ng·h/ml C_{max} = 3.22 ± 0.40 versus 2.03 ± 0.5 ng/ml *Hypericum* powder 2 g/day AUC = 32.9 ± 3.1 versus 27.1 ± 2.7 ng·h/ml C_{max} = 3.47 ± 0.2 versus 2.75 ± 0.60 ng/ml *Hypericum* powder 1 g/day AUC = 30.2 ± 4.2 versus 29.7 ± 5.7 ng·h/ml C_{max} = 3.53 ± 0.7 versus 3.25 ± 0.70 ng/ml *Hypericum* powder 0.5 g/day AUC = 29.1 ± 3.1 versus 29.3 ± 3.2 ng·h/ml C_{max} = 2.79 ± 0.5 versus 3.21 ± 0.60 ng/ml LI 160 AUC = 31.0 ± 0.4 versus 23.3 ± 1.8 ng·h/ml C_{max} = 3.17 ± 0.4 versus 2.0 ± 0.2 ng/ml ZE117 AUC = 34.5 ± 4.4 versus 32.6 ± 4.8 ng·h/ml C_{max} = 3.43 ± 0.59 versus 3.31 ± 0.69 ng/ml	[111]

(Continued)

Table 21.8 (*Continued*)

Compound	Male/female	Dose/day	Pharmacokinetic parameters without St John's Wort versus with St John's Wort	Reference
	15/13	120 mg/10 days	AUC = 24.2 (12.5–34.5) versus 22.0 (11.7–39.0) ng·h/ml C_{max} = 2.1 (1.3–2.8) versus 1.9 (1.1–3.3) ng/ml AUC = 6.2 (−1.0–16.6) versus 3.5 (0.5–11.5) ng·h/ml C_{max} = 0.5 (1.3–2.8) versus 0.2 (−0.6–0.8) ng/ml	[64]
	9/9	900 mg/14 days	ND	[74]
	8/0	900 mg/14 days	ND	[112]
Fexofenadine	9/3	900 mg/1 day	AUC = 965 ± 325 versus 1261 ± 507 μg·h/l CL/F = 77 ± 23 versus 62 ± 26 l/h C_{max} = 163 ± 43 versus 236 ± 96 μg/l $t_{1/2}$ = 3.5 ± 0.9 versus 3.6 ± 1.6 h	[75]
Gliclazide	9/3	900 mg/14 days	AUC = 965 ± 325 versus 871 ± 447 μg·h/l CL/F = 77 ± 23 versus 91 ± 32 l/h C_{max} = 163 ± 43 versus 154 ± 75 μg/l $t_{1/2}$ = 3.5 ± 0.9 versus 3.7 ± 1.2 h	[75]
	10/10	900 mg/12 days	C_{max} = 330 ± 144 versus 202 ± 101 ng/ml CL/F = 1961 ± 726 versus 3661 ± 1926 ml/min $t_{1/2}$ = 4.8 ± 1.3 versus 5.3 ± 2.0 h	[110]
	20/8	900 mg/10 days	CL/F = 77 ± 34 versus 132 ± 64 l/h	[83]
	15/6	900 mg/15 days	AUC = 67.2 (48.6–85.7) versus 43.6 (33.9–53.2) μg·h/ml C_{max} = 4.5 (3.9–5.0) versus 3.5 (3.0–4.0) μg/ml $t_{1/2}$ = 10.3 (9.1–11.4) versus 8.7 (7.8–9.6) h CL/F = 1.5 (1.2–1.8) versus 2.2 (1.9–2.6) l/h	[84]
Imatinib	6/6	900 mg/14 days	AUC = 34.5 ± 9.5 versus 24.2 ± 7.0 μg·h/ml C_{max} = 2153 ± 491 versus 1840 ± 489 ng/ml $t_{1/2}$ = 12.8 ± 3.2 versus 9.0 ± 2.3 h CL/F = 12.5 ± 3.6 versus 17.9 ± 5.6 l/h	[85]
Indinavir	10	900 mg/14 days	AUC = 28.9 (13.4–36.7) versus 19.7 (10.7–25.0) μg·h/ml C_{max} = 1.80 (0/88–2.6) versus 1.28 (0.92–2.0) μg/ml $t_{1/2}$ = 13.5 (10.8–18.1) versus 10.7 (9.1–13.5) h	[86]
	6/2	900 mg/16 days	AUC = 30.8 ± 8.4 versus 12.3 ± 4.7 μg·h/ml C_{max} = 12.3 ± 4.1 versus 8.9 ± 3.4 μg/ml	[52]

Mephenytoin	12/0	900 mg/14 days	4-OH mephenytoin (μmol) *2C19*1/*1* = 36 3 ± 9.3 versus 92.4 ± 45.4 *2C19*2/*2 and *3* = 26.5 ± 13.3 versus 28.0 ± 17.1	[109]
Mycophenolic acid	6/4	600 mg/14 days	AUC = 69.9 (56–81.7) versus 73.2 (54.8–86.6) ng·h/ml C_{max} = 19.7 (17.9–24.4) versus 19.8 (14.2–24.1) μg/ml	[113]
Midazolam	8/5	900 mg/1 day	intravenously AUC = 103.3 ± 42.5 versus 96.1 ± 38.1 μg·h/l CL = 34.2 ± 10.8 versus 37.3 ± 12.5 l/h $t_{1/2}$ = 3.1 ± 0.7 versus 2.9 ± 0.7 h *per os* AUC = 41.1 ± 34.5 versus 32.6 ± 23.5 μg·h/l C_{max} = 13.4 ± 6.3 versus 9.0 ± 4.0 μg/l CL/F = 121.8 ± 70.7 versus 152.8 ± 69.3 l/h $t_{1/2}$ = 0.75 (0.5–0.75) versus 1.0 (0.5–1.5) h	[78]
	8/5	900 mg/14 days	intravenously AUC = 103.3 ± 42.5 versus 81.2 ± 27.8 μg·h/l CL = 34.2 ± 10.8 versus 43.6 ± 15.8 l/h $t_{1/2}$ = 3.1 ± 0.7 versus 2.6 ± 0.6 h *per os* AUC = 41.1 ± 34.5 versus 19.6 ± 9.9 μg·h/l C_{max} = 13.4 ± 6 8 versus 7.7 ± 4.1 μg/l CL/F = 121.8 ± 70.7 versus 254.4 ± 127.8 l/h	[78]
	6/6	900 mg/28 days	ND	[71]
	10/10	900 mg/12 days	intravenously $t_{1/2}$ = 3.2 ± 1.4 versus 2.6 ± 1.0 h *per os* CL/F = 1182 ± 346 versus 3063 ± 809 ml/min C_{max} = 20.2 ± 6.6 versus 9.6 ± 3.2 ng/ml	[110]

(*Continued*)

Table 21.8 (Continued)

Compound	Male/female	Dose/day	Pharmacokinetic parameters without St John's Wort versus with St John's Wort	Reference
	0/12	900 mg/21 days	intravenously AUC = 93.2 ± 28.2 versus 87.5 ± 17.5 μg·h/l CL = 37.7 ± 11.3 versus 39.0 ± 10.3 l/h $t_{1/2}$ = 3.9 ± 1.1 versus 3.5 ± 1.1 h *per os* AUC = 68.3 ± 74.2 versus 40.0 ± 27.4 μg·h/l C_{max} = 1.40 ± 9.5 versus 11.1 ± 4.0 μg/l $t_{1/2}$ = 2.7 ± 0.6 versus 2.0 ± 0.6 h CL = 109.2 ± 47.9 versus 166.7 ± 81.3 h	[114]
	6/6	900 mg/28 days	hydroxymidazolam (OH-MDZ)/midazolam (MDZ) 0.379 (0.250–0.507) versus 0.914 (0.633–1.195)	[72]
	20/8	900 mg/10 days	intravenously CL = 16.4 ± 4.9 versus 24.5 ± 5.5 l/h *per os* CL = 88 ± 34 versus 248 ± 108 l/h	[83]
	42/0	14 days	*Hypericum* 2.7 g/day (ratio SJW/control) AUC = 0.79 (0.70–0.87) C_{max} = 0.61 (0.30–0.92) $t_{1/2}$ = 1.01 (0.73–1.28) *Hypericum* 1.8 g/day (ratio SJW/control) AUC = 0.62 (0.47–0.77) C_{max} = 0.70 (0.58–0.82) $t_{1/2}$ = 0.89 (0.81–0.96) *Hypericum* 1.2 g/day (ratio SJW/control) AUC = 0.68 (0.58–0.78) C_{max} = 0.66 (0.39–0.92) *Hypericum* 0.6 g/day (ratio SJW/control) AUC = 0.78 (0.63–0.95) C_{max} = 1.09 (0.63–1.55)	[115]

	20/0	[illegible]/14 days	AUC = 116.5 ± 57.4 versus 99.3 ± 49.4 ng·ml/h C_{max} = 48.5 ± 29.8 versus 45.1 ± 29.0 ng/ml $t_{1/2}$ = 2.54 ± 0.73 versus 2.36 ± 0.59 h CL/F = 1224 ± 514 versus 1420 ± 541 ml/min	[116]
	12	900 mg/14 days	AUC = 84.4 ± 8.0 versus 87.6 ± 5.7 ng·h/ml C_{max} = 28.2 ± 2.5 versus 28.5 ± 2.3 ng/ml $t_{1/2}$ = 1.84 ± 0.18 versus 1.86 ± 0.14 h CL/F = 65.3 ± 8.4 versus 59.7 ± 3.8 l/h	[117]
Nifedipine	5/5	900 mg/14 days	AUC = 339.8 ± 154.2 versus 207.9 ± 111.7 μg·l/h C_{max} = 47.5 ± 15.4 versus 28.3 ± 6.6 μg/l $t_{1/2}$ = 7.7 ± 3.0 versus 7.2 ± 2.3 h	[118]
Omeprazole	12/0	900 mg/14 days	*CYP2C19*1* AUC = 3.19 ± 0.85 versus 1.63 ± 0.40 μmol·l/h C_{max} = 1.64 ± 0.39 versus 0.76 ± 0.15 μmol/l *CYP2C19*2 and *3* AUC = 9.07 ± 1.72 versus 5.35 ± 0.93 μmol·l/h C_{max} = 4.23 ± 0.17 versus 2.64 ± 0.53 μmol/l	[109]
Oral contraceptive	0/12	900 mg/21 days	ethinylestradiol AUC = 2177 ± 1543 versus 1661 ± 1324 ng·h/l C_{max} = 97.3 ± 74.6 versus 103.6 ± 78.9 ng/l $t_{1/2}$ = 23.4 ± 19.5 versus 12.2 ± 7.1 h CL = 63.3 ± 71.6 versus 93.1 ± 127.9 l/h norethindrone AUC = 131.8 ± 35.1 versus 118.3 ± 41.1 ng·h/l C_{max} = 17.4 ± 5.1 versus 16.4 ± 5.2 ng/l $t_{1/2}$ = 12.6 ± 7.2 versus 12.1 ± 4.9 h CL = 8.2 ± 2.7 versus 9.5 ± 3.4 l/h	[114]

(Continued)

Table 21.8 (*Continued*)

Compound	Male/female	Dose/day	Pharmacokinetic parameters without St John's Wort versus with St John's Wort	Reference
	0/18	900 mg/21 days	ethinylestradiol cycle A AUC = 436.6 ± 185.4 versus 393.9124.8 pg·h/ml C_{max} = 53.7 ± 15.4 versus 53.2 ± 12.3 pg/ml $t_{1/2}$ = 45.5 ± 87.1 versus 23.4 ± 13.5 h cycle B AUC = 436.6 ± 185.4 versus 437.3 ± 137.2 pg·h/ml C_{max} = 53.7 ± 15.4 versus 55.6 ± 13.9 pg/ml $t_{1/2}$ = 45.5 ± 87.1 versus 36.2 ± 64.8 h 3-ketodesogestrel cycle A AUC = 31.2 ± 13.3 versus 17.7 ± 6.4 pg·h/ml C_{max} = 3.6 ± 1.3 versus 3.0 ± 0.9 pg/ml $t_{1/2}$ = 25.8 ± 7.8 versus 15.9 ± 10.1 h cycle B AUC = 31.2 ± 13.3 versus 18.4 ± 8.4 pg·h/ml C_{max} = 3.6 ± 1.3 versus 2.9 ± 1.0 pg/ml $t_{1/2}$ = 25.8 ± 7.8 versus 16.5 ± 7.4 h	[119]
	0/16	900 mg/8 weeks	norethindrone AUC = 113.2 (91.3–150.6) versus 98.9 (78.6–124.9) ng·h/ml C_{max} = 14.9 (12.2–18.4) versus 15.2 (10.9–19.3) ng/ml CL/F = 7.6 (6.6–9.8) versus 9.97 (8.0–12.0) l/h ethinylestradiol AUC = 994 (874–1118) versus 854 (712–1071) ng·h/ml C_{max} = 90 (82–98) versus 84 (73–98) ng/ml CL/F = 18.2 (15.4–20.9) versus 23.0 (18.7–26.6) l/h	[63]
Pravastatin	8/0	900 mg/14 days	AUC = 109.4 ± 17.4 versus 96.6 ± 13.4 ng·h/ml C_{max} = 36.5 ± 5.7 versus 30.8 ± 5.2 ng/ml	[120]
Prednisone	8/0	900 mg/28 days	AUC = 97 ± 23.5 versus 97.3 ± 11.0 µg·h/l C_{max} = 15.4 ± 4.19 versus 15.1 ± 3.42 µg/l $t_{1/2}$ = 3.85 ± 1.49 versus 5.11 ± 2.78 h CL/F = 2.48 ± 0.532 versus 2.21 ± 0.4991/h/kg	[121]

Quazepam	13/0	900 mg/14 days	AUC = 217 ± 28.7 versus 161 ± 25.2 ng·h/ml C_{max} = 30.5 ± 3.9 versus 21.8 ± 3.9 ng/ml $t_{1/2}$ = 8.8 ± 0.5 versus 8.4 ± 0.4 h	[122]
Simvastatin	8/0	900 mg/14 days	AUC = 11.9 ± 3.69 versus 5.77 ± 1.80 ng·h/ml C_{max} = 3.6 ± 1.0 versus 2.5 ± 1.7 ng/ml	[120]
Tacrolimus	6/4	900 mg/14 days	AUC = 180 (144–202) versus 75.9 (54.7–99.3) ng·h/ml C_{max} = 23 (17–28.3) versus 12.7 (9.5–16.6) ng/ml simvastatin hydroxy acid AUC = 14.64 ± 3.3 versus 5.54 ± 1.7 ng·h/ml	[113]
	8/2	900 mg/18 days	AUC = 306.9 ± 175.8 versus 198.7 ± 139.6 μg·h/l C_{max} = 29.0 ± 10.1 versus 22.4 ± 12.8 ng/ml $t_{1/2}$ = 29.6 ± 4.5 versus 27.8 ± 4.0 h CL/F = 349.0 ± 126.0 versus 586.4 ± 274.9 ml/h/kg	[123]
	9/0	900 mg/12 days	intravenously AUC = 1082 ± 228 versus 1007 ± 149 ng·h/ml $t_{1/2}$ = 6.4 ± 2.0 versus 5.5 ± 1.4 h CL = 485 ± 125 versus 506 ± 77 ml/min *per os* AUC = 944 ± 488 versus 651 ± 406 ng·h/ml C_{max} = 115.3 ± 64.6 versus 90.8 ± 64.4 ng/ml $t_{1/2}$ = 7.5 ± 2.4 versus 6.1 ± 3.1 h CL/F = 1254 ± 1057 versus 2423 ± 2434 ml/min	[124]
Theophylline	12/0	900 mg/15 days	AUC = 176.9 ± 34.0 versus 171.1 ± 25.7 μg·h/ml C_{max} = 7.5 ± 1.0 versus 7.4 ± 1.1 μg/ml $t_{1/2}$ = 9.7 ± 1.4 versus 9.1 ± 1.3 h CL/F = 0.037 ± 0.009 versus 0.038 ± 0.009 l/h/kg	[125]
Tolbutamide	8/5	900 mg/1 day	AUC = 684.1 ± 239.6 versus 678.9 ± 277 mg·h/l C_{max} = 51.0 ± 10.7 versus 49.6 ± 7.9 mg/l $t_{1/2}$ = 9.2 ± 2.2 versus 9.5 ± 3.2 h CL/F = 0.73 ± 0.26 versus 0.78 ± 0.25 l/h	[78]
Verapamil	8/5	900 mg/14 days	AUC = 684.1 ± 239.6 versus 678.5 ± 303.9 mg·h/l C_{max} = 51.0 ± 10.7 versus 51.4 ± 9.5 mg/l $t_{1/2}$ = 9.2 ± 2.2 versus 8.5 ± 3.5 h CL/F = 0.73 ± 0.26 versus 0.74 ± 0.32 l/h	[78]

(Continued)

Table 21.8 (*Continued*)

Compound	Male/female	Dose/day	Pharmacokinetic parameters without St John's Wort versus with St John's Wort	Reference
	8/0	900 mg/14 days	*R*-verapamil AUC = 2406 ± 1695 versus 420 ± 239 ng·ml/min C_{max} = 9.4 ± 7.0 versus 1.9 ± 1.3 ng/ml $t_{1/2}$ = 212 ± 36 versus 219 ± 66 min *S*-verapamil AUC = 413 ± 316 versus 56 ± 32 ng·ml/min C_{max} = 1.5 ± 1.3 versus 0.2 ± 0.1 ng/ml $t_{1/2}$ = 301 ± 119 versus 309 ± 179 h	[126]
Voriconazole	16/0	900 mg/1 day	AUC = 23.5 ± 15.6 versus 25.2 ± 16.2 μg·h/ml C_{max} = 2.56 ± 0.56 versus 3.13 ± 0.91 μg/ml $t_{1/2}$ = 8.18 ± 4.73 versus 6.37 ± 2.45 h CL/F = 390 ± 192 versus 371 ± 215 ml/min	[127]
	16/0	900 mg/14 days	AUC = 23.5 ± 15.6 versus 9.63 ± 6.03 μg·h/ml C_{max} = 2.56 ± 0.56 versus 1.87 ± 0.75 μg/ml $t_{1/2}$ = 8.18 ± 4.73 versus 4.95 ± 1.34 h CL/F = 390 ± 192 versus 952 ± 524 ml/min	[127]
Warfarin	12/0	2 weeks	*S*-warfarin AUC = 65.4 ± 13.8 versus 47.7 ± 8.3 μg·h/ml C_{max} = 1.89 ± 0.26 versus 1.82 ± 0.34 μg/l $t_{1/2}$ = 31.7 ± 4.5 versus 25.1 ± 4.3 h CL/F = 198 ± 38 versus 270 ± 44 ml/min *R*-warfarin AUC = 120.9 ± 32.9 versus 91.1 ± 15.4 μg·h/ml C_{max} = 1.92 ± 0.32 versus 1.84 ± 0.36 μg/l $t_{1/2}$ = 51.7 ± 9.6 versus 40.3 ± 3.9 h CL/F = 110 ± 25 versus 142 ± 29 ml/min	[128]

References

1 Nahrstedt, A. and Butterweck, V. (1997) Biologically active and other chemical constituents of the herb of *Hypericum perforatum* L. *Pharmacopsychiatry*, **30** (Suppl. 2), 129–134.

2 Butterweck, V. and Schmidt, M. (2007) St. John's wort: role of active compounds for its mechanism of action and efficacy. *Wien. Med. Wochenschr.*, **157**, 356–361.

3 Butterweck, V. (2003) Mechanism of action of St John's wort in depression: what is known? *CNS Drugs*, **17**, 539–562.

4 Saller, R., Melzer, J., and Reichling, J. (2003) [St. John's Wort (*Hypericum perforatum*): a plurivalent raw material for traditional and modern therapies]. *Forsch. Komplementarmed. Klass. Naturheilkd.*, **10** (Suppl. 1), 33–40.

5 Gaedcke, F. (2003) [The example: St. John's wort. Manufacturing and quality aspects of plant extracts]. *Pharm. Unserer Zeit*, **32**, 192–201.

6 Greeson, J.M., Sanford, B., and Monti, D.A. (2001) St. John's wort (*Hypericum perforatum*): a review of the current pharmacological, toxicological, and clinical literature. *Psychopharmacology*, **153**, 402–414.

7 Council of Europe (2001) *European Pharmacopoeia*, 6th edn, Council of Europe, Strasbourg, France.

8 Borrelli, F. and Izzo, A.A. (2009) Herb–drug interactions with St John's wort (*Hypericum perforatum*): an update on clinical observations. *AAPS J.*, **11**, 710–727.

9 Suzuki, O., Katsumata, Y., Oya, M., Bladt, S., and Wagner, H. (1984) Inhibition of monoamine oxidase by hypericin. *Planta Med.*, **50**, 272–274.

10 Demisch, L., Holzl, J., and Gollnik, B. (1989) Identification of selective MAO-type-A inhibitors in *Hypericum perforatum* L. (Hyperforat). *Pharmacopsychiatry*, **22**, 194.

11 Thiede, H.M. and Walper, A. (1994) Inhibition of MAO and COMT by hypericum extracts and hypericin. *J. Geriatr. Psychiatry Neurol.*, **7** (Suppl. 1), S54–S56.

12 Bennett, D.A., Jr, Phun, L., Polk, J.F., Voglino, S.A., Zlotnik, V., and Raffa, R.B. (1998) Neuropharmacology of St. John's Wort (hypericum). *Ann. Pharmacother.*, **32**, 1201–1208.

13 Bracher, A. (2001) Trial on HYP611 confirms effectiveness [HYP611 – Studie bestätigt Wirksamkeit]. *Ärztliche Praxis*, **51** (Suppl.), 3–4.

14 Gastpar, M., Singer, A., and Zeller, K. (2006) Comparative efficacy and safety of a once-daily dosage of hypericum extract STW3-VI and citalopram in patients with moderate depression: a double-blind, randomised, multicentre, placebo-controlled study. *Pharmacopsychiatry*, **39**, 66–75.

15 HDTSG (2002) Effect of *Hypericum perforatum* (St John's wort) in major depressive disorder: a randomized controlled trial. *JAMA*, **287**, 1807–1814.

16 Cott, J.M. (1997) *In vitro* receptor binding and enzyme inhibition by *Hypericum perforatum* extract. *Pharmacopsychiatry*, **30** (Suppl. 2), 108–112.

17 Nathan, P.J. (2001) *Hypericum perforatum* (St John's Wort): a non-selective reuptake inhibitor? A review of the recent advances in its pharmacology. *J. Psychopharmacol.*, **15**, 47–54.

18 Kalb, R., Trautmann-Sponsel, R.D., and Kieser, M. (2001) Efficacy and tolerability of hypericum extract WS 5572 versus placebo in mildly to moderately depressed patients. A randomized double-blind multicenter clinical trial. *Pharmacopsychiatry*, **34**, 96–103.

19 Kasper, S., Anghelescu, I.G., Szegedi, A., Dienel, A., and Kieser, M. (2006) Superior efficacy of St John's wort extract WS 5570 compared to placebo in patients with major depression: a randomized, double-blind, placebo-controlled, multi-center trial (ISRCTN77277298). *BMC Med.*, **4**, 14.

20 Hansgen, K. and Vesper, J. (1996) Antidepressive Wirksamkeit eines

hochdosierten *Hypericum*-Extraktes. *Munchener Medizinische Wochenschift.*, **138**, 29–33.

21 Laakmann, G., Schule, C., Baghai, T., and Kieser, M. (1998) St. John's wort in mild to moderate depression: the relevance of hyperforin for the clinical efficacy. *Pharmacopsychiatry*, **31** (Suppl. 1), 54–59.

22 Lecrubier, Y., Clerc, G., Didi, R., and Kieser, M. (2002) Efficacy of St. John's wort extract WS 5570 in major depression: a double-blind, placebo-controlled trial. *Am. J. Psychiatry*, **159**, 1361–1366.

23 Philipp, M., Kohnen, R., and Hiller, K.O. (1999) *Hypericum* extract versus imipramine or placebo in patients with moderate depression: randomised multicentre study of treatment for eight weeks. *BMJ*, **319**, 1534–1538.

24 Schrader, E., Meier, B., and Brattstrom, A. (1998) *Hypericum* treatment of mild moderate depression in a placebo-controlled study. A prospective, double-blind, randomized, placebo-controlled, multicentre study. *Hum. Psychopharmacol.*, **13**, 163–169.

25 Volz, H.P. and Laux, P. (2000) Potential treatment for subthreshold and mild depression: a comparison of St. John's wort extracts and fluoxetine. *Compr. Psychiatry*, **41** (Suppl. 1), 133–137.

26 Witte, B., Harrer, G., Kaptan, T., Podzuweit, H., and Schmidt, U. (1995) [Treatment of depressive symptoms with a high concentration hypericum preparation. A multicenter placebo controlled double-blind study]. *Fortschr. Med.*, **113**, 404–408.

27 Woelk, H. (2000) Comparison of St John's wort and imipramine for treating depression: randomised controlled trial. *BMJ*, **321**, 536–539.

28 Lavie, G., Mazur, Y., Lavie, D., and Meruelo, D. (1995) The chemical and biological properties of hypericin – a compound with a broad spectrum of biological activities. *Med. Res. Rev.*, **15**, 111–119.

29 Hadjur, C., Richard, M.J., Parat, M.O., Jardon, P., and Favier, A. (1996) Photodynamic effects of hypericin on lipid peroxidation and antioxidant status in melanoma cells. *Photochem. Photobiol.*, **64**, 375–381.

30 Behnke, K., Jensen, G.S., Graubaum, H.J., and Gruenwald, J. (2002) *Hypericum perforatum* versus fluoxetine in the treatment of mild to moderate depression. *Adv. Ther.*, **19**, 43–52.

31 Harrer, G., Schmidt, U., Kuhn, U., and Biller, A. (1999) Comparison of equivalence between the St. John's wort extract LoHyp-57 and fluoxetine. *Arzneimittelforschung*, **49**, 289–296.

32 Schrader, E. (2000) Equivalence of St John's wort extract (Ze 117) and fluoxetine: a randomized, controlled study in mild-moderate depression. *Int. Clin. Psychopharmacol.*, **15**, 61–68.

33 Szegedi, A., Kohnen, R., Dienel, A., and Kieser, M. (2005) Acute treatment of moderate to severe depression with hypericum extract WS 5570 (St John's wort): randomised controlled double blind non-inferiority trial versus paroxetine. *BMJ*, **330**, 503.

34 van Gurp, G., Meterissian, G.B., Haiek, L.N., McCusker, J., and Bellavance, F. (2002) St John's wort or sertraline? Randomized controlled trial in primary care. *Can. Fam. Physician*, **48**, 905–912.

35 Tang, J., Colacino, J.M., Larsen, S.H., and Spitzer, W. (1990) Virucidal activity of hypericin against enveloped and non-enveloped DNA and RNA viruses. *Antiviral Res.*, **13**, 313–325.

36 Hu, D., Gao, Y., Shao, C., Feng, Q., and Wang, R. (2008) Study on hypericin in *Hypericum perforatum* L and its interactions with human immunodeficiency virus-1 reverse transcriptase. *J. Mol. Sci.*, **24**, 280–283.

37 Cui, Y., Gurley, B., Ang, C.Y., and Leakey, J. (2002) Determination of hyperforin in human plasma using solid-phase extraction and high-performance liquid chromatography with ultraviolet detection. *J. Chromatogr. B*, **780**, 129–135.

38 Weiser, D. (1991) Pharmacokinetic von Hypericin nach oraler Einnahme des Johanniskraut Extraktes LI160. *Nervenheilkunde*, **10**, 318–319.

39 Graefe, E.U., Wittig, J., Mueller, S., Riethling, A.K., Uehleke, B., Drewelow, B., Pforte, H., Jacobasch, G., Derendorf,

H., and Veit, M. (2001) Pharmacokinetics and bioavailability of quercetin glycosides in humans. *J. Clin. Pharmacol.*, **41**, 492–499.

40 Day, A.J., Mellon, F., Barron, D., Sarrazin, G., Morgan, M.R., and Williamson, G. (2001) Human metabolism of dietary flavonoids: identification of plasma metabolites of quercetin. *Free Radic. Res.*, **35**, 941–952.

41 Castano, A., Demidova, T., and Hamblin, M. (2004) Mechanisms in photodynamic therapy: part one–photosensitizers, photochemistry and cellular localization. *Photodiagn. Photodyn. Ther.*, **1**, 279–293.

42 de Witte, P., Agostinis, P., Van Lint, J., Merlevede, W., and Vandenheede, J.R. (1993) Inhibition of epidermal growth factor receptor tyrosine kinase activity by hypericin. *Biochem. Pharmacol.*, **46**, 1929 1936.

43 Kubin, A., Wierrani, F., Burner, U., Alth, G., and Grunberger, W. (2005) Hypericin–the facts about a controversial agent. *Curr. Pharm. Des.*, **11**, 233–253.

44 Ishii, K., Furuta, T., and Kasuya, Y. (2001) Determination of rutin in human plasma by high-performance liquid chromatography utilizing solid-phase extraction and ultraviolet detection. *J. Chromatogr. B*, **759**, 161–168.

45 Komoroski, B.J., Zhang, S., Cai, H., Hutzler, J.M., Frye, R., Tracy, T.S., Strom, S.C., Lehmann, T., Ang, C.Y., Cui, Y.Y., and Venkataramanan, R. (2004) Induction and inhibition of cytochromes P450 by the St. John's wort constituent hyperforin in human hepatocyte cultures. *Drug Metab. Dispos.*, **32**, 512–518.

46 Chaloupka, R., Obsil, T., Plasek, J., and Sureau, F. (1999) The effect of hypericin and hypocrellin-A on lipid membranes and membrane potential of 3T3 fibroblasts. *Biochim. Biophys. Acta*, **1418**, 39–47.

47 Miccoli, L., Beurdeley-Thomas, A., De Pinieux, G., Sureau, F., Oudard, S., Dutrillaux, B., and Poupon, M.F. (1998) Light-induced photoactivation of hypericin affects the energy metabolism of human glioma cells by inhibiting hexokinase bound to mitochondria. *Cancer Res.*, **58**, 5777–5786.

48 Thomas, C., MacGill, R.S., Miller, G.C., and Pardini, R.S. (1992) Photoactivation of hypericin generates singlet oxygen in mitochondria and inhibits succinoxidase. *Photochem. Photobiol.*, **55**, 47–53.

49 Ruschitzka, F., Meier, P.J., Turina, M., Luscher, T.F., and Noll, G. (2000) Acute heart transplant rejection due to Saint John's wort. *Lancet*, **355**, 548–549.

50 Roby, C.A., Anderson, G.D., Kantor, E., Dryer, D.A., and Burstein, A.H. (2000) St John's Wort: effect on CYP3A4 activity. *Clin. Pharmacol. Ther.*, **67**, 451–457.

51 L'Homme, R.F., Dijkema, T., van der Ven, A.J., and Burger, D.M. (2006) Brief report: enzyme inducers reduce elimination half-life after a single dose of nevirapine in healthy women. *J. Acquir. Immune Defic. Syndr.*, **43**, 193–196.

52 Piscitelli, S.C., Burstein, A.H., Chaitt, D., Alfaro, R.M., and Falloon, J. (2000) Indinavir concentrations and St John's wort. *Lancet*, **355**, 547–548.

53 Prost, N., Tichadou, L., Rodor, F., Nguyen, N., David, J.M., and Jean-Pastor, M.J. (2000) [St. Johns wort–venlafaxine interaction]. *Presse Med.*, **29**, 1285–1286.

54 Bon, S., Hartmann, K., and Kubn, M. (1999) Johanniskraut: ein enzym induktor? *Schweitzer Apothekerzeitung*, **16**, 535–536.

55 Staffeldt, B., Kerb, R., Brockmoller, J., Ploch, M., and Roots, I. (1994) Pharmacokinetics of hypericin and pseudohypericin after oral intake of the *Hypericum perforatum* extract LI 160 in healthy volunteers. *J. Geriatr. Psychiatry Neurol.*, **7** (Suppl. 1), S47–S53.

56 Brockmoller, J., Reum, T., Bauer, S., Kerb, R., Hubner, W.D., and Roots, I. (1997) Hypericin and pseudohypericin: pharmacokinetics and effects on photosensitivity in humans. *Pharmacopsychiatry*, **30** (Suppl. 2), 94–101.

57 Kerb, R., Brockmoller, J., Staffeldt, B., Ploch, M., and Roots, I. (1996) Single-dose and steady-state

pharmacokinetics of hypericin and pseudohypericin. *Antimicrob. Agents Chemother.*, **40**, 2087–2093.
58 Noldner, M. and Schotz, K. (2002) Rutin is essential for the antidepressant activity of *Hypericum perforatum* extracts in the forced swimming test. *Planta Med.*, **68**, 577–580.
59 Beer, A.M. and Ostermann, T. (2001) [St. John's wort: interaction with cyclosporine increases risk of rejection for the kidney transplant and raises daily cost of medication]. *Med. Klin.*, **96**, 480–483.
60 Erlund, I., Alfthan, G., Siren, H., Ariniemi, K., and Aro, A. (1999) Validated method for the quantitation of quercetin from human plasma using high-performance liquid chromatography with electrochemical detection. *J. Chromatogr. B*, **727**, 179–189.
61 Hollman, P.C., van Trijp, J.M., Buysman, M.N., van der Gaag, M.S., Mengelers, M.J., de Vries, J.H., and Katan, M.B. (1997) Relative bioavailability of the antioxidant flavonoid quercetin from various foods in man. *FEBS Lett.*, **418**, 152–156.
62 Wentworth, J., Agostini, M., Love, J., Schwabe, J., and Chatterjee, V. (2000) St John's wort, a herbal antidepressant, activates the steroid X receptor. *J. Endocrinol.*, **166**, 11–16.
63 Murphy, P.A., Kern, S.E., Stanczyk, F.Z., and Westhoff, C.L. (2005) Interaction of St. John's Wort with oral contraceptives: effects on the pharmacokinetics of norethindrone and ethinyl estradiol, ovarian activity and breakthrough bleeding. *Contraception*, **71**, 402–408.
64 Arold, G., Donath, F., Maurer, A., Diefenbach, K., Bauer, S., Henneicke-von Zepelin, H.H., Friede, M., and Roots, I. (2005) No relevant interaction with alprazolam, caffeine, tolbutamide, and digoxin by treatment with a low-hyperforin St John's wort extract. *Planta Med.*, **71**, 331–337.
65 Johne, A., Schmider, J., Brockmoller, J., Stadelmann, A.M., Stormer, E., Bauer, S., Scholler, G., Langheinrich, M., and Roots, I. (2002) Decreased plasma levels of amitriptyline and its metabolites on comedication with an extract from St. John's wort (*Hypericum perforatum*). *J. Clin. Psychopharmacol.*, **22**, 46–54.
66 Obach, R.S. (2000) Inhibition of human cytochrome P450 enzymes by constituents of St. John's Wort, an herbal preparation used in the treatment of depression. *J. Pharmacol. Exp. Ther.*, **294**, 88–95.
67 Ito, K., Iwatsubo, T., Kanamitsu, S., Ueda, K., Suzuki, H., and Sugiyama, Y. (1998) Prediction of pharmacokinetic alterations caused by drug–drug interactions: metabolic interaction in the liver. *Pharmacol. Rev.*, **50**, 387–412.
68 Hennessy, M., Kelleher, D., Spiers, J.P., Barry, M., Kavanagh, P., Back, D., Mulcahy, F., and Feely, J. (2002) St Johns wort increases expression of P-glycoprotein: implications for drug interactions. *Br. J. Clin. Pharmacol.*, **53**, 75–82.
69 Wenk, M., Todesco, L., and Krahenbuhl, S. (2004) Effect of St John's wort on the activities of CYP1A2, CYP3A4, CYP2D6, *N*-acetyltransferase 2, and xanthine oxidase in healthy males and females. *Br. J. Clin. Pharmacol.*, **57**, 495–499.
70 Whitten, D.L., Myers, S.P., Hawrelak, J.A., and Wohlmuth, H. (2006) The effect of St John's wort extracts on CYP3A: a systematic review of prospective clinical trials. *Br. J. Clin. Pharmacol.*, **62**, 512–526.
71 Gurley, B.J., Gardner, S.F., Hubbard, M.A., Williams, D.K., Gentry, W.B., Cui, Y., and Ang, C.Y. (2002) Cytochrome P450 phenotypic ratios for predicting herb–drug interactions in humans. *Clin. Pharmacol. Ther.*, **72**, 276–287.
72 Gurley, B.J., Gardner, S.F., Hubbard, M.A., Williams, D.K., Gentry, W.B., Cui, Y., and Ang, C.Y. (2005) Clinical assessment of effects of botanical supplementation on cytochrome P450 phenotypes in the elderly: St John's wort, garlic oil, *Panax ginseng* and *Ginkgo biloba*. *Drugs Aging*, **22**, 525–539.
73 Mai, I., Bauer, S., Perloff, E.S., Johne, A., Uehleke, B., Frank, B., Budde, K., and Roots, I. (2004) Hyperforin content determines the magnitude of the St John's wort–cyclosporine drug

interaction. *Clin. Pharmacol. Ther.*, **76**, 330–340.

74 Gurley, B.J., Swain, A., Hubbard, M.A., Williams, D.K., Barone, G., Hartsfield, F., Tong, Y., Carrier, D.J., Cheboyina, S., and Battu, S.K. (2008) Clinical assessment of CYP2D6-mediated herb–drug interactions in humans: effects of milk thistle, black cohosh, goldenseal, kava kava, St. John's wort, and Echinacea. *Mol. Nutr. Food Res.*, **52**, 755–763.

75 Wang, Z., Hamman, M.A., Huang, S.M., Lesko, L.J., and Hall, S.D. (2002) Effect of St John's wort on the pharmacokinetics of fexofenadine. *Clin. Pharmacol. Ther.*, **71**, 414–420.

76 Roby, C.A., Dryer, D.A., and Burstein, A.H. (2001) St. John's wort: effect on CYP2D6 activity using dextromethorphan–dextrorphan ratios. *J. Clin. Psychopharmacol.*, **21**, 530 532.

77 Johne, A., Brockmoller, J., Bauer, S., Maurer, A., Langheinrich, M., and Roots, I. (1999) Pharmacokinetic interaction of digoxin with an herbal extract from St John's wort (*Hypericum perforatum*). *Clin. Pharmacol. Ther.*, **66**, 338–345.

78 Wang, Z., Gorski, J.C., Hamman, M.A., Huang, S.M., Lesko, L.J., and Hall, S.D. (2001) The effects of St John's wort (*Hypericum perforatum*) on human cytochrome P450 activity. *Clin. Pharmacol. Ther.*, **70**, 317–326.

79 Ereshefsky, B., Gewertz, N., Lam, Y., Vega, L., and Ereshelsky, L. (1999) Determination of St. John's wort differential metabolismDetermination of St. John's wort differential metabolism at CYP2D6 and CYP3A4 using dextromethorphan probe methodology. *Proceedings of the 39th Annual Meeting of the New Clinical Drug Evaluation Unit, Boca Raton. FL*, poster 1301.

80 Markowitz, J.S., DeVane, C.L., Boulton, D.W., Carson, S.W., Nahas, Z., and Risch, S.C. (2000) Effect of St. John's wort (*Hypericum perforatum*) on cytochrome P-450 2D6 and 3A4 activity in healthy volunteers. *Life Sci.*, **66**, PL133–PL139.

81 Zhou, S.F., Zhou, Z.W., Li, C.G., Chen, X., Yu, X., Xue, C.C., and Herington, A. (2007) Identification of drugs that interact with herbs in drug development. *Drug Discov. Today*, **12**, 664–673.

82 Will-Shahab, L., Bauer, S., Kunter, U., Roots, I., and Brattstrom, A. (2009) St John's wort extract (Ze 117) does not alter the pharmacokinetics of a low-dose oral contraceptive. *Eur. J. Clin. Pharmacol.*, **65**, 287–294.

83 Xie, R., Tan, L.H., Polasek, E.C., Hong, C., Teillol-Foo, M., Gordi, T., Sharma, A., Nickens, D.J., Arakawa, T., Knuth, D.W., and Antal, E.J. (2005) CYP3A and P-glycoprotein activity induction with St. John's Wort in healthy volunteers from 6 ethnic populations. *J. Clin. Pharmacol.*, **45**, 352–356.

84 Xu, H., Williams, K.M., Liauw, W.S., Murray, M., Day, R.O., and McLachlan, A.J. (2008) Effects of St John's wort and CYP2C9 genotype on the pharmacokinetics and pharmacodynamics of gliclazide. *Br. J. Pharmacol.*, **153**, 1579–1586.

85 Frye, R.F., Fitzgerald, S.M., Lagattuta, T.F., Hruska, M.W., and Egorin, M.J. (2004) Effect of St John's wort on imatinib mesylate pharmacokinetics. *Clin. Pharmacol. Ther.*, **76**, 323–329.

86 Smith, P., Bullock, J.M., Booker, B.M., Haas, C.E., Berenson, C.S., and Jusko, W.J. (2004) The influence of St. John's wort on the pharmacokinetics and protein binding of imatinib mesylate. *Pharmacotherapy*, **24**, 1508–1514.

87 Miller, L. (1998) Herbal medicinals: selected clinical considerations focusing on known or potential drug–herb interactions. *Arch. Intern. Med.*, **158**, 2200–2211.

88 Fugh-Berman, A. (2000) Herb–drug interactions. *Lancet*, **355**, 134–138.

89 Yue, Q.Y., Bergquist, C., and Gerden, B. (2000) Safety of St John's wort (*Hypericum perforatum*). *Lancet*, **355**, 576–577.

90 de Maat, M., Hoetelmans, R., van Gorp, E., Meenhorst, P., Mulder, J., and Beijnen, J. (2001) Drug interaction between St John's wort and nevirapine. *AIDS*, **15**, 420–421.

91 Barnes, J., Anderson, L., and Philipson, J. (2001) St John's wort (*Hypericum perforatum* L.): a review of its chemistry,

pharmacology and clinical properties. *J. Pharm. Pharmacol.*, **53**, 583–600.

92 Lantz, M.S., Buchalter, E., and Giambanco, V. (1999) St. John's wort and antidepressant drug interactions in the elderly. *J. Geriatr. Psychiatry Neurol.*, **12**, 7–10.

93 Barbenel, D.M., Yusufi, B., O'Shea, D., and Bench, C.J. (2000) Mania in a patient receiving testosterone replacement postorchidectomy taking St John's wort and sertraline. *J. Psychopharmacol.*, **14**, 84–86.

94 Breidenbach, T., Kliem, V., Burg, M., Radermacher, J., Hoffmann, M.W., and Klempnauer, J. (2000) Profound drop of cyclosporin A whole blood trough levels caused by St. John's wort (*Hypericum perforatum*). *Transplantation*, **69**, 2229–2230.

95 Breidenbach, T., Hoffmann, M.W., Becker, T., Schlitt, H., and Klempnauer, J. (2000) Drug interaction of St John's wort with cyclosporin. *Lancet*, **355**, 1912.

96 Rey, J.M. and Walter, G. (1998) *Hypericum perforatum* (St John's wort) in depression: pest or blessing? *Med. J. Aust.*, **169**, 583–586.

97 Barone, G.W., Gurley, B.J., Ketel, B.L., Lightfoot, M.L., and Abul-Ezz, S.R. (2000) Drug interaction between St. John's wort and cyclosporine. *Ann. Pharmacother.*, **34**, 1013–1016.

98 Mai, I., Kruger, H., Budde, K., Johne, A., Brockmoller, J., Neumayer, H.H., and Roots, I. (2000) Hazardous pharmacokinetic interaction of Saint John's wort (*Hypericum perforatum*) with the immunosuppressant cyclosporin. *Int. J. Clin. Pharmacol. Ther.*, **38**, 500–502.

99 Karliova, M., Treichel, U., Malago, M., Frilling, A., Gerken, G., and Broelsch, C.E. (2000) Interaction of *Hypericum perforatum* (St. John's wort) with cyclosporin A metabolism in a patient after liver transplantation. *J. Hepatol.*, **33**, 853–855.

100 Mandelbaum, A., Pertzborn, F., Martin-Facklam, M., and Wiesel, M. (2000) Unexplained decrease of cyclosporin trough levels in a compliant renal transplant patient. *Nephrol. Dial. Transplant.*, **15**, 1473–1474.

101 Turton-Weeks, S.M., Barone, G.W., Gurley, B.J., Ketel, B.L., Lightfoot, M.L., and Abul-Ezz, S.R. (2001) St John's wort: a hidden risk for transplant patients. *Prog. Transplant.*, **11**, 116–120.

102 Ahmed, S.M., Banner, N.R., and Dubrey, S.W. (2001) Low cyclosporin A level due to Saint John's wort in heart transplant patients. *J. Heart Lung Transplant.*, **20**, 795.

103 Moschella, C. and Jaber, B.L. (2001) Interaction between cyclosporine and *Hypericum perforatum* (St. John's wort) after organ transplantation. *Am. J. Kidney Dis.*, **38**, 1105–1107.

104 Alscher, D.M. and Klotz, U. (2003) Drug interaction of herbal tea containing St. John's wort with cyclosporine. *Transpl. Int.*, **16**, 543–544.

105 Bolley, R., Zulke, C., Kammerl, M., Fischereder, M., and Kramer, B.K. (2002) Tacrolimus-induced nephrotoxicity unmasked by induction of the CYP3A4 system with St John's wort. *Transplantation*, **73**, 1009.

106 Markowitz, J.S., Donovan, J.L., DeVane, C.L., Taylor, R.M., Ruan, Y., Wang, J.S., and Chavin, K.D. (2003) Effect of St John's wort on drug metabolism by induction of cytochrome P450 3A4 enzyme. *JAMA*, **290**, 1500–1504.

107 Andren, L., Andreasson, A., and Eggertsen, R. (2007) Interaction between a commercially available St. John's wort product (Movina) and atorvastatin in patients with hypercholesterolemia. *Eur. J. Clin. Pharmacol.*, **63**, 913–916.

108 Burstein, A.H., Horton, R.L., Dunn, T., Alfaro, R.M., Piscitelli, S.C., and Theodore, W. (2000) Lack of effect of St John's Wort on carbamazepine pharmacokinetics in healthy volunteers. *Clin. Pharmacol. Ther.*, **68**, 605–612.

109 Wang, L.S., Zhu, B., Abd El-Aty, A.M., Zhou, G., Li, Z., Wu, J., Chen, G.L., Liu, J., Tang, Z.R., An, W., Li, Q., Wang, D., and Zhou, H.H. (2004) The influence of St John's Wort on CYP2C19 activity with respect to genotype. *J. Clin. Pharmacol.*, **44**, 577–581.

110 Dresser, G.K., Schwarz, U.I., Wilkinson, G.R., and Kim, R.B. (2003) Coordinate induction of both cytochrome P4503A and MDR1 by St John's wort in healthy

subjects. *Clin. Pharmacol. Ther.*, **73**, 41–50.

111 Mueller, S.C., Uehleke, B., Woehling, H., Petzsch, M., Majcher-Peszynska, J., Hehl, E.M., Sievers, H., Frank, B., Riethling, A.K., and Drewelow, B. (2004) Effect of St John's wort dose and preparations on the pharmacokinetics of digoxin. *Clin. Pharmacol. Ther.*, **75**, 546–557.

112 Durr, D., Stieger, B., Kullak-Ublick, G.A., Rentsch, K.M., Steinert, H.C., Meier, P.J., and Fattinger, K. (2000) St John's Wort induces intestinal P-glycoprotein/MDR1 and intestinal and hepatic CYP3A4. *Clin. Pharmacol. Ther.*, **68**, 598–604.

113 Mai, I., Stormer, E., Bauer, S., Kruger, H., Budde, K., and Roots, I. (2003) Impact of St John's wort treatment on the pharmacokinetics of tacrolimus and mycophenolic acid in renal transplant patients. *Nephrol. Dial. Transplant.*, **18**, 819–822.

114 Hall, S.D., Wang, Z., Huang, S.M., Hamman, M.A., Vasavada, N., Adigun, A.Q., Hilligoss, J.K., Miller, M., and Gorski, J.C. (2003) The interaction between St John's wort and an oral contraceptive. *Clin. Pharmacol. Ther.*, **74**, 525–535.

115 Mueller, S.C., Majcher-Peszynska, J., Uehleke, B., Klammt, S., Mundkowski, R.G., Miekisch, W., Sievers, H., Bauer, S., Frank, B., Kundt, G., and Drewelow, B. (2006) The extent of induction of CYP3A by St. John's wort varies among products and is linked to hyperforin dose. *Eur. J. Clin. Pharmacol.*, **62**, 29–36.

116 Mueller, S.C., Majcher-Peszynska, J., Mundkowski, R.G., Uehleke, B., Klammt, S., Sievers, H., Lehnfeld, R., Frank, B., Thurow, K., Kundt, G., and Drewelow, B. (2009) No clinically relevant CYP3A induction after St. John's wort with low hyperforin content in healthy volunteers. *Eur. J. Clin. Pharmacol.*, **65**, 81–87.

117 Imai, H., Kotegawa, T., Tsutsumi, K., Morimoto, T., Eshima, N., Nakano, S., and Ohashi, K. (2008) The recovery time-course of CYP3A after induction by St John's wort administration. *Br. J. Clin. Pharmacol.*, **65**, 701–707.

118 Wang, X.D., Li, J.L., Su, Q.B., Guan, S., Chen, J., Du, J., He, Y.W., Zeng, J., Zhang, J.X., Chen, X., Huang, M., and Zhou, S.F. (2009) Impact of the haplotypes of the human pregnane X receptor gene on the basal and St John's wort-induced activity of cytochrome P450 3A4 enzyme. *Br. J. Clin. Pharmacol.*, **67**, 255–261.

119 Pfrunder, A., Schiesser, M., Gerber, S., Haschke, M., Bitzer, J., and Drewe, J. (2003) Interaction of St John's wort with low-dose oral contraceptive therapy: a randomized controlled trial. *Br. J. Clin. Pharmacol.*, **56**, 683–690.

120 Sugimoto, K., Ohmori, M., Tsuruoka, S., Nishiki, K., Kawaguchi, A., Harada, K., Arakawa, M., Sakamoto, K., Masada, M., Miyamori, I., and Fujimura, A. (2001) Different effects of St John's wort on the pharmacokinetics of simvastatin and pravastatin. *Clin. Pharmacol. Ther.*, **70**, 518–524.

121 Bell, E.C., Ravis, W.R., Chan, H.M., and Lin, Y.J. (2007) Lack of pharmacokinetic interaction between St. John's wort and prednisone. *Ann. Pharmacother.*, **41**, 1819–1824.

122 Kawaguchi, A., Ohmori, M., Tsuruoka, S., Nishiki, K., Harada, K., Miyamori, I., Yano, R., Nakamura, T., Masada, M., and Fujimura, A. (2004) Drug interaction between St John's Wort and quazepam. *Br. J. Clin. Pharmacol.*, **58**, 403–410.

123 Hebert, M.F., Park, J.M., Chen, Y.L., Akhtar, S., and Larson, A.M. (2004) Effects of St. John's wort (*Hypericum perforatum*) on tacrolimus pharmacokinetics in healthy volunteers. *J. Clin. Pharmacol.*, **44**, 89–94.

124 Schwarz, U.I., Hanso, H., Oertel, R., Miehlke, S., Kuhlisch, E., Glaeser, H., Hitzl, M., Dresser, G.K., Kim, R.B., and Kirch, W. (2007) Induction of intestinal P-glycoprotein by St John's wort reduces the oral bioavailability of talinolol. *Clin. Pharmacol. Ther.*, **81**, 669–678.

125 Morimoto, T., Kotegawa, T., Tsutsumi, K., Ohtani, Y., Imai, H., and Nakano, S. (2004) Effect of St. John's wort on the pharmacokinetics of theophylline in healthy volunteers. *J. Clin. Pharmacol.*, **44**, 95–101.

126 Tannergren, C., Engman, H., Knutson, L., Hedeland, M., Bondesson, U., and Lennernas, H. (2004) St John's wort decreases the bioavailability of *R*- and *S*-verapamil through induction of the first-pass metabolism. *Clin. Pharmacol. Ther.*, **75**, 298–309.

127 Rengelshausen, J., Banfield, M., Riedel, K.D., Burhenne, J., Weiss, J., Thomsen, T., Walter-Sack, I., Haefeli, W.E., and Mikus, G. (2005) Opposite effects of short-term and long-term St John's wort intake on voriconazole pharmacokinetics. *Clin. Pharmacol. Ther.*, **78**, 25–33.

128 Jiang, X., Williams, K.M., Liauw, W.S., Ammit, A.J., Roufogalis, B.D., Duke, C.C., Day, R.O., and McLachlan, A.J. (2004) Effect of St John's wort and ginseng on the pharmacokinetics and pharmacodynamics of warfarin in healthy subjects. *Br. J. Clin. Pharmacol.*, **57**, 592–599.

22
Food Components and Supplements

Alexandr Parlesak

22.1
Introduction

The major part of food consists of chemical compounds that can be used for energy production, biological synthesis, or maintenance of metabolic processes by the host. These components are defined as nutrients, and can be categorized into macronutrients (proteins, carbohydrates, triglycerides, and alcohol), minerals, and micronutrients. The latter category comprises 13 vitamins and numerous trace elements. Both macro- and micronutrients can interact with enzyme systems related to xenobiotic metabolism either by regulation of their expression or direct interference with their enzymatic activity.

During food consumption, we ingest a wide range of xenobiotics, either as an original part of food (e.g., secondary plant metabolites such as flavonoids), or as contaminants that enter the food chain at different stages. For these components, a wide spectrum of biological effects was observed that ranges from health-threatening impacts (e.g., polycyclic aromatic amines acting as carcinogens) to health-protective effects (e.g., flavonoids ameliorating detrimental effects of mitochondrial oxidative stress). Secondary plant metabolites along with vitamins, specific types of macronutrients and live bacteria (probiotics) as well as substances promoting the growth of these bacteria (prebiotics) are added to food to achieve health effects exceeding its pure nutritional function. Therefore, several of these effects are mediated by enzyme systems involved in xenobiotic and drug metabolism, and in some cases this might lead to undesired interactions with medication. The supplements and contaminants can compete directly with drug oxidation, induce or suppress the expression of xenobiotic-metabolizing enzymes, change the bioavailability of drugs, and, in the case of live bacteria, bring in their own xenobiotic metabolism, including cytochrome P450 (CYP) activity. In numerous cases, nutrients, food contaminants, and secondary plant metabolites can themselves become substrates for xenobiotic-metabolizing enzymes, resulting in health-promoting or health-threatening products.

Metabolism of Drugs and Other Xenobiotics, First Edition. Edited by Pavel Anzenbacher, Ulrich M. Zanger.

This chapter focuses on how important components of our daily nutrition and supplements can interfere with xenobiotic metabolism, and how knowledge of this interaction might be exploited to avoid unwanted nutrition–drug interactions, but also to promote bioavailability of poorly absorbed drugs. Moreover, important mechanisms of direct interactions between compounds found in food (nutrients, secondary plant metabolites, and contaminants) and the host's xenobiotic metabolism are pointed out. As some of the health-promoting effects of secondary plant metabolites and vitamins are caused by antagonizing adverse mechanisms of natural or artificial contaminants of food, this chapter starts with the role of the host's xenometabolism in the detrimental effects of these contaminants.

22.2 Food Contaminants

22.2.1 Polycyclic Aromatic Hydrocarbons and Polycyclic Aromatic Amines

Since the ground-breaking study by Wattenberg *et al.* [1], it has become clear that polycyclic aromatic hydrocarbons (PAHs) such as benzo[*a*]pyrene, phenanthrene, and others can chemically modify DNA in the living cell and induce malignant lesions (i.e., in the intestine). CYP1 enzymes (comprising CYP1A1, 1A2, and 1B1) are considered as a relevant detoxication system for these carcinogens. Today, it is clear that CYP1A1 (together with CYP1B1 and some CYP3A enzymes) is the key enzyme in metabolizing PAHs [2], while CYP1A2 instead converts heterocyclic aromatic amines [3]. The expression of CYP1 is under control of the cytosolic aryl hydrocarbon receptor (AhR) [4], which heterodimerizes upon ligand (e.g., PAH, dioxin) binding with the AhR nuclear translocator (ARNT). This heterodimer forms a high-affinity DNA binding complex that aligns to specific target DNA sequences known as dioxin-responsive elements (DREs) in the regulatory areas of the responsive CYP1 genes [5]. This regulatory mechanism deserves special attention as it stands in contrast to the regulation of all other CYPs, which depend on heterodimerization of ligand-recognizing receptors with the retinoid X receptor (RXR).

A passionately discussed question has been whether rather an inhibition or an enhancement of CYP1 activity is desirable to prevent arylalkylation of DNA and to reduce the associated genotoxicity. Metabolic activation, which is the generation of reactive intermediates (epoxides) capable of binding to DNA, was considered for decades to be the key procarcinogenic process [6]. However, without the intermediate generation of DNA-reactive epoxides, the hydroxylated phase I metabolites cannot be converted by phase II enzymes, leading finally to detoxication of carcinogenic PAH [7]. The concept of "toxication" of PAHs and polycyclic aromatic amines (PAAs) seemed substantiated by studies with mice overexpressing CYP1A1, which were more susceptible to cancers and genotoxicity when the PAH was brought in direct contact with the corresponding organs instead of oral, systemic application [8]. However, benzo[*a*]pyrene feeding (125 mg/kg/day) results in much higher acute toxicity, lethality, and formation of benzo[*a*]pyrene–DNA adducts in the gastrointestinal tract, liver, and other organs of mice that are deficient for CYP1A1 (*Cyp1a1*$^{-/-}$ mice) compared to wild-type animals [9]. Hence, in the intact animal (and presumably also in humans), intestinal CYP1A1 activity seems important in elimination and detoxification of PAHs and PAAs, and is, in all likelihood, an important factor in cancer prevention, especially when the activity of phase II enzymes is taken into consideration.

Based on the findings mentioned above, an intentional inhibition of CYP1A by secondary plant metabolites, which are also prevalent in numerous food supplements at high doses, should be considered with caution. Although the *in vitro* efficacy of, for example, resveratrol and other flavonoids in the inhibition of CYP1A has been proven [10], epidemiological evidence for the efficiency of isolated secondary plant metabolites in cancer prevention is missing.

22.2.2
Acrylamide

The amount of acrylamide (*n*-propenamide: CH_2=CH–CO–NH_2) consumed on a daily basis along with a westernized diet comprises approximately 50 μg/day/kg body weight [11]. In rodents, acrylamide was proven to be carcinogenic at doses of 2 mg/day/kg body weight or higher, and affected the thyroid gland and testicles in male rats, as well as the mammary gland, brain, thyroid gland, oral cavity, and uterus in female rats [12]. In humans, CYP2E1 accounts for approximately 25% of the formation of the chemically reactive epoxide glycidamide from acrylamide [13] and it is assumed that this epoxide is the reactive form of acrylamide, leading to DNA alkylation. An increased consumption of food with known CYP2E1 inhibitors such as diallylsulfide from garlic might contribute to a reduced formation of the active carcinogen [14], while an enhancement of CYP2E1 activity (e.g., by ethanol consumption) might promote its synthesis if one follows the "toxication" hypothesis that has also been claimed for PAHs. So far, the experimental evidence (e.g., comparative feeding acrylamide to wild-type and *Cyp2e1*$^{-/-}$ mice) for the toxifying effect is missing and further scientific evidence is needed before a general recommendation on a higher intake of secondary plant metabolites aiming at cancer prevention coming from acrylamide can be released.

Anyway, strong evidence for the causative role of acrylamide at doses consumed with our diet in cancer development has been cast in doubt as in cohort studies either no significant or even a negative correlation between the consumption of acrylamide-rich food and the incidence of, for example, colon cancer was found. This effect was explained by the parallel increase of fiber consumption, which is considered to prevent colon cancer [15]. Nevertheless, some authors continue to claim that single organs might be more susceptible to acrylamide-induced carcinogenesis than the colon and the potential protective effect from

CYP2E1-inhibiting supplements/food constituents such as diallylsulfide should be exploited [11].

22.2.3 Nitrosamines

In parallel to acrylamide, metabolic activation of *N*-nitroso compounds into DNA-reactive intermediates is achieved mainly by CYP2E1 and, to a lesser extent, by CYP2A6. As shown with CYP2E1-deficient mice, the capability of CYP2E1 to act as *N*-nitrosodimethyl-amine demethylase promoted the hepatocarcinogenic potential of this nitrosamine after treatment with diethylnitrosamine (10 mg/kg body weight) [16]. However, the relevance of dietary intake of nitrate/nitrite as a causative agent of nitrosamine-associated cancer development in humans has been questioned due to the comparably high formation of nitrite from Arg by endogenous nitric oxide synthase, the latter being approximately 30-times higher than the dietary intake of nitrate/nitrite. So far, no epidemiological evidence exists for an association between the increased intake of cured goods, which are rich in nitrite and nitrate, and cancer incidence [17]. Anyway, intending to reduce even the theoretical likelihood of carcinogen "toxification" by CYP2E1, an elevated intake of compounds that inhibit CYP2E1 activity seems desirable. This effect might be achieved by elevated consumption of, for example, garlic or its bioeffective components such as diallylsulfide [14].

22.2.4 Fungal Toxins

The best-known carcinogens in food of fungal origin are aflatoxins, which occur as green-fluorescing variants (aflatoxins G1/G2) and blue-fluorescing compounds (aflatoxins B1/B2). If cattle eat aflatoxin B1/B2-containing chow, these aflatoxins are transformed by the bovine metabolism into the M1/M2 form that can occasionally be found in milk.

The primarily affected organ by these carcinogens is the liver. Just as with other water-insoluble compounds, aflatoxins are metabolized by CYP (i.e., by CYP3A4) to give in a first step the *exo*-8,9-epoxide form of the corresponding aflatoxin (Figure 22.1) [18]. Apart from CYP3A4, also prostaglandin synthase and lipoxygenases can promote formation of the *exo*-8,9-epoxide of aflatoxin, which can effectively react with DNA. The resulting adduct is readily intercalated into the DNA helix. CYP1A2, which was suspected to be also a procarcinogenic activator of aflatoxin, seems rather to facilitate the formation of the *endo*-8,9-epoxide, which shows poor reactivity with DNA and plays a protective role in aflatoxin-induced hepatocarcinogenesis [19].

While epoxidases are considered to have a low efficacy in the detoxication of reactive aflatoxin metabolites, the glutathione *S*-transferase (GST) pathway is thought to play a dominant role in aflatoxin conjugation (Figure 22.1) [18]. As in

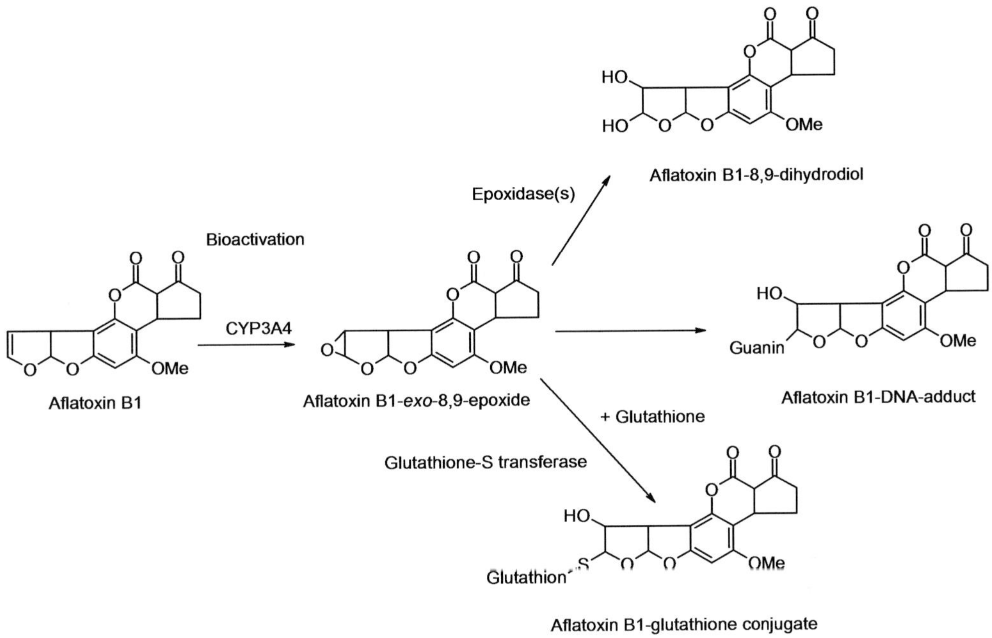

Figure 22.1 Bioactivation of aflatoxin B1 by CYP3A4 to its *exo*-8,9-epoxide and the three major pathways of this epoxide.

the case of acrylamide and nitrosamines, the bioactivation of the aflatoxin into the corresponding epoxide is seen as the critical step that enables the modification of DNA. Hence, drugs that can inhibit the activity of CYP3A4 (and other CYPs that form epoxides from aflatoxins) and compounds that can induce the conversion of aflatoxins by GST activity such as oltipraz are considered to be protective against cancer induced by these fungal toxins [20].

Apart from aflatoxins, trichothecenes such as ochratoxin, deoxynivalenol (DON), nivalenol, T-2, and HT-2 are major toxic contaminants of food generated by fungi. For small-grain cereals, maize, or related products, maximum concentrations in food were defined for aflatoxins, ochratoxin A, DON, zearalenone, and fumonisins. Reasons for setting limits for the concentrations of these food contaminants are based not only on their carcinogenic potential, but also on their acute toxicity leading to, for example, Balkan endemic nephropathy, which is caused by consumption of ochratoxin. In parallel to aflatoxins, ochratoxin experiences metabolic activation by CYPs (i.e., CYPs 2C11, 1A2, and 3A) [21]. Data on bioactivation of other fungus-borne toxins in food are scarce, but cell culture experiments indicate that a higher expression of CYP1A2 and CYP2E1 is linked to a higher acute cytotoxicity of ochratoxin A, while no dependency of DON cytotoxicity on CYP expression was found [22].

22.3
Vitamins

22.3.1
Vitamin A, Retinoic Acid, and Carotenoids

Apart from its function in the visual process, metabolites of the oxidized form of retinol (retinoic acid isomers) play an essential role in embryonic development and postnatal survival. Key enzymes related to the regulation of this hormone are members of the CYP26 family (CYP26A1, CYP26B1, and CYP26C1). CYP26A1 is considered mainly to limit cytoplasmic concentrations of retinoic acid by a negative feedback loop as response elements in the promoter region of CYP26A1 (retinoic acid response elements) are ligands for isoforms of heterodimers of the retinoic acid receptor and the retinoid X receptor (RXR), which binds 9-*cis*-retinoic acid (reviewed in [23]). This system has high importance in the life cycle because holo-RXR is also a partner for the formation of heterodimers receptors that are related to fatty acid metabolism (peroxisome proliferator-activated receptor (PPAR-α)), leukotriene/prostaglandin response (PPAR-γ), sexual hormone function (constitutive androstane receptor CAR), metabolism and excretion of xenobiotic substances (CAR, pregnane X receptor (PXR)), bile acid metabolism (farnesoid X receptor (FAR)), cholesterol and glucose homeostasis (liver X receptor (LXR)), energy metabolism (thyroid receptor), and vitamin D function (vitamin D receptor). A limited availability of retinoic acid can occur during embryonic development under alcohol exposure, as alcohol competes with retinol for oxidation by alcohol dehydrogenase [24]. This can have dramatic consequences for the healthy growth of the fetus, such as the fetal alcohol syndrome.

Main dietary sources of retinol are retinylesters (mainly from liver consumption) and carotenoids, which can be cleaved by intestinal dioxygenases to give retinal, which is consequently reduced to retinol. Within the cell, a small percentage of the retinol is oxidized to retinoic acid. Excess retinoic acid is oxidized by CYP26 mainly to 4-hydroxy-retinoic acid or 4-oxo-retinoic acid (Figure 22.2). The polar metabolites of retinoic acid are subjected to derivatization by UDP-glucuronosyltransferase (UGT) enzymes before excretion [25]. Of note, other CYPs such as CYP2C8 and CYP3A4 are also able to catabolize retinoic acid in the liver to its polar metabolites, including 18-hydroxy-retinoic acid. Although CYP2C8 has a higher activity in retinoic acid hydroxylation, the higher abundance of CYP3A4 equals the contribution of both CYPs to hepatic degradation of excess retinoic acid [26].

As retinoic acid is used as a drug for treatment of promyelocytic leukemia and skin diseases, its therapeutic efficacy can be increased by application of CYP26A1 inhibitors to prolong retinoic acid's half-life. Imidazole-based CYP inhibitors such as ketoconazole can slow down retinoic acid catabolism [27].

Retinoic acid is a substrate for CYP2C8 and its application leads to significant prolongation of the half-life of other drugs that are substrates of this enzyme, if those are applied in parallel. Prominent examples of these compounds are taxol,

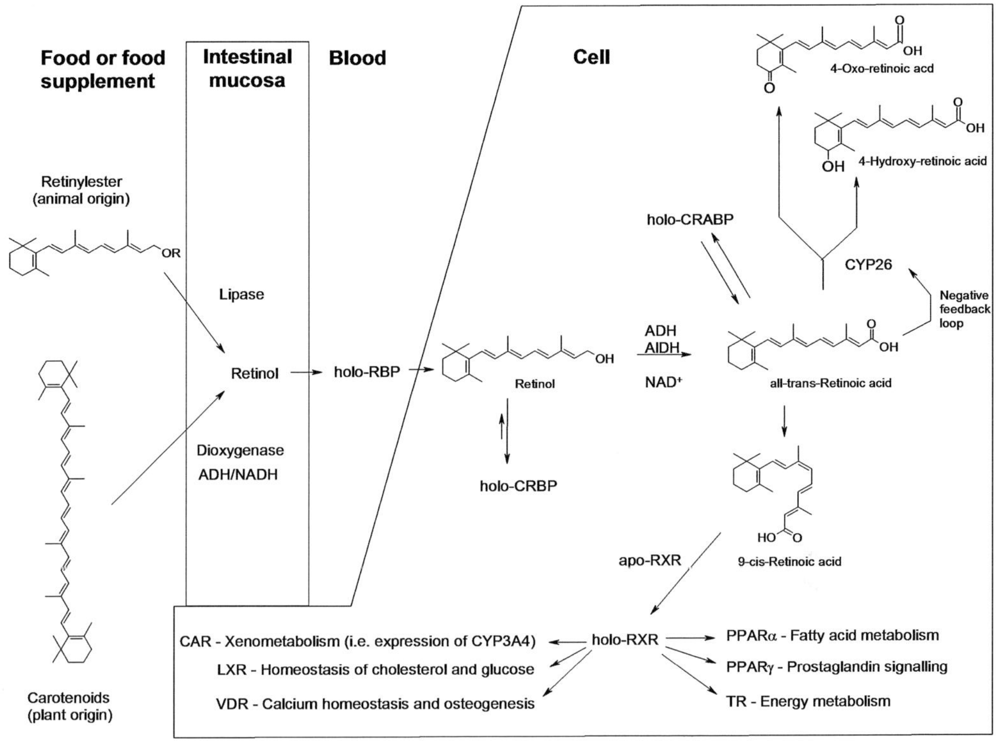

Figure 22.2 Uptake of vitamin A (retinol) from food or food supplements, intracellular metabolism of retinol to retinoic acid, and relevance of retinoic acid availability for some metabolic regulation pathways. While retinoic acid (in its 9-*cis* form) is relevant for the regulation of the metabolism of numerous drugs mainly via CYP3A4, it is also under regulation of CYP26 activity, which regulates the concentration of free retinoic acid by a negative feedback loop. Abbreviations: ADH, alcohol dehydrogenase; AlDH, acetaldehyde dehydrogenase; CRABP, cellular retinoic acid binding protein; CRBP, cellular retinol binding protein; RBP, retinol binding protein; PPAR, peroxisome proliferator-activated receptor; CAR, constitutive androstane receptor; LXR, liver X receptor; TR, thyroid receptor; VDR, vitamin D receptor.

tolbutamide, and warfarin [28]. However, retinoic acid, which is a drug requiring prescription, and retinol are almost never present in food supplements, in contrast to their precursors, the carotenoids. The interactions of carotenoids with drug-metabolizing enzymes are complex and hard to predict. In rat liver, feeding of astaxanthin–a carotenoid–can alter CYP1A activities by two different mechanisms, which seemingly impair each other: induction of protein expression and impairment of NADPH P450-reductase dependent electron transfer. In contrast, the activities of phase II enzymes (GSTs and UGTs) remain unchanged by this carotenoid [29]. Although more and more supplements are found on the market that contain carotenoids, the Food and Nutrition Board advises against supplementation with these micronutrients. One reason for this recommendation might be the results of the ATBC (α-tocopherol, β-carotene) study with more than 29 000 participants, in which a large number of Finns were supplemented with β-carotene. In this population, the risk of smokers developing small-cell lung carcinoma was elevated by a factor of 1.8 compared to the placebo group of smokers, which led to a premature end of the study [30]. Whether different CYP activities contributed to the observed risk elevation is unknown.

While with many other food constituents or food supplements the major concern is that their intake might affect drug metabolism, leading to undesired side-effects, the main issue with the quite sensitive retinoid homeostasis is that it might be deranged by drugs that interact with the enzymes involved. Ketoconazole impairs cellular retinoic acid oxidation, leading to a prolonged half-life of retinoic acid [31]. This interaction might cause "pseudo-hypervitaminosis"-like symptoms, which can become especially critical during pregnancy as an excess of retinoic acid, just like an inadequate availability of it, has strong teratogenic effects. Apart from the nonspecifically CYP-inhibiting, imidazole-based drugs, parathion (an insecticide) and quinidine (a heart antiarrhythmic drug) are also potent inhibitors of retinoic acid hydroxylation [32]. Other drugs that lower circulating concentrations of retinoic acid and its polar metabolites are anticonvulsant drugs, such as phentoin, carbamazepine, and valporate, and some antiepileptic drugs [23].

22.3.2 Vitamin D (Cholecalciferol and Ergocalciferol)

Two hydroxylation steps are necessary to convert the fat-soluble vitamin D (cholecalciferol and ergocalciferol) into calcitriol, which is the bioactive variant of vitamin D. Hydroxylation at C25 is catalyzed by mitochondrial (CYP27A1) and microsomal (human: CYP2R1, rat: CYP2J3) CYPs. Calcitriol (1α,25-$(OH)_2D_3$) is formed by 1α-hydroxylation through CYP27B1 [33]. Both 1α,25-$(OH)_2D_3$ and 25-$(OH)D_3$ are inactivated by CYP24A1 in a multistep oxidation procedure. Comparable to retinol/retinoic acid, the hormonal efficacy of this vitamin is regulated by a complex interplay of CYPs involving negative feedback loops. As with retinoic acid, both poor supplementation and excess doses have adverse effects on the individual's health, and some of these effects (i.e., teratogenicity) are common to both vitamins in the case of overdosing.

The CYP27B1-mediated bioactivation of vitamin D, which is considered to be a neurosteroid involved in nerve growth and differentiation, has attracted attention as both pseudo-hypovitaminosis D and genetic polymorphisms of CYP27B1 have been linked to autism and the Rett syndrome [34]. Moreover, intervention studies have shown that vitamin D supplementation lowers the risk of developing colon cancer and autism [35]. The incidence of these diseases in Westernized societies is steadily increasing. This tendency might be connected to the warning of the American Medical Association and other medical associations released in 1989 to avoid sunlight in order to prevent skin cancer, as approximately 90% of vitamin D are synthesized in the skin under exposure to UV radiation from sunlight.

Hence, vitamin D is one of the few vitamins considered worth being supplements, particularly in infants, toddlers, and aged persons (i.e., during wintertime).

Inhibition of CYP27B1 by drugs such as VID400 might be useful in diseases in which calcitriol is overproduced, such as sarcoidosis or nephrolithiasis [36]. Specific inhibitors of CYP24A1, such as ketoconazole, might be used to extend the half-life of $1\alpha,25\text{-}(OH)_2D_3$ or vitamin D analogs within target cells, especially in malignant cells that overexpress CYP24A1 and in which a differentiation by vitamin D is desired. A comparable effect is attributed to phytoestrogens such as genistein from soy, which seem to induce CYP27B1 and to suppress CYP24, thereby increasing the systemic availability of calcitriol [37].

Antifungal agents (ketoconazole), aromatase inhibitors applied in breast cancer (letrozole), and retinoic acid metabolism blockers used in prostate cancer (liarozole) can interfere with CYPs involved in vitamin D activation and catabolism [36]. Especially after prolonged application of these drugs, indicators of calcitriol efficacy such as hypo/hypercalcemia or bone density should be scrutinized.

22.3.3
Vitamin E (Tocopherol)

Vitamin E is a fat-soluble compound that is known to work as a radical scavenger by trapping single electrons from radicals, thereby preventing radical chain growth. Following the theory that cardiovascular and other ischemic diseases are caused by radicals and oxidative stress, vitamin E (α-tocopherol) has been praised as a magic bullet against these diseases. However, large intervention trials were rather disappointing with regard to prevention of these diseases [38]. On the contrary, meta-analyses indicate that high-dose supplementation of this vitamin is associated with a higher overall mortality [39, 40]. As a possible explanation for this phenomenon, the capability of α-tocopherol to induce CYP3A4 via PXR/RXR activation (see Section 22.3.1) and a resulting lower average plasma concentration of therapeutic drugs have been stressed. However, a recent study has shown that midazolam, which is a substrate for CYP3A4, was not metabolized faster in volunteers after a preceding supplementation with vitamin E [41]. In line with this finding, statin-receiving patients did not show a higher CYP3A4 activity if supplemented with vitamin E, as assessed by the ratio of cortisol to its metabolite 6β-hydroxycortisol [42]. Other drugs such as cyclosporine were shown to be less bioavailable in the case of parallel vitamin E intake, but this effect might also be based on an enhanced activity of P-glycoprotein (P-gp) [43].

Hence, the molecular mechanism of the higher mortality after supplementation with vitamin E remains obscure, although an increased blood pressure has been demonstrated after supplementation with α-tocopherol [44]. As the overall benefits of a high-dose supplementation with respect to cancer and cardiovascular disease/ ischemic stroke remain more than questionable, no scientific arguments exist for supplementation with this vitamin, especially in the face of its blood pressure-increasing properties.

22.3.4
Water-Soluble Vitamins (Thiamine and Riboflavin)

Inadequate availability of thiamine increases the activity of CYP2E1 and CYP2C8, and enhances the catabolism of drugs that are substrates of these enzymes [45]. A comparable effect was observed for riboflavin deficiency and enzymes related to benzo[*a*]pyrene hydroxylation, presumably CYP1 [46].

In general, information on the effects of an elevated intake of other water-soluble vitamins on the activity of drug-metabolizing enzymes is rather scarce and does not attract considerable scientific interest.

22.4
Macronutrients

Both the origin and the amount of any of the four macronutrients consumed can affect the expression of enzyme and transmembrane transport systems that are related to xenobiotic metabolism. In some cases, specific parts of macronutrients, such as polyunsaturated fatty acids, can become substrates for xenobiotic-metabolizing enzymes and can be converted into hormone-like mediators. The interaction of the intake of protein, fatty acids, and carbohydrates is dealt with subsequently, while the effect of alcohol consumption is described in Chapter 18.

22.4.1
Protein

In many clinically critical stages, a high-protein, low-carbohydrate diet is applied. Shifts in the protein intake, however, may affect the activity of, for example, anti-coagulants such as warfarin. It is assumed that a high protein intake increases CYP450 activity, leading to suboptimal plasma concentrations of warfarin mainly due to presystemic clearance. Therefore, shifts in the diet with abrupt changes of the protein content demand a control for the therapeutic efficacy of this drug [47]. Especially with drugs such as warfarin, it is difficult to narrow down the effects of the affected phase I enzymes as it is metabolized by at least three different CYPs (CYP1A2, CYP2D6, and CYP3A4) [48].

It was hypothesized that the origin of the supplemented protein might affect the differential expression of single CYPs. At least in rodents, hepatic CYP2E1 protein expression is reduced after supplementation with soy protein (i.e., after application of a diet inducing nonalcoholic steatohepatitis [49]), but the relevance of these findings needs clinical proof.

In a rodent model, soy protein was shown to enhance CYP3A expression up to 3-fold in comparison to caseine after coapplication of dexamethasone by a PXR-dependent pathway [50]. Although single transcription factors by which food protein of a particular origin influences the expression of single CYPs were identified recently, the prediction of which CYP will be induced or suppressed by the intake of a particular protein remains difficult. However, the potential of therapeutic protein supplementation along with small-molecule drugs has been recognized and more research can be expected in this field [51].

22.4.2
Fatty Acids

Metabolites of 20-carbon fatty acids with four (arachidonic acid) or five (eicosapentanoic acid) double bonds are important signaling molecules that regulate pain, fever, inflammation, thrombocyte aggregation, vasodilatation, and many other biological processes. These metabolites are part of complex signaling pathways that are initiated by mobilization of arachidonic acid from membrane phospholipids by phospholipase A_2 [52]. Prostaglandins and leukotrienes, which are synthesized by cyclooxygenases and lipoxygenases, respectively, are the best-known compounds emerging from these acids. However, arachidonic acid and eicosapentanoic acid are also substrates for CYPs that form two groups of substrates: ω-hydroxyeicosatetraenoic acids (HETEs), which are formed by ω-hydroxylases, and epoxyeicosatrienoic acids (EETs), which are generated primarily in endothelial cells from the activity of epoxygenases. CYP2J2 and CYP2C9 play a dominant role in the synthesis of EETs, together with CYP1A1 [53], and some proteins delineated from orphan genes coding for CYPs (CYP4X1 and CYP2U1) were shown to be capable of EET synthesis [54, 55]. EETs have an anti-inflammatory effect, and antagonize the adhesion and extravasation of leukocytes [56]. In contrast to EETs, HETEs are formed from arachidonic acid by CYP4A and CYP4F to autacoids such as 20-HETE, which is the principal isoform of this substance class, and has shown vasoconstrictory and proinflammatory activity [57].

Cardiovascular diseases along with cancer are the most important reasons for premature death in developed and many developing countries. As pointed out above, the balance of EETs and HETEs – and therefore also the balance of activities of EET- and HETE-producing CYPs – might play an important role in the development of both diseases. Due to the anti-inflammatory and vasodilatory properties of EETs, and proinflammatory and vasoconstrictory effects of HETEs, the intake of supplements that modulate the concentration ratio of these compounds via regulation of CYP activity, and thereby reduce cardiovascular risk, seem promising and so far unexploited [58]. In the case of cancer, the balance of EETs and HETEs seems of crucial importance for tumor growth, angiogenesis, and vascularization. Although some experimental data from animal studies are available, scientific data on the regulation of cancer development by EETs/HETEs is considered to be insufficient so far [59].

It can be presumed that at least some food components/supplements induce or inhibit some of the CYP activities affecting EET/HETE concentrations, but information on these interactions is scarce. Our group found recently that mice with a dysfunctional Toll-like receptor 2 (TLR2) do not express intestinal CYP1A1 and are incapable of PAH decomposition (unpublished results). Ligands for the heterodimers TLR1/TLR2 and TLR2/TLR6 are bacterial cell wall components of both

Gram-positive and Gram-negative bacteria. Hence, the composition of the intestinal flora might affect the intestinal activity of CYP1A1. CYP1A1 acts predominantly as a subterminal hydroxylase to give 19-HETE, but also 14,15-EET [53]. Based on these findings, shifting the intestinal flora by supplementation with probiotics might antagonize the development of both intestinal inflammation and cancer via the CYP1A1/EET/HETE pathway, but further studies are needed to prove this hypothesis.

22.4.3
Carbohydrates

In rats, a low carbohydrate intake was shown to induce CYP2E1 (and also moderately that of CYP2C11/6) and to increase the metabolism of substrates for this enzyme (e.g., toluene) up to 4-fold [60]. A change of the fat content of the applied chow (without changing the fatty acid composition) in this study remained without effect.

22.5
Secondary Plant Metabolites

22.5.1
Grapefruit Juice, Naringenin, and Presystemic Drug Clearance by CYP3A4

One of the first clinically relevant interactions noted between food and drug metabolism was the markedly increased availability of felodipine – a 1,4-dihydropyridine calcium entry blocker – in the case of coadministration of juice from grapefruit (*Citrus paradis*). This effect was paralleled by an enhancement of the pharmacological effects of the drug [61]. Basically, grapefruit juice interacts by inhibiting presystemic drug metabolism facilitated by CYP3A isoforms in the small bowel. One of the major grapefruit-specific flavonoids is naringin, which is the glycolysated form of naringenin – a polyphenol (Figure 22.3). Naringin can account for up to 10% of the edible dry mass of grapefruits. The suspected point of interaction between felodipine and naringenin is intestinal CYP3A4, the activity of which is inhibited by this secondary plant metabolite. Hence, the pharmacodynamics of the whole spectrum of drugs that are metabolized exclusively or partly by CYP3A4 (benzodiazepines such as midazolam, antihistamines such as terfenadine, immunosuppressive drugs such as cyclosporine, sexual hormones such as estradiol, etc.) might be affected significantly after extensive consumption of naringin-containing fruits or their juices [62].

Based on different reports, typical changes in plasma drug concentrations that can be expected after coadministration of grapefruit juice may range between a doubling and a tripling, which might narrow the therapeutic index of the drug in question. Apart from the drug groups mentioned above, the bioavailability of proteinase inhibitors (saquinavir) can also be enhanced considerably by grapefruit

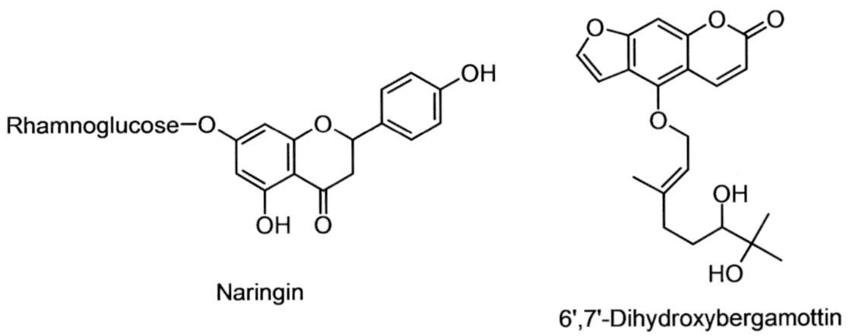

Figure 22.3 Chemical structures of naringin and 6′,7′-dihydroxybergamottin – the key pharmacologically relevant compounds in grapefruit.

juice, the unaffected presystemic clearance of which allows only a bioavailability of approximately 4%. Especially in the case of expensive drugs with a low bioavailability, the targeted application of grapefruit juice can help to increase bioavailability and to reduce associated costs [61].

22.5.2 Inhibition of Metabolic Activation of Drugs by CYP3A4

An undesired effect can occur in the case of the need for a presystemic metabolic activation of an initially noneffective drug. The histamine H_1 receptor antagonist terfenadin is biologically inactive with respect to its intended drug effect unless converted by CYP3A4 into the desired antihistaminicum. Unmetabolized terfenadin, which can cause cardiac arrhythmias, is usually not detectable in plasma. Parallel ingestion of terfenadin with grapefruit juice resulted in detectable plasma levels of this drug and prolonged QT intervals [63]. Moreover, it has been reported that naringin also inhibits the *N*-demethylation of caffeine – a process catalyzed by CYP1A2 [62] – whereas the conversion of theophylline remained unchanged.

22.5.3 Secondary Plant Metabolites, CYP Modulation, and Intestinal Inflammation

Bergamottin and 6′,7′-dihydroxybergamottin are two furanocoumarins that occur together with naringenin in grapefruit. Their inhibitory efficacy on CYP3A4 corresponds to that of the artificial CYP3A4 inhibitor SKF-525a [64]. Inhibition of CYP3A4 activity by these compounds is paralleled by a reduced expression of endothelial cell adhesion molecules (ECAMs), which are released by endothelial cells, and are relevant for the recruitment and extravasation of leukocytes and onset of inflammation. On the basis of these findings, a reduction of ECAM expression and leukocyte adhesion by natural CYP3A inhibitors was suggested in the clinical treatment of inflammatory bowel disease (IBD) [64]. More recent studies [65] indicate that also other, yet partly unknown compounds belonging to the coumarin/furanocoumarin substance class from grapefruit peel oil are also capable of CYP3A4 inhibition. Attempts to exploit possible health-promoting properties such as suppression of inflammation in the form of food supplements at this level can be foreseen.

22.5.4 Parallel Consumption of Drugs and Inhibitors of Intestinal Drug Metabolism–Threats and Chances

Recommendations on the parallel consumption of grapefruit juice and drug intake should in the first instance be directed towards avoiding adverse effects such as with terfenadin. They can be limited to avoid parallel consumption, as only a 2-h time difference between drug and grapefruit juice intake renders the effect of naringin negligible. However, a realistic prediction of the effect of grapefruit juice on drug metabolism under real-life conditions is difficult due to the high variance of patients' intestinal activity of CYP3A4, varying concentrations of CYP inhibitors in juice, and the irregularity of the consumption of these juices/fruits. Moreover, hepatic insufficiency and other pre-existing medical conditions might predispose to enhanced or otherwise abnormal drug effects in the case of parallel intake of grapefruit juice [66].

A bigger threat of a significantly changed drug metabolism than from food emerges from food supplements that contain secondary plant metabolites (i.e., polyphenols). Health claims that have been linked to an increased intake of these flavonoids concern mainly the reduction of risk for cardiovascular disease and cancer [67]. A daily intake recommendation of 500–1000 mg for this compound class in order to achieve the claims on health effects, which are in most cases clinically unproven, is common in commercially available over-the-counter products. Hence, the described effects on drug metabolism from one serving of polyphenol-containing food might be exacerbated considerably by supplements that comprise a 10- to 100-fold amount of these compounds.

Even in the case of compounds that formally belong to the same class, such as polyphenols, interactive effects can result in unforeseeable changes in the induction and suppression of drug-metabolizing enzymes. Hence, the parallel intake of such supplements with drugs should be avoided. Digging deeper into the molecular mechanisms of the regulation of CYP expression by flavonoids such as quercetin and kaempferol reveals a complex interaction between induction/enhancement of mRNA production of the corresponding CYP and direct inhibition of oxidation of the substrate/drug by these compounds. Thus, it may occur that a drug promotes mRNA production of a cytochrome in parallel to inhibiting its enzyme activity for one given substrate. This effect is valid not only for CYP3A, but also for other CYPs such as CYP1A1. Naphtoflavone, for instance, is a potent inducer of CYP1A1 expression, which is inhibited, however, by kaempferol, myricetin, and quercetin. In contrast, apigenin, chrysin, galangin, luteolin, and morin synergistically enhance naphthoflavone-induced CYP1A1 expression in primary mouse hepatocytes [68]. However, the acute inhibitory effect of CYP activity seems to prevail in clinical relevance compared to the induction of CYP protein synthesis and the associated elevation of CYP activity.

Quercetin and rutin are two flavonoids that are prevalent in many fruits, vegetables, and food supplements, and are substrates for both CYP3A4 and P-gp. Hence, two effects that can counteract each other may occur in parallel – inhibition of presystemic inactivation of drug-metabolizing enzymes (leading to increased bioavailability of the drug) and transport of the drug from the enterocyte cytoplasm into the intestinal lumen (decreasing the drug bioavailability). Recent experiments with rats show that the interaction with P-gp might be the more relevant one, as both quercetin and rutin inhibited the bioavailability of cyclosporine by about 50% [69].

22.5.5 Glucosinolates and Allylsulfides

Isothiocyanates, which can be found in cruciferous vegetables (Brassicaceae) such as broccoli, cauliflower, brussel sprouts, and cabbage, harbor the chemical group –N=C=S. They are produced from glucosinolates by the vegetable-intrinsic enzyme myrosinase after destruction of cellular membranes. Feeding with isothiocyanates (around 5–10 μmol/day), such as phenethyl isothiocyanate (PITC) and sulforaphane, has been shown to inhibit carcinogenesis in cancer-susceptible mice, thereby reaching steady-state levels of 120–250 nM sulforaphane [70] or up to 42 μM PITC [71] in plasma. Hence, micromolar plasma concentrations of isothiocyanates can be achieved *in vivo*.

Comparable to flavonoids, a dichotonic effect of isothiocyanates on CYP activity was noted. On the one hand, PITC dose-dependently upregulated the mRNA expression of CYP1A1 and 1A2 [72]. On the other hand, PITC competitively inhibited biochemical catalyses of CYP1A2, 2A6, 2B6, 2C9, 2C19, 2D6, 2E1, and 3A4 [73].

An even more relevant aspect of health-promoting properties of isothiocyanates might be their capability to induce phase II enzymes such as GST [74], which might explain the faster elimination of carcinogenic polycyclic amines (e.g., 2-amino-1-methyl-6-phenylimidazo[4,5-*b*]pyridine (PhIP)) from body tissues after both PITC and sulforaphane supplementation [75, 76]. PITC treatment has also been shown to strongly increase the expression of the antioxidant enzyme heme oxygenase-1, thereby lowering intracellular oxidative burden [77].

The final assessment of isothiocyanates seen from the health-promoting perspective remains difficult, based on their antagonizing effects on mRNA expression of CYPs on the one hand, and inhibition of their enzymatic activity on the other. Furthermore, the scientific community still disagrees on whether an enhanced activity of CYPs is rather procarcinogenic due to "bioactivation" of carcinogens (conversion of procarcinogens to carcinogens) [78] or anticarcinogenic by promoting targeted elimination of carcinogens [9]. However, large longitudinal epidemiological studies indicate that a high intake of isothiocyanate-containing food is associated with both a reduced cardiovascular disease incidence and overall mortality, but not cancer-related deaths [79]. These findings make isothiocyanates worth considering as food supplements for prevention of the biggest cause of death in industrialized countries.

22.5.6
Caffeine

A solid base of epidemiologic and experimental evidence exists for the fact that PAAs such as PhIP are potent inducers of cancer (e.g., breast cancer in women) [80]. PPAs are hydroxylated by CYP1A2 [3], which is a hydroxylase that is strongly induced (up to 16-fold) in rats by both coffee extract and caffeine [81]. Despite this induction and the corresponding higher conversion rate of PhIP to its DNA-reactive phase I intermediates after caffeine supplementation, no higher PhIP–DNA adduct formation in colon and pancreas was measured, while liver adducts decreased by 50% over control animals [81]. Hence, just as with PAH, the carcinogenicity of PAAs *in vivo* seems to be rather lowered by the induction of hydroxylases that handle carcinogenic compounds. This is in line with epidemiological findings that show that a high consumption of coffee is not associated with carcinogenesis of the digestive tract [82] and the fact that CYP1A2 produces the endoperoxide form of PAAs, which has a low tendency to react with DNA [19].

The considerable variation in metabolic activity of CYP1A2 that can be based on caffeine consumption may affect the catabolism of only a minority of applied drugs such as GTS-21, a selective α-7-nicotinic acetylcholine receptor partial agonist, the phosphodiesterase type IV inhibitor, YM-64227, and AC-3933, a central benzodiazepine receptor partial inverse agonist [83].

22.5.7
Cholesterol

Due to its central role in the development of cardiovascular diseases, cholesterol, which can originate from nutrition, but also from endogenous production, is one of the most-considered biological molecules. Along with triglycerides, cholesterol is transported from the liver to the periphery as part of apolipoprotein B-containing low-density lipoprotein (LDL) particles. Particularly in persons with high average LDL concentrations (hypercholesteremia), this lipoprotein can be oxidized and phagocytosed, which contributes to the formation of plaque-forming foam cells. This process – generally termed atherogenesis – can be antagonized by reverse cholesterol transport, which is facilitated by high-density lipoprotein (HDL) and the associated apolipoprotein A1. In general, the risk of developing cardiovascular disease decreases with increasing concentrations of HDL (cholesterol) and reduced concentrations of LDL (cholesterol). The standard pharmaceutical approach to reduce cardiovascular disease risk is to reduce endogenous cholesterol synthesis.

Cholesterol is a substrate for several CYPs, which therefore play an important role in cholesterol homeostasis (reviewed in [84]). Figure 22.4 depicts the role of

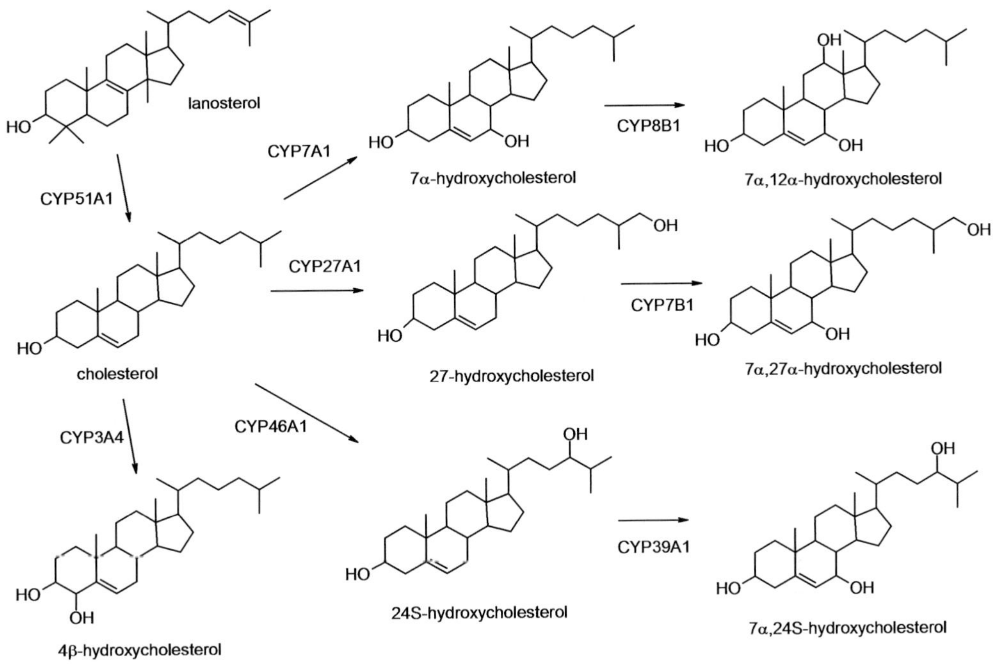

Figure 22.4 CYP enzymes in the metabolism of cholesterol and primary oxysterols (reviewed in detail, e.g., in [84, 85]).

eight different CYPs, seven of which contribute to cholesterol degradation to oxysterols (the cholesterol hydroxylases CYP7A1, CYP8B1, CYP27A1, CYP7B1, CYP46A1, CYP39A1, and CYP3A4) and one that facilitates cholesterol synthesis (lanosterol-14-demethylase CYP51A1). The main purpose of cholesterol hydroxylase products is primarily to contribute to metabolic pathways related to excess cholesterol secretion from the body, to bile acid synthesis, and to their detoxification.

Oxysterols function as ligands for LXRs and PPARs that regulate the activation of the ATP-binding cassette (ABC) transporter and other cholesterol-lowering genes that are involved in cellular cholesterol efflux and biliary secretion of cholesterol into the intestine [86, 87]. Elevation of systemic cholesterol concentrations leads to an endogenous induction of cholesterol hydroxylases along with the subsequent elevated generation of oxysterols and reduction of intestinal absorption of cholesterol. Hence, the reduction of systemic LDL-cholesterol levels facilitated by the increased activity of cholesterol hydroxylases might protect arteries from atherosclerosis, whereas inhibition of related CYPs blocks oxidative reactions, promotes cellular cholesterol accumulation, and enhances the atherosclerotic vascular process.

From the point of modulating CYP activity for cardiovascular disease prevention, two counteracting effects of CYP3A4 are of relevance: the reduction of circulating concentrations of LDL-cholesterol by enhanced CYP3A4 activity/oxysterol production, and the enhancement of the inflammatory status by CYP3A4, which might promote the phagocytosis of (oxidized) LDL particles and atherosclerosis. Clinical intervention studies with angiographic or ultrasonographic outcomes indicate that drugs inducing CYP (i.e., CYP3A4) activity, such as fibrates, statins, cholestyramine, thiazolidinedione, anticonvulsants, and alcohol, reduce atherosclerosis and also cardiovascular disease morbidity/mortality [88–90].

As mentioned above, secondary plant metabolites such as naringenin, bergamottin, and others are well-known inhibitors of CYP3A4. Based on the relevance of CYP3A4 (and other cholesterol hydroxylases) for systemic cholesterol concentrations, one could expect enhanced atherogenesis after elevated intake of such secondary plant metabolites. Obviously, the opposite holds true as an increased consumption of food containing such inhibitors (i.e., citrus fruits) is rather connected to a reduction of cardiovascular disease risk than to its enhancement [91]. Several possible explanations for the longevity-promoting role of a higher intake of secondary plant metabolites from citrus fruits and cruciferous vegetables [79] were suggested. (i) Secondary plant metabolites might activate phase II enzymes such as GSTs, which might lead to a faster elimination of carcinogens [92]. (ii) They might reduce the ratios of circulating HETEs, which are produced by CYP3A4 (i.e., 20-HETE), towards circulating EETs, which might lead to an upregulated production of apolipoprotein A1/A2 (and HDL) via PPAR-α [93]. (iii) The impaired production of proinflammatory HETEs by CYP3A4 might ameliorate the inflammatory status of the consumer.

Hence, the intake of food components and/or supplements that contain ligands for receptors triggering cholesterol hydroxylases seems to harbor potential to contribute to a reduction of cardiovascular disease morbidity and mortality.

22.6
Probiotics and Prebiotics in the Modulation of Drug Metabolism

Apart from the uptake of nutrients, one key function of the gastrointestinal tract is to prevent the permeation of bacterial compounds that can trigger an inflammatory response. A key signaling pathway in the induction of (transmucosal) inflammation is endotoxin (lipopolysaccharide (LPS)), which is recognized by the homodimeric TLR4, while further bacterial ligands for other TLRs such as TLR2 and TLR9 have either no proinflammatory or even an anti-inflammatory potential [94]. As the incidence of chronic inflammatory diseases such as IBD is constantly increasing in westernized countries, elaborate efforts have been made to counteract this development, also by means of probiotics (live microorganisms that exert health benefits) and prebiotics (fibers promoting the growth of such microorganisms in the intestine). There are at least three levels of interaction when it comes to enzymes involved in drug metabolism, the intestinal microflora, and the maintenance of the intestinal barrier.

Firstly, intestinal microorganisms have their own repertoire of CYPs (and other hydroxylating enzymes) that can metabolize drugs and other xenobiotics [95]. Only the fact that the upper small intestine of humans, where the majority of orally applied drugs are absorbed, is virtually free of microorganisms (usually less than 10^4–10^5 CFU/ml jejunal juice) avoids bacterial catabolism of these drugs. However, this condition might change after application of drugs that promote small intestinal bacterial overgrowth such as proton pump antagonists or after alcohol consumption.

In the case of biological activation of (expensive) drugs by CYPs such as terfenadin [63] or lovostatin [96], the parallel application of probiotics, which help to produce the biologically active variant, might be a future perspective to achieve a higher drug efficacy and cost reduction. Particularly effective in this context might be microorganisms with stably transfected CYPs with a presumed health-promoting activity [97].

Secondly, the presence of individual microorganisms can modulate the expression of intestinal (and presumably also hepatic) enzyme systems that are involved in the metabolism of xenobiotics such as CYP [98]. LPS decreases hepatic expression of CYP3A4 and prolongs the half-life of drugs such as telithromycin – the metabolism of which depends on CY3A4 [51]. Enteropathogens cause a downregulation of a wide variety of CYPs [99]. In addition, our group found that intestinal, but not hepatic, expression and activity of CYP1A1 strictly depends on the activation of TLR2, which recognizes lipoteichoic acid – a widespread constituent of bacterial cell walls (unpublished results).

Thirdly, numerous CYPs and also multidrug resistance gene-coded proteins such as P-gp are involved in hepatic secretion of bile acids into the intestinal lumen. Bile acids were shown to prevent the permeation of LPS through layers of intestinal mucosa cells and to antagonize transepithelial inflammation onset [100]. Hence, a higher activity of cholesterol-converting and bile acid-producing CYPs might not only promote the reduction of circulating cholesterol levels, but also ameliorate transepithelial permeability of bacterial immunostimulants and limit transepithelial inflammation processes.

References

1 Wattenberg, L.W., Leong, J.L., and Strand, P.J. (1962) Benzpyrene hydroxylase activity in the gastrointestinal tract. *Cancer Res.*, **22**, 1120–1125.

2 Uno, S., Dalton, T.P., Dragin, N., Curran, C.P., Derkenne, S., Miller, M.L., Shertzer, H.G., Gonzalez, F.J., and Nebert, D.W. (2006) Oral benzo[*a*]pyrene in Cyp1 knockout mouse lines: CYP1A1 important in detoxication, CYP1B1 metabolism required for immune damage independent of total-body burden and clearance rate. *Mol. Pharmacol.*, **69**, 1103–1114.

3 Butler, M.A., Iwasaki, M., Guengerich, F.P., and Kadlubar, F.F. (1989) Human P450PA (P450-1A2), the phenacetin *O*-deethylase, is primarily responsible for the hepatic 3-demethylation of caffeine and *N*-oxidation of carcinogenic amines. *Proc. Natl. Acad. Sci. USA*, **86**, 7696–7700.

4 Chiaro, C.R., Patel, R.D., Marcus, C.B., and Perdew, G.H. (2007) Evidence for an aryl hydrocarbon receptor-mediated cytochrome p450 autoregulatory pathway. *Mol. Pharmacol.*, **72**, 1369–1379.

5 Fukunaga, B.N. and Hankinson, O. (1996) Identification of a novel domain in the aryl hydrocarbon receptor required for DNA binding. *J. Biol. Chem.*, **271**, 3743–3749.
6 Grover, P.L. and Sims, P. (1968) Enzyme-catalysed reactions of polycyclic hydrocarbons with deoxyribonucleic acid and protein *in vitro*. *Biochem. J.*, **110**, 159–160.
7 Nebert, D.W., Dalton, T.P., Okey, A.B., and Gonzalez, F.J. (2004) Role of aryl hydrocarbon receptor-mediated induction of the CYP1 enzymes in environmental toxicity and cancer. *J. Biol. Chem.*, **279**, 23847–23850.
8 Conney, A.H. (2003) Enzyme induction and dietary chemicals as approaches to cancer chemoprevention: the Seventh DeWitt S. Goodman Lecture. *Cancer Res.*, **63**, 7005–7031.
9 Uno, S., Dalton, T.P., Derkenne, S., Curran, C.P., Miller, M.L., Shertzer, H.G., and Nebert, D.W. (2004) Oral exposure to benzo[*a*]pyrene in the mouse: detoxication by inducible cytochrome P450 is more important than metabolic activation. *Mol. Pharmacol.*, **65**, 1225–1237.
10 Piver, B., Berthou, F., Dreano, Y., and Lucas, D. (2001) Inhibition of CYP3A, CYP1A and CYP2E1 activities by resveratrol and other non volatile red wine components. *Toxicol. Lett.*, **125**, 83–91.
11 Hogervorst, J.G., Baars, B.J., Schouten, L.J., Konings, E.J., Goldbohm, R.A., and van den Brandt, P.A. (2010) The carcinogenicity of dietary acrylamide intake: a comparative discussion of epidemiological and experimental animal research. *Crit. Rev. Toxicol.*, **40**, 485–512.
12 Johnson, K.A., Gorzinski, S.J., Bodner, K.M., Campbell, R.A., Wolf, C.H., Friedman, M.A., and Mast, R.W. (1986) Chronic toxicity and oncogenicity study on acrylamide incorporated in the drinking water of Fischer 344 rats. *Toxicol. Appl. Pharmacol.*, **85**, 154–168.
13 Doroshyenko, O., Fuhr, U., Kunz, D., Frank, D., Kinzig, M., Jetter, A., Reith, Y., Lazar, A., Taubert, D., Kirchheiner, J., Baum, M., Eisenbrand, G., Berger, F.I., Bertow, D., Berkessel, A., Sörgel, F., Schömig, E., and Tomalik-Scharte, D. (2009) *In vivo* role of cytochrome P450 2E1 and glutathione-*S*-transferase activity for acrylamide toxicokinetics in humans. *Cancer Epidemiol. Biomarkers Prev.*, **18**, 433–443.
14 Taubert, D., Glöckner, R., Müller, D., and Schömig, E. (2006) The garlic ingredient diallyl sulfide inhibits cytochrome P450 2E1 dependent bioactivation of acrylamide to glycidamide. *Toxicol. Lett.*, **164**, 1–5.
15 Mucci, L.A. and Wilson, K.M. (2008) Acrylamide intake through diet and human cancer risk. *J. Agric. Food Chem.*, **56**, 6013–6019.
16 Kang, J.S., Wanibuchi, H., Morimura, K., Gonzalez, F.J., and Fukushima, S. (2007) Role of CYP2E1 in diethylnitrosamine-induced hepatocarcinogenesis *in vivo*. *Cancer Res.*, **67**, 11141–11146.
17 Wild, D. (2003) Cancer from nitrite-cured meat products? *Mitteilungsblatt BAFF*, **42** (**162**), 361–367.
18 Guengerich, F.P., Johnson, W.W., Shimada, T., Ueng, Y.F., Yamazaki, H., and Langouët, S. (1998) Activation and detoxication of aflatoxin B1. *Mutat. Res.*, **402**, 121–128.
19 Ueng, Y.F., Shimada, T., Yamazaki, H., and Guengerich, F.P. (1995) Oxidation of aflatoxin B1 by bacterial recombinant human cytochrome P450 enzymes. *Chem. Res. Toxicol.*, **8**, 218–225.
20 Roebuck, B.D., Liu, Y.L., Rogers, A.E., Groopman, J.D., and Kensler, T.W. (1991) Protection against aflatoxin B1-induced hepatocarcinogenesis in F344 rats by 5-(2-pyrazinyl)-4-methyl-1,2-dithiole-3-thione (oltipraz): predictive role for short-term molecular dosimetry. *Cancer Res.*, **51**, 5501–5506.
21 Pfohl-Leszkowicz, A., Pinelli, E., Bartsch, H., Mohr, U., and Castegnaro, M. (1998) Sex- and strain-specific expression of cytochrome P450s in ochratoxin A-induced genotoxicity and carcinogenicity in rats. *Mol. Carcinog.*, **23**, 76–85.
22 Lewis, C.W., Smith, J.E., Anderson, J.G., and Freshney, R.I. (1999) Increased cytotoxicity of food-borne mycotoxins

toward human cell lines *in vitro* via enhanced cytochrome P450 expression using the MTT bioassay. *Mycopathologia*, **148**, 97–102.
23 Ross, A.C. and Zolfaghari, R. (2011) Cytochrome p450s in the regulation of cellular retinoic acid metabolism. *Annu. Rev. Nutr.*, **31**, 65–87.
24 Parlesak, A., Menzl, I., Feuchter, A., Bode, J.C., and Bode, C. (2000) Inhibition of retinol oxidation by ethanol in the rat liver and colon. *Gut*, **47**, 825–831.
25 Samokyszyn, V.M., Gall, W.E., Zawada, G., Freyaldenhoven, M.A., Chen, G., Mackenzie, P.I., Tephly, T.R., and Radominska-Pandya, A. (2000) 4-Hydroxyretinoic acid, a novel substrate for human liver microsomal UDP-glucuronosyltransferase(s) and recombinant UGT2B7. *J. Biol. Chem.*, **275**, 6908–6914.
26 McCormick, A.M., Napoli, J.L., Schnoes, H.K., and DeLuca, H.F. (1978) Isolation and identification of 5,6-epoxyretinoic acid: a biologically active metabolite of retinoic acid. *Biochemistry*, **17**, 4085–4090.
27 Van Wauwe, J.P., Coene, M.C., Goossens, J., Cools, W., and Monbaliu, J. (1990) Effects of cytochrome P-450 inhibitors on the *in vivo* metabolism of all-*trans*-retinoic acid in rats. *J. Pharmacol. Exp. Ther.*, **252**, 365–369.
28 Yamazaki, H. (1999) Effects of arachidonic acid, prostaglandins, retinol, retinoic acid and cholecalciferol on xenobiotic oxidations catalysed by human cytochrome P450 enzymes. *Xenobiotica*, **29**, 231–241.
29 Ohno, M., Darwish, W.S., Ikenaka, Y., Miki, W., and Ishizuka, M. (2011) Astaxanthin can alter CYP1A-dependent activities via two different mechanisms: induction of protein expression and inhibition of NADPH P450 reductase dependent electron transfer. *Food Chem. Toxicol.*, **49**, 1285–1291.
30 Rautalahti, M., Albanes, D., Virtamo, J., Taylor, P.R., Huttunen, J.K., and Heinonen, O.P. (1997) Beta-carotene did not work: aftermath of the ATBC study. *Cancer Lett.*, **114**, 235–236.
31 Van Wauwe, J.P., Coene, M.C., Goossens, J., Van Nijen, G., Cools, W., and Lauwers, W. (1988) Ketoconazole inhibits the *in vitro* and *in vivo* metabolism of all-*trans*-retinoic acid. *J. Pharmacol. Exp. Ther.*, **245**, 718–722.
32 Nadin, L. and Murray, M. (1999) Participation of CYP2C8 in retinoic acid 4-hydroxylation in human hepatic microsomes. *Biochem. Pharmacol.*, **58**, 1201–1208.
33 Sakaki, T., Sugimoto, H., Hayashi, K., Yasuda, K., Munetsuna, E., Kamakura, M., Ikushiro, S., and Shiro, Y. (2011) Bioconversion of vitamin D to its active form by bacterial or mammalian cytochrome P450. *Biochim. Biophys. Acta*, **1814**, 249–256.
34 Currenti, S.A. (2010) Understanding and determining the etiology of autism. *Cell. Mol. Neurobiol.*, **30**, 161–171.
35 Lieberman, D.A., Prindiville, S., Weiss, D.G., Willett, W., and VA Cooperative Study Group 380 (2003) Risk factors for advanced colonic neoplasia and hyperplastic polyps in asymptomatic individuals. *JAMA*, **290**, 2959–2967.
36 Prosser, D.E. and Jones, G. (2004) Enzymes involved in the activation and inactivation of vitamin D. *Trends Biochem. Sci.*, **29**, 664–673.
37 Cross, H.S., Kállay, E., Lechner, D., Gerdenitsch, W., Adlercreutz, H., and Armbrecht, H.J. (2004) Phytoestrogens and vitamin D metabolism: a new concept for the prevention and therapy of colorectal, prostate, and mammary carcinomas. *J. Nutr.*, **134**, 1207S–1212S.
38 Vivekananthan, D.P., Penn, M.S., Sapp, S.K., Hsu, A., and Topol, E.J. (2003) Use of antioxidant vitamins for the prevention of cardiovascular disease: meta-analysis of randomized trials. *Lancet*, **361**, 2017–2023.
39 Bjelakovic, G., Nikolova, D., Gluud, L.L., Simonetti, R.G., and Gluud, C. (2007) Mortality in randomized trials of antioxidant supplements for primary and secondary prevention: systematic review and meta-analysis. *JAMA*, **297**, 842–857.
40 Miller, E.R., Pastor-Barriuso, R., Dalal, D., Riemersma, R.A., Appel, L.J., and Guallar, E. (2005) Meta-analysis:

high-dosage vitamin E supplementation may increase all-cause mortality. *Ann. Intern. Med.*, **142**, 37–46.

41 Clarke, M.W., Burnett, J.R., Wu, J.H., Hodgson, J.M., Ledowski, T., Puddey, I.B., and Croft, K.D. (2009) Vitamin E supplementation and hepatic drug metabolism in humans. *J. Cardiovasc. Pharmacol.*, **54**, 491–496.

42 Leonard, S.W., Joss, J.D., Mustacich, D.J., Blatt, D.H., Lee, Y.S., and Traber, M.G. (2007) Effects of vitamin E on cholesterol levels of hypercholesterolemic patients receiving statins. *Am. J. Health Syst. Pharm.*, **64**, 2257–2266.

43 Barany, P., Stenvinkel, P., Ottosson-Seeberger, A., Alvestrand, A., Morrow, J., Roberts, J.J., 2nd, and Salahudeen, A.K. (2001) Effect of 6 weeks of vitamin E administration on renal haemodynamic alterations following a single dose of neoral in healthy volunteers. *Nephrol. Dial. Transplant.*, **16**, 580–584.

44 Ward, N.C., Wu, J.H., Clarke, M.W., Puddey, I.B., Burke, V., Croft, K.D., and Hodgson, J.M. (2007) The effect of vitamin E on blood pressure in individuals with type 2 diabetes: a randomized, double-blind, placebo-controlled trial. *J. Hypertens.*, **25**, 227–234.

45 Yoo, J.S., Park, H.S., Ning, S.M., Lee, M.J., and Yang, C.S. (1990) Effects of thiamine deficiency on hepatic cytochromes P450 and drug-metabolizing enzyme activities. *Biochem. Pharmacol.*, **39**, 519–525.

46 Pangrekar, J., Krishnaswamy, K., and Jagadeesan, V. (1993) Effects of riboflavin deficiency and riboflavin administration on carcinogen–DNA binding. *Food Chem. Toxicol.*, **31**, 745–750.

47 Hornsby, L.B., Hester, E.K., and Donaldson, A.R. (2008) Potential interaction between warfarin and high dietary protein intake. *Pharmacotherapy*, **28**, 536–539.

48 Daly, A.K. and King, B.P. (2003) Pharmacogenetics of oral anticoagulants. *Pharmacogenetics*, **13**, 247–252.

49 Yang, H.Y., Tzeng, Y.H., Chai, C.Y., Hsieh, A.T., Chen, J.R., Chang, L.S., and Yang, S.S. (2011) Soy protein retards the progression of non-alcoholic steatohepatitis via improvement of insulin resistance and steatosis. *Nutrition*, **27**, 943–948.

50 Ronis, M.J., Chen, Y., Liu, X., Blackburn, M.L., Shankar, K., Landes, R.D., Fang, N., and Badger, T.M. (2011) Enhanced expression and glucocorticoid-inducibility of hepatic cytochrome P450 3A involve recruitment of the pregnane-X-receptor to promoter elements in rats fed soy protein isolate. *J. Nutr.*, **141**, 10–16.

51 Lee, J.I., Zhang, L., Men, A.Y., Kenna, L.A., and Huang, S.M. (2010) CYP-mediated therapeutic protein–drug interactions: clinical findings, proposed mechanisms and regulatory implications. *Clin. Pharmacokinet.*, **49**, 295–310.

52 Zeldin, D.C. (2001) Epoxygenase pathways of arachidonic acid metabolism. *J. Biol. Chem.*, **276**, 36059–36062.

53 Nebert, D.W. and Karp, C.L. (2008) Endogenous functions of the aryl hydrocarbon receptor (AHR): intersection of cytochrome P450 1 (CYP1)-metabolized eicosanoids and AHR biology. *J. Biol. Chem.*, **283**, 36061–36065.

54 Stark, K., Dostalek, M., and Guengerich, F.P. (2008) Expression and purification of orphan cytochrome P4504X1 and oxidation of anandamide. *FEBS J.*, **275**, 3706–3717.

55 Chuang, S.S., Helvig, C., Taimi, M., Ramshaw, H., Collop, A.H., Amad, M., White, J.A., Petkovich, M., Jones, G., and Korczak, B. (2004) CYP2U1, a novel human thymus- and brain-specific cytochrome P450, catalyzes omega- and (omega-1)-hydroxylation of fatty acids. *J. Biol. Chem.*, **279**, 6305–6314.

56 Node, K., Huo, Y., Ruan, X., Yang, B., Spiecker, M., Ley, K., Zeldin, D.C., and Liao, J.K. (1999) Anti-inflammatory properties of cytochrome P450 epoxygenase-derived eicosanoids. *Science*, **285**, 1276–1279.

57 Miyata, N. and Roman, R.J. (2005) Role of 20-hydroxyeicosatetraenoic acid (20-HETE) in vascular system. *J. Smooth Musc. Res.*, **41**, 175–193.

58 Fleming, I. (2008) Vascular cytochrome p450 enzymes: physiology and pathophysiology. *Trends Cardiovasc. Med.*, **18**, 20–25.

59 Panigrahy, D., Kaipainen, A., Greene, E.R., and Huang, S. (2010) Cytochrome P450-derived eicosanoids: the neglected pathway in cancer. *Cancer Metastasis Rev.*, **29**, 723–735.

60 Nakajima, T., Wang, R.S., and Murayama, N. (1993) Immunochemical assessment of the influence of nutritional, physiological and environmental factors on the metabolism of toluene. *Int. Arch. Occup. Environ. Health*, **65** (**1** Suppl.), S127–S130.

61 Bailey, D.G., Arnold, J.M., Munoz, C., and Spence, J.D. (1993) Grapefruit juice–felodipine interaction: mechanism, predictability and effect of naringin. *Clin. Pharmacol. Ther.*, **53**, 637–642.

62 Ameer, B. and Weintraub, R.A. (1997) Drug interactions with grapefruit juice. *Clin. Pharmacokinet.*, **33**, 103–121.

63 Benton, R.E., Honig, P.K., Zamani, K., Cantilena, L.R., and Woosley, R.L. (1996) Grapefruit juice alters terfenadine pharmacokinetics, resulting in prolongation of repolarization on the electrocardiogram. *Clin. Pharmacol. Ther.*, **59**, 383–388.

64 Sasaki, M., Elrod, J.W., Jordan, P., Itoh, M., Joh, T., Minagar, A., and Alexander, J.S. (2004) CYP450 dietary inhibitors attenuate TNF-alpha-stimulated endothelial molecule expression and leukocyte adhesion. *Am. J. Physiol. Cell. Physiol.*, **286**, C931–C939.

65 César, T.B., Manthey, J.A., and Myung, K. (2009) Minor furanocoumarins and coumarins in grapefruit peel oil as inhibitors of human cytochrome P450 3A4. *J. Nat. Prod.*, **72**, 1702–1704.

66 Hukkinen, S.K., Varhe, A., Olkkola, K.T., and Neuvonen, P.J. (1995) Plasma concentrations of triazolam are increased by concomitant ingestion of grapefruit juice. *Clin. Pharmacol. Ther.*, **58**, 127–131.

67 Hertog, M.G., Kromhout, D., Aravanis, C., Blackburn, H., Buzina, R., Fidanza, F., Giampaoli, S., Jansen, A., Menotti, A., Nedeljkovic, S., *et al.* (1995) Flavonoid intake and long-term risk of coronary heart disease and cancer in the seven countries study. *Arch. Intern. Med.*, **155**, 381–386.

68 Chatuphonprasert, W., Kondo, S., Jarukamjorn, K., Kawasaki, Y., Sakuma, T., and Nemoto, N. (2010) Potent modification of inducible CYP1A1 expression by flavonoids. *Biol. Pharm. Bull.*, **33**, 1698–1703.

69 Yu, C.P., Wu, P.P., Hou, Y.C., Lin, S.P., Tsai, S.Y., Chen, C.T., and Chao, P.D. (2011) Quercetin and rutin reduced the bioavailability of cyclosporine from neoral, an immunosuppressant, through activating P-glycoprotein and CYP 3A4. *J. Agric. Food Chem.*, **59**, 4644–4648.

70 Hu, R., Xu, C., Shen, G., Jain, M.R., Khor, T.O., Gopalkrishnan, A., Lin, W., Reddy, B., Chan, J.Y., and Kong, A.N. (2006) Identification of Nrf2-regulated genes induced by chemo-preventive isothiocyanate PEITC by oligonucleotide microarray. *Life Sci.*, **79**, 1944–1955.

71 Ji, Y., Kuo, Y., and Morris, M.E. (2005) Pharmacokinetics of dietary phenethyl isothiocyanate in rats. *Pharm. Res.*, **22**, 1658–1666.

72 Gross-Steinmeyer, K., Stapleton, P.L., Liu, F., Tracy, J.H., Bammler, T.K., Quigley, S.D., Farin, F.M., Buhler, D.R., Safe, S.H., Strom, S.C., and Eaton, D.L. (2004) Phytochemical-induced changes in gene expression of carcinogen-metabolizing enzymes in cultured human primary hepatocytes. *Xenobiotica*, **34**, 619–632.

73 Nakajima, M., Yoshida, R., Shimada, N., Yamazaki, H., and Yokoi, T. (2001) Inhibition and inactivation of human cytochrome P450 isoforms by phenethyl isothiocyanate. *Drug Metab. Dispos.*, **29**, 1110–1113.

74 Hu, R., Khor, T.O., Shen, G., Jeong, W.S., Hebbar, V., Chen, C., Xu, C., Reddy, B., Chada, K., and Kong, A.N. (2006) Cancer chemoprevention of

intestinal polyposis in ApcMin/+ mice by sulforaphane, a natural product derived from cruciferous vegetable. *Carcinogenesis*, **27**, 2038–2046.

75 Dingley, K.H., Ubick, E.A., Chiarappa-Zucca, M.L., Nowell, S., Abel, S., Ebeler, S.E., Mitchell, A.E., Burns, S.A., Steinberg, F.M., and Clifford, A.J. (2003) Effect of dietary constituents with chemopreventive potential on adduct formation of a low dose of the heterocyclic amines PhIP and IQ and phase II hepatic enzymes. *Nutr. Cancer*, **46**, 212–221.

76 Dinkova-Kostova, A.T., Fahey, J.W., Wade, K.L., Jenkins, S.N., Shapiro, T.A., Fuchs, E.J., Kerns, M.L., and Talalay, P. (2007) Induction of the phase 2 response in mouse and human skin by sulforaphane-containing broccoli sprout extracts. *Cancer Epidemiol. Biomarkers Prev.*, **16**, 847–851.

77 Xu, C., Yuan, X., Pan, Z., Shen, G., Kim, J.H., Yu, S., Khor, T.O., Li, W., Ma, J., and Kong, A.N. (2006) Mechanism of action of isothiocyanates: the induction of ARE-regulated genes is associated with activation of ERK and JNK and the phosphorylation and nuclear translocation of Nrf2. *Mol. Cancer Ther.*, **5**, 1918–1926.

78 Wogan, G.N., Hecht, S.S., Felton, J.S., Conney, A.H., and Loeb, L.A. (2004) Environmental and chemical carcinogenesis. *Semin. Cancer Biol.*, **14**, 473–486.

79 Zhang, X., Shu, X.O., Xiang, Y.B., Yang, G., Li, H., Gao, J., Cai, H., Gao, Y.T., and Zheng, W. (2011) Cruciferous vegetable consumption is associated with a reduced risk of total and cardiovascular disease mortality. *Am. J. Clin. Nutr.*, **94**, 240–246.

80 Sinha, R., Gustafson, D.R., Kulldorff, M., Wen, W.Q., Cerhan, J.R., and Zheng, W. (2000) 2-Amino-1-methyl-6-phenylimidazo[4,5-*b*]pyridine, a carcinogen in high-temperature-cooked meat, and breast cancer risk. *J. Natl. Cancer Inst.*, **92**, 1352–1354.

81 Turesky, R.J., Richoz, J., Constable, A., Curtis, K.D., Dingley, K.H., and Turteltaub, K.W. (2003) The effects of coffee on enzymes involved in metabolism of the dietary carcinogen 2-amino-1-methyl-6-phenylimidazo[4,5-*b*] pyridine in rats. *Chem. Biol. Interact.*, **145**, 251–265.

82 Rosenberg, L., Werler, M.M., Palmer, J.R., Kaufman, D.W., Warshauer, M.E., Stolley, P.D., and Shapiro, S. (1989) The risks of cancers of the colon and rectum in relation to coffee consumption. *Am. J. Epidemiol.*, **130**, 895–903.

83 Kamimura, H. (2006) Genetic polymorphism of cytochrome P450s in beagles: possible influence of CYP1A2 deficiency on toxicological evaluations. *Arch. Toxicol.*, **80**, 732–738.

84 Luoma, P.V. (2007) Cytochrome P450–physiological key factor against cholesterol accumulation and the atherosclerotic vascular process. *Ann. Med.*, **39**, 359–370.

85 Russell, D.W. (2000) Oxysterol biosynthetic enzymes. *Biochim. Biophys. Acta*, **1529**, 126–135.

86 Björkhem, I., Diczfalusy, U., and Lütjohann, D. (1999) Removal of cholesterol from extrahepatic sources by oxidative mechanisms. *Curr. Opin. Lipidol.*, **10**, 161–165.

87 Ory, D.S. (2004) Nuclear receptor signalling in the control of cholesterol homeostasis: have the orphans found a home. *Circ. Res.*, **95**, 660–670.

88 Frick, M.H., Syvänne, M., Nieminen, M.S., Kauma, H., Majahalme, S., Virtanen, V., Kesäniemi, Y.A., Pasternack, A., and Taskinen, M.R. (1997) Prevention of the angiographic progression of coronary vein-graft atherosclerosis by gemfibrozil after coronary by-pass surgery in men with low levels of HDL cholesterol. *Circulation*, **96**, 2137–2143.

89 Blankenhorn, D.H., Azen, S.P., Kramsch, D.M., Mack, W.J., Cashin-Hemphill, L., Hodis, H.N., *et al.*, and the MARS Research Group (1993) Coronary angiographic changes with lovastatin therapy: the Monitored Atherosclerosis Regression Study (MARS). *Ann. Intern. Med.*, **119**, 969–976.

90 Femia, R., Natali, A., L'Abbate, A., and Ferrannini, E. (2006) Coronary atherosclerosis and alcohol

consumption. Angiographic and mortality data. *Arterioscler. Thromb. Vasc. Biol.*, **26**, 1607–1612.

91 Yamada, T., Hayasaka, S., Shibata, Y., Ojima, T., Saegusa, T., Gotoh, T., Ishikawa, S., Nakamura, Y., and Kayaba, K. (2011) Frequency of citrus fruit intake is associated with the incidence of cardiovascular disease: the Jichi Medical School Cohort Study. *J. Epidemiol.*, **21**, 169–175.

92 Talalay, P. and Fahey, J.W. (2001) Phytochemicals from cruciferous plants protect against cancer by modulating carcinogen metabolism. *J. Nutr.*, **131**, 3027S–3033S.

93 Ng, V.Y., Huang, Y., Reddy, L.M., Falck, J.R., Lin, E.T., and Kroetz, D.L. (2007) Cytochrome P450 eicosanoids are activators of peroxisome proliferator-activated receptor alpha. *Drug Metab. Dispos.*, **35**, 1126–1134.

94 Baeuerlein, A., Ackermann, S., and Parlesak, A. (2009) Transepithelial activation of human leukocytes by probiotics and commensal bacteria: role of Enterobacteriaceae-type endotoxin. *Microbiol. Immunol.*, **53**, 241–250.

95 Agematu, H., Matsumoto, N., Fujii, Y., Kabumoto, H., Doi, S., Machida, K., Ishikawa, J., and Arisawa, A. (2006) Hydroxylation of testosterone by bacterial cytochromes P450 using the *Escherichia coli* expression system. *Biosci. Biotechnol. Biochem.*, **70**, 307–311.

96 Bailey, D.G., Malcolm, J., Arnold, O., and Spence, J.D. (1998) Grapefruit juice–drug interactions. *Br. J. Clin. Pharmacol.*, **46**, 101–110.

97 Garrait, G., Jarrige, J.F., Blanquet, S., Beyssac, E., and Alric, M. (2007) Recombinant *Saccharomyces cerevisiae* strain expressing a model cytochrome P450 in the rat digestive environment: viability and bioconversion activity. *Appl. Environ. Microbiol.*, **73**, 3566–3574.

98 Fukushima, K., Ogawa, H., Takahashi, K., Naito, H., Funayama, Y., Kitayama, T., Yonezawa, H., and Sasaki, I. (2003) Non-pathogenic bacteria modulate colonic epithelial gene expression in germ-free mice. *Scand. J. Gastroenterol.*, **38**, 626–634.

99 Morgan, E.T., Goralski, K.B., Piquette-Miller, M., Renton, K.W., Robertson, G.R., Chaluvadi, M.R., Charles, K.A., Clarke, S.J., Kacevska, M., Liddle, C., Richardson, T.A., Sharma, R., and Sinal, C.J. (2008) Regulation of drug-metabolizing enzymes and transporters in infection, inflammation, and cancer. *Drug Metab. Dispos.*, **36**, 205–216.

100 Parlesak, A., Schaeckeler, S., Moser, L., and Bode, C. (2007) Conjugated primary bile salts reduce permeability of endotoxin through intestinal epithelial cells and synergize with phosphatidylcholine in suppression of inflammatory cytokine production. *Crit. Care Med.*, **35**, 2367–2374.

Part Four
Metabolism of Unnatural Xenobiotics

23 Environmental Pollutants

Marie Stiborova

23.1 Introduction – An Overview

Environmental pollutants are the components of environmental pollution defined to be: "The contamination of the physical and biological components of the earth/atmosphere system to such an extent that normal environmental processes are adversely affected" [1]. In other words, environmental pollutants are constituent parts of the pollution process. They are the actual "executing agents" of environmental pollution. They can come in gaseous, solid, or liquid form. Environmental pollution takes place when the environment cannot process and neutralize harmful byproducts of human activities (e.g., poisonous gas emissions) without any structural or functional damage to its system. General characteristics of environmental pollutants [2] were identified as (i) pollutants do not recognize boundaries (i.e., they are transboundary), (ii) many environmental pollutants cannot be degraded by living organisms and therefore stay in the environment for many years, and (iii) they destroy the biota and habitat. Environmental pollutants from many different sources contaminate water, air, and land, putting humans and ecosystems at risk, and often pitting people against industry. By viewing competing interests and their implications within a broad ecosystem analysis, ecohealth approaches strive to protect health while balancing the needs of various stakeholders and contribute to safeguarding the ecosystem. Such compounds cause harm or discomfort to humans or other living organisms, or damage the components (habitats) of the environment, such as land, sea, fresh water, and atmosphere. Pollutants can be naturally occurring substances or energies, but are considered contaminants when in excess of natural levels (http://en.wikipedia.org/wiki/Pollution). Most environmental pollutants are, however, the products of anthropogenic activity, being compounds that are not naturally present in the environment, including living organisms. Such pollutants are also called "xenobiotics" and are understood as substances foreign to an entire biological system (i.e., artificial substances that did not exist in nature before their synthesis by humans). These environmental pollutants are present in the environment because, on the one hand, the natural

Metabolism of Drugs and Other Xenobiotics, First Edition. Edited by Pavel Anzenbacher, Ulrich M. Zanger.

environment does not know how to decompose the unnaturally generated elements (i.e., anthropogenic pollutants) and, on the other hand, there is a lack of knowledge on the part of humans about how to decompose these pollutants artificially. Humans are paying the price of these pollutants on many levels – from direct harm to health through cancer, neurological impairment, and other ailments, to contamination of the food chain and the failing capacity of ecosystems to absorb waste and provide the essentials for life. These complex and urgent problems require innovative, flexible, and action-oriented approaches to finding solutions.

It has been evaluated that there are more than 150 000 different chemicals in the marketplace (i.e., potential environmental pollutants (xenobiotics) that have been released into the air, water, and land on a regular basis), and their numbers and amounts are considered to still be increasing considerably. There are several ways by which xenobiotics are introduced into living organisms, the most important among them being (i) inhalation (also known as inspiration – the movement of air from the external environment, through the airways, and into the alveoli), (ii) oral administration (*per os* – a route of administration where a substance is taken through the mouth), and (iii) through the skin. Thereafter, the environmental pollutants are distributed among the tissues of organisms and transported into their cells. Depending on their biotransformation (metabolism), they can either be eliminated from these cells (being thereafter excreted from organisms) or accumulated in organisms.

23.1.1 Types of Environmental Pollutants

Environmental pollutants are grouped according to several characteristics. Depending on their biodegradability, the pollutants can be divided into biodegradable pollutants, pollutants that can be decomposed biologically, and nonbiodegradable pollutants. Biodegradable pollutants are those that can be broken down and processed by living organisms, including organic waste products, phosphates, and inorganic salts. For example, if a pollutant is organic, it can be used by a living organism to obtain energy and other material from carbohydrates, proteins, etc. Therefore, biodegradable pollutants are only "temporary nuisances" that can be neutralized and converted into harmless compounds. However, it is important to remember that they can be serious pollutants if released in large amounts in small areas, thus exceeding the natural capacity of the environment to "assimilate" them. Nonbiodegradable pollutants are those that cannot be decomposed by living organisms and therefore persist in the ecosphere for long periods of time. They include bottles, cans, plastics, metal, some pesticides and herbicides, and radioactive isotopes. Nonbiodegradable pollutants are dangerous because living organisms have neither the enzymes capable of processing these pollutants nor defensive systems against them. In addition to that, for example, fat-soluble (but not water-soluble) nonbiodegradable pollutants (such as chlorinated hydrocarbons, benzene, etc.) are not excreted with urine, but are accumulated in the fat of living organisms, because they cannot be metabolized. Likewise, some water-soluble nonbiodegradable pollutants (such as heavy metal ions) cannot be metabolized or detoxified, and are accumulated both in nonliving parts of the environment (i.e., water, soil) and in living organisms. Moreover, many of these pollutants are toxic (toxins, toxicants). Therefore, organisms retain 100% of these pollutants (xenobiotics, toxins). The xenobiotics (toxins) are then circulated throughout the food chains via the process of biomagnification. For example, plant-eating animals (herbivores) will eat intoxicated plants; meat-eating animals (carnivores, including humans) will eat herbivores and will absorb the toxins already accumulated in the herbivores' bodies. This is how humans can acquire high concentrations of toxins from their food sources, with all the negative consequences following such consumption.

Concerning their physicochemical properties, environmental pollutants are grouped into polar (hydrophilic) and nonpolar (hydrophobic) pollutants. Depending on the presence of pollutants in different components (parts) of the environment, they are grouped into air, water, and soil pollutants. Another characteristic that is utilized for grouping environmental pollutants is their source. According this feature, pollutants are grouped as agricultural, industrial, and biological pollutants. Furthermore, the most important property used for classifying environmental pollutants is their effect on organisms. The toxicity of environmental pollutants is one of the most important effects utilized for classifying these xenobiotic pollutants. Some of the most important biologically active environmental pollutants, including toxic ones, are discussed in this and additional chapters.

23.2 Overview of Environmental Pollutants

23.2.1 Air Pollutants

Oxides of sulfur and nitrogen, such as sulfur dioxide (SO_2) and NO_x (NO, NO_2), and ozone (O_3) are the most important gas environmental air pollutants. Other important gaseous pollutants are oxides of carbon (carbon monoxide (CO), a local pollutant important because of its high toxicity, and carbon dioxide (CO_2), important as a global environmental pollutant), numerous volatile organic compounds (organic compounds that evaporate easily), and persistent organic pollutants (organic compounds that are resistant to environmental degradation through chemical, biological, and photolytic processes; because of this, they have been observed to persist in the environment, to be capable of long-range transport, bioaccumulate in human and animal tissue, biomagnify in food chains, and to have a potential significant impact on human health and the environment) (http://www.chem.unep.ch/pops/ritter/en/ritteren.pdf). Ammonia and airborne particles are additional air environmental pollutants.

23.2.2
Water Pollutants

Both organic and inorganic compounds are water pollutants. Several of the most important groups of water pollutants are:

- A range of organohalides used as insecticides and pesticides.
- Volatile organic compounds including solvents and hydrocarbons.
- Chlorinated solvents.
- Detergents and chemical compounds found in cosmetics products.
- Heavy metals.
- Acidity caused from sulfur dioxide and/or oxides of nitrogen.
- Fertilizers from agricultural use.

23.2.3
Soil Pollutants

The most important groups of soil pollutants are hydrocarbons, solvents, pesticides, and heavy metals.

Here, we will describe some of the most important, most toxic, abundant, or otherwise interesting environmental pollutants. In particular, we will be considering two general features of the biological effects of environmental pollutants:

i) How pollutants (xenobiotics) can influence the intermediate metabolism of living organisms.
ii) How living organisms can influence the fate of xenobiotics in the environment, including their own metabolism.

Concerning both these features, the following subsections describe briefly the toxic effects and fate in organisms of selected pollutants. For practical reasons, the list is far from complete, but we hope that all significant compounds are included.

23.3
Toxic and Hazardous Environmental Pollutants Interacting with Drug Metabolism

23.3.1
Acetaldehyde

Acetaldehyde is an environmental pollutant occurring widely in nature. It is produced industrially on a large -scale. It is also generated in humans endogenously, by oxidation of ethanol. It is a Group 1 human carcinogen [3–5] and http://www.epa.gov/iris/subst/0290.htm). Acetaldehyde is oxidized by acetaldehyde dehydrogenase and catalase into acetic acid, and further metabolized in the citric acid cycle.

23.3.2 Acetonitrile

Acetonitrile is produced mainly as a byproduct of acrylonitrile manufacture. It is metabolized to produce hydrogen cyanide, which is the source of its toxic effects [6]. The symptoms include breathing difficulties, slow pulse rate, nausea, and vomiting. It is metabolized by the cytochrome P450 (CYP) enzyme CYP2E1 to glyconitrile that undergoes a spontaneous decondensation to give hydrogen cyanide and formaldehyde [7, 8].

23.3.3 2-Acetylaminofluorene

2-Acetylaminofluorene was intended for use as a pesticide, but it has never been marketed because of its carcinogenicity to experimental animals ([9] and http://toxnet.nlm.nih.gov/cgi-bin/sis/htmlgen?HSDB). It is, however, frequently used as a positive control by toxicologists to study the carcinogenicity and mutagenicity of aromatic amines. 2-Acetylaminofluorene is a carcinogen inducing carcinomas of the liver and the urinary bladder, testicular mesotheliomas, and Zymbal gland tumors [10]. No data are available to evaluate the carcinogenicity of 2-acetylaminofluorene in humans. 2-Acetylaminofluorene is oxidized by CYP enzymes such as CYP1A2 to *N*-hydroxy-2-acetylaminofluorene, which is a proximal carcinogen and is more potent than the parent molecule. This metabolite can be *O*-acetylated by cytosolic *N*-acetyltransferase (NAT) enzymes to yield *N*-acetyl-*N*-acetoxyaminofluorene. This intermediate can spontaneously rearrange to form the nitrenium and carbenium ions, forming DNA adducts.

23.3.4 Acrolein

Connections have been found between acrolein in the smoke from tobacco cigarettes and the risk of lung cancer [11, 12]. Acrolein is not only an environmental pollutant, but it is also formed as a toxic metabolite of cyclophosphamide – a cytotoxic chemotherapy agent (activated by CYP2B6 and CYP2C19 [13]) – and results in hemorrhagic cystitis. *N*-acetylcysteine or MESNA (2-mercaptoethane sulfonate sodium) are used to counteract acrolein.

23.3.5 Acrylamide

Acrylamide is a pollutant produced by the chemical industry. It is of concern as a probable human carcinogen (Group 2A) [14]. It is used to synthesize polyacrylamide, which finds many uses, and also occurs in many fried and baked starchy foods [15]. Cigarette smoking is also an important acrylamide source [16]. Increased risks of postmenopausal endometrial and ovarian cancer with increasing dietary acrylamide intake were found [17]. A connection was also found between acrylamide intake and colorectal cancer [18]. Acrylamide decomposes nonthermally to form ammonia, and thermal decomposition produces carbon monoxide, carbon dioxide, and oxides of nitrogen. Acrylamide, as well as its metabolite – the carcinogenic epoxide glycidamide – are conjugated with glutathione (probably by glutathione *S*-transferase (GST) enzymes). Acrylamide conversion to glycidamide is catalyzed by CYP2E1 [19], which hence takes part in the activation of this chemical.

23.3.6
4-Aminobiphenyl

4-Aminobiphenyl is produced by the chemical industry; it is used to manufacture azo dyes. It is a carcinogen inducing tumors in a number of species, predominantly in the urinary bladder [20, 21] and also in the liver. According the International Agency for Research on Cancer (IARC), 4-aminobiphenyl is a Group 1 human carcinogen, inducing urinary bladder tumors [20]. It is activated via *N*-hydroxylation by CYP1A2 liver enzymes [22], and subsequently through *O*-sulfation and *O*-acetylation of its *N*-hydroxy derivative by phenol sulfating SULT1A1 and arylamine NAT2, respectively [23]. The *N*-hydroxylamine metabolite and its conjugates can spontaneously rearrange to form the nitrenium and carbenium ions, forming DNA adducts.

23.3.7
o-Anisidine

o-Anisidine is a pollutant produced by industrial manufacturing dyes. It is a potent carcinogen, causing tumors of the urinary bladder in rats and mice [24]. The IARC has classified *o*-anisidine as a Group 2B carcinogen [24], which is possibly carcinogenic to humans. It also exhibits other toxic effects, including hematological changes, anemia, and nephrotoxicity [24]. This compound is oxidatively activated by *N*-hydroxylation with CYP2E1 to form nitrenium and carbenium ions generating DNA adducts that persist in the urinary bladder [25, 26]. Its detoxication occurs via *O*-demethylation [26].

23.3.8
Acrylonitrile (2-Propenenitrile)

Acrylonitrile is a pollutant used as an important monomer for the manufacture of useful plastics. It has been classified by the IARC as a Class 2B carcinogen (possibly carcinogenic to humans) [27]. In rats and mice, increased incidences of glial cell tumors of the central nervous system were found, and it also increases the formation of malignant mammary tumors, Zymbal gland carcinomas, benign and malignant hepatocellular tumors, and extrahepatic angiosarcomas. It is metabolized to the reactive cyanoethylene oxide (CEO) (also called glycidonitrile), mainly by CYP2E1, but also by other forms of human CYP [27, 28]. CEO is a substrate for glutathione conjugation and is excreted in the form of mercapturic acids [29].

23.3.9 Arsenic and Arsenic Compounds

These pollutants enter the environment mainly by their use as pesticides, weed killers, and wood preservatives. The IARC recognizes arsenic and arsenic compounds as Group 1 carcinogens (carcinogenic to human). Depending on the route of administration they induce tumors of several human tissues [20, 30, 31]. Arsenic and its compounds also influence many metabolic processes in organisms via their high affinity for thiols present in the form of Cys residues situated at the active sites of many important enzymes [32]. Arsenic readily reacts with sulfhydryl groups in GSH and Cys [33, 34]. The complex between arsenic and vicinal sulfhydryl reagent is particularly strong. Arsenic alters heme biosynthesis via inhibition of δ-aminolevulinic acid dehydratase [35]. It also disrupts ATP production through several mechanisms. At the level of the citric acid cycle, arsenic inhibits lipoic acid, which is a cofactor for pyruvate dehydrogenase–a lipoic acid-dependent enzyme [36]. By competing with phosphate it also uncouples oxidative phosphorylation, thus inhibiting energy-linked reduction of NAD^+, mitochondrial respiration, and ATP synthesis. Hydrogen peroxide production is also increased, which might form reactive oxygen species and oxidative stress that might be the cause of its carcinogenic effect [31]. Inorganic arsenic and its compounds, upon entering the food chain, are progressively metabolized through a process of methylation. Arsenic metabolism is characterized in many species by two main types of reactions: (i) reduction of pentavalent to trivalent arsenic, and (ii) oxidative methylation reactions in which trivalent forms of arsenic are sequentially methylated to form mono-, di-, and trimethylated products using *S*-adenosylmethionine as the methyl donor and glutathione as an essential cofactor [37, 38].

23.3.10 Asbestos

Asbestos is a set of six naturally occurring silicate minerals–the serpentine class chrysotile, and the amphibole class amosite, crocidolite, tremolite, anthophyllite, and actinolite. Asbestos use became widespread because of its properties such as sound absorption, average tensile strength, and its resistance to heat, electrical, and chemical damage. The inhalation of asbestos fibers can cause serious illnesses, including malignant lung cancer, mesothelioma (a formerly rare cancer strongly associated with exposure to amphibole asbestos), and asbestosis (a type of pneumoconiosis) [39]. Therefore, asbestos and all commercial forms of asbestos (including chrysotile asbestos) are classified to be human carcinogens based on sufficient evidence of carcinogenicity to humans (Group 1 carcinogens) [39–41]. Asbestos fibers may act at multiple stages of the carcinogenic process by both genetic and epigenetic mechanisms [39, 42]. Recently, it has been pointed out that there is probably a cross-talk between transcription factors regulating CYP pulmonary metabolism and those associated with asbestos and tobacco smoking [43].

23.3.11
Antimony Compounds

The main use of antimony is in the form of antimony trioxide and it is used in the production of flame-proofing compounds. Antimony compounds are also used in the chemical industry (polymerization processes). Antimony trioxide has suspected carcinogenic potential for humans (a Class 2B carcinogen, possibly carcinogenic) [44, 45].

23.3.12
Benzene

Benzene is both an industrial environmental pollutant, and a component of cigarette smoke, gasoline, and automotive emissions. The IARC has rated benzene as "known to be carcinogenic to humans" (Group 1) [20]. Long-term exposure to excessive levels of benzene in the air causes leukemia – a potentially fatal cancer of the blood-forming organs – in susceptible individuals. In particular, acute myeloid leukemia or acute nonlymphocytic leukemia is not disputed to be caused by benzene [20]. Metabolism is a prerequisite for the development of benzene-mediated myelotoxicity. The CYP2E1 enzyme, and perhaps other CYPs, can generate H_2O_2 when acting as oxidases of NADPH. The hydroxyl radical formed from H_2O_2 can hydroxylate benzene to yield phenol. An alternative mechanism for phenol formation is designed to reflect the fate of the benzene oxide–oxepin system. When benzene oxide is the first product, it can rearrange nonenzymatically to form phenol. Alternatively, benzene oxide can be hydrated via epoxide hydrolase to yield 1,2-benzene dihydrodiol, which can in turn to form catechol. The reaction of benzene oxide with glutathione catalyzed by GST leads to the formation of premercapturic acid. It is likely that benzene oxide or its oxepin are precursors to ring opening [46]. Phenol can be further hydroxylated to form hydroquinone or catechol. In theory, 1,2,4-benzenetriol may be formed by the hydroxylation of either hydroquinone or catechol; however, Inoue *et al.* [47] suggested that catechol is not a precursor of 1,2,4-benzenetriol in humans. Benzene oxide also equilibrates spontaneously with the corresponding oxepine valence tautomer, which can ring open to yield a reactive α,β-unsaturated aldehyde – *trans-trans*-muconaldehyde (MCA). Further reduction or oxidation of MCA gives rise to either 6-hydroxy-*trans-trans*-2,4-hexadienal or 6-hydroxy-*trans-trans*-2,4-hexadienoic acid and the residue of a covalently bound DNA adduct (i.e., N^7-phenylguanine) [46]. Benzene forms DNA adducts also through its metabolites such as *p*-benzoquinone and hydroquinone. *N*(2)-(4-hydroxyphenyl)-2′-deoxyguanosine is the principal adduct identified *in vivo* [48]. Furthermore, histones are bone marrow targets of benzene, although the identity of the reactive metabolite(s) giving rise to these adducts remains unknown. Although the fate of benzene oxide is known in remarkable detail, coupling this information to the site and mechanism of action remains to be established [46].

23.3.13 Benzidine

Benzidine was used in manufacturing dyes, but it has been withdrawn from use in most industries because of its carcinogenicity. Benzidine has been classified by the IARC to be a human carcinogen (Group 1 carcinogen), inducing urinary bladder tumor formation [20]. Benzidine initiation of bladder cancer is complex, involving multiple organs (i.e., liver, kidney, and bladder) and metabolic pathways (i.e., *N*-acetylation, *N*-glucuronidation, peroxidation, and reactive nitrogen oxygen species). CYP1A-mediated activation of benzidine leads to its *N*-hydroxylated metabolite, which itself or after its conjugation forms reactive species generating DNA adducts. Benzidine is also *N*-acetylated by NAT1 and NAT2. The major *in vivo* adduct was identified as *N*-(deoxyguanosin-8-yl)-*N′*-acetyl-benzidine – a product derived either directly from *N*-hydroxy-*N′*-acetyl-benzidine or after *O*-esterification of this *N*-hydroxy arylamine. Formation of *N*-(deoxyguanosin-8-yl)-benzidine, *N*-(deoxyguanosin-8-yl)-*N,N′*-diacetyl-benzidine, and *N*-(deoxyguanosin-*N2*-yl)-benzidine is also mediated by peroxidase-catalyzed reactions. These enzymes also form an *N*,3-(deoxyguanosin-*N7*,*C*8-yl)-benzidine derivative [49, 50]

23.3.14 1,3-Butadiene (Vinyl Ethylene)

1,3-Butadiene is a chemical made from the processing of petroleum. Most of the 1,3-butadiene manufactured is used in the production of synthetic rubber. The IARC has classified 1,3-butadiene in Group 2A (probable human carcinogen) based on limited evidence in humans and sufficient evidence in animals [51]. 1,3-Butadiene induces tumors at multiple organ sites in mice and rats [52]. 1,3-Butadiene is oxidized by human CYP2A6 and 2E1 to 1,2-epoxy-3-butene (butadiene monoepoxide) [53], which is an activation metabolite of this carcinogen. The *N*-1-(2,3,4-trihydroxybutyl)adenine adduct formation was found to be induced by 1,3-butadiene and was detected in lymphocytes of workers occupationally exposed to this carcinogen [54].

23.3.15 Cadmium Compounds

Cadmium was used for corrosion-resistant plating on steel, and cadmium compounds were used to stabilize plastic and in nickel/cadmium batteries and cadmium/telluride solar panels. Owing to their toxicities, their use is now decreasing. Cadmium and cadmium compounds are classified as Group 1 carcinogens (carcinogenic to human) [55]. There has been research linking exposure to cadmium and its compounds to lung, prostate, kidney, and bladder cancer [56–59]. Most studies indicate cadmium is poorly mutagenic and probably acts through indirect or epigenetic mechanisms, potentially including aberrant activation of oncogenes and suppression of apoptosis [60]. In addition to producing a variety of toxic manifestations, cadmium is known to accumulate in certain "target" organs, including the liver and kidney, where histological and functional damage becomes apparent. Cadmium accumulates in the kidney proximal tubular epithelium cells and causes damage. Thereafter, development of chronic kidney disease occurs. One of the causative mechanisms of chronic kidney disease is thought to be oxidative stress [61]. Cadmium also inhibits heme biosynthesis, carbohydrate metabolism, and drug-metabolizing enzymes in the liver of animals via interaction with enzymes containing either SH groups of Cys or the imidazole residue of His that are essential for their activities and that participate in these processes (i.e., glyceraldehyde 3-phosphate dehydrogenase, δ-aminolevulinate dehydratase) [62, 63]. Cadmium also induces metallothionein in the liver and kidney that decreases the actual cadmium ion concentrations [64].

23.3.16 Carbon Tetrachloride

Carbon tetrachloride pollution evolved from its former widespread use in fire extinguishers, as a precursor to refrigerants, and as a cleaning agent. Chronic exposure to carbon tetrachloride as well as chloroform can cause liver [65, 66] and kidney damage, and could result in cancer [67]. It has been classified by the IARC as a Group 2B carcinogen (possible human carcinogen) [27]. Activation of chloroform by CYP2E1, CYP2B1, and possibly CYP3A enzymes leads to the trichloromethyl radical, which binds to cellular macromolecules and lipids. Moreover, it can be converted further to hydroxy or peroxy trichloromethyl radicals, which are active in lipid peroxidation [68]. Similar processes are active in the dehalogenation of volatile anesthetics such as halothane.

23.3.17 Carbon Monoxide

Carbon monoxide is an air pollutant produced from the partial oxidation of carbon-containing compounds. Carbon monoxide mainly causes adverse effects in humans by combining with hemoglobin to form carboxyhemoglobin in the blood. This prevents oxygen binding to hemoglobin, reducing the oxygen-carrying capacity of the blood and leading to hypoxia. The main manifestations of acute poisoning develop in those organ systems most dependent on oxygen use–the central nervous system and the heart [69]. The affinity between hemoglobin and carbon monoxide is approximately 230 times stronger than the affinity between hemoglobin and oxygen. Thereafter, carbon monoxide binds to hemoglobin in preference to oxygen [70]. Carboxyhemoglobin can revert to hemoglobin, but the recovery takes time because the carboxyhemoglobin complex is fairly stable. Oxygen works as an antidote as it increases the removal of carbon monoxide from hemoglobin, in turn providing the body with normal levels of oxygen [71]. Additionally, myoglobin and mitochondrial cytochrome *c* oxidase are thought to be adversely affected by carbon monoxide. In the case of myoglobin, carbon monoxide also has a higher affinity for myoglobin–about 60 times greater than that of oxygen [72]. Carbon monoxide binds to cytochrome *c* oxidase with less affinity than oxygen, so it is possible that it requires significant intracellular hypoxia before binding. This binding interferes with aerobic metabolism and efficient ATP synthesis. Cells respond by switching to anaerobic metabolism, causing anoxia, lactic acidosis, and eventual cell death. The rate of dissociation between carbon monoxide and cytochrome *c* oxidase is slow, causing a relatively prolonged impairment of oxidative metabolism [73, 74]. Carbon monoxide also causes brain lipid peroxidation [75]. Thereafter, it causes endothelial cell and platelet release of nitric oxide, and the formation of oxygen free radicals, including peroxynitrite [73]. In the brain this causes further mitochondrial dysfunction, capillary leakage, leukocyte sequestration, and apoptosis [76]. The result of these effects is lipid peroxidation, which causes delayed reversible demyelinization of white matter in the central nervous system that can lead to edema and necrosis within the brain [77].

23.3.18 Chloroform

Chloroform is used as a solvent and as a reagent for the synthesis of several chloroform chemicals. Chronic exposure to this compound can damage the liver (where chloroform is metabolized to phosgene) and the kidneys. Furthermore, some people develop sores when their skin is immersed in chloroform. The IARC has classified chloroform as possibly carcinogenic to humans–a Group 2B designation [78]. It has been most readily associated with hepatocellular carcinoma; CYPs are known to participate in the activation processes (see also Section 23.3.16 and [68]).

23.3.19 Chloroprene

Chloroprene is a pollutant introduced into the environment from its use in the production of the polymer polychloroprene. It has been classified by the IARC as possibly carcinogenic to humans (Group 2B), but is carcinogenic to animals [78]. In mice and rats it produced neoplasia in several tissues, such as the lung, Harderian gland, thyroid gland mammary gland, liver, kidney, skin, mesentery, forestomach, and Zymbal gland [78]. The toxicological profile of chloroprene *in vivo* depends on the balance between oxidative metabolism by CYPs (predominantly by CYP2E1 and 2A6) [79], leading to epoxides (predominantly to (1-chloroethenyl)oxirane and α,β-unsaturated carbonyl compounds), and the detoxications by hydrolysis and conjugation with glutathione. The reaction of (1-chloroethenyl)oxirane with 2′- deoxyguanosine gave one major adduct – *N*7-(3-chloro-2-hydroxy-3-buten-1-yl)-guanine – and several minor adducts. The metabolite (*Z*)-2-chlorobut-2-en-1-al is a reactive α,β-unsaturated aldehyde that has been shown to form etheno adducts (etheno derivatives of 2′-deoxyadenosine) [80].

23.3.20
Cr (VI) Compounds

Emissions of chromium compounds to air and water occur mainly from the chemical manufacturing industry (dyes, rubber, pharmaceuticals and plastic products), from the metal finishing industry, from electrical and aircraft manufacturers, and from the combustion of oil and coal. Hexavalent chromium compounds are listed as IARC Group 1 carcinogens (carcinogenic to human) [81]. There is sufficient evidence in humans for the carcinogenicity of Cr(VI) compounds as encountered in chromate production, chromate pigment production, and chromium plating industries [81]. Chronic inhalation of hexavalent chromium compounds increases the risk of lung cancer (lungs are especially vulnerable, followed by fine capillaries in the kidneys and intestine). Hexavalent chromium compounds are genotoxic carcinogens. The damage from Cr(VI) compounds is caused by hydroxyl radicals, produced during reoxidation of pentavalent chromium by hydrogen peroxide molecules present in the cell. Namely, hexavalent chromium is transported into cells via the sulfate transport mechanisms, taking advantage of the similarity of sulfate and chromate with respect to their structure and charge. Trivalent chromium, which is the more common variety of chromium compounds, is not transported into cells. Inside the cell, Cr(VI) is reduced first to the metastable pentavalent chromium (Cr(V)) and then to trivalent chromium Cr(III). Reductases such as NAD(P)H : quinone oxidoreductase as well as vitamin C and other reducing agents combine with chromate to give Cr(III) products inside the cell [82, 83]. Strontium chromate is the strongest carcinogen of the chromates used in industry. Soluble compounds, like chromic acid, are much weaker carcinogens [83].

23.3.21
Cobalt and Cobalt Compounds

Cobalt and its compounds are local environmental pollutants produced mainly by the chemical industry (used as catalysts), production of batteries, and as a colorant (pigment). Although cobalt is an essential element for health in animals in low amounts as a component of vitamin B_{12}, it also exhibits toxic effects [84]. Cobalt and cobalt compounds are classified by the IARC to be possibly carcinogenic to humans (Group 2B). However, cobalt metal with tungsten carbide is classified probably carcinogenic to humans (Group 2A) [85]. A number of working group members supported an evaluation in Group 1 because as a transition element, cobalt shares a number of chemical properties with iron and thus it has been suggested that it may catalyze the decomposition of hydrogen peroxide by a Fenton-like mechanism. While several studies have indeed indicated that reactive oxygen species are formed in the presence of a mixture of Co(II) ions and hydrogen peroxide [85–87], the exact nature of the radicals formed is still a matter of speculation. These free radicals have been proposed to account for several toxic properties of cobalt compounds, including their genotoxic activity.

23.3.22 1,4-Dichlorobenzene

The IARC has classified 1,4-dichlorobenzene, which is used as a pesticide, a deodorant, and a precursor in the production of the polymer poly(*p*-phenylene sulfide), as possibly carcinogenic to humans (Group 2B). However, it is carcinogenic to animals [20, 78]. After oral administration, it increased the incidence of adenomas and carcinomas of the liver in male and female mice, and of renal tubular carcinomas in male rats. 1,4-Dichlorobenzene is oxidized by CYP2E1 mainly to 2,5-dichlorophenol that is excreted through the urine as the sulfate and glucuronide conjugates. Another biotransformation pathway for 1,4-dichlorobenzene may be postulated, leading to the urinary excretion of a mercapturic acid of 1,4-dichlorobenzene or chlorophenol [88].

23.3.23 1,3-Dichloropropene

Utilization of 1,3-dichloropropene as a pesticide causes its presence in the environment. The IARC has determined that 1,3-dichloropropene is possibly carcinogenic to humans (Group 2B) [20]. Nevertheless, there is adequate evidence of its carcinogenicity in animals. Technical-grade 1,3-dichloropropene (containing 1.0% epichlorohydrin), when given by gavage, produced tumors of the urinary bladder, lung, and forestomach in mice, and of the liver and forestomach in rats. Inhalation exposure produced an increase in the incidence of bronchioalveolar adenomas in mice. It is an alkylation agent that reacts with glutathione. This conjugation is the principle metabolic pathway of 1,3-dichloropropene, which leads to its elimination as mercapturic acids [20]. Apart from this major route of 1,3-dichloropropene metabolism (conjugation with glutathione), it is also oxidized to carbon dioxide. An additional, minor route of metabolism proposed for this compound involves epoxidation catalyzed by CYP1A to the corresponding 1,3-dichloropropene oxide, which results in acute hepatic injury [89, 90].

23.3.24 Dichloromethane

Dichloromethane, which is widely used as a paint stripper, is metabolically converted to carbon monoxide mostly by CYP2E1 in the liver, resulting in elevation of blood carboxyhemoglobin levels and potentially leading to carbon monoxide poisoning [91, 92]. Dichloromethane is a carcinogenic compound, as it has been linked to cancer of the lungs and liver in laboratory animals [4]. The IARC has determined that dichloromethane is possibly carcinogenic to humans (Group 2B) [4]. Two alternative pathways involving CYP2E1 and GSTs are considered to be responsible for the activation metabolism of dichloromethane [93, 94]. Dichloromethane-derived DNA–glutathione adducts, rather than formation of formaldehyde via a GST pathway [95], are responsible for the carcinogenic effects of dichloromethane [93, 94].

23.3.25 1,1-Dimethylhydrazine

1,1-Dimethylhydrazine is used as a component of jet and rocket fuels, and is an intermediate for chemical synthesis. The IARC has classified this chemical as a possibly carcinogenic compound to humans (Group 2B); however, it is a carcinogen for experimental animals [4, 96]. When administered by gavage, 1,1-dimethylhydrazine increased the incidence of lung and colon tumors in mice. When administered in drinking water, 1,1-dimethylhydrazine induced high incidences of angiosarcomas in various organs and tumors of the kidney, lung, and liver in mice. The same route of administration induced liver carcinomas in rats [4, 20, 96]. Oxidation of 1,1-dimethylhydrazine leads to its activation to form DNA adducts [97]. The increased expression of CYP2E1 induced by chronic ethanol consumption promotes the development of 1,1-dimethylhydrazine-induced colon cancer in rats, indicating a role CYP2E1 in its activation [98].

23.3.26 Ethylene Oxide

Ethylene oxide is one of the most important raw materials used in the large-scale chemical production with a high potential for human exposure. Ethylene oxide is an alkylating agent, a direct acting mutagen, and carcinogen. The IARC has classified ethylene oxide into Group 1, as a chemical carcinogenic to humans [14]. There is evidence that this alkylation agent is associated with the incidence breast and bone cancer [99, 100]. Positive exposure-response trends for lymphoid tumors were also found, but for males only [100]. Ethylene oxide metabolism occurred primarily via cytosolic GST-mediated glutathione conjugation, with highest activity in the liver [101]. The mutagenicity and carcinogenicity of ethylene oxide is attributed to reaction with DNA, which leads to the formation of multiple 2-hydroxyethyl DNA adducts [102].

23.3.27 Formaldehyde

Occupational exposure to formaldehyde by inhalation is mainly from three types of sources: thermal or chemical decomposition of formaldehyde-based resins, formaldehyde emission from aqueous solutions, and the production of formaldehyde resulting from the combustion of a variety of organic compounds. Formaldehyde can be toxic, allergenic, and carcinogenic [103]. The primary exposure concern is for the workers in the industries producing or using formaldehyde. The IARC has classified formaldehyde as a known human carcinogen (Group 1), associated with nasal sinus cancer and nasopharyngeal cancer, and possibly with leukemia [103]. The current data indicate that both genotoxicity and cytotoxicity of formaldehyde play important roles in the carcinogenesis produced by formaldehyde in nasal tissues. DNA–protein cross-links provide a potentially useful marker of genotoxicity [104]. Formaldehyde is also formed during demethylation reactions catalyzed by CYPs; however, the levels are relatively low and do not pose any harm to the organism.

23.3.28 Heptachlor

Heptachlor is a persistent organic pollutant used as an insecticide. It is lipophilic compound, thus it tends to accumulate in the body fat of humans and animals. Humans are exposed to heptachlor through drinking water and foods, including breast milk [105]. Heptachlor epoxide is derived from a pesticide that was banned in several countries. It is still found in soil and water supplies, and can turn up in food and be passed along in breast milk. The IARC has classified the compound as a possible human carcinogen that is carcinogenic to experimental animals (Group 2B) [106]. Increased incidences of hepatocellular neoplasms (including carcinomas) were seen in experimental animals; also, heptachlor is a known endocrine disruptor (see Chapter 24). In the case of technical-grade heptachlor, thyroid follicular cell adenomas and carcinomas were seen in rats.

23.3.29 Hexachlorobenzene

Hexachlorobenzene is a persistent organic pollutant used as a fungicide that was banned from use in several countries. Hexachlorobenzene is lipophilic, accumulates in humans, and is excreted as a Cys conjugate of pentachlorobenzene. In rats, hexachlorobenzene has been shown to follow several metabolic pathways, which include the formation of pentachlorobenzene, tetrachlorobenzene, and tri- and tetrachlorophenol. Human CYP3A4 was found to catalyze hexachlorobenzene metabolism [107]. The IARC has classified hexachlorobenzene as a Group 2B carcinogen (possibly carcinogenic to humans), but it is carcinogenic to experimental animals [20, 106, 108, 109]. It produced liver cell tumors and renal tubular tumors in experimental animals. After perinatal administration, it also increased the incidences of parathyroid adenomas, hemangioendotheliomas, and thyroid follicular cell adenomas [20, 106, 108–110]. Accidental consumption by humans of a large quantity of hexachlorobenzene resulted in a liver disease (porphyria cutanea tarda), neurological effects, and skin changes, which were persistent. Chronic oral exposure in humans has been shown to also give rise to a porphyria cutanea tarda, as well as skin lesions, ulceration, thyroid effects, and bone effects. Neurological changes have been reported in rodents exposed to hexachlorobenzene. Hexachlorobenzene can also cause embryolethality and teratogenic effects [106]. In the livers of experimental animals, hexachlorobenzene induced CYP enzymes (CYP1A and 2B), NAD(P)H:quinone oxidoreductase, and GST, and inhibited uroporphyrinogen decarboxylase, iron accumulation, and oxidative damage. Some of these effects are believed to be involved in the production of hepatic tumors [111, 112].

23.3.30 Hydrazine

Exposure to hydrazine may occur in its production, and in the production of chemical blowing agents, agricultural chemicals, and in water treatment. Human exposure to hydrazine has resulted in severe effects upon the central nervous system, liver, and kidneys. In rats, hydrazine is hepatotoxic, causing accumulation of triglycerides, inhibition of protein synthesis, and the formation of macromitochondria [4]. Most urinary elimination of hydrazine was as unchanged hydrazine, with acetylhydrazine being the main metabolite, but a minor elimination product. Tissue retention was longest in kidney, mainly due to the presence of acetylhydrazine. Hydrazine is metabolized and detoxified by at least three microsomal CYP enzymes in the liver (CYP2E1, CYP2B, and CYP1A), ultimately yielding molecular nitrogen [113, 114]. The IARC has classified hydrazine as a Group 2B carcinogen (possibly carcinogenic to humans), but is carcinogenic to experimental animals [4]. Hydrazine was tested for carcinogenicity by oral administration to experimental animals, producing liver, nasal, and mammary and lung tumors. In hamsters, it produced liver tumors and thyroid adenomas following oral or inhalation exposure [4]. It is a genotoxic carcinogen; *in vivo* treatment of experimental animals results in the formation of N^7-methylguanine and O^6-methylguanine in liver DNA [4].

23.3.31 Lead and Lead Compounds

Since lead has been used widely for centuries, the effects of exposure are worldwide [115]. Lead and other heavy metals create reactive radicals that damage cell structures, including DNA and cell membranes [116] Lead also interferes with DNA transcription, enzymes that help in the synthesis of vitamin D, and enzymes that maintain the integrity of the cell membrane. Anemia may result when the cell membranes of red blood cells become more fragile as a result of damage to their membranes [117]. Lead also interferes with the normal metabolism of calcium in cells and causes it to build up within them [118]. The primary cause of lead's toxicity is its interference with a variety of enzymes because it binds to sulfhydryl groups of Cys of many enzymes. Part of lead's toxicity results from its ability to mimic other metals that take part in biological processes, which act as cofactors in many enzymatic reactions, displacing them at the enzymes on which they act. Lead is capable of binding to and interacting with many of the same enzymes as these metals; however, due to its differing chemistry, it does not properly function as a cofactor, thus interfering with the enzyme's ability to catalyze its normal reactions. Among the essential metals with which lead interacts are calcium, iron, and zinc [119]. One of the main causes of the pathology of lead is that it interferes with the activity of an essential enzyme called δ-aminolevulinic acid dehydratase, which is an intermediate in the biosynthesis of heme – the prosthetic group or cofactor of, for example, hemoglobin, cytochromes, and heme enzymes. Lead also inhibits the enzyme ferrochelatase – another enzyme involved in the formation of heme (for review, see [120–122]).

23.3.32 Lindane (All Isomers)

Lindane and its isomers belong among the persistent organic pollutants: they are relatively long-lived in the environment and bioaccumulate in food chains. Most of the adverse human health effects reported for lindane have been related to agricultural uses and chronic, occupational exposure of seed treatment workers. Exposure to large amounts of lindane can harm the nervous system [123]. Lindane interferes with γ-aminobutyric acid (GABA) neurotransmitter function by interacting with the GABA-A receptor–chloride channel complex at the picrotoxin binding site. In humans, lindane affects the nervous system, liver, and kidneys, and may be a carcinogen [20, 108, 109]. Based primarily on evidence from animal studies, most evaluations of lindane have concluded that it may possibly cause cancer. In 1987, the IARC classified lindane as a Group 2B possible human carcinogen [20, 108, 109], carcinogenic to experimental animals, which may be related to its inductive effect on activities of CYP enzymes known to activate carcinogens (CYP1A, CYP2E1, and CYP2B) [124].

23.3.33 Mercury Compounds

The consumption of fish is by far the most significant source of ingestion-related mercury exposure in humans and animals, although plants and livestock also contain mercury due to bioaccumulation of mercury from soil, water, and atmosphere, and due to biomagnification by ingesting other mercury-containing organisms [125, 126]. Mercury is such a highly reactive toxic agent that it is difficult to identify its specific mechanism of damage and much remains unknown about the mechanism [127]. It causes damage to the central nervous system, endocrine system, kidneys, and other organs, and adversely affects the mouth, gums, and teeth. Exposure over long periods of time or heavy exposure to mercury vapor can result in brain damage [127]. Compounds of mercury tend to be much more toxic than the element itself, and organic compounds of mercury are often extremely toxic and have been implicated in causing brain and liver damage. The most dangerous mercury compound is dimethylmercury. Methylmercury is the major source of organic mercury for all individuals. It works its way up the food chain through bioaccumulation in the environment, reaching high concentrations among populations of some species [128]. Both methylmercury and inorganic mercury bind to various thiol-containing compounds and proteins (glutathione, Cys, albumin, etc.). The binding and dissociation of these mercury–thiol complexes are believed to control the movement of mercury and its toxic effects in the body [127, 128].

23.3.34 NO_x

NO_x is a term for the mono-nitrogen oxides NO (nitrogen monoxide, nitric oxide) and NO_2 (nitrogen dioxide). They are produced from the reaction of nitrogen and oxygen gases in the air during combustion, especially at high temperatures. In areas of high motor vehicle traffic, such as in large cities, the amount of nitrogen oxides emitted into the atmosphere as air pollution can be quite significant. In atmospheric chemistry, the term NO_x means the total concentration of NO and NO_2. Nitrogen dioxide inflames the lining of the lungs and it can reduce immunity to lung infections. This can cause problems such as wheezing, coughing, colds, flu, and bronchitis. Increased levels of nitrogen dioxide can have a significant impact on people with asthma, because it can cause more frequent and more intense attacks. Children with asthma and older people with heart disease are most at risk. NO_x react to form smog and acid rain. NO_x also react with volatile organic compounds in the presence sunlight to form ozone, and later with common organic chemicals and ozone, to form a wide variety of toxic products: nitroarenes, nitrosamines, and also nitrate radicals, some of which may cause biological mutations [129]. Nitric oxide is produced also as an endogenous molecule (acting in neurotransmission, regulation of vascular tone, and host defense). It was implicated in the downregulation of CYPs (e.g., during inflammation) [130].

23.3.35 Ozone

Low-level ozone (or tropospheric ozone) is an atmospheric pollutant. It is formed by the reaction of sunlight on air containing hydrocarbons and nitrogen oxides, which react to form ozone directly at the source of the pollution or many kilometers down wind [131]. Ozone photolysis by UV light leads to production of hydroxyl radicals and these plays a part in the removal of hydrocarbons from the air, but this is also the first step in the creation of components of smog such as peroxyacyl nitrates that can be powerful eye irritants [131]. Interestingly, in a recent study it has been shown that aryl hydrocarbon receptor (AhR) is an ozone sensor in human skin; this leads to increased mRNA expression of CYP1A1, CYP1A2, and CYP1B1 [132].

23.3.36 Parathion

Parathion is one of the most dangerous pesticides [133]. It is a cholinesterase inhibitor–disrupting the nervous system by inhibiting the acetylcholinesterase

[133, 134]. Parathion is a substrate of human CYP3A4 and 2B6 [135]; its toxic metabolite – paraoxon – should be further hydrolyzed to *p*-nitrophenol and diethylphosphate by paraoxonase (see also Chapter 6) [136].

23.3.37
Phthalates

Phthalates are manufactured chemicals that are commonly added as plasticizers to make plastics more flexible. The IARC has downgraded its former classification of di-(2-ethyl-hexyl)-phthalate (DEHP) as a potential human carcinogen. In January 2000, an IARC working group decided in the light of a large body of other relevant data, including evidence from genetically engineered mice, that the chemical should instead be described as "not classifiable as to carcinogenicity to humans." DEHP was initially classified as a potential carcinogen following rodent studies, in which it was found to cause liver tumors through a mechanism called peroxisome proliferation when administered at high doses. It should be mentioned here that so-called peroxisome proliferators are known to induce enzymes of the CYP4 family and may induce many other processes involved in lipid homeostasis. The IARC has now ruled that the mechanism by which DEHP increases the incidence of liver tumors in rats and mice is not relevant to humans [137]. Based on animal studies, long-term exposure may cause liver and kidney damage. Phthalates also act as endocrine disruptors. The phthalate di(*n*-butyl) phthalate or its metabolite monobutyl phthalate suppress steroidogenesis by fetal-type Leydig cells in primates as in rodents [138]. In an epidemiological study it was "suggested that male reproductive development in humans could be affected by prenatal exposure to environmentally relevant levels of phthalates" [139]. It should be noted, however, that for such effects, exposure to a combination of phthalates and antiandrogenic pesticides is needed [140]. Mono-ethyl-hexyl-phthalate – a metabolite of DEHP – has been found to interact with all three peroxisome proliferator-activated receptors, which might be related to its function as a metabolic disruptor [141]. In general, the exposure of children to phthalates is greater than that of adults.

23.3.38
Polycyclic Aromatic Hydrocarbons

Polycyclic aromatic hydrocarbons (PAHs), formed by the incomplete combustion of coal, oil, petrol, wood, tobacco, charbroiled meats, garbage, or other organic materials, are potent atmospheric pollutants. The toxicity of PAHs is dependent on their structures, with types of compound varying from being nontoxic to being extremely toxic. Thus, highly carcinogenic PAHs may be small or large. One PAH compound – benzo[*a*]pyrene – is notable for being the first chemical carcinogen to be discovered (and is one of many carcinogens found in cigarette smoke). The IARC has classified some PAHs such as benzo[*a*]anthracene, benzo[*a*]pyrene, benzo[*b*]fluoranthene, benzo[*k*]fluoranthene, chrysene, dibenz[*a*,*h*]anthracene, and indeno[1,2,3-*cd*]pyrene as probable or possible human carcinogens (Group 2A and 2B) [20, 142–146]. PAHs known for their carcinogenic, mutagenic, and teratogenic properties are benzo[*a*]anthracene and chrysene, benzo[*b*]fluoranthene, benzo[*j*]fluoranthene, benzo[*k*]fluoranthene, benzo[*a*]pyrene, benzo[*ghi*]perylene, coronene, dibenz[*a,h*]anthracene, indeno[1,2,3-*cd*]pyrene, and ovalene [147]. Genotoxic properties of PAHs depend on their enzymatic activation catalyzed by many CYPs, predominantly by CYPs of the 1A subfamily.

23.3.39 Polychlorinated Biphenyls

Polychlorinated biphenyls (PCBs) have been widely used for many applications, especially as dielectric fluids in transformers, capacitors, and coolants [148]. Due to the toxicity and stability of PCBs they are classified as persistent organic pollutants. Concerns about the toxicity of PCBs are largely based on compounds within this group that share a structural similarity and toxic mode of action with dioxin. The toxicity of PCBs varies considerably among congeners. The coplanar PCBs, known as non-*ortho*-PCBs because they are not substituted at the ring positions *ortho* to (next to) the other ring, tend to have dioxin-like properties and generally are among the most toxic congeners. Studies in workers exposed to PCBs have shown changes in blood and urine that may indicate liver damage [148]. The IARC has determined that PCBs are probably carcinogenic to humans (Group 2A) [20, 96, 149]. PCBs exhibit a wide range of toxic effects. These effects may vary depending on the specific PCB. Similar to dioxin, toxicity of coplanar PCBs and mono-*ortho*-PCBs is thought to be primarily mediated via binding to AhR [150–152]–the receptor that is highly conserved in an evolutionary sense and functions in the same way in humans as in experimental animals. As AhR is a transcription factor, abnormal activation may disrupt cell function by altering the transcription of genes. The concept of toxic equivalency factors (TEF) is based on the ability of a PCB to activate AhR. However, not all effects may be mediated by AhR, and PCBs do not alter estrogen concentrations to the same degree as other ligands of AhR such as polychlorinated dibenzo-*p*-dioxins (PCDDs) and polychlorinated dibenzofurans (PCDFs), possibly reflecting the reduced potency of PCBs to induce CYP1A1 and CYP1B1 [153]. Examples of other actions of PCBs include di-*ortho*-substituted noncoplanar PCBs interfering with intracellular signal transduction dependent on calcium; this may lead to neurotoxicity [154]. *Ortho*-PCBs may disrupt thyroid hormone transport by binding to transthyretin [155].

23.3.40 Polychlorinated Dioxins and Furans

PCDDs and PCDFs belong among the persistent organic pollutants, and are ubiquitous in soil, sediment, and air. PCDFs are formed as inadvertent byproducts in the production and use of polychlorinated biphenyls, and, in combination with PCDDs, in the production of chlorophenols [156–158]. 2,3,7,8-Tetrachlorodibenzo-

p-dioxin (TCDD) has been evaluated by the IARC as carcinogenic to humans, causing tumors of liver and lung (IARC Group 1 classification) [159, 160]. TCDD is also a multisite carcinogen in experimental animals and has been shown by several lines of evidence to act through a mechanism involving the AhR. Tissue concentrations of TCDD are similar in heavily exposed human populations in which an increased overall cancer risk was observed and in exposed rats that developed tumors in carcinogenicity tests. Other PCDDs, the nonchlorinated dibenzo-*p*-dioxin, and PCDFs were evaluated as not classifiable as to their carcinogenicity to humans (Group 3) [159, 160].

23.3.41 **Styrene and Styrene Oxide**

Styrene is the precursor to manufacture polystyrene and several copolymers [161]. It is rapidly distributed throughout the body. A large percentage of absorbed styrene is excreted as urinary mandelic and phenylglyoxylic acids, with glutathione conjugates forming a minor fraction of the metabolites. The predominant first metabolite is styrene-7,8-oxide–the formation of which appears to be catalyzed mainly by CYP2B6 and also by CYP2E1 and 1A2 in humans. Exposure of humans to styrene leads to the formation of both protein and DNA adducts in human and experimental animals such as rats and mice. The levels of the *N*-terminal Val adduct of hemoglobin – *N*-(1-hydroxy-2-phenylethyl)valine–have been found to be 4 times higher in styrene-exposed workers than in controls, and the levels of the DNA adduct–O^6-(2-hydroxy-1-phenylethyl)-2′-deoxy-guanosine-3′-monophosphate–have been found to be about 5 times higher than in controls [162]. Although styrene is only weakly toxic, it has been classified by the IARC as possibly carcinogenic to humans (Group 2B) and carcinogenic to experimental animals (mice) [163]. An increase in the incidence of pulmonary tumors and hepatocellular adenomas in mice was found. A major metabolite of styrene–styrene-7,8-oxide (styrene oxide)–has been classified as probably carcinogenic to humans (Group 2A) and carcinogenic to experimental animals [164]. Styrene-7,8-oxide given by oral intubation induced a high incidence of both benign and malignant tumors of the forestomach in experimental animals (rats and mice) [164, 165].

23.3.42 **Sulfur Dioxide**

Sulfur dioxide is produced in various industrial processes. Since coal and petroleum often contain sulfur compounds, their combustion generates sulfur dioxide. Further oxidation of SO_2 leads via SO_3 to H_2SO_4 production that causes acid rain [166]. Sulfur dioxide is a component of reduction smog (London smog). Inhaling sulfur dioxide is associated with increased respiratory symptoms and disease, difficulty in breathing, and premature death [166]. With experimental animals (rats) it has been also shown that inhalation of sulfur dioxide leads to diminishing activity of CYP2B and CYP2E1 in the lung, and CYP2B in the liver [167].

23.3.43
Tetrachloroethylene (Tetrachloroethene, Perchloroethylene)

Tetrachloroethylene (tetrachloroethene) – a volatile organic compound and an excellent solvent for organic materials – has been the predominant solvent used by the dry-cleaning industry for many years. It is a common soil contaminant. The IARC has classified tetrachloroethene as a Group 2A carcinogen, which means that it is probably carcinogenic to humans and carcinogenic to experimental animals [168]. Like many chlorinated hydrocarbons, tetrachloroethene is a central nervous system depressant and can enter the body through respiratory or dermal exposure [169]. This compound is known to be nephrotoxic (after activation by GST) and toxic in the human liver after activation by CYPs of the 2B family after conversion to an epoxide; here, reactive species formed by this reaction may bind to proteins and form neoantigens [170].

23.3.44
Vinyl Chloride

Vinyl chloride is used almost exclusively by the plastics industry to produce polyvinyl chloride and copolymers. It is released into the environment in emissions and effluents from the plastics industry. Vinyl chloride is known to be a human carcinogen based on sufficient evidence of carcinogenicity to humans (Group 1) [20]. The evidence that vinyl chloride causes cancer in humans is based on numerous epidemiological studies. These studies show its association with a very rare tumor – angiosarcoma of the liver. Exposure to vinyl chloride also causes cancer at other tissue sites, including the liver (tumors other than angiosarcoma), brain, lung, lymphatic system, and hematopoietic system (organs and tissues involved in production of blood) [20]. There is sufficient evidence for the carcinogenicity of vinyl chloride to experimental animals, causing malignant and benign tumors at multiple tissue sites, including angiosarcoma of the liver, lung tumors, mammary gland tumors, angiosarcoma (blood vessel tumors), Zymbal gland tumors, and kidney tumors (nephroblastoma) [20, 171]. This compound is a genotoxic carcinogen that is oxidized by CYP enzymes to chloroethylene oxide, which can undergo spontaneous rearrangement to form chloracetaldehyde; both of these metabolites can bind to DNA forming etheno adducts. These adducts can cause mutations, for example, in the *p53* tumor-suppressor gene and the *ras* protooncogene initiating formation of tumors in human liver (angiosarcoma of the liver [172].

23.4
Summary

The overview of pollutants interacting with drug-metabolizing enzymes, as presented above, is of course far from complete; however, we hope it covers the most important and biochemically interesting compounds from the innumerable plethora of existing chemicals and (at least potential) pollutants to our environment.

References

1 Kemp, D.D. (1998) *The Environment Dictionary*, Routledge, London.

2 Santos, M.A. (1990) *Managing Planet Earth: Perspectives on Population, Ecology, and the Law*, Bergin & Garvey, Westport, CT.

3 IARC (1985) *Allyl Compounds, Aldehydes, Epoxides, and Peroxides. IARC Monographs on the Evaluation of Carcinogenic Risk of Chemicals to Humans*, vol. 36, International Agency for Research on Cancer, Lyon.

4 IARC (1999) *Re-Evaluation of Some Organic Chemicals, Hydrazine, and Hydrogen Peroxide. IARC Monographs on the Evaluation of Carcinogenic Risk of Chemicals to Humans*, vol. 71, International Agency for Research on Cancer, Lyon.

5 IARC (2009) International agency for research on Cancer Monograph Working Group, special report: policy a review of human carcinogens – Part E: tobacco, areca nut, alcohol, coal smoke, and salted fish. *Lancet*, **10**, 1033–1034.

6 Caravati, E.M. and Litovitz, T. (1988) Pediatric cyanide intoxication and death from an acetonitrile-containing cosmetic. *J. Am. Med. Assoc.*, **260**, 3470–3473.

7 International Programme on Chemical Safety (1993) *Environmental Health Criteria 154: Acetonitrile*, World Health Organization, Geneva.

8 Feierman, D.E., Cederbaum, A.I., Feierman, D.E., and Cederbaum, A.I. (1998) Role of cytochrome P-450 IIE1 and catalase in the oxidation of acetonitrile to cyanide. *Chem. Res. Toxicol.*, **2**, 359–366.

9 Sittig, M. (1991) *Handbook of Toxic and Hazardous Chemicals and Carcinogens*, 3rd edn, Noyes, Park Ridge, NJ.

10 Cabral, J.R. and Neal, G.E. (1983) Testicular mesotheliomas in rats exposed to *N*-2-fluorenylacetamide (FFA). *Tumori*, **69**, 195–199.

11 Feng, Z., Hu, W., Hu, Y., and Tang, M. (2006) Acrolein is a major cigarette-related lung cancer agent: preferential binding at p53 mutational hotspots and inhibition of DNA repair. *Proc. Natl. Acad. Sci. USA*, **103**, 15404–15409.

12 Kehrer, J.P. and Biswal, S.S. (2000) The molecular effects of acrolein. *Toxicol. Sci.*, **57**, 6–15.

13 Wang, H. and Tompkins, L.M. (2008) CYP2B6: new insights into a historically overlooked cytochrome P450 isozyme. *Curr. Drug Metab.*, **9**, 598–610.

14 IARC (1995) *Some Industrial Chemicals. IARC Monographs on the Evaluation of Carcinogenic Risk of Chemicals to Humans*, vol. 60, International Agency for Research on Cancer, Lyon.

15 Tareke, E., Rydberg, P., Karlsson, P., Eriksson, S., and Törnqvist, M. (2002) Analysis of acrylamide, a carcinogen formed in heated foodstuffs. *J. Agric. Food. Chem.*, **50**, 4998–5006.

16 Vesper, H.W., Bernert, J.T., Ospina, M., Mezera, T., Ingham, L., Smith, A., Gary, L., and Myers, G.L. (2007) Assessment of the relation between biomarkers for smoking and biomarkers for acrylamide exposure in humans. *Cancer Epidemiol. Biomarkers Prev.*, **16**, 2471–2478.

17 Hogervorst, J.G., Schouten, L.J., Konings, E.J., Goldbohm, R.A., and Van Den Brandt, P.A. (2007) A prospective study of dietary acrylamide intake and the risk of endometrial, ovarian, and breast cancer. *Cancer Epidemiol. Biomarkers Prev.*, **16**, 2304–2013.

18 Larsson, S.C., Åkesson, A., Bergkvist, L., and Wolk, A. (2009) Dietary acrylamide intake and risk of colorectal cancer in a prospective cohort of men. *Eur. J. Cancer*, **45**, 513–516.

19 Doroshyenko, O., Fuhr, U., Kunz, D., Frank, D., Kinzig, M., Jetter, A., Reith, Y., Lazar, A., Taubert, D., Kirchheiner, J., Baum, M., Eisenbrand, G., Berger, F.I., Bertow, D., Berkessel, A., Sörgel,

F., Schömig, E., and Tomalik-Scharte, D. (2009) *In vivo* role of cytochrome P450 2E1 and glutathione *S*-transferase activity for acrylamide toxicokinetics in humans. *Cancer Epidemiol. Biomarkers Prev.*, **18**, 433–443.

20 IARC (1987) *Overall Evaluations of Carcinogenicity. An Updating of IARC Monographs Volumes 1 to 42. IARC Monographs on the Evaluation of Carcinogenic Risk of Chemicals to Humans, Supplement 7*, International Agency for Research on Cancer, Lyon.

21 Feng, Z., Hu, W., Rom, W.N., Beland, F.A., and Tang, M.S. (2002) 4-aminobiphenyl is a major etiological agent of human bladder cancer: evidence from its DNA binding spectrum in human *p53* gene. *Carcinogenesis*, **23**, 1721–1727.

22 Yu, M.C., Skipper, P.L., Tannenbaum, S.R., Chan, K.K., and Ross, R.K. (2002) Arylamine exposures and bladder cancer risk. *Mutat. Res.*, **506–507**, 21–28.

23 Ozawa, S., Katoh, T., Inatomi, H., Imai, H., Kuroda, Y., Ichiba, M., and Ohno, Y. (2002) Association of genotypes of carcinogen-activating enzymes, phenol sulfotransferase SULT1A1 (ST1A3) and arylamine *N*-acetyltransferase NAT2, with urothelial cancer in a Japanese population. *Int. J. Cancer*, **102**, 418–421.

24 IARC (1982) *Some Aromatic Amines, Anthraquinones and Nitroso Compounds, and Inorganic Fluorides. IARC Monographs on the Evaluation of the Carcinogenic Risk of Chemicals to Humans*, vol. 27, International Agency for Research on Cancer, Lyon.

25 Stiborová, M., Mikšanová, M., Šulc, M., Rýdlová, H., Schmeiser, H.H., and Frei, E. (2005) Identification of a genotoxic mechanism for the carcinogenicity of the environmental pollutant and suspected human carcinogen *o*-anisidine. *Int. J. Cancer*, **116**, 667–678.

26 Naiman, K., Dračínská, H., Martínková, M., Šulc, M., Dračínský, M., Kejíková, L., Hodek, P., Hudeček, J., Liberda, J., Schmeiser, H.H., Frei, E., and Stiborová, M. (2008) Redox cycling in the metabolism of the environmental pollutant and suspected human carcinogen *o*-anisidine by rat and rabbit hepatic microsomes. *Chem. Res. Toxicol.*, **21**, 1610–1621.

27 Wang, H., Chanas, B., and Ghanayem, B.I. (2002) Cytochrome P450 2E1 (CYP2E1) is essential for acrylonitrile metabolisms to cyanide: comparative studies using CYP2E1-null and wild-type mice. *Drug Metab. Dispos.*, **30**, 911–917.

28 Kedderis, G.L. and Batra, R. (1993) Species differences in the hydrolysis of 2-cyanoethylene oxide, the epoxide metabolite of acrylonitrile. *Carcinogenesis*, **14**, 685–689.

29 Kedderis, G.L., Batra, R., and Turner, M.J. (1995) Conjugation of acrylonitrile and 2-cyanoethylene oxide with hepatic glutathione. *Toxicol. Appl. Pharmacol.*, **135**, 9–17.

30 IARC (1980) *Some Metals and Metallic Compounds. IARC Monographs on the Evaluation of the Carcinogenic Risk of Chemicals to Humans*, vol. 23, International Agency for Research on Cancer, Lyon.

31 IARC (2002) *Some Drinking-Water Disinfectants and Contaminants, Including Arsenic. IARC Monographs on the Evaluation of Carcinogenic Risks to Humans*, vol. 84, International Agency for Research on Cancer, Lyon.

32 Grund, S.C., Hanusch, K., and Wolf, H.U. (2008) Arsenic and arsenic compounds, in *Ullmann's Encyclopedia of Industrial Chemistry*, Wiley-VCH Verlag GmbH, Weinheim.

33 Scott, N., Hatelid, K.M., MacKenzie, N.E., and Carter, D.E. (1993) Reactions of arsenic(III) and arsenic(V) species with glutathione. *Chem. Res. Toxicol.*, **6**, 102–106.

34 Delnomdedieu, M., Basti, M.M., Otvos, J.D., and Thomas, D.J. (1994) Complexation of arsenic species in rabbit erythrocytes. *Chem. Res. Toxicol.*, **7**, 621–627.

35 Woods, J.S. and Fowler, B.A. (1978) Altered regulation of mammalian hepatic heme biosynthesis and urinary porphyrin excretion during prolonged exposure to sodium arsenate. *Toxicol. Appl. Pharmacol.*, **43**, 361–371.

36 Szinicz, L. and Forth, W. (1988) Effects of As_2O_3 on gluconeogenesis. *Arch. Toxicol.*, **61**, 444–449.

37 Styblo, M., Delnomdedieu, M., and Thomas, D.J. (1995) Biological mechanisms and toxicological consequences of the methylation of arsenic, in *Toxicology of Metals – Biochemical Aspects* (eds R.A. Goyer and M.G. Cherian), Springer, Berlin, pp. 407–433.

38 Vahter, M. (1999) Methylation of inorganic arsenic in different mammalian species and population groups. *Sci. Prog.*, **82**, 69–88.

39 Berman, D.W. and Crump, K.S. (2008) Update of potency factors for asbestos-related lung cancer and mesothelioma. *Crit. Rev. Toxicol.*, **38** (Suppl. 1), 1–47.

40 IARC (1973) *Some Inorganic and Organometallic Compounds. IARC Monographs on the Evaluation of Carcinogenic Risk of Chemicals to Humans*, vol. 2, International Agency for Research on Cancer, Lyon.

41 IARC (1977) *Asbestos. IARC Monographs on the Evaluation of Carcinogenic Risk of Chemicals to Humans*, vol. 14, International Agency for Research on Cancer, Lyon.

42 Barrett, J.C. (1994) Cellular and molecular mechanisms of asbestos carcinogenicity: implications for biopersist. *Environ. Health Perspect.*, **102**, 19–23.

43 Anttila, S., Raunio, H., and Hakkola, J. (2011) Cytochrome P450 mediated pulmonary metabolism of carcinogens: regulation and cross-talk in lung carcinogenesis. *Am. J. Respir. Cell. Mol. Biol.*, **44**, 583–590.

44 Grund, S.C., Hanusch, K., Breunig, H.J., and Wolf, H.U. (2006) Antimony and antimony compounds, in *Ullmann's Encyclopedia of Industrial Chemistry*, Wiley-VCH Verlag GmbH, Weinheim.

45 IARC (1989) *Antimony Trioxide and Antimony Trisulfide. IARC Monographs on the Evaluation of Carcinogenic Risk of Chemicals to Humans*, vol. 47, International Agency for Research on Cancer, Lyon.

46 Monks, T.J., Butterworth, M., and Lau, S.S. (2010) The fate of benzene-oxide. *Chem. Biol. Interact.*, **184**, 201–206.

47 Inoue, O., Kanno, E., Kakizaki, M., Watanabe, T., Higashikawa, K., and Ikeda, M. (2000) Urinary phenylmercapturic acid as a marker of occupational exposure to benzene. *Ind. Health*, **38**, 195–204.

48 Rodriguez, B., Yang, Y., Guliaev, A.B., Chenna, A., and Hang, B. (2010) Benzene-derived *N*2-(4-hydroxyphenyl)-deoxyguanosine adduct: UvrABC incision and its conformation in DNA. *Toxicol. Lett.*, **193**, 26–32.

49 Yamazoe, Y., Zenser, T.V., Miller, D.W., and Kadlubar, F.F. (1988) Mechanism of formation and structural characterization of DNA adducts derived from peroxidative activation of benzidine. *Carcinogenesis*, **9**, 1635–1641.

50 Zenser, T.V., Lakshmi, V.M., Hsu, F.F., and Davis, B.B. (2002) Metabolism of *N*-acetylbenzidine and initiation of bladder cancer. *Mutat. Res.*, **506–507**, 29–40.

51 IARC (2008) *1,3-Butadiene, Ethylene Oxide and Vinyl Halides (Vinyl Fluoride, Vinyl Chloride and Vinyl Bromide). IARC Monographs on the Evaluation of Carcinogenic Risk of Chemicals to Humans*, vol. 97, International Agency for Research on Cancer, Lyon.

52 Csanidy, G.A., Guengerich, F.P., and Bond, J.A. (1992) Comparison of the biotransformation of 1,3-butadiene and its metabolite, butadiene monoepoxide, by hepatic and pulmonary tissues from humans, rats and mice. *Carcinogenesis*, **13**, 1143–1153.

53 Duescher, R.J. and Elfarra, A.A. (1994) Human liver microsomes are efficient catalysts of 1,3-butadiene oxidation: evidence for major roles by cytochromes P450 2A6 and 2E1. *Arch. Biochem. Biophys.*, **311**, 342–349.

54 Zhao, C., Vodicka, P., Šrám, R.J., and Hemminki, K. (2000) Human DNA adducts of 1,3-butadiene, an important environmental carcinogen. *Carcinogenesis*, **21**, 107–111.

55 IARC (1993) *Beryllium, Cadmium, Mercury and Exposures in the Glass Manufacturing Industry. IARC Monographs on the Evaluation of Carcinogenic Risk of Chemicals to Humans*, vol. 58, International Agency for Research on Cancer, Lyon.

56 Mandel, J.S., McLaughlin, J.K., Schlehofer, B., Mellemgaard, A., Helmert, U., Lindblad, P., McCredie, M., and Adami, H.O. (1995) International renal-cell cancer study. IV. Occupation. *Int. J. Cancer*, **61**, 601–605.

57 Siemiatycki, J.R., Dewar, R., Nadon, L., and Gerin, M. (1994) Occupational risk factors for bladder cancer: results from a case-control study in Montreal, Quebec, Canada. *Am. J. Epidemiol.*, **140**, 1061–1080.

58 Sorahan, T., Lister, A., Gilthorpe, M.S., and Harrington, J.M. (1995) Mortality of copper cadmium alloy workers with special reference to lung cancer and non-malignant diseases of the respiratory system, 1946–92. *Occup. Environ. Med.*, **52**, 804–812.

59 van der Gulden, J.W., Kolk, J.J., and Verbeek, A.L. (1995) Work environment and prostate cancer risk. *Prostate*, **27**, 250–257.

60 Waalkes, M.P. (2003) Cadmium carcinogenesis. *Mutat. Res.*, **533**, 107–120.

61 Gobe, G. and Crane, D. (2010) Mitochondria, reactive oxygen species and cadmium toxicity in the kidney. *Toxicol. Lett.*, **198**, 49–55.

62 Mounaji, K., Vlassi, M., Erraiss, N.E., Wegnez, M., Serrano, A., and Soukri, A. (2003) *In vitro* effect of metal ions on the activity of two amphibian glyceraldehyde-3-phosphate dehydrogenases: potential metal binding sites. *Comp. Biochem. Physiol. B*, **135**, 241–254.

63 Luchese, C., Zeni, G., Rocha, J.B., Nogueira, C.W., and Santos, F.W. (2007) Cadmium inhibits delta-aminolevulinate dehydratase from rat lung *in vitro*: interaction with chelating and antioxidant agents. *Chem. Biol. Interact.*, **165**, 127–137.

64 Nordberg, M., Jin, T., and Nordberg, G.F. (1992) Cadmium, metallothionein and renal tubular toxicity. *IARC Sci. Publ.*, **118**, 293–297.

65 Recknagel, R.O. (1967) Carbon tetrachloride hepatotoxicity. *Pharmacol. Rev.*, **19**, 145–208.

66 Masuda, Y. (2006) [Learning toxicology from carbon tetrachloride-induced hepatotoxicity]. *Yakugaku Zasshi*, **126**, 885–899.

67 Rood, A.S., McGavran, P.D., Aanenson, J.W., and Till, J.E. (2001) Stochastic estimates of exposure and cancer risk from carbon tetrachloride released to the air from the rocky flats plant. *Risk Anal.*, **21**, 675–695.

68 Weber, L.W., Boll, M., and Stampfl, A. (2003) Hepatotoxicity and mechanism of action of haloalkanes: carbon tetrachloride as a toxicological model. *Crit. Rev. Toxicol.*, **33**, 105–136.

69 Kao, L.W. and Nañagas, K.A. (2006) Toxicity associated with carbon monoxide. *Clin. Lab. Med.*, **26**, 99–125.

70 Townsend, C.L. and Maynard, R.L. (2002) Effects on health of prolonged exposure to low concentrations of carbon monoxide. *Occup. Environ. Med.*, **59**, 708–711.

71 Omaye, S.T. (2002) Metabolic modulation of carbon monoxide toxicity. *Toxicology*, **180**, 139–150.

72 Nelson, L.H. (2002) Carbon monoxide, in *Goldfrank's Toxicologic Emergencies*, 7th edn, McGraw-Hill, New York, pp. 1689–1704.

73 Hardy, K.R. and Thom, S.R. (1994) Pathophysiology and treatment of carbon monoxide poisoning. *J. Toxicol. Clin. Toxicol.*, **32**, 613–629.

74 Alonso, J.R., Cardellach, F., Lopez, S., Casademont, J., and Miro, O. (2003) Carbon monoxide specifically inhibits cytochrome *c* oxidase of human mitochondrial respiratory chain. *Pharmacol. Toxicol.*, **93**, 142–146.

75 Weaver, L.K. (2009) Clinical practice. Carbon monoxide poisoning. *N. Engl. J. Med.*, **360**, 1217–1225.

76 Blumenthal, I. (2001) Carbon monoxide poisoning. *J. R. Soc. Med.*, **94**, 270–272.

77 Gorman, D., Drewry, A., Huang, Y.L., and Sames, C. (2003) The clinical toxicology of carbon monoxide. *Toxicology*, **187**), 25–38.

78 IARC (1999) *Some Chemicals That Cause Tumours of the Kidney or Urinary Bladder in Rodents and Some Other Substances. IARC Monographs on the Evaluation of Carcinogenic Risk of Chemicals to Humans, Chloroform*, vol. 73,

International Agency for Research on Cancer, Lyon.

79 Himmelstein, M.W., Carpenter, S.C., Hinderliter, P.M., Snow, T.A., and Valentine, R. (2001) The metabolism of β-chloroprene: preliminary in-vitro studies using liver microsomes. *Chem. Biol. Interact.*, **135–136**, 267–284.

80 Munter, T., Cottrell, L., Ghai, R., Golding, B.T., and Watson, W.P. (2007) The metabolism and molecular toxicology of chloroprene. *Chem. Biol. Interact.*, **166**, 323–331.

81 IARC (1990) *Chromium, Nickel, and Welding. IARC Monographs on the Evaluation of Carcinogenic Risk of Chemicals to Humans*, vol. 49, International Agency for Research on Cancer, Lyon.

82 De Flora, S., Morelli, A., Basso, C., Romano, M., Serra, D., and De Flora, A. (1985) Prominent role of DT-diaphorase as a cellular mechanism reducing chromium(VI) and reverting its mutagenicity. *Cancer Res.*, **45**, 3188–3196.

83 Salnikow, K. and Zhitkovich, A. (2008) Genetic and epigenetic mechanisms in metal carcinogenesis and cocarcinogenesis: nickel, arsenic, and chromium. *Chem. Res. Toxicol.*, **21**, 28–44.

84 Donaldson, J.D. and Beyersmann, D. (2005) Cobalt and cobalt compounds, in *Ullmann's Encyclopedia of Industrial Chemistry*, Wiley-VCH Verlag GmbH, Weinheim.

85 IARC (1991) *Cobalt and Cobalt Compounds. IARC Monographs on the Evaluation of Carcinogenic Risk of Chemicals to Humans*, vol. 52, International Agency for Research on Cancer, Lyon.

86 Moorhouse, C.P., Halliwell, B., Grootveld, M., and Gutteridge, J.M.C. (1985) Cobalt(II) ion as a promoter of hydroxyl radical and possible "crypto-hydroxyl" radical formation under physiological conditions. Differential effects of hydroxyl radical scavengers. *Biochim. Biophys. Acta*, **843**, 261–268.

87 Lison, D. and Lauwerys, R. (1993) Evaluation of the role of reactive oxygen species in the interactive toxicity of carbide–cobalt mixtures on macrophages in culture. *Arch. Toxicol.*, **67**, 347–351.

88 Hissinka, A.M., Dunnewijk, R., van Ommen, B., and van Bladeren, P.J. (1997) Kinetics and metabolism of 1,4-dichlorobenzene in male Wistar rats: no evidence for quinone metabolites. *Chem. Biol. Interact.*, **103**, 17–33.

89 Secodin, L., Maso, S., and Trevisan, A. (1999) Different effects of (CIS+TRANS) 1,3-dichloropropene in renal cortical slices derived from male and female rats. *Hum. Exp. Toxicol.*, **18**, 106–110.

90 Bartels, M.J., Brzak, K.A., Mendrala, A.L., and Stott, W.T. (2000) Mechanistic aspects of the metabolism of 1,3-dichloropropene in rats and mice. *Chem. Res. Toxicol.*, **13**, 1096–1102.

91 Fagin, J., Bradley, J., and Williams, D. (1980) Carbon monoxide poisoning secondary to inhaling methylene chloride. *Br. Med. J.*, **281**, 1461.

92 Kim, S.N., Seo, J.Y., Jung, D.W., Lee, M.Y., Jung, Y.S., and Kim, Y.C. (2007) Induction of hepatic CYP2E1 by a subtoxic dose of acetoaminophen in rats: increase in dichloromethane metabolism and carboxyhemoglobin elevation. *Drug Metab. Dispos.*, **35**, 1754–1758.

93 Watanabe, K., Liberman, R.G., Skipper, P.L., Tannenbaum, S.R., and Guengerich, F.P. (2007) Analysis of DNA adducts formed *in vivo* in rats and mice from 1,2-dibromoethane, 1,2-dichloroethane, dibromomethane, and dichloromethane using HPLC/accelerator mass spectrometry and relevance to risk estimates. *Chem. Res. Toxicol.*, **20**, 1594–1600.

94 Anders, M.W., Andersen, M.E., Clewell, H.J., 3rd, Gargas, M.L., Guengerich, F.P., and Reitz, R.H. (2010) Comment on M.V. Evans and J.C. Caldwell: evaluation of two different metabolic hypotheses for dichloromethane toxicity using physiologically based pharmacokinetic modeling of *in vivo* gas uptake data exposure in female B6C3F1 mice. *Toxicol. Appl. Pharmacol.*, **244**, 280–290. *Toxicol. Appl. Pharmacol.*, **248**, 63–64.

95 Casanova, M., Bell, D.A., and Heck, H.D. (1997) Dichloromethane metabolism to formaldehyde and

reaction of formaldehyde with nucleic acids in hepatocytes of rodents and humans with and without glutathione S-transferase *T1* and *M1* genes. *Toxicol. Sci.*, **37**, 168–180.

96 IARC (1974) *Some Aromatic Amines, Hydrazine and Related Substances, N-Nitroso Compounds and Miscellaneous Alkylating Agents. IARC Monographs on the Evaluation of Carcinogenic Risk of Chemicals to Humans*, vol. 4, International Agency for Research on Cancer, Lyon.

97 Sedgwick, B. (1992) Oxidation of methylhydrazines to mutagenic methylating derivatives and inducers of the adaptive response of *Escherichia coli* to alkylation damage. *Cancer Res.*, **52**, 3693–3697.

98 Hayashi, N., Tsutsumi, M., Fukura, M., Yano, H., Tsuchishima, M., and Takase, S. (2007) Effect of chronic dietary ethanol consumption on colonic cancer in rats induced by 1,1-dimethylhydrazine. *Alcohol. Clin. Exp. Res.*, **31** (**1** Suppl.), S72–S76.

99 Steenland, K., Whelan, E., Deddens, J., Stayner, L., and Ward, E. (2003) Ethylene oxide and breast cancer incidence in a cohort study of 7576 women (United States). *Cancer Causes Control*, **14**, 531–539.

100 Steenland, K., Stayner, L., and Deddens, J. (2004) Mortality analyses in a cohort of 18 235 ethylene oxide exposed workers: follow up extended from 1987 to 1998. *Occup. Environ. Med.*, **61**, 2–7.

101 Brown, C.D., Wong, B.A., and Fennell, T.R. (1996) *In vivo* and *in vitro* kinetics of ethylene oxide metabolism in rats and mice. *Toxicol. Appl. Pharmacol.*, **136**, 8–19.

102 Tompkins, E.M., McLuckie, K.I., Jones, D.J., Farmer, P.B., and Brown, K. (2009) Mutagenicity of DNA adducts derived from ethylene oxide exposure in the pSP189 shuttle vector replicated in human Ad293 cells. *Mutat. Res.*, **67**, 129–137.

103 IARC (2006) *Formaldehyde, 2-Butoxyethanol and 1-Tert-Butoxypropan-2-ol. IARC Monographs on the Evaluation of Carcinogenic Risks to Humans*, vol. 88, International Agency for Research on Cancer, Lyon.

104 Zhang, L., Freeman, L.E., Nakamura, J., Hecht, S.S., Vandenberg, J.J., Smith, M.T., and Sonawane, B.R. (2010) Formaldehyde and leukemia: epidemiology, potential mechanisms, and implications for risk assessment. *Environ. Mol. Mutagen.*, **51**, 181–191.

105 Metcalf, R.L. (2002) Insect control, in *Ullmann's Encyclopedia of Industrial Chemistry*, Wiley-VCH Verlag GmbH, Weinheim.

106 IARC (2001) *Chlordane and Heptachlor. IARC Monographs on the Evaluation of Carcinogenic Risks to Humans*, vol. 79, International Agency for Research on Cancer, Lyon.

107 Mehmood, Z., Williamson, M.P., Kelly, D.E., and Kelly, S.L. (1996) Metabolism of organochlorine pesticides: the role of human cytochrome P450 3A4. *Chemosphere*, **33**, 759–769.

108 IARC (1979) *Some Halogenated Hydrocarbons. IARC Monographs on the Evaluation of Carcinogenic Risk of Chemicals to Humans*, vol. 20, International Agency for Research on Cancer, Lyon.

109 IARC (1982) *Chemicals, Industrial Processes and Industries Associated with Cancer in Humans. IARC Monographs on the Evaluation of Carcinogenic Risk of Chemicals to Humans, Supplement 4*, International Agency for Research on Cancer, Lyon.

110 Smith, A.G. and Cabral, J.R. (1980) Liver-cell tumours in rats fed hexachlorobenzene. *Cancer Lett.*, **11**, 169–172.

111 Smith, A.G., Carthew, P., Francis, J.E., Cabral, J.R., and Manson, M.M. (1993) Enhancement by iron of hepatic neoplasia in rats caused by hexachlorobenzene. *Carcinogenesis*, **14**, 1381–1387.

112 Franklin, M.R., Phillips, J.D., and Kushner, J.P. (1997) Cytochrome P450 induction, uroporphyrinogen decarboxylase depression, porphyrin accumulation and excretion, and gender influence in a 3-week rat model of porphyria cutanea tarda. *Toxicol. Appl. Pharmacol.*, **147**, 289–299.

113 Delaney, J. and Timbrell, J.A. (1995) Role of cytochrome P450 in hydrazine toxicity in isolated hepatocytes *in vitro*. *Xenobiotica*, **25**, 1399–1410.

114 Mörike, K., Koch, M., Fritz, P., Urban, W., and Eichelbaum, M. (1996) Identification of N_2 as a metabolite of acetylhydrazine in the rat. *Arch. Toxicol.*, **70**, 300–305.

115 Payne, M. (2008) Lead in drinking water. *Can. Med. Assoc. J.*, **179**, 253–254.

116 Flora, S., Mittal, M., and Mehta, A. (2008) Heavy metal induced oxidative stress and its possible reversal by chelation therapy. *Indian J. Med. Res.*, **128**, 501–523.

117 Yu, M.H. (2005) *Environmental Toxicology: Biological and Health Effects of Pollutants*, 2nd edn, CRC Press, Boca Raton, FL.

118 Chisolm, J.J. (2004) Lead poisoning, in *Oski's Essential Pediatrics*, 2nd edn (eds M. Crocetti, M.A. Barone, and F.A. Oski), Lippincott Williams & Wilkins, Baltimore, MD, pp. 221–222.

119 Kosnett, M.J. (2006) Lead, in *Poisoning and Drug Overdose*, 5th edn (ed. K.R. Olson), Lange/McGraw-Hill, New York, p. 238.

120 Fujita, H., Nishitani, C., and Ogawa, K. (2002) Lead, chemical porphyria, and heme as a biological mediator. *Tohoku J. Exp. Med.*, **196**, 53–64.

121 Barbosa, F.J.R., Tanus-Santos, J.E., Gerlach, R.F., and Parsons, P.J. (2005) A critical review of biomarkers used for monitoring human exposure to lead: advantages, limitations, and future needs. *Environ. Health Perspect.*, **113**, 1669–1674.

122 Patrick, L. (2006) Lead toxicity, a review of the literature. Part 1: exposure, evaluation, and treatment. *Alternat. Med. Rev.*, **11**, 2–22.

123 Singal, A. and Thami, G.P. (2006) Lindane neurotoxicity in childhood. *Am. J. Ther.*, **13**, 277–280.

124 Johri, A., Yadav, S., Dhawan, A., and Parmar, D. (2007) Overexpression of cerebral and hepatic cytochromes P450 altersbehavioral activity of rat offspring following prenatal exposure to lindane. *Toxicol. Appl. Pharmacol.*, **225**, 278–292.

125 Davidson, P.W., Myers, G.J., and Weiss, B. (2004) Mercury exposure and child development outcomes. *Pediatrics*, **113** (4 Suppl.), 1023–1029.

126 Clifton, J.C., 2nd (2007) Mercury exposure and public health. *Pediatr. Clin. North Am.*, **54**, 237–269.

127 Clarkson, T.W. and Magos, L. (2006) The toxicology of mercury and its chemical compounds. *Crit. Rev. Toxicol.*, **36**, 609–662.

128 Mozaffarian, D. and Rimm, E.B. (2006) Fish intake, contaminants, and human health: evaluating the risks and the benefits. *JAMA*, **296**, 1885–1899.

129 Galloway, J.N., Townsend, A.R., Erisman, J.W., Bekunda, M., Cai, Z., Freney, J.R., Martinelli, L.A., Seitzinger, S.P., and Sutton, M.A. (2008) Transformation of the nitrogen cycle: recent trends, questions, and potential solutions. *Science*, **320**, 889–892.

130 Vuppugalla, R. and Mehvar, R. (2004) Short-term inhibitory effects of nitric oxide on cytochrome P450-mediated drug metabolism. *Drug Metab. Dispos.*, **32**, 1446–1454.

131 Jerrett, M., Burnett, R.T., Pope, C.A., 3rd, Ito, K., Thurston, G., Krewski, D., Shi, Y., Calle, E., and Thun, M. (2009) Long-term ozone exposure and mortality. *N. Engl. J. Med.*, **360**, 1085–1095.

132 Afaq, F., Zaid, M.A., Pelle, E., Khan, N., Syed, D.N., Matsui, M.S., Maes, D., and Mukhtar, H. (2009) Aryl hydrocarbon receptor is an ozone sensor in human skin. *J. Invest. Dermatol.*, **129**, 2396–2403.

133 Eyer, F., Meischner, V., Kiderlen, D., Thiermann, H., Worek, F., Haberkorn, M., Felgenhauer, N., Zilker, T., and Eyer, P. (2003) Human parathion poisoning. A toxicokinetic analysis. *Toxicol. Rev.*, **22**, 143–163.

134 Eyer, P., Worek, F., Thiermann, H., and Eddleston, M. (2010) Paradox findings may challenge orthodox reasoning in acute organophosphate poisoning. *Chem. Biol. Interact.*, **187**, 270–278.

135 Butler, A.M. and Murray, M. (2012) Biotransformation of parathion in human liver: participation of CYP3A4 and its inactivation during microsomal

parathion oxidation. *J. Pharmacol. Exp. Ther.*, **280**, 966–973.

136 Furlong, C.E., Suzuki, S.M., Stevens, R.C., Marsillach, J., Richter, R.J., Jarvik, G.P., Checkoway, H., Samii, A., Costa, L.G., Griffith, A., Roberts, J.W., Yearout, D., and Zabetian, C.P. (2010) Human PON1, a biomerker of risk disease and exposure. *Chem. Biol. Interact.*, **187**, 355–361.

137 IARC (2000) *Di-(2-ethylhexyl) Phthalate. IARC Monographs on the Evaluation of Carcinogenic Risk of Chemicals to Humans*, vol. 77, International Agency for Research on Cancer, Lyon.

138 Hallmark, N., Walker, M., McKinnell, C., Mahood, I.K., Scott, H., Bayne, R., Coutts, S., Anderson, R.A., Greig, I., Morris, K., and Sharpe, R.M. (2007) Effects of monobutyl and di(*n*-butyl) phthalate *in vitro* on steroidogenesis and Leydig cell aggregation in fetal testis explants from the rat: comparison with effects *in vivo* in the fetal rat and neonatal marmoset and *in vitro* in the human. *Environ. Health Perspect.*, **115**, 390–396.

139 Tilson, H.A. (2008) EHP Papers of the Year, 2008. *Environ. Health Perspect.*, **116**, A234.

140 Toppari, J., Virtanen, H., Skakkebaek, N.E., and Main, K.M. (2006) Environmental effects on hormonal regulation of testicular descent. *J. Steroid Biochem. Mol. Biol.*, **102**, 184–186.

141 Desvergne, B., Feige, J., and Casals-Casas, C. (2009) PPAR-mediated activity of phthalates: a link to the obesity epidemic? *Mol. Cell. Endocrinol.*, **304**, 43.

142 IARC (1973) *Some Polycyclic Aromatic Hydrocarbons and Heterocyclic Compounds. IARC Monographs on the Evaluation of Carcinogenic Risk of Chemicals to Humans*, vol. 3, International Agency for Research on Cancer, Lyon.

143 IARC (1983) *Polynuclear Aromatic Compounds, Part 1. Chemical, Environmental and Experimental Data. IARC Monographs on the Evaluation of Carcinogenic Risk of Chemicals to Humans*, vol. 32, International Agency for Research on Cancer, Lyon.

144 IARC (1984) *Polynuclear Aromatic Compounds, Part 3. Industrial Exposures in Aluminum Production, Coal Gasification, Coke Production, and Iron and Steel Founding. IARC Monographs on the Evaluation of Carcinogenic Risk of Chemicals to Humans*, vol. 34, International Agency for Research on Cancer, Lyon.

145 IARC (1985) *Polynuclear Aromatic 4. Bitumens, Coal Tars and Derived Products, Shale Oils and Soots. IARC Monographs on the Evaluation of Carcinogenic Risk of Chemicals to Humans*, vol. 35, International Agency for Research on Cancer, Lyon.

146 IARC (2010) *Some Non-Heterocyclic Polycyclic Aromatic Hydrocarbons and Some Related Exposures. IARC Monographs on the Evaluation of Carcinogenic Risks to Humans*, vol. 92, International Agency for Research on Cancer, Lyon.

147 Luch, A. (2005) *The Carcinogenic Effects of Polycyclic Aromatic Hydrocarbons*, Imperial College Press, London.

148 Rudel, R.A., Seryak, L.M., and Brody, J.G. (2008) PCB-containing wood floor finish is a likely source of elevated PCBs in resident's blood, household air and dust: a case study of exposure. *Environ. Health*, **7**, 2.

149 IARC (1978) *Polychlorinated Biphenyls and Polybrominated Biphenyls. IARC Monographs on the Evaluation of Carcinogenic Risk of Chemicals to Humans*, vol. 18, International Agency for Research on Cancer, Lyon.

150 Safe, S. and Hutzinger, O. (1984) Polychlorinated biphenyls (PCBs) and polybrominated biphenyls (PBBs): biochemistry, toxicology, and mechanism of action. *Crit. Rev. Toxicol.*, **13**, 319–395.

151 Safe, S., Bandiera, S., Sawyer, T., Robertson, L., Safe, L., Parkinson, A., Thomas, P.E., Ryan, D.E., Reik, L.M., and Levin, W. (1985) PCBs: structure–function relationships and mechanism of action. *Environ. Health Perspect.*, **60**, 47–56.

152 Safe, S. (2000) Endocrine disruptors and human health – is there a problem? An update. *Environ. Health Perspect.*, **108**, 487–493.

153 Wang, S.L., Chang, Y.C., Chao, H.R., Li, C.M., Li, L.A., Lin, L.Y., and Päpke, O. (2006) Body burdens of polychlorinated dibenzo-*p*-dioxins, dibenzofurans, and biphenyls and their relations to estrogen metabolism in pregnant women. *Environ. Health Perspect.*, **114**, 740–745.

154 Simon, T., Britt, J.K., and James, R.C. (2007) Development of a neurotoxic equivalence scheme of relative potency for assessing the risk of PCB mixtures. *Regul. Toxicol. Pharmacol.*, **48**, 148–170.

155 Chauhan, K.R., Kodavanti, P.R., and McKinney, J.D. (2000) Assessing the role of *ortho*-substitution on polychlorinated biphenyl binding to transthyretin, a thyroxine transport protein. *Toxicol. Appl. Pharmacol.*, **162** (**1**), 10–21.

156 Vos, J.G., Koeman, J.H., van der Maas, H.L., ten Noever de Braun, M.C., and de Vos, R.H. (1970) Identification and toxicological evaluation of chlorinated dibenzofuran and chlorinated naphthalene in two commercial polychlorinated biphenyls. *Food Cosmet. Toxicol.*, **8**, 625–633.

157 Rappe, C., Buser, H.-R., and Bosshardt, H.-P. (1978) Identification and quantification of polychlorinated dibenzo-*p*-dioxins (PCDDs) and dibenzofurans (PCDFs) in 2,4,5-T ester formulations and Herbicide Orange. *Chemosphere*, **7**, 431–438.

158 Rappe, C., Gara, A., and Buser, H.-R. (1978) Identification of polychlorinated dibenzofurans (PCDFs) in commercial chlorophenol formulations. *Chemosphere*, **7**, 981–991.

159 IARC (1997) *Polychlorinated Dibenzo-Para-Dioxins and Polychlorinated Dibenzofurans. IARC Monographs on the Evaluation of Carcinogenic Risks to Humans*, vol. 69, International Agency for Research on Cancer, Lyon.

160 McGregor, D.B., Partensky, C., Wilbourn, J., and Rice, J.M. (1998) An IARC evaluation of polychlorinated dibenzo-*p*-dioxins and polychlorinated dibenzofurans as risk factors in human carcinogenesis. *Environ. Health Perspect.*, **106** (Suppl. 2), 755–760.

161 Denis, H. and Castor, J.W.M. (2005) Styrene, in *Ullmann's Encyclopedia of Industrial Chemistry*, Wiley-VCH Verlag GmbH, Weinheim.

162 IARC (1994) *Styrene. IARC Monographs on the Evaluation of Carcinogenic Risk of Chemicals to Humans*, vol. 60, International Agency for Research on Cancer, Lyon.

163 IARC (2002) *Styrene. IARC Monographs on the Evaluation of Carcinogenic Risk of Chemicals to Humans*, vol. 82, International Agency for Research on Cancer, Lyon.

164 IARC (1994) *Styrene-7,8-Oxide. IARC Monographs on the Evaluation of Carcinogenic Risk of Chemicals to Humans*, vol. 60, International Agency for Research on Cancer, Lyon.

165 Lijinsky, W. (1986) Rat and mouse forestomach tumors induced by chronic oral administration of styrene oxide. *J. Natl. Cancer Inst.*, **77**, 471–476.

166 Holleman, A.F. and Wiberg, E. (2001) *Inorganic Chemistry*, Academic Press, San Diego, CA.

167 Quin, G. and Meng, Z. (2012) Effect of sulfur dioxide inhalation on CYP2B1/2 and CYP2E1 in rat liver and lung. *Inhal. Toxicol.*, **18**, 581–588.

168 IARC (1995) *Tetrachloroethylene. IARC Monographs on the Evaluation of Carcinogenic Risk of Chemicals to Humans*, vol. 63, International Agency for Research on Cancer, Lyon.

169 Schreiber, J.S., Hudnell, H.K., Geller, A.M., House, D.E., Aldous, K.M., Force, M.S., Langguth, K., Prohonic, E.J., and Parker, J.C. (2002) Apartment residents' and day care workers' exposures to tetrachloroethylene and deficits in visual contrast sensitivity. *Environ. Health Perspect.*, **110**, 655–664.

170 White, I.N.H. and De Matteis, F. (2001) The role of CYP forms in the metabolism and metabolic activation of

HCFC and other halocarbons. *Toxicol. Lett.*, **124**, 121–128.

171 IARC (1979) *Some Monomers, Plastics, and Synthetic Elastomers, and Acrolein. IARC Monographs on the Evaluation of Carcinogenic Risk of Chemicals to Humans*, vol. 19, International Agency for Research on Cancer, Lyon.

172 Kielhorn, J., Melber, C., Wahnschaffe, U., Aitio, A., and Mangelsdorf, I. (2000) Vinyl chloride: still a cause for concern. *Environ. Health Perspect.*, **108**, 579–588.

24
Environmental Estrogens

Miroslav Machala and Jan Vondráček

24.1
Introduction

Endocrine disrupting chemicals (EDCs) – drugs, environmental contaminants, and dietary constituents – are compounds that, by their definition, interfere with normal endocrine functions. They may disrupt endocrine regulation at several steps, which include alterations of hormonal biosynthesis, transport, binding, action, or elimination of natural hormones in the body, as well as deregulation of hormone-specific nuclear receptor-mediated gene expression or nongenomic signaling [1]. EDCs usually have a potential to disrupt multiple endocrine systems at the same time, and a given compound may, for example, affect simultaneously estrogen-, androgen-, and thyroid-regulated processes, which are generally considered the most sensitive targets of EDC exposure. Both decreased and increased activities of hormones and/or their respective receptors and associated proteins may negatively affect normal endocrine functions. This may in turn lead to a range of effects, including reproductive and neurodevelopmental defects associated with impaired fertility, neurobehavioral effects (including also deficits in learning and memory abilities), and further adverse processes, such as carcinogenicity [2–4]. During recent years, numerous studies have also indicated that EDCs, including environmental estrogens, may affect the cardiovascular system and metabolism, thus contributing to the development of obesity and associated metabolic disorders, including type 2 diabetes mellitus [5–10]. This, together with their possible association with hormone-dependent cancer or developmental/reproductive disturbances in wildlife [11, 12], has led to increased attention being paid to both estrogenic and antiestrogenic activities of xenobiotics [13]. This

Metabolism of Drugs and Other Xenobiotics, First Edition. Edited by Pavel Anzenbacher, Ulrich M. Zanger.

chapter will therefore primarily focus on EDCs with estrogenic/antiestrogenic modes of action.

24.2
Estrogen Receptor Signaling Pathways

The two estrogen receptors (ERs) – ER-α and ER-β – mediate the biological effects of estrogens. These two ligand-dependent transcription factors control gene expression in response to estrogen exposure and they regulate numerous physiological processes, including development, reproduction, metabolism, homeostasis in bone tissue, and cardiovascular regulation [14, 15]. Both ERs have in part unique and partly overlapping roles, which largely depend on cellular context and tissue-specific expression of both receptor proteins and associated coregulators [15, 16]. Although both ER-α and ER-β show similar affinities for 17β-estradiol, for other types of ligands, ligand-selective binding and/or transactivation of ERs have often been observed in various *in vivo* and *in vitro* systems [17, 18]. Activated ERs regulate transcription of target genes through direct binding to ER element sequences [15]. In some cases, however, the ER is tethered to DNA through other transcription factors such as specificity protein-1 (Sp-1) or activator protein-1 (AP-1) [19].

Although in the past the majority of the action of xenoestrogens has been considered to be mediated primarily via nuclear ERs, several recent studies suggest that also the ability of environmental estrogens to trigger signaling through membrane ERs should be taken into account (for a recent review, see [20]). The nongenomic ER signaling pathway leads to a rapid activation of intracellular kinase signaling cascades [21]. Two alternative models of estrogen action have been proposed, which are involved in such "rapid responses." (i) The rapid membrane events could be mediated by the membrane-localized ER-α or ER-β, which initiate kinase signaling cascades (including mitogen-activated protein kinases, such as extracellular signal-regulated kinases 1/2 (ERK1/2)) through their association with further membrane signaling modules, including G-proteins, caveolins, and receptor tyrosine kinases. (ii) ER-α is not directly involved and the response to estrogen is expected to be mediated by another membrane-associated estrogen-binding protein (G-protein-coupled receptor GPR30) [22].

ER activity can also be regulated in a ligand-independent manner, as in the case of ER-α, via phosphorylation of specific Ser or Tyr residues in the activation function-1 region of ER-α by ERK1/2, protein kinase A, or other protein kinases [21]. These kinases provide a link between activation of various growth factors and estrogenic signaling, and thus contribute to the complexity of ER regulation. As outlined below, ER-α and ER-β also interact with various other transcription factors, which may both interfere with their function and modulate metabolism of endogenous ER ligands, such as 17β-estradiol. These include important mediators of toxicity of environmental compounds, such as the aryl hydrocarbon receptor (AhR) or constitutive androstane receptor (CAR) [23–25]. Various chemicals identi-

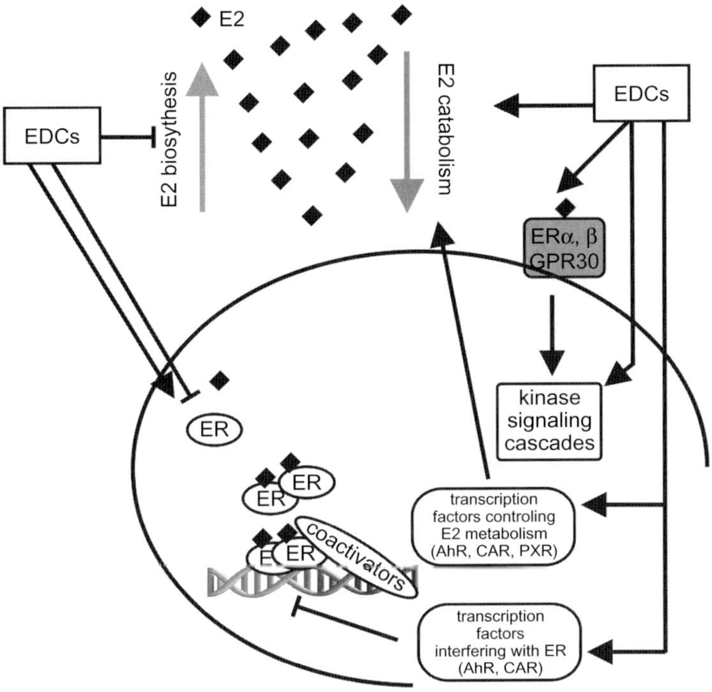

Figure 24.1 Interactions of EDCs with estrogen signaling.

fied as estrogens or antiestrogens may thus affect ER activation and function at various steps of ER signaling pathway (Figure 24.1).

24.3
Agonistic/Antagonistic Effects of Xenobiotics on ERs

The adverse effects of many EDCs are primarily associated with their direct interaction with ligand-binding domains of ER-α and ER-β. Some synthetic ER agonists, such as diethylstilbestrol (DES) and 17α-ethinylestradiol (EE2), show high ER affinity and a high potency to transactivate ERs. DES was the first synthetic estrogen widely administered to pregnant women prior to the discovery of its teratogenic and oncogenic effects [26]. DES is a strong estrogen, which can also induce a rapid nongenomic ER signaling, leading to activation of phosphoinositide 3-kinase/Akt pathway and histone methylation [27, 28]. Today, it is primarily used as a model experimental compound, which due its high estrogenic potency can model adverse effects of EDCs on the endocrine system, including their impact on reproduction, development, and carcinogenesis [29].

An important class of ER agonists and antagonists is comprised of selective ER modulators, which elicit tissue-specific effects [30]. Some of them became important therapeutics, while others are again frequently used as model compounds in experimental studies. A classic example thereof is tamoxifen – an effective therapeutic antagonist of ER-α in mammary cells inhibiting ER-α-dependent breast cancer progression, which acts, at the same time, as an ER-α agonist in the endometrium [31]. Selective ER ligands may induce conformations recruiting specific nuclear receptor cofactors, such as steroid receptor coactivator-1 (SRC-1/NCOA1), responsible for differential ER responses (reviewed in [11]). SRC-1 is involved in differential ER responses in mammary and endometrial cells; it is expressed at high levels in the endometrium and its knockdown prevents the proliferation of endometrial cells [32].

In contrast to pharmaceuticals, environmental EDCs, such as organochlorine pesticides dieldrin, endosulfan, methoxychlor, dichlorodiphenyltrichloroethane (DDT), or their metabolites, are often relatively weak modulators of ER-mediated activity (primarily due to much lower binding affinities to ERs than 17β-estradiol itself) [11, 20]. Interestingly, these compounds may differentially affect both ER receptors; methoxychlor and its metabolite are agonists of ER-α and antagonists of ER-β, respectively [33]. It is important to note that there are still large knowledge gaps concerning the effects of EDCs on ER-β signaling, as compared to ER-α [34]. It is necessary to point out that only relatively high doses of DDT or methoxychlor stimulate estrogenic responses *in vivo*, such as uterine proliferation and impairment of normal follicle development [35]. Similarly, some polycyclic aromatic hydrocarbons, produced by incomplete combustion processes, have been shown to be estrogenic at relatively high doses *in vivo* [36, 37].

Many industrial chemical contaminants, including bisphenol A and its analogs, alkylphenols, dialkyl phthalates, and brominated flame retardants also elicit estrogenic activity *in vitro* and *in vivo* [11, 13, 34]. Similarly to organochlorine pesticides, their relative potencies to transactivate ERs are rather low, compared to 17β-estradiol or DES. Therefore, there is a controversy regarding their potencies to impair normal estrogen functions [38]. Parabens and benzophenone derivatives have been also found to be weakly estrogenic in various *in vitro* assays, and they exhibit estrogenic potency several orders of magnitude lower that 17β-estradiol (reviewed in [39]). Weak antiestrogenic potencies of several polycyclic musk compounds have also been reported, with a preference for ER-β [40]. Importantly, hydroxy metabolites of EDCs possess generally higher potencies to induce ER-dependent gene expression. Therefore, a role of drug-metabolizing enzymes, especially cytochrome P450 (CYP) enzymes, should be taken into account (e.g., as shown for brominated diphenyl ethers and their major hydroxy metabolites) [41].

The induction equivalency approach has been successfully applied to estimate a relative contribution of EDCs to the total estrogenic activity of abiotic environmental samples. In this approach, relative effective potencies (REPs) of individual compounds, based on established *in vitro* assays, are multiplied by their concentrations. Due to low REP values of major environmental contaminants, it is perhaps not surprising that the natural estrogens 17β-estradiol and estrone have been reported to be principle contributors to the estrogenic activity of complex abiotic environmental samples [42, 43]. Similar findings that estrone and, partly, 17β-estradiol are major estrogenic compounds present in river sediments have been reported using "effect-directed analysis" of their bioactive fractions. Industrial contaminants such as alkylphenols, anthraquinone, benz[*a*]anthracene-7,12-dione, bisphenol A, and musk compounds may thus only weakly contribute to the overall ER-mediated activity in such complex environmental samples [44]. Nevertheless, it should be noted that additivity, as well as activation of alternative signaling pathways (such as nongenomic ER activity), may potentiate effects of even weakly estrogenic compounds present in environmental mixtures [45].

Many plant secondary metabolites, including dietary flavonoids, are phytoestrogens – another category of nonphysiological estrogens. The daily phytoestrogen intake can be up to several orders higher than the expected intake of industrial contaminants and pesticide residues. Although phytoestrogens have relatively weak estrogenic activities, their serum levels may reach up to micromolar concentrations; therefore, their estrogenic and/or antiestrogenic activities have been hypothesized to affect both normal endocrine functions and they have been suggested to be employed therapeutically [46, 47]. Phytoestrogens may disturb estrogen biosynthesis and either positively or negatively modulate ER transactivation. Both estrogenic and antiestrogenic activities have been reported for some phytoestrogens, dependent on concentration/dose and the specific tissue involved [48]. Some phytoestrogens have a strict ER subtype selectivity. Genistein – a major soy flavonoid – shows a high binding affinity and selectivity for ER-β, and it recruits the SRC-2 (GRIP-1) coactivator to ER-β, which may contribute to its transcriptional selectivity [49, 50]. Additionally, determination of ER-mediated activities of silybins – silymarin constituents (a mixture of flavonolignans from *Silybum marianum*) – showed that natural compounds may activate ER-α in a stereospecific manner [51]. Thus, phytoestrogens may both positively and negatively affect ER signaling, and therefore their beneficial and potential adverse effects should be appreciated when evaluating their impact on human health [48].

As suggested above, the negative impact of EDCs on estrogen signaling can be mediated by other transcription factors or signaling pathways being activated by such EDCs. Polychlorinated dibenzo-*p*-dioxins, polychlorinated dibenzofurans, and related AhR ligands have been shown to induce a range of antiestrogenic effects in various cell and tissue types [25]. Several mechanisms have been proposed to contribute to antiestrogenicity of persistent AhR ligands. These may include enhanced metabolism of endogenous estrogens, as discussed below, competition for common transcriptional coactivators, direct AhR–ER interaction at gene promoters, or binding to inhibitory dioxin-responsive elements blocking expression of ER-target genes (extensively reviewed in [25, 52]). Other possible mechanisms may involve the AhR protein partner – the AhR nuclear translocator (ARNT). ARNT has been shown to enhance the transcriptional capacity of ERs and its sequestration by activated AhR may lead to a decreased ER activity [53]. Finally, AhR has been reported to act as an E3 ubiquitin ligase targeting both ER-α and ER-β for proteasomal degradation [52, 54]. Nevertheless, it should be noted that ER-α may also repress AhR-dependent transcription, which adds to the complexity of AhR–ER interactions [55]. Several authors have also indicated that antiestrogenic effects of AhR ligands are markedly stronger on ER-β than on ER-α receptor [34, 53]. Other nuclear receptors activated by xenobiotics, such as CAR, may also impair ER activity by competing for limiting coactivators, including p160 coactivator [23]. However, unlike the case of AhR, these interactions have so far received significantly less attention in our understanding of the molecular mechanisms of EDCs action.

24.4
Effects of EDCs on Biosynthesis and Metabolism of Estrogens

EDCs may affect ER signaling indirectly through modification of steroidogenesis and metabolism of natural estrogens [56, 57]. Expression of aromatase (CYP19) is a key regulatory step in the biosynthesis of estrogens. Atrazine and other triazine herbicides, as well as chlordane and methoxychlor, induce aromatase activity, and consequently enhance estrogen synthesis and estrogenic responses [58, 59]. Opposite (antiestrogenic) effects of various phytoestrogens mediated by competitive binding to aromatase protein, and thus preventing normal estrogen synthesis, have also been reported [60]. Hydroxy metabolites of 2,2′,4,4′-tetrabromodiphenyl ether (BDE-47) and 2,2′,4,4′,5-penta-BDE (BDE-99) have been found to inhibit aromatase activity at low micromolar concentrations in H295R human adrenocortical carcinoma cells [61], and 6-hydroxy-BDE-47 effectively suppressed also expression of other steroidogenic genes such as *CYP11B* and *StAR* (steroidogenic acute regulatory protein) in H295R cells at concentrations as low as 0.025 μM [62]. This suggests that not only the modulation of expression or activity of CYP19, but also the effects of other steroidogenic enzymes may significantly affect estrogen signaling.

Steroid hormones are inactivated and eliminated through hydroxylations by CYP enzymes, followed by conjugation with glucuronide and sulfate [63]. A number of CYP enzymes possess steroid hydroxylase activity, and a systematic characterization of oxidative metabolism of 17β-estradiol and estrone has been reported, using selectively expressed human CYP isoforms [64]. CYP1A1, CYP1A2, and CYP3A4 catalyzed hydroxylation of estrogens mainly to 2-hydroxy-17β-estradiol and 2-hydroxyestrone, with only a minor production of 4-hydroxy metabolites. Additionally, 4-, 6α-, 6β-, 7α-, 15α-, 16α-, and 16β-hydroxy derivatives and several others were detected, albeit at low levels [64]. CYP1B1 mainly catalyzed the formation of 4-hydroxyestrogens and catechol estrogens; however, total CYP1B1 activity was significantly lower compared with CYP1A and CYP3A activities [64]. Other CYP enzymes, such as CYP2B6, CYP2C19, CYP3A5, and CYP3A7, have also been reported to participate in hydroxylation of estrogens [65].

Enhanced 17β-estradiol metabolism may lead to the suppression of estrogenic action and/or formation of reactive 17β-estradiol metabolites. Although 16α-hydroxyestrogens have been shown to exhibit estrogenic activities similar to 17β-estradiol, 2-hydroxyestrogens are only weak ER agonists and some may even antagonize ERs [66]. The 4-hydroxy-17β-estradiol is of particular toxicological concern, since its formation leads to production of 3,4-catechol/quinone metabolites, reactive oxygen species production, and DNA damage [67, 68]. Therefore, induction or high basal expression of CYP1B1 in transformed breast epithelial cells is associated with higher risk in breast cancer, while in normal epithelial cells, the contribution of CYP1B1 to hydroxylation of estrogens is relatively low [68].

Sulfotransferases (SULTs) and UDP-glucuronosyltransferases (UGTs) are major classes of phase II biotransformation enzymes conjugating hydroxyestrogens. Estrogen SULT2E1 is more preferential to estrogen metabolites than hydroxysteroid SULT2A1. Further, UGT2B isoforms are also significantly involved in the conjugation of steroid hydroxy metabolites [63].

Many xenobiotics, including important EDCs acting as agonists of AhR, CAR, or pregnane X receptor (PXR), may cause antiestrogenic effects by enhancing steroid catabolism, even without their direct interactions with ERs. CYP1A1, CYP1A2, and CYP1B1 are highly inducible by AhR agonists such as dioxins or polycyclic aromatic hydrocarbons [69]. Both CYP2B and CYP3A isoforms are induced via CAR/PXR by a variety of xenobiotics, such as DDT, methoxychlor, atrazine, polybrominated diphenyl ethers, and others [70–74]. Similarly, different isoforms of SULT and UGT display differential responses to xenobiotic inducers [75–77]. The rat hepatic UGT2B1 – a main isoform involved in steroid metabolism in the rat – was increased after treatment with pregnenolone-16α-carbonitrile and phenobarbital [63]. Therefore, although elevated clearance of steroid hormones may be to some extent compensated by a feedback increase of hormone production [78], xenobiotics may generally suppress both systemic or local steroid hormone levels, including estrogens.

24.5 Case of Polychlorinated Biphenyls

The complexity of mechanisms underlying the estrogenic/antiestrogenic of EDCs can be illustrated by looking at the effects of polychlorinated biphenyls (PCBs) on estrogen signaling. PCBs are a group of synthetic organochlorine chemicals that became globally distributed in the environment as complex mixtures. PCBs are known to elicit either estrogenic or antiestrogenic activities *in vitro* and *in vivo*. In general, lower-chlorinated PCBs have been shown to induce ER-dependent gene expression and estrogenic responses [79]. In a marked contrast, higher-chlorinated (penta- to octa-chlorinated) congeners, which are predominant constituents of both industrial and environmental mixtures, are antiestrogenic [79–81]. The dioxin-like PCBs with a coplanar structure, which are potent AhR agonists, are generally antiestrogenic and this activity has been related to activation of AhR. Their AhR-dependent modes of action on estrogen-sensitive cells may include repression of ER-dependent gene expression [25], inhibition of 17β-estradiol-induced cell cycle regulators, and mitogenesis [82] or effects of PCBs on 17β-estradiol metabolism [83, 84], as discussed above. Importantly, in reporter gene assays, PCB congeners are most effective at micromolar concentrations,

and biomedical applications. *Med. Res. Rev.*, **31**, 364–442.

19 Safe, S. and Kim, K. (2008) Non-classical genomic estrogen receptor (ER)/specificity protein and ER/activating protein-1 signaling pathways. *J. Mol. Endocrinol.*, **41**, 263–275.

20 Watson, C.S., Jeng, Y.J., and Kochukov, M.Y. (2010) Nongenomic signaling pathways of estrogen toxicity. *Toxicol. Sci.*, **115**, 1–11.

21 Hall, J.M., Couse, J.F., and Korach, K.S. (2001) The multifaceted mechanisms of estradiol and estrogen receptor signaling. *J. Biol. Chem.*, **276**, 36869–36872.

22 Hewitt, S.C., Deroo, B.J., and Korach, K.S. (2005) Signal transduction. A new mediator for an old hormone? *Science*, **307**, 1572–1573.

23 Min, G., Kim, H., Bae, Y., Petz, L., and Kemper, J.K. (2002) Inhibitory cross-talk between estrogen receptor (ER) and constitutively activated androstane receptor (CAR). CAR inhibits ER-mediated signaling pathway by squelching p160 coactivators. *J. Biol. Chem.*, **277**, 34626–34633.

24 Pascussi, J.M., Gerbal-Chaloin, S., Duret, C., Daujat-Chavanieu, M., Vilarem, M.J., and Maurel, P. (2008) The tangle of nuclear receptors that controls xenobiotic metabolism and transport: crosstalk and consequences. *Annu. Rev. Pharmacol. Toxicol.*, **48**, 1–32.

25 Safe, S. and Wormke, M. (2003) Inhibitory aryl hydrocarbon receptor-estrogen receptor alpha cross-talk and mechanisms of action. *Chem. Res. Toxicol.*, **16**, 807–816.

26 Mittendorf, R. (1995) Teratogen update: carcinogenesis and teratogenesis associated with exposure to diethylstilbestrol (DES) *in utero*. *Teratology*, **51**, 435–445.

27 Bredfeldt, T.G., Greathouse, K.L., Safe, S.H., Hung, M.C., Bedford, M.T., and Walker, C.L. (2010) Xenoestrogen-induced regulation of EZH2 and histone methylation via estrogen receptor signaling to PI3K/AKT. *Mol. Endocrinol.*, **24**, 993–1006.

28 Nadal, A., Ropero, A.B., Laribi, O., Maillet, M., Fuentes, E., and Soria, B. (2000) Nongenomic actions of estrogens and xenoestrogens by binding at a plasma membrane receptor unrelated to estrogen receptor alpha and estrogen receptor beta. *Proc. Natl. Acad. Sci. USA*, **97**, 11603–11608.

29 Ma, L. (2009) Endocrine disruptors in female reproductive tract development and carcinogenesis. *Trends Endocrinol. Metab.*, **20**, 357–363.

30 Katzenellenbogen, B.S. and Frasor, J. (2004) Therapeutic targeting in the estrogen receptor hormonal pathway. *Semin. Oncol.*, **31**, 28–38.

31 Swaby, R.F., Sharma, C.G., and Jordan, V.C. (2007) SERMs for the treatment and prevention of breast cancer. *Rev. Endocr. Metab. Disord.*, **8**, 229–239.

32 Shang, Y. and Brown, M. (2002) Molecular determinants for the tissue specificity of SERMs. *Science*, **295**, 2465–2468.

33 Gaido, K.W., Leonard, L.S., Maness, S.C., Hall, J.M., McDonnell, D.P., Saville, B., and Safe, S. (1999) Differential interaction of the methoxychlor metabolite 2,2-bis-(*p*-hydroxyphenyl)-1,1,1-trichloroethane with estrogen receptors alpha and beta. *Endocrinology*, **140**, 5746–5753.

34 Swedenborg, E., Pongratz, I., and Gustafsson, J.A. (2010) Endocrine disruptors targeting ERbeta function. *Int. J. Androl.*, **33**, 288–297.

35 Tiemann, U. (2008) *In vivo* and *in vitro* effects of the organochlorine pesticides DDT, TCPM, methoxychlor, and lindane on the female reproductive tract of mammals: a review. *Reprod. Toxicol.*, **25**, 316–326.

36 Kummer, V., Mašková, J., Zralý, Z., Neča, J., Šimečková, P., Vondráček, J., and Machala, M. (2008) Estrogenic activity of environmental polycyclic aromatic hydrocarbons in uterus of immature Wistar rats. *Toxicol. Lett.*, **180**, 212–221.

37 Abdelrahim, M., Ariazi, E., Kim, K., Khan, S., Barhoumi, R., Burghardt, R., Liu, S., Hill, D., Finnell, R., Wlodarczyk, B., Jordan, V.C., and Safe, S. (2006) 3-Methylcholanthrene and other aryl hydrocarbon receptor agonists directly activate estrogen receptor alpha. *Cancer Res.*, **66**, 2459–2467.

38 Vandenberg, L.N., Maffini, M.V., Sonnenschein, C., Rubin, B.S., and Soto, A.M. (2009) Bisphenol-A and the great divide: a review of controversies in the field of endocrine disruption. *Endocr. Rev.*, **30**, 75–95.

39 Witorsch, R.J. and Thomas, J.A. (2010) Personal care products and endocrine disruption: a critical review of the literature. *Crit. Rev. Toxicol.*, **40** (Suppl. 3), 1–30.

40 van der Burg, B., Schreurs, R., van der Linden, S., Seinen, W., Brouwer, A., and Sonneveld, E. (2008) Endocrine effects of polycyclic musks: do we smell a rat? *Int. J. Androl.*, **31**, 188–193.

41 Hamers, T., Kamstra, J.H., Sonneveld, E., Murk, A.J., Kester, M.H., Andersson, P.L., Legler, J., and Brouwer, A. (2006) *In vitro* profiling of the endocrine-disrupting potency of brominated flame retardants. *Toxicol. Sci.*, **92**, 157–173.

42 Houtman, C.J., Van Houten, Y.K., Leonards, P.E., Brouwer, A., Lamoree, M.H., and Legler, J. (2006) Biological validation of a sample preparation method for ER-CALUX bioanalysis of estrogenic activity in sediment using mixtures of xeno-estrogens. *Environ. Sci. Technol.*, **40**, 2455–2461.

43 Kinani, S., Bouchonnet, S., Creusot, N., Bourcier, S., Balaguer, P., Porcher, J.M., and Ait-Aissa, S. (2010) Bioanalytical characterisation of multiple endocrine- and dioxin-like activities in sediments from reference and impacted small rivers. *Environ. Pollut.*, **158**, 74–83.

44 Lübcke-von Varel, U., Machala, M., Ciganek, M., Neča, J., Pěnčíková, K., Pálková, L., Vondráček, J., Löffler, I., Streck, G., Reifferscheid, G., Flückiger-Isler, S., Weiss, J.M., Lamoree, M., and Brack, W. (2011) Polar compounds dominate *in vitro* effects of sediment extracts. *Environ. Sci. Technol.*, **45**, 2384–2390.

45 Kortenkamp, A. (2007) Ten years of mixing cocktails: a review of combination effects of endocrine-disrupting chemicals. *Environ. Health Perspect.*, **115** (Suppl. 1), 98–105.

46 Mense, S.M., Hei, T.K., Ganju, R.K., and Bhat, H.K. (2008) Phytoestrogens and breast cancer prevention: possible mechanisms of action. *Environ. Health Perspect.*, **116**, 426–433.

47 Virk-Baker, M.K., Nagy, T.R., and Barnes, S. (2010) Role of phytoestrogens in cancer therapy. *Planta Med.*, **76**, 1132–1142.

48 Patisaul, H.B. and Jefferson, W. (2010) The pros and cons of phytoestrogens. *Front. Neuroendocrinol.*, **31**, 400–419.

49 Kuiper, G.G., Lemmen, J.G., Carlsson, B., Corton, J.C., Safe, S.H., van der Saag, P.T., van der Burg, B., and Gustafsson, J.A. (1998) Interaction of estrogenic chemicals and phytoestrogens with estrogen receptor beta. *Endocrinology*, **139**, 4252–4263.

50 Nakajima, M., Cooney, M.J., Tu, A.H., Chang, K.Y., Cao, J., Ando, A., An, G.J., Melia, M., and de Juan, E., Jr (2001) Normalization of retinal vascular permeability in experimental diabetes with genistein. *Invest. Ophthalmol. Vis. Sci.*, **42**, 2110–2114.

51 Plíšková, M., Vondráček, J., Křen, V., Gažák, R., Sedmera, P., Walterová, D., Psotová, J., Šimánek, V., and Machala, M. (2005) Effects of silymarin flavonolignans and synthetic silybin derivatives on estrogen and aryl hydrocarbon receptor activation. *Toxicology*, **215**, 80–89.

52 Ohtake, F., Fujii-Kuriyama, Y., and Kato, S. (2009) AhR acts as an E3 ubiquitin ligase to modulate steroid receptor functions. *Biochem. Pharmacol.*, **77**, 474–484.

53 Ruegg, J., Swedenborg, E., Wahlström, D., Escande, A., Balaguer, P., Pettersson, K., and Pongratz, I. (2008) The transcription factor aryl hydrocarbon receptor nuclear translocator functions as an estrogen receptor beta-selective coactivator, and its recruitment to alternative pathways mediates antiestrogenic effects of dioxin. *Mol. Endocrinol.*, **22**, 304–316.

54 Ohtake, F., Baba, A., Takada, I., Okada, M., Iwasaki, K., Miki, H., Takahashi, S., Kouzmenko, A., Nohara, K., Chiba, T., Fujii-Kuriyama, Y., and Kato, S. (2007) Dioxin receptor is a ligand-dependent E3 ubiquitin ligase. *Nature*, **446**, 562–566.

55 Beischlag, T.V. and Perdew, G.H. (2005) ER alpha–AHR–ARNT protein–protein interactions mediate estradiol-dependent

transrepression of dioxin-inducible gene transcription. *J. Biol. Chem.*, **280**, 21607–21611.
56 Sanderson, J.T. (2006) The steroid hormone biosynthesis pathway as a target for endocrine-disrupting chemicals. *Toxicol. Sci.*, **94**, 3–21.
57 Tsuchiya, Y., Nakajima, M., and Yokoi, T. (2005) Cytochrome P450-mediated metabolism of estrogens and its regulation in human. *Cancer Lett.*, **227**, 115–124.
58 Laville, N., Balaguer, P., Brion, F., Hinfray, N., Casellas, C., Porcher, J.M., and Ait-Aissa, S. (2006) Modulation of aromatase activity and mRNA by various selected pesticides in the human choriocarcinoma JEG-3 cell line. *Toxicology*, **228**, 98–108.
59 Sanderson, J.T., Boerma, J., Lansbergen, G.W., and van den Berg, M. (2002) Induction and inhibition of aromatase (CYP19) activity by various classes of pesticides in H295R human adrenocortical carcinoma cells. *Toxicol. Appl. Pharmacol.*, **182**, 44–54.
60 Kao, Y.C., Zhou, C., Sherman, M., Laughton, C.A., and Chen, S. (1998) Molecular basis of the inhibition of human aromatase (estrogen synthetase) by flavone and isoflavone phytoestrogens: a site-directed mutagenesis study. *Environ. Health Perspect.*, **106**, 85–92.
61 Canton, R.F., Sanderson, J.T., Letcher, R.J., Bergman, A., and van den Berg, M. (2005) Inhibition and induction of aromatase (CYP19) activity by brominated flame retardants in H295R human adrenocortical carcinoma cells. *Toxicol. Sci.*, **88**, 447–455.
62 Song, R., Duarte, T.L., Almeida, G.M., Farmer, P.B., Cooke, M.S., Zhang, W., Sheng, G., Fu, J., and Jones, G.D. (2009) Cytotoxicity and gene expression profiling of two hydroxylated polybrominated diphenyl ethers in human H295R adrenocortical carcinoma cells. *Toxicol. Lett.*, **185**, 23–31.
63 You, L. (2004) Steroid hormone biotransformation and xenobiotic induction of hepatic steroid metabolizing enzymes. *Chem. Biol. Interact.*, **147**, 233–246.
64 Lee, A.J., Cai, M.X., Thomas, P.E., Conney, A.H., and Zhu, B.T. (2003) Characterization of the oxidative metabolites of 17beta-estradiol and estrone formed by 15 selectively expressed human cytochrome p450 isoforms. *Endocrinology*, **144**, 3382–3398.
65 Zhu, B.T. and Lee, A.J. (2005) NADPH-dependent metabolism of 17beta-estradiol and estrone to polar and nonpolar metabolites by human tissues and cytochrome P450 isoforms. *Steroids*, **70**, 225–244.
66 Gupta, M., McDougal, A., and Safe, S. (1998) Estrogenic and antiestrogenic activities of 16alpha- and 2-hydroxy metabolites of 17beta-estradiol in MCF-7 and T47D human breast cancer cells. *J. Steroid Biochem. Mol. Biol.*, **67**, 413–419.
67 Bolton, J.L. and Thatcher, G.R. (2008) Potential mechanisms of estrogen quinone carcinogenesis. *Chem. Res. Toxicol.*, **21**, 93–101.
68 Cavalieri, E., Chakravarti, D., Guttenplan, J., Hart, E., Ingle, J., Jankowiak, R., Muti, P., Rogan, E., Russo, J., Santen, R., and Sutter, T. (2006) Catechol estrogen quinones as initiators of breast and other human cancers: implications for biomarkers of susceptibility and cancer prevention. *Biochim. Biophys. Acta*, **1766**, 63–78.
69 Nebert, D.W. and Dalton, T.P. (2006) The role of cytochrome P450 enzymes in endogenous signalling pathways and environmental carcinogenesis. *Nat. Rev. Cancer*, **6**, 947–960.
70 Jones, S.A., Moore, L.B., Shenk, J.L., Wisely, G.B., Hamilton, G.A., McKee, D.D., Tomkinson, N.C., LeCluyse, E.L., Lambert, M.H., Willson, T.M., Kliewer, S.A., and Moore, J.T. (2000) The pregnane X receptor: a promiscuous xenobiotic receptor that has diverged during evolution. *Mol. Endocrinol.*, **14**, 27–39.
71 Li, H.C., Dehal, S.S., and Kupfer, D. (1995) Induction of the hepatic CYP2B and CYP3A enzymes by the proestrogenic pesticide methoxychlor and by DDT in the rat. Effects on methoxychlor metabolism. *J. Biochem. Toxicol.*, **10**, 51–61.

72 Moore, L.B., Parks, D.J., Jones, S.A., Bledsoe, R.K., Consler, T.G., Stimmel, J.B., Goodwin, B., Liddle, C., Blanchard, S.G., Willson, T.M., Collins, J.L., and Kliewer, S.A. (2000) Orphan nuclear receptors constitutive androstane receptor and pregnane X receptor share xenobiotic and steroid ligands. *J. Biol. Chem.*, **275**, 15122–15127.

73 Ugazio, G., Bosio, A., Nebbia, C., and Soffietti, M.G. (1991) Age- and sex-related effects on hepatic drug metabolism in rats chronically exposed to dietary atrazine. *Res. Commun. Chem. Pathol. Pharmacol.*, **73**, 231–243.

74 Wyde, M.E., Bartolucci, E., Ueda, A., Zhang, H., Yan, B., Negishi, M., and You, L. (2003) The environmental pollutant 1,1-dichloro-2,2-bis (*p*-chlorophenyl)ethylene induces rat hepatic cytochrome P450 2B and 3A expression through the constitutive androstane receptor and pregnane X receptor. *Mol. Pharmacol.*, **64**, 474–481.

75 Liu, L. and Klaassen, C.D. (1996) Regulation of hepatic sulfotransferases by steroidal chemicals in rats. *Drug Metab. Dispos.*, **24**, 854–858.

76 Runge-Morris, M., Rose, K., Falany, C.N., and Kocarek, T.A. (1998) Differential regulation of individual sulfotransferase isoforms by phenobarbital in male rat liver. *Drug Metab. Dispos.*, **26**, 795–801.

77 Vansell, N.R. and Klaassen, C.D. (2002) Increase in rat liver UDP-glucuronosyltransferase mRNA by microsomal enzyme inducers that enhance thyroid hormone glucuronidation. *Drug Metab. Dispos.*, **30**, 240–246.

78 Xie, W., Yeuh, M.F., Radominska-Pandya, A., Saini, S.P., Negishi, Y., Bottroff, B.S., Cabrera, G.Y., Tukey, R.H., and Evans, R.M. (2003) Control of steroid, heme, and carcinogen metabolism by nuclear pregnane X receptor and constitutive androstane receptor. *Proc. Natl. Acad. Sci. USA*, **100**, 4150–4155.

79 Plíšková, M., Vondráček, J., Canton, R.F., Neča, J., Kočan, A., Petrík, J., Trnovec, T., Sanderson, T., van den Berg, M., and Machala, M. (2005) Impact of polychlorinated biphenyls contamination on estrogenic activity in human male serum. *Environ. Health Perspect.*, **113**, 1277–1284.

80 Bonefeld-Jørgensen, E.C., Andersen, H.R., Rasmussen, T.H., and Vinggaard, A.M. (2001) Effect of highly bioaccumulated polychlorinated biphenyl congeners on estrogen and androgen receptor activity. *Toxicology*, **158**, 141–153.

81 Hamers, T., Kamstra, J.H., Cenijn, P.H., Pěnčíková, K., Pálková, L., Šimečková, P., Vondráček, J., Andersson, P.L., Stenberg, M., and Machala, M. (2011) *In vitro* toxicity profiling of ultrapure non-dioxin-like polychlorinated biphenyl congeners and their relative toxic contribution to PCB mixtures in humans. *Toxicol. Sci.*, **121**, 88–100.

82 Buchanan, D.L., Ohsako, S., Tohyama, C., Cooke, P.S., and Iguchi, T. (2002) Dioxin inhibition of estrogen-induced mouse uterine epithelial mitogenesis involves changes in cyclin and transforming growth factor-beta expression. *Toxicol. Sci.*, **66**, 62–68.

83 Takemoto, K., Nakajima, M., Fujiki, Y., Katoh, M., Gonzalez, F.J., and Yokoi, T. (2004) Role of the aryl hydrocarbon receptor and Cyp1b1 in the antiestrogenic activity of 2,3,7,8-tetrachlorodibenzo-*p*-dioxin. *Arch. Toxicol.*, **78**, 309–315.

84 van Duursen, M.B., Sanderson, J.T., van der Bruggen, M., van der Linden, J., and van den Berg, M. (2003) Effects of several dioxin-like compounds on estrogen metabolism in the malignant MCF-7 and nontumorigenic MCF-10A human mammary epithelial cell lines. *Toxicol. Appl. Pharmacol.*, **190**, 241–250.

85 Richthoff, J., Rylander, L., Jonsson, B.A., Akesson, H., Hagmar, L., Nilsson-Ehle, P., Stridsberg, M., and Giwercman, A. (2003) Serum levels of 2,2′,4,4′,5,5′-hexachlorobiphenyl (CB-153) in relation to markers of reproductive function in young males from the general Swedish population. *Environ. Health Perspect.*, **111**, 409–413.

86 Hany, J., Lilienthal, H., Sarasin, A., Roth-Harer, A., Fastabend, A., Dunemann, L., Lichtensteiger, W., and Winneke, G. (1999) Developmental exposure of rats to a reconstituted PCB

mixture or aroclor 1254: effects on organ weights, aromatase activity, sex hormone levels, and sweet preference behavior. *Toxicol. Appl. Pharmacol.*, **158**, 231–243.

87 Badawi, A.F., Cavalieri, E.L., and Rogan, E.G. (2000) Effect of chlorinated hydrocarbons on expression of cytochrome P450 1A1, 1A2 and 1B1 and 2- and 4-hydroxylation of 17beta-estradiol in female Sprague-Dawley rats. *Carcinogenesis*, **21**, 1593–1599.

88 Hayes, C.L., Spink, D.C., Spink, B.C., Cao, J.Q., Walker, N.J., and Sutter, T.R. (1996) 17 Beta-estradiol hydroxylation catalyzed by human cytochrome P450 1B1. *Proc. Natl. Acad. Sci. USA*, **93**, 9776–9781.

89 Yamazaki, H., Shaw, P.M., Guengerich, F.P., and Shimada, T. (1998) Roles of cytochromes P450 1A2 and 3A4 in the oxidation of estradiol and estrone in human liver microsomes. *Chem. Res. Toxicol.*, **11**, 659–665.

90 Petersen, M.S., Halling, J., Damkier, P., Nielsen, F., Grandjean, P., Weihe, P., and Brosen, K. (2007) Polychlorinated biphenyl (PCB) induction of CYP3A4 enzyme activity in healthy Faroese adults. *Toxicol. Appl. Pharmacol.*, **224**, 202–206.

91 Kester, M.H., Bulduk, S., Tibboel, D., Meinl, W., Glatt, H., Falany, C.N., Coughtrie, M.W., Bergman, A., Safe, S.H., Kuiper, G.G., Schuur, A.G., Brouwer, A., and Visser, T.J. (2000) Potent inhibition of estrogen sulfotransferase by hydroxylated PCB metabolites: a novel pathway explaining the estrogenic activity of PCBs. *Endocrinology*, **141**, 1897–1900.

92 van den Hurk, P., Kubiczak, G.A., Lehmler, H.J., and James, M.O. (2002) Hydroxylated polychlorinated biphenyls as inhibitors of the sulfation and glucuronidation of 3-hydroxy-benzo[*a*] pyrene. *Environ. Health Perspect.*, **110**, 343–348.

25
Biotransformation of Insecticides

Corie A. Ellison, Alice L. Crane, and James R. Olson

25.1
Introduction to Insecticides

An insecticide is a chemical used to kill or control populations of unwanted insects. There are several different categories of insecticides that work by a number of different mechanisms, such as inhibiting cholinesterase activity (organophosphates and carbamates), disrupting sodium channel activity (pyrethroids), altering insect behavior (*N,N*-diethyl-*m*-toluamide (DEET)), or mimicking insect hormones (juvenile hormone analogs). Today, the majority of insecticides used around the world belong to one of three categories: organophosphate, pyrethroid, or carbamate. This chapter will focus on the biotransformation of insecticides from the three major classes with an emphasis on recent advances in insecticide biotransformation research. For a more historical and comprehensive review of insecticides, the authors suggest Krieger [1], Knaak *et al.* [2, 3], and Chambers and Levi [4].

25.1.1
Organophosphate Insecticides

Organophosphate insecticides – a large and diverse class of chemicals – possess a central phosphorous atom that has three single-bound constituents and a coordinated covalent bound to sulfur or oxygen (Figure 25.1). There are several different subclasses of organophosphate insecticides, which are based on the constituents bound to the phosphorus atom. The insecticidal activity of organophosphates is attributed to their ability to inhibit cholinesterase activity through an irreversible phosphorylation reaction that results in overexcitation of the nervous system. The primary neurotoxic target for organophosphate insecticides is acetylcholinesterase, but both butyrylcholinesterase and carboxylesterase can also be inhibited, and are more sensitive targets at lower-level organophosphate exposures. Some organophosphates (e.g., chlorpyrifos, parathion, and diazinon) contain a P=S moiety and require oxidative desulfuration to form an oxon metabolite (i.e., a compound with

Metabolism of Drugs and Other Xenobiotics, First Edition. Edited by Pavel Anzenbacher, Ulrich M. Zanger.

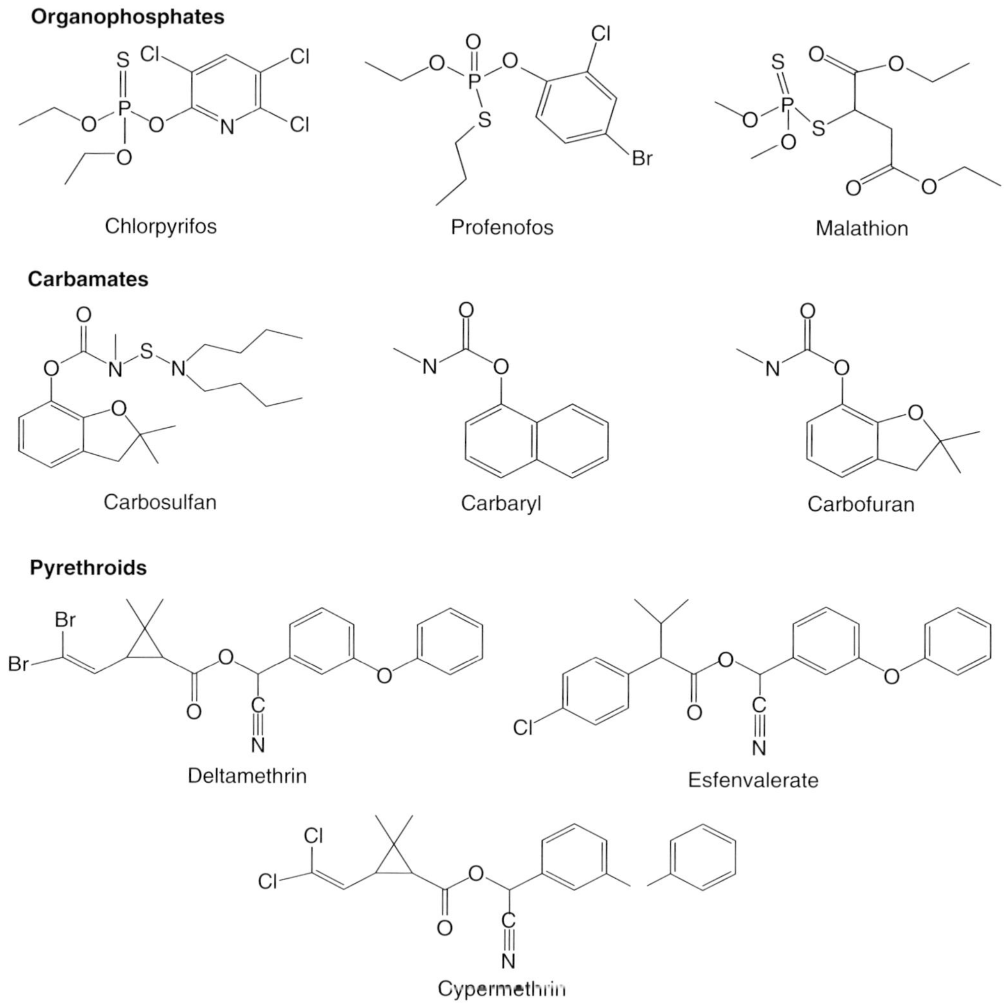

Figure 25.1 Chemical structures of select insecticides.

a P=O moiety) capable of inhibiting cholinesterase activity, while other compounds (e.g., profenofos) contain a P=O moiety and are biologically active in their parent form. The mammalian toxicity of organophosphate insecticides varies widely, with compounds like dicrotophos and disulfoton being highly toxic to mammals, while malathion and trichlorfon are considered relatively safe. Generally speaking, organophosphate insecticides are not persistent within the environment, and hydrolysis of the compounds increases with pH, temperature, and UV light. Elimination in humans is also fairly quick, with urinary excretion half-lives usually ranging between 3 and 30 h [5]. A more comprehensive discussion of organophosphate insecticides can be found in chapters 64–6 of [1].

25.1.2
Carbamate Insecticides

Carbamate insecticides are esters derived from carbamic acid, and have the general formula ROC(=O)NHCH$_3$ for *N*-methylcarbamates and ROC(=O)N(CH$_3$)$_2$ for dimethylcarbamates (Figure 25.1). Similar to organophosphates, their insecticidal activity is attributed to inhibition of acetylcholinesterase; however, most carbamates produce less mammalian toxicity than organophosphates. The lower mammalian toxicity of carbamates is due to a transient and reversible inhibition of acetylcholinesterase, which is generally resolved within several hours. Carbamate insecticides are biologically active in their parent form and do not require metabolic activation for cholinesterase inhibition, although some may be metabolized to more active structures. The magnitude of toxicity to mammals varies with the chemical, with compounds like aldicarb and carbofuran being more potent than carbaryl and thiodicarb; however, most carbamates are generally considered "safe" to humans with toxicity rarely occurring outside of accidental exposures and self-poisonings. There is little evidence for bioaccumulation of carbamates in humans since these compounds are quickly metabolized and eliminated in urine [5, 6]. More detailed information on carbamate chemistry and toxicity can be found in chapters 73–75 of [1].

25.1.3
Pyrethroid Insecticides

Pyrethroid insecticides originated from the naturally occurring insecticides in the pyrethrum extracts of chrysanthemum flowers, which contains a mixture of six different compounds: pyrethrin I and II, cinerin I and II, and jasmolin I and II. To improve the chemical effectiveness and stability of these insecticides, several different synthetic analogs have been formed by modifying the alcohol and/or acid moiety of the compounds (Figure 25.1). Most pyrethroid insecticides can be classified as a first- or second-generation pyrethroid. First-generation pyrethroids are mainly used indoors due to their sensitivity to light, air, and temperature, and include the compounds resmethrin and tetramethrin. Second-generation pyrethroids are much more stable and are used widely for agricultural pests, and include the compounds cypermethrin, deltamethrin, and permethrin. Pyrethroids are active in their parent form and do not require metabolic activation for insecticidal activity. Pyrethroids cause paralysis in insects by disrupting the kinetics of voltage-sensitive sodium channels, which results in an increased sodium permeability of the nerve membrane. In general, pyrethroids have low acute toxicity in mammals [7]; however, the potential for neurotoxicity following exposure is still of interest. The low acute mammalian toxicity of pyrethroids has been attributed to faster metabolism, higher body temperature, and lower sensitivity in mammals. Elimination in humans is fairly quick, with 50% or more of the compound generally being excreted in urine within 36 h [8–12]. More detailed information on specific pyrethroids can be found in chapters 76 and 77 of [1].

25.1.4
Organochlorine Insecticides

Organochlorine insecticides such asdichlorodiphenyltrichloroethane (DDT) were heavily used during and after World War II due to their broad spectrum of insecticidal activity and low mammalian toxicity. However, their resistance to breakdown in the environment resulted to undesirable effects such as bioaccumulation in animals and humans, which eventually led to their ban in most areas of the world. Interestingly, even though DDT has not been used for several decades, measurable amounts of the DDT metabolite, dichlorodiphenyldichloroethylene (DDE), can still be found in most human studies due to the widespread use and persistence of DDT/DDE in the body and environment. Further information on organochlorine insecticides can be found in [1] and will not be further discussed in this chapter.

25.2
Metabolism of Insecticides

The liver is regarded as the primary organ responsible for insecticide metabolism, although it should be noted that metabolism can also occur extrahepatically. Generally speaking, insecticide metabolism occurs in two phases. Phase I reactions involve oxidation, reduction, or hydrolyses of an insecticide, and can lead to activation and/or detoxification of the parent compound. Phase II reactions involve the combination of phase I metabolites with an endogenous molecule to form a molecule that can be more readily excreted. This section will discuss the major enzymes involved in phase I and phase II metabolism of insecticides.

25.2.1
Hepatic Phase I Enzymes Involved in Biotransformation of Insecticides

25.2.1.1 Cytochrome P450s

Cytochrome P450s (CYPs) have been the primary focus of insecticide metabolism and as such a large amount of information is available for review. Hepatic microsomes contain many forms of CYPs, making them ideal for assessing combinatorial CYP-mediated metabolism of insecticides. The metabolism of organophosphate insecticides like chlorpyrifos [13–18], parathion [13, 14, 17, 19, 20], diazinon [14, 17, 21], malathion [22], profenofos [23], dimethoate [24], and fenthion [25] has been characterized using liver microsomes from human, rat, and/or mouse. The metabolism of carbamate insecticides like carbosulfan [26, 27], carbaryl [28], and carbofuran [29], and the metabolism of pyrethroids like deltamethrin [30, 31], esfenvalerate [31], and permethrin [32], has also been characterized using liver microsomes from various species. Table 25.1 summarizes kinetic parameters for metabolite formation from pooled human liver microsomes for several different organophosphate and carbamate insecticides. Pyrethroid insecticides were omitted

Table 25.1 Kinetic parameters for CYP-mediated metabolism of some insecticides by pooled human liver microsomes.

	Metabolite 1			Metabolite 2			Metabolite 3			References
	V_{max}	K_m	CL_{int}	V_{max}	K_m	CL_{int}	V_{max}	K_m	CL_{int}	
Organophosphates										
Chlorpyrifos[a)]	0.346	2.5	138	0.453	16.2	28.0	–	–	–	[13]
Parathion[b)]	0.790	17.7	44.6	0.588	25.1	23.4	–	–	–	[13]
Carbamates										
Carbosulfan[c)]	5	269	18.6	2	32	62.5	–	–	–	[26]
Carbaryl[d)]	0.04	349	0.115	0.87	349	2.49	0.57	81	7.04	[28]

V_{max} values expressed as nmol/min/mg protein; K_m values expressed as μM; CL_{int} values expressed as μl/min/mg protein.

a) Metabolite 1, chlorpyrifos oxon; Metabolite 2, 3,4,5-trichloropyrindinol.

b) Metabolite 1, paraoxon; Metabolite 2, *p*-nitrophenol.

c) Metabolite 1, carbosulfan sulfinamide; Metabolite 2, dibutylamine.

d) Metabolite 1, 5-hydroxycarbaryl; Metabolite 2, 4-hydroxycarbaryl; Metabolite 3, carbaryl methylol.

from Table 25.1 since metabolism assays for pyrethroids often examine the disappearance of the parent compound rather than the formation of metabolites due to the fact that numerous metabolites are formed from a single parent compound.

A limitation of using microsomes for metabolism assays is the lack of CYP-specific information. To overcome this, some researchers have used microsomes from animals pretreated with a CYP inducer, such as phenobarbital [19, 33]; however, CYP induction is not specific to only one isoform. Others have used immunoinhibition assays that compare insecticide metabolism in the presence and absence of a CYP-specific antibody [14, 22]. Another indirect approach is to use a known chemical inhibitor of CYP activity that is often semispecific for a CYP isoform or family. This approach has been used in assessing the metabolism of several organophosphate insecticides like chlorpyrifos [17] diazinon [17, 21], dimethoate [24], fenthion [25], malathion [22], and parathion [17].

The most direct way of assessing CYP-specific metabolism of insecticides is the use of recombinant CYP enzymes. This approach provides metabolism data on a CYP-specific basis and allows for the identification of major CYPs involved in insecticide metabolism. Several studies have taken this approach for assessing metabolism of organophosphate, carbamate, and pyrethroid insecticides. Through this approach, CYP2B6, CYP2C19, and CYP3A4 have been identified as being the major human CYPs involved in organophosphate insecticide metabolism [13, 18, 21]. For some organophosphates, individual CYPs preferentially mediate metabolism for one pathway over another. For example, as illustrated in Figure 25.2, CYP2B6 favors metabolic activation of the organophosphate insecticide chlorpyrifos to chlorpyrifos oxon, while CYP2C19 favors detoxification [13], thus showing how CYP isoforms can preferentially aid in the activation or detoxification

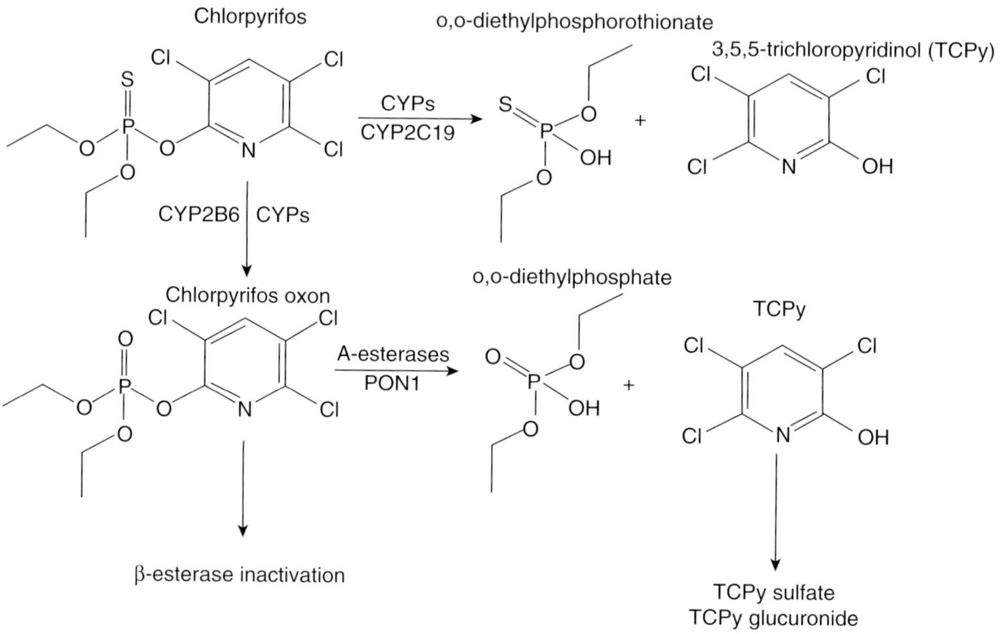

Figure 25.2 Primary human enzymes contributing to the metabolism of the organophosphate insecticide chlorpyrifos, as reported by Foxenberg *et al.* [13].

of an insecticide. For carbamate metabolism, CYP1A1, CYP1A2, CYP2B6, CYP2C19, and CYP3A4 have been identified as the primary human CYPs involved in metabolism for a variety of compounds [27–29]. Table 25.2 summarizes kinetic parameters for the metabolism of several organophosphate and carbamate insecticides from recombinant human CYP2B6, CYP2C19, and CYP3A4. For pyrethroids, CYP2C8, CYP2C9, CYP2C19, CYP3A4, and CYP3A5 have been identified as the human CYPs involved in metabolism, while CYP1A1, CYP1A2, CYP2C6, CYP2C11, CYP3A1, and CYP3A2 are the rat CYPs involved in metabolism [30–32, 34]. Further information on the CYPs involved in metabolism for a specific insecticide can be found in chapter 38 of [1].

CYP2B6, CYP2C19, and CYP3A4 are all actively involved in the metabolism of several different insecticides, but the kinetic values vary among the different CYPs (see Table 25.2). For the compounds shown in Table 25.2, CYP2B6 and CYP2C19 consistently have a lower K_m value for metabolite formation compared to CYP3A4, indicating that both CYP2B6 and CYP2C19 have a higher affinity for the different insecticide compounds. The low K_m value of CYP2B6 and CYP2C19 suggests that these CYPs play a predominate role in insecticide metabolism at low-level real-world exposures. CYP3A4 has the largest V_{max} value for metabolite formation for several of the compounds in Table 25.2, indicating a higher metabolic capacity of CYP3A4 relative to CYP2B6 and CYP2C19. When assessing the contribution of a

Table 25.2 Kinetic values for some insecticides metabolized by recombinant human CYP2B6, CYP2C19, and CYP3A4.

	CYP2B6			CYP2C19			CYP3A4			References
	V_{max}	K_m	CL_{int}	V_{max}	K_m	CL_{int}	V_{max}	K_m	CL_{int}	
Organophosphates										
Chlorpyrifos										
chlorpyrifos oxon	12.5	0.81	15 432	2.47	1.2	2058	11.9	27	441	[13]
3,4,5-trichloropyrindinol	1.55	2.1	738	13.1	1.6	8187	12.7	33	385	
Parathion										
paraoxon	4.83	0.61	7 918	4.88	0.56	8714	14.0	66	212	[13]
p-nitrophenol	1.80	0.74	2 432	2.34	0.60	3900	15.7	31	506	
Carbamates										
Carbosulfan										
carbosulfan sulfinamide	26.9	28	961	11.6	93	125	25.3	171	148	[27]
Carbaryl										
5-hydroxycarbaryl	0.29	110	2.6	0.99	62	16	2.34	281	8.3	[28]
4-hydroxycarbaryl	0.80	11	73	2.21	44	50	5.81	235	25	
carbaryl methylol	15.5	45	344	3.46	15	231	1.47	156	9.4	

V_{max} values expressed as nmol/min/nmol P450; K_m values expressed as μM; CL_{int} values expressed as μl/min/nmol CYP.

CYP isoform to the total hepatic metabolism of an insecticide it is also important to consider the relative CYP abundance of each CYP isoform within the liver. While CYP2B6 and CYP2C19 are more catalytically active (as represented by CL_{int}) than CYP3A4 towards several insecticides (see Table 25.2), their hepatic content is about 8–9 times lower than CYP3A4 content [35, 36] and thus CYP3A4 may become important in overall hepatic metabolism due to its sheer abundance, even if its activity is lower than other CYPs.

25.2.1.2 Flavin-Containing Monooxygenases

Insecticide substrates for flavin-containing monooxygenases (FMOs) include organophosphates, such as phorate, disulfoton, sulprofos, and fenthion [25, 37, 38], and the carbamates methiocarb and aldicarb [37, 38]. Little is known about the specific isoforms of FMOs involved in insecticide metabolism. FMO1 is the most active FMO involved in metabolism of phorate, disulfoton, sulprofos, fenthion, and methiocarb [25, 37]; however, it is essentially absent in adult human liver [39]. FMO3 is expressed in adult liver and is the second most catalytically active FMO involved in insecticide metabolism, but compared to hepatic CYP-mediated metabolism of the insecticides its contribution is likely to be small [37].

25.2.1.3 Others

Carboxylesterases – broad-spectrum Ser hydrolases involved in drug and xenobiotic metabolism – are widely distributed in mammalian tissue, with the highest concentrations being found in the liver. Recent work has shown that carboxylesterases are involved in the metabolism of a number of pyrethroid insecticides in both humans and rodents [30, 31, 40–42] as well as metabolism of the organophosphate insecticide, malathion [43].

Paraoxonase 1 (PON1) is a high-density lipoprotein-associated enzyme that is synthesized in the liver and secreted into the plasma where it hydrolyzes lipid peroxides. In addition to hydrolyzing lipid peroxides, PON1 has received a great deal of attention for its ability to detoxify the oxon metabolite of organophosphate insecticides [44–46]. The *in vitro* catalytic efficacy of PON1 is substrate-dependent, with activity being relatively high towards diazinon oxon, moderate towards chlorpyrifos oxon, and low towards paraoxon [47]. PON1 knockout mice are extremely sensitive to diazinon oxon and chlorpyrifos oxon, but do not show increased sensitivity to paraoxon. Intraperitoneal injection of purified PON1 into PON1 knockout mice provides protection against the toxicity of diazinon oxon and chlorpyrifos oxon, but not against paraoxon [48–50]. These *in vivo* observations support the *in vitro* observations that PON1 activity is substrate-dependent and suggest that the *in vitro* catalytic efficiency of PON1 determines the *in vivo* efficacy for detoxifying organophosphate insecticides [48].

25.2.2
Phase II Metabolism of Insecticides

Phase II metabolism of insecticides generally involves the reaction of the primary metabolite with endogenous agents to form secondary metabolites. A common phase II reaction involves the tripeptide glutathione (GSH), resulting in sulfation via glutathione *S*-transferases. Glutathione conjugates can be formed directly from the parent compound or from the reactive intermediates, resulting in a variety of metabolites. Studies looking at metabolites in human urine following chlorpyrifos poisoning as well as animal studies with similar compounds lend evidence that this pathway may be important in the *in vivo* metabolism of organophosphates [49, 50]. Phase II metabolism is generally considered less important than phase I with regard to determining the relative toxicity of the compound, since most of the metabolites of insecticides are already detoxified. However, for the organophosphate metabolite prothiophos oxon, it has been suggested that conjugation with glutathione forms a metabolite capable of inhibiting acetylcholinesterase [3]. Therefore, in some cases, phase II metabolism may play a role in bioactivation of the parent compound.

In addition to glutathione conjugation reactions, sulfide and glucuronide conjugates, catalyzed by sulfotransferases and glucuronosyltransferases, respectively, are formed by conjugation with organophosphate primary metabolites. Carbamates are principally metabolized via phase I oxidation and hydrolysis, and this is followed by phase II conjugation of some of the resulting cleaved products [51]. Glucuronide and sulfate derivatives of the aryl substituents are the major products found in the urine. Glutathione conjugates may be excreted in bile or recycled back into systemic circulation to be transformed into more hydrophilic products to be excreted in the urine. Pyrethroids can be excreted in urine following conjugation with glucuronic acid, sulfuric acid, or amino acids, or they can be excreted in bile following conjugation with cholesterol, bile acid, or triglyceride.

Phase II reactions are generally regarded as being important for aiding in excretion of insecticide metabolites, but indirect effects of phase II metabolism may have an influence on insecticide toxicity. For instance, depletion of glutathione has been observed in both human and animals exposed to certain organophosphates and pyrethroid compounds, which can contribute to oxidative stress and DNA damage [52–54].

25.3
Extrahepatic Metabolism of Insecticides

Biotransformation of insecticides occurs mainly in the liver, but can also occur in extrahepatic tissues such as the gastrointestinal tract, skin, lungs, kidney, blood, and brain. Important enzymes found in the blood and throughout all tissues include PON1, an A-esterase that detoxifies the active oxon metabolites of organophosphates, B-esterases acetylcholinesterase and butyrylcholinesterase, which can metabolize the active P=O moiety of organophosphates, but are inhibited in the process, and carboxylesterases which can metabolize pyrethroids. In addition to these enzymes, the CYP and FMO systems are found in many extrahepatic tissues, and may play an important role in insecticide metabolism. CYP3A4 – an important CYP in organophosphate, pyrethroid, and carbamate metabolism – makes up approximately 82% of intestinal CYP isoforms in humans [55]. FMO1 is essentially absent in adult human liver, but is expressed in the human kidney and intestine [56], suggesting that FMO1 may play a role in renal and intestinal metabolism of insecticides [57].

Dermal exposure is often the main route of exposure to insecticides and potentially plays a role in insecticide biotransformation prior to the agents reaching the liver. CYPs are known to be expressed in human skin with the majority being found in basal layer keratinoctyes [58]. Metabolism of several different insecticides, including parathion, has been examined in mouse skin microsomes and by using the porcine skin flap model [59, 60]. Certain pyrethroids, carbamates, and organophosphates are also known to be metabolized throughout the respiratory tract, where nasal passage and different types of alveolar cells contain CYPs, FMO, phase II enzymes, and carboxylesterases [61].

Considering that neurotoxicity is an important toxic endpoint for most insecticides, there are surprisingly only a few animal metabolism studies conducted in brain tissue [62–68], with little or no published research available on the metabolism of insecticides in human brain tissue. A small amount of toxic metabolite formed at this target site of toxicity may have a greater impact on systemic toxicity than the greater magnitude of toxic metabolite formed at the liver, which may not reach the brain or other sites of action. Therefore, there is a great need to study insecticide metabolism in the brain, particularly for the subset of organophosphate compounds that are bioactivated to neurotoxic metabolites at specific cellular and subcellular sites of toxicity. CYP2B6, which is primarily responsible for activation of certain organophosphate insecticides, is located in most regions of the human brain [69–71]. Knowledge of the kinetics of insecticide metabolism in the brain would also greatly improve the current physiologically based pharmacokinetic/pharmacodynamic models available for these agents.

25.4 Factors Affecting Metabolism

There are many factors that may alter the predicted metabolism of insecticides, making it difficult to extrapolate data from *in vitro* systems to *in vivo* systems and between animal models and humans. Many of these factors also contribute to interindividual variability in metabolism and therefore contribute to the uncertainty involved in human risk assessment. This section will focus on the underlying mechanisms of variations in interspecies and interindividual metabolism of insecticides.

25.4.1 Route of Exposure

The route of exposure as well as the amount and duration of exposure can affect the disposition and resulting metabolism of an insecticide. The oral route of exposure will favor first-pass metabolism in the liver, which will detoxify and/or bioactivate the insecticide. First-pass metabolism will be avoided if exposure occurs via dermal absorption or inhalation, although the insecticide may still undergo some metabolism extrahepatically before entering the bloodstream, as previously discussed. Depending on the chemical and physical properties of the insecticide, the disposition and rate and extent of metabolism will vary following dermal, inhalation, and oral exposures. For example, marked differences in the metabolites recovered from the pyrethroid compound cypermethrin were evident depending on oral or dermal exposure [8]. Furthermore, inherent physiological differences can alter insecticide metabolism for these routes of exposure, including organ CYP content, FMO content, microbial make-up in the gut, skin thickness, and body mass index.

25.4.2
Interaction of Xenobiotics

Human exposure to insecticides does not occur in isolation, and pharmacological agents, other toxins, and diet can induce or suppress xenobiotic metabolism. An important consideration in CYP-mediated metabolism of insecticides is the fact that several insecticides have the potential to both inhibit and induce certain CYP isoforms. Many organophosphate compounds release a highly reactive sulfur during oxidative desulfuration, which then interacts with the heme iron of CYPs inhibiting CYP activities in an isoform-specific manner. In addition to inhibiting xenobiotic metabolism, this can inhibit metabolism of endogenous CYP substrates such as steroid hormones [72, 73]. Pyrethroids and carbamates have also been shown to be inhibitors of certain CYPs [74]. Organophosphates, in addition to being able to inhibit CYPs, have also been shown to induce a number of CYP isoforms [75, 76]. For example, chlorpyrifos has been shown to induce CYP1A1, CYP1A2, CYP3A4, CYP1B1, and CYP2B6 mRNA *in vitro*, and also increased the enzymatic activity of CYP1A1, CYP2B6, and CYP3A4 [76]. Uniquely, the carbamate carbaryl has been shown to induce the CYP1A family via interaction with the aryl hydrocarbon receptor [77]. Other toxins in addition to insecticides can also influence CYP levels. For example, alcohol and nicotine have been shown to induce CYP2B6 – one of the most important CYPs in chlorpyrifos bioactivation – in the liver and the brain [78].

Different formulations of insecticides can impact metabolism depending on the composition and delivery method [79]. Piperonyl butoxide – a potent CYP inhibitor – is often used as an insecticide synergist in pyrethroid and carbamate formulations, by preventing detoxification of the insecticides [80, 81]. Furthermore, especially in the occupational setting, exposure to insecticides most commonly consists of exposure to a combination of different compounds that have the potential to potentiate each other's action or act synergistically. For instance the organophosphate chlorpyrifos has been shown to inhibit the metabolism of the carbamate, carbaryl [28]. Additionally, the oxon metabolites of organophosphates are potent inhibitors of human carboxylesterases, which are important in the metabolism of pyrethroids [41].

25.4.3
Impact of Age, Gender, Species, and Pathology

Differences in the extent of metabolism and ultimate toxicity of each compound may vary by age, gender, species, and underlying pathology. Fetuses and young animals are often more sensitive to the toxic effects of insecticides due to lower levels of xenobiotic-metabolizing enzymes, more permeable blood–brain barriers, and other factors. Important fetal xenobiotic-metabolizing proteins are often different than those in the adult. For instance, FMO1 is the predominate FMO enzyme in the fetal liver, while FMO1 is poorly expressed in adults [82]. Metabolism of insecticides may also vary by gender, and differences in CYP activity between males and females can arise due to differences in sex hormones. CYP3A4, which participates in the metabolism of many insecticides, has been shown to be expressed 2-fold higher in women than in men [83]. Interspecies variability in insecticide metabolism also provides a challenge when extrapolating metabolic pathways and rate constants from rodents to humans. Studies in liver microsomes of different species have shown that rodents have an increased metabolic activity towards organophosphate and carbamate insecticides as compared to humans [18, 29]. Additionally, the relative abundance of different phase II metabolites varies widely in studies conducted in different species. Lastly, underlying pathology can have a large effect on the metabolism of an insecticide by an individual. Liver and kidney disease can affect the ability to metabolize xenobiotics, leading to increased circulating levels of the parent compound, which can either increase or decrease the toxicity of the insecticide depending on the relative potency of the parent compound and metabolites.

25.4.4
Interindividual Genetic Variability

A large part of interindividual variability in metabolism may stem from genetic polymorphisms in important insecticide-metabolizing enzymes. Two common polymorphisms in PON1 have been identified: (i) a Leu/Met amino acid polymorphism at position 55 ($PON1_{L55M}$) and (ii) a Gln/Arg amino acid polymorphisms at position 192 ($PON1_{Q192R}$) [84]. The $PON1_{55}$ polymorphism affects PON1 mRNA [85] and plasma protein levels [86], which ultimately influence PON1 activity. $PON1_{55L}$ is associated with higher PON1 plasma protein concentrations compared to the $PON1_{55M}$ isoform [86]. The $PON1_{192}$ polymorphism has been shown to affect PON1 enzyme activity towards organophosphates in a substrate-specific manner [47]. The $PON1_{192R}$ allele hydrolyzes paraoxon *in vitro* faster than the $PON1_{192Q}$ allele; however, the $PON1192_{Q}$ allele hydrolyzes diazoxon, sarin, and soman faster than the $PON1_{192R}$ allele [47]. These findings have been disputed by O'Leary *et al.* [87] who found that the $PON1_{192R}$ allele hydrolyzes diazoxon faster than the $PON1_{192Q}$ allele. However, in both cases, the $PON1_{192QR}$ genotype showed an intermediate activity towards diazoxon compared to $PON1_{192RR}$ and $PON1_{192QQ}$. *In vivo* studies utilizing PON1 knockout mice showed that intraperitoneal injection of $PON1_{192R}$ or $PON1_{192Q}$ both provided a similar degree of protection against diazoxon, while $PON1_{192R}$ provided better protection against chlorpyrifos oxon than $PON1_{192Q}$ [48], thus demonstrating the importance of the $PON1_{192}$ allele in determining organophosphate sensitivity. The status of PON1 includes both the amount of PON1 protein present (influenced by $PON1_{55}$ polymorphism) and the efficacy of the enzyme (influenced by $PON1_{192}$ polymorphism). Thus, the PON1 genotype and phenotype of an individual may serve as a biomarker for organophosphate susceptibility [88].

For insecticides that undergo CYP-isoform-specific metabolism, genetic variability may hold similar importance in the field of toxicology. Dai *et al.* [89] reported that the metabolism of chlorpyrifos by CYP3A4*3 and CYP3A4*19 is comparable to wild-type CYP3A4, while CYP3A4*18 has significantly increased metabolism of chlorpyrifos and CYP3A4*17 has significantly decreased metabolism of chlorpyrifos. The CYP2C9*2 variant is not active in metabolizing chlorpyrifos, unlike wild-type CYP2C9 [18]. The CYP2C19 variants CYP2C19*5, CYP2C19*6, and CYP2C19*8 have no detectable desulfuration activity (i.e., activation) and very limited dearylation activity (i.e., detoxification) of chlorpyrifos, relative to wild-type CYP2C19 [18]. Additionally, CYP2C19 has a common polymorphism (CYP2C19*2) that results in a null phenotype (i.e., no active protein) and is in a relatively high prevalence (around 20%) in several populations [90, 91]. CYP2B6 – the most active CYP for the bioactivation of several organophosphates – is also polymorphic and there is a need to study the effect of these isoforms on organophosphate metabolism. Polymorphisms in any CYP can potentially shift the balance between bioactivation and detoxification of an organophosphate insecticide *in vivo*, which could potentially affect the compound's toxicity.

25.5 Conclusions

Metabolism of insecticides is complex, and in order to improve our current risk assessment models and understanding of human metabolism, gaps in our knowledge that need to be filled include:

- The need to understand CYP-specific metabolism (activation and/or detoxification) of insecticides in humans at exposures encountered occupationally and environmentally.
- The need to better understand factors regulating metabolism and disposition to target sites, and the role of extrahepatic metabolism, especially in the brain.
- The need to better understand the potential of insecticides to alter the metabolism and resulting toxicity of other endogenous and exogenous substrates.
- The need to identify human biomarkers of exposure, effect, and susceptibility to better assess the risk of insecticides – alone and in combination – on human health.

Note

The first two authors contributed equally to this work.

References

1 Krieger, R.I. (2010) *Hayes' Handbook of Pesticide Toxicology*, 3rd edn, Academic Press, San Diego, CA.

2 Knaak, J.B., *et al.* (2008) Parameters for carbamate pesticide QSAR and PBPK/PD models for human risk assessment.

Rev. Environ. Contam. Toxicol., **193**, 53–212.
3 Knaak, J.B., *et al.* (2004) Physicochemical and biological data for the development of predictive organophosphorus pesticide QSARs and PBPK/PD models for human risk assessment. *Crit. Rev. Toxicol.*, **34**, 143–207.
4 Chambers, J.E. and Levi, P.E. (1992) *Organophosphates: Chemistry, Fate, and Effects*, Academic Press, San Diego, CA.
5 Feldmann, R.J. and Maibach, H.I. (1974) Percutaneous penetration of some pesticides and herbicides in man. *Toxicol. Appl. Pharmacol.*, **28**, 126–132.
6 Sams, C., Patel, K., and Jones, K. (2010) Biological monitoring for exposure to pirimicarb: method development and a human oral dosing study. *Toxicol. Lett.*, **192**, 56–60.
7 Soderlund, D.M., *et al.* (2002) Mechanisms of pyrethroid neurotoxicity: implications for cumulative risk assessment. *Toxicology*, **171**, 3–59.
8 Woollen, B.H., *et al.* (1992) The metabolism of cypermethrin in man: differences in urinary metabolite profiles following oral and dermal administration. *Xenobiotica*, **22**, 983–991.
9 Eadsforth, C.V., Bragt, P.C., and van Sittert, N.J. (1988) Human dose–excretion studies with pyrethroid insecticides cypermethrin and alphacypermethrin: relevance for biological monitoring. *Xenobiotica*, **18**, 603–614.
10 Challis, I.R. and Adcock, J.W. (1981) The metabolism of the carbamate insecticide bendiocarb in the rat and in man. *Pestic. Sci.*, **12**, 638–644.
11 Leng, G., Kuhn, K.H., and Idel, H. (1997) Biological monitoring of pyrethroids in blood and pyrethroid metabolites in urine: applications and limitations. *Sci. Total Environ.*, **199**, 173–181.
12 Tomalik-Scharte, D., *et al.* (2005) Dermal absorption of permethrin following topical administration. *Eur. J. Clin. Pharmacol.*, **61**, 399–404.
13 Foxenberg, R.J., *et al.* (2007) Human hepatic cytochrome p450-specific metabolism of parathion and chlorpyrifos. *Drug Metab. Dispos.*, **35**, 189–193.
14 Buratti, F.M., *et al.* (2003) CYP-specific bioactivation of four organophosphorothioate pesticides by human liver microsomes. *Toxicol. Appl. Pharmacol.*, **186**, 143–154.
15 Choi, K., *et al.* (2006) Metabolism of chlorpyrifos and chlorpyrifos oxon by human hepatocytes. *J. Biochem. Mol. Toxicol.*, **20**, 279–291.
16 Poet, T.S., *et al.* (2003) *In vitro* rat hepatic and intestinal metabolism of the organophosphate pesticides chlorpyrifos and diazinon. *Toxicol. Sci.*, **72**, 193–200.
17 Sams, C., Mason, H.J., and Rawbone, R. (2000) Evidence for the activation of organophosphate pesticides by cytochromes P450 3A4 and 2D6 in human liver microsomes. *Toxicol. Lett.*, **116**, 217–221.
18 Tang, J., *et al.* (2001) Metabolism of chlorpyrifos by human cytochrome P450 isoforms and human, mouse, and rat liver microsomes. *Drug Metab. Dispos.*, **29**, 1201–1204.
19 Kim, D.O., *et al.* (2005) Role of metabolism in parathion-induced hepatotoxicity and immunotoxicity. *J. Toxicol. Environ. Health A*, **68**, 2187–2205.
20 Mutch, E., *et al.* (2003) Do multiple cytochrome P450 isoforms contribute to parathion metabolism in man? *Arch. Toxicol.*, **77**, 313–320.
21 Kappers, W.A., *et al.* (2001) Diazinon is activated by CYP2C19 in human liver. *Toxicol. Appl. Pharmacol.*, **177**, 68–76.
22 Buratti, F.M., *et al.* (2005) Malathion bioactivation in the human liver: the contribution of different cytochrome p450 isoforms. *Drug Metab. Dispos.*, **33**, 295–302.
23 Abass, K., *et al.* (2007) *In vitro* metabolism and interaction of profenofos by human, mouse and rat liver preparations. *Pestic. Biochem. Physiol.*, **87**, 238–247.
24 Buratti, F.M. and Testai, E. (2007) Evidences for CYP3A4 autoactivation in the desulfuration of dimethoate by the human liver. *Toxicology*, **241**, 33–46.
25 Leoni, C., Buratti, F.M., and Testai, E. (2008) The participation of human hepatic P450 isoforms, flavin-containing monooxygenases and aldehyde oxidase in

the biotransformation of the insecticide fenthion. *Toxicol. Appl. Pharmacol.*, **233**, 343–352.

26 Abass, K., *et al.* (2009) Metabolism of carbosulfan. I. Species differences in the *in vitro* biotransformation by mammalian hepatic microsomes including human. *Chem. Biol. Interact.*, **181**, 210–219.

27 Abass, K., *et al.* (2010) Metabolism of carbosulfan II. Human interindividual variability in its *in vitro* hepatic biotransformation and the identification of the cytochrome P450 isoforms involved. *Chem. Biol. Interact.*, **185**, 163–173.

28 Tang, J., *et al.* (2002) *In vitro* metabolism of carbaryl by human cytochrome P450 and its inhibition by chlorpyrifos. *Chem. Biol. Interact.*, **141**, 229–241.

29 Usmani, K.A., Hodgson, E., and Rose, R.L. (2004) *In vitro* metabolism of carbofuran by human, mouse, and rat cytochrome P450 and interactions with chlorpyrifos, testosterone, and estradiol. *Chem. Biol. Interact.*, **150**, 221–232.

30 Anand, S.S., *et al.* (2006) Characterization of deltamethrin metabolism by rat plasma and liver microsomes. *Toxicol. Appl. Pharmacol.*, **212**, 156–166.

31 Godin, S.J., *et al.* (2007) Identification of rat and human cytochrome p450 isoforms and a rat serum esterase that metabolize the pyrethroid insecticides deltamethrin and esfenvalerate. *Drug Metab. Dispos.*, **35**, 1664–1671.

32 Nakamura, Y., *et al.* (2007) The *in vitro* metabolism of a pyrethroid insecticide, permethrin, and its hydrolysis products in rats. *Toxicology*, **235**, 176–184.

33 Ma, T. and Chambers, J.E. (1995) A kinetic analysis of hepatic microsomal activation of parathion and chlorpyrifos in control and phenobarbital-treated rats. *J. Biochem. Toxicol.*, **10**, 63–68.

34 Scollon, E.J., *et al.* (2009) *In vitro* metabolism of pyrethroid pesticides by rat and human hepatic microsomes and cytochrome p450 isoforms. *Drug Metab. Dispos.*, **37**, 221–228.

35 Shimada, T., *et al.* (1994) Interindividual variations in human liver cytochrome P-450 enzymes involved in the oxidation of drugs, carcinogens and toxic chemicals: studies with liver microsomes of 30 Japanese and 30 Caucasians. *J. Pharmacol. Exp. Ther.*, **270**, 414–423.

36 Yeo, K.R., Rostami-Hodjegan, A., and Tucker, G.T. (2004) Abundance of cytochromes P450 in human liver: a meta-analysis. *Br. J. Clin. Pharmacol.*, **57**, 687–688.

37 Usmani, K.A., *et al.* (2004) *In vitro* sulfoxidation of thioether compounds by human cytochrome P450 and flavin-containing monooxygenase isoforms with particular reference to the CYP2C subfamily. *Drug Metab. Dispos.*, **32**, 333–339.

38 Tynes, R.E. and Hodgson, E. (1985) Catalytic activity and substrate specificity of the flavin-containing monooxygenase in microsomal systems: characterization of the hepatic, pulmonary and renal enzymes of the mouse, rabbit, and rat. *Arch. Biochem. Biophys.*, **240**, 77–93.

39 Phillips, I.R., *et al.* (1995) The molecular biology of the flavin-containing monooxygenases of man. *Chem. Biol. Interact.*, **96**, 17–32.

40 Godin, S.J., *et al.* (2006) Species differences in the *in vitro* metabolism of deltamethrin and esfenvalerate: differential oxidative and hydrolytic metabolism by humans and rats. *Drug Metab. Dispos.*, **34**, 1764–1771.

41 Ross, M.K., *et al.* (2006) Hydrolytic metabolism of pyrethroids by human and other mammalian carboxylesterases. *Biochem. Pharmacol.*, **71**, 657–669.

42 Crow, J.A., *et al.* (2007) Hydrolysis of pyrethroids by human and rat tissues: examination of intestinal, liver and serum carboxylesterases. *Toxicol. Appl. Pharmacol.*, **221**, 1–12.

43 Buratti, F.M. and Testai, E. (2005) Malathion detoxification by human hepatic carboxylesterases and its inhibition by isomalathion and other pesticides. *J. Biochem. Mol. Toxicol.*, **19**, 406–414.

44 Povey, A.C. (2010) Gene–environmental interactions and organophosphate toxicity. *Toxicology*, **278**, 294–304.

45 Furlong, C.E., *et al.* (2005) Paraoxonase 1 (PON1) status and risk of insecticide exposure. *J. Biochem. Mol. Toxicol.*, **19**, 182–183.

46 Costa, L.G. (2006) Current issues in organophosphate toxicology. *Clin. Chim. Acta*, **366**, 1–13.

47 Davies, H.G., *et al.* (1996) The effect of the human serum paraoxonase polymorphism is reversed with diazoxon, soman and sarin. *Nat. Genet.*, **14**, 334–336.

48 Li, W.F., *et al.* (2000) Catalytic efficiency determines the in-vivo efficacy of PON1 for detoxifying organophosphorus compounds. *Pharmacogenetics*, **10**, 767–779.

49 Bicker, W., *et al.* (2005) A case study of acute human chlorpyrifos poisoning: novel aspects on metabolism and toxicokinetics derived from liquid chromatography-tandem mass spectrometry analysis of urine samples. *Toxicol. Lett.*, **159**, 235–251.

50 Fujioka, K. and Casida, J.E. (2007) Glutathione *S*-transferase conjugation of organophosphorus pesticides yields *S*-phospho-, *S*-aryl-, and *S*-alkylglutathione derivatives. *Chem. Res. Toxicol.*, **20**, 1211–1217.

51 Ecobichon, D.J. and Joy, R.M. (1994) *Pesticides and Neurological Diseases*, 2nd edn, CRC Press, Boca Raton, FL.

52 Pena-Llopis, S., Ferrando, M.D., and Pena, J.B. (2003) Fish tolerance to organophosphate-induced oxidative stress is dependent on the glutathione metabolism and enhanced by *N*-acetylcysteine. *Aquat. Toxicol.*, **65**, 337–360.

53 Falcioni, M.L., *et al.* (2010) The primary role of glutathione against nuclear DNA damage of striatum induced by permethrin in rats. *Neuroscience*, **168**, 2–10.

54 Banerjee, B.D., Seth, V., and Ahmed, R.S. (2001) Pesticide-induced oxidative stress: perspectives and trends. *Rev. Environ. Health*, **16**, 1–40.

55 Paine, M.F., *et al.* (2006) The human intestinal cytochrome P450 “pie”. *Drug Metab. Dispos.*, **34**, 880–886.

56 Yeung, C.K., *et al.* (2000) Immunoquantitation of FMO1 in human liver, kidney, and intestine. *Drug Metab. Dispos.*, **28**, 1107–1111.

57 Furnes, B. and Schlenk, D. (2005) Extrahepatic metabolism of carbamate and organophosphate thioether compounds by the flavin-containing monooxygenase and cytochrome P450 systems. *Drug Metab. Dispos,*, **33**, 214–218.

58 Baron, J.M. and Skazik, C. (2010) Research in practice: the second barrier of the human skin. *J. Dtsch. Dermatol. Ges.*, **8**, 155–158.

59 Venkatesh, K., *et al.* (1992) The flavin-containing monooxygenase in mouse lung: evidence for expression of multiple forms. *J. Biochem. Toxicol.*, **7**, 163–169.

60 Williams, P.L., Carver, M.P., and Riviere, J.E. (1990) A physiologically relevant pharmacokinetic model of xenobiotic percutaneous absorption utilizing the isolated perfused porcine skin flap. *J. Pharm. Sci.*, **79**, 305–311.

61 Dahl, A.R. and Gerde, P. (1994) Uptake and metabolism of toxicants in the respiratory tract. *Environ. Health Perspect.*, **102** (Suppl. 11), 67–70.

62 Yadav, S., *et al.* (2006) Regional specificity in deltamethrin induced cytochrome P450 expression in rat brain. *Toxicol. Appl. Pharmacol.*, **217**, 15–24.

63 Soranno, T.M. and Sultatos, L.G. (1992) Biotransformation of the insecticide parathion by mouse brain. *Toxicol. Lett.*, **60**, 27–37.

64 Johri, A., *et al.* (2006) Long lasting effects of prenatal exposure to deltamethrin on cerebral and hepatic cytochrome P450s and behavioral activity in rat offspring. *Eur. J. Pharmacol.*, **544**, 58–68.

65 Forsyth, C.S. and Chambers, J.E. (1989) Activation and degradation of the phosphorothionate insecticides parathion and EPN by rat brain. *Biochem. Pharmacol.*, **38**, 1597–1603.

66 de Lima, J.S., *et al.* (1996) Methyl parathion activation by a partially purified rat brain fraction. *Toxicol. Lett.*, **87**, 53–60.

67 Chambers, J.E. and Chambers, H.W. (1989) Oxidative desulfuration of chlorpyrifos, chlorpyrifos-methyl, and leptophos by rat brain and liver. *J. Biochem. Toxicol.*, **4**, 201–203.

68 Albores, A., *et al.* (2001) Cytochrome P450 2B (CYP2B)-mediated activation of

methyl-parathion in rat brain extracts. *Toxicol. Lett.*, **124**, 1–10.

69 Bhagwat, S.V., Boyd, M.R., and Ravindranath, V. (2000) Multiple forms of cytochrome P450 and associated monooxygenase activities in human brain mitochondria. *Biochem. Pharmacol.*, **59**, 573–582.

70 Bieche, I., *et al.* (2007) Reverse transcriptase-PCR quantification of mRNA levels from cytochrome (CYP)1, CYP2 and CYP3 families in 22 different human tissues. *Pharmacogenet. Genomics*, **17**, 731–742.

71 Gervot, L., *et al.* (1999) Human CYP2B6: expression, inducibility and catalytic activities. *Pharmacogenetics*, **9**, 295–306.

72 Halpert, J., Hammond, D., and Neal, R.A. (1980) Inactivation of purified rat liver cytochrome P-450 during the metabolism of parathion (diethyl *p*-nitrophenyl phosphorothionate). *J. Biol. Chem.*, **255**, 1080–1089.

73 Hodgson, E. and Rose, R.L. (2006) Organophosphorus chemicals: potent inhibitors of the human metabolism of steroid hormones and xenobiotics. *Drug Metab. Rev.*, **38**, 149–162.

74 Abass, K., Turpeinen, M., and Pelkonen, O. (2009) An evaluation of the cytochrome P450 inhibition potential of selected pesticides in human hepatic microsomes. *J. Environ. Sci. Health B*, **44**, 553–563.

75 Rose, R.L. and Hodgson, E. (2005) Pesticide metabolism and potential for metabolic interactions. *J. Biochem. Mol. Toxicol.*, **19**, 276–277.

76 Das, P.C., *et al.* (2008) Enzyme induction and cytotoxicity in human hepatocytes by chlorpyrifos and *N,N*-diethyl-*m*-toluamide (DEET). *Drug Metabol. Drug Interact.*, **23**, 237–260.

77 Boronat, S., *et al.* (2007) Modulation of aryl hydrocarbon receptor transactivation by carbaryl, a nonconventional ligand. *FEBS J.*, **274**, 3327–3339.

78 Miksys, S., *et al.* (2003) Smoking, alcoholism and genetic polymorphisms alter CYP2B6 levels in human brain. *Neuropharmacology*, **45**, 122–132.

79 Axelrad, J.C., Howard, C.V., and McLean, W.G. (2002) Interactions between pesticides and components of pesticide formulations in an *in vitro* neurotoxicity test. *Toxicology*, **173**, 259–268.

80 Hodgson, E. and Philpot, R.M. (1974) Interaction of methylenedioxyphenyl (1,3-benzodioxole) compounds with enzymes and their effects on mammals. *Drug Metab. Rev.*, **3**, 231–301.

81 Ryu, D.Y., Levi, P.E., and Hodgson, E. (1995) Regulation of cytochrome P-450 isozymes CYP1A1, CYP1A2 and CYP2B10 by three benzodioxole compounds. *Chem. Biol. Interact.*, **96**, 235–247.

82 Dolphin, C.T., *et al.* (1996) Differential developmental and tissue-specific regulation of expression of the genes encoding three members of the flavin-containing monooxygenase family of man, FMO1, FMO3 and FM04. *Eur J Biochem*, **235**, 683–689.

83 Wolbold, R., *et al.* (2003) Sex is a major determinant of CYP3A4 expression in human liver. *Hepatology*, **38**, 978–988.

84 Adkins, S., *et al.* (1993) Molecular basis for the polymorphic forms of human serum paraoxonase/arylesterase: glutamine or arginine at position 191, for the respective A or B allozymes. *Am. J. Hum. Genet.*, **52**, 598–608.

85 Leviev, I., Negro, F., and James, R.W. (1997) Two alleles of the human paraoxonase gene produce different amounts of mRNA. An explanation for differences in serum concentrations of paraoxonase associated with the (Leu–Met54) polymorphism. *Arterioscler. Thromb. Vasc. Biol.*, **17**, 2935–2939.

86 Garin, M.C., *et al.* (1997) Paraoxonase polymorphism Met–Leu54 is associated with modified serum concentrations of the enzyme. A possible link between the paraoxonase gene and increased risk of cardiovascular disease in diabetes. *J. Clin. Invest.*, **99**, 62–66.

87 O'Leary, K.A., *et al.* (2005) Genetic and other sources of variation in the activity of serum paraoxonase/diazoxonase in humans: consequences for risk from exposure to diazinon. *Pharmacogenet. Genomics*, **15**, 51–60.

88 Li, W.F., Costa, L.G., and Furlong, C.E. (1993) Serum paraoxonase status: a major factor in determining resistance to organophosphates. *J. Toxicol. Environ. Health*, **40**, 337–346.

89 Dai, D., *et al.* (2001) Identification of variants of CYP3A4 and characterization of their abilities to metabolize testosterone and chlorpyrifos. *J. Pharmacol. Exp. Ther.*, **299**, 825–831.

90 Shimizu, T., *et al.* (2003) Bioinformatics research on inter-racial difference in drug metabolism II. Analysis on relationship between enzyme activities of CYP2D6 and CYP2C19 and their relevant genotypes. *Drug Metab. Pharmacokinet.*, **18**, 71–78.

91 Bozina, N., Bradamante, V., and Lovric, M. (2009) Genetic polymorphism of metabolic enzymes P450 (Cyp) as a susceptibility factor for drug response, toxicity, and cancer risk. *Arh. Hig. Rada Toksikol.*, **60**, 217–242.

Index

Page numbers in *italics* refer to figures, those in **bold** refer to tables.

Metabolism of Drugs and Other Xenobiotics, First Edition. Edited by Pavel Anzenbacher, Ulrich M. Zanger.

d

f

g

n

o